Plant and Animal Proteins in Health and Disease Prevention

This book explores the vital role of proteins in human health through 40 in-depth chapters organized into four comprehensive sections, which include "Introductory Concepts," "Foods of Animal Origin," "Foods of Plant Origin," and "Resources." The book delves into the biochemical processes behind protein metabolism and its influence on a wide range of health conditions. Aimed at educating readers on the diverse sources and types of protein, it provides valuable insights into how both plant and animal proteins contribute to disease prevention and overall wellness.

Features:

- Chapters feature subsections titled "Effects of Other Proteins" to aid in comparative interpretation.
- Each chapter contains a Mini Dictionary of Terms and Summary Points to facilitate clear understanding.
- Highly illustrated with figures and multiple tables in each chapter.
- Chapter contributors represent global coverage.

Plant and Animal Proteins in Health and Disease Prevention is written for nutritionists, food scientists, healthcare professionals, research scientists and practitioners, and policy makers. It is also designed for professors, students, and libraries.

Plant and Animal Proteins in Health and Disease Prevention

Edited by
Victor R. Preedy

CRC Press
Taylor & Francis Group
Boca Raton London New York

CRC Press is an imprint of the
Taylor & Francis Group, an **informa** business

Designed cover image: Shutterstock

First edition published 2026
by CRC Press
2385 NW Executive Centre Drive, Suite 320, Boca Raton FL 33431

and by CRC Press
4 Park Square, Milton Park, Abingdon, Oxon, OX14 4RN

CRC Press is an imprint of Taylor & Francis Group, LLC

ISBN: 9781032982885 (hbk)
ISBN: 9781032982939 (pbk)
ISBN: 9781003597926 (ebk)

DOI: 10.1201/9781003597926

Typeset in Times
by Deanta Global Publishing Services, Chennai, India

Contents

Preface

Dietary proteins are an important component of health and wellbeing. Their compositional amino acids provide biochemical precursors and contribute to structural components of tissue systems via macromolecule formation. Protein requirements vary across the lifespan and different needs must be met in scenarios of ill health. However, diets low in protein can have a detrimental impact, as can diets very high in protein. Furthermore, there are many different types of dietary proteins, and, across populations, their intake varies in terms of amount, source, and quality. Also, there are significant variations in the extent to which each protein type is consumed. There is an ongoing dialogue to discover new sources of dietary protein or determine what optimal intakes are. However, some material on protein intakes and different protein sources fail to address the academic diversity of the reader or include comparative information. Moreover, information on dietary protein is scattered throughout the literature. These limitations are met in *Plant and Animal Proteins in Health and Disease Prevention*. Coverage includes introductory chapters, low-protein diets and intakes, metabolic disorders and diseases, protein quality, metabolism, effects on organs, high protein diets and intakes, the life span, childhood, aging and other areas. This serves as a comprehensive resource on the biomedical and nutritional aspects of dietary protein.

- Book 1: *Protein Intake in Health and Disease*
- Book 2: *Plant and Animal Proteins in Health and Disease Prevention*

Plant and Animal Proteins in Health and Disease Prevention has the following sections:

SECTION 1: SETTING THE SCENE AND INTRODUCTORY CHAPTERS

Chapter 1 Planetary Health and Animal and Plant Dietary Proteins
Chapter 2 Plant and Animal Protein Intake and Their Metabolic Differential Effects
Chapter 3 Dietary Plant and Animal Proteins and Satiety
Chapter 4 Role of Animal and Plant Protein on Child Health Outcomes
Chapter 5 Dietary Plant and Animal Protein–Phenolic Interactions: Effects of Gastrointestinal Digestion and Gut Microbiota

SECTION 2: FOODS OF ANIMAL ORIGIN

Chapter 6 Amino Acid Quality of Meat Proteins
Chapter 7 Animal Protein and Its Impact on Adiposity
Chapter 8 Red Meat Protein and Links with Disease: A Focus on Diabetes
Chapter 9 Animal Protein Intake and Cancer Risk
Chapter 10 Bovine Milk Proteins: A Compositional Profile
Chapter 11 Dairy Protein and the Risk of Non-Alcoholic Fatty Liver Disease
Chapter 12 Dairy Proteins and Metabolic Health: A Focus on Bioactive Peptides
Chapter 13 Dairy Protein and Gut Microbiota
Chapter 14 Dairy Proteins in the Diet and Skeletal Muscle Metabolism in Adults
Chapter 15 Antioxidant Peptides from Hydrolysis of Whey Protein
Chapter 16 Using Whey Protein Concentrate and Curcumin as a Combinational Approach
Chapter 17 Whey Protein and Impact on Obesity
Chapter 18 Use of Whey Protein in Children with Autism
Chapter 19 Fish Protein and Peptides: Impact on Health

SECTION 3: FOODS OF PLANT ORIGIN

SECTION 4: RESOURCES

Each chapter has the following subsections:

The Effects of Other Proteins
Mini Dictionary of Terms
Summary Points

These subsections encompass unique features in the book, which bridge the transintellectual and transdisciplinary divides. The section *The Effects of Other Proteins* ensures there is comparative information within chapters. The *Mini Dictionary of Terms* aids the novice reader. The *Summary Points* encapsulates the entire chapter in succinct sentences.

Contributors include international and national experts, from respected institutions. Leaders in the field and trendsetters are also contributors. Furthermore, emerging fields of protein nutrition are also incorporated in *Nutritional Aspects of Dietary Protein.*

This book is essential reading for nutritionists, food scientists, health care professionals, research scientists, the medical professions, and other practitioners, policy makers, and institutional or governmental departments. It is also designed for teachers and lecturers, undergraduates, graduates, post-graduates, professors, and libraries.

The Editor

Acknowledgements

I wish to acknowledge the professionalism and dedication of Tom Connelly, who helped throughout the preparation and production of this book.

I am also very grateful to Randy Brehm for her guidance and support, from when the ideas for this book were first proposed to the completion of the project.

The Editor

About the Editor

Victor R. Preedy BSc, PhD, DSc, FRSB, FRSPH, FRCPath, FRSC is Honorary Professor in the Department of Clinical Biochemistry at King's College Hospital, Emeritus Professor in Faculty of Life Sciences and Medicine at King's College London, and Visiting Professor at the University of Suffolk, UK. Professor Preedy graduated with an honours degree in Biology and Physiology with Pharmacology. He gained his University of London, UK, PhD on the biochemical measurements in protein metabolism and gained a second doctoral degree for his outstanding contribution to protein metabolism in health and disease. Professor Preedy was elected as a Fellow of the Royal Society of Medicine in 2022. He is also a Fellow of the Royal Society of Biology, The Royal College of Pathologists, The Royal Society for Public Health, and The Royal Society of Chemistry. He was the founding Director of the Genomics Centre at King's College London and held the post from 2006 to 2020. In his career, Professor Preedy has carried out research at the Cardiothoracic Institute, National Heart Hospital (part of Imperial College London), The School of Pharmacy (now part of University College London), and the MRC Centre at Northwick Park Hospital. He has collaborated with research groups in Finland, Japan, Australia, USA, and Germany. He is a leading expert on the science of health. To his credit, Professor Preedy has published over 750 articles, which include peer-reviewed manuscripts based on original research, abstracts, symposium presentations, reviews, and numerous books and volumes.

Contributors

Ioanna Alexandropoulou
Department of Rheumatology and Clinical Immunology
University Hospital of Larissa
Larissa, Greece
and
Faculty of Medicine
University of Thessaly, Biopolis,
Larissa, Greece

Peter Uchenna Amadi
Department of Pediatrics, Faculty of Medicine and Dentistry
University of Alberta
Edmonton, Alberta, Canada

Kiran Ambatipudi
Department of Biosciences and Bioengineering
Indian Institute of Technology Roorkee
Roorkee, India

Vahid Reza Askari
Clinical Research Development Unit, Imam Reza Hospital, Faculty of Medicine
Mashhad University of Medical Sciences
Mashhad, Iran

Burcu Ateş Özcan
Department of Nutrition and Dietetics, Faculty of Health Sciences
Marmara University
Istanbul, Turkey

Margarete Almeida Freitas de Azevedo
Postgraduate Program in Food and Nutrition
Federal University of Piauí
Teresina, Brazil

Anida Maria Băbţan
Department of Oral Rehabilitation, Faculty of Dental Medicine
Iuliu Haţieganu University of Medicine and Pharmacy
Cluj-Napoca, Romania

Jamie I. Baum
Department of Food Science, Center for Human Nutrition
University of Arkansas System Division of Agriculture
Fayetteville, Arkansas, USA

Marina del Rosario Bettiol
Multidisciplinary Institute for Agri-Food and Biotechnology Research and Transfer (IMITAB), National Scientific and Technical Research Council (CONICET)
National University of Villa María
Córdoba, Argentina

Diana Bogueva
Curtin University Sustainability Policy Institute
Curtin University
Perth, Australia

Adina Bianca Boşca
Department of Histology, Faculty of Medicine
Iuliu Haţieganu University of Medicine and Pharmacy
Cluj-Napoca, Romania

Maarten C. Bosland
Department of Pathology, College of Medicine
University of Illinois at Chicago
Chicago, Illinois, USA

Esra Capanoglu
Department of Food Engineering
Istanbul Technical University
Istanbul, Turkey

Cristina Capittini
Department of Medicine
University of Pavia
Pavia, Italy

Cara L. Cargo-Froom
Department of Animal Biosciences
University of Guelph
Guelph, Ontario, Canada

Vanessa Brito Lira de Carvalho
Postgraduate Program in Food and Nutrition
Federal University of Piauí
Teresina, Brazil

Ana Maria Castejon
Department of Pharmaceutical Sciences, Barry and Judy Silverman College of Pharmacy
Nova Southeastern University
Fort Lauderdale, Florida, USA

Subhiksha Chandrasekaran
Department of Food Science and Human Nutrition
University of Illinois Urbana-Champaign
Urbana, Illinois, USA

Ranjitha Chandrashekar
Department of Nutritional Sciences
Oklahoma State University
Stillwater, Oklahoma, USA

Maria Carmen Collado
Department of Biotechnology
Institute of Agrochemistry and Food Technology
Valencia, Spain

Daniel A. Columbus
Prairie Swine Centre, Inc.
Saskatoon, Saskatchewan, Canada

Ali Ebrahimi Dabagh
Department of Nutrition Sciences
Mashhad University of Medical Sciences
Mashhad, Iran

Arpita Das
Department of Biosciences and Bioengineering
Indian Institute of Technology Roorkee
Roorkee, India

Maria do Carmo de Carvalho e Martins
Department of Biophysics and Physiology
Federal University of Piauí
Teresina, Brazil
and
Professor at the UNIFAESF University Center
Foriano, Brazil

Elvira Gonzalez de Mejia
Department of Food Science and Human Nutrition
University of Illinois Urbana-Champaign
Urbana, Illinois, USA

Ayşe Betül Demirbaş
Department of Nutrition and Dietetics, Faculty of Health Sciences
Atlas University
Istanbul, Turkey

Richard Deth
Barry and Judy Silverman College of Pharmacy
Nova Southeastern University
Fort Lauderdale, Florida, USA

Vermont P. Dia
Department of Food Science
The University of Tennessee Knoxville
Knoxville, Tennessee, USA

Kelly Aparecida Dias
Laboratory of Vitamin Analysis, Department of Nutrition and Health
Universidade Federal de Viçosa
Viçosa, Brazil

Michele Di Stefano
Department of Medicine
University of Pavia
Pavia, Italy

Ingrid Elisia
BC Cancer Research Centre
Vancouver, British Columbia, Canada

Natalia S. Fanelli
Division of Nutritional Sciences
University of Illinois Urbana-Champaign
Urbana, Illinois, USA

Anca Corina Farcas
Department of Food Science
University of Agricultural Sciences and Veterinary Medicine Cluj-Napoca
Cluj-Napoca, Romania

Constantinos Giagkinis
Department of Food Science and Nutrition, School of Environment
University of the Aegean
Limnos, Greece

Kalliopi K. Gkouskou
Laboratory of Biology, School of Medicine
National and Kapodistrian University of Athens
Athens, Greece

Andrea Gomes Santana de Melo
Coordination of the Nutrition Course
Federal University of Piauí
Picos, Brazil

Maria G. Grammatikopoulou
Department of Rheumatology and Clinical Immunology
University Hospital of Larissa
and
Faculty of Medicine
University of Thessaly, Biopolis,
Larissa, Greece

Jimmy Gutman
Immunotec Research Inc.
Blainville, Quebec, Canada

Reza Hakkak
Department of Dietetics and Nutrition, College of Health Professions
Department of Pediatric, College of Medicine
University of Arkansas For Medical Sciences
Little Rock, Arkansas, USA
and
Arkansas Children's Research Institute
Little Rock, Arkansas, USA

Patrick Hardigan
Dr. Kiran C. Patel College of Allopathic Medicine
Nova Southeastern University
Fort Lauderdale, Florida, USA

Aubree L. Hawley
Department of Food Science, Center for Human Nutrition
University of Arkansas System Division of Agriculture
Fayetteville, Arkansas, USA

Aranka Ilea
Department of Oral Rehabilitation, Faculty of Dental Medicine
Iuliu Hațieganu University of Medicine and Pharmacy
Cluj-Napoca, Romania

Ayushi Kapoor
Department of Biosciences and Bioengineering
Indian Institute of Technology Roorkee
Roorkee, India

Keita Kanzaki
Department of Clinical Nutrition, Faculty of Health Science and Technology
Kawasaki University of Medical Welfare
Okayama, Japan

Yıldırım Kayacan
Faculty of Yaşar Doğu Sport Sciences
University of Ondokuz Mayıs
Samsun, Turkey

Deniz Günal-Köroğlu
Department of Food Engineering
Istanbul Technical University
Istanbul, Turkey

Gerald Krystal
BC Cancer Research Centre
Vancouver, British Columbia, Canada

Yu-Jin Kwon
Department of Family Medicine
Yonsei University College of Medicine
Seoul, South Korea

Moattar Latif
Department of Pediatrics, Faculty of Medicine and Dentistry
University of Alberta
Edmonton, Alberta, Canada

Jun-Hyuk Lee
Department of Family Medicine, Nowon Eulji Medical Center
Eulji University School of Medicine
Seoul, South Korea

Ana Lemus Conejo
Functional Food Research and Development Center (CIDAF)
Granada, Spain

Wei Li
Department of Dietetics and Nutrition, College of Health Professions
University of Arkansas for Medical Sciences
Little Rock, Arkansas, USA

Laís Lima de Castro Abreu
Coordination of the Nutrition Course
Federal University of Piauí
Picos, Brazil

Joyce Lopes Macedo
Postgraduate Program in Biotechnology
Federal University of Piauí
Teresina, Brazil

José M. Lou-Bonafonte
Department of Pharmacology, Physiology and Legal and Forensic Medicine
University of Zaragoza
Zaragoza, Spain

Ceres Mattos Della Lucia
Laboratory of Vitamin Analysis, Department of Nutrition and Health
Universidade Federal de Viçosa
Viçosa, Brazil

Christopher P.F. Marinangeli
Protein Industries Canada
Regina, Saskatchewan, Canada

Dora Marinova
Curtin University Sustainability Policy Institute
Curtin University
Perth, Australia

Roberto Martínez-Beamonte
Department of Biochemistry and Molecular and Cellular Biology
University of Zaragoza
Zaragoza, Spain

Maria E. Martin-Rubio
Department of Cell Biology, Faculty of Biology
University of Seville
Seville, Spain

Masako Matsunaga
Department of Quantitative Health Sciences
John A. Burns School of Medicine
University of Hawaii at Manoa
Honolulu, Hawaii, USA

Carmen Mihaela Mihu
Department of Histology, Faculty of Medicine
Iuliu Hațieganu University of Medicine and Pharmacy
Cluj-Napoca, Romania

Maria C. Millan Linares
Food and Health Department
Instituto de la Grasa (CSIC)
Seville, Spain

Carla Forte Maiolino Molento
Animal Science Department
Federal University of Parana
Curitiba, Brazil

Mariana Angélica Montenegro
Multidisciplinary Institute for Agri-Food and Biotechnology Research and Transfer (IMITAB), National Scientific and Technical Research Council (CONICET)
National University of Villa María
Córdoba, Argentina

Bharath Kumar Mulakala
Texas A&M AgriLife Institute for Advancing Health Through Agriculture
College Station, TX
and Microbiome and Metabolism Research Unit
Arkansas Children's Nutrition Center
Little Rock, Arkansas, USA

María Angeles Navarro
Department of Biochemistry and Molecular and Cellular Biology
University of Zaragoza
Zaragoza, Spain

Oana Raluca Negrean
Department of Food Science
University of Agricultural Sciences and Veterinary Medicine Cluj-Napoca
Cluj-Napoca, Romania

Matthew G. Nosworthy
Agriculture and Agri-Food Canada
Guelph Research and Development Centre
Guelph, Ontario, Canada

Masaru Ochiai
Department of Animal Science, School of Veterinary Medicine
Kitasato University
Towada, Japan

Lívya Alves Oliveira
Laboratory of Vitamin Analysis, Department of Nutrition and Health
Universidade Federal de Viçosa
Viçosa, Brazil

Jesús Osada
Department of Biochemistry and Molecular and Cellular Biology
University of Zaragoza
Zaragoza, Spain

Sousana K. Papadopoulou
Department of Nutritional Sciences and Dietetics, Faculty of Health Sciences
International Hellenic University
Thessaloniki, Greece

Vinood B. Patel
School of Life Sciences
University of Westminster
London, UK

Stavros Pellios
1st Orthopaedic Department
424 General Military Hospital
and
Academic Orthopaedic Department, Papageorgiou General Hospital
Aristotle University Medical School,
Thessaloniki, Greece

Izabela Cristina Pereira de Araújo
Postgraduate Program in Biotechnology
Federal University of Piauí
Teresina, Brazil

Stephanie Michelin Santana Pereira
Laboratory of Vitamin Analysis, Department of Nutrition and Health
Universidade Federal de Viçosa
Viçosa, Brazil

Clive Julian Christie Phillips
Curtin University Sustainability Policy Institute
Curtin University
Perth, Australia
and
Institute of Veterinary Medicine and Animal Science
Estonia University of Life Sciences
Tartu, Estonia

Julianne Viana Freire Portela
Coordination of the Nutrition Course
Federal University of Piauí
Picos, Brazil

Victor R. Preedy
School of Life Course and Population Sciences
Faculty of Life Science and Medicine
King's College London
London, UK

Vafa Baradaran Rahimi
Department of Cardiovascular Diseases, Faculty of Medicine
Mashhad University of Medical Sciences
Mashhad, Iran

Rajkumar Rajendram
Department of Medical Education, College of Medicine
King Saud bin Abdulaziz University for Health Sciences
Riyadh, Saudi Arabia

Jolene R. Rearick
Microbiome and Metabolism Research Unit
Arkansas Children's Nutrition Center
Little Rock, Arkansas, USA

Fernando Rivero-Pino
Department of Medical Biochemistry, Molecular Biology, and Immunology
University of Seville
Seville, Spain

Samantha Robertson
Department of Comparative Biosciences
University of Wisconsin–Madison
Madison, Wisconsin, USA

Chetanjot Kaur Romana
Department of Food Science, Center for Human Nutrition
University of Arkansas System Division of Agriculture
Fayetteville, Arkansas, USA

Yanina Estefanía Rossi
Multidisciplinary Institute for Agri-Food and Biotechnology Research and Transfer (IMITAB), National Scientific and Technical Research Council (CONICET)
National University of Villa María
Córdoba, Argentina

Irina Rozenfeld
Dr Kiran C. Patel College of Osteopathic Medicine
Nova Southeastern University
Fort Lauderdale, Florida, USA

Kübra Şahin
Department of Nutrition and Dietetics, Faculty of Health Sciences
Üsküdar University
Istanbul, Turkey

Nurit Sheinberg
Department of Clinical and School Psychology, College of Psychology
Nova Southeastern University
Fort Lauderdale, Florida, USA

Tiago Soares
Coordination of the Nutrition Course
Federal University of Piauí
Picos, Brazil

Sonia Ancuta Socaci
Department of Food Science
University of Agricultural Sciences and Veterinary Medicine Cluj-Napoca
Cluj-Napoca, Romania

Maria Spanoudaki
Dietetics and Nutrition Department
424 General Military Hospital
and
Department of Nutritional Sciences and Dietetics, Faculty of Health Sciences
International Hellenic University
Thessaloniki, Greece

Jordan Ashley Spaw
Barry and Judy Silverman College of Pharmacy
Nova Southeastern University
Fort Lauderdale, Florida, USA

Hans H. Stein
Division of Nutritional Sciences
University of Illinois Urbana-Champaign
Urbana, Illinois, USA

Masatoshi Suzuki
Department of Comparative Biosciences and The Stem Cell and Regenerative Medicine Center
University of Wisconsin–Madison
Madison, Wisconsin, USA

Rabia Syed
Tennessee Department of Agriculture
Nashville, Tennessee, USA

Giovanni Tulipano
Department of Molecular and Translational Medicine
University of Brescia
Brescia, Italy

Aparna Verma
Department of Biosciences and Bioengineering
Indian Institute of Technology Roorkee
Roorkee, India

Ana Paula Vico
Multidisciplinary Institute for Agri-Food and Biotechnology Research and Transfer (IMITAB), National Scientific and Technical Research Council (CONICET)
National University of Villa María
Córdoba, Argentina

Nayara Vieira do Nascimento Monteiro
Postgraduate Program in Food and Nutrition
Federal University of Piauí
Teresina, Brazil

Masanobu Wada
Graduate School of Humanities and Social Sciences
Hiroshima University
Hiroshima, Japan
and
Faculty of Human Health Science
Hiroshima Bunka Gakuen University
Hiroshima, Japan

Daiki Watanabe
Graduate School of Health and Sport Sciences
Osaka University of Health and Sport Sciences
Osaka, Japan

Ying Wu
Department of Food and Animal Sciences
Tennessee State University
Nashville, Tennessee, USA

Hayrullah Yazar
Faculty of Medicine, Department of Biochemistry
University of Sakarya
Sakarya, Turkey

Laxmi Yeruva
Microbiome and Metabolism Research Unit
Arkansas Children's Nutrition Center
Little Rock, Arkansas, USA

Jihyun Yoon
Department of Family Medicine, Anam Hospital
Korea University College of Medicine
Seoul, South Korea

Jianmei Yu
Department of Family and Consumer Sciences
North Carolina Agricultural and Technical State University
Greensboro, North Carolina, USA

1 Planetary Health and Animal and Plant Dietary Proteins

Clive Julian Christie Phillips, Carla Forte Maiolino Molento, Diana Bogueva, and Dora Marinova

ABBREVIATIONS

BSE	Bovine spongiform encephalopathy
CO_2e	Carbon dioxide equivalent
DM	Dry matter
US, USA	United States of America

INTRODUCTION

The Earth's limited resources are under increasing pressure to provide food for an expanding global population that is also shifting its dietary preferences with economic development. Although the share of proteins in the human diet has remained relatively constant between 8% and 16% (Carpenter et al. 2023), their source has changed from predominantly plant-based to increasingly animal-sourced over the centuries. As living standards and income levels across the world increase, so does the desire for animal-derived proteins. This poses significant challenges as, according to scientific evidence, animal-sourced proteins have more negative environmental health impacts than proteins derived from plants (Marinova and Bogueva 2022). Among these environmental impacts are higher generated greenhouse gas emissions as well as increased water and land usage (Godfray et al. 2018), pollution, inefficient resource use, destruction of native habitats and biodiversity loss. Unless the planet's ecosystems are maintained or restored, all progress humanity has made in improving its living standards will be threatened by deteriorating planetary health. The interrelated factors and relationships between population health and environmental well-being are seriously affected by human protein choices.

It is important to recognise that both animal and plant proteins can deliver a balanced diet for humans. Enhancing understanding of the factors that influence protein selection is vital for identifying alternative approaches to reduce the reliance on animal-derived proteins and promoting the adoption of plant-rich diets.

An additional stimulus for a shift may come from radical innovation, as it seems easier to change the way food of animal origin is produced than to reduce the human appetite for meat, dairy, fish and eggs. Thus, biotechnological advances, such as precision fermentation and cellular agriculture, bring new possibilities for sustainable and ethical protein production for the benefit of humans, animals and the planet.

This chapter explores the field of animal and plant proteins by first describing the global trends and drivers in human protein consumption. Then, the extant animal and plant production systems are discussed, stating the need for a protein transition to more plant-based choices to achieve food security and a healthier planet. Finally, new options for dietary protein supply for humans are outlined, which provide alternative and more sustainable animal food choices.

DOI: 10.1201/9781003597926-1

GLOBAL TRENDS IN PLANT AND ANIMAL PROTEIN INTAKE

Nowadays, many people are consuming more protein than their actual nutritional needs. The global average protein intake exceeds the average daily requirement for adults by more than one-third, amounting to roughly 68 g per person per day (Ranganathan and Waite 2016). In the world's most affluent regions, protein consumption is even higher. This trend towards overconsumption of protein is influenced by various factors, including dietary preferences, marketing and misconceptions about protein needs. Furthermore, protein intake is rising in developing and emerging economies aspiring to reach the levels present in the Western world. Such excessive protein intake can lead to health concerns and nutrient imbalances, with consequences for human health (Willett et al. 2019).

Plant and animal protein intake are experiencing various degrees of nutritional transition within evolving food systems. This transition involves progressively replacing plant proteins with various animal proteins, particularly from poultry, but also beef, pork, lamb, eggs, dairy, fish and seafood, depending on geographic location, religion, culture and availability. Diets, particularly in low- and middle-income countries, traditionally centred primarily on grains, legumes, staple starchy crops and root vegetables. Now, these diets are increasingly characterised by the consumption of animal products newly available to the more affluent consumer, as well as highly processed foods and increased amounts of added sugars and fats. For some consumers in the West, however, diets built around high levels of meat consumption typical of the Western world are giving way to more plant-based products – the flexitarianism trend, showing intention to reduce meat consumption or add food variety. Another change is the modernisation of customary eating habits in extended food distribution networks, shifts in food retailing and a higher frequency of dining away from home (HLPE 2017).

Drivers for Animal Protein Consumption

The recent rising trend of animal protein intake shows no sign of abating, and only a few countries have reached peak meat consumption (Whitton et al. 2021). In some cases, meat is a staple due to the limited availability of plant-based foods, such as in traditional Inuit communities in the Arctic (Godfray et al. 2018) or populations living in deserts or semi-desert environments characterised by sparse vegetation and limited nutritional options (Funghi et al. 2020; Joshi et al. 2023). However, this is not the norm, as protein consumption is linked not only to food system sustainability but also to many economic, socio-cultural, environmental, health and animal welfare issues. These include societal acceptance and approval of meat-rich diets (Ederer and Leroy 2023), ranging from traditional cultures to cultural perceptions linking meat to masculinity in the West (Bogueva and Phau 2016) to rising consumption as a result of increased incomes and urbanisation in many emerging economies (Milford et al. 2019).

In many food environments, adopting plant-based dietary choices might not be feasible. Particularly in low-income nations, access to affordable and year-round nutritious plant-based foods can be limited. Additionally, for many impoverished households, animal farming serves as a crucial source of income (Ederer and Leroy 2023). There is a pressing need for further investigation into methods of encouraging technological and behavioural shifts while effectively addressing sustainability trade-offs.

Drivers for a Shift to Plant Protein Consumption

For individuals with diets rich in meat and dairy products, transitioning towards diets with a larger proportion of plant-based foods, fungi and algae can substantially alleviate the environmental strain imposed by animal agriculture (Marinova and Bogueva 2022). This shift can lead to reduced greenhouse gas emissions, decreased land and water use and a more sustainable approach to food production, thus contributing positively to environmental conservation and regenerative efforts. Many drivers can encourage individuals to shift towards diets with a greater emphasis on plant-based foods, grouped as incorporating health consciousness, environmental concerns and animal welfare (Figure 1.1). Health consciousness, including concerns about health and well-being, such as reducing the risk of chronic diseases like heart disease, type 2 diabetes and certain cancers, can positively motivate people to opt for plant-rich diets. A growing awareness of the ecological impact of meat production, including deforestation, water usage and greenhouse gas emissions, may encourage individuals to choose plant-based options for a lower environmental footprint. Ethical concerns about the treatment of animals in the meat industry drive some individuals to implement plant-rich diets, as plant proteins do not involve the same level of animal exploitation.

Derivatives of the main drivers are cultural and social influences, economic factors, accessibility, taste and variety and government policies, as well as environmental activism, the media, celebrities, social movements and influencers. The availability of tasty and diverse food choices based on plants, fungi and algae, including substitutes or analogues that mimic the taste and texture of meat, is one of the options currently explored and offered to make it more appealing for people to switch to plant-rich diets. Cultural and social factors, including peer pressure, family choices and cultural or religious beliefs, play a significant role in encouraging dietary changes, including shifts towards more plant-based dietary choices. Within this, cultural traditions and dietary habits often dictate which foods are considered "normal" or "appropriate" in a particular community. People may be more inclined to adopt plant-rich diets if their cultural heritage or traditions include plant-based dishes or if they are exposed to such foods within their socio-cultural environment.

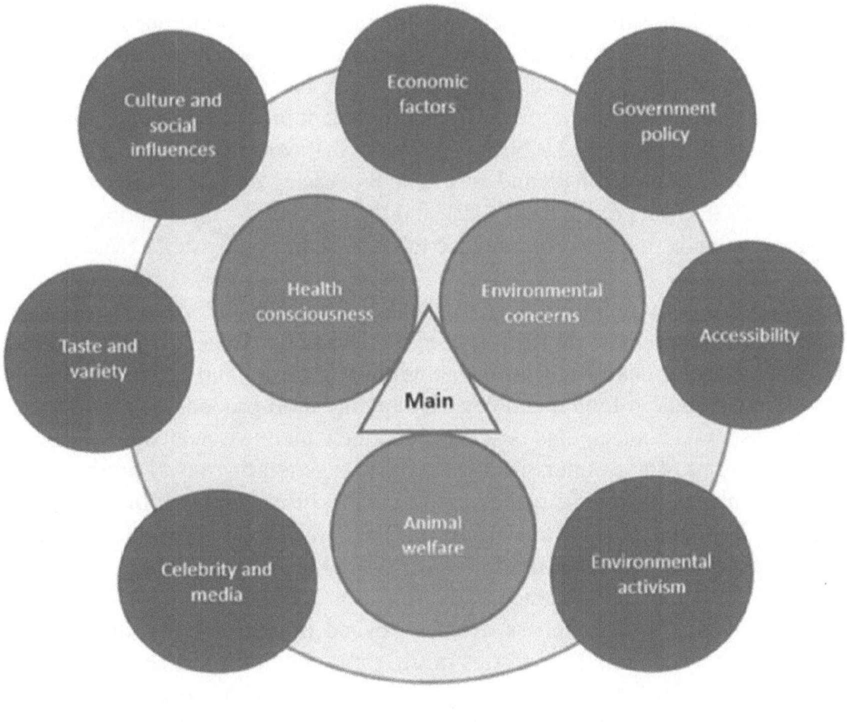

FIGURE 1.1 Drivers towards a plant-rich dietary shift. The drivers moving people towards more plant-based foods centre on health consciousness, environmental concerns and animal welfare. Numerous other factors influencing this transition include social factors, economic situations, government intervention, access to plant-based foods, environmental activism, media involvement and the attractiveness of plant-based foods. Source: Authors.

Family dynamics, habits and the influence of relatives on dietary choices are also significant, especially if they are supportive or already follow similar dietary patterns. Conversely, familial resistance or cultural expectations to consume certain foods can pose challenges to dietary change. Similar impacts are attributed to peers and the effect of social norms followed during social gatherings and dining with friends. Social pressure and the desire to fit in with peers can affect dietary choices. People may feel more comfortable adopting plant-rich diets if they have a supportive social circle that also embraces or respects their choices.

Economic factors are similarly important. The cost-effectiveness of plant-rich diets can make them attractive to meat-eaters, especially when compared to the rising costs of meat and dairy products. Government initiatives, such as dietary guidelines promoting reduced meat consumption or subsidies for plant-based agriculture, can encourage dietary shifts. Furthermore, improved availability and accessibility of plant-based foods in mainstream supermarkets, restaurants and fast-food outlets can make it more convenient for people to incorporate them into their diets. Celebrities, social movements, influencers and media are similarly important drivers nowadays. Their public endorsement of the benefits of practising certain diets, such as vegan or vegetarian, can influence public perceptions and choices. Likewise, advocacy and awareness campaigns by environmental organisations and activists, such as Sea Shepherd, can inspire individuals and sway opinions and practices related to food choices. Documentaries and films exposing agricultural and manufacturing practices used in the production of meat and animal-based foodstuffs can sway people's attitudes away from these protein sources.

Drivers for Plant Protein Consumption

Despite the dominant desire for meat, dairy and fish in consumer preferences, plant proteins continue to play a major role in human diets. A popular trend in Western countries is transitioning to protein-rich, plant-based products, such as nuts, soya, peas, beans, chickpeas and other legumes, as well as tofu, tempeh, seitan and plant milks. The global plant proteins market is forecasted to reach US$17.4 billion in 2027 from US$12.2 billion in 2022 (Shahbandeh 2022). This comes in addition to the strong growth of the global fruit and vegetable processing market, which is expected to reach US$530 billion in 2028 (Facts & Factors 2022), and the expanding consumption of fresh fruits and vegetables, whose value is projected to increase to US$211 billion by 2028 (Market Data Forecast 2023).

The desire among a growing minority of consumers for products for plant protein is strong and projected to substantially escalate over the upcoming decade due to health and environmental concerns, with many adopting flexitarianism or including vegetarian and vegan options. This shift is facilitated by developments in food technology and plant-based products, with the next generation of food innovations and advancements described as a new technological wave (Tziva et al. 2020). The intensifying interest of consumers in plant protein is generating novel prospects that embrace the functional advantages of diverse proteins, the variety of proteins within diets and innovative sources of protein. It is catalysing a transformative shift in the food industry, leading to the exploration of novel prospects and initiatives in protein consumption.

Many consumers are now more attuned to the functional advantages, health and nutritional benefits of diverse proteins. This awareness extends beyond protein content alone, with a growing emphasis on the unique functional properties of different plant proteins central to new alternative proteins manufacturing. For example, legumes like lentils and chickpeas offer protein as well as fibre and essential micronutrients, while nuts and seeds provide healthy fats along with high protein content. This awareness has led to a more nuanced approach to nutrition, where consumers seek a variety of plant proteins to meet their dietary needs. The interest in plant protein has encouraged people to diversify their diets, moving away from relying solely on a single source of protein, such as meat or dairy products, and incorporating a wider range of proteins based on plants, fungi and algae into their meals, including practising flexitarianism. This shift towards dietary diversity has many positive implications for nutrition overall, as different plant proteins bring distinct nutritional profiles and health benefits to consumers. Less conventional sources, such as hemp, algae and fungi, are also being explored.

Factors contributing to the surge in favour of plant proteins include the potential positive impacts on health associated with higher plant consumption. Furthermore, as demand for plant-based protein grows, a surge in food innovation has started to bring novel and unconventional sources of protein that potentially offer distinct characteristics and new flavours and tastes. Consumers' apprehensions about potential negative health repercussions from diets rich in animal protein, including heightened saturated fat intake, are another reason for change. While plant-based meat alternatives generate significant interest as potentially more sustainable choices, holding a promise for health and environmental benefits, many consumers exhibit hesitancy in fully substituting meat with these alternatives. Some aspects of their impact on nutrition, health and the environment still require additional investigation (Rubio et al. 2020) – a sentiment that echoes similar concerns related to cultured meat and synthetic milk.

Ethical concerns related to animal treatment are further driving consumers to perceive plant protein as a beneficial option. Also, the increased awareness among consumers about the necessity of enhancing the environmental sustainability of food production is considered an important factor by many. Although food production vastly varies across the world, it is important to understand some of the fundamental differences between animal and plant protein production systems and how they impact planetary health.

ANIMAL AND PLANT PROTEIN PRODUCTION SYSTEMS

Protein content in human food varies considerably: 1–3% in vegetables, 3% in milk, 15% in eggs, 10–20% in meat, 8–25% in nuts and seeds and 20–36% in legumes (WCRF and AICR 1997). Traditional diets in developing nations contain a much greater proportion of dietary protein from plants, but economic growth has increased animal protein preferences (Whitton et al. 2021). As animal production is associated with global concerns about environmental pollution, zoonotic diseases and inefficient land and water use leading to low food security, it can be argued that developed nations are offsetting some of the true cost of their reliance on animal proteins to developing countries. Animal proteins are highly digestible and have a good amino acid balance, which is beneficial if food intake is limited. However, in excess, animal protein consumption has been linked to many non-communicable diseases, including obesity, cardiovascular disease, type 2 diabetes and certain cancers. These diseases are prevalent in population groups adhering to Western-type diets rich in animal-derived proteins. The environmental impacts of such food choices, however, are felt by the entire global human population, irrespective of the ecological footprints of individual diets.

ANIMAL PROTEIN PRODUCTION SYSTEMS

Animal protein production systems are responsible for much larger negative environmental impacts than plant-based food production. This is partly because of their inherent inefficiency, requiring high-quality feed for farm animals, which convert the feed into meat, milk or eggs. A major part of the feed is used to sustain the animals, the so-called maintenance component. With the genetic "improvement" of farm animals over the last 200 years, the acceleration of growth, milk and egg output and reproduction requires increased nutrient density in feed. Hence, farm animal feeds compete directly with human food, whereas previously, less productive animals could rely more on poor-quality feed grown on less fertile soil that could not produce human food directly.

Plant-Based Animal Feed

High-protein animal feeds from plants are transported long distances after large-scale intensive monocultural production, mainly in the Americas (mostly Brazil and the USA), e.g. soya to Europe and alfalfa to China. Soya requires warmer conditions to grow than those in Europe (Chojnacka et al. 2021). Food security in the European Union (EU) is therefore limited by dependence on imported feed for animals, despite the EU's Common Agricultural Policy's fundamental objective of increased security. The massive scale of meat production in China, particularly pork, makes the industries dependent on imported animal feed. Chickens, dairy cows and pigs rely extensively on soyabean meal, maize, and distillers' and brewers' grains for protein. Extrusion applies high temperatures, 150–160°C and high pressure to break down the antinutritive components in soya (trypsin, haemagglutinin and saponin), which reduce protein digestibility in monogastric and young animals. Mineral availability may also decline following extrusion due to degradation of phytase, requiring extra minerals to be added to the feed. Amino acids, particularly lysine and methionine, may be supplemented to improve the efficiency of protein utilisation. Antinutritive components in soya are often treated by heat processing. The polysaccharides in soyabean meal are poorly digested by monogastric animals, such as pigs and poultry, and supplementary enzymes are added to improve digestion. Oilseed meals are also used as high-quality supplements in animal diets, available after oil (in the case of rape, canola, sunflowers, etc.) or fibre (in the case of cotton) extraction for human use. Most of the imported soyabeans in China are converted into animal feed. All these processes are energy-intensive and ecologically inefficient compared to the production of plant proteins for direct human consumption.

In addition to concentrated, cereal-based feed, cattle and sheep obtain substantial protein from herbage, either fresh or conserved as hay and silage, using their ability to digest cellulose by microorganisms in their rumen. Legumes, such as clovers, improve soil fertility due to their symbiotic relationship with bacteria that fix nitrogen in their roots. Although this may appear as an environmentally benign option to supply animal proteins, the competition for land use is immense. Currently, 27% of the planet's land mass is used by the farm animal industries compared to only 7% for crops for direct human consumption (Ritchie and Roser 2019). Land clearing for agricultural purposes is also destroying native habitats, driving biodiversity loss and species extinctions.

Animal By-Products

Animal by-products, such as blood, feathers and meat and bone meal, provide high-quality protein in animal diets; however, there are restrictions on their use due to the risk of transmissible diseases, including zoonotic diseases such as bovine encephalopathy, classical swine fever and avian influenza. Some by-products are banned for ruminant feed, while others require extensive processing (e.g., rendering). A range of animal by-products, such as offal, can be suitable for human consumption, but safety concerns and cultural restrictions, including disgust, prevent the Western consumer at large from using them. The large volume of by-products produced and the restrictions on their use manifest significant inefficiencies in animal protein production that come at an environmental cost.

The portion of slaughtered animals available for use ranges from 32% for chickens to 38% for pigs and 46–48% for cattle and sheep (Alm 2012), with the remainder classified as by-products. Failure to use these by-products constitutes a major source of inefficiency in human food protein production, yet the risk to human health is often considered sufficient to lead to stringent restrictions. These were imposed during the bovine spongiform encephalopathy (BSE) outbreak in the 1990s but were relaxed soon after, particularly for aquacultural purposes (Jędrejek et al. 2016). Unused by-products have to be safely disposed of as fertiliser, biofuel or landfill waste, contributing to air and land pollution.

Fishmeal, sourced from wild-caught by-catch, aquacultural trimmings and purpose-grown fish, is produced by the major fish-producing countries, Peru, Chile and the Nordic countries, and is widely used in aquaculture, pig and chicken feed (Jędrejek et al. 2016). This appears to be an efficient use of ecological resources; however, intensive industrial fishing with the preference for larger species and the large volumes of by-catch (in some cases up to 90%) impact the natural balance of the world's oceans.

Plant Protein Production Systems

Traditionally, although their protein content is not high, cereal crops provide about 46% of global food protein (De Ron et al. 2017). Regional staples include rice in Asia, wheat in Europe, maize in the Americas and a variety of cereal crops including sorghum and millet in Africa. Globally, wheat and its products supply the most protein, 16 g/person/day, followed by rice (10 g), and maize (4 g) (Poutanen et al. 2022). As climate change accelerates, drought-resistant crops such as amaranth will be increasingly used to produce human and animal food. Higher food production potential still can be realised with aquatic plants, such as duckweed (Lemnaceae species), which can produce 100 t DM/ha/year with 30% crude protein (Pagliuso et al. 2022). However, these require extensive management and are likely to be most useful in small farms.

Plant-derived proteins have a consistently lower environmental footprint than animal proteins. They require substantially less land per 100 g of protein (Figure 1.2). For example, grain cultivation requires 40 times less land than lamb. While 100 g of protein from beef and lamb requires a land area of 164–185 m^2, peas and grains produce this amount of protein on only 3.4–4.6 m^2 (Poore and Nemecek 2018). Proteins sourced from meat and dairy are associated with much higher greenhouse gas emissions (Figure 1.3). Grain-derived protein emits only 2.7 kg CO_2e per 100 g compared to 50 kg for beef, 18 kg for farmed prawns and 9.5 kg for cow's milk. Notwithstanding the large variations around the world, major cereals, peas, bananas and nuts generate far less greenhouse gas emissions (Poore and Nemecek 2018). Increasing the share of animal-based proteins in the human diet leads to a wide range of planetary health challenges, and they represent an inefficient way of providing food for the global population.

Efficiency of Protein Production

Animal protein production is inherently inefficient because of the nutrient costs of maintaining the livestock. In the case of ruminant animals, micro-organisms contribute to greenhouse gas emissions through enteric fermentation and the release of methane. Improving the efficiency of animal protein production will be much less successful in maximising food security than increasing the plant-based content in human diets or converting to plant-based options. It must be acknowledged that

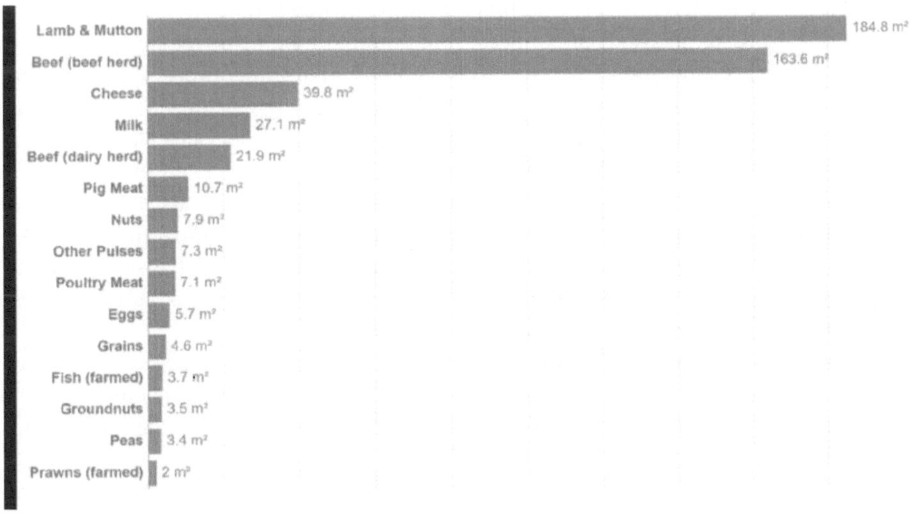

FIGURE 1.2 Land use per 100 g of protein The data is derived from an analysis of 1530 studies and data from 139 authors. Finally, 570 studies were included from approximately 38700 commercial farms in 119 countries, representing about 90% of world protein consumption. Source: Poore and Nemecek 2018; Ritchie et al. 2022; free of copyright restrictions.

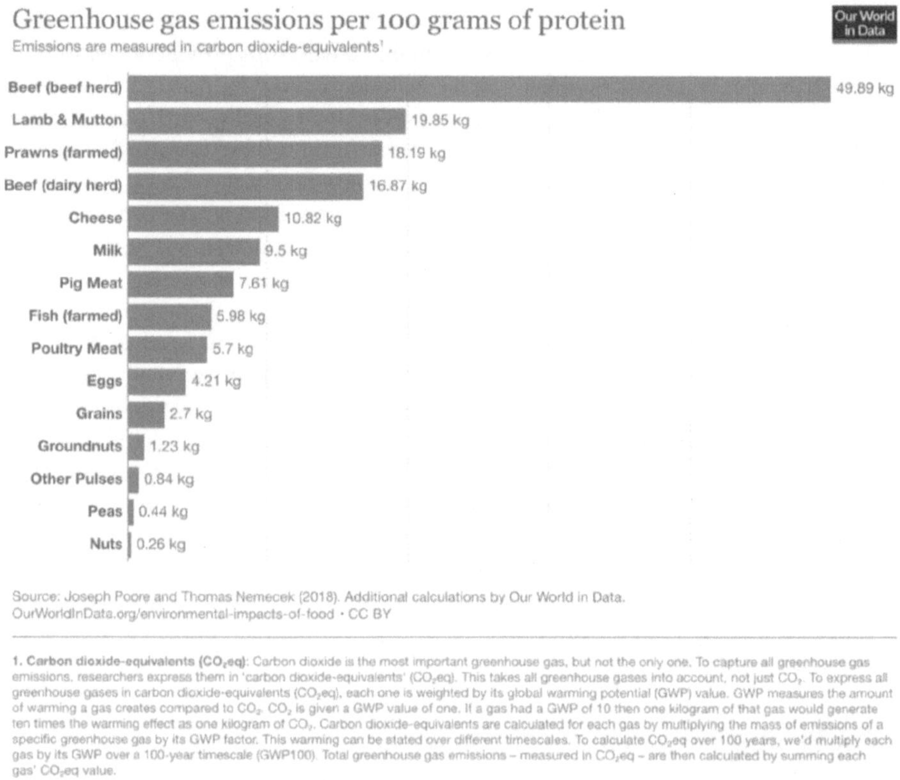

FIGURE 1.3 Greenhouse gas emissions per 100 g of protein The data is derived from an analysis of 1530 studies and data from 139 authors. Finally, 570 studies were included from approximately 38700 commercial farms in 119 countries, representing about 90% of world protein consumption. Source: Poore and Nemecek 2018; Ritchie et al. 2022; free of copyright restrictions.

sheep and beef cattle can be reared on land that would be difficult, though not usually impossible, to grow crops on. However, methods of using marginal land are being developed, such as drought-resistant crops, which are valuable in drought-prone regions, and timber crops, which can be grown on land too steep for traditional cropping. Furthermore, preserving natural habitats for wildlife is similarly important for human well-being, spiritual needs, ecosystem services and planetary health.

Protein is one of the most expensive components in food and feed. If animal protein demand continues to increase, maximising protein utilisation when feeding animals will be increasingly important to improve efficiency. For example, ensuring the feed composition and feed availability enable animals to grow at their genetic potential is crucial. This may involve supplementing with synthetic amino acids, enzymes, phytases, minerals, etc. An imbalance of nutrients means that some are wasted, being voided from the animal in their excreta.

With the major advances in genetic potential that have occurred, rapid growth leads to welfare issues that are of serious concern to the public. For example, in rapidly growing chickens, tibial dyschondroplasia impairs walking and causes painful bone breakages during catching and transport after the growth period (Pines and Reshef 2015).

Fertiliser for animal and plant production is a major source of pollutants to the atmosphere, both in the manufacturing process and from animals consuming the plants. Farmed animals, particularly cattle, release a potent greenhouse gas, methane, in significant quantities and contribute to acidification and eutrophication, biodiversity loss and zoonotic risks (Gerber et al. 2013).

Most importantly, eating animal-based proteins is a very inefficient method of protein conversion (Figure 1.4). In the case of beef, 96.2% of the proteins in the feed are lost, and only 3.8%

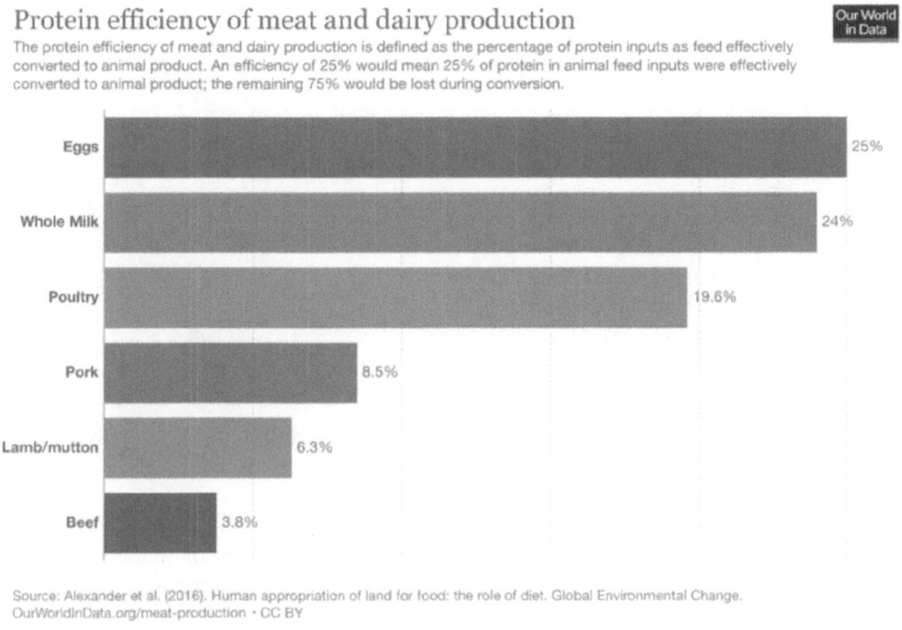

FIGURE 1.4 Protein efficiency of meat and dairy production. The data is derived from an analysis of 1530 studies and data from 139 authors. Finally, 570 studies were included from approximately 38700 commercial farms in 119 countries, representing about 90% of world protein consumption. Source: Poore and Nemecek 2018; Ritchie 2021; free of copyright restrictions.

are efficiently converted for human consumption. At 25% efficiency, eggs have one of the highest protein conversions among the animal-derived foods. These low rates of protein conversion put excessive pressure on the planet and its soils, pushing farmers to grow more crops and use synthetic fertilisers in an ever-accelerating cycle. Pollution from high levels of nitrogen fertiliser not only transgresses national boundaries (Richardson et al. 2023) but also reduces nutrient cycling efficiency by increasing the presence of this element in urine, atmospheric emissions, accumulation in the soil and leachate from agrarian areas.

Given the myriad of problems generated by the human preference for animal-sourced proteins – environmental and human health-related – a protein transition to plant-rich diets is a necessary priority (Poulain 2021). Driven by concerns for human health, climate action, ecological regeneration, habitat conservation and animal welfare, sustainability-conscious individuals in food-secure societies are shifting towards plant proteins (Marinova et al. 2022). New options for dietary protein supply are facilitating these changes while assisting in achieving global food security.

New Options for Dietary Protein for Humans

It is alarming that human food security remains unresolved. Humanity has come a long way since the agricultural Green Revolution and has been implementing incremental innovation in food production for more than seventy years. While it is true that humanity's ability to produce food has increased significantly, there are "elephants in the room" (Figure 1.5). The strategies employed to improve food production have created the absurd reality where food for more than 80 billion farm animals globally is produced in an effort to feed 8 billion humans. There are also the "elephants" of forest destruction for pasture and crops to feed farm animals, greenhouse gas emissions, water use and waste management problems, openly acknowledged by the Food and Agriculture Organisation of the United Nations decades ago (FAO 2006). Another "elephant" trumpeting since the 1960s is the unfair treatment of animals in intensive production systems (Harrison 1964). There is also the

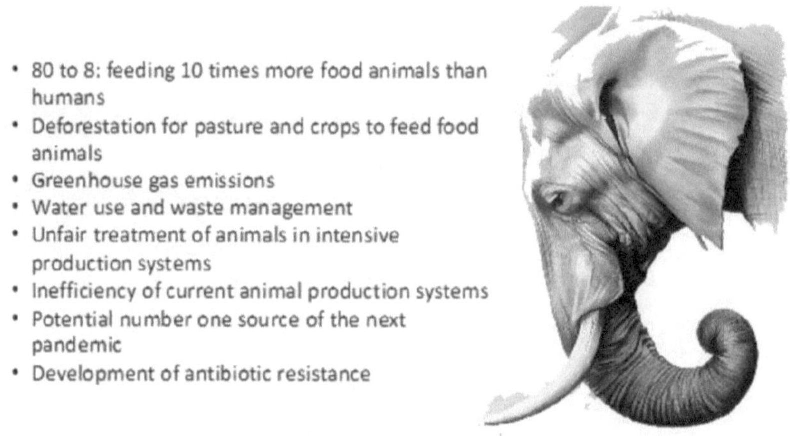

FIGURE 1.5 Issues with conventional animal protein production. The "elephant in the room" refers to the problems associated with conventional animal protein production. These include the facts that 80 billion farm animals are fed to feed 8 billion humans, an 80:8 ratio, and that deforestation is continuing at an unprecedented level to achieve that. The inefficient animal production systems used involve cruelty, and they have considerable greenhouse gas emissions, water use and waste problems. They are also a major source of antibiotic resistance and probably the next pandemic. Image available for free download from www.hiclipart.com/free-transparent-background-png-clipart-ielxb/download.

"elephant" representing the inefficiency of the current animal production systems as compared to new technologies. The health "elephants" signal the risk of novel pandemics (UNEP 2020) and intensive animal production's major contribution to the development of antibiotic resistance by pathogens (Wang et al. 2023) that may leave medicine in a state similar to the pre-antibiotic era. Indeed, a whole herd of "elephants" is in the room, while in nature, wild animals are disappearing at an unprecedented rate as more and more of the Earth's carbon atoms are sequestered by human and, mostly, farm animal bodies (Heidemann et al. 2020).

Considering all issues involved, current animal food production and human food security challenges suggest that insisting on incremental improvements based on the same paradigms may not be the best approach. Although alternative consumption diets such as vegetarianism and veganism exist, the estimates for global meat demand remain on a steadily increasing pathway. This progressive increase in meat demand comes mostly from predictions of increased per capita meat consumption in Asian countries as a result of a process termed "meatification" (Hansen and Jakobsen 2020). It is not that a reversal of this trend is impossible, but it would require a long time, especially considering the vested interests that have resulted in a powerful pro-meat consumption rhetoric (Hannan 2020). Thus, if animal proteins bring many problems with them and if consumption trends appear to be against a fast transition away from animal proteins, are there any other strategies? This current context is highly conducive to disruptive innovation and a new food technological wave with what has been termed "alternative proteins". These proteins differ from traditional animal and plant proteins as they are not simply grown but produced through technological means. They are expected to shape a new food landscape that is environmentally friendlier and offers better prospects for the human population.

Disruptive innovation has replaced some animal products before (Figure 1.6). For example, the introduction of petroleum-based products on the market was a significant factor in reducing the demand for whale oil (McCollough and Check Jr 2010). Although plant-based milks and oils have been used for millennia as alternatives to cow's milk and animal fats, their recent resurgence and

A

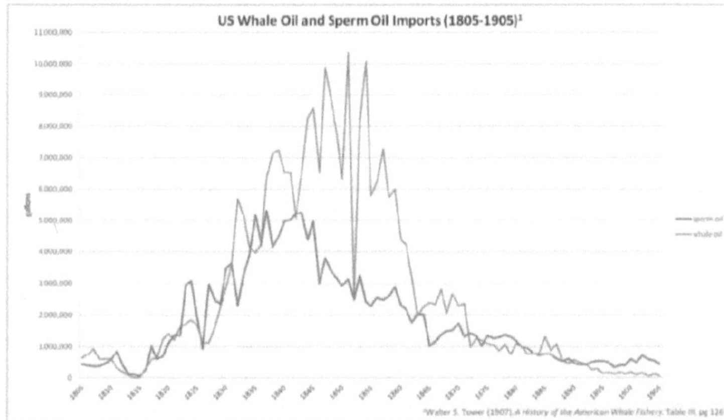

B

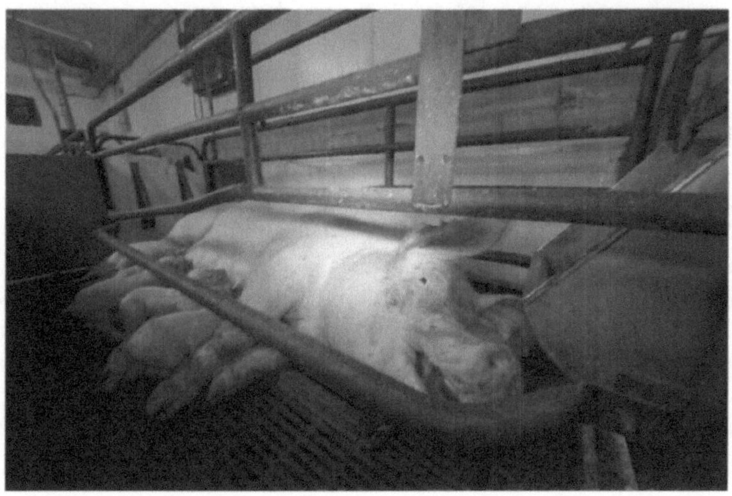

FIGURE 1.6 Animals rescued by disruptive innovation in the past (A – whales used for oil production) and potentially in the future (B – sow and piglets in a current intensive pig production barn).

diversification are creating disruptive new commercial opportunities. Radical innovation in producing the animal protein itself seems to be on the verge of becoming disruptive, as new technologies for creating meat, dairy, egg and fish proteins without animals involved gain important momentum in solving human food challenges. Radical innovation occurs when an existing technological paradigm shifts and new technological pathways are launched (Morais-da-Silva et al. 2022a; Tziva et al. 2020). Alternative proteins produced through precision fermentation and cell cultivation represent such new trajectories within the context of human food production. The market share of alternative proteins will likely increase as their quality improves and their price falls, in a movement called the great meat revolution (Biscarra-Bellio et al. 2023).

The innovation brought by cellular agriculture requires new ways of thinking. For instance, whether cell-based meat is vegan is not a straightforward issue, as its production is uncoupled from animal suffering and animal killing (Heidemann et al. 2020). However, it is probably not vegetarian, as it is composed of real animal cells. Alternative proteins are also a new story as healthy food items. Regulations to ensure their safety are under development and at different stages across the world. There is also the issue of their value as highly customised food items. For example, a cell-based steak can be produced with precisely defined levels of fat, pre-modelled in their distribution as, for instance, a specifically determined marbling pattern. Other possibilities relate to hybrid products, made of animal muscle cells mixed with plant fats. Such products can bring the amino acid profile of animal proteins without the disadvantages of animal fat, such as high cholesterol levels. Thus, alternative protein products can be tailored to human health needs as well as desires.

Many questions, however, remain about the environmental footprint of these new proteins. Although some claim that it is at least 90% smaller than that of animal-derived proteins (Bryant 2022), there is the potential to further decrease greenhouse gas emissions if renewable energy sources are used. Transparency and safety in the production processes are concerns raised specifically by younger consumers, who are not prepared to add another suite of problems created by previous generations (Bogueva and Marinova 2022).

As with previous paradigm shifts, the changes do not occur only regarding technological aspects, but social impacts are usually implicated as well. The social aspects of a shift towards alternative proteins have been increasingly discussed in recent years, and while there are relatively persistent challenges, high levels of engagement with the new protein production systems are coupled with increased advantages (Morais-da-Silva et al. 2022b). In addition, new technologies are limited in the scope of the advances they can bring, while the problems with food security are multifactorial, with a high level of complexity that crosses the boundaries between biotechnological, social and political systems. Even then, there seem to be good reasons to believe that alternative proteins will provide a valuable contribution towards food security, human and animal well-being and the sustainability of food production systems.

CONCLUSIONS

Concerns about planetary health are shaping the food production environment, with increasing awareness about the higher costs of animal proteins compared to plant proteins. While consumers are navigating this space, responding to a myriad of economic, environmental, human health, animal welfare, cultural and marketing drivers, the global trends indicate that people are not prepared to give up their love for animal-derived proteins. Despite abundant evidence about the detrimental impacts of increased consumption of animal proteins, people are very slow to embrace more plant-rich diets while the planet is boiling and burning, with many other species lost or on the brink of extinction.

In challenging situations when things appear bleak and are heading towards a precipice, humanity finds ways to rediscover its strength and creativity by shifting to new technological trajectories. Are we in such a moment in time when the dichotomy between animal and plant proteins is being transformed into new ways of supplying nutrition to the human species? The new proteins are lurking in scientific labs, entrepreneurial start-ups and people's imaginations. However, if normal meat and cow's milk gradually become stranger and cultured meat and synthetic milk develop as the more normal options (van der Weele and Driessen 2019), such a food transition has the potential to increase the hope for a change that is gentler to the natural world and leaves no one behind.

SUMMARY POINTS

- Animal-based protein is increasing in popularity worldwide.
- Feeding the human population with animal protein is inefficient in the use of scarce land and other resources.
- Feeding the human population with animal protein contributes significantly to global climate change.
- Overconsuming animal protein has some serious health consequences.
- Many drivers encourage plant-derived proteins, despite global growth in meat consumption.
- Cultivated meat is becoming available, which may reduce reliance on farmed animals.

- A transition to better food choices is required to reduce the environmental, ethical and health burdens of the current food systems.
- The dynamic changes in human protein consumption need to be better managed nationally and internationally.

MINI DICTIONARY OF TERMS

- **Alternative protein:** Protein that is derived from plants and/or produced through technological means.
- **Animal by-product:** Material obtained from dead or live animals not intended for human consumption.
- **By-catch:** Marine animals caught and discarded by industrial fishers.
- **Elephant in the room:** A metaphor for an obvious but difficult problem people do not want to talk about.
- **Environmental footprint:** The environmental impact of a human activity.
- **Fishmeal:** An animal feed product made predominantly of fish-derived material.
- **Flexitarian:** A person following flexitarianism.
- **Flexitarianism:** A semi-vegetarian diet where the consumer deliberately reduces the intake of meat and other animal-based products.
- **Incremental innovation:** An innovation that involves making gradual improvements and refinements to existing products, services or processes.
- **Meatification:** A shift to meat-rich dietary preferences in countries with traditionally low meat consumption.
- **New protein:** A broad category of types of proteins that are not used traditionally in the human diet, including new technological food products, such as cultured/cellular meat and synthetic milk.
- **Plant-rich diet:** A diet with a significant amount of plant-based products, including vegetables, fruits, nuts, legumes, seeds and vegetable oils.
- **Protein conversion:** Animal-based transformation of protein into protein for human consumption.
- **Radical innovation:** An innovation that involves significant and transformative changes, creating new paradigms or new ways of providing products, services or processes.
- **Technological trajectory:** Technology development follows a particular pattern of technological choices.

REFERENCES

Alm, M. 2012. Review of the EU feed ban on non-ruminant processed animal proteins: Outlook of the European Fat Processors and Renderers Association (EFPRA). Paper presented at the TAIEX Workshop, Russia. http://www.fefac.eu/ file.pdf?FileID=42256&CacheMode=Fresh (accessed September 11, 2023).

Biscarra-Bellio, J. C., G. B. de Oliveira, M. C. P. Marques and C. F. M. Molento. 2023. Demand changes meat as changing meat reshapes demand: The great meat revolution. *Meat Science* 196:109040. https://doi.org/10.1016/j.meatsci.2022.109040

Bogueva, D. and D. Marinova. 2022. Australian generation Z and the nexus between climate change and alternative proteins. *Animals* 12:2512. https://doi.org/10.3390/ ani12192512

Bogueva, D. and I. Phau 2016. Meat myths and marketing. In *Impact of meat consumption on health and environmental sustainability*, edited by T. Raphaely and D. Marinova, pp. 264–276. Hershey, PA: IGI Global.

Bryant, C. J. 2022. Plant-based animal product alternatives are healthier and more environmentally sustainable than animal products. *Future Foods* 6:100174. https://doi.org/10.1016/j.fufo.2022.100174

Carpenter, K., D. W. Kent-Jones, A. S. Truswell and J. Weininger. 2023. *Human nutrition*. Encyclopedia Britannica. https://www.britannica.com/science/human-nutrition/BMR-and-REE-energy-balance (accessed October 5, 2023).

Chojnacka, K., K. Mikula, G. Izydorczyk, D. Skrzypczak, A. Witek-Krowiak, A. Gersz, K. Moustakas, J. Iwaniuk, M. Grzędzicki and M. Korczyński. 2021. Innovative high digestibility protein feed materials reducing environmental impact through improved nitrogen-use efficiency in sustainable agriculture. *Journal of Environmental Management* 291:112693. https://doi.org/10.1016/j.jenvman.2021.112693 .Enzymes

De Ron, A., F. Sparvoli, J. J. Pueyo and D. Bazile. 2017. Protein crops: Food and feed for the future. *Frontiers in Plant Science* 8. https://doi.org/10.3389/fpls.2017.00105

Ederer, P. and F. Leroy. 2023. The societal role of meat—what the science says. *Animal Frontiers* 13(2):3–8. https://doi.org/10.1093/af/vfac098

Facts & Factors. 2022. Global fruit & vegetable processing market size expected to reach USD 530 billion by 2028. https://www.fnfresearch.com/news/global-fruit-vegetable-processing-market (accessed October 5, 2023).

Food and Agriculture Organisation of the United Nations (FAO). 2006. *Livestock's long shadow: Environmental issues and options*. Rome: FAO. ftp://ftp.fao.org/docrep/fao/010/a0701e/A0701E00.pdf.

Funghi, C., R. H. J. Heim, W. Schuett, S. C. Griffith and J. Oldeland. 2020. Estimating food resource availability in arid environments with Sentinel 2 satellite imagery. *PeerJ* 8:e9209. https://doi.org/10.7717/peerj.9209

Gerber, P. J., H. Steinfeld, B. Henderson, A. Mottet, C. Opio, J. Dijkman, A. Falcucci and G. Tempio. 2013. *Tackling climate change through livestock: A global assessment of emissions and mitigation opportunities. Rome*: Food and Agriculture Organization of the United Nations (FAO).

Godfray, H. C. J., P. Aveyard, T. Garnett, J. W. Hall, T. J. Key, J. Lorimer, R. T. Pierrehumbert, P. Scarborough, M. Springmann and S. A. Jebb. 2018. Meat consumption, health, and the environment. *Science* 361:eaam5324. https/doiorg/10.1126/science.aam5324

Hannan, J. 2020. *Meatsplaining: The Animal agriculture industry and the rhetoric of denial*. Sydney: Sydney University Press.

Hansen, A. and J. Jakobsen. 2020. Meatification and everyday geographies of consumption in Vietnam and China. *Geografiska Annaler: Series B, Humanan Geography* 102(1):21–39. https://doi.org/10.1080/04353684.2019.1709217

Harrison, R. 1964. *Animal machines*. London: Vincent Stuart Publishers.

Heidemann, M. S., C. F. M. Molento, G. G., Reis and C. J. C. Philips. 2020. Uncoupling meat from animal slaughter and its impacts on human-animal relationships. *Frontiers in Psychology* 11:1824. https://doi.org/10.3389/fpsyg.2020.01824

High Level Panel of Experts on Food Security and Nutrition (HLPE). 2017. *Nutrition and food systems*. Rome: Committee on World Food Security. http://www.fao.org/3/a-i7846e.pdf.

Jędrejek, D., J. Levic, J. Wallace and W. Oleszek. 2016. Animal by-products for feed: Characteristics, European regulatory framework, and potential impacts on human and animal health and the environment. *Journal of Animal and Feed Sciences* 25(3):189–202. https://doi.org/10.22358/jafs/65548/2016

Joshi, T., P. R. Deepa, M. Joshi and P. K. Sharma. 2023. Matters of the desert: A perspective on achieving food and nutrition security through plants of the (semi) arid regions. *Journal of Agriculture and Food Research* 14:100725. https://doi.org/10.1016/j.jafr.2023.100725

Marinova, D. and D. Bogueva 2022. *Food in a planetary emergency*. Singapore: Springer Nature.

Marinova, D., D. Bogueva, Y. Wu and X. Guo. 2022. China and changing food trends: A sustainability transition perspective. *Ukrainian Food Journal* 11(1):126–47. https://doi.org/ 10.24263/2304- 974X-2022-11- 1-13

Market Data Forecast. 2023. Fresh fruits and vegetables market. https://www.marketdataforecast.com/market-reports/fresh-fruits-and-vegetables-market (accessed October 5, 2023).

McCollough, J. and H. F. Check Jr. 2010. The baleen whales' saving grace: The introduction of petroleum based products in the market and its impact on the whaling industry. *Sustainability* 2:3142–57. https//doi.org/10.3390/su2103142

Milford, A. B., C. Le Mouël, B. L. Bodirsky and S. Rolinski. 2019. Drivers of meat consumption. *Appetite* 141:104313. https://doi.org/10.1016/j.appet.2019.06.005

Morais-da-Silva, R. L., G. G. Reis, H. Sanctorum and C. F. M. Molento. 2022a. The social impact of cultivated and plant-based meats as radical innovations in the food chain: Views from Brazil, the United States and Europe. *Frontiers in Sustainable Food Systems* 6:1056615. https//doi.org/10.3389/fsufs.2022.1056615

Morais-da-Silva, R. L., G. G. Reis, H. Sanctorum and C. F. M. Molento. 2022b. The social impacts of a transition from conventional to cultivated and plant-based meats: Evidence from Brazil. *Food Policy* 111:102337. https://doi.org/10.1016/j.foodpol.2022.102337

Pagliuso, D., A. Grandis, J. S. Fortirer, P. Camargo, E. I. S. Floh and M. S. Buckeridge. 2022. Duckweeds as promising food feedstocks globally. *Agronomy* 12:796. https://doi.org/10.3390/agronomy12040796

Pines, M., and R. Reshef, 2015. Poultry bone development and bone disorders. In *Sturkie's Avian physiology*, 6th ed., edited by C. G. Scanes. Elsevier. https://www.sciencedirect.com/science/article/abs/pii/B9780124071605000154

Poore, J. and T. Nemecek. 2018. Reducing food's environmental impacts through producers and consumers. *Science* 360(6392):987–992. https://doi.org/10.1126/science.aaq021

Poulain J.-P. 2021. Food in transition: The place of food in the theories of transition. *The Sociological Review Monographs* 69(3):702–24. https://doi.org/101177/00380261211009092

Poutanen, K. S., A. O. Kårlund, C. Gómez-Gallego, D. P. Johansson, N. M. Scheers, I. M. Marklinder, A. K. Eriksen et al. 2022. Grains – a major source of sustainable protein for health. *Nutrition Reviews* 80(6):1648–63. https://doi.org/10.1093/nutrit/nuab084

Ranganathan, J. and R. Waite 2016. *Sustainable diets: What you need to know in 12 charts.* World Research Institute. https://www.wri.org/insights/sustainable-diets-what-you-need-know-12-charts (accessed October 7, 2023).

Richardson, K., W. Steffen, W. Luch, J. Bendtsen, S. E. Cornell, J. F. Donges, M. Drüke et al. 2023. Earth beyond six of nine boundaries. *ScienceAdvances* 9(37). https//doi.org/10.1126/sciadv.adh2458

Ritchie, H. 2021. *If the world adopted a plant-based diet we would reduce global agricultural land use from 4 to 1 billion hectares.* Our World in Data. https://ourworldindata.org/land-use-diets (accessed October 7, 2023).

Ritchie, H., P. Rosado and M. Roser 2022. *Environmental impacts of food production.* Our World in Data. https://ourworldindata.org/environmental-impacts-of-food (accessed October 7, 2023)

Ritchie, H. and M. Roser 2019. *Land use.* Our World in Data. https://ourworldindata.org/land-use#citation (accessed October 5, 2023).

Rubio, N. R., N. Xiang and D. L. Kaplan. 2020. Plant-based and cell-based approaches to meat production. *Nature Communication* 11:6276. https://doi.org/10.1038/s41467-020-20061-y

Shahbandeh, M. 2022. Global plant protein market value 2022–2027. *Statista.* https://www.statista.com/statistics/658619/global-plant-protein-market-value/_(accessed October 5, 2023).

Tziva, M., S. O. Negro, A. Kalfagianni and M. P. Hekkert. 2020. Understanding the protein transition: The rise of plant-based meat substitutes. *Environmental Innovation and Societal Transitions*, 35:217–31. https://doi.org/10.1016/j.eist.2019.09.004

United Nations Environment Programme (UNEP) and International Livestock Research Institute 2020. Preventing the next pandemic: Zoonotic diseases and how to break the chain of transmission. https://www.unep.org/resources/report/preventing-future-zoonotic-disease-outbreaks-protecting-environment-animals-and (accessed October 5, 2023).

van der Weele, C. and C. Driessen. 2019. How normal meat becomes stranger as cultured meat becomes more normal: Ambivalence and ambiguity below the surface of behavior. *Frontiers in Sustainable Food Systems* 3:69. https://doi.org/10.3389/fsufs.2019.00069

Wang, H., J. F. Qi, R. Qin, K. Ding, D. W Graham and Y.-G. Zhu. 2023. Intensified livestock farming increases antibiotic resistance genotypes and phenotypes in animal feces. *Communications Earth & Environment* 4:123. https://doi.org/10.1038/s43247-023-00790-w

Whitton, C., D. Bogueva, D. Marinova and C. J. C. Phillips. 2021. Are we approaching peak meat consumption? Analysis of meat consumption from 2000 to 2019 in 35 countries and its relationship to gross domestic product. *Animals* 11(12):3466. https://doi.org/10.3390/ani11123466

Willett, W., J. Rockstrõm, B. Loken, M. Springmann, T. Lang, S. Vermeulen T. Garnett et al. 2019 Food in the anthropocene: The EAT–lancet commission on healthy diets from sustainable food systems. *The Lancet* 393(10170):447–92. https://doi.org/10.1016/S0140-6736(18)31788-4

World Cancer Research Fund (WCRF) and American Institute for Cancer Research (AICR). 1997. *Food, nutrition and the prevention of cancer: A global perspective.* Washington, DC: BANTA Book Group.

2 Plant and Animal Protein Intake and Their Metabolic Differential Effects

Masako Matsunaga

ABBREVIATIONS

AP	Animal protein
BMI	Body mass index
BP	Blood pressure
CRP	C-reactive protein
DBP	Diastolic blood pressure
DIAAS	Digestible indispensable amino acid scores
FFQ	Food frequency questionnaire
FG	Fasting plasma or serum glucose
HbA1c	Glycated hemoglobin
HDL-C	High-density lipoprotein cholesterol
HOMA-IR	Homeostasis model assessment for insulin resistance
hs-CRP	High-sensitivity C-reactive protein
LCD	Low-carbohydrate diet
LDL-C	Low-density lipoprotein cholesterol
MDA	Malondialdehyde
MetS	Metabolic syndrome
NCEP/ATP III	National Cholesterol Education Program's Adult Treatment Panel III
NHANES	National Health and Nutrition Examination Survey
PDCAAS	Protein digestibility-corrected amino acid scores
PP	Plant protein
RCT	Randomized clinical trial
SBP	Systolic blood pressure
T2DM	Type 2 diabetes mellitus
TC	Total cholesterol
TG	Triglycerides
TNF-α	Tumor necrosis factor-α

INTRODUCTION

Proteins are the major functional and structural components of all the cells in the body. The human body needs adequate intakes of dietary proteins to maintain cellular integrity and function for health and reproduction (Institute of Medicine 2006). Animal proteins (APs) and plant proteins (PPs) are the primary dietary sources. Common AP sources among US adults include meat, poultry, seafood, dairy, and eggs (Hoy et al. 2022). Most PPs come from grains (e.g., yeast bread and rolls/buns), while beans, peas, and nuts/seeds contribute less to total protein consumption (Pasiakos et al. 2015).

DOI: 10.1201/9781003597926-2

Amid the rising popularity of plant-based diets, studies exploring the benefits of PP-rich diets have increased dramatically over the past decade. Several focus specifically on the effects of PP intake on managing or preventing metabolic syndrome (MetS), a complex risk factor for cardiovascular diseases and type 2 diabetes mellitus (T2DM). This chapter discusses the current understanding of MetS, nutritional differences between PP and AP foods, and findings from past epidemiological studies and randomized controlled trials regarding PP-rich and AP-rich diets' associations with metabolic-related biomarkers. Finally, it explores the effects of other protein types on these biomarkers.

METABOLIC SYNDROME

MetS is a precursor of metabolic diseases, such as T2DM and cardiovascular diseases (Wilson et al. 2005). It is also associated with developing non-alcoholic fatty liver disease (NAFLD) and chronic kidney diseases (Markova et al. 2017; Zhang and Lerman 2017). MetS is characterized by abdominal obesity, abnormal levels of blood pressure (BP), fasting glucose (FG), triglycerides (TG), and high-density lipoprotein cholesterol (HDL-C) (Alberti et al. 2009) (Figure 2.1). Previously, the diagnostic criteria for MetS were inconsistent across organizations. In 2009, six organizations (the International Diabetes Federation Task Force on Epidemiology and Prevention; National Heart, Lung, and Blood Institute; American Heart Association; World Heart Federation; International Atherosclerosis Society; and International Association for the Study of Obesity) reached a harmonized definition, establishing that MetS diagnosis requires at least three or more abnormal findings out of these five MetS characteristics (Figure 2.1) (Alberti et al. 2009). The prevalence of MetS among US adults assessed with the National Cholesterol Education Program's Adult Treatment Panel III (NCEP/ATP III), which is similar to the criteria above, was 35% based on the National

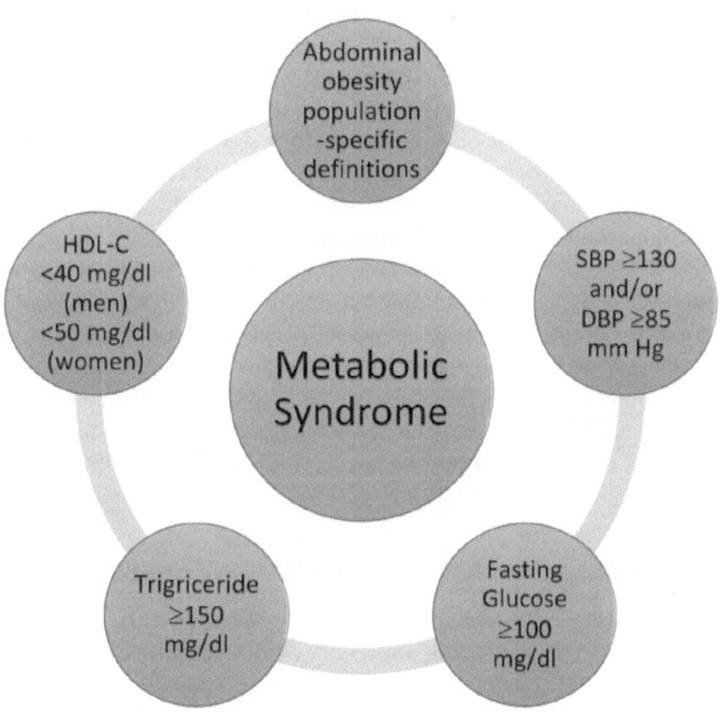

FIGURE 2.1 Components of metabolic syndrome according to the Joint Interim Statement (Albert et al., 2009). *Abbreviations*: HDL-C: high-density lipoprotein concentration. SBP: systolic blood pressure. DBP diastolic blood pressure.

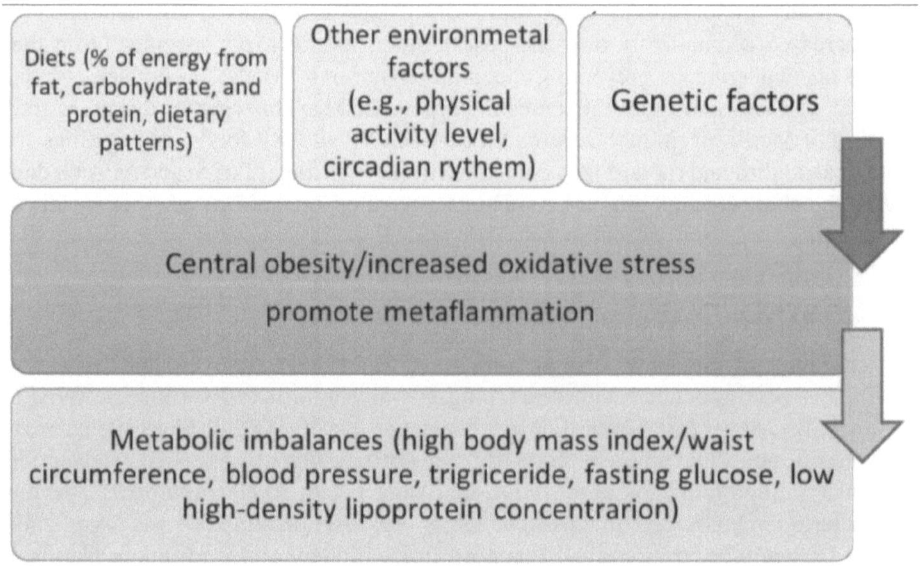

FIGURE 2.2 Factors contributing to the development of metabolic imbalances.

Health and Nutrition Examination Survey (NHANES) 2011–2016 data (Hirode and Wong 2020). The prevalence remained stable in older adults but increased in younger adults. In the Asia-Pacific region, a study conducted in urban Pakistan reported a high prevalence (49%) based on the modified NECP/ATP III criteria (Hydrie et al. 2009). The Philippines appears to have a low prevalence (12%) based on the NECP/ATP III criteria with the 2003–2004 national survey study (Morales et al. 2008). A review study reported that about 20% or more of the Asia-Pacific adult population was affected by MetS, with a secular increase in prevalence (Ranasinghe et al. 2017).

Although the mechanism of MetS development is still being explored, past studies reported evidence suggesting the involvement of proinflammatory states and oxidative stress (Figure 2.2). An imbalance between energy intake and output is a well-known risk factor for obesity (Reilly and Saltiel 2017). Chronic inflammation, also known as metaflammation, can occur in obese individuals, which is one of the important factors contributing to MetS. Specifically, the expansion of adipose tissues is susceptive to increased inflammatory responses through adipocyte death, hypoxia, and interactions between the cells and extracellular matrix (Reilly and Saltiel 2017). Consequently, the chronic proinflammatory status disrupts the pancreas β-cell function, leading to insulin resistance (Yang et al. 2023). Obesity is also associated with hypertension, hypertriglyceridemia, and dyslipidemia, and these are increasing risks for oxidative stress and proinflammatory status (Safaei et al. 2021; Silveira Rossi et al. 2022). Recent studies also suggest a link between circadian rhythm and MetS, as MetS is highly prevalent among those with shift work (Deota and Panda 2021; Alqaderi et al. 2023).

BIOMARKERS OF INFLAMMATION AND OXIDATIVE STRESS

Besides traditional biomarkers of metabolic diseases (e.g., BP, FG, TG), inflammation biomarkers, such as C-reactive protein (CRP) and proinflammatory cytokines, have also been measured in MetS studies (Silveira Rossi et al. 2022; Monserrat-Mesquida et al. 2020).

CRP is a protein synthesized in the liver, and the CRP level in the blood rises in response to acute and chronic inflammation. High-sensitivity CRP (hs-CRP) assays are more sensitive than regular CRP tests and have been used to detect low-grade inflammation, with normal levels <0.3 mg/dL (or <3 mg/L) in healthy individuals. Minor elevations (0.3–1.0 mg/dL or 3–10 mg/L) are detected in pregnant women and individuals with diabetes, depression, the common cold, gingivitis, periodontitis, cigarette smoking, and genetic predispositions, and various reasons can further elevate hs-CRP levels (Nehring et al. 2023). Hs-CRP has also been used as an indicator of future cardiovascular disease risks. A hs-CRP level <1.0 mg/L is considered low risk, and >3.0 mg/L is considered high risk (Ridker 2003).

Metaflammation is also characterized by an increase of proinflammatory cytokines, such as interleukin (IL)-1β, IL-6, and tumor necrosis factor-α (TNF-α). IL-1 and TNF-α are generated from chronically inflamed adipose tissue; IL-6 is produced by adipocytes and other cell types (Silveira Rossi et al. 2022). Molecules modified by reactive oxygen species have been used as biomarkers of oxidative stress. For example, a high level of malondialdehyde (MDA), a final product of polyunsaturated fatty acid peroxidation in cells, suggests a higher intensity of oxidative stress (Gaweł et al. 2004). Protein carbonylation, the oxidation of side chains of proteins promoted by reactive oxygen species (Suzuki et al. 2010), has also been used as an oxidative stress biomarker. Nitrotyrosine, a product of tyrosine nitration mediated by peroxynitrite, indicates nitrosative stress (Pacher and Szabó 2006; Pinchuk et al. 2019).

PLANT PROTEIN FOOD VS. ANIMAL PROTEIN FOOD

Adequate protein intake is correlated with satiety, glycemic response, gastric emptying rate, and insulin secretion (Jamshidi et al. 2022). These associations suggest benefits for metabolic balance. While various protein foods are available, their quality depends on several factors (Figure 2.3).

Amino acid profile is one factor in protein quality. Proteins consist of amino acids linked by peptide bonds. Generally, APs include all essential amino acids (those not synthesized in mammals), while PPs have lower levels of essential amino acids – particularly branched-chain amino acids (leucine, isoleucine, and valine) and the sulfur-containing amino acid methionine. Digestibility is another factor of protein quality. PPs are less digestible than APs due to their high content in β-sheet conformation and low α-helix amount in the protein secondary structure (Carbonaro et al. 2012). The digestibility of dietary protein can be expressed by a protein digestibility-corrected amino acid score (PDCAAS) ranging from 0 to 1 (or 0–100%) (Leser 2013). For example, PDCAAS values are 92% for red meat, 100% for cow's milk and eggs, but less than 100% for most PP foods (Hoffman

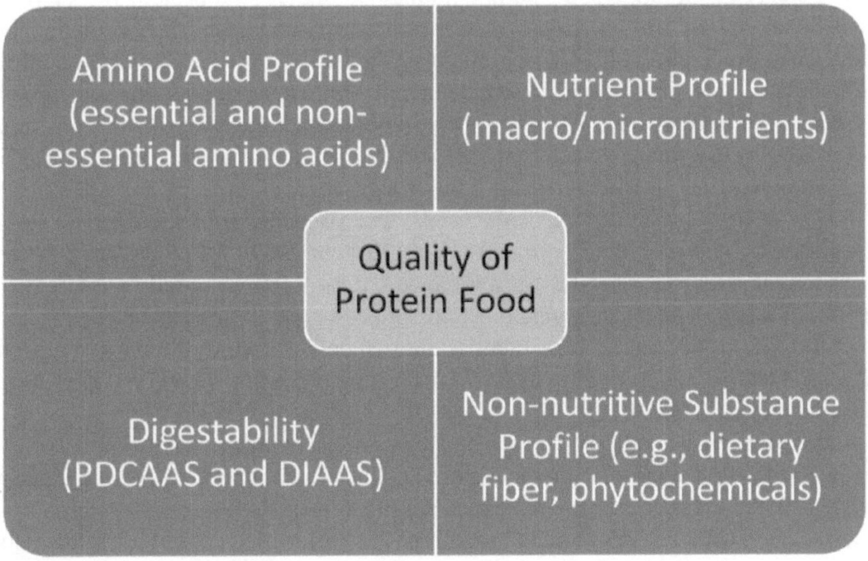

FIGURE 2.3 Factors contributing to protein food quality.

and Falvo 2004). While PDCAAS is based on digestibility at the total digestive tract, digestible indispensable amino acid scores (DIAAS) are based on digestibility at the end of the small intestine (Food and Agriculture Organization 2013). DIAAS is not truncated at 100, providing more accurate assessments than PDCAAS. The DIAAS is greater than 100 for most meats, milk, and eggs, aside from some processed meats, but falls below 100 for most PP foods (Berrazaga et al. 2019).

The overall nutrient profile of protein foods is another important factor in determining their quality. A recent study reported differences in overall nutrient intakes across quartiles of PP intake among US adults (Marinangeli et al. 2023). The study found that the group with the highest PP intake (Q4) had a higher intake of dietary fiber, folate, iron, and zinc but a lower intake of vitamins B12 and D compared to the group with the lowest PP intake (Q1). Another study examined the differences across quintiles of total protein from AP among US adults (Hoy et al. 2023). The study reported that many in the group with lowest AP intake (Q1) more often met recommended intakes for folate, vitamin C, saturated fat, cholesterol, and fiber compared to the group with the highest AP intake (Q5). However, they consumed less protein and failed to meet recommended intakes for vitamins A, B12, choline, zinc, and calcium. These findings suggest that PP-rich diets provide various nutrients but may result in inadequate protein and certain nutrients abundant in APs.

PP foods also contain phytochemicals with antioxidant properties. For example, soybeans and soy products contain various phytochemicals, such as phenolic acids, flavonoids, isoflavones, and saponins (Luthria et al. 2007). Buckwheat is a rich source of flavonoids and phenolic acids (Multari et al. 2016). Thus, phytochemicals via PP intake may also help prevent and manage MetS (Cicero and Colletti 2016; Santa et al. 2023),

EPIDEMIOLOGICAL STUDIES OF PLANT PROTEIN-RICH DIETS AND METABOLISM

Several epidemiological studies examined associations between dietary protein sources and various metabolic-related outcomes (Table 2.1). Jamshidi et al. (2022) examined associations between dietary protein sources and the risk of MetS in Iranian adults. Study participants were categorized into quintiles of total, AP, and PP intake for each sex based on their responses to a 125-item food frequency questionnaire (FFQ). In this study, 40% of women and 25% of men had MetS. After adjusting for potential confounders, the authors found that higher total protein and PP intakes were negatively associated with MetS diagnosis (lower prevalence) and each MetS component (abdominal obesity, BP, FG, TG, and HDL-C) in both sexes. Higher AP intake was also negatively associated with MetS diagnosis in men. However, among MetS components, higher AP Intake was negatively associated only with abdominal obesity in both sexes and TG in men.

Chen et al. (2018) examined associations between adherence to a plant-based diet and insulin resistance, one of the MetS characteristics, using longitudinal data from non-diabetic adult participants in a prospective study in the Netherlands. The participants' adherence to a plant-based diet was assessed by applying their responses to a 170-item FFQ to a plant-based dietary index. Homeostatic model assessment for insulin resistance (HOMA-IR) was used to assess their insulin resistance status: a higher level indicates more insulin resistance. After adjusting for sociodemographic and lifestyle factors and other potential confounders, the study found that a higher index score was associated with a lower level of HOMA-IR, supporting the benefits of greater adherence to a plant-based diet.

Meng et al. (2021) examined associations between protein intake and cardiometabolic risk factors among Chinese adults using the China Health and Nutrition Survey 2009 data. This cross-sectional study estimated the percentage of energy from PP and AP from three 24-hour dietary recalls. Biomarkers included CRP and glycated hemoglobin (HbA1c), which indicates average blood sugar levels over the past 2–3 months. The study found that a higher intake of PP was associated with a lower LDL-C/HDL-C ratio and higher HDL-C and HbA1c after adjusting for potential confounders.

TABLE 2.1
Epidemiological Studies Examining Associations between Plant and/or Animal Protein-Rich Diets and Metabolic-Related Outcomes

Authors and Publication Year	Study Design/Population	Protein Food/Sources	Study Findings of Metabolic-Related Outcomes
Jamshidi et al. 2022	Cross-sectional study with Iranian adults (the Fasa Cohort Study in the Prospective Epidemiological Research Study in Iran, n = 8922)	Quintiles of total protein/AP/PP intake (g/kg of body weight)	Higher consumption of total/PP was negatively associated with a prevalence of MetS and its components.
Chen et al. 2018	Longitudinal study with adults in the Netherlands (the Rotterdam Study, n = 6798)	Scores of dietary index to assess adherence to a plant-based diet	A higher score on the plant-based dietary index was associated with lower insulin resistance (HOMA-IR) and lower T2DM risk.
Meng et al. 2021	Cross-sectional study with Chinese adults (China Health and Nutrition Survey 2009, n = 7886)	Quintiles of total protein/AP/PP intake (% of total energy)	AP was positively associated with total cholesterol, LDL-C, non-HDL-C, and uric acid. PP was inversely associated with non-HDL-C and LDL-C/HDL-C ratio and positively associated with HDL-C and glycated hemoglobin.
Vallianou et al. 2013	Cross-sectional study with adults in Greece (n = 490)	Tertiles of non-heme protein/heme protein/PP intake (% of total energy)	Heme AP intake was positively associated with hemoglobin and hematocrit.
Hruby and Jacques 2019	Longitudinal study with adults predominantly Caucasian Americans (Framingham Heart Study, n = 2061)	Quartiles of the energy-adjusted average intake of AP/PP (g/day)	PP was inversely associated with changes in inflammation and oxidative stress score.

Abbreviations: AP: animal protein, PP: plant protein, HDL-C: high-density lipoprotein cholesterol, HOMA-IR: homeostasis model assessment for insulin resistance, LDL-C: low-density lipoprotein cholesterol, MetS: metabolic syndrome, T2DM: type 2 diabetes mellitus.

On the other hand, a higher AP intake was associated with a higher level of low-density lipoprotein (LDL-C) and uric acid. However, neither protein source was associated with CRP.

Vallianou et al. (2013) investigated associations between dietary protein sources and various biomarkers, including CRP, among healthy adults in Greece. In this cross-sectional study, dietary intake was evaluated by a 76-item FFQ, and participants were categorized in tertiles based on the percentages of energy from three protein sources: non-heme AP (i.e., dairy products, eggs), heme AP (i.e., meat, fish, seafood), and PP. After adjusting for potential factors that affect associations (age, sex, dietary quality, and other lifestyle factors), the study found positive associations between heme AP intake and hematological biomarkers (hemoglobin and hematocrit). However, none of the three protein sources were associated with CRP in this study.

Hruby and Jacques (2019) examined associations between PP and AP intakes and changes in biomarkers of inflammation and oxidative stress among participants in Framingham Heart Study Offspring cohort. Participants were categorized into quartiles based on the energy-adjusted average

PP and AP intakes estimated from their responses to a 126-item FFQ. An inflammation and oxidate stress score was calculated from nine biomarkers, including hs-CRP and serum IL-6, for each individual: a higher score indicates a higher degree of inflammation and oxidative stress. The study found that higher PP intake was associated with less increased score, suggesting PP-rich diets are beneficial in managing inflammation and oxidative stress.

EPIDEMIOLOGICAL STUDIES OF PLANT PROTEIN-RICH DIETS AND METABOLISM IN NHANES

Several studies have examined cross-sectional associations between protein sources and metabolic-related biomarkers among US adults using the NHANES data (Table 2.2). NHANES collected 24-hour dietary recalls, What We Eat in America, essential data for assessing dietary intake among the US population. Berryman et al. (2016) examined differences in anthropometric measures and cardiometabolic and renal biomarkers by deciles of PP and AP intakes among adults. The researchers found that both protein sources were associated with cardiometabolic benefits, particularly for abdominal obesity: higher intake was inversely associated with body weight, body mass index (BMI), and waist circumference after adjusting for potential confounders. However, higher AP intake was associated with higher FG and blood urea nitrogen. In contrast, higher PP intake was associated with lower blood urea nitrogen and creatinine.

Hong et al. (2022) investigated associations between PP intakes and maternal insulin resistance among pregnant women. This study found that higher PP intake was associated with lower insulin and HOMA-IR levels. The study also conducted animal experiments with pregnant rats fed 100% PP, 50% PP/AP, and 100% AP and found similar associations. Additionally, the animal experiment found differences in endogenous metabolites (e.g., amino acids, vitamins, and their derivatives) and metabolic pathways (FoxO and mTOR signaling pathways) between the PP and AP groups. The authors concluded that PP intake was inversely associated with maternal insulin resistance, potentially influenced by amino acids and other metabolites and pathways induced by different protein sources.

Another cross-sectional study found beneficial associations between intake patterns of protein foods and hs-CRP levels among adults (Matsunaga et al. 2021). The study used dietary index components for protein food groups from the Healthy Eating Index-2015 (total proteins, seafood and PPs) and the calorie-based Dietary Approaches to Stop Hypertension (DASH) dietary index (APs, PPs) to assess the quality of protein food intake patterns. A higher component score indicates better adherence to the recommended dietary pattern. The authors found that poorer adherence to the HEI-2015 seafood and PPs, DASH PPs, and DASH APs (<80% of the maximum score) was associated with an elevated hs-CRP level (>3.0 mg/L). They also found that individuals with diabetes who had a low score on these three components were more likely to have an elevated hs-CRP level than those without diabetes who had a high score (≥80% of the maximum score).

Huang et al. (2023) examined associations between the quality of low-carbohydrate diets (LCDs) and cardiometabolic biomarkers among adults. Healthy and unhealthy LCD scores were calculated by the percentage of energy from each macronutrient and their subcategories related to healthy and unhealthy dietary patterns. The study described the healthy LCD as a diet emphasizing unsaturated fat, PP, and fewer low-quality carbohydrates and the unhealthy LCD as emphasizing saturated fat, AP, and fewer high-quality carbohydrates. After adjusting for potential confounders, the researchers found that the healthy LCD was associated with lower levels of insulin, HOMA-IR, CRP, and TG and higher levels of HDL-C. The unhealthy LCD was associated with higher levels of insulin, HOMA-IR, CRP, and LDL-C.

TABLE 2.2
Epidemiological Studies Examining Cross-Sectional Associations between Plant/Animal Protein-Rich Diets and Metabolic-Related Biomarkers in NHANES

Authors and Publication Year	Study Population	Protein Food/Sources	Study Findings of Metabolic-Related Biomarkers
Berryman et al. 2016	US adults (NHANES 2007–2010, n = 11,111)	Deciles of total/AP/PP intake (g/kg of body weight)	Diets higher in AP and PP are associated with cardiometabolic benefits, particularly for abdominal obesity, and no apparent kidney function impairment.
Hong et al. 2022	US pregnant women (NHANES 1999–2018, n = 1034)	Tertiles of AP/PP intake (g/day) and the ratio of AP/PP	PP intake was negatively associated with insulin and HOMA-IR.
Matsunaga et al. 2021	US adults (NHANES 2005–2010, n = 12,070)	Low or high scores of index components (HEI-2015: total protein, seafood and PPs; DASH index: APs, PPs)	A low score for seafood and PPs, APs, and PPs was associated with elevated hs-CRP. Those with diabetes and a low score were more likely to have elevated hs-CRP than those without diabetes who had a high score.
Huang et al. 2023	US adults (NHANES 2003–2018, n = range 16,301–34,359)	Quartiles of healthy LCD scores (high in PP). Quartiles of unhealthy LCD scores (high in AP)	Healthy LCD was inversely associated with insulin, HOMA-IR, CRP, and TG and positively associated with HDL-C. Unhealthy LCD was positively associated with insulin, HOMA-IR, CRP, and LDL-C.

Abbreviations: AP: animal protein, CRP: C-reactive protein, PP: plant protein, HDL-C: high-density lipoprotein cholesterol, HOMA-IR: homeostasis model assessment for insulin resistance, hs-CRP: high sensitivity C-reactive protein, LDL-C: low-density lipoprotein cholesterol, LCD: low-carbohydrate diet.

RANDOMIZED CLINICAL TRIAL STUDIES WITH INDIVIDUALS WITH DIABETES

Past epidemiological studies suggest beneficial associations between PP-rich diets and MetS-related biomarkers. However, they also show inconsistent results for metabolic-related biomarkers. Randomized clinical trials (RCTs) have the advantage of eliminating biases that observational studies often encounter. In RCTs examining the effects of PP-rich diets (Table 2.3), participants' adherence to assigned diets and physical activity levels were monitored.

Jamilian and Asemi (2015) examined the effects of soy protein-rich diets on metabolic-related biomarkers among women with gestational diabetes mellitus in Iran. In this parallel RCT, participants followed a soy protein diet (35% soy protein, 35% other PP, and 30% AP) or a control diet (70% AP, 30% PP) for six weeks. Both diets provided about 15% of energy from protein. Mean dietary intakes were similar for energy and carbohydrates but differed for total fat, saturated fat, polyunsaturated fatty acids, cholesterol, and dietary fiber. The researchers found differences in interactions between time and treatment for FG, insulin, HOMA-IR, TG, very low-density lipoprotein cholesterol, quantitative insulin sensitivity check index, and biomarkers for oxidative stress (plasma total antioxidant capacity, plasma total glutathione, and plasma MDA), suggesting beneficial effects of the soy-protein diet.

Researchers in Germany studied the effect of high-protein PP and AP diets on metabolic-related biomarkers in adults with T2DM who adhered to either diet for six weeks (Sucher et al. 2017;

TABLE 2.3
Randomized Clinical Trials Examining Associations between Plant/Animal Protein-Rich Diets and Metabolic-Related Biomarkers

Authors and Publication Year	Study Design and Subjects	Protein Food/Sources	Study Findings of Metabolic-Related Biomarkers
Jamilian and Asemi 2015	A randomized parallel clinical trial with women with gestational diabetes mellitus in Iran (n = 68)	Soy diet (0.8 g/kg protein, 35% AP, 35% soy protein, 30% other PP) vs. control diet (0.8 g/kg protein, 70% AP, 30% PP) for six weeks	Control group: increased serum insulin, HOMA-IR, TG, very LDL-C, and TC/HDL-C ratio. Soy diet group: decreased FG and increased quantitative insulin resistance index, total antioxidant capacity, total glutathione, and MDA. Soy diet improved glucose homeostasis parameters, TG, biomakers of oxidative stress.
Sucher et al. 2017; Markova et al. 2017; Pivovarova-Ramich et al. 2020	A randomized open-label, parallel clinical trial with adult patients with T2DM in Germany (n = 37)	AP or PP high-protein isocaloric diet (30% protein, 40% carbohydrate, 10% saturated fat, 10% monounsaturated fat, 10% polyunsaturated fat) for six weeks	Decreased hepatic enzymes, inflammation biomarkers (MDA and protein carbonyls), and increased insulin sensitivity and nitrotyrosine.
Kahleova et al. 2018	A randomized, open-label parallel clinical trial with overweight or obese adults in the US (n = 75)	Plant-based diet (low-fat vegan diet) or usual diet (control), and no change in physical activity in both the diet groups for 16 weeks	Treatment group: decreased body weight, visceral fat volume, and HOMA-IR. The decrease in fat mass was positively associated with PP intake and negatively associated with AP intake. After adjusting for changes in BMI and energy intake, a decrease in fat mass was associated with a decreased % leucine intake, and a decrease in HOMA-IR was associated with a decreased % histidine intake.
Roussell et al. 2012	A four-period, randomized, crossover, controlled feeding clinical trial with hypercholesterolemic participants in the US (n = 36)	Healthy American diet (HAD), DASH diet (PP-rich), BOLD diet (AP-rich), or BOLD+ diet (high-protein AP-rich) for five weeks each. Each diet was rich in fruits, vegetables, and lean meats with similar amounts of total fat, fat types, and cholesterol.	TC and LDL-C decreased after DASH, BOLD, and BOLD+. Apolipoprotein A-I, C-III, and C-III bound to apolipoprotein A1 particles decreased after BOLD and BOLD+. Apolipoprotein B decreased after BOLD+. In those with a baseline CRP of <1 mg/L, TC decreased after all diets, and LDL-C decreased after DASH, BOLD, and BOLD+ diets. In those with a baseline CRP of >1 mg/L, LDL-C and TC decreased after BOLD and BOLD+.

Abbreviations: AP: animal protein, BD: blood pressure, BMI: body mass index, CRP: C-reactive protein, DBP: diastolic blood pressure, FG: fasting glucose, HbA1c: glycated hemoglobin, HDL-C: high-density lipoprotein cholesterol, HOMA-IR: homeostasis model assessment for insulin resistance, hs-CRP: high-sensitivity CRP, LDL-C: low-density lipoprotein cholesterol, MDA: malondialdehyde, PP: plant protein, SBP: systolic blood pressure, T2DM: type 2 diabetes mellitus, TC: total cholesterol, TG: triglycerides: TNF-α: tumor necrosis factor-α.

Markova et al. 2017; Pivovarova-Ramich et al. 2020). The diets were isocaloric with the same percent of energy from protein (30%), carbohydrate (40%), and fat (30%). Postprandial plasma tests found higher branched-chain amino acids and methionine levels in the AP group and higher arginine and asparagine levels in the PP group (Markova et al. 2017). Both diets provided similar improvements in total cholesterol (TC), LDL-C, and systolic BP (SBP). Uric acid also decreased in both, but the AP group reduced more than the PP group. There were no differences in other biomarkers. However, the PP group improved HbA1c, diastolic BP (DBP), and fasting non-esterified fatty acid levels, while the AP group improved insulin sensitivity, CRP, and FG (Sucher et al. 2017). The researchers also examined the dietary effects on biomarkers of hepatic conditions (Markova et al. 2017). Both groups reduced liver fat, independently of body weight but correlating with FG, insulin, and insulin sensitivity improvements. The reductions also correlated with the index of de novo lipogenesis, a metabolic pathway involved in the endogenous synthesis of fatty acids, which is associated with cardiometabolic diseases (Ameer et al. 2014). Both groups decreased inflammatory makers: proinflammatory cytokines (IL18) decreased in the AP group and TNF-α decreased in the PP group. Fibroblast growth factor 21, a metabolic regulator of energy homeostasis (Tezze et al. 2019), decreased by 50% in both groups, correlating with liver fat loss. (Markova et al. 2017). In the study focused on the effects on oxidative stress and antioxidant status (Pivovarova-Ramich et al. 2020), researchers found both groups reduced plasma levels of MDA and protein carbonyls and increased nitrotyrosine. The study concluded that the isocaloric diets high in PP and AP similarly improved oxidative stress among adults with T2DM.

RANDOMIZED CLINICAL TRIAL STUDIES WITH OVERWEIGHT/OBESE INDIVIDUALS

Dietary effects on metabolic biomarkers may be more pronounced in individuals with T2DM who already have abnormal levels. Also, test diets for T2DM are high in protein, which may not be practical for those without T2DM. Since the development of MetS occurs before the onset of T2DM, RCTs using those at risk for MetS (e.g., without T2DM) may identify effective MetS prevention strategies (Table 2.3).

Kahleova et al. (2018) examined the effect of a plant-based diet on body composition and insulin resistance among overweight or obese adults. This open-label, parallel RCT instructed participants to follow a plant-based vegan diet (treatment) or practice a usual diet (control) for 16 weeks. Compared to the baseline, the total protein and amino acid intake and percent of energy from protein decreased in the treatment group but not in the control group. Over the study period, the treatment group reduced body weight, visceral fat volume, and HOMA-IR. After adjusting for changes in BMI and energy intake, the study found that reductions in fat mass and HOMA-IR were associated with decreased intake of leucine and histidine, respectively, both abundant in AP. The researchers concluded that the quality and quantity of dietary protein are associated with improvements in body weight/composition and insulin resistance in overweight individuals.

Roussell et al. (2012) examined the effect of PP- or AP-rich diets on cardiometabolic biomarkers in hypercholesterolemic adults (mean BMI = 25.7 kg/m^2). This crossover controlled feeding study provided participants with four diets for five weeks each: Healthy American diet (HAD; 17% of energy from protein), DASH diet (18% of energy from protein, higher in PP than HAD), Beef in an Optimal Lean diet (BOLD; 19% of energy from protein, higher in AP than HAD), and BOLD plus additional protein (BOLD+, 27% of energy from protein, higher in total protein and AP than HAD). DASH, BOLD, and BOLD+ were higher in fiber and lower in cholesterol than HAD. A prior study reported that US adults derive about 16% of energy from protein on average (Huang et al. 2023), making BOLD+ the only high-protein diet in this study. The researchers found that TC, LDL-C, and HDL-C decreased after DASH, BOLD, and BOLD+ but not after HAD. The study found no effect on CRP. However, among participants with CRP <1 mg/L at baseline, TC decreased after all diets, and LDL-C decreased after DASH, BOLD, and BOLD+. For those with baseline CRP ≥ 1mg/L, TC and LDL-C decreased only after BOLD and BOLD+, suggesting AP-rich diets can help manage metabolic balance when fatty meats are excluded.

PREVENTION AND MANAGEMENT OF METABOLIC SYNDROME

Past studies suggest adequate protein intake helps manage metabolic balance, but protein source significantly affects outcomes. PP foods provide amino acids, nutrients, and phytochemicals that help manage metabolic balance. However, their lower essential amino acid density and digestibility increase the risks of inadequate protein and essential amino acid intake. AP foods provide all essential amino acids and are rich in the nutrients lacking in PP, but habitual overconsumption of high-fat AP may promote weight gain and elevate LDL-C. However, lean AP foods paired with plant foods are still beneficial for metabolic balance.

The 2020–2025 Dietary Guidelines for Americans, based on scientific evidence on diet and health, recommend including a variety of protein foods from both animal and plant sources (US Department of Agriculture and US Department of Health and Human Services 2020). According to the dietary reference intakes by the Food and Nutrition Board of the Institute of Medicine (Institute of Medicine 2006), the recommended amount of protein intake is 0.8 g/kg body weight/day of high-quality protein for most individuals to meet dietary requirements. Further research is needed to find optimal PP/AP ratios for omnivores and PP types and quantities for vegetarians to ensure adequate protein and essential amino acid intake.

THE EFFECTS OF OTHER PROTEINS

This chapter focuses on the differential metabolic effects of PP and AP, but other proteins warrant consideration. Dairy proteins are also part of our diets and come from both animal and plant sources. Cow's milk is the most common source of dairy products and contains whey, casein, albumin, and transferrin, all rich in essential amino acids (Koirala et al. 2023). Studies assessing postprandial responses to milk protein digestion show that milk proteins benefit vascular function independently of BP and glycemic homeostasis (Fekete Á et al. 2016). A review highlights milk-derived bioactive peptides' potential antioxidative, anti-inflammatory, and antihypertensive roles in MetS management (Koirala et al. 2023).

Cow's milk is also a good source of riboflavin, vitamin B12, vitamin D, potassium, pantothenic acids, magnesium, selenium, and calcium. Fermented dairy products offer probiotics, which support metabolic balances (Torres et al. 2019). Low-fat dairy products from cow's milk are generally recommended because full-fat dairy products are high in saturated fat. Fortified plant-based milk and milk products may be less nutritious but are still great alternatives for those intolerant or sensitive to lactose. Further research is needed to study the effects of animal- and plant-based dairy products on metabolic balance.

MINI DICTIONARY OF TERMS

- **Adipose tissue:** Also known as body fat; regulates metabolism by communicating with other organs and the nervous system through hormonal signals. An adipocyte is a cell that stores fat.
- **Baseline:** The starting point of a study. Data at baseline are obtained prior to or at the onset of a study.
- **Crossover study:** A type of clinical study where participants receive multiple treatments sequentially.
- **Lacto-ovo vegetarian:** A diet including plant foods, eggs, and dairy foods.
- **Omnivore:** Consumes both plant and animal foods.

- **Parallel study:** Clinical trial where participants remain in one treatment arm throughout.
- **Pescatarian:** A diet excluding all meat except fish and seafood.
- **Postprandial:** After eating.
- **Vegetarian:** Excludes meat; subtypes include vegan (plants only).

SUMMARY POINTS

- This chapter compares the metabolic effects of plant (PP) and animal protein (AP) foods.
- Metabolic syndrome is a condition of metabolic imbalance: abdominal obesity and abnormal blood pressure, triglycerides, fasting glucose, and high-density lipoprotein cholesterol.
- Inflammation and oxidative stress are involved in the development of metabolic syndrome.
- PP foods are lower in branched-chain amino acids and methionine and less digestible than AP but rich in fiber and antioxidant phytochemicals.
- PP-rich diets show preventative and therapeutic potential for metabolic balance.
- AP-rich diets benefit metabolic balance when combined with nutrient-dense plant foods.
- Both protein sources are beneficial for managing metabolic balance if selected wisely based on quality.

REFERENCES

Alberti, K. G., R. H. Eckel, et al. 2009. Harmonizing the metabolic syndrome: A joint interim statement of the international diabetes federation task force on epidemiology and prevention; national heart, lung, and blood institute; American heart association; world heart federation; international atherosclerosis society; and international association for the study of obesity. *Circulation* 120 (16):1640–5.

Alqaderi, H., A. Abdullah, et al. 2023. The relationship between sleep and salivary and serum inflammatory biomarkers in adolescents. *Front Med* 10:1175483.

Ameer, F., L. Scandiuzzi, et al. 2014. De novo lipogenesis in health and disease. *Metabolism* 63 (7):895–902.

Berrazaga, I., V. Micard, et al. 2019. The role of the anabolic properties of plant- versus animal-based protein sources in supporting muscle mass maintenance: A critical review. *Nutrients* 11 (8):1825.

Berryman, C. E., S. Agarwal, et al. 2016. Diets higher in animal and plant protein are associated with lower adiposity and do not impair kidney function in US adults. *Am J Clin Nutr* 104 (3):743–9.

Carbonaro, M., P. Maselli, et al. 2012. Relationship between digestibility and secondary structure of raw and thermally treated legume proteins: A Fourier transform infrared (FT-IR) spectroscopic study. *Amino Acids* 43 (2):911–21.

Chen, Z., M. G. Zuurmond, et al. 2018. Plant versus animal based diets and insulin resistance, prediabetes and type 2 diabetes: The Rotterdam Study. *Eur J Epidemiol* 33 (9):883–93.

Cicero, A. F., and A. Colletti. 2016. Role of phytochemicals in the management of metabolic syndrome. *Phytomedicine* 23 (11):1134–44.

Deota, S., and S. Panda. 2021. New horizons: Circadian control of metabolism offers novel insight into the cause and treatment of metabolic diseases. *J Clin Endocrinol Metab* 106 (3):e1488–93.

Fekete Á, A., D. I. Givens, et al. 2016. Can milk proteins be a useful tool in the management of cardiometabolic health? An updated review of human intervention trials. *Proc Nutr Soc* 75 (3):328–41.

Food and Agriculture Organization. 2013. *Dietary Protein Quality Evaluation in Human Nutrition: Report of an FAO Expert Consultation*. Rome: Food and Agriculture Organzation of the United Nations Rome.

Gaweł, S., M. Wardas, et al. 2004. Malondialdehyde (MDA) as a lipid peroxidation marker. *Wiad Lek* 57 (9–10):453–5.

Hirode, G., and R. J. Wong. 2020. Trends in the prevalence of metabolic syndrome in the United States, 2011–2016. *JAMA* 323 (24):2526–28.

Hoffman, J. R., and M. J. Falvo. 2004. Protein – which is best? *J Sports Sci Med* 3 (3):118–30.

Hong, Yuting, Chen Yang, et al. 2022. Dietary plant protein intake can reduce maternal insulin resistance during pregnancy. *Nutrients* 14 (23):5039.

Hoy, M. K., T. Murayi, et al. 2023. Effect of animal protein intake on meeting recommendations for nutrient intake among US adults, What We Eat in America, NHANES 2015–2018. *Curr Dev Nutr* 7 (2):100027.

Hoy, M. Katherine, Theophile Murayi, et al. 2022. Diet quality and food intakes samong US adults by level of animal protein intake, What We Eat in America, NHANES 2015–2018. *Curr Dev Nutr* 6 (5):nzac035.

Hruby, A., and P. F. Jacques. 2019. Dietary protein and changes in biomarkers of inflammation and oxidative stress in the Framingham heart study offspring cohort. *Curr Dev Nutr* 3 (5):nzz019.

Huang, Y., X. Li, et al. 2023. Healthy and unhealthy low-carbohydrate diets and plasma markers of cardiometabolic risk. *Br J Nutr* 130 (1):137–46.

Hydrie, M. Z., A. S. Shera, et al. 2009. Prevalence of metabolic syndrome in urban Pakistan (Karachi): Comparison of newly proposed International Diabetes Federation and modified Adult Treatment Panel III criteria. *Metab Syndr Relat Disord* 7 (2):119–24.

Institute of Medicine. 2006. *Dietary Reference Intakes: The Essential Guide to Nutrient Requirements.* Edited by Jennifer Pitzi Hellwig Jennifer J. Otten, and Linda D. Meyers. Washington, DC: National Academies Press.

Jamilian, M., and Z. Asemi. 2015. The effect of soy intake on metabolic profiles of women with gestational diabetes mellitus. *J Clin Endocrinol Metab* 100 (12):4654–61.

Jamshidi, A., M. Farjam, et al. 2022. Evaluating type and amount of dietary protein in relation to metabolic syndrome among Iranian adults: Cross-sectional analysis of Fasa Persian cohort study. *Diabetol Metab Syndr* 14 (1):42.

Kahleova, H., R. Fleeman, et al. 2018. A plant-based diet in overweight individuals in a 16-week randomized clinical trial: Metabolic benefits of plant protein. *Nutr Diabetes* 8 (1):58.

Koirala, P., M. Dahal, et al. 2023. Dairy milk protein-derived bioactive peptides: Avengers against metabolic syndrome. *Curr Nutr Rep* 12 (2):308–26.

Leser, S. 2013. The 2013 FAO report on dietary protein quality evaluation in human nutrition: Recommendations and implications: FAO dietary protein report. *Nutrition Bulletin* 38 (4):421–28.

Luthria, Devanand L., Ronita Biswas, et al. 2007. Comparison of extraction solvents and techniques used for the assay of isoflavones from soybean. *Food Chem* 105 (1):325–33.

Marinangeli, C. P. F., K. Miller, et al. 2023. Effect of increasing plant protein intake on protein quality and nutrient intake of US adults. *Appl Physiol Nutr Metab* 48 (1):49–61.

Markova, M., O. Pivovarova, et al. 2017. Isocaloric diets high in animal or plant protein reduce liver fat and inflammation in individuals with type 2 diabetes. *Gastroenterology* 152 (3):571–85.e8.

Matsunaga, Masako, Eric L. Hurwitz, et al. 2021. Adequate intake of plant protein foods and moderate intake of animal protein foods are inversely associated with C-reactive protein in US adults with diabetes: A cross-sectional study with national health and nutrition examination survey. *Nutrition* 89:111276.

Meng, S., Z. Cui, et al. 2021. Associations between dietary animal and plant protein intake and cardiometabolic risk factors-A cross-sectional study in China health and nutrition survey. *Nutrients* 13 (2):336.

Monserrat-Mesquida, Margalida, Magdalena Quetglas-Llabrés, et al. 2020. Metabolic syndrome is associated with oxidative stress and proinflammatory state. *Antioxidants* 9 (3):236.

Morales, D. D., F. E. Punzalan, et al. 2008. Metabolic syndrome in the Philippine general population: Prevalence and risk for atherosclerotic cardiovascular disease and diabetes mellitus. *Diab Vasc Dis Res* 5 (1):36–43.

Multari, S., M. Neacsu, et al. 2016. Nutritional and phytochemical content of high-protein crops. *J Agric Food Chem* 64 (41):7800–811.

Nehring, S. M., A. Goyal, et al. 2023. C Reactive protein. In *StatPearls*. Treasure Island, FL: StatPearls Publishing LLC.

Pacher, P., and C. Szabó. 2006. Role of peroxynitrite in the pathogenesis of cardiovascular complications of diabetes. *Curr Opin Pharmacol* 6 (2):136–41.

Pasiakos, Stefan M., Sanjiv Agarwal, et al. 2015. Sources and amounts of animal, dairy, and plant protein intake of US adults in 2007–2010. *Nutrients* 7 (8):7058–69.

Pinchuk, I., D. Weber, et al. 2019. Gender- and age-dependencies of oxidative stress, as detected based on the steady state concentrations of different biomarkers in the MARK-AGE study. *Redox Biol* 24:101204.

Pivovarova-Ramich, O., M. Markova, et al. 2020. Effects of diets high in animal or plant protein on oxidative stress in individuals with type 2 diabetes: A randomized clinical trial. *Redox Biol* 29:101397.

Ranasinghe, P., Y. Mathangasinghe, et al. 2017. Prevalence and trends of metabolic syndrome among adults in the asia-pacific region: A systematic review. *BMC Public Health* 17 (1):101.

Reilly, S. M., and A. R. Saltiel. 2017. Adapting to obesity with adipose tissue inflammation. *Nat Rev Endocrinol* 13 (11):633–43.

Ridker, P. M. 2003. Clinical application of C-reactive protein for cardiovascular disease detection and prevention. *Circulation* 107 (3):363–9.

Roussell, M. A., A. M. Hill, et al. 2012. Beef in an optimal lean diet study: Effects on lipids, lipoproteins, and apolipoproteins. *Am J Clin Nutr* 95 (1):9–16.

Safaei, M., E. A. Sundararajan, et al. 2021. A systematic literature review on obesity: Understanding the causes & consequences of obesity and reviewing various machine learning approaches used to predict obesity. *Comput Biol Med* 136:104754.

Santa, K., Y. Kumazawa, et al. 2023. Prevention of metabolic syndrome by phytochemicals and vitamin D. *Int J Mol Sci* 24 (3):2627.

Silveira Rossi, J. L., S. M. Barbalho, et al. 2022. Metabolic syndrome and cardiovascular diseases: Going beyond traditional risk factors. *Diabetes Metab Res Rev* 38 (3):e3502.

Sucher, S., M. Markova, et al. 2017. Comparison of the effects of diets high in animal or plant protein on metabolic and cardiovascular markers in type 2 diabetes: A randomized clinical trial. *Diabetes Obes Metab* 19 (7):944–52.

Suzuki, Y. J., M. Carini, et al. 2010. Protein carbonylation. *Antioxid Redox Signal* 12 (3):323–5.

Tezze, C., V. Romanello, et al. 2019. FGF21 as modulator of metabolism in health and disease. *Front Physiol* 10:419.

Torres, S., E. Fabersani, et al. 2019. Adipose tissue inflammation and metabolic syndrome: The proactive role of probiotics. *Eur J Nutr* 58 (1):27–43.

U.S. Department of Agriculture and U.S. Department of Health and Human Services. 2020. *Dietary Guidelines for Americans, 2020–2025*. 9th ed. https://www.dietaryguidelines.gov/, accessed 3 March.

Vallianou, N. G., V. P. Bountziouka, et al. 2013. Influence of protein intake from haem and non-haem animals and plant origin on inflammatory biomarkers among apparently-healthy adults in Greece. *J Health Popul Nutr* 31 (4):446–54.

Wilson, P. W., R. B. D'Agostino, et al. 2005. Metabolic syndrome as a precursor of cardiovascular disease and type 2 diabetes mellitus. *Circulation* 112 (20):3066–72.

Yang, S. H., G. Tao, et al. 2023. Dietary phytochemical and metabolic disease prevention: Focus on plant proteins. *Front Nutr* 10:1089487.

Yki-Järvinen H. 2014. Non-alcoholic fatty liver disease as a cause and a consequence of metabolic syndrome. *The Lancet Diabetes & Endocrinology* 2 (11):901–10. https://doi.org/10.1016/S2213-8587(14)70032-4

Zhang, X., and L. O. Lerman. 2017. The metabolic syndrome and chronic kidney disease. *Transl Res* 183:14–25.

3 Dietary Plant and Animal Proteins and Satiety

Ioanna Alexandropoulou, Kalliopi K. Gkouskou, and Maria G. Grammatikopoulou

ABBREVIATIONS

AA	amino acid
AgRP	agouti-related peptide
α-MSH	α-melanocyte-stimulating hormone
cAMP	cyclic adenosine monophosphate
CART	cocaine- and amphetamine-regulated transcript
CCK	cholecystokinin
CNS	central nervous system
DIT	diet-induced thermogenesis
FFM	fat-free mass
GABA	γ-aminobutyric acid
GI	gastrointestinal
GIP	glucose-dependent insulinotropic polypeptide
GLP-1	glucagon-like peptide-1
GLP-1R	glucagon-like peptide-1 receptor
LepR	leptin receptor
MC4R	melanocortin-4 receptor
NPY	neuropeptide Y
PKA	protein kinase A
POMC	pro-opiomelanocortin
PP	pancreatic polypeptide
PYY	peptide YY
REE	resting energy expenditure
T2DM	type 2 diabetes mellitus
TEI	total energy intake

INTRODUCTION

The homeostasis of appetite and satiety is regulated through a variety of afferent and efferent peripheral pathways, including complex interactions between hormones, peptides, genes, oral and psychological factors (hedonic/reward systems), motivational state, meal characteristics (size, cooking method, content, and form), and acquired responses (Mook 1989; Dalton et al. 2013; Braden, Gwin, and Leidy 2023; Amin and Mercer 2016; McLeod et al. 2022). The hypothalamus of the brain serves as the main control center for hunger and satiety through the interaction of hormones and peptides received from peripheral organs and those produced by its neurons (Austin and Marks 2008). Many hormones and peptides interact with target organs to achieve a balance in energy homeostasis. Some of these macromolecules carry messages from the periphery to the brain (mainly the hypothalamus),

DOI: 10.1201/9781003597926-3

while others convey messages from the brain to various organs. Any changes that may occur altering the balance between these molecules lead to a modification of energy regulation and possible pathological conditions (Yeung and Tadi 2023).

Peptides with different and competing functions are secreted from neurons of the infundibular nucleus/arcuate nucleus of the brain's hypothalamus. Some tend to stimulate appetite, leading to increased food intake and weight gain; these include neuropeptide Y (NPY) and agouti-related peptide (AgRP). On the other hand, other peptides inhibit appetite and promote weight loss, such as pro-opiomelanocortin (POMC) and cocaine- and amphetamine-regulated transcript (CART) (Austin and Marks 2008; Suzuki, Jayasena, and Bloom 2011).

APPETITE-STIMULATING PEPTIDES

NPY and AgRP

Neurons that secrete NPY and AgRP also secrete the neurotransmitter γ-aminobutyric acid (GABA). They project to other hypothalamic nuclei associated with the regulation of metabolism and are among the first to receive the peripheral signals of food intake and energy consumption reaching the brain. They influence energy homeostasis via the autonomic and endocrine systems, increasing food intake, decreasing energy consumption, and initiating ketogenesis. NPY- and AgRP-secreting neurons express both insulin and leptin receptors, allowing them to receive signals from the periphery about glucose and lipid metabolic status while simultaneously being inhibited by glucose (Huang et al. 2011).

NPY is included in the peptides that stimulate food intake. It was isolated in 1982 and shows 70% homology with peptide YY (PYY) and 50% with the pancreatic polypeptide (PP). Its secretion is regulated by many factors, inhibited by leptin and insulin, and stimulated by ghrelin and glucocorticoids. It is among the most abundant peptides in the hypothalamus (Austin and Marks 2008; H. Huang, Xu, and van den Pol 2011), stimulating appetite through its receptors belonging to the G protein-coupled receptors called Y (1 to 6), mainly Y1 and Y5.

AgRP is also secreted in the same neurons. In humans, the agouti gene is similar to its counterpart in mice. Its function lies in regulating the differential production of melanin pigments in the skin of mice. It acts paracrinely and not directly inside the melanocytes. It causes changes in cAMP levels, antagonizing α-melanocyte-stimulating hormone (α-MSH) in its binding to the melanocortin 1 receptor. This action occurs on the surface of melanocytes in the hair bulb (Miltenberger et al. 1997). In mice, inhibition of α-MSH binding to the melanocortin 1 receptor by increasing AgRP protein secretion leads to yellow coat color and long body length. At the same time, mice show insulin resistance, hyperglycemia, and obesity because the same protein acts as an antagonist of melanocortin 3 and 4 receptors and stimulates appetite (Austin and Marks 2008).

Ghrelin

Peptides that also stimulate appetite are produced and secreted in the periphery. Perhaps the most important of these is ghrelin. It is a 28-amino acid (AA) peptide discovered in 1999 (Alamri et al. 2016). The gene is produced and secreted mainly by the fundus endocrine cells in the gastric mucosa, type X/A cells. However, it can be produced in smaller quantities by other cells, such as those of the intestine, kidney, ovary, lung, pancreatic islets, ovary, and testis, but also brain (pituitary and hypothalamus) cells (Austin and Marks 2008). Ghrelin leads to the release of growth hormone, as it binds to the receptor that leads to its secretion. This receptor is coupled to a G protein and is secreted from various parts of the body, including the islets of the pancreas and various areas of the central nervous system (CNS). Receptor binding occurs in the hypothalamus and peripheral organs, such as the endocrine portion of the pancreas, sites where appetite and energy balance are regulated (Alamri et al. 2016). Ghrelin increases before meals, stimulating appetite, and decreases after food intake. It is considered a meal initiator (Cummings et al. 2001), enhancing appetite by stimulating the lateral hypothalamus area, which is responsible for hunger. It also participates in glucose metabolism regulation (reducing glucose tolerance) and taste regulation and minimizes glucose-induced insulin release, causing insulin resistance (Yeung and Tadi 2023; Alamri et al. 2016). Ghrelin levels inversely correlate with body weight, being high in lean individuals and decreased in obesity (Austin and Marks 2008).

APPETITE-SUPPRESSANT PEPTIDES

POMC/CART

As we mentioned above, the hypothalamus plays a central role in regulating energy expenditure and satiety through the secretion of peptides from POMC/CART neurons (Anderson et al. 2016). CART is an important neuropeptide crucial in the control of appetite and energy homeostasis, increasing energy expenditure and decreasing food intake (Lau et al. 2018). CART mRNA levels in the arcuate nucleus are regulated by leptin (Elias et al. 2001). POMC, known for its effect on energy metabolism, is converted to α-MSH in the hypothalamus and binds to the melanocortin-4 receptor (MC4R) in the paraventricular nucleus and other CNS circuitries to suppress appetite (Biglari et al. 2021). Agouti protein blocks the binding of α-MSH antagonistically to MC4R (Lu et al. 1994).

In a recent review, the authors report that POMC neurons of the arcuate nucleus expressing leptin's receptor affect glucose regulation rather than energy balance. Recent models suggest that leptin, specifically its high levels reaching the hypothalamus, activates POMC neurons, directly targeting the regulation of glucose metabolism and indirectly influencing energy homeostasis through the activation of GABAergic neurons (Lavoie, Michael, and Caron 2023).

Cholecystokinin (CCK)

Besides the CNS, peripheral organs also produce peptides that inhibit appetite and induce satiety. Cholecystokinin (CCK) appears to be the first peptide found to be associated with the regulation of food intake. It is produced in many areas of the gastrointestinal (GI) system but mainly in the small intestine (duodenum and jejunum). It has a short half-life in blood plasma, and its levels increase in the fourth quarter after meals (Suzuki, Jayasena, and Bloom 2011). It inhibits food intake and stomach motility while stimulating pancreatic secretion and bowel motility. There are two types of receptors, G protein-coupled 1 and 2. Inhibition is mainly due to the type 1 receptor located in the posterior regions of the brain on neurons of the vagus nerve. Additionally, CCK prevents ghrelin from stimulating hypothalamic neurons, stimulates pancreatic β cells to proliferate, and reduces insulin-dependent increases in food intake (Chandra and Liddle 2007). Its secretion is stimulated by the presence of food in the intestine, mainly fat, proteins, and AAs. There are many different forms of CCK produced by post-translational modifications from the same gene (Liddle et al. 1985).

Leptin

Leptin is a hormone produced and secreted mostly by subcutaneous white and brown adipose tissue in various organs. The gene that produces it is also called the obesity gene (ob) and is located on chromosome 7. Its levels in the blood are proportional to the size of the adipose tissue. Information about the body's energy is communicated by leptin to the CNS. Leptin's secretion follows a circadian rhythm but can change depending on nutritional status (Münzberg and Morrison 2015). Numerous factors regulate its secretion, including adipose tissue, physical exercise, dietary restriction, sex, and diet type. Hormonal factors, such as insulin, estradiol, testosterone, growth hormone, and glucocorticoids, also influence its secretion (Dagogo-Jack 2005).

Leptin receptors, classified as class I cytokines, are designated LepR (or Ob-R). Alternative splicing of the diabetes gene db (now called LepR) RNA produces six isoforms (LepR1–6). Receptors are categorized as long, secretory, or short (Gorska et al. 2010). Short receptors can transport leptin across the blood-brain barrier (Austin and Marks 2008). All isoforms share the same leptin binding domain but differ in their intracellular regions. LepR1, 2, 3, 4, and 6 are transmembrane receptors with the structure to bind Janus kinase 2 (JAK2), while 5 is soluble and binds circulating leptin, preventing its central transport.

Long-form LepR2 is the key brain receptor for leptin's effects on energy status and other functions. Its intracellular domain contains a long chain with three tyrosines phosphorylated by JAK2 in the context of signaling (Münzberg and Morrison 2015). LepR2 is expressed in the lateral hypothalamus and several hypothalamic nuclei, including the arcuate, paraventricular, and dorsal. Leptin binding to these receptors initiates chain reactions leading to inhibition of appetite-stimulating peptides NPY and AgRP and stimulation of appetite-suppressing peptides (Austin and Marks 2008).

Incretin Hormones

Incretin hormones include glucose-dependent insulinotropic polypeptide (GIP) and glucagon-like peptide-1 (GLP-1). Their plasma levels begin to increase after nutrient intake, particularly glucose and carbohydrates, and to a lesser extent with protein intake. These hormones stimulate insulin secretion, causing the so-called incretin effect, in which oral glucose administration elicits greater insulin secretion than intravenous administration, even when achieving identical plasma glucose levels. Incretins are produced in the intestine, with GIP specifically secreted by K cells in the duodenum and upper jejunum (Nauck and Meier 2018).

The GIP hormone is a 48-AA peptide originally isolated from pigs due to its ability to inhibit gastric acid secretion. For this reason, it was originally called "gastric inhibitory peptide." It was later found to act on the islets of the pancreas and stimulate insulin secretion. Food intake, especially glucose, stimulates GIP secretion, which leads to insulin secretion, pancreatic β cells and osteoblast proliferation, and energy storage in adipose tissue (Seino, Fukushima, and Yabe 2010).

GLP-1 is produced in several places: L cells in the small and large intestine, α-cells in the endocrine part of the pancreas, neurons in the hypothalamus, and brainstem cells, specifically in the caudate region. Gene transcription in all cell types produces a common proglucagon mRNA (Baggio and Drucker 2007). Pancreatic gene expression is stimulated by fasting and hypoglycemia and inhibited by insulin. Stimulation occurs through activation of the protein kinase C signaling pathway, which increases proglucagon mRNA levels, while the cyclic adenosine monophosphate (cAMP)/protein kinase A (PKA) pathway is also activated, stimulating transcription of the same gene. Transcription is stimulated due to an increase in cAMP, responding to a gene promoter element. Similarly, the activation of the GLP-1 gene in the intestine corresponds to the activation of the cAMP/PKA pathway (Baggio and Drucker 2007). In the hypothalamus, there are POMC neurons expressing GLP-1 receptors (GLP-1R) that control energy metabolism (Lavoie, Michael, and Caron 2023).

BEYOND SENSORY CUES: GENES AND APPETITE

The regulation of appetite by the CNS is susceptible to various sensory and environmental influences, contributing to overstimulation and generating signals beyond the brain's complete control (Alonso-Alonso and Pascual-Leone 2007). Recent research has shed light on the vulnerability of certain individuals to these signals, with genetics playing a significant role in shaping responses to food stimuli. Monogenic obesity, affecting a small proportion of the population, is mainly characterized by mutations in the leptin-melanocortin pathway, increasing appetite and reducing energy expenditure, thus dramatically elevating the risk of obesity (Nordang et al. 2017). Twin studies indicate that polygenic obesity, which affects a broader population, also impacts appetite (Schur and

Carnell 2017). Early investigations suggest that obesity-associated genes, such as FTO and MC4R, primarily influence the regulation of food intake, affecting appetite, satiety responsiveness, and binge eating (Horstmann et al. 2013; Willer et al. 2008; Micali et al. 2015; Den Hoed et al. 2009).

A meta-analysis involving nearly 340,000 individuals confirmed that genes linked to common obesity are primarily active in the brain and the CNS (Turcot et al. 2017). Recognizing these genetic traits as potential targets in obesity treatment and prevention, researchers suggest that genetic information can aid health professionals in formulating more personalized approaches (Gkouskou et al. 2024). Proposed interventions include dietary pattern changes that can modify eating behaviors. The impact of dietary protein on appetite and body weight gain can vary significantly among individuals. For example, FTO risk allele carriers can reduce food cravings and appetite when adhering to a hypocaloric, high-protein weight-loss diet (T. Huang et al. 2017), while carriers of the MC4R risk alleles may exhibit more pronounced increases in appetite and food cravings when adopting a high-protein diet (T. Huang et al. 2017). These examples highlight the individualized nature of dietary responses based on genetic variations, particularly regarding protein intake and its effects on appetite regulation.

PROTEIN AND APPETITE: WEIGHING THE EVIDENCE

Research consistently shows that meals with greater protein content reduce hunger and result in greater satiety and fullness ratings compared to lower protein preloads (Nielsen et al. 2018; M. Veldhorst et al. 2008; Dhillon et al. 2016; Rigamonti et al. 2020). The mechanisms behind protein-induced satiety are considered nutrient-specific, focusing primarily on the AA content and amount of each protein type (M. Veldhorst et al. 2008). Westerterp-Plantenga suggested that protein-induced satiety may actually result from the oxidation of AAs consumed in excess as part of diets incorporating primarily incomplete proteins (lacking at least one essential AA) (Westerterp-Plantenga et al. 2009). The consumption of complete proteins induces larger increases in energy expenditure compared to lower-quality proteins, thus promoting weight loss (Westerterp-Plantenga et al. 2009). Consequently, the consumption of different proteins seems to induce distinct nutrient-related responses in satiety hormones. Nonetheless, according to Dhillon et al. (Dhillon et al. 2016), trials of isolated proteins or AAs often adhere to proof-of-principle designs, administering supraphysiological doses and using controls that do not always relate to customary eating practices.

Research indicates that protein-induced satiety increases GLP-1 and PYY concentrations (M. Veldhorst et al. 2008). Most importantly, protein-induced satiety plays a crucial role in achieving and maintaining weight loss (M. Veldhorst et al. 2008; Westerterp-Plantenga et al. 2009).

Timing of Protein Intake

In addition to protein type, the timing of protein intake (acute or longitudinal) affects satiety and hunger. According to a recent meta-analysis (Kohanmoo, Faghih, and Akhlaghi 2020), acute protein ingestion acts as an appetite suppressant, reducing circulating ghrelin levels while augmenting CCK and GLP-1 concentrations. Nonetheless, the results of long-term trials are inconclusive, and more research is needed to understand the longitudinal effects of protein consumption on satiety (Kohanmoo, Faghih, and Akhlaghi 2020).

Increased Protein Intake and Appetite-Related Health Outcomes

Elevated protein intake (18–59% of the total energy intake [TEI]) has been shown to reduce body weight by approximately 1.6 kg compared to a standard protein diet (Hansen, Astrup, and Sjödin 2021). Furthermore, patients with prediabetes appear to benefit more from a high-protein diet compared to normoglycemic individuals, as do carriers of the obesity risk allele (AA genotype) compared to those with the AG and GG genotypes (Hansen, Astrup, and Sjödin 2021).

TABLE 3.1
Plausible Biological Mechanisms Explaining the Increased Protein-Induced Thermogenesis

1	The body's inability to store elevated protein intake, resulting in protein metabolism, thereby increasing thermogenesis
2	The increased energy cost associated with protein metabolism, including urea production and gluconeogenesis
3	The elevated ATP cost of peptide bond formation
4	The energy required to transport protons from the mitochondrial matrix to the inter-membrane space (proton-pump activity) in liver cells following the consumption of a high-protein meal
5	Protein intake prevents FFM degradation, which regulates REE, inducing increased FFM and higher REE with greater protein consumption
6	High protein intake results in elevated AA concentrations, increased hepatic gluconeogenesis and ketogenesis, and improved glucose homeostasis, all of which contribute to an increased satiety sensation

AA, amino acid; ATP, adenosine triphosphate; FFM, fat-free mass; REE, resting energy expenditure.

Clinical trials lasting 6–12 months have shown that a high-protein diet not only induces weight loss but can also prevent weight regain after successful weight loss is achieved (Moon and Koh 2020). As elevated protein intake is associated with increased satiety signaling and, by inference, lower food intake, the biological explanation for this weight loss is easily understood. Additionally, elevated protein diets are associated with diet-induced thermogenesis (DIT), as proteins have a greater DIT compared to fats and carbohydrates (Moon and Koh 2020; Halton and Hu 2004). The plausible biological mechanisms explaining the greater protein DIT and energy expenditure are detailed in Table 3.1 (Dehnavi et al. 2023).

Vegetarian versus Animal Proteins and Energy Expenditure

Since vegetarian and animal proteins have different AA content, they induce different postprandial responses (Dehnavi et al. 2023). Overall, animal proteins have been shown to induce increased postprandial resting energy expenditure (REE), substrate oxidation, and DIT compared to plant proteins (Dehnavi et al. 2023). This increased REE associated with the consumption of animal proteins has been attributed to the higher DIT of specific essential AAs in animal products compared with those observed in plant products (Mikkelsen, Toubro, and Astrup 2000). Furthermore, animal proteins are deemed to have greater nutritional value than plant proteins – due to the variety of essential AAs – and greater digestibility in the human GI tract (Kaur et al. 2022).

Vegetarian versus Animal Proteins for Satiety

A plethora of research has compared the effect of animal versus plant proteins on appetite sensations. Some trials (Neacsu et al. 2014; Nielsen et al. 2018) have suggested similar ad libitum energy intake, satiety, and hunger sensations – either as subjective measures or as gut hormone profiles – following the consumption of vegetarian and animal protein meals and diets, indicating that both can be effective in appetite control during weight loss interventions (Table 3.2). Kristensen and associates also showed that a vegetable-based meal with low protein content was as satiating and palatable as an animal-based meal with high protein content (Kristensen et al. 2016), suggesting that the fiber content of the vegetable meals was responsible for the fullness and satiety observed in this group. However, even when vegetarian and animal protein meals of similar fiber content were consumed, ad libitum energy intake, hunger, satiety, fullness, prospective food consumption, and composite appetite scores were not significantly different (Nielsen et al. 2018). To further examine

TABLE 3.2
Randomized Controlled Trials Comparing the Effect of Animal versus Plant Proteins on Appetite and Satiety

Author	Origin	Blinding, Design	Participants	Interventions	Duration	Outcomes	Results
Abou-Samra et al. (2011)	Switzerland	Single-blind, cross-over	N = 32 male volunteers	Preload (30 min before an ad libitum meal) containing: 1) 20 g of casein, 2) 20 g whey, 3) 20 g pea protein, 4) 20 g egg albumin, 5) 20 g maltodextrin, 6) water	Acute	Food intake (30 min later), subjective appetite (VAS), Glu	Food intake was lower only after casein and pea protein compared to the water control. Feelings of satiety were higher post-casein and pea protein compared to other preloads. Glu meal response was lower post-whey protein, compared to other preloads.
Abou-Samra et al. (2011)	Switzerland	Single-blind, cross-over	N = 32 male volunteers	Preload (starter during an *ad libitum* meal) containing: 1) 20 g of casein, 2) 20 g of pea protein, 3) 20 g of whey protein, or 4) water	Acute	Satiety	No difference was noted between preloads on *ad libitum* intake. Intake was higher after caloric preloads compared to water intake.
Belinova et al. (2014)	Czech Republic	Cross-over	N = 50 men with T2DM and N = 50 healthy men	Two standardized isocaloric meals: 1) a processed hamburger meat meal rich in protein and saturated fat (Pro-meal) and 2) a vegan meal rich in CHO (CHO-meal)	Acute	GI hormones (GIP, PYY, PP, GHR)	The Pro-meal increased persistent postprandial hyperinsulinemia in patients with T2DM. Plasma peak Glu levels were higher after the CHO-meal. GIP, PYY, and PP were higher, and GHR concentration was lower after the Pro-meal in healthy subjects. In contrast, GIP, PYY, and PP were lower after the Pro-meal in patients with T2DM patients.

(*Continued*)

TABLE 3.2 (CONTINUED)
Randomized Controlled Trials Comparing the Effect of Animal versus Plant Proteins on Appetite and Satiety

Author	Origin	Blinding, Design	Participants	Interventions	Duration	Outcomes	Results
Braden, Gwin, and Leidy (2023)	USA	Parallel	N = 32 adults	Four energy and protein-matched beverages (250 kcal, 24 g protein) with: 1) whey protein, 2) soy protein, 3) pea protein, or 4) micellar casein, followed by an ad libitum breakfast on the 5th day	4 days	Appetite (VAS), PYY, energy intake of subsequent meal	Casein and pea reduced 4 hr appetite and increased PYY compared with soy protein. Whey did not induce any changes. No differences in *ad libitum* energy intake were noted.
Douglas, Lasley, and Leidy (2015)	USA	Double-blind, cross-over	N = 21 adults (normal weight)	1) 400 kcal fiber-matched (FM) lunches (24 g beef or 24 g soy protein), 2) 400 kcal serving size-matched (SS) lunch with one serving of beef (24 g protein/1 g fiber) or soy (14 g protein/5 g fiber)	Acute	Appetite (PYY, GLP-1 levels) and neural activation (MRI)	Dinner was requested approximately 250 ± 20 min post-lunch, with no differences observed between beef versus soy within the matched meals. No differences were recorded in hunger, satiety, PYY, or GLP-1 responses post-beef versus post-soy lunches within matched conditions. However, the SS beef meal led to reductions in anterior cingulate and insular activation compared to soy. The serving size resulted in lower dinner energy intake.
Kahleova et al. (2021)	Czech Republic	Cross-over	N = 20 men with T2DM, N = 20 overweight/obese men, and N = 20 healthy men	Two energy- and macronutrient-matched meals: 1) a processed meat and cheese meal (M-meal) and 2) a vegan meal with tofu (V-meal)	Acute	Brain activity (ASL), GI hormones, and satiety (VAS)	Thalamus perfusion was the highest in men with T2DM and the lowest in those with obesity. Thalamus perfusion decreased post-M-meal in men with T2DM and overweight/obesity, and it decreased after the V-meal among healthy controls. Postprandial secretion of active GLP-1 increased (42%) after the V-meal compared to the M-meal in participants with T2DM and by 41% in healthy controls. Changes in thalamus perfusion after both test meals correlated with changes in satiety, fasting plasma Ins, C-peptide, and amylin.

(Continued)

TABLE 3.2 (CONTINUED)
Randomized Controlled Trials Comparing the Effect of Animal versus Plant Proteins on Appetite and Satiety

Author	Origin	Blinding, Design	Participants	Interventions	Duration	Outcomes	Results
Kahleova et al. (2019)	Czech Republic	Cross-over	N = 20 men with T2DM	Two energy- and macronutrient-matched meals: 1) a standard meat meal (M-meal) and 2) a vegan meal (V-meal)	Acute	Postprandial incretin (Glu, C-peptide, GLP-1, amylin, and GIP) and Ins secretion	Postprandial plasma glucose responses were similar after either meal. However, an increase in the secretion of Ins, C-peptide, GLP-1, and amylin was noted post-V-meal. Additionally, several β-cell function parameters increased post-V-meal.
Klementova et al. (2019)	Czech Republic	Cross-over	N = 20 men with T2DM, N = 20 obese men and N = 20 healthy men	Two energy- and macronutrient-matched meals: 1) a processed meat and cheese meal (M-meal) and 2) a vegan meal with tofu (V-meal)	Acute	Satiety (VAS), plasma concentrations of GLP-1, PYY, and amylin	Postprandial GLP-1 secretion increased after the V-meal in both T2DM and healthy controls. Plasma amylin levels increased in all groups after the V-meal. An increase in postprandial PYY levels followed the V-meal in healthy controls. Satiety was greater in all groups after the V-meal intake.
Kristensen et al. (2016)	Denmark	Double-blind, Cross-over	N = 43 healthy, normal weight, young men	1) HP-Meat (veal and pork) meal with 19% protein, 53% CHO, and 6 g fiber/100 g 2) HP-legumes (beans and peas) meal, with 19% protein, 53% CHO, and 25 g fiber/100 g 3) LP-legumes meal, with 9% protein, 62% CHO, and 10 g fiber/100 g	Acute	Subjective appetite sensations	HP-Legume induced reduced appetite, hunger, prospective intake, and higher fullness compared to HP-Meat and LP-Legume. Satiety was improved after HP-Legume than HP-Meat. When adjusted for palatability, HP-Legume reduced appetite, hunger, prospective intake, and increased fullness compared to HP-Meat. HP-Legume induced greater fullness than LP-Legume. EI was reduced by 12% and 13% post-HP-Legume compared to HP-Meat or LP-Legume.

(Continued)

TABLE 3.2 (CONTINUED)
Randomized Controlled Trials Comparing the Effect of Animal versus Plant Proteins on Appetite and Satiety

Author	Origin	Blinding, Design	Participants	Interventions	Duration	Outcomes	Results
Medawar et al. (2023)	Germany	Pooled, parallel	N = 16,379 adults	1) A single plant-based (vegetarian and vegan) meal and 2) an animal-based (animal flesh) meal	Acute	Satiety, mood, and stress	Meal intake induced satiety and improved mood status. However, plant-based meal choices failed to explain differences in post-meal hunger sensations. Protein content marginally mediated post-meal satiety, while taste rating and gender had a strong effect on both satiety and reported mood.
Neacsu et al. (2014)	UK	Cross-over	N = 20 men with obesity	1) Vegetarian (Soy-HPWL), 2) meat-based HPWL. Both diets were hypocaloric, with 30% protein, 30% fat, and 40% CHO	2 weeks	BW and motivation to eat, as well as plasma satiety biomarkers	Over the 2 weeks, subjects lost on average 2.41 and 2.27 kg with consumption of the Soy- and Meat-HPWL diets. Subjective hunger, fullness, desire to eat, preservation of LBM, and loss of % FM did not differ. There were differences in absolute concentrations of GHR and PYY between the two HPWL diets, although the response as AUC was not different.
Nielsen et al. (2018)	Denmark	Cross-over	N = 35 healthy men	1) Meal with fava beans and split peas (28.5 g fiber), 2) meal with pork/veal or eggs supplemented with pea fiber (28.5 g fiber), 3) meal with eggs without fiber supplementation (6.0 g fiber). All meals had a similar TEI (~3550 kJ), with 19% of TEI from protein	Acute	Subjective appetite sensations	No differences were noted in *ad libitum* TEI across test meals. No differences were found across meals for hunger, satiety, fullness, prospective food intake, or composite appetite score.

(Continued)

TABLE 3.2 (CONTINUED)
Randomized Controlled Trials Comparing the Effect of Animal versus Plant Proteins on Appetite and Satiety

Author	Origin	Blinding, Design	Participants	Interventions	Duration	Outcomes	Results
Veldhorst, Nieuwenhuizen, Hochstenbach-Waelen, van Vught et al. (2009)	The Netherlands	Single-blind	N = 25 healthy subjects	1) Breakfast: custard with casein, 2) breakfast: custard with soy, 3) breakfast: custard with whey protein. Meals either had normal protein content (10% TEI) or HP (25% TEI)	Acute	Appetite profile (VAS) and AA levels for 4 hr, as well as plasma Glu, Ins, active GLP-1, and active ghrelin concentrations	At normal protein intake (10%), whey reduced hunger more than casein or soy, coinciding with greater TRP, LEU, isoleucine, LYS, and THR responses. At HP, no differences in appetite were recorded. Whey triggered the strongest responses in levels of GLP-1 and Ins compared with casein and/or soy.
Veldhorst, Nieuwenhuizen, Hochstenbach-Waelen, Westerterp et al. (2009)	The Netherlands	Single-blind	N = 24 healthy subjects	1) Breakfast: custard with casein, 2) breakfast: custard with soy, 3) breakfast: custard with whey-GMP, 4) breakfast: custard with α-lactalbumin, 5) breakfast: custard with gelatin, 6) breakfast: custard with gelatin and TRP as protein source. Meals either had normal protein content (10% TEI) or HP (25% TEI)	Acute	Appetite (VAS) and EI	At normal and HP, TEI at lunch was ~20% lower after an a-lactalbumin or gelatin (+TRP) breakfast, compared with after a casein, soy, or whey-GMP breakfast. Different proteins (α-lactalbumin, gelatin, gelatin + TRP) that are approximately 40% more satiating than other proteins (casein, soy, whey, whey-GMP) induce a related ~20% reduction of energy intake in subsequent meal.

AA, amino acid; ASL, arterial spin labeling functional brain imaging; AUC, area under the curve; BF, body fat; BW, body weight; CHO, carbohydrates; TEI, total energy intake; Ins, insulin; GI, gastrointestinal; GIP, gastric inhibitory peptide; GHR, ghrelin; GLP-1, Glucagon-like Peptide 1; Glu, glucose; GMP, glycomacropeptide; HP, high-protein; HPWL, high-protein weight loss; Ins, insulin; LBM, lean body mass; LEU, leucine; LP, low-protein; LYS, Lysine; MRI, magnetic resonance imaging; PP, pancreatic polypeptide; PYY, peptide YY; T2DM, type 2 diabetes mellitus; THR, threonine; TRP, tryptophan; VAS, visual analog scale.

this hypothesis, Douglas et al. (Douglas, Lasley, and Leidy 2015) compared lunches of similar fiber content (soy- or beef-based) to lunch meals of similar serving sizes (soy- or beef-based). No differences were noted in hunger and satiety responses or PYY or GLP-1 concentrations after the beef or soy lunches under meal-matched conditions. However, serving-size-matched beef lunches led to reductions in anterior cingulate and insular activation in comparison to soy lunches. Furthermore, serving-size-matched meals reduced dinner energy intake, regardless of their protein source, more than fiber-matched meals. These findings suggest that the volume of consumed protein might be more important to satiety and subsequent energy intake than protein source or fiber content.

Consuming different protein types as a meal preload may also affect subsequent energy intake. Braden et al. compared the effects of isocaloric protein-preload beverages (with 24 g protein each), varying in protein source (whey, soy, pea protein isolates, or micellar casein), on appetite and subsequent energy intake (Braden, Gwin, and Leidy 2023). The results revealed that casein and pea reduced 4-hour appetite and increased PYY concentrations compared with soy protein. Abou-Samra et al. (2011) showed that when consumed as preloads, casein and pea protein reduce food intake compared to whey protein. However, this impact was only apparent when the preloads were consumed 30 minutes before the meal.

Other studies focus on the effect of specific AA intake. Veldhorst et al. (2009) compared the effect of three different breakfast meals with casein, soy, or whey protein, with normal or higher protein content, on the appetite profile of apparently healthy subjects. Their results showed that irrespective of protein source, differences in appetite ratings were apparent only when certain AAs exceeded or fell below particular threshold values. Specifically, greater leucine, tryptophan, isoleucine, lysine, and threonine responses were associated with an increased feeling of satiety. In a subsequent trial, the same research team suggested that some proteins appear to be approximately 40% more satiating than others, inducing a ~20% reduction in the energy intake of the subsequent meal (Veldhorst, Nieuwenhuizen, Hochstenbach-Waelen, Westerterp et al. 2009).

Some researchers, however, have also suggested that depending on the underlying pathology of the participants, vegan/vegetarian meals may induce a greater satiety response. In an early study, Belinova et al. (2014) showed that when an animal protein meal is consumed by healthy participants, GIP, PYY, and PP are increased, while ghrelin concentration is reduced. In contrast, when patients with type-2 diabetes mellitus (T2DM) consume the same meal, concentrations of GIP, PYY, and PP are reduced, indicating an opposite response (Belinova et al. 2014). In a recent trial, Klementova et al. (2019) revealed an increase in satiety and incretin concentrations following the consumption of a single plant-based meal with tofu compared to an energy- and macronutrient-matched processed meat and cheese meal in healthy men, men with T2DM, or obesity. However, it is evident that an energy-matched meal for normal-weight participants might well be a hypocaloric one for patients with T2DM or obesity. In this manner, hunger and satiety cues might be affected by the smaller stomachs of normal-weight participants and the level of energy intake. Similarly, Kahleova et al. (Kahleova et al. 2019; Klementova et al. 2019) revealed an increase in postprandial incretin and insulin secretion following the consumption of a vegan meal in T2DM. Furthermore, the increased post-meal GLP-1 secretion coincided with greater reported satiety and changes in thalamus perfusion, indicating that plant-based meals may be beneficial for treating T2DM and improving β-cell function (Kahleova et al. 2019; Klementova et al. 2019).

CONCLUSIONS

In summary, research appears unanimous on the increased satiety, elevated DIT, and energy expenditure following the consumption of high-protein meals. As for animal- and plant-based or alternative proteins, their different AA content appears to mediate, at least in part, distinct postprandial responses. The health status or underlying pathology of the consumer, the timing of the protein intake, and the serving size seem to affect post-meal satiety regulation.

MINI DICTIONARY OF TERMS

- **Alternative proteins:** Plant-based alternatives to animal proteins.
- **Diet-induced thermogenesis:** The amount of energy required for the metabolism of each meal.
- **Incretins:** Hormones released after the consumption of a meal, lowering blood glucose levels.

SUMMARY POINTS

- Meals with greater protein content reduce hunger and result in greater satiety compared to lower protein meals.
- Meals with greater protein content induce greater energy expenditure compared to lower protein meals.
- High-protein meals are associated with greater diet-induced thermogenesis, especially when complete proteins are consumed.
- Postprandial responses to animal versus plant-based proteins depend on the AA content and the health status of the consumer.
- Greater leucine, tryptophan, isoleucine, lysine, and threonine post-meal responses have been associated with an increased feeling of satiety.

REFERENCES

Abou-Samra, Rania, Lian Keersmaekers, Dino Brienza, Rajat Mukherjee, and Katherine Macé. 2011. "Effect of Different Protein Sources on Satiation and Short-Term Satiety When Consumed as a Starter." *Nutrition Journal* 10 (1): 139. https://doi.org/10.1186/1475-2891-10-139.

Alamri, Bader N., Kyungsoo Shin, Valerie Chappe, and Younes Anini. 2016. "The Role of Ghrelin in the Regulation of Glucose Homeostasis." *Hormone Molecular Biology and Clinical Investigation* 26 (1): 3–11. https://doi.org/10.1515/HMBCI-2016-0018.

Alonso-Alonso, Miguel, and Alvaro Pascual-Leone. 2007. "The Right Brain Hypothesis for Obesity." *JAMA* 297 (16): 1819–22. https://doi.org/10.1001/JAMA.297.16.1819.

Amin, Tehmina, and Julian G. Mercer. 2016. "Hunger and Satiety Mechanisms and Their Potential Exploitation in the Regulation of Food Intake." *Current Obesity Reports* 5 (1): 106–12. https://doi.org/10.1007/S13679-015-0184-5.

Anderson, Erica J. P., Isin Çakir, Sheridan J. Carrington, Roger D. Cone, Masoud Ghamari-Langroudi, Taneisha Gillyard, Luis E. Gimenez, and Michael J. Litt. 2016. "60 YEARS OF POMC: Regulation of Feeding and Energy Homeostasis by α-MSH." *Journal of Molecular Endocrinology* 56 (4): T157–74. https://doi.org/10.1530/JME-16-0014.

Austin, Juliana, and Daniel Marks. 2008. "Hormonal Regulators of Appetite." *International Journal of Pediatric Endocrinology* 2009 (1): 1–9. https://doi.org/10.1155/2009/141753.

Baggio, Laurie L., and Daniel J. Drucker. 2007. "Biology of Incretins: GLP-1 and GIP." *Gastroenterology* 132 (6): 2131–57. https://doi.org/10.1053/J.GASTRO.2007.03.054.

Belinova, Lenka, Hana Kahleova, Hana Malinska, Ondrej Topolcan, Jindra Vrzalova, Olena Oliyarnyk, Ludmila Kazdova, Martin Hill, and Terezie Pelikanova. 2014. "Differential Acute Postprandial Effects of Processed Meat and Isocaloric Vegan Meals on the Gastrointestinal Hormone Response in Subjects Suffering from Type 2 Diabetes and Healthy Controls: A Randomized Crossover Study." *PloS One* 9 (9): e107561. https://doi.org/10.1371/JOURNAL.PONE.0107561.

Biglari, Nasim, Isabella Gaziano, Jonas Schumacher, Jan Radermacher, Lars Paeger, Paul Klemm, Weiyi Chen, et al. 2021. "Functionally Distinct POMC-Expressing Neuron Subpopulations in Hypothalamus Revealed by Intersectional Targeting." *Nature Neuroscience* 24 (7): 913–29. https://doi.org/10.1038/S41593-021-00854-0.

Braden, Morgan L., Jess A. Gwin, and Heather J. Leidy. 2023. "Protein Source Influences Acute Appetite and Satiety but Not Subsequent Food Intake in Healthy Adults." *The Journal of Nutrition* 153 (6): 1825–33. https://doi.org/10.1016/J.TJNUT.2023.04.001.

Chandra, Rashmi, and Rodger A. Liddle. 2007. "Cholecystokinin." *Current Opinion in Endocrinology, Diabetes, and Obesity* 14 (1): 63–67. https://doi.org/10.1097/MED.0B013E3280122850.

Cummings, David E., Jonathan Q. Purnell, R. Scott Frayo, Karin Schmidova, Brent E. Wisse, and David S. Weigle. 2001. "A Preprandial Rise in Plasma Ghrelin Levels Suggests a Role in Meal Initiation in Humans." *Diabetes* 50 (8): 1714–19. https://doi.org/10.2337/DIABETES.50.8.1714.

Dagogo-Jack, Samuel. 2005. "Human Leptin Regulation and Promise in Pharmacotherapy." *Current Drug Targets* 2 (2): 181–95. https://doi.org/10.2174/1389450013348623.

Dalton, Michelle, Graham Finlayson, Emma Esdaile, and Neil King. 2013. "Appetite, Satiety, and Food Reward in Obese Individuals: A Behavioral Phenotype Approach." *Current Nutrition Reports* 2 (4): 207–15. https://doi.org/10.1007/S13668-013-0060-4/FIGURES/1.

Dehnavi, Zahra, Hanieh Barghchi, Ali Jafarzadeh Esfehani, Mehdi Barati, Zahra Khorasanchi, Farima Farsi, Andisheh Norouzian Ostad, et al. 2023. "Animal and Plant-Based Proteins Have Different Postprandial Effects on Energy Expenditure, Glycemia, Insulinemia, and Lipemia: A Review of Controlled Clinical Trials." *Food Science & Nutrition* 11 (8): 4398–408. https://doi.org/10.1002/FSN3.3417.

Dhillon, Jaapna, Bruce A. Craig, Heather J. Leidy, Akua F. Amankwaah, Katherene Osei-Boadi Anguah, Ashley Jacobs, Blake L. Jones, et al. 2016. "The Effects of Increased Protein Intake on Fullness: A Meta-Analysis and Its Limitations." *Journal of the Academy of Nutrition and Dietetics* 116 (6): 968–83. https://doi.org/10.1016/J.JAND.2016.01.003.

Douglas, Steve M., Tyler R. Lasley, and Heather J. Leidy. 2015. "Consuming Beef vs. Soy Protein Has Little Effect on Appetite, Satiety, and Food Intake in Healthy Adults." *The Journal of Nutrition* 145 (5): 1010–16. https://doi.org/10.3945/JN.114.206987.

Elias, Carol F., Charlotte E. Lee, Joseph F. Kelly, Rexford S. Ahima, Michael Kuhar, Clifford B. Saper, and Joel K. Elmquist. 2001. "Characterization of CART Neurons in the Rat and Human Hypothalamus." *The Journal of Comparative Neurology* 432 (1): 1–19. https://doi.org/10.1002/CNE.1085.

Gkouskou, Kalliopi K., Maria G. Grammatikopoulou, Evgenia Lazou, Theodora Vasilogiannakopoulou, Despina Sanoudou, and Aristides G. Eliopoulos. 2024. "A Genomics Perspective of Personalized Prevention and Management of Obesity." *Human Genomics* 18 (1): 1–13. https://doi.org/10.1186/S40246-024-00570-3.

Gorska, Elzbieta, K. Popko, A. Stelmaszczyk-Emmel, O. Ciepiela, A. Kucharska, and M. Wasik. 2010. "Leptin Receptors." *European Journal of Medical Research* 15 (2): 50–54. https://doi.org/10.1186/2047-783X-15-S2-50/FIGURES/3.

Halton, Thomas L., and Frank B. Hu. 2004. "The Effects of High Protein Diets on Thermogenesis, Satiety and Weight Loss: A Critical Review." *Journal of the American College of Nutrition* 23 (5): 373–85. https://doi.org/10.1080/07315724.2004.10719381.

Hansen, Thea Toft, Arne Astrup, and Anders Sjödin. 2021. "Are Dietary Proteins the Key to Successful Body Weight Management? A Systematic Review and Meta-Analysis of Studies Assessing Body Weight Outcomes after Interventions with Increased Dietary Protein." *Nutrients* 13 (9): 3193. https://doi.org/10.3390/NU13093193/S1.

Hoed, Marcel Den, Margriet S. Westerterp-Plantenga, Freek G. Bouwman, Edwin C. M. Mariman, and Klaas R. Westerterp. 2009. "Postprandial Responses in Hunger and Satiety Are Associated with the Rs9939609 Single Nucleotide Polymorphism in FTO." *The American Journal of Clinical Nutrition* 90 (5): 1426–32. https://doi.org/10.3945/AJCN.2009.28053.

Horstmann, Annette, Peter Kovacs, Stefan Kabisch, Yvonne Boettcher, Haiko Schloegl, Anke Tönjes, Michael Stumvoll, Burkhard Pleger, and Arno Villringer. 2013. "Common Genetic Variation near MC4R Has a Sex-Specific Impact on Human Brain Structure and Eating Behavior." *PLoS One* 8 (9): e74362. https://doi.org/10.1371/JOURNAL.PONE.0074362.

Huang, Hao, Youfen Xu, and Anthony N. van den Pol. 2011. "Nicotine Excites Hypothalamic Arcuate Anorexigenic Proopiomelanocortin Neurons and Orexigenic Neuropeptide Y Neurons: Similarities and Differences." *Journal of Neurophysiology* 106 (3): 1191–202. https://doi.org/10.1152/JN.00740.2010.

Huang, Tao, Yan Zheng, Adela Hruby, Donald A. Williamson, George A. Bray, Yiru Shen, Frank M. Sacks, and Lu Qi. 2017. "Dietary Protein Modifies the Effect of the MC4R Genotype on 2-Year Changes in Appetite and Food Craving: The POUNDS Lost Trial." *The Journal of Nutrition* 147 (3): 444. https://doi.org/10.3945/JN.116.242958.

Kahleova, Hana, Jaroslav Tintera, Lenka Thieme, Jiri Veleba, Marta Klementova, Michaela Kudlackova, Hana Malinska, et al. 2021. "A Plant-Based Meal Affects Thalamus Perfusion Differently than an Energy- and Macronutrient-Matched Conventional Meal in Men with Type 2 Diabetes, Overweight/Obese, and Healthy Men: A Three-Group Randomized Crossover Study." *Clinical Nutrition (Edinburgh, Scotland)* 40 (4): 1822–33. https://doi.org/10.1016/J.CLNU.2020.10.005.

Kahleova, Hana, Andrea Tura, Marta Klementova, Lenka Thieme, Martin Haluzik, Renata Pavlovicova, Martin Hill, and Terezie Pelikanova. 2019. "A Plant-Based Meal Stimulates Incretin and Insulin Secretion More Than an Energy- and Macronutrient-Matched Standard Meal in Type 2 Diabetes: A Randomized Crossover Study." *Nutrients* 11 (3): 486. https://doi.org/10.3390/NU11030486.

Kaur, Lovedeep, Boning Mao, Akashdeep Singh Beniwal, Abhilasha, Ramandeep Kaur, Feng Ming Chian, and Jaspreet Singh. 2022. "Alternative Proteins vs Animal Proteins: The Influence of Structure and Processing on Their Gastro-Small Intestinal Digestion." *Trends in Food Science & Technology* 122 (April): 275–86. https://doi.org/10.1016/J.TIFS.2022.02.021.

Klementova, Marta, Lenka Thieme, Martin Haluzik, Renata Pavlovicova, Martin Hill, Terezie Pelikanova, and Hana Kahleova. 2019. "A Plant-Based Meal Increases Gastrointestinal Hormones and Satiety More Than an Energy- and Macronutrient-Matched Processed-Meat Meal in T2D, Obese, and Healthy Men: A Three-Group Randomized Crossover Study." *Nutrients* 11 (1): 157. https://doi.org/10.3390/NU11010157.

Kohanmoo, Ali, Shiva Faghih, and Masoumeh Akhlaghi. 2020. "Effect of Short- and Long-Term Protein Consumption on Appetite and Appetite-Regulating Gastrointestinal Hormones, a Systematic Review and Meta-Analysis of Randomized Controlled Trials." *Physiology & Behavior* 226 (November): 113123. https://doi.org/10.1016/J.PHYSBEH.2020.113123.

Kristensen, Marlene D., Nathalie T. Bendsen, Sheena M. Christensen, Arne Astrup, and Anne Raben. 2016. "Meals Based on Vegetable Protein Sources (Beans and Peas) Are More Satiating than Meals Based on Animal Protein Sources (Veal and Pork) – a Randomized Cross-over Meal Test Study." *Food & Nutrition Research* 60: 1–9. https://doi.org/10.3402/FNR.V60.32634.

Lau, Jackie, Aitak Farzi, Yue Qi, Regine Heilbronn, Mario Mietzsch, Yan Chuan Shi, and Herbert Herzog. 2018. "CART Neurons in the Arcuate Nucleus and Lateral Hypothalamic Area Exert Differential Controls on Energy Homeostasis." *Molecular Metabolism* 7 (January): 102–18. https://doi.org/10.1016/J.MOLMET.2017.10.015.

Lavoie, Olivier, Natalie Jane Michael, and Alexandre Caron. 2023. "A Critical Update on the Leptin-Melanocortin System." *Journal of Neurochemistry* 165 (4): 467–86. https://doi.org/10.1111/JNC.15765.

Liddle, R. A., I. D. Goldfine, M. S. Rosen, R. A. Taplitz, and J. A. Williams. 1985. "Cholecystokinin Bioactivity in Human Plasma. Molecular Forms, Responses to Feeding, and Relationship to Gallbladder Contraction." *The Journal of Clinical Investigation* 75 (4): 1144–52. https://doi.org/10.1172/JCI111809.

Lu, Dongsi, Derril Willard, Indravadan R. Patel, Sue Kadwell, Laurie Overton, Tom Kost, Michael Luther, et al. 1994. "Agouti Protein Is an Antagonist of the Melanocyte-Stimulating-Hormone Receptor." *Nature* 371 (6500): 799–802. https://doi.org/10.1038/371799A0.

McLeod, C. J., G. M.W. Mycock, A. Twells, L. J. James, J. M. Brunstrom, and G. L. Witcomb. 2022. "Current Appetite Influences Relative Differences in the Expected Satiety of Foods for Momentary, but Not Hypothetical, Expected Satiety Assessments." *Appetite* 178 (November): 106159. https://doi.org/10.1016/J.APPET.2022.106159.

Medawar, Evelyn, Marie Zedler, Larissa de Biasi, Arno Villringer, and A. Veronica Witte. 2023. "Effects of Single Plant-Based vs. Animal-Based Meals on Satiety and Mood in Real-World Smartphone-Embedded Studies." *NPJ Science of Food* 7 (1). https://doi.org/10.1038/S41538-022-00176-W.

Micali, Nadia, Alison E. Field, Janet L. Treasure, and David M. Evans. 2015. "Are Obesity Risk Genes Associated with Binge Eating in Adolescence?" *Obesity* 23 (8): 1729–36. https://doi.org/10.1002/OBY.21147.

Mikkelsen, Per B., Søren Toubro, and Arne Astrup. 2000. "Effect of Fat-Reduced Diets on 24-h Energy Expenditure: Comparisons between Animal Protein, Vegetable Protein, and Carbohydrate." *The American Journal of Clinical Nutrition* 72 (5): 1135–41. https://doi.org/10.1093/AJCN/72.5.1135.

Miltenberger, Rosalynn J., Randall L. Mynatt, J. Erby Wilkinson, and Richard P. Woychik. 1997. "The Role of the Agouti Gene in the Yellow Obese Syndrome." *The Journal of Nutrition* 127 (9): 1902S–7S. https://doi.org/10.1093/JN/127.9.1902S.

Mook, Douglas G. 1989. "Oral Factors in Appetite and Satiety." *Annals of the New York Academy of Sciences* 575 (1): 265–80. https://doi.org/10.1111/J.1749-6632.1989.TB53249.X.

Moon, Jaecheol, and Gwanpyo Koh. 2020. "Clinical Evidence and Mechanisms of High-Protein Diet-Induced Weight Loss." *Journal of Obesity & Metabolic Syndrome* 29 (3): 166–73. https://doi.org/10.7570/JOMES20028.

Münzberg, Heike, and Christopher D. Morrison. 2015. "Structure, Production and Signaling of Leptin." *Metabolism – Clinical and Experimental* 64 (1): 13–23. https://doi.org/10.1016/J.METABOL.2014.09.010.

Nauck, Michael A., and Juris J. Meier. 2018. "Incretin Hormones: Their Role in Health and Disease." *Diabetes, Obesity and Metabolism* 20 (February): 5–21. https://doi.org/10.1111/DOM.13129.

Neacsu, Madalina, Claire Fyfe, Graham Horgan, and Alexandra M. Johnstone. 2014. "Appetite Control and Biomarkers of Satiety with Vegetarian (Soy) and Meat-Based High-Protein Diets for Weight Loss in Obese Men: A Randomized Crossover Trial." *The American Journal of Clinical Nutrition* 100 (2): 548–58. https://doi.org/10.3945/AJCN.113.077503.

Nielsen, Lone V., Marlene D. Kristensen, Lars Klingenberg, Christian Ritz, Anita Belza, Arne Astrup, and Anne Raben. 2018. "Protein from Meat or Vegetable Sources in Meals Matched for Fiber Content Has Similar Effects on Subjective Appetite Sensations and Energy Intake—A Randomized Acute Cross-Over Meal Test Study." *Nutrients* 10 (1). https://doi.org/10.3390/NU10010096.

Nordang, Gry B. N., Øyvind L. Busk, Kristian Tveten, Hans Ivar Hanevik, Anne Kristin M. Fell, Jøran Hjelmesæth, Øystein L. Holla, and Jens K. Hertel. 2017. "Next-Generation Sequencing of the Monogenic Obesity Genes LEP, LEPR, MC4R, PCSK1 and POMC in a Norwegian Cohort of Patients with Morbid Obesity and Normal Weight Controls." *Molecular Genetics and Metabolism* 121 (1): 51–56. https://doi.org/10.1016/J.YMGME.2017.03.007.

Rigamonti, Antonello E., Roberto Leoncini, Alessandra De Col, Sofia Tamini, Sabrina Cicolini, Laura Abbruzzese, Silvano G. Cella, and Alessandro Sartorio. 2020. "The Appetite–Suppressant and GLP-1-Stimulating Effects of Whey Proteins in Obese Subjects Are Associated with Increased Circulating Levels of Specific Amino Acids." *Nutrients* 12 (3): 775. https://doi.org/10.3390/NU12030775.

Schur, Ellen, and Susan Carnell. 2017. "What Twin Studies Tell Us About Brain Responses to Food Cues." *Current Obesity Reports* 6 (4): 371–79. https://doi.org/10.1007/S13679-017-0282-7/TABLES/1.

Seino, Yutaka, Mitsuo Fukushima, and Daisuke Yabe. 2010. "GIP and GLP-1, the Two Incretin Hormones: Similarities and Differences." *Journal of Diabetes Investigation* 1 (1–2): 8–23. https://doi.org/10.1111/J.2040-1124.2010.00022.X.

Suzuki, Keisuke, Channa N. Jayasena, and Stephen R. Bloom. 2011. "The Gut Hormones in Appetite Regulation." *Journal of Obesity*. https://doi.org/10.1155/2011/528401.

Turcot, Valérie, Yingchang Lu, Heather M. Highland, Claudia Schurmann, Anne E. Justice, Rebecca S. Fine, Jonathan P. Bradfield, et al. 2017. "Protein-Altering Variants Associated with Body Mass Index Implicate Pathways That Control Energy Intake and Expenditure in Obesity." *Nature Genetics* 50 (1): 26–41. https://doi.org/10.1038/s41588-017-0011-x.

Veldhorst, M. A. B., Arie G. Nieuwenhuizen, Ananda Hochstenbach-Waelen, Anneke J. A. H. van Vught, Klaas R. Westerterp, Marielle P. K. J. Engelen, Robert Jan M. Brummer, Nicolaas E. P. Deutz, and Margriet S. Westerterp-Plantenga. 2009. "Dose-Dependent Satiating Effect of Whey Relative to Casein or Soy." *Physiology & Behavior* 96 (4–5): 675–82. https://doi.org/10.1016/J.PHYSBEH.2009.01.004.

Veldhorst, Margriet A. B., Arie G. Nieuwenhuizen, Ananda Hochstenbach-Waelen, Klaas R. Westerterp, Marielle P. K. J. Engelen, Robert Jan M. Brummer, Nicolaas E. P. Deutz, and Margriet S. Westerterp-Plantenga. 2009. "A Breakfast with Alpha-Lactalbumin, Gelatin, or Gelatin + TRP Lowers Energy Intake at Lunch Compared with a Breakfast with Casein, Soy, Whey, or Whey-GMP." *Clinical Nutrition* 28 (2): 147–55. https://doi.org/10.1016/J.CLNU.2008.12.003.

Veldhorst, M. A. B., A. Smeets, S. Soenen, A. Hochstenbach-Waelen, R. Hursel, K. Diepvens, M. Lejeune, N. Luscombe-Marsh, and M. Westerterp-Plantenga. 2008. "Protein-Induced Satiety: Effects and Mechanisms of Different Proteins." *Physiology & Behavior* 94 (2): 300–307. https://doi.org/10.1016/J.PHYSBEH.2008.01.003.

Westerterp-Plantenga, M. S., A. Nieuwenhuizen, D. Tomé, S. Soenen, and K. R. Westerterp. 2009. "Dietary Protein, Weight Loss, and Weight Maintenance." *Annual Review of Nutrition* 29 (August): 21–41. https://doi.org/10.1146/ANNUREV-NUTR-080508-141056.

Willer, Cristen J., Elizabeth K. Speliotes, Ruth J. F. Loos, Shengxu Li, Cecilia M. Lindgren, Iris M. Heid, Sonja I. Berndt, et al. 2008. "Six New Loci Associated with Body Mass Index Highlight a Neuronal Influence on Body Weight Regulation." *Nature Genetics* 41 (1): 25–34. https://doi.org/10.1038/ng.287.

Yeung, Anthony Y., and Prasanna Tadi. 2023. "Physiology, Obesity Neurohormonal Appetite And Satiety Control." *StatPearls*, January.

4 Role of Animal and Plant Protein on Child Health Outcomes

Ranjitha Chandrashekar, Bharath Kumar Mulakala, Jolene R. Rearick, Maria Carmen Collado, and Laxmi Yeruva

ABBREVIATIONS

AA	Amino acids
AAP	American Academy of Pediatrics
BMI	Body mass index
ESPGHAN	European Society for Pediatric Gastroenterology, Hepatology, and Nutrition
EAA	Essential amino acids
LAZ scores	Length-for-age z-scores
LMICs	Low- and middle-income countries
MAL-ED	Malnutrition and enteric diseases
WHO	World Health Organization

INTRODUCTION

The role of nutrition in early childhood is paramount, as it sets the stage for a child's growth and development. Exclusive breastfeeding for the first 6 months of life, as recommended by the World Health Organization (WHO), the American Academy of Pediatrics (AAP), and European member states (Bagci Bosi et al. 2016), provide infants with essential nutrients and bioactive components crucial for their well-being. Human milk, with its unique macronutrient composition – 7% carbohydrates, 1% protein, and 3.8% fat – is not only a source of sustenance but also a complex blend of bioactive components (Carr et al. 2021). These components, including human milk oligosaccharides (HMO), cytokines, hormones, immunoglobulins, microRNA, and microbiota, play a multifaceted role in supporting infants (Carr et al. 2021). They aid in growth and development, play a pivotal role in programming metabolic processes, and facilitate the maturation of healthy microbiota, strengthening the infant's immune function, which is particularly vital in the early stages of life. However, when human milk feeding is not possible, milk formulas, often cow's milk-based (80%) or soy-based (12%), serve as nutritional alternatives. But what happens when we move beyond the exclusively milk-based diet and introduce complementary foods?

This chapter examines the impact of neonatal diet on child health outcomes, focusing on dietary protein sources. Specifically, it explores how animal protein versus plant protein intake affects children transitioning to complementary foods and its potential long-term health effects. Understanding how these dietary choices shape children's health trajectories is crucial for promoting optimal growth and development in early life. This chapter aims to elucidate this important aspect of pediatric nutrition and its broader implications for child health.

 DOI: 10.1201/9781003597926-4

NEONATAL DIET IS CRITICAL TO CHILDREN'S GROWTH AND DEVELOPMENT

Epidemiological studies indicate lower risks of respiratory infections, ear infections, gastrointestinal infections, asthma, and obesity in breastfed infants. Studies to date have compared breastfed versus formula-fed (cow's milk or plant-based formulas) infants. Recent reviews show increased weight gain in infants fed cow's milk infant formula with higher protein (2.0g/100kcal) compared to lower protein content (<1.8g/100kcal), while hydrolyzed casein formula reduced weight gain (Wallingford and Barber 2019; Ren et al. 2022). Previously, soy-based infant formula was recommended for infants with cow's milk allergy. National Health and Nutrition Examination Survey (NHANES) data indicate soy formula use in the US from 2003 to 2010, with no significant difference in infant growth. Interestingly, soy formulas disappeared from the European market due to concerns about isoflavones, phytoestrogen, and beany flavor. Recently, several other plant-based formulas have become more popular than cow's milk formulas (Vandenplas et al. 2021). For example, hydrolyzed rice formula has been shown to be tolerated by infants with no adverse outcomes and is nutritionally comparable to cow's milk and soy formula. Infants on this formula showed normal growth, comparable to soy infant formula or casein hydrolysate formula groups, and normal serum parameters for plasma total protein, albumin, minerals (calcium, magnesium), and alkaline phosphatase. Other formulas, such as Baby's Only Organic Plant-Based Pea Protein Formula and Sprout Organic Plant-Based Infant Formula, are also available. Scientific literature comparing child growth on these formulas to other formulas or breastfeeding is lacking.

Research also demonstrates the benefits of breastfeeding over formula feeding for various physiological systems. Breastfed infants have higher composite intelligence scores, language scores, and verbal intelligence scores between 3 and 5 years of age compared to infants fed cow's milk or soy formula (Bellando et al. 2020). After adjusting for variation in background and anthropometric data, no significant differences in development were observed between the formula-fed groups, but cognitive development was slightly higher in breastfed infants (Andres et al. 2012). In addition, breastfed infants had higher bone mineral content than soy formula-fed infants at 3 months. At 6 months, the soy formula-fed group showed enhanced bone metabolism compared to milk formula and breastfed groups (Chen et al. 2023). However, by 12 months, soy formula-fed infants had higher bone mineral content than the breastfed group. Body composition profiles differed across the three diet groups, with soy formula-fed infants showing a leaner body phenotype throughout the first year of life compared to breastfed or milk formula-fed infants (Andres et al. 2013). Moreover, breastfed infants showed the lowest fecal microbiota diversity up to 1 year of age and had higher levels of tryptophan pathway metabolites compared to those fed cow's milk or soy formula (Brink et al. 2020). In a preclinical model, no growth differences or organ development and health outcomes were observed between piglets fed cow's milk formula and plant-based Else formula (containing almonds and buckwheat as the primary sources) (Rosa et al. 2022; Gurung et al. 2023). These studies suggest similar health outcomes from cow's milk and plant-based formula intake. However, formulas vary, and recent evidence links infant anthropometrics to variations in the macronutrient composition of infant formulas (Young 2020). Furthermore, no randomized controlled trials during the infancy period (first 6 months) provide empirical evidence on animal versus plant protein intake's impact on infant health outcomes. As infant formulas contain components beyond protein, literature should be interpreted cautiously regarding animal versus plant protein intake and infant health outcomes. The following sections focus on the introduction of solid foods during infancy, particularly animal versus plant protein intake in early life, and its association with child health outcomes (Figure 4.1).

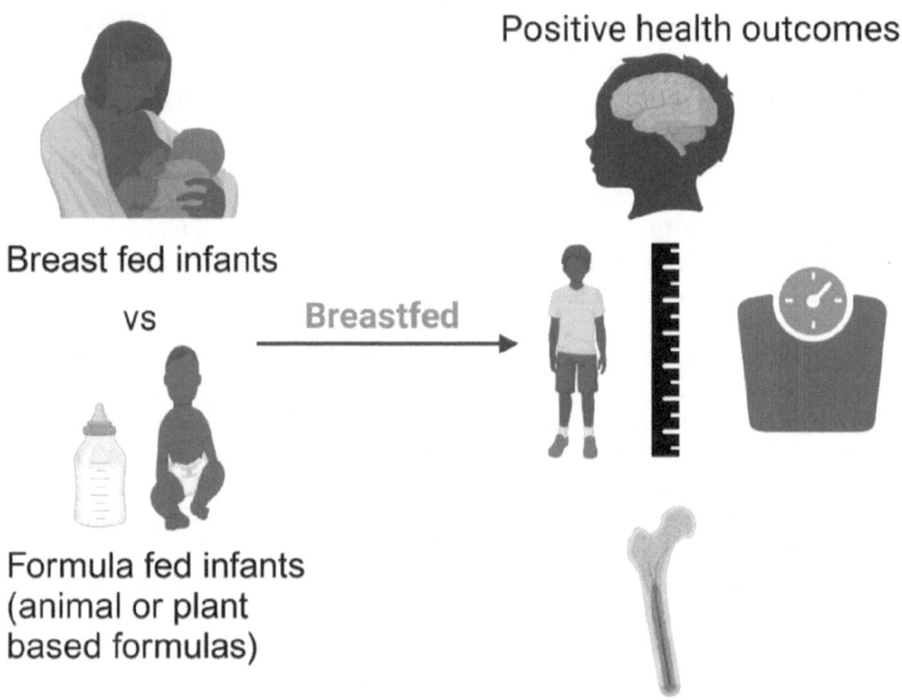

FIGURE 4.1 Neonatal diet (breast milk versus formula) plays a role in child health and development. In comparison to formula feeding, human milk feeding is associated with positive health outcomes such as bone quality, cognition, growth, and development. (Figure created using the BioRender online tool.)

COMPLEMENTARY DIET IN INFANTS PROMOTES GROWTH, METABOLIC HEALTH, AND COGNITION IN CHILDREN

As infants grow beyond 6 months of age, a breast milk or formula diet alone no longer meets their nutritional needs. To bridge this nutritional gap, complementary feeding becomes essential. The WHO and AAP recommend introducing appropriate complementary foods alongside breastfeeding up to 2 years of age. This balanced approach not only supports optimal growth but also contributes to the prevention of acute and chronic diseases in early and later life. Conversely, the European Society for Pediatric Gastroenterology, Hepatology, and Nutrition (ESPGHAN) suggests that complementary foods should not be introduced to infants before 4 months of age, but they should also not be delayed beyond 6 months of age. Despite these recommendations, there is still a discrepancy between the guidelines and practice. In addition, food allergies pose a significant health challenge during childhood. Allergic diseases are on the rise in Western societies, prompting a shift towards prioritizing prevention over treatment. The gut contains a significant load of antigens; thus, it is reasonable to consider the timing of exposure to solid foods during infancy, which could impact the likelihood of developing or being predisposed to allergic disorders. Most food allergies – over 90% – stem from eggs, peanuts, shellfish, fish, wheat, soy, and nuts. It has been reported that 5–6% of children by the age of 3 years suffer from food allergies.

Among the various dietary determinants of growth and development for infants, protein is an important dietary component that helps in tissue building and growth. Numerous studies focusing on infants and children have explored the connection between their consumption of animal-based foods and childhood nutrition, particularly in terms of linear growth. The study population included people from different countries. Infants and young children undergo various physiological states, including routine infections and rapid growth phases, which increase their amino acid (AA) requirements. Studies have revealed that even after adjusting for factors like essential amino acid composition, digestibility, energy deficits, and infections, up to 50% of the population in some countries may not have adequate protein intake (Parikh et al. 2022). Evidence comes from observational and intervention studies of the population's intake of various animal protein sources (i.e., red meat, eggs, chicken, dairy). The following sections will describe the evidence from various studies on the role of animal protein versus plant protein on growth, metabolic health, and cognition.

Animal Protein Intake Associates with Children's Growth

Physical growth and length have been indicators of children's well-being. Several studies, described below, provide evidence on this topic. A study conducted by Tang et al. focused on how dairy or meat complementary diets can influence the growth and development of formula-fed infants aged 5 to 12 months. Results showed that infants eating meat as complementary food had increased linear growth compared to those with dairy intake; however, the weight-for-length score increased in dairy groups compared to meat groups, suggesting distinct growth patterns (Tang, Hendricks, and Krebs 2018) based on protein source.

A randomized controlled trial by Chipili et al. demonstrated that adding fish powder to infants' diets increased their linear growth compared to control groups or those consuming sorghum powder (Chipili et al. 2022). Data from the Melbourne InFANT program, an observational prospective cohort study conducted between 2008 and 2013 with 345 children from 9 months to 5-year follow-up visits (Zheng et al. 2021), revealed that each additional 1 g or 1% increase in total protein intake at 9 months was associated with a corresponding rise of 0.016 units (95% CI 0.003 to 0.029) or 0.034 units (95% CI 0.005 to 0.063) in BMI z-score at 5 years. Notably, researchers found no significant evidence of a link between BMI z-score and dairy or plant proteins, including milk, yogurt, cheese, breast milk, and infant formula. Furthermore, the data suggest that elevated total protein and non-dairy animal protein intake during infancy are connected to higher BMI z-scores in early childhood. The MAL-ED (Malnutrition and Enteric Diseases) Birth Cohort Study in Dhaka, Bangladesh, examined the relationship between dietary components and the growth patterns of infants and toddlers and found that dietary animal protein exhibited a positive correlation with LAZ scores (length-for-age z-scores) (Das et al. 2020). Another study on infants aged 4–18 months following a cow's milk protein elimination diet showed lower weight values according to z-score for weight-for-age, weight-for-height, and BMI-for-age, but their height was similar to the control group (Frizzo et al. 2022). Conversely, Nordic Nutrition Recommendations revealed that high protein intake in infancy and early childhood led to increased growth and higher body mass index (BMI) later in adolescence (Arnesen et al. 2022).

In addition, another systematic review revealed that a higher intake of animal protein, especially from dairy products, is associated with growth, whereas vegetable protein does not show a similar effect (Arnesen et al. 2022). For example, in Malawian communities (Kaimila et al. 2019), higher animal protein intake in Limera resulted in improved growth in children compared to those in the Masenjere region, who consumed less animal protein. Although both regions predominantly relied on plant-based diets with maize as the staple food, the differences in growth outcomes were attributed to the quality of protein consumed. While most children met their daily protein requirements, the low quality and bioavailability of protein, mainly from plant sources, contributed to poor growth outcomes in the region with higher plant food consumption. This study underscores the significance of the quality of protein intake, particularly from animal sources, in early childhood. In conclusion, the research highlights the positive impact of animal-based protein consumption on children's growth and development, particularly in regions with predominantly plant-based diets, demonstrating that higher consumption of animal-based protein in infants increases the height-for-age z-score (Kaimila et al. 2019). However, not all studies support these findings. For example, a large cluster randomized efficacy trial conducted across the Democratic Republic of Congo, Zambia, Guatemala, and Pakistan, involving over 1,000 subjects, found no positive impact on preventing linear growth

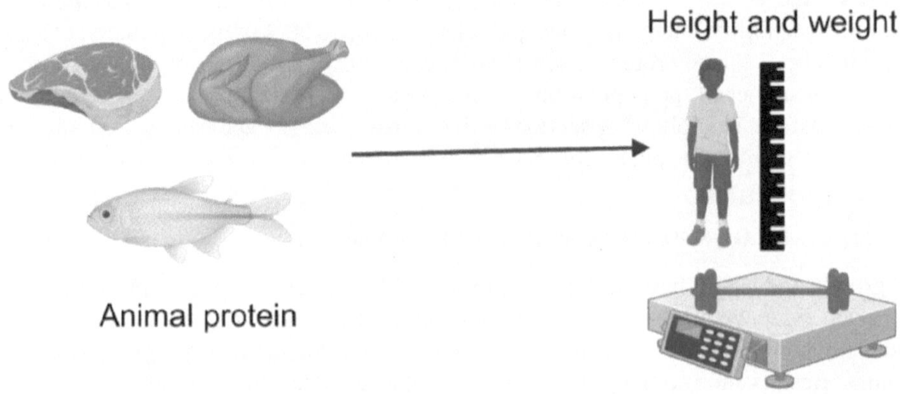

FIGURE 4.2 Animal protein intake is associated with children's height and weight. The recommended amount of animal protein intake in toddlers appears to promote optimal height and weight in children. (Figure created using the BioRender online tool.)

faltering when comparing the daily provision of lyophilized beef with micronutrient-fortified rice-soy cereal from 6 to 18 months of age (Krebs et al. 2012). These conflicting results suggest that the published literature varies in its recommendations for the intake of animal versus plant protein with complementary feeding for growth outcomes (Figure 4.2).

Animal Protein Intake Associates with Muscle Mass and Fat Mass

In rural Uganda, a study evaluated the effects of egg supplementation on the growth of primary school children (aged 6 to 9 years) participating in a school feeding program for 6 months. Children receiving two eggs per day showed greater increases in height, weight, and mid-upper-arm circumference, indicating significant gains in muscle mass compared to those receiving one egg per day or no eggs (Baum, Miller, and Gaines 2017). Researchers observed similar outcomes in a study from Kenya, where supplementing meat, milk, or energy over two academic years led to an increased mid-upper-arm muscle area in Kenyan school children aged 6 to 14 years, with the meat group experiencing the least increase in mid-upper-arm fat area (Neumann et al. 2013).

In addition, US cross-sectional studies have revealed that higher total protein and animal protein intake, rather than plant protein intake, is positively associated with indicators of muscle mass such as muscle mass index and leg lean mass (Sahni et al. 2015). Furthermore, longitudinal studies have demonstrated that increased consumption of total protein and animal protein is linked to a reduced loss of lean mass over a 3-year follow-up period (Liu et al. 2023). An observational longitudinal study conducted in Germany by Gunther et al. demonstrated that higher animal protein (i.e., dairy) intake at 12 months of age appears to be associated with higher fat mass at age 7 (Gunther et al. 2007).

A longitudinal cohort study investigated the relationship between a vegetarian diet and growth, micronutrient stores, and serum lipids among healthy children aged 6 months to 8 years. The researchers also sought to understand whether cow's milk consumption influences these relationships. The study reported no significant association between a vegetarian diet and z-score BMI, height, serum ferritin, 25OHD, or serum lipids. However, they found an association between lower mean z-score height and a vegetarian diet. Further analysis revealed that a vegetarian diet was closely associated with increased odds of children being underweight but showed no significant association with overweight or obesity. The study also focused on iron and vitamin D consumption in a vegetarian diet, which the researchers hypothesized to be low. Cow's milk consumption was associated with higher levels of non-high-density lipoprotein cholesterol and total cholesterol.

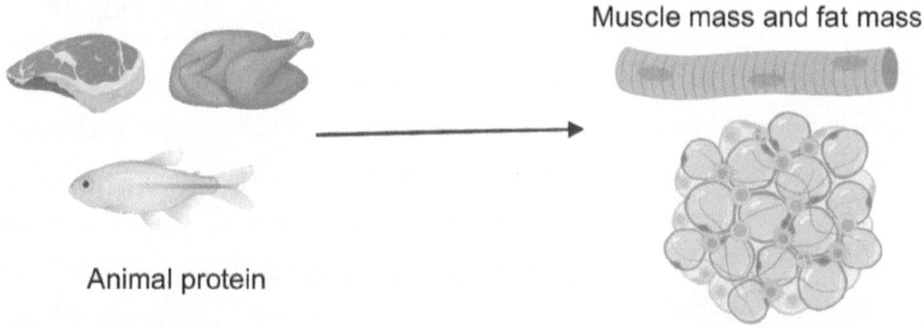

FIGURE 4.3 Animal protein intake is associated with muscle and fat mass in children. Animal protein intake in toddlers, as per recommendations, improves muscle and fat mass. (Figure created using the BioRender online tool.)

Ultimately, this study was not able to conclusively identify the differences in growth and biochemical measures in children following a vegetarian diet. Thus, it is possible that the source of animal protein might make a difference in muscle and fat mass outcomes (Figure 4.3).

Animal Protein Intake Associates with Metabolism and Cognitive Development

Recent research across various non-Western geographic locations, including Peru, Bangladesh, and Tanzania, has identified consistent metabolic changes associated with age in infants, suggesting a common metabolic maturation process. These changes involve a decline in certain amino acids, such as tryptophan and glutamine, in the blood and an increase in the urinary excretion of gut bacterial-host metabolites related to amino acids, such as tryptophan, tyrosine, and phenylalanine. These metabolic signatures appear to vary depending on the children's growth trajectories. In children with growth constraints, such as stunting, these urinary metabolites are excreted in larger quantities, indicating metabolic immaturity. This immaturity can be observed from as early as 3 months of age and may persist into the second year of life (Giallourou et al. 2020). Additionally, stunted children exhibit higher levels of metabolites related to the breakdown of tryptophan, which are linked to increased enzyme activity in response to infections and inflammation (Mayneris-Perxachs et al. 2016). Studies have also reported lower concentrations of essential amino acids (EAAs) in stunted children compared to healthy children. The low levels of EAAs have been attributed to factors such as poor protein quality in diets, reduced gut microbiome capacity to produce EAAs, and increased gut microbiome proteolytic activity (Kumar et al. 2018; Giallourou et al. 2020).

Animal protein intake has also been shown to correlate with improved cognitive development (Kaimila et al. 2019). Research from various countries has shown that children who consume diets rich in animal protein exhibit higher cognitive scores and better cognitive performance, which underscores the importance of early nutrition for long-term cognitive development. It emphasizes the significance of introducing nutrient-dense animal-source foods, such as fish, into young children's diets to address growth challenges and promote optimal cognitive development. Both linear growth and neurocognitive development are regulated by the mTORC1 pathway, a master regulator of growth and development influenced by AAs. Therefore, nutritional deficiencies during this critical phase can impact both physical growth and cognitive development simultaneously (Figure 4.4).

Animal Protein Intake Has a Role in Mitigating Stunting

In low- and middle-income countries (LMICs), where diets predominantly consist of staple foods like rice, wheat, maize, and tubers, there's a high likelihood of inadequate essential amino acids and

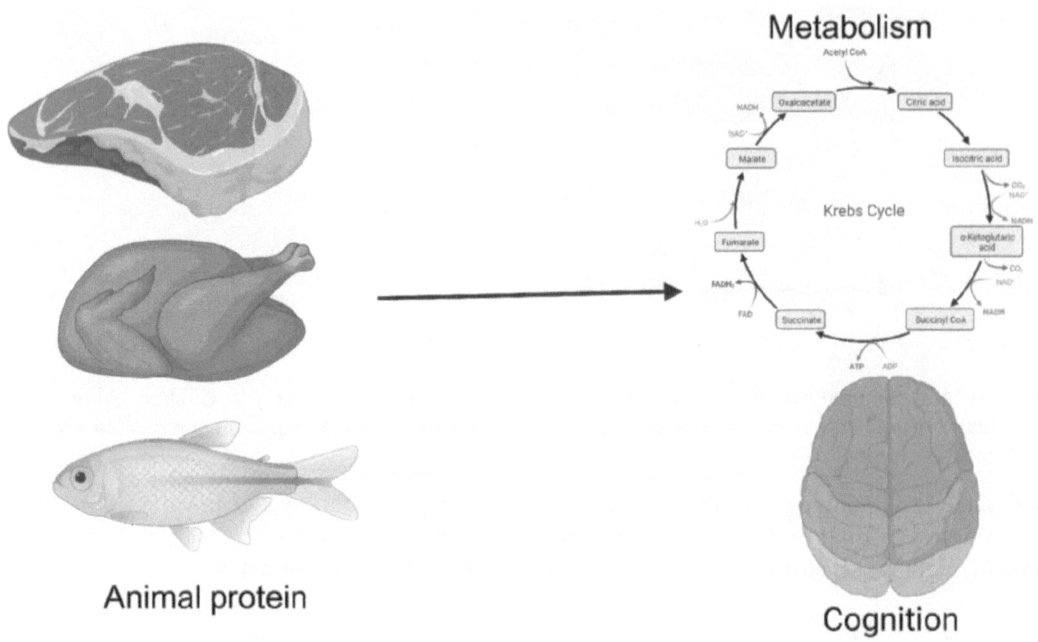

FIGURE 4.4 Animal protein plays a role in children's metabolism and cognition. Animal protein consumption with complementary feeding benefits cognitive development. (Figure created using the BioRender online tool.)

usable dietary protein, resulting in stunting. Stunting is associated with various adverse outcomes, including increased mortality and morbidity, impaired cognitive and motor development, poor school performance, and decreased economic productivity (De Sanctis et al. 2021). For instance, a cross-sectional study involving 3,150 infants and toddlers across several countries found that consuming meat and fish was associated with a lower likelihood of stunting and wasting, even after adjusting for potential confounding factors (Krebs et al. 2011). Another household survey conducted with over 2,500 Indian children indicated that children born to mothers who did not consume milk or dairy products at least once a week during pregnancy were 60% more likely to experience severe stunting. Additionally, low egg consumption was linked to a twofold increase in the odds of childhood stunting (Aguayo et al. 2016). Similarly, the SEANUTS study examined the impact of dairy consumption on the nutritional status of more than 12,000 children in several Asian countries. It found that the prevalence of stunting was nearly twice as high in children who did not consume dairy regularly compared to those who did (21.4% versus 10%) (Nguyen Bao et al. 2018). Furthermore, a review encompassing data from 74,548 children aged 6–23 months across 39 countries revealed that children who did not include any animal-based foods in their diet had a 44% higher likelihood of being stunted compared to those who consumed a balanced mix of animal-based foods, including meat, eggs, and dairy (Krasevec et al. 2017).

The observational studies align with intervention research; however, there have been relatively few high-quality randomized controlled trials investigating the impact of supplementing children's diets with animal-based foods on their growth and body composition. Most of these trials have taken place in African nations, with limited data available from Asian countries. For instance, a randomized controlled trial conducted in Ecuador involving children aged 6–9 months demonstrated that daily egg supplementation for 6 months reduced the prevalence of stunting by 47% and underweight by 74% compared to non-supplemented children (Iannotti et al. 2017). Furthermore, a systematic review assessing the impact of dairy product supplementation on physical growth estimated an additional annual growth benefit of about 0.4 cm for every 245 mL of daily milk consumed; however, most studies in this review were conducted in developed countries, with limited data from

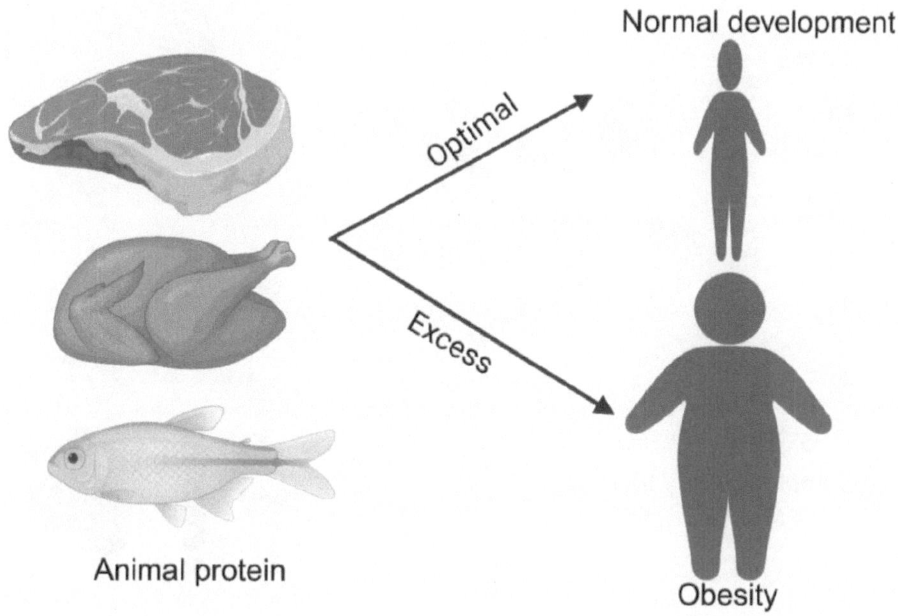

FIGURE 4.5 Excess animal protein results in obesity. Higher animal protein intake appears to increase the risk of obesity in children in Westernized countries, while it mitigates stunting among those living in low-middle-income countries. (Figure created using the BioRender online tool.)

developing nations (de Beer 2012). In conclusion, animal protein intake appears to prevent stunting in children (Figure 4.5).

Excess Animal Protein Intake Increases Risk of Obesity Later in Life

On the spectrum of protein intake, elevated consumption of animal protein – particularly during toddlerhood – has been linked to increased weight gain and a higher risk of obesity in developed countries (Jochum et al., 2022). Although the protein content in cow's milk infant formula has been reduced over time, significant protein intake can still occur with complementary foods, especially those containing dairy protein. The Dortmund Nutritional and Anthropometric Longitudinally Designed study suggests that critical periods during early childhood, specifically at 12 months and 5–6 years, are associated with a heightened risk of obesity later in life due to increased animal protein intake. This is consistent with the early protein hypothesis proposed by Koletzko et al., which suggests that excessive protein intake in early life may lead to metabolic mal-programming by triggering insulin and insulin-like growth factor (IGF-1) secretion, promoting early weight gain and adipogenesis (Gunther et al. 2007; Jochum et al. 2022). Clinical trials comparing low-protein infant formulas to high-protein formulas support these conclusions, revealing that elevated protein levels in formula are linked to an increased risk of childhood obesity characterized by higher BMI, significant weight gain, and excess body fat (Weber et al. 2014). In conclusion, early detection of growth trajectories and weight gain patterns is crucial for mitigating later obesity risk through targeted nutrition interventions (Figure 4.6).

SUMMARY POINTS

- This chapter focuses on animal versus plant protein as dietary sources.
- The literature highlights the positive impact of animal-source protein consumption on children's growth and development, particularly in regions with predominantly plant-based diets.

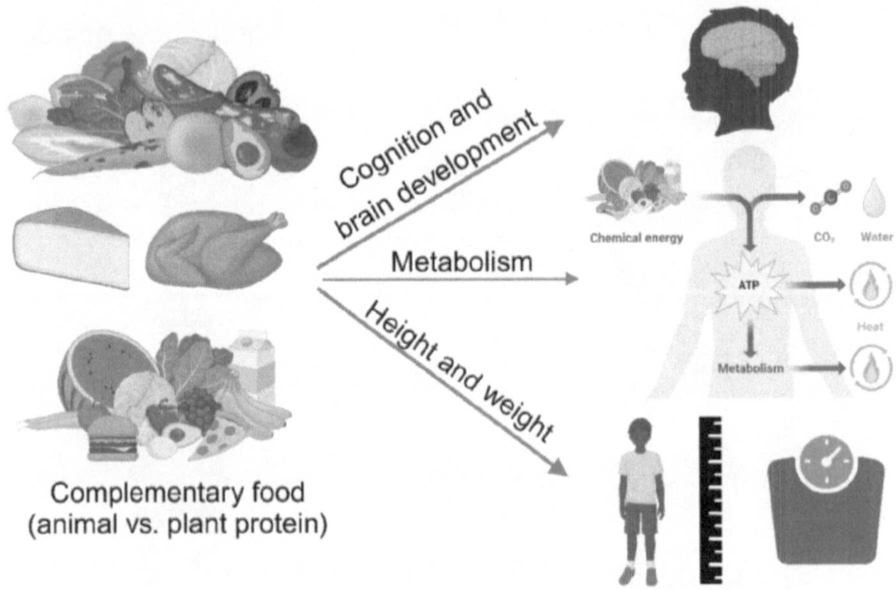

FIGURE 4.6 Combination of plant- and animal-based proteins will be optimal nutritional support for children. Combining plant- and animal-based foods at recommended levels leads to the programming of physiological systems that support healthy child development. (Figure created using the BioRender online tool.)

- It emphasizes introducing nutrient-dense animal-source foods like fish, eggs, and meat into young children's diets to address growth challenges while promoting optimal cognitive development.
- In LMICs, most children do not consume sufficient animal-based foods, and this is associated with higher rates of stunting. Among these foods, dairy proteins appear particularly beneficial for linear growth outcomes.
- Interestingly, excess animal protein intake beyond recommended levels is associated with body weight gain and increased obesity risks later in life among children from developed countries.
- Effective nutritional interventions should consider various factors, including energy content and the composition of micronutrients and macronutrients.
- Ideally, a balanced combination of plant- and animal-based foods should be developed to provide sustainable and culturally acceptable nutritional support for children (Figure 4.6).

ACKNOWLEDGMENTS

All figures were created with BioRender.com. We want to thank Jolene R. Rearick for the literature search.

REFERENCES

Aguayo, V. M., R. Nair, N. Badgaiyan, and V. Krishna. 2016. "Determinants of stunting and poor linear growth in children under 2 years of age in India: an in-depth analysis of Maharashtra's comprehensive nutrition survey." *Matern Child Nutr* 12 (Suppl 1):121–40. doi: 10.1111/mcn.12259.

Andres, A., P. H. Casey, M. A. Cleves, and T. M. Badger. 2013. "Body fat and bone mineral content of infants fed breast milk, cow's milk formula, or soy formula during the first year of life." *J. Pediatr* 163 (1):49–54. doi: S0022-3476(12)01556-9 [pii];10.1016/j.jpeds.2012.12.067 [doi].

Andres, A., M. A. Cleves, J. B. Bellando, R. T. Pivik, P. H. Casey, and T. M. Badger. 2012. "Developmental status of 1-year-old infants fed breast milk, cow's milk formula, or soy formula." *Pediatrics* 129 (6):1134–40. doi: peds.2011-3121 [pii];10.1542/peds.2011-3121 [doi].

Arnesen, E. K., B. Thorisdottir, C. Lamberg-Allardt, L. Barebring, B. Nwaru, J. Dierkes, A. Ramel, and A. Akesson. 2022. "Protein intake in children and growth and risk of overweight or obesity: a systematic review and meta-analysis." *Food Nutr Res* 66. doi: 10.29219/fnr.v66.8242.

Bagci Bosi, A. T., K. G. Eriksen, T. Sobko, T. M. Wijnhoven, and J. Breda. 2016. "Breastfeeding practices and policies in WHO European region member states." *Public Health Nutr* 19 (4):753–64. doi: 10.1017/S1368980015001767.

Baum, J. I., J. D. Miller, and B. L. Gaines. 2017. "The effect of egg supplementation on growth parameters in children participating in a school feeding program in rural Uganda: a pilot study." *Food Nutr Res* 61 (1):1330097. doi: 10.1080/16546628.2017.1330097.

Bellando, J., G. McCorkle, B. Spray, C. R. Sims, T. M. Badger, P. H. Casey, H. Scott, S. R. Beall, S. T. Sorensen, and A. Andres. 2020. "Developmental assessments during the first 5 years of life in infants fed breast milk, cow's milk formula, or soy formula." *Food Sci Nutr* 8 (7):3469–78. doi: 10.1002/fsn3.1630.

Brink, L. R., K. E. Mercer, B. D. Piccolo, S. V. Chintapalli, A. Elolimy, A. K. Bowlin, K. S. Matazel, L. Pack, S. H. Adams, K. Shankar, T. M. Badger, A. Andres, and L. Yeruva. 2020. "Neonatal diet alters fecal microbiota and metabolome profiles at different ages in infants fed breast milk or formula." *Am J Clin Nutr* 111 (6):1190–202. doi: 10.1093/ajcn/nqaa076.

Carr, L. E., M. D. Virmani, F. Rosa, D. Munblit, K. S. Matazel, A. A. Elolimy, and L. Yeruva. 2021. "Role of human milk bioactives on infants' gut and immune health." *Front Immunol* 12:604080. doi: 10.3389/fimmu.2021.604080.

Chen, J. R., H. A. Samuel, J. Shlisky, C. R. Sims, O. P. Lazarenko, D. K. Williams, A. Andres, and T. M. Badger. 2023. "A longitudinal observational study of skeletal development between ages 3 mo and 6 y in children fed human milk, milk formula, or soy formula." *Am J Clin Nutr* 117 (6):1211–18. doi: 10.1016/j.ajcnut.2023.04.002.

Chipili, G., A. Van Graan, C. J. Lombard, and E. Van Niekerk. 2022. "The efficacy of fish as an early complementary food on the linear growth of infants aged 6-7 months: a randomised controlled trial." *Nutrients* 14 (11). doi: 10.3390/nu14112191.

Das, S., J. J. Sanchez, A. Alam, A. Haque, M. Mahfuz, T. Ahmed, and K. Z. Long. 2020. "Dietary magnesium, Vitamin D, and animal protein intake and their association to the linear growth trajectory of children from birth to 24 months of age: results from MAL-ED birth cohort study conducted in Dhaka, Bangladesh." *Food Nutr Bull* 41 (2):200–10. doi: 10.1177/0379572119892408.

de Beer, H. 2012. "Dairy products and physical stature: a systematic review and meta-analysis of controlled trials." *Econ Hum Biol* 10 (3):299–309. doi: 10.1016/j.ehb.2011.08.003.

De Sanctis, V., A. Soliman, N. Alaaraj, S. Ahmed, F. Alyafei, and N. Hamed. 2021. "Early and long-term consequences of nutritional stunting: from childhood to adulthood." *Acta Biomed* 92 (1):e2021168. doi: 10.23750/abm.v92i1.11346.

Frizzo, J., V. C. C. Rodrigues, P. G. L. Speridiao, and M. B. Morais. 2022. "Evaluation of the complementary feeding practices, dietary intake, and nutritional status of infants on a cow's milk protein elimination diet." *J Pediatr (Rio J)* 98 (3):256–63. doi: 10.1016/j.jped.2021.06.005.

Giallourou, N., F. Fardus-Reid, G. Panic, K. Veselkov, B. J. J. McCormick, M. P. Olortegui, T. Ahmed, E. Mduma, P. P. Yori, M. Mahfuz, E. Svensen, M. M. M. Ahmed, J. M. Colston, M. N. Kosek, and J. R. Swann. 2020. "Metabolic maturation in the first 2 years of life in resource-constrained settings and its association with postnatal growths." *Sci Adv* 6 (15):eaay5969. doi: 10.1126/sciadv.aay5969.

Gunther, A. L., T. Remer, A. Kroke, and A. E. Buyken. 2007. "Early protein intake and later obesity risk: which protein sources at which time points throughout infancy and childhood are important for body mass index and body fat percentage at 7 y of age?" *Am J Clin Nutr* 86 (6):1765–72. doi: 10.1093/ajcn/86.5.1765.

Gurung, M., F. Rosa, B. Yelvington, N. Terry, Q. D. Read, B. D. Piccolo, B. Moody, P. Tripp, H. E. Pittman, 3rd, B. L. Fay, T. J. Ross, J. D. Sikes, J. B. Flowers, R. Fox, T. LeRoith, R. Talatala, F. Bar-Yoseph, and L. Yeruva. 2023. "Evaluation of a plant-based infant formula containing almonds and buckwheat on gut microbiota composition, intestine morphology, metabolic and immune markers in a neonatal piglet model." *Nutrients* 15 (2). doi: 10.3390/nu15020383.

Iannotti, L. L., C. K. Lutter, C. P. Stewart, C. A. Gallegos Riofrio, C. Malo, G. Reinhart, A. Palacios, C. Karp, M. Chapnick, K. Cox, and W. F. Waters. 2017. "Eggs in early complementary feeding and child growth: a randomized controlled trial." *Pediatrics* 140 (1). doi: 10.1542/peds.2016-3459.

Jochum, F., M. Abdellatif, A. Adel, A. Alhammadi, A. Alnemri, E. Alohali, K. AlSarraf, K. Al Said, M. Elzalabany, H. M. A. Isa, S. Kalyanasundaram, N. A. Reheim, and O. Saadah. 2022. "Burden of early life obesity and its relationship with protein intake in infancy: the middle east expert consensus." *Pediatr Gastroenterol Hepatol Nutr* 25 (2):93–108. doi: 10.5223/pghn.2022.25.2.93.

John, C. Wallingford, and Cynthia Barber 2019. "A review of studies on the growth of infants fed infant formula." *Current Developments in Nutrition* 3 (9):1–12.

Kaimila, Y., O. Divala, S. E. Agapova, K. B. Stephenson, C. Thakwalakwa, I. Trehan, M. J. Manary, and K. M. Maleta. 2019. "Consumption of animal-source protein is associated with improved height-for-age z scores in rural Malawian children aged 12(-)36 months." *Nutrients* 11 (2). doi: 10.3390/nu11020480.

Krasevec, J., X. An, R. Kumapley, F. Begin, and E. A. Frongillo. 2017. "Diet quality and risk of stunting among infants and young children in low- and middle-income countries." *Matern Child Nutr* 13 (Suppl 2). doi: 10.1111/mcn.12430.

Krebs, N. F., M. Mazariegos, E. Chomba, N. Sami, O. Pasha, A. Tshefu, W. A. Carlo, R. L. Goldenberg, C. L. Bose, L. L. Wright, M. Koso-Thomas, N. Goco, M. Kindem, E. M. McClure, J. Westcott, A. Garces, A. Lokangaka, A. Manasyan, E. Imenda, T. D. Hartwell, and K. M. Hambidge. 2012. "Randomized controlled trial of meat compared with multimicronutrient-fortified cereal in infants and toddlers with high stunting rates in diverse settings." *Am J Clin Nutr* 96 (4):840–7. doi: 10.3945/ajcn.112.041962.

Krebs, N. F., M. Mazariegos, A. Tshefu, C. Bose, N. Sami, E. Chomba, W. Carlo, N. Goco, M. Kindem, L. L. Wright, K. M. Hambidge, and Group Complementary Feeding Study. 2011. "Meat consumption is associated with less stunting among toddlers in four diverse low-income settings." *Food Nutr Bull* 32 (3):185–91. doi: 10.1177/156482651103200301.

Kumar, M., B. Ji, P. Babaei, P. Das, D. Lappa, G. Ramakrishnan, T. E. Fox, R. Haque, W. A. Petri, F. Backhed, and J. Nielsen. 2018. "Gut microbiota dysbiosis is associated with malnutrition and reduced plasma amino acid levels: Lessons from genome-scale metabolic modeling." *Metab Eng* 49:128–42. doi: 10.1016/j.ymben.2018.07.018.

Liu, Z. M., Q. Huang, H. H. Long, S. Y. Li, Y. Wu, S. J. Zhang, X. Y. Tang, and Y. M. Chen. 2023. "Increased dietary intakes of total protein, animal protein and white meat protein were associated with reduced bone loss-a prospective analysis based on guangzhou health and nutrition cohort, South China." *Nutrients* 15 (6). doi: 10.3390/nu15061432.

Mayneris-Perxachs, J., A. A. Lima, R. L. Guerrant, A. M. Leite, A. F. Moura, N. L. Lima, A. M. Soares, A. Havt, S. R. Moore, R. Pinkerton, and J. R. Swann. 2016. "Urinary N-methylnicotinamide and beta-aminoisobutyric acid predict catch-up growth in undernourished Brazilian children." *Sci Rep* 6:19780. doi: 10.1038/srep19780.

Neumann, C. G., L. Jiang, R. E. Weiss, M. Grillenberger, C. A. Gewa, J. H. Siekmann, S. P. Murphy, and N. O. Bwibo. 2013. "Meat supplementation increases arm muscle area in Kenyan schoolchildren." *Br J Nutr* 109 (7):1230–40. doi: 10.1017/S0007114512003121.

Nguyen Bao, K. L., S. Sandjaja, B. K. Poh, N. Rojroongwasinkul, C. N. Huu, E. Sumedi, J. N. Aini, S. Senaprom, P. Deurenberg, M. Bragt, I. Khouw, and Seanuts Study Group. 2018. "The consumption of dairy and its association with nutritional status in the South East Asian Nutrition Surveys (SEANUTS)." *Nutrients* 10 (6). doi: 10.3390/nu10060759.

Parikh, P., R. Semba, M. Manary, S. Swaminathan, E. Udomkesmalee, R. Bos, B. K. Poh, N. Rojroongwasinkul, J. Geurts, R. Sekartini, and T. T. Nga. 2022. "Animal source foods, rich in essential amino acids, are important for linear growth and development of young children in low- and middle-income countries." *Matern Child Nutr* 18 (1):e13264. doi: 10.1111/mcn.13264.

Ren, Q., K. Li, H. Sun, C. Zheng, Y. Zhou, Y. Lyu, W. Ye, H. Shi, W. Zhang, Y. Xu, and S. Jiang. 2022. "The association of formula protein content and growth in early infancy: a systematic review and meta-analysis." *Nutrients* 14 (11). doi: 10.3390/nu14112255.

Rosa, F., B. Yelvington, N. Terry, P. Tripp, H. E. Pittman, 3rd, B. L. Fay, T. J. Ross, J. D. Sikes, J. B. Flowers, F. Bar-Yoseph, and L. Yeruva. 2022. "Evaluation of the safety of a plant-based infant formula containing almonds and buckwheat in a neonatal piglet model." *Nutrients* 14 (7). doi: 10.3390/nu14071499.

Sahni, S., K. M. Mangano, M. T. Hannan, D. P. Kiel, and R. R. McLean. 2015. "Higher protein intake is associated with higher lean mass and quadriceps muscle strength in adult men and women." *J Nutr* 145 (7):1569–75. doi: 10.3945/jn.114.204925.

Tang, M., A. E. Hendricks, and N. F. Krebs. 2018. "A meat- or dairy-based complementary diet leads to distinct growth patterns in formula-fed infants: a randomized controlled trial." *Am J Clin Nutr* 107 (5):734–42. doi: 10.1093/ajcn/nqy038.

Vandenplas, Y., N. De Mulder, E. De Greef, and K. Huysentruyt. 2021. "Plant-based formulas and liquid feedings for infants and toddlers." *Nutrients* 13 (11). doi: 10.3390/nu13114026.

Weber, M., V. Grote, R. Closa-Monasterolo, J. Escribano, J. P. Langhendries, E. Dain, M. Giovannini, E. Verduci, D. Gruszfeld, P. Socha, B. Koletzko, and Group European Childhood Obesity Trial Study. 2014. "Lower protein content in infant formula reduces BMI and obesity risk at school age: follow-up of a randomized trial." *Am J Clin Nutr* 99 (5):1041–51. doi: 10.3945/ajcn.113.064071.

Young, B. 2020. "Variation in infant formula macronutrient ingredients is associated with infant anthropometrics." *Nutrients* 12 (11). doi: 10.3390/nu12113465.

Zheng, M., H. J. Yu, Q. Q. He, B. L. Heitmann, A. Rangan, S. A. McNaughton, and K. J. Campbell. 2021. "Protein intake during infancy and subsequent body mass index in early childhood: results from the melbourne InFANT program." *J Acad Nutr Diet* 121 (9):1775–84. doi: 10.1016/j.jand.2021.02.022.

5 Dietary Plant and Animal Protein–Phenolic Interactions

Effects of Gastrointestinal Digestion and Gut Microbiota

Deniz Günal-Köroğlu and Esra Capanoglu

ABBREVIATIONS

α-La	α-lactalbumin
β-Lg	β-lactoglobulin
ECG	Epicatechin gallate
EGC	Epigallocatechin
EGCG	Epigallocatechin gallate
SPI	Soy protein isolate

INTRODUCTION

Protein–phenolic interactions are primarily classified as covalent or non-covalent. Non-covalent interactions are more prevalent through hydrogen bonding, hydrophobic interactions, Van der Waals forces, and ionic interactions, forming complexes (Zhou et al. 2020; Ozdal, Capanoglu, and Altay 2013). Covalent interactions take place between functional groups of proteins (amine or amide groups) and quinone products of phenolic oxidation (highly reactive nucleophilic compounds) as a result of enzymatic reactions (e.g., polyphenol oxidase, laccase, tyrosinase) or non-enzymatic processes (e.g., alkaline reactions or free radical grafting), forming conjugates (Ozdal, Capanoglu, and Altay 2013). The binding mechanism and the effects of different factors on protein–phenolic interactions are summarized in Figure 5.1.

Many foods naturally contain both proteins and phenolic compounds. However, phenolic compounds are mostly compartmentalized in vacuoles, limiting interaction with other macronutrients until cellular disruption occurs. In the course of food processing or gastrointestinal digestion, these compounds come into contact with intracellular or extracellular molecules as the structural integrity of plant tissue is destroyed. Protein–phenolic interactions can occur with food proteins during food processing, with food proteins or enzymes during gastrointestinal breakdown, with blood plasma proteins after absorption, and with proteins in target organs (Rohn 2014).

The mechanical, chemical, and enzymatic processes, including forces, flow patterns, salts, mucins, proteins, pH, and digestive enzymes, are unique to each region of the gastrointestinal tract: mouth, esophagus, stomach, small intestine, and colon (Tan, Zhou, and McClements 2022). Simulated in vitro digestion methods provide information about the bioaccessibility of bioactive compounds; these methods are faster, cheaper, and avoid ethical issues compared to in vivo studies. The method consists of three different stages – mouth, gastric, and intestinal – mimicking in vivo conditions. In addition, each stage is performed under constant conditions (Minekus et al. 2014).

 DOI: 10.1201/9781003597926-5

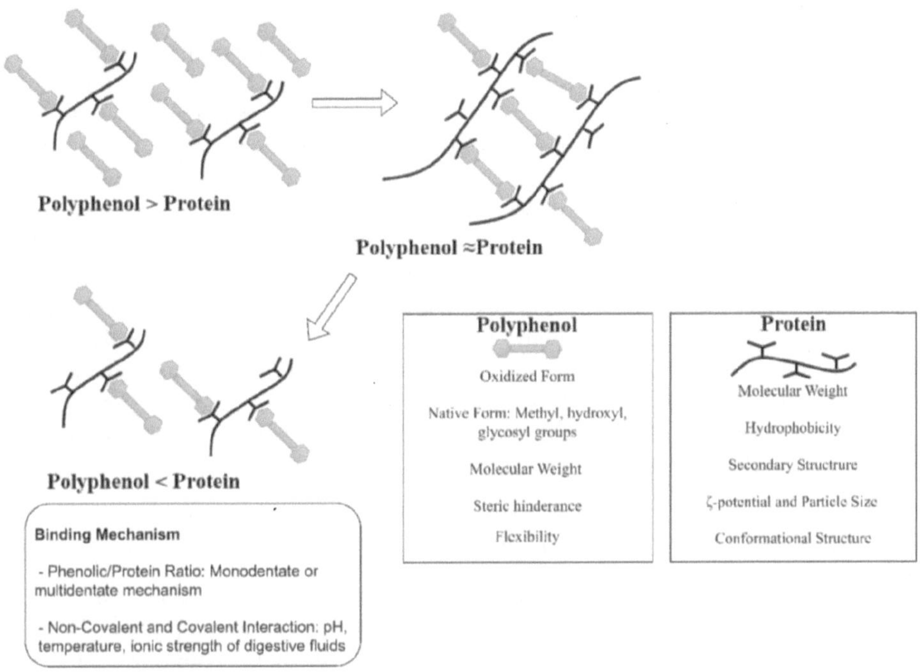

FIGURE 5.1 The mechanism of protein–phenolic interactions and the effects of different factors, adapted from D. Günal-Köroğlu, Lorenzo, and Capanoglu (2023).

Protein–phenolic interaction is known to affect protein digestibility. Proteins may be better digested when forming complexes or conjugates with phenolics due to structural and conformational changes that expose more protease target sites, enhancing enzymatic reactions by proteases (Xue et al. 2022). However, protein bioaccessibility can decrease when phenolics delay or prevent digestion by shielding enzymatic target sites on proteins, which prolongs the lifetime of intact proteins in digestive fluids (Stojadinovic et al. 2013).

IN VITRO STUDIES ON DAIRY PROTEIN INTERACTIONS

Whey and casein are the two main milk proteins. The primary proteins in whey are β-lactoglobulin (β-Lg; 18.2 kDa) and α-lactalbumin (α-La; 14.2 kDa). Studies have shown that green tea, black tea, coffee, and cocoa phenolic extracts slow down the gastric digestibility of β-Lg. However, intestinal digestion is slowed only by cocoa and coffee phenolic extracts compared to black tea extract due to their stronger binding affinity and greater destabilizing effects on protein structure (Stojadinovic et al. 2013). Phenolic extracts are mixtures of phenolic compounds; thus, it is important to determine which specific phenolic compound interacts predominantly with proteins or assess the overall effect of the mixture. Lai et al. (2012) discovered that gallic acid caused methionine oxidation in β-Lg peptides and decreased the degree of β-Lg hydrolysis after trypsin digestion. On the other hand, it was also shown that pepsin digestion of β-Lg was accelerated in the presence of green tea catechins (Tantoush et al. 2012). Khalifa et al. (2022) reported that cyanidin 3-glucoside and cyanidin 3-rutinoside facilitated β-Lg digestion through covalent conjugation, with cyanidin 3-rutinoside showing higher protein hydrolysis levels than other anthocyanins.

Phenolic concentration significantly affects protein digestion. Yu et al. (2016) found that grape seed polyphenol extracts above a concentration of 0.04 mg/mL slowed gastric breakdown of casein considerably but had no effect on whey or egg white protein. Jiang et al. (2018) observed that increasing concentrations of chlorogenic acid altered whey and casein digestibility during complexation.

Moreover, covalent chlorogenic acid conjugation improved the digestibility of whey compared to native whey (Xu et al. 2019). Wang et al. (2022) reported lower intestinal digestibility for whey via non-covalent or covalent interaction with rose anthocyanin extract; however, no noticeable alterations were observed during gastric digestion. Phenolic compounds may interact with enzymes in pancreatin to alter their structure, reducing catalytic activity and whey digestibility (Wang et al. 2022). Furthermore, Li et al. (2022) found that microwave heating enhanced protein digestibility and hydrolysis degree in α-La–safflower yellow complexes, while safflower yellow had a slight inhibitory effect on both properties without heating. Another study by Tantoush et al. (2012) determined that laccase–polymerized green tea catechins had a significant hindering impact on the pepsin digestion of α-La. Although α-La was unable to last even one minute in the presence of pepsin, it was able to endure more than three hours in the presence of oxidized and polymerized green tea catechins. Essentially, this occurs because additional interaction areas are exposed due to the opening of the protein's structure, especially in alkaline or thermal treatments (covalent interaction circumstances), especially oxidized phenolic compounds with a large molecular structure like anthocyanins (Günal-Köroğlu, Lorenzo, and Capanoglu 2023).

IN VITRO STUDIES ON EGG PROTEIN INTERACTIONS

Eggs are widely consumed for their high nutritional value. Ovalbumin (45 kDa) is the main protein in egg white (He et al. 2019), comprising approximately 60–65% of all the proteins in chicken egg whites (Lu et al. 2018; Shen et al. 2014). Ovotransferrin, a major iron-binding protein, accounts for around 12% of egg white proteins (Wei and Huang 2019). Studies have shown higher overall digestibility for ovalbumin–epigallocatechin gallate (EGCG) conjugates (He et al. 2019). In another study, ovotransferrin nanofibril–gallic acid complexes formed via non-covalent interactions exhibited greater digestibility compared to their covalent counterparts (Wei and Huang 2019).

Xue et al. (2022) determined that heated egg white protein–tea polyphenol complexes exhibited increased digestibility regardless of tea polyphenol concentration at moderate levels (85°C for 20 minutes). However, excessive polyphenol concentrations (>0.02%) formed dense network structures that blocked protease target sites, reducing enzymatic hydrolysis efficiency. The protein/phenolic ratio also influences the complex formation and may have different effects on the digestive system. Before saturation, intermolecular bridges between proteins are generated directly between interaction sites of the protein and phenolics at low phenolic concentrations (a multidentate mechanism). The contact sites of the protein chain become saturated at high phenolic concentrations, and many phenolics interact with one protein (a monodentate mechanism) (Günal-Köroğlu, Lorenzo, and Capanoglu 2023).

Ma et al. (2020) reported little effect from cyanidin-3-glucoside on pepsin digestion of ovalbumin but a significant inhibitory effect on intestinal digestion. Additionally, it was revealed that the hydrogen bonding sites of cyanidin-3-glucoside partially overlap with trypsin cleavage sites in ovalbumin rather than being close to the pepsin cleavage sites, which could hinder intestinal digestion. Similarly, Shen et al. (2014) observed that the conjugation of tea polyphenols provided quicker gastric digestion of ovalbumin or lysozyme; in contrast, it had a reverse effect on intestinal digestion.

IN VITRO STUDIES ON OTHER ANIMAL-BASED PROTEIN INTERACTIONS

Research on other animal-based proteins is limited. In a study by Cheng et al. (2023), it was revealed that the hydrolysis degree of pork myofibrillar protein increased from 55.4% to 64.0% after polyphenol modification, and the molecular weight of digested proteins decreased significantly. However, Xu et al. (2021) reported no appreciable changes in the overall digestibility of oxidized pork myofibrillar protein via interaction with epicatechin.

Han et al. (2021) found that the peptic digestion of scallop gonad proteins was improved with increasing concentrations of catechin's galloylated derivatives (ECG, EGC, EGCG). While EGCG significantly enhanced the peptic digestion of scallop gonad proteins, as indicated by increased peptide release during gastric digestion, it actually reduced tryptic and chymotryptic digestion in the intestinal phase. In contrast, ECG and EGC had only minor effects on protein digestibility throughout both digestion stages.

IN VITRO STUDIES ON PLANT-BASED PROTEIN INTERACTIONS

Plant-based protein sources have become increasingly preferred by consumers in recent years and are widely used in food formulations. In these formulations, bioactive ingredients are often added to increase nutritive value, creating functional foods. Therefore, studying the effect of plant-based protein–phenolic interactions on bioavailability is essential to determine whether these formulations meet their intended purpose as functional foods. Current studies on plant-based protein–phenolic interactions generally focus on soy protein, but studies evaluating other plant-based proteins are limited.

It has been highlighted that the interaction of soy protein isolate (SPI) with curcumin (Chen, Li, and Tang 2015), anthocyanin-rich black rice extracts (Zhang et al. 2018), or black soybean seed coat extract (Ren et al. 2018) facilitated enzymatic action on the protein, increasing hydrolysis rates regardless of thermal treatment. Moreover, non-covalent complexes of SPI with catechin or EGCG (at pH 7) enhanced protein digestibility compared to covalent conjugates, which were formed under alkaline conditions (pH 9). SPI was covalently crosslinked to form a stable protein structure with an anti-digestive effect associated with higher concentrations of anthocyanin-rich black rice extract powder, catechin, or EGCG – the higher the polyphenol content, the greater the effect (Dai et al. 2023; Zhou et al. 2020).

On the other hand, non-covalent complexes of pea protein with chlorogenic acid, resveratrol, and EGCG exhibited higher protein hydrolysis compared to native pea protein due to structural changes induced by complexation (Hao et al. 2022). Ma et al. (2022) reported that complexation with mulberry anthocyanins accelerated SPI digestion during intestinal digestion but somewhat delayed SPI digestion by pepsin, particularly for the α subunit of β-conglycinin (7S) and the basic subunit of glycinin (11S). Different interactions (hydrogen bonding, hydrophobic interactions, etc.) and variations in protein structure are influenced by differences in the number of phenolic hydroxyl groups in polyphenols (Zhou et al. 2020). Larger molecular sizes of polyphenols (e.g., tannins, anthocyanins) or galloylated forms (e.g., EGCG, ECG) are more potent and primarily bind to protein (Rohn 2014; Günal-Köroğlu, Lorenzo, and Capanoglu 2023). Therefore, even when using the same protein source, different phenolics can have varying effects on digestibility.

Taylor et al. (2007) examined lower digestibility in sorghum kafirin species due to interactions with condensed tannins. However, a complex of γ-kafirin and condensed tannins was marginally more digestible than total kafirin or residual kafirin complexes. This may be because γ-kafirin has a somewhat more open structure than bound total or bound residual kafirin due to its repetitive proline sequences (Taylor et al. 2007). The presence of more proline groups in proteins supports the protein–phenolic interaction. Proline-rich proteins have open and flexible conformations and allow hydrophobic interactions and hydrogen bonding with polyphenols (Rohn 2014).

IN VITRO STUDIES ON TRYPSIN AND GLUCOSIDASE INTERACTIONS

Phenolics interact with both food matrix proteins and proteolytic enzymes in the digestive system, causing changes in protein digestibility, bioaccessibility, and solubility. Trypsin primarily cleaves peptide chains at the carboxyl side of lysine or arginine residues; as a serine protease found in the digestive systems of many vertebrates, it can also trigger other pancreatic enzymes' activity (Xiao et al. 2015). According to Yu et al. (2016), trypsin's ability to digest whey protein and egg white was slightly improved by grape seed polyphenol extract. However, Zhou et al. (2020) stated that EGCG concentration and binding mechanisms (covalent and non-covalent) with SPI had only a slight impact on trypsin activity, indicating that EGCG inhibits trypsin activity to some extent. Trypsin's reaction site is usually a peptide bond close to arginine or lysine, meaning its effectiveness depends not only on amino acid composition but also on how polyphenols occupy these residues during interaction (Zhou et al. 2020). It has also been suggested that a potent inhibitor of α-glucosidase should have a modest inhibitory effect on trypsin and a strong inhibitory effect on α-glucosidase. Tannic acid's inhibitory pattern against trypsin and α-glucosidase was reported to involve both competitive and non-competitive inhibition mechanisms; tannic acid appears to be a potent α-glucosidase inhibitor with poor inhibitory activity for trypsin (Xiao et al. 2015).

α-Amylase and α-glucosidase are exo-acting glycoside hydrolase enzymes (glucosidases) essential for the breakdown of carbohydrates (e.g., starch) within the digestive tract. Inhibition of these enzymes decreases the postprandial impact of starch ingestion on blood glucose levels by slowing the passage of glucose from complex dietary carbs into the blood. For diabetics, glucosidase inhibitors are frequently used to lessen postprandial hyperglycemia brought on by the small intestine's starch digestion (Yilmazer-Musa et al. 2012).

Due to their low cost, relative safety, and lack of major gastrointestinal side effects, plants, and plant-based supplements may be a more palatable source of α-glucosidase inhibitors (Yilmazer-Musa et al. 2012). The inhibition of some enzymes, such as α-amylase, α-glucosidase, pepsin, lipase, and trypsin, is thought to be advantageous for obesity, type II diabetes, or gastroesophageal reflux disease (Zhou et al. 2018). Chen et al. (2020) revealed that cyanidin strongly inhibited the activity of α-glucosidase, whereas cyanidin-3-rutinoside and cyanidin-3-O-glucoside did not. Cyanidin's inhibitory activity exceeded that of acarbose – the most commonly used medication for postprandial glycemia control. Yilmazer-Musa et al. (2012) demonstrated that grape seed extract had equivalent or much greater potency than acarbose in substantially inhibiting both α-amylase and α-glucosidase activities. Tea extracts and catechin gallates (ECG or EGCG) were powerful inhibitors of α-glucosidase but less efficient in inhibiting α-amylase, while non-galloylated catechins (catechin, epicatechin) had no impact on either enzyme. Aleixandre et al. (2022) noted that phenolic acids with one hydroxyl group or one hydroxyl group plus one or two methoxy groups (e.g., *p*-coumaric acid, syringic acid, or vanillic acid), which are less polar, demonstrated better α-glucosidase inhibitory effects than phenolic acids with multiple hydroxyl groups (e.g., caffeic acid or protocatechuic acid). Conversely, phenolic acids with more hydroxyl groups (e.g., chlorogenic acid or gallic acid) demonstrated stronger α-amylase inhibitory effects than those with fewer hydroxyl groups like vanillic or syringic acids.

IN VITRO STUDIES ON OTHER DIGESTIVE ENZYME INTERACTIONS

Zhou et al. (2018) stated that the anti-digestion properties of grape seed procyanidins with different degrees of polymerization were dose-dependent and became stronger with higher molecular weights. The lipase-inhibiting properties of procyanidin fractions were the strongest, followed by those of α-amylase and pepsin. You et al. (2011) revealed that the anthocyanin extracts of muscadine grape, cyanidin, and cyanidin 3,5-diglucoside acted in a competitive mode against α-glucosidase and pancreatic lipase. Anthocyanins may have stronger inhibitory actions once they are digested, as cyanidin exhibited substantially stronger antidiabetic activity than cyanidin 3,5-diglucoside.

Stamogiannou et al. (2021) classified phenolics into three classes according to their effects on cellulase activity: activators (ferulic acid, syringic acid, sinapic acid, vanillic acid), non-inhibitors (*p*-coumaric acid, rutin), and inhibitors (quercetin, kaempferol, trans-cinnamic acid, luteolin, ellagic acid). This observation was linked to the phenolic compound's structure, particularly the activating effect of the methoxy group (-OCH_3). Tejirian et al. (2011) found that oligomeric phenolics had a greater ability than simple phenolics to inhibit enzymatic cellulolysis. Reversibly complexing oligomeric phenolics with cellulases could render them inactive. By adhering to cellulose, simple and oligomeric phenolics may also prevent enzymatic cellulolysis.

IN VIVO STUDIES ON PROTEIN-PHENOLIC INTERACTIONS

In vivo methods on animals or humans have also been used to investigate the bioavailability of different bioactive compounds reported in the literature. The apparent digestibility of crude protein and ruminal ammoniacal nitrogen concentration were significantly reduced by 0.3% and 0.6% tannic acid supplementation, respectively, while the level of total volatile fatty acids in the rumen increased in Xiangdong black goats (Wang et al. 2022). It is interesting to note that a complete meal with phenolic extract, but not one with a fruit and vegetable mixture, markedly reduced the rate and effectiveness of protein digestion in minipigs (Dufour et al. 2018). Li et al. (2020) reported that weaned piglets receiving dietary supplements of grape seed extract showed dose-dependent inhibition of lipase and α-amylase activity in the pancreas and duodenum, although this had no impact on trypsin activities in either location.

Petzke et al. (2005) reported that true nitrogen digestibility was much lower in rats fed an intense covalent conjugate of β-Lg and chlorogenic acid (higher phenolic ratio) compared to those fed a moderate conjugate of β-Lg and chlorogenic acid (lower phenolic ratio). This reduction was attributed to lower levels of methionine, cysteine, lysine, and tryptophan in rats fed a 10% protein diet. However, the conjugation of β-Lg with chlorogenic acid did not cause an extra shortage of essential amino acids because net protein utilization remained unchanged. A similar study by Rohn et al. (2006) revealed that rats fed a 10% protein diet containing conjugates of soy-protein with chlorogenic acid or quercetin demonstrated increased fecal and urine nitrogen excretion, which was linearly related to the phenolic ratio. True nitrogen digestibility, biological value, and net protein utilization were negatively impacted. Lysine, tryptophan, and sulfur-containing amino acids had lower protein digestibility-corrected amino acid scores than other amino acids. It was stated that the consequences of covalent protein–phenolic interaction were more pronounced with plant-based proteins, such as soy protein, compared to whey protein (Rohn et al. 2006; Petzke et al. 2005).

THE EFFECT OF PROTEIN-PHENOLIC INTERACTIONS ON GUT MICROBIOTA

Polyphenols significantly affect the bioaccessibility of other food components due to their interactions. By altering their physical and chemical properties through interactions with proteins, polyphenols are protected from oxidation and enzymatic hydrolysis during gastrointestinal digestion, resulting in improved biological activity, target-specific delivery, and bioaccessibility rates. The upper digestive tract cannot absorb most polyphenols, which are instead processed by enzymes produced by intestinal flora in the colon (Li et al. 2021). de Almeida et al. (2020) stated that an increase in caffeic acid content after gut fermentation was observed in bread with green coffee infusion and enzymatically processed bread containing green coffee infusion. According to molar concentrations throughout the same time frame, gut bacteria supported the hydrolysis of caffeoylquinic acid, and dicaffeoylquinic acid, accounting for 40% of caffeic acid release. The gut microbiota's influence on the dissociation of protein–phenolic complexes, which are formed in bread, may account for the remaining 60%. Further, enzymatic bioprocessing accelerated the release of ferulic acid during gut fermentation, whereas adding green coffee infusion increased bioaccessibility for all phenolic components. Moreover, Cheng et al. (2023) examined in vitro gut fermentation of myofibrillar protein–mulberry polyphenol complexes reaching the colon after digestion; these complexes contributed to the proliferation of *Lactobacillus* and encouraged the formation of short-chain fatty acids, demonstrating the potential to improve intestinal health.

On the other hand, Wu et al. (2020) declared that soy protein, whey protein, or gelatin encapsulation of blueberry anthocyanin extract dramatically decreased the composition and number of *Firmicutes* while increasing *Bacteroidetes* levels in gut microbiota populations. Additionally, anthocyanin extract microcapsules, particularly those encapsulated via soy protein isolate, triggered the gut microbiota to produce short-chain fatty acids. Lyu et al. (2023) reported that casein–cyanidin-3-glucoside complexes can increase the number of some beneficial microorganisms while decreasing some opportunistic pathogenic bacteria, restoring the quantity and variety of the gut microbiota. Casein–cyanidin-3-glucoside complexes regulated gut microbiota disruptions, therefore protecting against obesity and liver damage brought on by high-fat diets in mice. Zhou et al. (2023) demonstrated that probiotics such as *Bacteroides*, *Akkermansia*, and *Parabacteroides* became more prevalent while opportunistic pathogens like *Enterococcus* and *Staphylococcus* were suppressed following myofibrillar protein–chlorogenic acid complex reconstruction of the gut microbiota in type II diabetic rats. The complex also dramatically decreased secondary bile acids while significantly increasing the concentrations of intestinal metabolites such as butyric acid.

It has been established that polyphenols' bioaccessibility, digestibility, or antioxidant activity may be affected by their structure, content, and co-digestion of certain food components. Tamargo et al. (2022) stated that co-digestion of wine with food matrices such as glucose or whey protein considerably boosted total short- and medium-chain fatty acid synthesis, particularly butyric acid, and promoted intestinal health-related taxa like *Akkermansia* or *Bifidobacterium*. The presence of wine and whey protein in colonic medium reduced the production of ammonia ions. This reduction may be related to the decrease in colonic protein fermentation and amino acid metabolism.

DIETARY PROTEIN-PHENOLIC INTERACTIONS IN MODEL FOOD MATRICES

Polyphenols can be transported to the small intestine and colon by proteins, which serve as effective transporters by protecting polyphenols from enzymatic and oxidative breakdown during digestive processes. Polyphenols can be preserved in the digestive system by applications such as encapsulation, especially with macromolecules like proteins (Li et al. 2021). The structural characteristics of polyphenols, their precise roles during digestion, concentrations, the form of the phenolic source (pure, extracted, or encapsulated), and the complexity of the food matrix are all contributing factors to the contradictory outcomes reported in the literature (Khalifa et al. 2021; Günal-Köroğlu, Turan, and Capanoglu 2023). The structural profile and conformation of the food matrix, its associations with other food components such as dietary fibers and proteins, and food processing operations – including thermal, chemical, or mechanical treatments – all play significant roles in the effectiveness and release of phenolic constituents from the food matrix (Zahid et al. 2022).

Protein-rich foods are frequently consumed in combination with foods high in phenolic compounds, such as milk chocolate, coffee or tea with milk, or soy milk combined with fruit juice (Rohn et al. 2006). Coffee is one of the most consumed beverages in the world. Decaffeinated espresso and espresso with milk inhibited pancreatic lipase activity more effectively than regular espresso, possibly due to higher polyphenol content and milk-induced interactions (Jurema Soares et al. 2022). Adding a phenolic source could improve dairy protein digestibility. A model beverage of fruit juice and milk protein was investigated via pasteurization (63°C for 30 minutes) or sterilization (121°C for 10 minutes) of neutral and acidic solutions containing chlorogenic acid or catechin with whey protein by He et al. (2015). Gastric digestibility of unheated beverages was not statistically affected by phenolic concentration or presence, whereas intestinal protein digestion was more delayed by phenolic concentrations or catechin presence. However, whey digestibility was unaffected by phenolic compounds in any heat-treated samples. Additionally, blue honeysuckle juice added to fermented goat milk was reported to accelerate protein digestion in vitro (Ma et al. 2022).

Several studies have been conducted on model systems using real food matrices as references for component levels and profiles, including proteins and phenolics, in complex food matrices such as chocolate. Considering the amounts of whey and catechin/epicatechin mixtures in a real chocolate matrix, Accardo et al. (2023) reported that despite slight interactions with proteins, flavonoids didn't hinder or modify protein solubility, degree of hydrolysis, or peptide profiles during enzymatic digestion.

Yogurt is a well-known and efficient delivery system for plant-derived phenolic compounds, but the health-promoting effects of these compounds depend on their source and how they are incorporated into the yogurt (Zygmantaitė et al. 2021). Protein–phenolic interactions that result in indigestible proteins and inhibition of digestive enzymes were thought to be the cause of reduced in vitro protein digestibility in yogurt fortified with 1–5% pomegranate juice powder (Pan et al. 2019). Cranberry pomace added to yogurt before fermentation slowed protein digestion compared to plain yogurt and constrained phenol release after digestion (Zygmantaitė et al. 2021). Tlais et al. (2023) claimed that fermenting whey and fruit mix smoothies with *Lactiplantibacillus plantarum* significantly increased the release of anthocyanins.

In a study on different food matrices, Budryn et al. (2013) found that adding green coffee extract to a control matrix did not significantly alter protein pepsin digestibility beyond a 3% difference despite higher amino acid losses. Khalifa et al. (2018) reported that encapsulating mulberry anthocyanins with whey protein in energy balls led to decomposition of the β-Lg and α-La bands more easily in a concentration-dependent manner. Smaller polyphenols, unlike tannins, were found to have no detrimental effects on protein digestibility. Furthermore, mulberry anthocyanins improved the intestinal digestibility of energy balls after 45 days of storage by shielding the cleavage sites from the glycation reactions of the digestive enzymes, which mostly affect the lysine residues. On the other hand, soluble protein levels decreased due to protein aggregation during storage caused by glycation reactions and protein–protein interactions. After digesting wheat or lentil crackers prepared with onion skin powder, onion skin phenolic extract, or quercetin, free amino group levels were lower than those in plain crackers, except for lentil crackers co-digested with quercetin (Günal-Köroğlu, Turan, and Capanoglu 2023).

CONCLUSION

Phenolics are not digested in the upper gastrointestinal tract but are more extensively metabolized by the gut microbiota in the colon. Proteins can act as carriers for phenolics to reach the gut microbiota in the colon, increasing the bioaccessibility of these compounds. However, this interaction also affects protein digestibility. Changes in digestibility – and their positive or negative effects on proteins or phenolic compounds – have been extensively studied in the literature. Applications using model systems (solutions containing protein and phenolic sources) have employed either phenolic extracts or phenolic compounds. It should be noted that phenolic extracts typically contain mixtures of various phenolic compounds; thus, dominant compounds within an extract may drive overall effects on the protein digestibility within a system. This variability explains why results from studies using extracts may not align with those using pure phenolic compounds.

Other reasons for inconsistent results include differences in protein/phenolic ratios within systems, covalent versus non-covalent interactions, molecular size variations among phenolics, and differences in protein structures. Digestion of protein–phenolic conjugates or complexes in the gastric and intestinal phases also varies due to differing digestive fluid conditions across these stages. Phenolics may exert effects exclusively during the gastric phase, the intestinal phase, or both phases. This may ultimately alter digestion outcomes. Therefore, more detailed research is needed on this subject to better understand how these interactions influence digestibility.

Determining how protein-phenolic interactions affect digestibility within complex food matrices is challenging due to the numerous interacting components within foods. From a nutritional perspective, these effects are not easily measurable and generalizable. The form of protein-phenolic complexes within foods, or the co-digestion of these nutrients, can alter protein digestibility outcomes by stabilizing or destabilizing enzyme activities or modifying protein structure during gastrointestinal digestion through covalent and non-covalent interactions. The effect of protein-phenolic interactions on the digestibility of proteins during gastrointestinal digestion can be observed and interpreted as the overall result of all these effects.

MINI DICTIONARY OF TERMS

- **Acarbose:** A widely used medicine for postprandial glycemia; an α-glucosidase inhibitor.
- **Bioaccessibility:** The release of nutrients from the food matrix during gastrointestinal digestion, making them available for absorption.
- **Bioavailability:** The percentage of a nutrient that the human body can store or use for various physiological and metabolic processes; includes bioaccessibility and bioactivity.
- **Digestibility:** The proportion of a specific nutrient that an animal can absorb through its digestive system for sustaining life.
- **Phenolic compounds:** Secondary plant metabolites, including flavonoids (e.g., flavonols, flavanones, isoflavones, anthocyanins) and non-flavonoids (e.g., stilbenes, phenolic acids, tannins).

SUMMARY POINTS

- The effect of dietary protein–phenolic interaction on protein digestibility depends on factors such as proteins or phenolic compound structure, covalent or non-covalent interactions, protein/phenolic ratio, and environmental conditions like temperature or pH.
- Studies have focused extensively on milk proteins and soy proteins in pure solutions under different conditions.
- Protein digestibility can be interpreted as the overall result of (1) activation or inactivation of digestive enzymes or (2) changes in enzyme-interacting regions due to protein–phenolic interactions.
- Since the food matrix has a complex structure, protein–phenolic complexes have different effects specific to each food.
- These complexes may positively affect the gut microbiota and inhibit pathogenic bacteria.
- Although many studies exist on the digestion of proteins as a result of protein–phenolic interactions, more comparative or detailed studies are still required.

REFERENCES

Accardo, Francesca, Barbara Prandi, Francesca Terenziani, Tullia Tedeschi, and Stefano Sforza. 2023. "Evaluation of in Vitro Whey Protein Digestibility in a Protein-Catechins Model System Mimicking Milk Chocolate: Interaction with Flavonoids Does Not Hinder Protein Bioaccessibility." *Food Research International* 169: 112888. https://doi.org/https://doi.org/10.1016/j.foodres.2023.112888.

Aleixandre, Andrea, José Vicente Gil, Jorge Sineiro, and Cristina M. Rosell. 2022. "Understanding Phenolic Acids Inhibition of α-Amylase and α-Glucosidase and Influence of Reaction Conditions." *Food Chemistry* 372: 131231. https://doi.org/10.1016/j.foodchem.2021.131231.

Almeida, Suellen Silva de, Gabriela Bouça Marques da Costa, Maysa Silva Barreto, Denise Maria Guimarães Freire, Leandro Araújo Lobo, Regina Maria Cavalcanti Pilotto Domingues, Nathália Moura-Nunes, Mariana Monteiro, and Daniel Perrone. 2020. "Bioaccessibility and Gut Metabolism of Phenolic Compounds of Breads Added with Green Coffee Infusion and Enzymatically Bioprocessed." *Food Chemistry* 333: 127473. https://doi.org/10.1016/j.foodchem.2020.127473.

Budryn, Grażyna, E. Nebesny, D. Rachwal-Rosiak, and J. Oracz. 2013. "Fatty Acids, Essential Amino Acids, and Chlorogenic Acids Profiles, in Vitro Protein Digestibility and Antioxidant Activity of Food Products Containing Green Coffee Extract." *International Food Research Journal* 20 (5): 2133–44.

Chen, Fei Ping, Bian Sheng Li, and Chuan He Tang. 2015. "Nanocomplexation between Curcumin and Soy Protein Isolate: Influence on Curcumin Stability/Bioaccessibility and in Vitro Protein Digestibility." *Journal of Agricultural and Food Chemistry* 63 (13): 3559–69. https://doi.org/10.1021/acs.jafc.5b00448.

Chen Ji guang, Shao fu Wu, Qing feng Zhang, Zhong ping Yin, and Lu Zhang. 2020. "α-Glucosidase Inhibitory Effect of Anthocyanins from Cinnamomum Camphora Fruit: Inhibition Kinetics and Mechanistic Insights through in Vitro and in Silico Studies." *International Journal of Biological Macromolecules* 143: 696–703. https://doi.org/10.1016/J.IJBIOMAC.2019.09.091.

Cheng, Jingrong, Daobang Tang, Huaigu Yang, Xuping Wang, Yaosheng Lin, and Xueming Liu. 2023. "The Effects of Mulberry Polyphenols on the Digestibility and Absorption Properties of Pork Myofibrillar Protein in Vitro." *Meat Science* 202: 109205. https://doi.org/10.1016/J.MEATSCI.2023.109205.

Dai, Shicheng, Peilong Liao, Yilun Wang, Tian Tian, Xiaohong Tong, Bo Lyu, Lin Cheng, et al. 2023. "Soy Protein Isolate-Catechin Non-Covalent and Covalent Complexes: Focus on Structure, Aggregation, Stability and in Vitro Digestion Characteristics." *Food Hydrocolloids* 135: 108108. https://doi.org/10.1016/j.foodhyd.2022.108108.

Dufour, Claire, Michèle Loonis, Mylène Delosière, Caroline Buffière, Noureddine Hafnaoui, Véronique Santé-Lhoutellier, and Didier Rémond. 2018. "The Matrix of Fruit & Vegetables Modulates the Gastrointestinal Bioaccessibility of Polyphenols and Their Impact on Dietary Protein Digestibility." *Food Chemistry* 240: 314–22. https://doi.org/10.1016/j.foodchem.2017.07.104.

Günal-Köroğlu, D., J. M. Lorenzo, and E. Capanoglu. 2023. "Plant-Based Protein-Phenolic Interactions: Effect on Different Matrices and in Vitro Gastrointestinal Digestion." *Food Research International* 173 (1): 113269. https://doi.org/https://doi.org/10.1016/j.foodres.2023.113269.

Günal-Köroğlu, Deniz, Semra Turan, and Esra Capanoglu. 2023. "Protein-Phenolic Interactions in Lentil and Wheat Crackers with Onion Skin Phenolics: Effects of Processing and in Vitro Gastrointestinal Digestion." *Food and Function* 14 (8): 3538. https://doi.org/10.1039/d2fo02885a.

Hao, Linlin, Jinwei Sun, Mengqi Pei, Guofang Zhang, Chun Li, Chunmei Li, Xinkai Ma, Sixuan He, and Libo Liu. 2022. "Impact of Non-Covalent Bound Polyphenols on Conformational, Functional Properties and in Vitro Digestibility of Pea Protein." *Food Chemistry* 383: 132623. https://doi.org/10.1016/J.FOODCHEM.2022.132623.

Han, J., Y. Du, J. Yan, X. Jiang, H. Wu, and B. Zhu. 2021. "Effect of Non-Covalent Binding of Phenolic Derivatives with Scallop (Patinopecten yessoensis) Gonad Protein Isolates on Protein Structure and in Vitro Digestion Characteristics." *Food Chemistry* 357:129690. https://doi.org/10.1016/j.foodchem.2021.129690.

He, Weiyi, Haoxie Xu, Yuqin Lu, Tingting Zhang, Shuiming Li, Xiao Lin, Bingqi Xu, and Xuli Wu. 2019. "Function, Digestibility and Allergenicity Assessment of Ovalbumin–EGCG Conjugates." *Journal of Functional Foods* 61: 103490. https://doi.org/10.1016/J.JFF.2019.103490.

He, Zhiyong, Bo Yuan, Maomao Zeng, Guanjun Tao, and Jie Chen. 2015. "Effect of Simulated Processing on the Antioxidant Capacity and in Vitro Protein Digestion of Fruit Juice-Milk Beverage Model Systems." *Food Chemistry* 175: 457–64. https://doi.org/10.1016/J.FOODCHEM.2014.12.007.

Jiang, Jiang, Zhipeng Zhang, Jing Zhao, and Yuanfa Liu. 2018. "The Effect of Non-Covalent Interaction of Chlorogenic Acid with Whey Protein and Casein on Physicochemical and Radical-Scavenging Activity of in Vitro Protein Digests." *Food Chemistry* 268: 334–41. https://doi.org/10.1016/j.foodchem.2018.06.015.

Jurema Soares, Maiara, Marcela de Souza Figueira, Geni Rodrigues Sampaio, Rosana Aparecida Manólio Soares-Freitas, Ana Clara da Costa Pinaffi-Langley, and Elizabeth Aparecida Ferraz da Silva Torres. 2022. "Coffee Simulated Inhibition of Pancreatic Lipase and Antioxidant Activities: Effect of Milk and Decaffeination." *Food Research International* 160: 111730. https://doi.org/10.1016/j.foodres.2022.111730.

Khalifa, Ibrahim, José M. Lorenzo, Sneh Punia Bangar, Osama M. Morsy, Asad Nawaz, Noman Walayat, and Remah Sobhy. 2022. "Effect of the Non-Covalent and Covalent Interactions between Proteins and Mono- or Di-Glucoside Anthocyanins on β-Lactoglobulin-Digestibility." *Food Hydrocolloids* 133: 107952. https://doi.org/10.1016/J.FOODHYD.2022.107952.

Khalifa, Ibrahim, Rongzu Nie, Zhenzhen Ge, Kaikai Li, and Chunmei Li. 2018. "Understanding the Shielding Effects of Whey Protein on Mulberry Anthocyanins: Insights from Multispectral and Molecular Modelling Investigations." *International Journal of Biological Macromolecules* 119: 116–24. https://doi.org/10.1016/J.IJBIOMAC.2018.07.117.

Khalifa, Ibrahim, Wei Zhu, Asad Nawaz, Kaikai Li, and Chunmei Li. 2021. "Microencapsulated Mulberry Anthocyanins Promote the in Vitro-Digestibility of Whey Proteins in Glycated Energy-Ball Models." *Food Chemistry* 345: 128805. https://doi.org/10.1016/J.FOODCHEM.2020.128805.

Lai, Ping, Atsushi Okazawa, Yoshihiro Izumi, Takeshi Bamba, Eiichiro Fukusaki, Masaaki Yoshikawa, and Akio Kobayashi. 2012. "Gallic Acid Oxidizes Met Residues in Peptides Released from Bovine β-Lactoglobulin by in Vitro Digestion." *Journal of Bioscience and Bioengineering* 114 (3): 297–305. https://doi.org/10.1016/J.JBIOSC.2012.04.019.

Li, Jinzhe, Yue Liu, Tianqi Li, Munkh Amgalan Gantumur, Abdul Qayum, Akhunzada Bilawal, Zhanmei Jiang, and Lizhe Wang. 2022. "Non-Covalent Interaction and Digestive Characteristics between α-Lactalbumin and Safflower Yellow: Impacts of Microwave Heating Temperature." *LWT* 159 (April): 113206. https://doi.org/10.1016/j.lwt.2022.113206.

Li, Q. H., H. S. Yan, H. Q. Li, J. J. Gao, and R. R. Hao. 2020. "Effects of Dietary Supplementation with Grape Seed Procyanidins on Nutrient Utilisation and Gut Function in Weaned Piglets." *Animal* 14 (3): 491–98. https://doi.org/10.1017/S1751731119002234.

Li Yuting, Dong He, Bing Li, Marianne N. Lund, Yifan Xing, Yi Wang, Fuxiang Li, et al. 2021. "Engineering Polyphenols with Biological Functions via Polyphenol-Protein Interactions as Additives for Functional Foods." *Trends in Food Science & Technology* 110: 470–82. https://doi.org/10.1016/J.TIFS.2021.02.009.

Lu, Yuqin, Shuiming Li, Haoxie Xu, Tingting Zhang, Xiao Lin, and Xuli Wu. 2018. "Effect of Covalent Interaction with Chlorogenic Acid on the Allergenic Capacity of Ovalbumin." *Journal of Agricultural and Food Chemistry* 66 (37): 9794–9800. https://doi.org/10.1021/acs.jafc.8b03410.

Lyu, Qiyan, Hongting Deng, Shunxin Wang, Hesham El-Seedi, Hui Cao, Lei Chen, and Hui Teng. 2023. "Dietary Supplementation with Casein/Cyanidin-3-O-Glucoside Nanoparticles Alters the Gut Microbiota in High-Fat Fed C57BL/6 Mice." *Food Chemistry* 412: 135494. https://doi.org/10.1016/j.foodchem.2023.135494.

Ma, Jiage, Yusi Miao, Jinzhe Li, Yue Ma, Mengguo Wu, Wan Wang, Cong Xu, Zhanmei Jiang, and Juncai Hou. 2022. "Incorporation of Blue Honeysuckle Juice into Fermented Goat Milk: Physicochemical, Sensory and Antioxidant Characteristics and In Vitro Gastrointestinal Digestion." *Foods* 11 (19): 3065. https://doi.org/10.3390/foods11193065.

Ma, Zhen, Jing Cheng, Shunshan Jiao, and Pu Jing. 2022. "Interaction of Mulberry Anthocyanins with Soybean Protein Isolate: Effect on the Stability of Anthocyanins and Protein in Vitro Digestion Characteristics." *International Journal of Food Science and Technology* 57 (4): 2267–76. https://doi.org/10.1111/ijfs.15576.

Ma, Zhen, Govindarajan Prasanna, Linlei Jiang, and Pu Jing. 2020. "Molecular Interaction of Cyanidin-3-O-Glucoside with Ovalbumin: Insights from Spectroscopic, Molecular Docking and in Vitro Digestive Studies." *Journal of Biomolecular Structure and Dynamics* 38 (6): 1858–67. https://doi.org/10.1080/07391102.2019.1618735.

Minekus, M, M Alminger, P Alvito, S Ballance, T Bohn, C Bourlieu, F Carriere, et al. 2014. "A Standardised Static in Vitro Digestion Method Suitable for Food – an International Consensus." *Food & Function* 5 (6): 1113–24. https://doi.org/10.1039/C3FO60702J.

Ozdal, Tugba, Esra Capanoglu, and Filiz Altay. 2013. "A Review on Protein–Phenolic Interactions and Associated Changes." *Food Research International* 51 (2): 954–70. https://doi.org/10.1016/j.foodres.2013.02.009.

Pan, Li Hua, Fei Liu, Shui Zhong Luo, and Jian ping Luo. 2019. "Pomegranate Juice Powder as Sugar Replacer Enhanced Quality and Function of Set Yogurts: Structure, Rheological Property, Antioxidant Activity and in Vitro Bioaccessibility." *LWT* 115: 108479. https://doi.org/10.1016/j.lwt.2019.108479.

Petzke, Klaus J., Stefane Schuppe, Sascha Rohn, Harshadrai M. Rawel, and Jürgen Kroll. 2005. "Chlorogenic Acid Moderately Decreases the Quality of Whey Proteins in Rats." *Journal of Agricultural and Food Chemistry* 53 (9): 3714–20. https://doi.org/10.1021/jf048186z.

Ren, Cong, Wenfei Xiong, Dengfeng Peng, Yun He, Peiyuan Zhou, Jing Li, and Bin Li. 2018. "Effects of Thermal Sterilization on Soy Protein Isolate/Polyphenol Complexes: Aspects of Structure, in Vitro Digestibility and Antioxidant Activity." *Food Research International* 112: 284–90. https://doi.org/10.1016/j.foodres.2018.06.034.

Rohn, Sascha. 2014. "Possibilities and Limitations in the Analysis of Covalent Interactions between Phenolic Compounds and Proteins." *Food Research International* 65: 13–19. https://doi.org/10.1016/j.foodres.2014.05.042.

Rohn, Sascha, Klaus J. Petzke, Harshadrai M. Rawel, and Jürgen Kroll. 2006. "Reactions of Chlorogenic Acid and Quercetin with a Soy Protein Isolate – Influence on the in Vivo Food Protein Quality in Rats." *Molecular Nutrition and Food Research* 50 (8): 696–704. https://doi.org/10.1002/mnfr.200600043.

Shen, Fei, Fuge Niu, Junhua Li, Yujie Su, Yuntao Liu, and Yanjun Yang. 2014. "Interactions between Tea Polyphenol and Two Kinds of Typical Egg White Proteins—Ovalbumin and Lysozyme: Effect on the Gastrointestinal Digestion of Both Proteins in Vitro." *Food Research International* 59: 100–7. https://doi.org/10.1016/J.FOODRES.2014.01.070.

Stamogiannou, Ioanna, John Van Camp, Guy Smagghe, Davy Van de Walle, Koen Dewettinck, and Katleen Raes. 2021. "Impact of Phenolic Compound as Activators or Inhibitors on the Enzymatic Hydrolysis of Cellulose." *International Journal of Biological Macromolecules* 186: 174–80. https://doi.org/10.1016/j.ijbiomac.2021.07.052.

Stojadinovic, Marija, Jelena Radosavljevic, Jana Ognjenovic, Jelena Vesic, Ivana Prodic, Dragana Stanic-Vucinic, and Tanja Cirkovic Velickovic. 2013. "Binding Affinity between Dietary Polyphenols and β-Lactoglobulin Negatively Correlates with the Protein Susceptibility to Digestion and Total Antioxidant Activity of Complexes Formed." *Food Chemistry* 136 (3–4): 1263–71. https://doi.org/j.foodchem.2012.09.040.

Tamargo, Alba, Carolina Cueva, Mariana Silva, Natalia Molinero, Beatriz Miralles, Begoña Bartolomé, and M. Victoria Moreno-Arribas. 2022. "Gastrointestinal Co-Digestion of Wine Polyphenols with Glucose/Whey Proteins Affects Their Bioaccessibility and Impact on Colonic Microbiota." *Food Research International* 155: 111010. https://doi.org/10.1016/j.foodres.2022.111010.

Tan, Yunbing, Hualu Zhou, and David Julian McClements. 2022. "Application of Static in Vitro Digestion Models for Assessing the Bioaccessibility of Hydrophobic Bioactives: A Review." *Trends in Food Science and Technology* 122: 314–27. https://doi.org/10.1016/j.tifs.2022.02.028.

Tantoush, Ziyad, Danijela Apostolovic, Bojana Kravic, Ivana Prodic, Luka Mihajlovic, Dragana Stanic-Vucinic, and Tanja Cirkovic Velickovic. 2012. "Green Tea Catechins of Food Supplements Facilitate Pepsin Digestion of Major Food Allergens, but Hampers Their Digestion If Oxidized by Phenol Oxidase." *Journal of Functional Foods* 4 (3): 650–60. https://doi.org/10.1016/j.jff.2012.04.006.

Taylor, Janet, Scott R. Bean, Brian P. Ioerger, and John R.N. Taylor. 2007. "Preferential Binding of Sorghum Tannins with γ-Kafirin and the Influence of Tannin Binding on Kafirin Digestibility and Biodegradation." *Journal of Cereal Science* 46 (1): 22–31. https://doi.org/10.1016/j.jcs.2006.11.001.

Tejirian, Ani, and Feng Xu. 2011. "Inhibition of Enzymatic Cellulolysis by Phenolic Compounds." *Enzyme and Microbial Technology* 48 (3): 239–47. https://doi.org/10.1016/j.enzmictec.2010.11.004.

Tlais, Ali Zein Alabiden, Elisabetta Trossolo, Stefano Tonini, Pasquale Filannino, Marco Gobbetti, and Raffaella Di Cagno. 2023. "Fermented Whey Ewe's Milk-Based Fruit Smoothies: Bio-Recycling and Enrichment of Phenolic Compounds and Improvement of Protein Digestibility and Antioxidant Activity." *Antioxidants* 12 (5): 1091. https://doi.org/10.3390/antiox12051091.

Wang, Yun, Cheng Yang, Jian Zhang, and Lianfu Zhang. 2022. "Interaction between Whey Protein Isolate and Rose Anthocyanin Extracts at Different PHs: Structure, Emulsification and Digestibility of Complexes." *Food Bioscience* 49: 101888. https://doi.org/10.1016/j.fbio.2022.101888.

Wang, Zuo, Lei Yin, Lei Liu, Xinyi Lan, Jianhua He, Fachun Wan, Weijun Shen, Shaoxun Tang, Zhiliang Tan, and Yanming Yang. 2022. "Tannic Acid Reduced Apparent Protein Digestibility and Induced Oxidative Stress and Inflammatory Response without Altering Growth Performance and Ruminal Microbiota Diversity of Xiangdong Black Goats." *Frontiers in Veterinary Science* 9: 1004841. https://doi.org/10.3389/fvets.2022.1004841.

Wei, Zihao, and Qingrong Huang. 2019. "Modulation of Formation, Physicochemical Properties, and Digestion of Ovotransferrin Nanofibrils with Covalent or Non-Covalent Bound Gallic Acid." *Journal of Agricultural and Food Chemistry* 67 (35): 9907–15. https://doi.org/10.1021/acs.jafc.9b02630.

Wu, Yue, Yongbin Han, Yang Tao, Dandan Li, Guangjie Xie, Pau Loke Show, and Sze Ying Lee. 2020. "In Vitro Gastrointestinal Digestion and Fecal Fermentation Reveal the Effect of Different Encapsulation Materials on the Release, Degradation and Modulation of Gut Microbiota of Blueberry Anthocyanin Extract." *Food Research International* 132: 109098. https://doi.org/10.1016/j.foodres.2020.109098.

Xiao, Huizhi, Benguo Liu, Haizhen Mo, and Guizhao Liang. 2015. "Comparative Evaluation of Tannic Acid Inhibiting α-Glucosidase and Trypsin." *Food Research International* 76 (3): 605–10. https://doi.org/10.1016/j.foodres.2015.07.029.

Xu, Haoxie, Tingting Zhang, Yuqin Lu, Xiao Lin, Xiaopeng Hu, Lizhong Liu, Zhendan He, and Xuli Wu. 2019. "Effect of Chlorogenic Acid Covalent Conjugation on the Allergenicity, Digestibility and Functional Properties of Whey Protein." *Food Chemistry* 298: 125024. https://doi.org/10.1016/j.foodchem.2019.125024.

Xu, M., M. Sun, C. Lu, Y. Han, X. Yao, X. Niu, … and Q. Zhu. 2021. "Influence of Epicatechin on Oxidation-Induced Physicochemical and Digestibility Changes in Porcine Myofibrillar Proteins during Refrigerated Storage." *Journal of the Science of Food and Agriculture* 101(2): 746–53. https://doi.org/10.1002/jsfa.10687.

Xue, Hui, Guowen Zhang, Tianfeng Han, Ruiling Li, Huilan Liu, Binghong Gao, Yonggang Tu, and Yan Zhao. 2022. "Improvement of Gel Properties and Digestibility of the Water-Soluble Polymer of Tea Polyphenol-Egg White under Thermal Treatment." *Food Chemistry* 372: 131319. https://doi.org/10.1016/j.foodchem.2021.131319.

Yilmazer-Musa, Meltem, Anneke M. Griffith, Alexander J. Michels, Erik Schneider, and Balz Frei. 2012. "Grape Seed and Tea Extracts and Catechin 3-Gallates Are Potent Inhibitors of α-Amylase and α-Glucosidase Activity." *Journal of Agricultural and Food Chemistry* 60:8924–29. https://doi.org/10.1021/jf301147n.

You, Qi, Feng Chen, Xi Wang, Pengju G. Luo, and Yueming Jiang. 2011. "Inhibitory Effects of Muscadine Anthocyanins on α-Glucosidase and Pancreatic Lipase Activities." *Journal of Agricultural and Food Chemistry* 59 (17): 9506–11. https://doi.org/10.1021/jf201452v.

Yu, Jianmei, Yang Mi, and Shuang Ji. 2016. "In Vitro Evaluating the Influence of Grape Seed Polyphenol Extract on the Digestibility of Macronutrients." *Journal of Health Sciences* 4: 167–76. https://doi.org/10.17265/2328-7136/2016.04.001.

Zahid, Hafza Fasiha, Akhtar Ali, Chaminda Senaka Ranadheera, Zhongxiang Fang, Frank R. Dunshea, and Said Ajlouni. 2022. "In Vitro Bioaccessibility of Phenolic Compounds and Alpha-Glucosidase Inhibition Activity in Yoghurts Enriched with Mango Peel Powder." *Food Bioscience* 50: 102011. https://doi.org/10.1016/j.fbio.2022.102011.

Zhang, Yan, Si Chen, Baokun Qi, Xiaonan Sui, and Lianzhou Jiang. 2018. "Complexation of Thermally-Denatured Soybean Protein Isolate with Anthocyanins and Its Effect on the Protein Structure and in Vitro Digestibility." *Food Research International* 106: 619–25. https://doi.org/10.1016/j.foodres.2018.01.040.

Zhou, Peiyu, Lingmin Zhang, Wei Li, Shuting Zhang, Lanxin Luo, Jian Wang, and Baoshan Sun. 2018. "In Vitro Evaluation of the Anti-Digestion and Antioxidant Effects of Grape Seed Procyanidins According to Their Degrees of Polymerization." *Journal of Functional Foods* 49: 85–95. https://doi.org/10.1016/j.jff.2018.08.001.

Zhou, Si Duo, Yan Fei Lin, Xiao Xu, Ling Meng, and Ming Sheng Dong. 2020. "Effect of Non-Covalent and Covalent Complexation of (–)-Epigallocatechin Gallate with Soybean Protein Isolate on Protein Structure and in Vitro Digestion Characteristics." *Food Chemistry* 309: 125718. https://doi.org/10.1016/j.foodchem.2019.125718.

Zhou, Zhiwei, Dan Wang, Xinyi Xu, Jin Dai, Guangjie Lao, Senlin Zhang, Xiaofang Xu, András Dinnyés, Youling Xiong, and Qun Sun. 2023. "Myofibrillar Protein-Chlorogenic Acid Complexes Ameliorate Glucose Metabolism via Modulating Gut Microbiota in a Type 2 Diabetic Rat Model." *Food Chemistry* 409: 135195. https://doi.org/10.1016/j.foodchem.2022.135195.

Zygmantaitė, Gabrielė, Milda Keršienė, Ina Jasutienė, Aušra Šipailienė, Petras Rimantas Venskutonis, and Daiva Leskauskaitė. 2021. "Extract Isolated from Cranberry Pomace as Functional Ingredient in Yoghurt Production: Technological Properties and Digestibility Studies." *LWT – Food Science and Technology* 148: 111751. https://doi.org/10.1016/J.LWT.2021.111751.

6 Amino Acid Quality of Meat Proteins

Natalia S. Fanelli and Hans H. Stein

ABBREVIATIONS

AA	Amino acid
DIAA	Digestible indispensable amino acid
DIAAS	Digestible indispensable amino acid score
FAO	Food and Agriculture Organization
IAA	Indispensable amino acid
SID	Standardized ileal digestibility
USDA	US Department of Agriculture

INTRODUCTION

Meat derived from different animal species, such as poultry, pigs, cattle, and sheep, is an essential component of many cuisines around the world, offering a variety of cuts with different flavors, textures, and cooking properties suitable for a wide range of applications. However, within each type of meat, there may be distinctions based on specific cuts or preparation methods that may influence protein quality (Bailey et al. 2020a). Cultural, historical, geographical, socio-economic, and ethical factors also play a role in shaping the preferences and practices related to meat consumption and what is considered meat (Wahlqvist 2007).

Meat, in general, refers to the flesh edible part of animals (typically domesticated), including muscles, fat, ligaments, and tendons (Food and Agriculture Organization [FAO] 2021). Commonly consumed meats include poultry (including broiler chickens, laying hens, turkeys, ducks, and geese), pork, beef (including cows, steers, calves, heifers, and bulls), and lamb or mutton (from sheep). Although not widely consumed, game meat is another protein in this category and comprises meat from wild animals that are typically hunted, such as deer, boar, elk, rabbit, and game birds (quail and pheasant), among others (FAO 2018).

Several cuts are available, each with its own level of tenderness, recommended cooking methods, and nutrient contents, including amino acids (AA) and fat concentrations. Broiler chicken is the most widely consumed type of poultry and has lean flesh and mild flavor, providing cuts such as breasts, thighs, wings, and drumsticks. White meat from the breast and wings is leaner and more tender, whereas dark meat from thighs and drumsticks is richer in flavor and often juicier (Bihan-Duval et al. 2008). Beef can be divided into various cuts, the most common being rib, chuck (shoulder), brisket (chest), round (legs, thigh, and butt), tenderloin, and sirloin (rear of the animal). Meat obtained from young calves is called veal (US Department of Agriculture [USDA] and Food Safety and Inspection Service [FSIS] 2013). Similar to beef, pork can be categorized into cuts such as shoulder, ribs, loin, belly (high fat), and leg. Common cuts of pork include loin, bacon, ham, chops, and tenderloin (Bailey et al. 2020b). Lamb and mutton are meats that differ in terms of the age of the animal. Common cuts from sheep include chops, leg, loin, shoulder, and rack. Lamb refers to meat from young sheep, while mutton comes from mature animals (USDA 2022).

DOI: 10.1201/9781003597926-6

Animal-based proteins, including meats, are excellent sources of protein in human diets (Bender 1992). Proteins, more specifically indispensable amino acids (IAA), are required for muscle growth, development, and the overall health of the human body. As a result, the AA quality of animal proteins is important because it impacts the nutritional value of protein and its ability to provide IAA required for body protein synthesis and various physiological functions in humans (Bender 1992). The objective of this chapter is to provide information about AA concentration, digestibility, protein quality, and how processing affects protein quality in different meat cuts.

NUTRIENT CONCENTRATIONS

Meat is a valuable dietary source of protein and contains all the required amino acids (AA) as well as other important nutrients. Nutrient content may differ among meat cuts due to inherent physiological and anatomical variables such as muscle composition, fat distribution, and connective tissue. Nutrient concentrations also vary depending on the specific breed of the animal, age, feeding practices, and cooking methods (Bender 1992). Lean cuts have greater protein concentrations, whereas cuts with more connective tissue or fat contains less protein. The presence of IAA, contributes to the role of meat in muscle protein synthesis and the overall protein quality of meals. The type of muscle fiber in meat also affects the concentration of IAA (Franco 2010). Therefore, understanding the variations in protein concentrations and AA profiles is critical for optimizing nutritional intake and meeting dietary requirements.

Fat is an important component of meat, particularly as a source of essential polyunsaturated fatty acids, contributing to its sensory attributes and nutritional value (Wyness 2016). Generally, cuts from lean steaks, tend to have the least concentration of fat. In contrast, cuts from muscles with higher intramuscular fat deposition may have greater fat concentrations (Bender 1992). As an example, ribeye or T-bone steaks from beef are known for their marbling, indicating a greater fat content and enhanced flavor. Lean cuts, on the other hand, such as chicken breast or pork tenderloin, contain less fat (Bender 1992).

Table 6.1 contains examples of IAA and fat concentrations in various cuts of meat.

Regardless of species or cooking methods, lysine is the IAA present at the greatest concentration, whereas tryptophan is present at the least concentration. Other nutrients in meats not commonly present in plant-based foods include vitamins B_{12} and B_6, as well as iron, zinc, and selenium (Bender 1992).

DIGESTIBILITY OF PROTEIN AND AA

The digestibility of protein and AA in meat cuts can vary depending on animal species, muscle type, protein structure, and individual variations due to gut microbiota composition, enzyme activity, and overall intestinal health (Stein et al. 2007). Tender cuts with less connective tissue, such as fillets or loins, are usually more easily digestible than tougher cuts requiring longer cooking times or additional tenderization techniques. Proper cooking methods can also enhance the digestibility of meat proteins, ensuring optimal utilization of the AA by the body (Bender 1992).

Because of the similarities in the digestive systems between humans and pigs, the standardized ileal digestibility (SID) of AA in human foods determined in pigs is in agreement with values determined in humans (Rowan et al. 1994; Hodgkinson et al. 2022). Generally, meat proteins are highly digestible, with an average digestibility of 90–95%. As an example, values for the SID of protein and IAA in pork products such as pork loin, bacon, ground pork, porcine heart hydrolysate, raw belly, and ham ranged from 83 to 100% (Bailey et al. 2020b; Bindari et al. 2018; Fanelli et al. 2022). Ground beef, ribeye roast, topside beef steak, and bovine muscle hydrolysate yielded SID values ranging from 88 to 100% (Bailey et al. 2020a; Bindari et al. 2018; Fanelli et al. 2022; Hodgkinson et al. 2018).

TABLE 6.1
Concentration of Protein, Fat, and Indispensable Amino Acids (IAA) of Some Meat Cuts, g/100g (% of portion)[1,2]

Item	Protein	Fat	Histidine	Isoleucine	Leucine	Lysine	Methionine	Phenylalanine	Threonine	Tryptophan	Valine
Poultry[3]											
Raw chicken breast	20.8	9.2	0.6	1.0	1.5	1.7	0.6	0.8	0.9	0.2	1.0
Cooked chicken breast	29.8	7.8	0.9	1.5	2.2	2.5	0.8	1.2	1.2	0.3	1.5
Raw chicken thigh	16.6	14.6	0.4	0.7	1.3	1.4	0.4	0.6	0.7	0.2	0.7
Cooked chicken thigh	23.3	14.7	0.7	1.0	1.9	2.1	0.6	0.9	1.0	0.2	1.1
Raw chicken wing	17.5	12.8	0.7	0.9	1.5	1.80	0.5	0.7	0.8	0.2	0.9
Cooked chicken wing	23.8	16.9	0.9	1.2	2.0	2.3	0.6	1.0	1.1	0.3	1.2
Raw chicken drumstick	9.6	44.2	0.2	0.3	0.5	0.5	0.2	0.3	0.3	0.0	0.3
Cooked chicken drumstick	16.6	44.0	0.3	0.5	0.9	0.9	0.3	0.5	0.5	0.1	0.6
Beef											
Raw beef ribs	21.3	6.8	0.8	0.9	1.6	1.7	0.7	0.8	0.8	0.2	0.9
Cooked beef ribs	27.2	9.7	1.0	1.1	2.0	2.2	0.9	1.1	1.0	0.3	1.2
Raw beef tenderloin	21.0	6.9	0.8	0.9	1.6	1.7	0.7	0.8	0.8	0.2	0.9
Cooked beef tenderloin	27.3	8.1	1.0	1.3	2.4	2.6	0.7	1.1	1.3	0.3	1.4

(Continued)

TABLE 6.1 (CONTINUED)
Concentration of Protein, Fat, and Indispensable Amino Acids (IAA) of Some Meat Cuts, g/100g (% of portion)[1,2]

Item	Protein	Fat	Histidine	Isoleucine	Leucine	Lysine	Methionine	Phenylalanine	Threonine	Tryptophan	Valine
Raw beef brisket	14.7	14.9	0.5	0.6	1.1	1.1	0.3	0.5	0.6	0.1	0.6
Cooked beef brisket	18.2	19.0	0.6	0.8	1.4	1.5	0.5	0.7	0.7	0.2	0.9
Raw veal	18.6	13.1	0.7	0.9	1.5	1.5	0.4	0.7	0.8	0.2	1.0
Cooked veal	24.3	7.6	0.9	1.2	1.9	2.0	0.6	1.0	1.1	0.3	1.3
Pork											
Raw pork ribs	19.3	11.8	0.8	1.0	1.7	1.8	0.5	0.8	0.9	0.2	1.0
Cooked pork ribs	27.0	14.7	1.1	1.3	2.2	2.4	0.7	1.1	1.2	0.3	1.4
Raw pork chops	20.7	9.0	0.9	1.0	1.8	1.9	0.6	0.9	0.9	0.2	1.1
Cooked pork chops	25.6	11.1	1.1	1.3	2.2	2.4	0.7	1.1	1.2	0.3	1.3
Cured bacon[4]	33.9	35.1	1.4	1.6	2.8	3.0	0.9	1.4	1.5	0.4	1.7
Raw pork tenderloin	20.4	2.1	0.9	1.0	1.7	1.9	0.6	0.9	0.9	0.2	1.1
Cooked pork tenderloin	26.0	4.0	1.1	1.3	2.2	2.4	0.7	1.1	1.2	0.3	1.4
Sheep											
Raw lamb loin	15.4	26.2	0.3	0.7	1.2	1.3	0.5	0.6	0.7	0.2	0.8

(Continued)

TABLE 6.1 (CONTINUED)
Concentration of Protein, Fat, and Indispensable Amino Acids (IAA) of Some Meat Cuts, g/100g (% of portion)[1,2]

Item	Protein	Fat	Histidine	Isoleucine	Leucine	Lysine	Methionine	Phenylalanine	Threonine	Tryptophan	Valine
Cooked lamb loin	21.1	21.0	0.4	0.9	1.6	1.8	0.7	0.8	1.0	0.2	1.1
Raw lamb leg	18.6	14.5	0.4	0.8	1.4	1.6	0.6	0.7	0.9	0.2	0.9
Cooked lamb leg	24.8	15.6	0.8	1.2	1.9	2.1	0.6	1.0	1.0	0.3	1.3
Raw lamb shoulder	16.2	22.9	0.3	0.7	1.3	1.4	0.5	0.6	0.8	0.2	0.8
Cooked lamb shoulder[5]	20.9	23.4	0.4	0.9	1.6	1.8	0.7	0.8	1.0	0.2	1.1

[1]Values were obtained from the USDA Food Database 2023.
[2]Cooked refers to the roasting process.
[3]Meat and skin.
[4]Pan-fried.
[5]Slow-roasted.

Because AA are present alongside fat molecules in meats, and because fat influences the digestibility and availability of AA (Li and Sauer 1994; Cervantes-Pahm and Stein 2008), the concentration of fat may affect the SID of AA in specific cuts of meat. Fats can form complexes with proteins, potentially affecting the access of digestive enzymes to protein molecules and reduce AA digestibility. In contrast, fat may also slow gastric emptying and therefore increase SID of AA.

PROTEIN QUALITY

Meats are considered high-quality proteins due to the presence of IAA and greater digestibility when compared with other foods. However, this varies depending on the cut and the composition of AA (Fanelli et al. 2022; Hodgkinson et al. 2018). Cuts with connective tissue and marbling may have the least protein concentration, but cuts with greater marbling may have greater digestibility of AA, and all types of meat usually increase the protein quality of mixed meals.

Several methods have been developed to determine protein quality in human foods. The current method recommended by the FAO to assess protein quality is called the digestible indispensable amino acid score (DIAAS; FAO 2013). This method recommends using pigs as a model when humans are unavailable because of their digestive similarities (FAO 2013; Hodgkinson et al. 2020). The DIAAS is calculated using the protein and AA composition of a food and their respective SID values. Digestible indispensable amino acid (DIAA) reference ratios are used to compare results with human AA patterns for infants, children, adolescents, and adults. The least reference ratio (first limiting AA) is then determined as DIAAS. Cut-off values are based on values ranging from 75 to 99 for foods with "good" protein quality and values of 100 or more for foods with "excellent" protein quality (FAO 2013). However, no claims can be made for foods with a DIAAS less than 75.

Protein quality in a number of different cuts of meat has been reported (Table 6.2). Generally, protein quality in meat proteins depends on cooking techniques and intrinsic individual differences.

PROCESSING

Different processing methods such as heat treatment, dehydrating, curing, smoking, fermenting, aging, and mechanical processing can impact protein quality of meats (Bailey et al. 2020a; Hodgkinson et al. 2018). Effects of processing on protein quality can vary based on the specific cut, processing conditions, and the type and amount of added ingredients. Heat treatment, such as cooking, roasting, or grilling, is essential to improve sensory characteristics, but it can also change protein structure and impact protein quality, either positively or negatively (Santé-Lhoijtellierv et al. 2008). Both overheating and underheating of meats can have a negative impact on protein quality and overall sensory attributes of the meat (Santanu et al. 2014).

Overcooking or excessive heat exposure may lead to protein denaturation, which causes changes in the three-dimensional structure and protein degradation (Yu et al. 2017). Although protein denaturation in meat at temperatures around 70°C may increase the digestibility of AA, temperatures over 100°C may cause protein aggregation and cross-linking, resulting in a more rigid and less tender meat texture as well as reduced digestibility of AA and protein quality (Di Luccia et al. 2015; Gatellier et al. 2010; Li et al. 2017). As an example, overcooked ground beef reduced protein quality by 22%, and grilling and roasting topside steak reduced protein quality by 17% and 6%, respectively, demonstrating that some meats (and processes used) may have heat damage at different levels of heating (Bailey et al. 2020a; Hodgkinson et al. 2018).

Lysine is the AA most affected by overheating because of the exposed epsilon amino group that can easily combine with a reducing sugar in the Maillard reaction, thereby preventing its use in protein synthesis. However, depending on the time and temperature used to cook, lysine in meat is often not affected by cooking or processing because of the lack of reducing sugars in meat (Bailey et al. 2020a; Hodgkinson et al. 2018). Overheating can also cause lipid oxidation, which can result in formation of potentially indigestible compounds that can impair AA availability, promote the

TABLE 6.2
Protein Quality of Different Meat Cuts as Indicated by the Digestible Indispensable Amino Acid (DIAAS) Method[1,2,3]

	DIAAS		
Item	**Infants (0 to 6 Months)**	**Children (6 Months to 3 Years)**	**Older Children, Adolescents, and Adults**
Porcine plasma hydrolysate[4]	60 (Isoleucine)	87 (Sulfur AA)	102 (Sulfur AA)
Porcine muscle hydrolysate[4]	21 (Tryptophan)	42 (Tryptophan)	54 (Tryptophan)
Porcine heart hydrolysate[4]	38 (Tryptophan)	76 (Tryptophan)	87 (Isoleucine)
Pork raw belly[5]	—	111	119
Smoked bacon[5]	—	109	117
Smoked-cooked bacon[5]	—	126	142
Non-cured ham[5]	—	115	124
Cured ham[5]	—	117	126
Raw pork loin[6]	55 (Histidine)	78 (Histidine)	97 (Histidine)
Roasted pork loin[5,6]	60 (Tryptophan)	107–129	117–139
Grilled pork loin[6]	61 (Tryptophan)	112	123
Fried pork loin[6]	69 (Tryptophan)	112	126
Salami[7]	—	107	120
Back ribs[8]	63 (Aromatic AA)	106	114
Shoulder butt[8]	64 (Aromatic AA)	107	115
Tenderloin[8]	66 (Aromatic AA)	115	124
Coppa[8]	63 (Aromatic AA)	115	128
Prosciutto[8]	70 (Aromatic AA)	127	137
Speck[8]	72 (Tryptophan)	111	119
Chorizo sausage[8]	65 (Tryptophan)	99 (Sulfur AA)	113
Italian sausage[8]	72 (Tryptophan)	113	122
Bratwurst sausage[8]	64 (Tryptophan)	101	117
Raw ground beef[7]	—	111	121
Cooked ground beef[7]	—	92 (Leucine)	99 (Leucine)
Ground pork 80% lean, burger[9]	—	111	119
Ground beef 80% lean, burger[9]	—	102	110
Ground beef 93% lean, burger[9]	—	111	119
Bologna[7]	—	118	128
Bovine muscle hydrolysate[4]	32 (Tryptophan)	63 (Tryptophan)	81 (Tryptophan)
Ribeye roast[7]	—	99 (Leucine)–121	107–130
Beef jerky[7]	—	102	120
Raw beef topside steak[10]	—	97 (Valine)	—
Boiled beef topside steak[10]	—	99 (Valine)	—
Grilled beef topside steak[10]	—	80 (Valine)	—
Pan-fried beef topside steak[10]	—	98 (Valine)	—
Roasted beef topside steak[10]	—	91 (Valine)	—

(*Continued*)

TABLE 6.2 (CONTINUED)
Protein Quality of Different Meat Cuts as Indicated by the Digestible Indispensable Amino Acid (DIAAS) Method[1,2,3]

	DIAAS		
Item	**Infants (0 to 6 Months)**	**Children (6 Months to 3 Years)**	**Older Children, Adolescents, and Adults**
Roasted beef tenderloin[8]	—	120	—
Roasted turkey breast[8]	—	111	—

[1]Values are DIAAS followed by first-limiting amino acid (AA) in parentheses. If DIAAS values >100, no limiting AA is present.
[2]The DIAAS values were determined using pig as the animal model.
[3]Values not reported are noted by "-".
[4]Bindari et al. 2018.
[5]Bailey et al. 2020b.
[6]Mathai 2018.
[7]Bailey et al. 2020a.
[8]Fanelli et al. 2024.
[9]Fanelli et al. 2022.
[10]Hodgkinson et al. 2018.

Maillard reaction, and have negative effects on flavor, as well as potentially form harmful compounds. Overcooking can also cause moisture loss from the meat, resulting in a dry and less succulent texture (Bender 1992).

Undercooking meats may result in insufficient protein denaturation, leaving the proteins in their native state. This can lead to a chewy and rubbery texture due to the lack of protein breakdown and tenderization (Bender 1992). Undercooked meat may also have reduced protein digestibility due to the presence of enzymes or protein structures that are more resistant to digestion and can fail to eliminate harmful bacteria that may be present in raw meat (Bender 1992). Nevertheless, when appropriate processing is used, the digestibility of IAA and protein quality are increased, as demonstrated when ribeye was heated to 64°C (Bailey et al. 2020a). Therefore, to ensure optimal protein quality, it is important to cook meats properly and avoid both overheating and underheating (Hodgkinson et al. 2018). The ideal cooking temperature and cooking time vary depending on the type of meat, cut, and desired doneness, which can vary among individuals and cultures. Using cooking methods that allow for precise temperature control (i.e., the use of a thermometer) can help achieve the desired level of doneness while preserving protein quality.

EFFECTS OF OTHER PROTEINS

In this chapter, AA quality of meat proteins was discussed regarding nutrient concentrations, AA digestibility, protein quality, and processing. However, consideration must be given to other proteins, such as soy and milk proteins. The digestibility of AA and quality of proteins, including soy protein isolate, soy flour, whey protein isolate, milk protein concentrate, whey protein concentrate, and skim milk powder, are relatively close to the quality of meat proteins (Fanelli et al. 2022; Mathai et al. 2017). However, most plant-based proteins, including proteins from corn, peas, oats, rice, beans, and wheat, have reduced protein quality compared with meats because of concentrations of limiting AA and the extensive processing that is sometimes applied to these types of foods (Mathai et al.

2017; Rutherfurd et al. 2015). Because proteins are usually consumed together with other foods in combined meals, the excellent protein quality of meat can compensate for the low-quality proteins in plant-based ingredients. As an example, burgers are usually consumed with burger buns. Thus, if animal-based burgers are combined with a burger bun, this combination can provide enough digestible AA for individuals older than three years old, although the protein quality of the burger bun is very poor (Fanelli et al. 2022). However, if a pea-based burger was combined with a burger bun, complementarity was less than with animal-based burgers, and sulfur AA was still limiting in the combined diet (Fanelli et al. 2022). In addition, milk can complement lower-quality cereal-based proteins such as cornflakes and oats in traditional breakfast-style porridge combinations and provide an AA-balanced meal (Fanelli et al. 2021).

CONCLUSIONS

Meat supplies not only high-quality protein but also IAA, vitamins, and minerals that are essential for human health. The many cuts and varieties of meats that are available provide a wide range of culinary possibilities. Meat generally has excellent protein quality due to greater digestibility of AA than in plant-based foods, but the quality can be influenced by processing methods and fat content. The protein quality of meat, as evaluated by the DIAAS method, also varies depending on the specific cut and cooking techniques. Cooking and processing procedures must be considered when evaluating protein quality because they affect protein digestion and overall meat quality. Therefore, understanding the effects of processing procedures on protein quality is necessary for retaining the nutritional value of meat.

MINI DICTIONARY OF TERMS

- **Connective tissue:** Structural tissue that supports and connects different components of an animal, which are made up of collagen.
- **Flesh:** Soft, edible part of an animal's body, typically referring to the muscle tissue consumed as food.
- **Marbling:** The distribution of fat within muscle fibers contributes to the tenderness and juiciness of specific cuts.
- **Tenderness:** The degree of softness or ease with which the meat can be chewed or cut.
- **Texture:** Physical consistency and mouthfeel of the meat.

SUMMARY POINTS

- Each type of meat has distinct cuts that affect protein quality.
- Factors such as culture and ethics influence meat preferences.
- Meat usually provides IAA for human growth and health.
- Individuals can maximize the benefits of nutrients that meat provides as part of a well-balanced diet by carefully selecting and preparing meat pieces.
- All meat cuts have much greater protein quality than most plant proteins, and meat will, therefore, contribute to a well-balanced diet if consumed in combination with lower-quality plant proteins.
- Lean cuts have greater protein concentrations, whereas cuts with more connective tissue have lower protein content.
- Protein quality is affected by the type of cuts, animal species, cooking procedures, and intrinsic characteristics of a food.
- Overheating can result in protein degradation, whereas undercooking may result in insufficient protein denaturation.

REFERENCES

Bailey, H. M., J. K. Mathai, E. P. Berg and H. H. Stein. 2020a. Most meat products have digestible indispensable amino acid scores that are greater than 100, but processing may increase or reduce protein quality. *British Journal of Nutrition* 124:14–22.

Bailey, H. M., J. K. Mathai, E. P. Berg and H. H. Stein. 2020b. Pork products have digestible indispensable amino acid scores (DIAAS) that are greater than 100 when determined in pigs, but processing does not always increase DIAAS. *The Journal of Nutrition* 150:475–482.

Bender, A. 1992. *Meat and meat products in human nutrition in developing countries.* FAO food and nutrition paper 53. Food and Agriculture Organization of the United Nations. Rome. http://www.fao.org/docrep/t0562e/T0562E00.htm (accessed June 18, 2023).

Bihan-Duval, L., M. Debut, C. M. Berri, N. Sellier, V. Santé-Lhoutellier, Y. Jégo and C. Beaumont. 2008. Chicken meat quality: Genetic variability and relationship with growth and muscle characteristics. *BMC Genetics* 9:1–6.

Bindari, Y. R., H. N. Lærke, and J. V. Nørgaard. 2018. Standardized ileal digestibility and digestible indispensable amino acid score of porcine and bovine hydrolyzates in pigs. *Journal of the Science of Food and Agriculture* 98:2131–2137.

Cervantes-Pahm, S. K. and H. H. Stein. 2008. Effect of dietary soybean oil and soybean protein concentration on the concentration of digestible amino acids in soybean products fed to growing pigs. *Journal of Animal Science* 86:1841–1849.

Di Luccia, A., B. La Gatta, A. Nicastro, G. Petrella, C. Lamacchia and G. Picariello. 2015. Protein modifications in cooked pork products investigated by a proteomic approach. *Food Chemistry* 172:447–455.

Fanelli, N. S., H. M. Bailey, L. V. Guardiola and H. H. Stein. 2021. Values for digestible indispensable amino acid score (DIAAS) determined in pigs are greater for milk than for breakfast cereals, but DIAAS values for individual ingredients are additive in combined meals. *The Journal of Nutrition* 151:540–547.

Fanelli, N. S., H. M. Bailey, T. W. Thompson, R. Delmore, M. N. Nair and H. H. Stein. 2022. Digestible indispensable amino acid score (DIAAS) is greater in animal-based burgers than in plant-based burgers if determined in pigs. *European Journal of Nutrition* 61:461–475.

Fanelli, N. S., J. C. F. R. Martins and H. H. Stein. 2024. The digestible indispensable amino acid scores (DIAAS) in pork cuts, hams, and sausages is close to or above 100 and pork ingredients can complement ingredients with lower protein quality. *Journal of the Science in Food and Agriculture Reports* 4:326–335.

FAO. 2013. *Dietary protein quality evaluation in human nutrition: Report of an FAO expert group.* FAO food and nutrition paper 92. Food and Agriculture Organization of the United Nations. http://www.fao.org/3/a-i3124e.pdf (accessed June 21, 2023).

FAO. 2018. *Game meat – production and trade in the UNECE region.* The United Nations Economic Commission for Europe. https://unece.org/fileadmin/DAM/timber/meetings/2018/20180321/game-meat-draft-2018-03.pdf (accessed June 18, 2023).

FAO. 2021. *Indicator 10: Individual average daily consumption of meat.* Milan Urban Food Policy Pact. https://www.fao.org/3/CB4058EN/CB4058EN.pdf (accessed June 18, 2023).

Franco, D., L. Gonzalez, E. Bispo, P. Rodriguez, J. I. Garabal and T. Moreno. 2010. Study of hydrolyzed protein composition, free amino acid, and taurine content in different muscles of Galician blonde beef. *Journal of Muscle Foods* 21:769–784.

Gatellier, P., A. Kondjoyan, S. Portanguen and V. Sante-Lhoutellier. 2010. Effect of cooking on protein oxidation in n-3 polyunsaturated fatty acids enriched beef. Implication on nutritional quality. *Meat Science* 85:645–650.

Hodgkinson, S. M., C. A. Montoya, P. T. Scholten, S. M. Rutherfurd and P. J. Moughan. 2018. Cooking conditions affect the true ileal digestible amino acid content and digestible indispensable amino acid score (DIAAS) of bovine meat as determined in pigs. *The Journal of Nutrition* 148:1564–1569.

Hodgkinson, S. M., H. H. Stein, S. de Vries, W. H. Hendriks and P. J. Moughan. 2020. Determination of true ileal amino acid digestibility in the growing pig for calculation of digestible indispensable amino acid score (DIAAS). *The Journal of Nutrition* 150:2621–2623.

Hodgkinson, S. M., N. Stroebinger, N. van der Wielen, C. Montoya, W. H. Hendriks, H. H. Stein and P. J. Moughan. 2022. Comparison of true ileal amino acid digestibility between adult humans and growing pigs. *The Journal of Nutrition* 152:1635–1646.

Li, L., Y. Liu, X. Zou, J. He, X. Xu, G. Zhou and C. Li. 2017. In vitro protein digestibility of pork products is affected by the method of processing. *Food Research International* 92:88–94.

Li, S. and W. C. Sauer. 1994. The effect of dietary fat content on amino acid digestibility in young pigs. *Journal of Animal Science* 72:1737–1743.

Mathai, J. K. 2018. *Digestible indispensable amino acid scores (DIAAS) for various food proteins and assessment of intra-experiment variation of DIAAS*. PhD diss. University of Illinois at Urbana-Champaign. https://www.ideals.illinois.edu/items/109804 (accessed June 22, 2023).

Mathai, J. K., Y. Liu and H. H. Stein. 2017. Values for digestible indispensable amino acid scores (DIAAS) for some dairy and plant proteins may better describe protein quality than values calculated using the concept for protein digestibility-corrected amino acid scores (PDCAAS). *British Journal of Nutrition* 117:490–499.

Rowan, A. M., P. J. Moughan, M. N. Wilson, K. Maher and C. Tasman-Jones. 1994. Comparison of the ileal and faecal digestibility of dietary amino acids in adult humans and evaluation of the pig as a model animal for digestion studies in man. *British Journal of Nutrition* 71:29–42.

Rutherfurd, S. M., A. C. Fanning, B. J. Miller and P. J. Moughan. 2015. Protein digestibility-corrected amino acid scores and digestible indispensable amino acid scores differentially describe protein quality in growing male rats. *The Journal of nutrition* 145:372–379.

Santanu, D. C., S. Haines, D. Harland, S. Clerens, C. van Koten and J. Dyer 2014. Effect of cooking on meat proteins: mapping hydrothermal protein modification as a potential indicator of bioavailability. *Journal Agricultural Food Chemistry* 62:8187–8196.

Santé-Lhoijtellier, V., T. Astrijc, P. Marinova, E. Greve and P. Gatellier. 2008. Effect of meat cooking on physicochemical state and in vitro digestibility of myofibrillar proteins. *Journal Agricultural Food Chemistry* 56:1488–1494.

Stein, H. H., B. Sève, M. F. Fuller, P. J. Moughan and C. F. M. De Lange. 2007. Invited review: Amino acid bioavailability and digestibility in pig feed ingredients: Terminology and application. *Journal of Animal Science* 85:172–180.

USDA. 2022. *Sheep, lamb and mutton*. U.S. Department of Agriculture. https://www.ers.usda.gov/topics/animal-products/sheep-lamb-mutton/ (accessed June 18, 2023).

USDA and FSIS. 2013. *Veal from farm to table*. U.S. Department of Agriculture and Food Safety and Inspection Service. https://www.fsis.usda.gov/food-safety/safe-food-handling-and-preparation/meat/veal-farm-table (accessed June 18, 2023).

USDA Food Database. 2023. https://fdc.nal.usda.gov/index.html (accessed June 19, 2023).

Wahlqvist, M. L. 2007. Regional food culture and development. *Asia Pacific Journal of Clinical Nutrition* 16:2.

Wyness, L. 2016. The role of red meat in the diet: Nutrition and health benefits. *Proceedings of the Nutrition Society* 75:227–232.

Yu, T. Y., J. D. Morton, S. Clerens and J. M. Dyer. 2017. Cooking-induced protein modifications in meat. *Comprehensive Reviews in Food Science and Food Safety* 16:141–159.

7 Animal Protein and Its Impact on Adiposity

Laís Lima de Castro Abreu, Julianne Viana Freire Portela, Andrea Gomes Santana de Melo, Tiago Soares, and Maria do Carmo de Carvalho e Martins

ABBREVIATIONS

BCAAs	branched-chain amino acids
BMI	body mass index
BMIz	body mass index for age
CBAs	bioactive compounds
CNCDs	chronic non-communicable diseases
IGF-1	insulin-like growth factor-1
IM	intestinal microbiota
LDL-c	low-density lipoprotein
SCAAs	sulphur-containing amino acids
TEV	total energy value
WHR	waist-to-hip ratio

INTRODUCTION

Proteins play a crucial role in biological functions, serving as essential nutrients that contribute to the creation, supplementation and support of body tissues. In addition, they are vital for metabolic processes and immune system functioning, as indicated by the Food and Agriculture Organization (FAO 2015).

Complete proteins are derived from sources such as meat, milk, eggs, fish and poultry, which contain all essential amino acids in appropriate quantities to meet the body's needs. Partially incomplete proteins, on the other hand, provide amino acids in quantities sufficient only for basic maintenance, such as those obtained from legumes, oilseeds and cereals (Cozzolino 2012).

The fundamental difference between animal and vegetable protein sources lies in their amino acid composition, which affects the availability of essential amino acid chains (Hevia-Larraín 2019). The composition of essential amino acids in the source is directly linked to the biological value and quality of the protein (Van Vliet, Burd, and Van Loon 2015).

Proteins of animal origin tend to be of higher quality than plant-based proteins. This is due to their easier digestibility and ability to provide all the essential nutrients needed to promote muscle protein properties and maintain muscle health (Reid 2022; Olaniyan 2021).

Thanks to significant investments in technology aimed at improving product quality and promoting competitiveness in the market, Brazil became the second-largest beef producer in the world in 2019, accounting for around 15.92% of global production. In addition, in 2018, Brazil was recognized as the largest exporter of chicken meat, contributing 32.81% of global exports. In the pork sector, the country ranked fourth in terms of production, with a global share of 3.33% (Embrapa 2019).

 DOI: 10.1201/9781003597926-7

Although animal proteins are known for their superior digestibility and quality, their consumption has been linked to an increased risk of cardiovascular disease (Colby et al. 2018; Rouhani et al. 2014; Weber et al. 2016; Wright et al. 2017). Cardiovascular diseases account for the majority of deaths related to non-communicable diseases, affecting more than 17.9 million people annually, according to the World Health Organization 2018.

This chapter will explore basic information about proteins, including their chemical and nutritional composition, food sources and daily consumption recommendations. It will also examine the nutritional effects of animal protein on adipose tissue and its potential consequences for human health. With these considerations in mind, this study aims to analyze the effects of animal protein consumption on adiposity.

PROTEINS OF ANIMAL ORIGIN

The human body is extremely complex, consisting of a wide variety of molecules, including proteins. Proteins are polymeric biomolecules present in all cells and perform diverse functions across various biological processes (Nelson and Cox 2018).

The monomeric precursors of proteins are 20 amino acids – eight essential ones that must be obtained from food and 12 non-essential ones that are synthesized by the body. Structurally, amino acids feature a functional carbon atom linked in a tetrahedral arrangement to a carboxyl group (-COOH), an amino group (-NH2), a hydrogen atom (-H) and a radical (-R), which differs between amino acids. Glycine is an exception because it has a hydrogen atom as a radical side group (Belitz et al. 2004).

Amino acids have two stereoisomers: L-amino acids (with the amino group on the left) and D-amino acids (with the amino group on the right). In humans, only L-amino acids are absorbed by the gastrointestinal tract. However, some proteins exposed to high temperatures may have amino acid residues in the D-form, reducing their nutritional value.

Amino acids form peptide bonds by condensing the carboxyl group of one amino acid and the amino group of another, releasing a water molecule in the process. This creates peptides with an amino-terminal end on the left and a carboxyl-terminal end on the right.

Some proteins consist solely of amino acids (simple proteins); others include non-protein chemical groups called prosthetic groups, which are permanently attached to conjugated proteins. The classification of conjugated proteins depends on the chemical nature of their prosthetic groups, resulting in proteins with unique properties and activities (Nelson and Cox 2018).

Protein functions include structural support, enzymatic activity, immunological defense, extracellular matrix formation, motor functions, transportation, hormonal regulation, construction and maintenance of muscles, bones, skin, tissues, body functions and protein synthesis (Reynolds et al. 2015). Proteins also play critical roles in food technology, influencing texture, consistency, foaming properties and emulsification.

Proteins have four structural levels: primary, secondary, tertiary and quaternary. The three-dimensional structure of a protein is stabilized mainly by non-covalent interactions. The primary structure represents a specific sequence of amino acid residues joined by peptide bonds or disulfide bonds into polypeptide chains. This sequence determines the protein's function. The secondary structure involves arrangements of amino acid residues stabilized by hydrogen bonds, forming α-helixes or pleated β-sheet conformations. The tertiary structure refers to three-dimensional arrangements of all the atoms in a protein, formed by peptide bonds, hydrogen bonds, ionic interactions, disulfide bridges and hydrophobic interactions. The quaternary structure results from combining two or more polypeptide chains stabilized by aggregated apolar side chains, hydrogen bonds and disulfide bonds (Nelson and Cox 2018).

Animal protein is categorized into dairy-based sources (e.g., casein, whey proteins) or non-dairy sources such as meat (e.g., collagen, gelatin and bovine plasma protein), poultry, eggs (e.g., egg albumin, conalbumin, ovomucoid and avidin) and fish (Xiong 2004), as shown in Figure 7.1. In

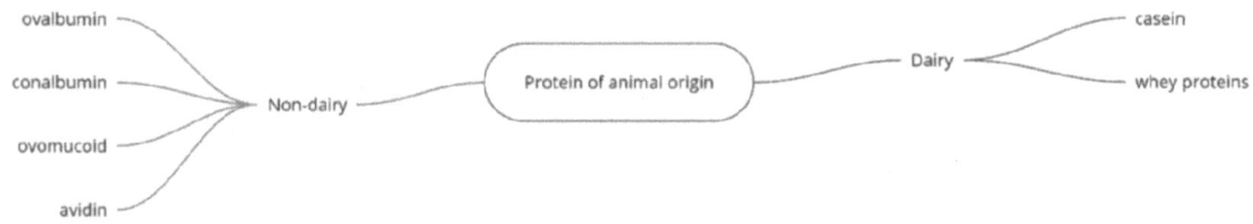

FIGURE 7.1 Animal protein is classified as non-dairy and dairy.

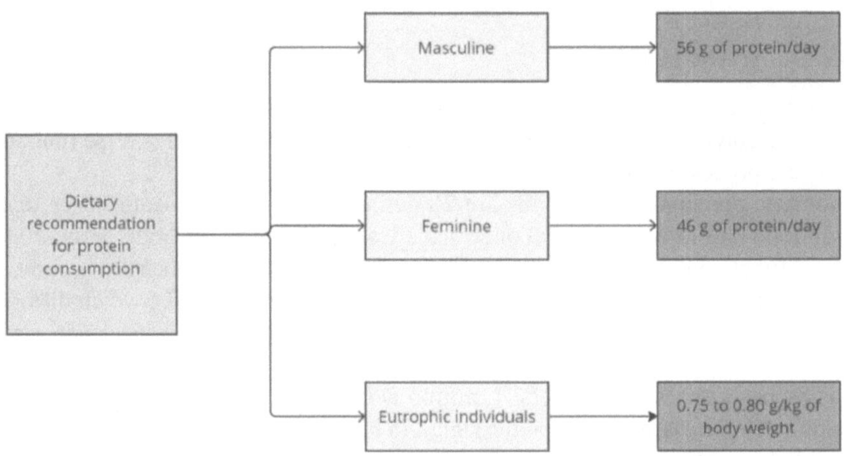

FIGURE 7.2 Daily protein recommendation according to sex and nutritional status.

terms of protein content, beef is known to contain 23.20%, lamb 21.9%, mutton 21.5% and chicken and fish 21% (Christudas et al. 2020). Dairy contains about 3.6% protein, while egg whites contain approximately 10.5%.

Proteins are among the most important nutrients for maintaining vital cellular processes essential for the metabolism and function of living beings. The recommended daily intake is 56 g/day for men and 46 g/day for women (Reynolds et al. 2005). On average, individuals should consume 0.75–0.80 g/kg body weight daily (FAO 2015), as illustrated in Figure 7.2.

CONSEQUENCES OF ADIPOSITY

Adipose tissue is a connective tissue divided into two types: brown and white. The former specializes in thermogenesis, producing heat and regulating temperature, while the latter provides thermal insulation and mechanical protection against shocks and trauma without compromising the integrity and functionality of the tissue. White adipose tissue is also the body's main energy reservoir (Fonseca-Alaniz et al. 2006), with adipocytes responsible for storing lipids in the form of triacylglycerol.

The distribution of this tissue and its accumulation in the body are indicative of health-related risks (Fonseca-Alaniz et al. 2006). Adiposity refers to excess fat in stored adipose tissue and is physiologically defined as an accumulation of fat cells in specific areas. This process is triggered by genetic factors, a sedentary lifestyle, eating habits and other lifestyle factors (Gonçalves et al. 2020).

Excess fat in adipose tissue is strongly linked to the emergence of metabolic disorders, especially visceral adiposity, which manifests as central obesity. Central obesity is associated with various

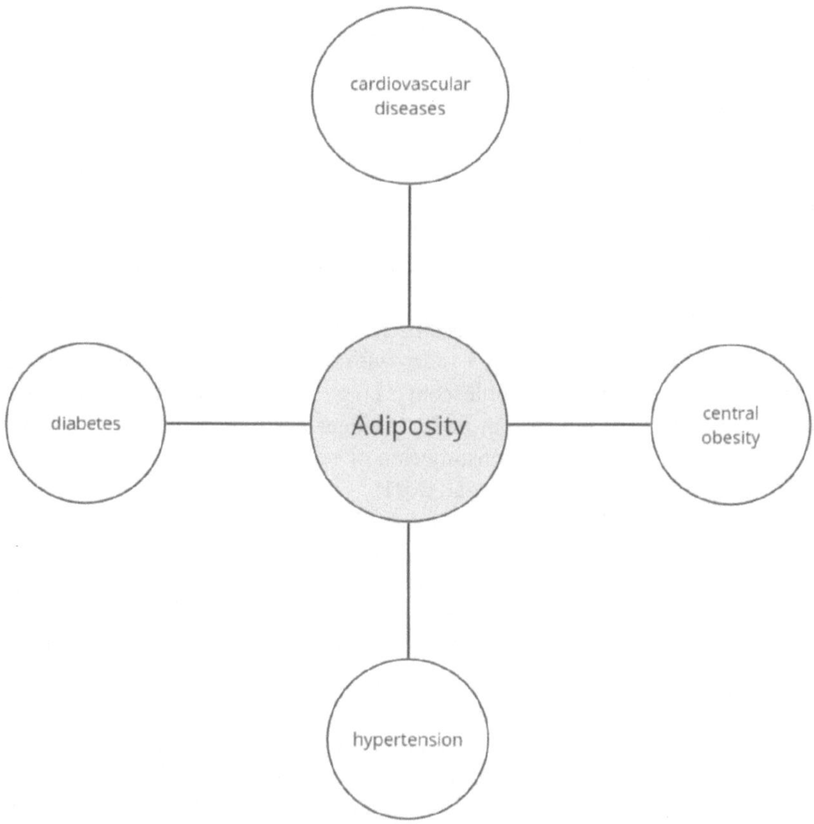

FIGURE 7.3 Central obesity is associated with several morbidities and comorbidities, including leading to the emergence and maintenance of cardiometabolic diseases, such as diabetes, hypertension and cardiovascular events.

morbidities and comorbidities, including cardiometabolic diseases such as diabetes, hypertension and cardiovascular events (Huang and Geng 2019), as illustrated in Figure 7.3.

Adiposity and its consequences are a major public health problem due to high morbidity and mortality rates, as well as reduced life expectancy. On the other hand, the implications of adiposity go beyond biology and physiology, causing psychological and social changes that negatively impact an individual's quality of life (Barbosa et al. 2021). From an economic point of view, adiposity contributes to a considerable increase in healthcare costs (OECD 2019).

Among the various factors influencing adiposity, diet plays an important and modifiable role, especially the consumption of animal protein. However, the mechanism underlying this relationship remains unclear. A study by Segovia-Siapco et al. (2020) on adolescents revealed a positive link between higher intakes of animal protein, total protein, branched-chain amino acids (BCAAs), methionine and cysteine with body adiposity and fat mass. This association was particularly evident among overweight and obese adolescents who consumed higher amounts of animal protein. According to these authors, further studies are needed to better document the relationship between animal protein consumption and adiposity, given that protein is an essential nutrient that performs several important functions in the body.

Dor et al. (2022), in a study of Israeli adolescents, found that a high daily intake of non-dairy proteins – specifically an increment of 10 g from meat and poultry – was significantly associated with overweight and obesity. However, no such association was found for proteins derived from dairy products (except butter) regarding weight or body composition changes. These authors noted that while their research found a stimulating effect of certain protein sources on body weight gain, the mechanism of action is unclear. Some studies have suggested that animal protein increases the stimulation of insulin-like growth factor-1 (IGF-1), triggering body adiposity process. Additionally, consumption of red meat, processed meats and poultry has been associated with higher body weight. Even so, further research is needed to establish causality between these findings.

A study by Lotfi et al. (2022) on obese Iranian adolescents classified as metabolically healthy and unhealthy found that substituting carbohydrates with higher intakes of either animal or vegetable protein reduced the likelihood of being metabolically unhealthy. According to these authors, animal proteins often contain significant amounts of saturated fats, which can have negative effects on human health. Thus, healthier dietary choices – such as fish, eggs, dairy products, nuts and other low-fat foods – can help reduce metabolic obesity among adolescents.

Studies carried out over a period of 6.5 years with European adult men and women produced similar findings to those observed in adolescents: consumption of animal protein was associated with weight gain regardless of gender but had a stronger association among women. This finding was attributed to the higher long-term consumption of red meat, processed meat and poultry compared to fish or dairy products (Halkjaer et al. 2011).

The relationship between meat intake and body adiposity distribution was examined by Khodayari et al. (2022) in adult Iranian individuals. The study found a greater likelihood of central adiposity among those consuming ultra-processed meats; however, no direct association was observed between red meat, fish, offal consumption and general obesity. Kim et al. (2015) suggested that ultra-processed meats have higher levels of saturated fatty acids, sodium concentrations and nitrosamines, which are considered to induce obesity (Zhu et al. 2019; Lee et al. 2016).

The multicenter ELSA-Brazil survey of adults aged 35–74 years found secondary results indicating that participants consuming higher amounts of red meat or processed meats had greater abdominal adiposity (Aprelini et al. 2019). According to Clifton (2012), routine meat consumption increases obesity risk; however, some findings remain contradictory due to individual differences such as genetics, health status, cultural influences or lack of standardization regarding red meat classifications (Khodayari et al. 2022).

NUTRITIONAL REPERCUSSIONS OF ANIMAL PROTEIN CONSUMPTION AND ITS RELATIONSHIP WITH ADIPOSITY

Obesity is characterized by the excessive accumulation of adipose tissue, resulting from a prolonged positive energy balance. This state of adipocyte hyperplasia and hypertrophy leads to significant metabolic alterations, including insulin resistance, dyslipidemia and chronic low-grade inflammation. Central adiposity, in particular, is strongly associated with an exacerbated inflammatory profile, increasing the risk of cardiovascular and metabolic diseases. In addition, the development of obesity results from multiple factors, including genetic predisposition, environmental influences and dietary imbalances (Narciso et al. 2019). Among dietary factors, the role of dietary protein in the development of obesity is still controversial. Although it is essential for cell growth and maintenance (Stang and Story 2005), recommendations on the quantity and quality of protein intake throughout life vary, reflecting divergences in the scientific literature. Studies show that protein intake and its amino acid composition may be associated with adiposity, but the findings differ between adults, children and adolescents. Elevated plasma levels of branched-chain amino acids (BCAAs: leucine, isoleucine and valine) in hypercaloric diets have been linked to pediatric obesity and insulin resistance, increasing the risk of developing type 2 diabetes (Guevara-Aguirre and Rosenbloom 2019). In a study of healthy individuals aged between 8 and 18 years, high plasma concentrations of BCAAs were found to be positively associated with age-adjusted body mass index (BMIz) (McCormack et al. 2013). However, there is controversy over the direct relationship between dietary intake of BCAAs and plasma levels of these amino acids, as other metabolic mechanisms may influence this correlation (Nagata et al. 2013). Studies conducted with healthy adults in East Asia and Western countries have shown an inverse association between dietary intake of BCAAs and overweight/obesity (Qin et al. 2011). Sulphur-containing amino acids (SCAAs: methionine and cysteine) have been linked to body weight regulation. Experimental studies indicate that increased cysteine intake can promote weight gain, while methionine restriction reduces visceral fat mass (Malloy et al. 2006). Observational investigations in humans have reported similar associations to those observed in animal models, with plasma cysteine concentration being a more robust indicator of adiposity than dietary intake (Virtanen et al. 2006). However, there are still gaps in the literature on the consumption of BCAAs and SCAAs by healthy adolescents and their relationship with body composition.

A study conducted by Segovia-Siapco et al. (2020) assessed whether the intake of protein (animal, vegetable and total), BCAAs and SCAAs is associated with general and central obesity as well as the body composition of healthy adolescents aged 12–18. Participants answered a questionnaire on diet, physical activity, lifestyle habits and demographic data. Anthropometric data such as weight, height, waist and hip circumference were also evaluated, along with body composition by bioimpedance. The analysis included 530 participants, 56% of whom were girls, with an average age of 15 years. Of these, 26% were vegetarians; the majority had a body mass index (BMI) within the normal range, while 22% were classified as overweight/obese. Around 20% were abdominally obese, with the majority being girls. The girls had more body fat and less muscle mass than the boys, which was expected. Adolescents classified as overweight/obese – both body and central – had a higher intake of fats, a lower intake of carbohydrates, less time spent in vigorous physical activity and more fat and muscle mass than their peers in the normal BMI range. The average protein intake was 16% of the total energy value (TEV), with 45% coming from animal sources and 55% from plant sources. Boys consumed a higher percentage of protein than girls, while those classified as overweight/obese consumed more protein than those within the normal BMI range.

In addition, the intake of amino acid-containing residues (AACRs) and SCAAs was lower in the group classified as being within the normal range, and these, as well as those with a normal waist-to-hip ratio (WHR), also ate more protein from plant sources than those classified as overweight/obese. The proportion of SCAAs in the total protein intake was also lower in the normal WHR group. Adolescents classified as overweight/obese consumed more red meat and chicken but less soy and legumes compared to those within the normal range. Higher intakes of total protein, animal protein, AACRs and SCAAs were significantly associated with higher BMI and body fat levels, while higher intakes of animal protein and SCAAs were positively associated with WHR.

Thus, the authors concluded that higher intakes of total protein, animal protein, AACRs and SCAAs were associated with higher overall adiposity and fat mass in healthy adolescents. In addition, there was a positive association between animal protein and SCAA intake and abdominal obesity. Adolescents with higher BMIs consumed more total and animal protein but fewer vegetables, with the exception of grains. The intake of AACRs and SCAAs was also slightly higher in overweight/obese people.

In a prospective study among adults who took part in the Diet, Genes and Obesity (Diogenes) project of the European Prospective Investigation into Cancer and Nutrition, it was found that total protein intake from foods of animal origin was positively associated with weight gain but did not alter waist circumference. Plant protein, however, was not associated with overall body obesity or central adiposity (Halkjaer et al. 2011). Another prospective study among adults found that animal protein intake increased obesity risk and vegetable protein reduced it (Bujnowski et al. 2011). Similar results were found in the GINIplus and LISAplus studies, which followed children into adolescence; these studies found that exposure to red meat during childhood was associated with increased fat mass during adolescence (Harris et al. 2016).

Previous research has examined possible mechanisms linking animal protein intake to increased obesity risk and, thus, to the degree of adiposity. Although unlikely to be the sole contributor to

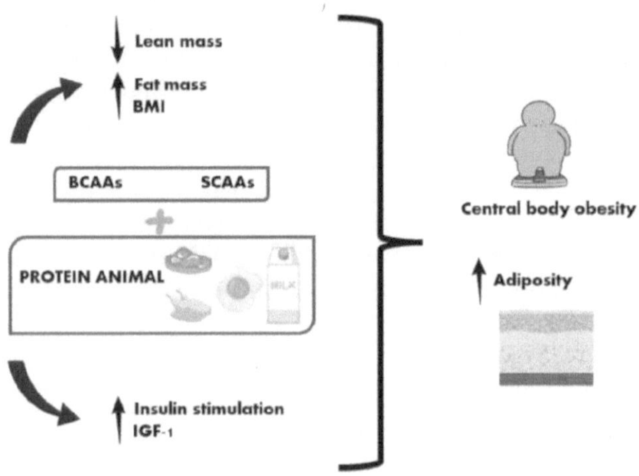

FIGURE 7.4 SCAAs – sulphur-containing amino acids; BCAAs – branched-chain amino acids; IGF-1 – insulin-like growth factor-1; BMI – body mass index.

obesity, red meat and its products are energy-rich foods, which may explain their association with overweight/obesity (Arango-Angarita et al. 2019; Rouhani et al. 2014). Meat is frequently consumed in the Western diet, especially by adolescents, and its potential health effects could therefore be significant. The positive link between animal protein intake and obesity may be related to the possible increase in insulin stimulation (World Health Organization 2018) and IGF-1 (Hoppe et al. 2004). Although IGF-1 plays an important role in regulating human growth, it has also been associated with the proliferation and differentiation of adipocytes. On the other hand, plant-based diets (particularly vegan diets) have been associated with lower circulating levels of total IGF-1 and higher levels of IGF-binding proteins, suggesting a lower intake of proteins high in essential amino acids and lower levels of IGF-1 (Allen et al. 2002), as illustrated in Figure 7.4.

Despite the many studies reporting the deleterious effects of animal protein, studies have shown that animal protein supplementation can improve adiposity, limit lean mass loss and promote visceral fat loss, as well as modulate gut microbial functions by impacting the amino acid metabolism of the gut microbiota (IM) (Bel Lassen et al. 2021). Perhaps the role of protein in the development of obesity, and consequently its relationship with the degree of adiposity, has been overlooked due to the fact that this macronutrient is essential for growth and development. Although there is still a scarcity of studies, there is growing evidence that protein intake – particularly the type of protein ingested – and certain amino acid groups are linked to overweight/obesity; however, more studies investigating this relationship are needed.

EFFECTS OF OTHER PROTEINS

The realization that diets rich in vegetables, such as those of the contemporary Mediterranean and Asian populations, reduce the risk of chronic non-communicable diseases (CNCDs) has prompted research that has identified nutrient and non-nutrient substances that act on specific physiological targets, thereby interfering with the pathogenic processes of these diseases, such as adiposity (Bastos et al. 2009). This evidence has led to changes in dietary guidelines, which now recommend eating more fruit and vegetables. Plant-based foods are well-known sources of energy, protein, vitamins and minerals, as well as the primary or sole source of vitamin C, folate, fiber and bioactive compounds (CBAs), all of which are essential for human metabolism.

Studies have also shown that the metabolism of proteins by intestinal microbiota (IM) can link obesity to the development of adiposity and its metabolic complications. Interactions between diet and IM can regulate energy metabolism (Bel Lassen et al. 2021). Thus, protein supplementation has been used as a strategy to improve diet composition; however, individual characteristics of the IM, food sources and industrial processing influence the rate of absorption and the effect of these proteins. In general, proteins from plant sources are less digestible than proteins of animal origin, and lower protein digestibility results in a greater presence of undigested peptides in the colon, which will be metabolized by bacteria (Alvarez Calatayud et al. 2018).

In the distal intestine, undigested peptides contribute to the production of short-chain fatty acids, ammonia, sulphur-containing metabolites (e.g., hydrogen sulfide and methanethiol) and neuroactive compounds (e.g., tryptamine, serotonin, phenethylamine and histamine). Some of these metabolites are related to deleterious health effects; for example, ammonia and hydrogen sulphide favor the development of colon cancer and inflammatory bowel disease, while others, such as branched-chain amino acids, can have beneficial effects (Pereira 2019), as can be seen in Figure 7.5.

Depending on their nature, protein-rich diets can have a direct effect on the composition of the intestinal bacterial community by increasing the abundance of bile-tolerant microorganisms (such as *Alistipes*, *Bilophila* and *Bacteroides*) and decreasing the levels of *Firmicutes* that metabolize dietary plant polysaccharides (such as *Roseburia*, *Eubacterium rectale*, *Bifidobacteria* and *Ruminococcus bromii*) (Bel Lassen et al. 2021). Despite the promising findings regarding protein supplementation, it is important to consider that IM responds differently to dietary interventions, and its composition can condition the host's response. In this sense, genetic assessment of bacterial composition and function can help predict responses to specific dietary interventions, opening the door to personalized nutrition based on the gut microbiota.

For overweight/obese individuals, a protein intake similar to that recommended for the general population is advised, with an emphasis on plant-based proteins (e.g., 100 g soy contains 1.3 g saturated fat and 0 mg cholesterol) and fish (2.9 g saturated fat and 68 mg cholesterol per 100 g on average). This approach aims to reduce the intake of saturated fats and cholesterol, since red

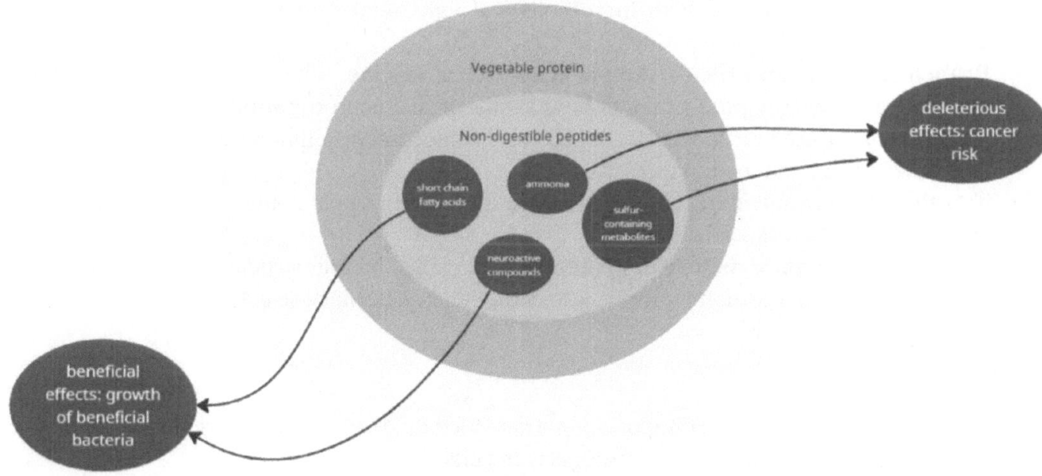

FIGURE 7.5 The consumption of vegetable proteins is associated with several beneficial health effects, including improved lipid profile, reduced cardiovascular risk, modulation of the intestinal microbiota and reduced systemic inflammation.

meat has higher levels (7.3 g saturated fat and 85 mg cholesterol per 100 g on average) (NCEP 2001). Replacing animal protein with soy protein lowers blood concentrations of total cholesterol and LDL-c in hypercholesterolemic individuals (NCEP 2002). Diets low in saturated fats and cholesterol containing 25 g/day of soy protein can reduce serum LDL-c concentrations by up to 5% (NCEP 2001, 2002). In summary, there is a consensus that protein intake should correspond to 15% of the TEV.

FINAL CONSIDERATIONS

Protein is present in various foods in varying quantities and is indispensable in the human diet. The foods with the highest protein content are meat, eggs, dairy products and grains. Protein of animal origin is made up of essential amino acids. Proteins of plant origin, on the other hand, must be combined with foods from the same group to obtain full nutritional value, as they lack some essential amino acids. The nutritional and biological value of a food varies according to the amount of amino acids present. However, as a secondary energy source, protein's role in obesity has been overlooked.

Although these animal protein sources are known for their better digestibility and quality, their consumption has been linked to an increased risk of CNCDs, such as obesity and cardiovascular diseases. In this context, the intake of protein, especially animal protein – including BCAAs and SCAAs – has been associated with central body obesity and changes in body composition characterized by a reduction in lean mass and an increase in fat mass in healthy adolescents.

Obesity is a disease caused by various factors, including genetic, psychological and nutritional. It is characterized by excess fat in the adipose tissue, leading to adiposity, which is caused by excessive calorie intake with lower energy expenditure. Changing one's diet is one of the first steps towards controlling weight and obesity, and it's a long and laborious process. However, it's important to note that this diet must be adapted to each individual's needs.

Replacing animal proteins – especially processed red meats – with plant-based proteins can confer substantial long-term health benefits. Public health recommendations should, therefore, focus on improving the choice of protein sources.

MINI DICTIONARY OF TERMS

- **Adiposity:** Excess fat in the body.
- **Animal protein:** Proteins with high biological value and which have all the essential amino acids in sufficient quantities.
- **Branched-chain amino acids:** Amino acids such as leucine, isoleucine and valine, which are involved in energy production, protein synthesis and neurotransmitters.
- **Sulphur-containing amino acids:** Amino acids that contain sulphur, such as cysteine and its oxidized form and methionine.
- **Tetrahedral arrangement:** The organization of atoms in a pentatomic molecule with four atoms attached to a central atom.
- **Three-dimensional structure of proteins:** Determined by four structural levels: primary structure, secondary structure, tertiary structure and quaternary structure.

SUMMARY POINTS

- Proteins are one of the most important nutrients for the functioning of organisms and are responsible for coordinating vital processes in cells.
- The recommended protein intake is 0.75–0.80 g/kg body weight.
- Diet plays an important and modifiable role in body adiposity; animal proteins are particularly implicated, although the mechanism of action is still unclear.

- Consumption of amino acid-containing residues and sulphur-containing amino acids is associated with a higher risk of general adiposity and increased fat mass.
- There is growing evidence that protein intake – particularly specific types of protein and certain amino acid groups – may contribute to overweight/obesity risks. However, more studies investigating this relationship are needed.

REFERENCES

Aguirre, J. G. and Rosenbloom, A. L. 2019 Branched chain and aromatic amino acids are associated with insulin resistance during pubertal development in girls. *J. Adolesc. Health.* 65, 313–314.

Alaniz, M. H. F.; Takada, J.; Vale, M. I. C, A. and Lima, F. B. 2006. O tecido adiposo como centro regulador do metabolismo / The adipose tissue as a regulatory center of the metabolismo. *Arq. Bras. Endocrinol. Metab.* 50(2), 216–229.

Allen, N. E. et al. 2002. The associations of diet with sérum insulin-like growth factor I and its main binding proteins in 292 women meat-eaters, vegetarians, and vegans. *Cancer Epidemiol. Biomark. Prev.* 11(11), 1441–1448.

Aprelini, C. M. O.; Luft, V. C.; Meléndez, G. V.; Schmidt, M. I.; Mill, J. G. and Molina, M. D. C. B. 2019. Consumption of red and processed meat, insulin resistance, and diabetes in the Brazilian longitudinal study of adult health (ELSA-Brasil). *Rev. Panam. Salud. Publica.* 3(43), e40.

Arango-Angarita, A.; Levy, S. T. and Ramírez, R. S. 2019. Dietary energy density is associated with body mass index-for-age in Mexican adolescents. *Matern. Child. Nutr.* 15, e12664.

Barbosa, I. A.; Silveira, M. F.; Fonseca, A. D. G.; Brito, M. F. S. F.; Pinho, L. D. and Silva, C. S. D. O. 2021. Qualidade de vida e adiposidade em adolescentes: Efeitos diretos e indiretos. *Ciência & Saúde Coletiva.* 26, 5661–5670.

Bastos, D. H. M.; Rogero, M. M. and Arêas, J. A. G. 2009. Mecanismos de ação de compostos bioativos dos alimentos no contexto de processos inflamatórios relacionados à obesidade. *Arq. Bras. Endocrinol Metab.* 53, 5.

Belitz, H. D.; Grosch, W. and Shieberle, P. 2004. Amino acids, pepetides, proteins. *Food Chemistry.* 8, 88.

Bujnowski, D.; Xun, P.C.; Daviglus, M.L.; Van Horn, L.; He, K. and Stamler, J. 2011. Longitudinal association between animal and vegetable protein intake and obesity among men in the united states: The Chicago Western Electric study. *J. Am. Die. Assoc.* 111, 1150–1155.

Calatayud, A. G. et al. 2018. Dieta y microbiota. Impacto en la salud. *Nutri. hospitalaria.* 35, 11–15.

Christudas, S.; Devaraj, R. and Xu, B. 2020. Different impacts of plant proteins and animal proteins on human health through altering gut microbiota. *Funct. Foods in Health and Dis.* 10(5), 228–241.

Clifton, P. 2012. Effects of a high protein diet on body weight and comorbidities associated with obesity. *Br J Nutri.* 108(2), S122–S129.

Colby, S. et al. 2018. Low protein intake among college males is associated with increased bmi. *Top. Clin. Nutr.* 33, 219–226.

Cozzolino, S. M. F. 2012. *Biodisponibilidade de nutrientes*, 4th ed. Barueri, SP: Manole.

Dor, C.; Stark, A. H.; Dichtiar, R.; Keinan-Boker, L. and Sinai, T. 2022. Non-Dairy animal protein consumption is positively associated with overweight and obesity in israeli adolescents. *Foods (Basel, Switzerland).* 11(14), 2072.

Embrapa: Empresa Brasileira de Pesquisa Agropecuária. 2019. *Participação da Produção Brasileira no Mundo – 2018.* Disponível em. https://www.embrapa.br/suinos-eaves/cias/mapas.

Expert Panel on Detection, Evaluation. 2001. Executive summary of the third report of the National Cholesterol Education Program (NCEP) expert panel on detection, evaluation, and treatment of high blood cholesterol in adults (adult treatment panel III). *JAMA.* 285(19), 2486–2497.

FAO. 2015. The state of food insecurity in the world 2015. Meeting the 2015 International Hung.

Gonçalves, M. F.; Rosa, A. N. and Lima, F. V. 2020. Tratamento do fibro edema geloide no glúteo com a utilização da radiofrequência e endermoterapia. *Health and Bioscienc.* 1(2), 1–11.

Guevara-Aguirre, J.; Rosenbloom, A.L. 2019. Branched chain and aromatic amino acids are associated with insulin resistance during pubertal development in girls. *J. Adolesc. Health.* 65, 313–314.

Halkjaer, J. et al. 2011. Intake of total, animal and plant protein and subsequent changes in weight or waist circumference in European men and women: The Diogenes project. *Int. J. Obes.* 35, 1104–1113.

Harris, C. et al. 2016. Prospective associations of meat consumption during childhood with measures of body composition during adolescence: Results from the GINIplus and LISAplus birth cohorts. *Nutr. J.* 15, 101.

Hoppe, C.; Udam, T. R.; Lauritzen, L.; Molgaard, C.; Juul, A. and Michaelsen, K. F. 2004. Animal protein intake, sérum insulin-like growth factor i, and growth in healthy 2.5-y-old Danish children. *Am. J. Clin. Nutr.* 80, 447–452.

Huang, T.; Geng, T. T. 2019. Central obesity and all-cause and cause specific mortality: A systematic review and dose-response meta-analysis of prospective studies. *Circulation.* 139, AP219.

Khodayari, S.; Sadeghi, O.; Safabakhsh, M. and Khosravi, H, M. 2022. Meat consumption and the risk of general and central obesity: The Shahedieh study. *BMC Research Notes.* 15(1), 339.

Kim, Y.; Keogh, J. and Clifton, P. 2015. A review of potential metabolic etiologies of the observed association between red meat consumption and development of type 2 diabetes mellitus. *Metabolism.* 64(7), 768–779.

Larraín, V. M. A. H. 2019. *Influência de fonte proteica da dieta nas adaptações crônicas ao treinamento de força.* Dissertação de Mestrado. Escola de Educação Física e Esporte da Universidade de São Paulo. São Paulo.

Lassen, B. P. et al. 2021. Protein supplementation during an energy-restricted diet induces visceral fat loss and gut microbiota amino acid metabolism activation: A randomized trial. *Scien. Rep.* 11(1), 15620.

Lee, S. K. and Kim, M. K. 2016. Relationship of sodium intake with obesity among Korean children and adolescents: Korea national health and nutrition examination survey. *Br J Nutr.* 115(5), 834–841.

Lotfi, K. S. et al. 2022. Dietary total, plant and animal protein intake in relation to metabolic health status in overweight and obese adolescents. *Sci Rep.* 12, 10055.

Malloy, V. L.; Krajcik, R. A.; Bailey, S. J.; Hristopoulos, G.; Plummer, J. D. and Orentreich, N. 2006. Methionine restriction decreases visceral fat mass and preserves insulin action in aging male Fischer 344 rats independent of energy restriction. *Aging Cell.* 5, 305–314.

McCormack, S. E.; Shaham, O.; McCarthy, M. A. et al. 2013. Circulating branched-chain amino acid concentrations are associated with obesity and future insulin resistance in children and adolescents. *Pediatr. Obes.* 8, 52–61.

Nagata, C.; Nakamura, K.; Wada, K.; Tsuji, M.; Tamai, Y.; Kawachi, T. 2013. Branched-chain amino acid intake and the risk of diabetes in a Japanese community: The Takayama study. *Am. J. Epidemiol.* 178, 1226–1232.

Narciso, J.; Silva, A. J.; Rodrigues, V. et al. 2019. Behavioral, contextual and biological factors associated with obesity during adolescence: A systematic review. *PLoS One.* 14, e0214941.

National Cholesterol Education Program (US). 2002. *Expert Panel on Detection, and Treatment of High Blood Cholesterol in Adults.* Third report of the National Cholesterol Education Program (NCEP) Expert Panel on detection, evaluation, and treatment of high blood cholesterol in adults (Adult Treatment Panel III). No. 2. The Program.

Nelson, D. L. and Cox, M. M. 2018. *Princípios de bioquímica de Lehninger.* Porto Alegre-Artmed. 7th ed.

OCDE. 2019. *O fardo pesado da obesidade: a economia da prevenção; Organização para a Cooperação e Desenvolvimento Econômico.* Paris: França.

Olaniyan, E. T.; O'Halloran, F. and McCarthy, A. L. 2021. Considerações sobre proteínas dietéticas para síntese de proteínas musculares e preservação da massa muscular em idosos. *Nutr Res Rev.* 34, 147–157.

Pereira, C. A. P. 2019. Microbiota intestinal humana y dieta. *Ciencia y Tecnología.* 12(1), 31–42.

Qin, L. Q.; Xun, P.; Bujnowski, D.; Daviglus, M.L.; Van Horn, L.; Stamler, J. and He, K. 2011. Higher branched-chain amino acid intake is associated with a lower prevalence of being overweight or obese in middle-aged East Asian andWestern adults. *J. Nutr.* 141, 249–254.

Reid-McCann, R. J.; Brennan, S. F.; McKinley, M. C. and McEvoy, C. T. 2022. O efeito da proteína animal versus vegetal na massa muscular, força muscular, desempenho físico e sarcopenia em adultos: protocolo para uma revisão sistemática. *Rev. do sistema.* 11, 64.

Reynolds, C. M.; Gray, C.; Li, M.; Segovia, S. A. and Vickers, M. H. 2015. Early life nutrition and energy balance disorders in offspring in later life. *Nutrients.* 7(9), 8090–8111.

Rouhani, M. H.; Abargouei, A. S.; Surkan, P. J. and Azadbakht, L. 2014. Is there a relationship between red or processed meat intake and obesity? A systematic review and meta-analysis of observational studies. *Obes. Rev.* 15, 740–748.

Segovia-Siapco, G. S.; Khayef, G.; Pribis, P.; Oda, K.; Haddad, E. and Sabaté, J. 2020. Animal protein intake is associated with general adiposity in adolescents: The teen food and development study. *Nutrients.* 12(1), 1–36.

Stang, J. and Story, M. 2005. Nutrition needs of adolescents. In *Guidelines for Adolescent Nutrition Services*, edited by J. Stang and M. Story, 21–34. Minneapolis, MN: University of Minnesota.

Van, V. S.; Burd, N. A. and Van, L. L. J. 2015. The skeletal muscle anabolic response to plantversus animal-based protein consumption. *J Nutr.* 145(9), 1981–1991.

Virtanen, J. K.; Voutilainen, S.; Rissanen, T. H. et al. 2006. High dietary methionine intake increases the risk of acute coronary events in middle-aged men. *Nutr. Metab. Cardiovas. Dis.* 161, 113–120.

Weber, M.; Luque, V.; Escribano, J. et al. 2016. E_ect of early protein supply on body fat deposition during infancy and childhood: A randomized trial. *J. Ped. Gastroent Nutr.* 62, 668–669.

World Health Organization. 2018. *Enfermedades no transmisibles.* OMS. [acessado em 01 de setembro de 2022]. Disponível em: https://www.who.int/es/news-room/fact-sheets/detail/noncommunicable-diseases. Pages/overweight-obesity-statistics.aspx

Wright, M.; Sotres-Alvarez, D.; Mendez, M. A. and Adair, L. 2017. The association of trajectories of protein intake and age-specific protein intakes from 2 to 22 years with BMI in early adulthood. *Br. J. Nutr.* 117, 750–758.

Xiong, Y. L. 2004. Muscle proteins. In *Proteins in Food Processing*, edited by R. Y. Yada. Cambridge, UK: Woodhead Publishing.

Zhu, J.; Kong, Y. Yu, J. et al. 2019. Consumption of drinking water N-Nitrosamines mixture alters gut microbiome and increases the obesity risk in young male rats. *Environ. Pollut.* 248, 388–396.

8 Red Meat Protein and Links with Disease

A Focus on Diabetes

Margarete Almeida Freitas de Azevedo, Nayara Vieira do Nascimento Monteiro, and Maria do Carmo de Carvalho e Martins

ABBREVIATIONS

ACL	ATP-citrate lyase
AGEs	Advanced glycation end products
AKT	Protein kinase B
BCAA	Branched-chain amino acid
BCAT	Branched-chain aminotransferase
BCKAs	Branched-chain ketoacids
BCKDH	Branched-chain ketoacid dehydrogenase complex
BDK	Alpha-branched-chain ketoacid dehydrogenase kinase complex
BMI	Body mass index
DM	Diabetes mellitus
EDCs	Endocrine-disrupting compounds
HOMA-IR	Homeostatic index model assessment for insulin
hs-CRP	High-sensitivity C-reactive protein
IKK	Inhibitor of kappa B serine kinase
IL-1β	Interleukin 1β
IL-6	Interleukin 6
IR	Insulin resistance
IRS	Insulin receptor substrate
IRS-1	Insulin receptor substrate 1
IRS-2	Insulin receptor substrate 2
JNK	c-Jun NH2-terminal kinase
MCP-1	Monocyte chemotactic protein-1
mTOR1	Mammalian target of rapamycin complex 1
mTOR2	Mammalian target of rapamycin complex 2
NF-κB	Nuclear factor kappa beta
PAI-1	Plasminogen activator inhibitor-1
PI3K	Phosphoinositide 3-kinase
PKC	Protein kinase C
PKCδ	Protein kinase Cδ
PPM1K	Protein phosphatase dependent on Mg^{2+}/Mn^{2+} 1K
Rag GTPases	Ras-related GTP-binding proteins
ROS	Reactive oxygen species

DOI: 10.1201/9781003597926-8

S6k1	S6 ribosomal protein kinase 1
SFA	Saturated fatty acid
SHBG	Sex hormone-binding globulin
SICI	Continuous insulin infusion
SMCG	Continuous glucose monitoring system
TMAO	Trimethylamine N-oxide
TNF-α	Tumor necrosis factor-alpha

INTRODUCTION

Great emphasis has been placed on the effects of a high biological value protein diet on human health, particularly in terms of the possible benefits for body weight control, metabolism and healthy aging (Huang et al. 2020). However, substantial evidence indicates that the source of protein, and not just the amount consumed, is important (Zheng et al. 2022).

Despite the evidence and interest in the beneficial effects of dietary protein on health, there are still no recommendations about the food sources of this macronutrient (Huang et al. 2020). According to Al-Shaar et al. (2020), a substantial body of evidence from randomized trials and observational studies indicates that high red meat consumption is associated with an increased risk of morbidity and mortality from major chronic diseases such as cardiovascular disease, diabetes mellitus, metabolic syndrome and cancer.

Red meat is a source of protein with high biological value and is a good source of branched-chain amino acids (BCAAs) and B vitamins. On the other hand, processed red meat in particular contains relatively high levels of saturated fat, sodium and preservatives (e.g., nitrites), which can exacerbate inflammation, trigger oxidative stress and contribute to the development of insulin resistance (IR) (Struijk et al. 2022).

Estimates suggest that a global shift from current diets to plant-based diets could reduce the risk of premature mortality from chronic non-communicable diseases by 18–21% (Neufingerl and Eilander 2021). Dietary protein and amino acids are essential modulators of glucose metabolism; however, high protein intake has detrimental effects on glucose homeostasis, resulting in insulin resistance and increased gluconeogenesis (Tremblay et al. 2007). A comparison of the amount of protein and essential amino acids in foods of plant and animal origin can be seen in Table 8.1.

Several mechanisms have been proposed from longitudinal observational studies to explain why the combined intake of red meats can increase the risk of cardiometabolic diseases, such as cardiovascular disease and type 2 diabetes mellitus (O'Connor et al. 2021) (Figure 8.1).

Diabetes mellitus (DM) is a metabolic disorder characterized by persistent hyperglycemia due to a deficiency in the production and/or action of insulin. DM is classifiedbased on its etiopathogenesis into type 1 diabetes (DM1), type 2 diabetes (DM2), gestational diabetes or other forms (Rodacki et al. 2023).

DM1 results from the destruction of the beta cells in the pancreatic islets – which may involve autoimmune processes – while DM2, the most prevalent type, is greatly influenced by environmental factors such as diet, sedentary lifestyle, insulin resistance or variations in the levels of secretion of this hormone (Golbert et al. 2019).

Given the growing interest in understanding how red meat consumption contributes to disease development – as well as the important role of dietary factors in preventing DM2 – the aim of this chapter is to describe the impact of red meat protein on DM2.

TABLE 8.1
Composition of Essential Amino Acids and Protein Content in Beef, Poultry and Chickpeas per 100g

Amino Acid	Bovine (g/100g)*	Poultry (g/100g)*	Chickpea (g/100g)**
Isoleucine	10.4	9.5	0.36
Leucine	16.3	15.4	0.48
Histidine	7.5	6.2	0.24
Lysine	18.5	18.4	0.91
Methionine	5.5	4.9	0.12
Phenylalanine	9.1	9.2	0.42
Threonine	9.4	8.5	0.06
Tryptophan	2.6	2.3	-
Total Protein***	32.8	32.0	21.2

*Agroceres (2021); **Meurer (2019); ***TACO (2011).

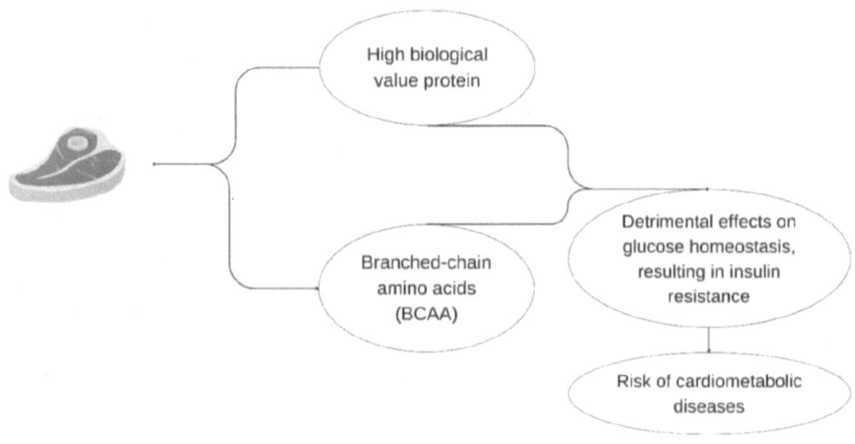

FIGURE 8.1 Cardiometabolic diseases associated with red meat consumption.

ASSOCIATION BETWEEN RED MEAT PROTEIN CONSUMPTION AND DIABETES MELLITUS

With regard to the relationship between red meat protein consumption and DM, Schwingshackl (2017) reported from a systematic review with a meta-analysis the existence of a relationship between the intake of 12 main food groups and the risk of DM2. The meta-evidence was classified as high for the consumption of red meat, processed meat and sugary drinks in relation to the increased risk of developing diabetes mellitus.

Red meat consumption has been associated with a pro-inflammatory state and, consequently, a higher risk of DM2 and metabolic syndromes, but the mechanisms involved in this association are not fully defined (Mazidi et al. 2021). However, it is known that the metabolic disorders associated with insulin resistance are widespread, involving not only carbohydrate and fat metabolism but also protein metabolism (Adeva et al. 2011).

High dietary protein intake can negatively affect glucose homeostasis, contributing to insulin resistance and increased gluconeogenesis (Tian et al. 2017). An analysis conducted across three prospective cohort studies (Nurses' Health Study, Nurses' Health Study II and Health Professionals Follow-up Study), covering more than four million person-years of follow-up, suggested that a higher intake of animal protein was associated with an increased risk of DM2, while a higher intake of vegetable protein was associated with a modestly reduced risk (Malik et al. 2016) (Figure 8.2).

Furthermore, in a cohort study carried out with Danish women, Ibsen et al. (2021) showed that replacing red meat with eggs can reduce the risk of DM2 in middle-aged adults. Replacing red meat with milk, yogurt, whole grains or refined grains was also associated with a reduction in the risk of this disease.

Wittenbecher et al. (2015), in a nested case-cohort study with a sample of 2,681 people, including 688 incident cases of diabetes, found that increased ferritin values, as well as low glycine values and changes in serum concentrations of liver-specific lipid metabolites (lysophosphatidylcholines, sphingomyelins, diacyl phosphatidylcholines and acyl-alkyl phosphatidylcholines), were associated with total red meat consumption and, independently of red meat, linked to diabetes risk. In contrast, Lajous et al. (2011), in the prospective study analyzing processed and unprocessed red meat consumption among 66,118 French women, found a direct association only for processed red meat.

A positive correlation between the intake of red and processed meat and the risk of DM2 was found in four meta-analyses of prospective studies. Red and processed meats contain components such as saturated fatty acids (SFAs), advanced glycation end products (AGEs), BCAAs, heme iron, trimethylamine N-oxide (TMAO) and endocrine-disrupting compounds (EDCs), which may contribute to insulin resistance. In the case of heme iron, an increase in its stock can contribute to the oxidation of fatty acids, increasing the production of free radicals, which act to damage pancreatic beta cells (Kim et al. 2015). Aune et al. (2009) identified 12 cohort studies showing the relative risk (RR) for DM2 as follows: for total meat, RR = 1.17 (95% CI: 0.92–1.48); for red meat, RR = 1.21 (95% CI: 1.07–1.38); for processed meat, RR = 1.41 (95% CI: 1.25–1.60). A second meta-analysis concluded that eating red meat was not associated with DM2 (n = 5; RR = 1.16; 95% CI: 0.92–1.46; P = 0.25); however, eating processed meat was associated with a 19% higher risk (n = 7; RR = 1.19; 95% CI: 1.11–1.27; P = <0.001) (Micha et al. 2010).

Pan et al. (2011) confirmed these findings in a meta-analysis involving 442,101 participants and 28,228 cases of diabetes: for unprocessed red meat, RR = 1.19 per 100 g/day (95% CI: 1.04–1.37), and for processed red meat, RR = 1.51 per 50 g/day (95% CI: 1.25–1.83). Feskens et al. (2013) corroborated these results by showing that processed meats are associated with a potentially higher risk

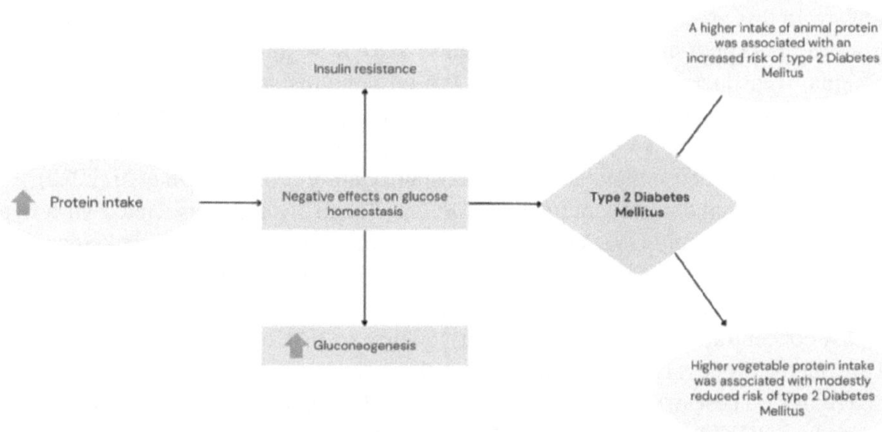

FIGURE 8.2 Dietary protein intake and the risk of type 2 diabetes development.

of DM2 and coronary heart disease compared to unprocessed red meats, although the latter still pose a significant risk for these conditions.

An association between the consumption of red and processed meat and the development of IR and DM was also found in the Longitudinal Study of Adult Health (ELSA-Brazil), which included 15,105 civil servants aged 35–74 years from public universities or research institutions across Brazil (Aprelini et al. 2019). The authors showed that high red meat consumption increased the likelihood of new DM cases by 40% among men and women (95% CI: 1.04–1.96); only high processed meat consumption increased IR risk – a precursor to DM and cardiovascular disease.

In another cohort study of 53,163 participants from the Danish Diet, Cancer and Health study – where there were 6,879 incident cases of DM2 – totally replacing red meat with fish or poultry reduced DM2 risk; replacing processed red meats with unprocessed ones also lowered risks (Ibsen et al. 2019).

POSSIBLE RELATIONSHIP BETWEEN RED MEAT PROTEIN BCAAS AND THE RISK OF DIABETES MELLITUS

High protein intake in the diet has negative effects on glucose homeostasis, facilitating insulin resistance and increasing gluconeogenesis by activating the mammalian target of rapamycin complex 1 (mTOR1), a nutrient sensor that operates a negative feedback loop towards insulin receptor substrate 1 (IRS-1) signaling. This involves serine phosphorylation that inhibits tyrosine phosphorylation and blocks the ectopic expression and translocation of glucose transporters, resulting in insulin resistance (Tian et al. 2017; Ye et al. 2020).

BCAAs are particularly sensitive to the action of insulin, and their metabolism is profoundly altered in IR states (Adeva et al. 2011). The BCAA leucine activates mTOR1 similarly to insulin while also activating S6 ribosomal protein kinase 1 (S6K1), which, when persistently activated, leads to the phosphorylation of IRS-1 serine, inhibiting it. This interruption in signaling can result in the targeting of proteolysis via a proteasomal pathway (Kim et al. 2015).

In pancreatic islet beta cells, this negative regulation mediated by mTOR1/S6K1 constitutes an intracellular mechanism that suppresses excessive insulin signaling and the mammalian target of rapamycin 2 complex (mTOR2) under physiological conditions and contributes to the control of cell growth and homeostasis (Nakamura et al. 2022). However, chronic hyperactivation of mTOR1/S6K1, when induced by obesity and overnutrition, can attenuate insulin and mTOR2 signaling, resulting in decreased beta cell function and the development of DM2 (Figure 8.3).

The activation of the mTOR1 pathway by leucine via constituents of the Ras-related GTP-binding proteins (Rag GTPases) family is considered an important mechanism in the impaired insulin signaling pathway. In this process, serum branched-chain ketoacids (BCKAs) inhibit insulin signaling by inhibiting the phosphorylation of protein kinase B (AKT), an important and universal factor in insulin signal transduction. When activated, the tyrosine residues of substrates 1 and 2 of the insulin receptors (IRS-1 and IRS-2) are phosphorylated by the insulin receptors, binding them to the enzyme phosphoinositide 3-kinase (PI3K). This activation triggers AKT and protein kinase C (PKC), which regulate glucose metabolism by phosphorylating proteins (Du et al. 2022).

BCAAs, such as leucine, isoleucine and valine, have been strongly associated with hyperinsulinemia, insulin resistance and DM due to the inhibition of the α-branched-chain ketoacid dehydrogenase complex (BCKDH) via insulin. This inhibition leads to decreased catabolism of BCAAs (Bawadi et al. 2022) (Figure 8.4). However, controversy remains as to whether the increase in plasma BCAA concentrations is a cause or a consequence of IR (Rousseau et al. 2019). BCKAs are produced during the process of BCAA metabolism through deamination by branched-chain aminotransferase (BCAT). These α-keto acids undergo irreversible oxidative decarboxylation by the mitochondrial enzyme BCKDH, which is inhibited by the α-ketoacid dehydrogenase branched-chain

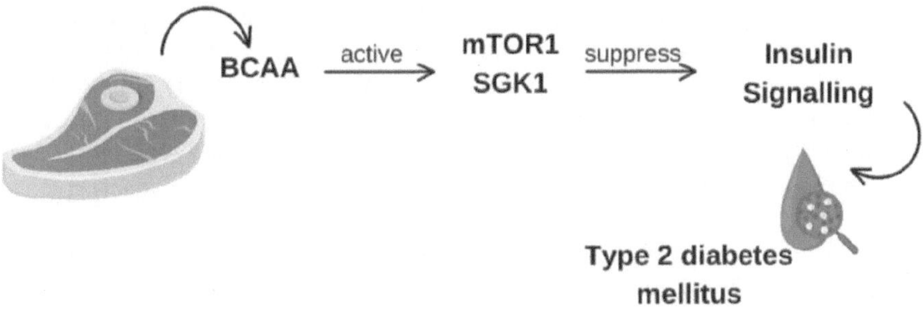

FIGURE 8.3 BCAA-induced activation of mTOR1/S6K1 is associated with obesity and overnutrition.

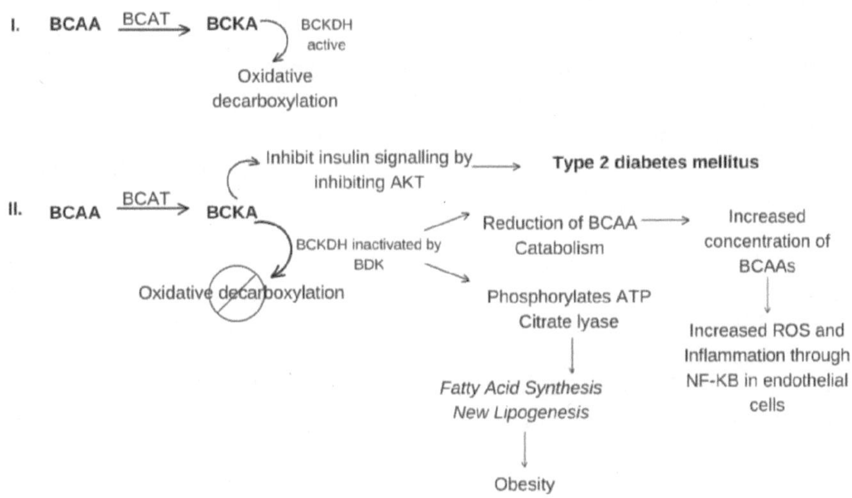

FIGURE 8.4 BCAA metabolism processes and the production of branched-chain ketoacids (BCKAs).

kinase (BDK) complex and is activated by the Mg2+/Mn2+-dependent protein phosphatase 1K (PPM1K) (White et al. 2021).

It is plausible that the loss of BCAA catabolizing enzyme function could increase BCKA concentration in skeletal muscle and disrupt downstream metabolism, including insulin signaling (Biswas et al. 2020). However, it is still unclear whether defects in the expression and activity of the muscle BCAA-catabolizing enzyme precede or follow obesity-induced IR.

Decreased metabolization of BCAAs contributes to another important aspect of obesity. For instance, it has been proposed that BDK may increase obesity risk by inhibiting BCAA metabolism in obese animals. Inflammation may also negatively regulate BCAA catabolism and lipogenesis in visceral adipose tissue, partly through the nuclear factor kappa beta (NF-κB) pathway. Additionally, endoplasmic reticulum stress may also negatively regulate the BCAA metabolism pathway (Du et al. 2022).

The relationship between BCAA and IR in cases of excess adipose tissue was discussed by Zhou et al. (2019). Through integrated genomic analyses, these authors revealed a unique association between the expression of the gene responsible for BCAA catabolism – specifically those encoding BCKDH subunits – and IR, which was observed only in individuals with obesity among human and mouse populations. This suggests an adiposity-dependent relationship between the BCAA catabolic pathway and IR.

In experimental models of obesity and IR in rodents, it has been shown that obesity impairs BCAA catabolism by negatively regulating multiple enzymes of the BCAA catabolic pathway at the transcriptional level, including BCAT and BCKDH (White et al. 2021). This relationship with obesity is still unclear, but defects in BCAA catabolism may lead to increased fatty acid synthesis, as BDK may not only regulate BCAA metabolism but also phosphorylate ATP-citrate lyase (ACL), a critical enzyme in fatty acid synthesis, as well as regulate the de novo lipogenesis pathway (Du et al. 2022) (Figure 8.4).

It is important to note that a similar negative transcriptional regulation of BCAA catabolic enzymes is observed in the white adipose tissue of humans with obesity, which is reversed by bariatric surgery. It has been shown that bariatric surgery in individuals with obesity and DM2 causes more robust reductions in BCAA and related metabolites than those observed with behavioral intervention when the two groups are matched for the amount of weight loss (Laferrère et al. 2011).

In addition, amino acids affect glucose metabolism by stimulating insulin and glucagon secretion, and by serving as substrates for gluconeogenesis. Although stimulating insulin secretion is expected to prevent hyperglycemia resulting from increased gluconeogenesis, this process may not be sufficiently compensated for in individuals with impaired insulin secretion (Sluijs et al. 20109). Considering that BCAAs are modulators of insulin secretion, another possible mechanism by which hyperaminoacidemia could contribute to the development of DM would be through hyperinsulinemia, a condition that leads to the exhaustion of pancreatic beta cells and a consequent reduction in insulin synthesis and release (Wang et al. 2011).

When evaluating the direct effects of high levels of BCAA and the possible mechanisms involved in the generation of reactive oxygen species (ROS) and inflammation in human endothelial cells, Zhenyukh et al. (2018) observed that high concentrations of BCAAs can trigger oxidative stress and inflammation through the activation of the NF-κB pathway in endothelial cells and the vasculature, probably contributing to endothelial dysfunction and cardiovascular disease often found in different pathological conditions associated with the presence of high BCAA levels, which may be in line with the role of overactivation of the AKT-mTOR1 axis and the resulting metabolic diseases such as DM2 (Figure 8.4).

Regarding the relationship between BCAAs and DM2, a study of a large cohort of racially and ethnically diverse postmenopausal women in the United States showed that higher meat intake increased the risk of DM2 by 4% in postmenopausal women, and that the association between BCAAs and diabetes risk was attenuated but remained positive after adjusting for meat intake, suggesting that BCAA intake is partly, but not entirely, contributing to the association of meat with DM2 risk (Isanejad et al. 2017). In view of the results found, the authors of the aforementioned study stated that the increased risk of DM2 associated with higher meat consumption can be explained in part by the contribution of meat to BCAA intake and/or possibly by the increase in heme iron load.

OTHER COMPOUNDS PRESENT IN RED MEAT AND THEIR POSSIBLE RELATIONSHIP WITH THE RISK OF DIABETES MELLITUS

Components present in red meat, such as iron, have been shown to increase the formation of ROS, which could possibly affect the function of pancreatic islet beta cells (Sanders et al. 2022). Iron overload in the body can act as a strong pro-oxidant and trigger oxidative stress, producing damage to cells in different organs, such as pancreatic beta cells, resulting in reduced insulin synthesis and secretion and impaired insulin signaling for proper glycemic control (Esfandiar et al. 2019).

In addition, red meat contains bioavailable heme iron, which has the potential to increase the storage of iron and advanced glycation end products, as well as increase the generation of free radicals (O'Connor et al. 2021). The high iron content in red meat has also been linked to the induction of inflammation by stimulating the release of pro-inflammatory cytokines such as interleukin 6 (IL-6), interleukin 1β (IL-1β) and tumor necrosis factor-α (TNF-α) (Shiraseb et al. 2022). However, most humans seem to have an innate biological ability to regulate circulating iron concentrations when dietary iron fluctuates, which is therefore able to minimize the generation of free radicals and inflammation related to excess iron, and it is unlikely that this chronic inflammation can explain the positive associations between red meat intake and the risk of DM (O'Connor et al. 2021).

However, it is possible that the body's iron-binding capacity may be exceeded by the consumption of processed meat containing large amounts of heme iron, triggering oxidative stress as a result of the increase in free iron and acting as a pro-inflammatory agent (Shiraseb et al. 2022).

Another possible explanation is that high protein intake in the diet can worsen glycemic control due to the ability of amino acids to impair glucose synthesis by inhibiting glucose transport and phosphorylation, leading to insulin resistance (Bawadi et al. 2022). In addition, excessive intake of red meat can increase the chances of abnormalities in lipid metabolism and induce inflammatory changes (Sun et al. 2022). For instance, Shiraseb et al. (2022) assessed the relationship between red, white and processed meat consumption and inflammatory and metabolic biomarkers in overweight and obese women. They showed that red meat intake positively associated with levels of plasminogen activator inhibitor-1 (PAI-1), high-sensitivity C-reactive protein (hs-CRP) and monocyte chemoattractant protein-1 (MCP-1).

High circulating concentrations of fatty acids can also interfere with insulin signal transduction by regulating inflammation and oxidative stress, leading to IR. Fatty acids can influence IRS activity by regulating IRS protein phosphorylation or act at the IRS transcriptional level through histone acetylation. In adipocytes, fatty acids activate protein kinase Cδ (PKCδ), leading to the activation of inhibitor of serine kinase kappa B (IKK) and c-Jun NH2-terminal kinase (JNK), which catalyze the phosphorylation of IRS-1, ultimately reducing insulin-induced glucose uptake (Ye et al. 2020).

Red meat has also been associated with weight gain and body fat accumulation, which increases inflammatory processes and further explains its association with an increased risk of developing DM (Chai et al. 2017). Obesity is characterized by low levels of chronic inflammation and is linked to changes in insulin sensitivity, systemic arterial hypertension, atherosclerosis and even some cancers (Khanna et al. 2022). Obese people have high levels of pro-inflammatory adipokines (cytokines) such as angiotensinogen, TNF-α, IL-6, leptin, MCP-1 and resistin (Dias et al. 2017; Ellulu et al. 2017; Fernández-Sánchez et al. 2011). This chronic inflammation is another mechanism proposed to explain the positive associations between red meat consumption and DM risk, as both BCAAs and fatty acids play a crucial role in regulating metabolic homeostasis (O'Connor et al. 2021; Ye et al. 2020).

In processed red meat, another plausible explanation for its association with DM2 risk involves nitrites and nitrates used during processing. These substances are converted into nitrosamines in the gastrointestinal tract, which are toxic to pancreatic beta cells, increasing the DM risk (Tong et al. 2009). However, red meat intake has no independent influence on the risk of cardiometabolic diseases in the short term (O'Connor et al. 2021) (Figure 8.5).

Evidence suggests that replacing red meat with other protein sources helps reduce the risk of chronic non-communicable diseases such as DM. For example, Ley et al. (2014) showed that isocaloric replacement of red meat with alternative protein foods like poultry, fish, legumes and nuts was associated with a favorable profile of biomarkers of inflammation and glycemic control in a cross-sectional study with female participants without diabetes from the Nurses' Health Study. Thus, for those who choose to consume red meat, similar to what is recommended for all other protein-rich foods, it should be consumed in the context of a healthy dietary pattern, including adequate intake of fruit, vegetables and whole grains, as well as respecting energy needs to reduce cardiometabolic risk.

THE EFFECTS OF OTHER PROTEINS

Red meat protein intake has been associated with an increased risk of developing chronic non-communicable diseases, such as DM. Several mechanisms may explain this relationship, most notably mechanisms involving the role of BCAAs in the development of insulin resistance. However,

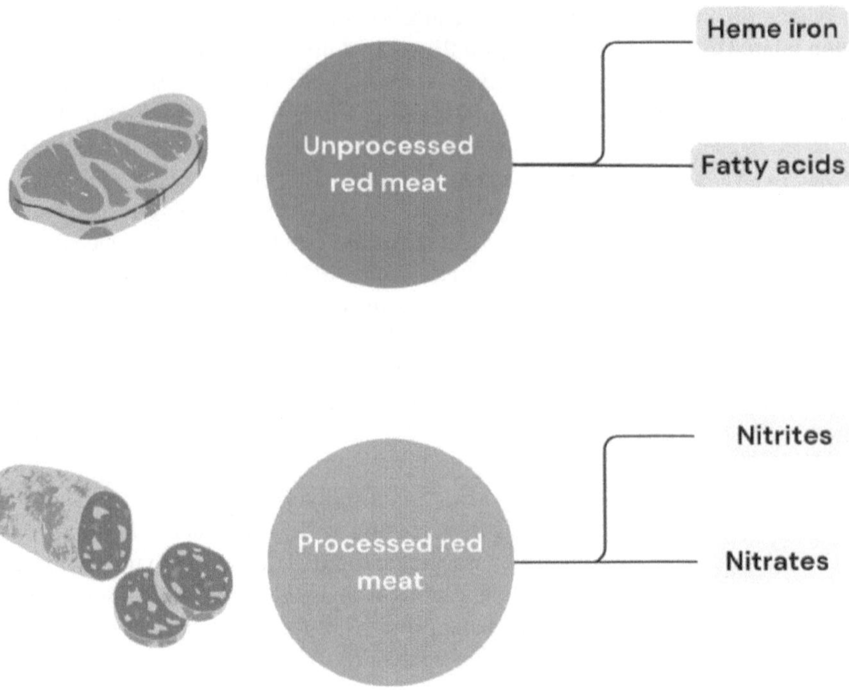

FIGURE 8.5 Other compounds in red meat associated with diabetes mellitus.

long-term follow-up studies are needed to produce conclusive evidence about these effects in humans. Such studies could demonstrate the importance of lifestyle and dietary strategies that replace red meat with other protein sources, such as poultry or fish, for diabetes prevention and management. Plant-based products – such as soy protein, wheat, chickpeas and lentils – are used because they have a high protein content (Luz et al. 2022). Meat analogs are also gaining prominence in the market, but improvements are needed, especially in sensory aspects, such as texture, appearance and flavor (Evangelista 2022).

MINI DICTIONARY OF TERMS

- **ATP-citrate lyase:** A key enzyme in the de novo synthesis of fatty acids, responsible for generating cytosolic acetyl-CoA and oxaloacetate.
- **Branched-chain amino acids:** Essential amino acids leucine, valine and isoleucine, which have a branched aliphatic side chain. They are called "essential" because the body does not have the enzymes needed to synthesize them.
- **De novo lipogenesis:** A biological process by which carbon atoms from carbohydrates (glucose, fructose, lactose, etc.) are transformed into lipids (fatty acids).
- **Endocrine disruptors:** Exogenous (non-natural) chemical substances, or mixtures of chemical substances, that interfere with any aspect of hormonal action.
- **GIP** (Gastric Inhibitory Peptide or Glucose-Dependent Insulinotropic Peptide) is an incretin hormone produced by K cells in the small intestine (primarily in the duodenum and jejunum). It is released in response to the ingestion of nutrients, especially carbohydrates and fats.
- **Heme iron:** Iron found in the hemoglobin molecules of foods of animal origin; it is considered the most nutritionally important because it is highly bioavailable.
- **Insulin receptor substrate 1:** A protein involved in insulin signal transduction.

- **Trimethylamine N-oxide:** An intestinal metabolite derived from the microbiota when digesting food of animal origin.

KEY FACTS ABOUT RED MEAT PROTEIN AND DIABETES

- High dietary protein intake has negative effects on glucose homeostasis by activating the mammalian target of rapamycin complex 1 (mTOR1).
- Amino acids affect glucose metabolism by stimulating insulin and glucagon secretion while serving as substrates for gluconeogenesis.
- High consumption of BCAAs, substances that modulate insulin secretion, may increase the risk of developing DM due to hyperinsulinemia, which could result in the exhaustion of pancreatic beta cells and a reduction in insulin synthesis.
- Components present in red meat, such as iron, can act as strong pro-oxidants and trigger oxidative stress, causing damage to cells in different organs, such as pancreatic beta cells, resulting in reduced insulin synthesis and secretion and impaired insulin signaling for proper glycemic control.
- Excessive intake of red meat can increase the chances of abnormalities in lipid metabolism and inflammatory alterations, as the high presence of fatty acids can interfere with insulin signal transduction by regulating inflammation and oxidative stress, leading to IR.

SUMMARY POINTS

- Red meat consumption has been associated with a pro-inflammatory state and, consequently, a higher risk of DM2 and metabolic syndromes. Nowadays, protein metabolism, not just carbohydrate and fat metabolism, has also been associated with metabolic disorders such as insulin resistance. Other components present in red meat, such as saturated fatty acids, iron and sodium, may also be factors related to the increased risk of developing diabetes mellitus.
- BCAAs are involved in modulating insulin signaling pathways and controlling glucose homeostasis, so altered metabolism of these amino acids can result in the development of insulin resistance. BCAAs, such as leucine, isoleucine and valine, have been strongly associated with hyperinsulinemia, insulin resistance and diabetes mellitus. However, it remains controversial whether the increase in plasma BCAA concentrations is a cause or a consequence of IR.

REFERENCES

Adeva MM, Calviño J, Souto G, Donapetry C. Insulin resistance and the metabolism of branched-chain amino acids in humans. *Amino Acids*. 2011 Oct 8;43(1):171–81.

Al-Shaar L, Satija A, Wang DD, et al. Red meat intake and risk of coronary heart disease among US men: prospective cohort study. *BMJ*. 2020;371:m4141.

Aprelini CMO, Luft VC, Meléndez GV, Schmidt MI, Mill JG, Molina MCB. Consumo de carne vermelha e processada, resistência insulínica e diabetes no Estudo Longitudinal de Saúde do Adulto (ELSA-Brasil). *Rev Panam Salud Publica*. 2019;43:e40.

Aune D, Ursin G, Veierød MB. Meat consumption and the risk of type 2 diabetes: a systematic review and meta-analysis of cohort studies. *Diabetologia*. 2009;52:2277–2287.

Bawadi H, Al-Bayyari N, Tayyem R, Shi Z. A ingestão de proteínas entre os pacientes com diabetes tratados com insulina está ligada a um mau controlo glicémico: Findings of NHANES data. *Diabetes Metab Syndr Obes*. 2022 Mar 8;15:767–775.

Biswas D, Dao KT, Mercer A, Cowie AM, Duffley L, El Hiani Y, Kienesberger PC, Pulinilkunnil T. Branched-chain ketoacid overload inhibits insulin action in the muscle. *J Biol Chem*. 2020 Nov 13;295(46):15597–15621.

Chai W, Morimoto Y, Cooney RV, Franke AA, Shvetsov YB, Le Marchand L, Haiman CA, Kolonel LN, Goodman MT, Maskarinec G. Dietary red and processed meat intake and markers of adiposity and inflammation: the multiethnic cohort study. *J Am Coll Nutr.* 2017 Jul;36(5):378–385.

Dias PC, Henriques P, Anjos LA dos, Burlandy L. Obesity and public policies: conceptions and strategies adopted by the Brazilian government. *Cad Saude Publica.* 2017;33(7):1–12.

Du C, Liu WJ, Yang J, Zhao SS, Liu HX. The role of branched-chain amino acids and branched-chain α-Keto acid dehydrogenase kinase in metabolic disorders. Front Nutr. 2022;9:932670.

Ellulu MS, Patimah I, Khaza'ai H, Rahmat A, Abed Y. Obesity and inflammation: the linking mechanism and the complications. *Arch Med Sci.* 2017 Jun; 4(13): 851–863.

Esfandiar Z, Hosseini-Esfahani F, Mirmiran P, Habibi-Moeini AS, Azizi F. Red meat and dietary iron intakes are associated with some components of metabolic syndrome: Tehran Lipid and Glucose Study. *J Transl Med.* 2019;17:1–9.

Evangelista TADO. Plant-Based: uma revisão sobre proteínas alternativas como substitutos da carne. 2022. Available from: https://monografias.ufop.br/bitstream/35400000/4635/6/MONOGRAFIA_Prote%c3%adnasAlternativasSubstitutos.pdf

Fernández-Sánchez A, Madrigal-Santillán E, Bautista M, Esquivel-Soto J, Morales-Gonzalez A, Esquivel-Chirino C, et al. Inflammation, oxidative stress, and obesity. *Int J Mol Sci.* 2011 May;12(5):3117–3132.

Feskens EJM, Sluik D, Van Woudenbergh GJ. Meat consumption, diabetes, and its complications. *Curr Diab Rep* [Internet]. 2013;13(2):298–306.

Golbert A, Vasques ACJ, Faria ACRA, Lottenberg AMP, Joaquim AG, Vianna AGD, et al. Diretrizes da Sociedade Brasileira de Diabetes 2019-2020. São Paulo: Clannad; 2019, pp. 19–20.

Huang J, Liao LM, Weinstein SJ, Sinha R, Graubard BI, Albanes D. Association between plant and animal protein intake and overall and cause-specific mortality. JAMA Intern Med. 2020;180(9):1173–1184.

Ibsen D B, Jakobsen MU, Halkjær J., Tjønneland A., Kilpeläinen TO, Parner ET, & Overvad K. Replacing red meat with other nonmeat food sources of protein is associated with a reduced risk of type 2 diabetes in a danish cohort of middle-aged adults. *J Nutr.* 2021;151(5):1241–1248.

Ibsen, DB, Warberg, CK, Würtz, AML et al. Replacement of red meat with poultry or fish and risk of type 2 diabetes: a Danish cohort study. *Eur J Nutr.* 2019;58:2705–2712.

Isanejad M, LaCroix AZ, Thomson CA, Tinker L, Larson JC, Qi Q, Qi L, Cooper-DeHoff RM, Phillips LS, Prentice RL, Beasley JM. Branched-chain amino acid, meat intake and risk of type 2 diabetes in the women's health initiative. *Br J Nutr.* 2017 Jun;117(11):1523–1530.

Khanna D, Khanna S, Khanna P, Kahar P, Patel BM. Obesity: A chronic low-grade inflammation and its markers. *Cureus.* 2022 Feb 28;14(2):e22711.

Kim Y, Keogh J, Clifton P. A review of potential metabolic etiologies of the observed association between red meat consumption and development of type 2 diabetes mellitus. *Metabolism.* 2015 Jul;64(7):768–779.

Laferrère B, Reilly D, Arias S, Swerdlow N, Gorroochurn P, Bawa B, Bose M, Teixeira J, Stevens RD, Wenner BR, Bain JR, Muehlbauer MJ, Haqq A, Lien L, Shah SH, Svetkey LP, Newgard CB. Differential metabolic impact of gastric bypass surgery versus dietary intervention in obese diabetic subjects despite identical weight loss. *Sci Transl Med.* 2011 Apr 27;3(80):80re2.

Lajous M, Tondeur L, Fagherazzi G, de Lauzon-Guillain B, Boutron-Ruaualt MC. Clavel-chapelon F. Processed and unprocessed red meat consumption and incident type 2 diabetes among french women. *Diabetes Care.* 2011 Nov 18;35(1):128–130.

Ley SH, Sun Q, Willett WC, Eliassen AH, Wu K, Pan A, Grodstein F, Hu FB. Associations between red meat intake and biomarkers of inflammation and glucose metabolism in women. *Am J Clin Nutr.* 2014 Feb;99(2):352–360.

Luz GM, Pallone JAL. Alimentos à base de plantas: dietas, tendências de mercado, composição nutricional e ensaios in vitro de bioacessibilidade e biodisponibilidade de minerais. *Avanços em Ciência e Tecnologia de Alimentos.* 2022;6:12–29. Available from: https://downloads.editoracientifica.org/articles/220207845.pdf

Malik VS, Li Y, Tobias DK, Pan A, Hu FB. Dietary protein intake and risk of type 2 diabetes in US men and women. *Am J Epidemiol.* 2016 Apr 15;183(8):715–728.

Mazidi M, Kengne A, George E, Siervo M. The association of red meat intake with inflammation and circulating intermediate biomarkers of type 2 diabetes is mediated by central adiposity. *Br J Nutr.* 2021;125(9):1043–1050.

Meurer MC. Efeitos do ultrassom nas propriedades tecnológicas da água de cozimento do grão-de-bico (aquafaba). lumeufrgsbr [Internet]. 2019 [cited 2024 Mar 22]. Available from: https://lume.ufrgs.br/handle/10183/193024

Micha R, Wallace SK, Mozaffarian D. Red and processed meat consumption and risk of incident coronary heart disease, stroke, and diabetes mellitus: a systematic review and meta-analysis. *Circulation.* 2010;121(21):2271–2283.

Nakamura M, Satoh N, Horita S, Nangaku M. Insulin-induced mTOR signaling and gluconeogenesis in renal proximal tubules: a mini-review of current evidence and therapeutic potential. *Front Pharmacol* [Internet]. 2022;13:1015204.

Neufingerl N, Eilander A. Nutrient intake and status in adults consuming plant-based diets compared to meat-eaters: a systematic review. *Nutrients.* 2021 Dec 23;14(1):29.

O'Connor LE, Kim JE, Clark CM, Zhu W, Campbell WW. Effects of total red meat intake on glycemic control and inflammatory biomarkers: a meta-analysis of randomized controlled trials. *Adv Nutr.* 2021 Feb 1;12(1):115–127.

Pan A, Sun Q, Bernstein AM, Schulze MB, Manson JE, Willett WC, et al. Red meat consumption and risk of type 2 diabetes: 3 cohorts of US adults and an updated meta-analysis. *Am J Clin Nutr* [Internet]. 2011 Aug 10;94(4):1088–1096.

Rousseau M, Guénard F, Garneau V, Allam-Ndoul B, Lemieux S, Pérusse L, Vohl MC. Associations between dietary protein sources, Plasma BCAA and short-chain acylcarnitine levels in adults. *Nutrients.* 2019 Jan 15;11(1):173.

Sanders LM, Wilcox ML, Maki KC. Red meat consumption and risk factors for type 2 diabetes: a systematic review and meta-analysis of randomized controlled trials. *Eur J Clin Nutr.* 2022;77(2):156–165.

Schwingshackl L, Hoffmann G, Lampousi AM, Knüppel S, Iqbal K, Schwedhelm C, et al. Food groups and risk of type 2 diabetes mellitus: a systematic review and meta-analysis of prospective studies. *Eur J Epidemiol* [Internet]. 2017;32(5):363–375.

Rodacki M, Teles M, Gabbay M, Montenegro R, Bertoluci M, Lamounier R. Classificação do diabetes. Diretriz Oficial da Sociedade Brasileira de Diabetes. 2023. doi:10.29327/557753.2022-1.

Shiraseb F, Hosseininasab D, Mirzababaei A, Bagheri R, Wong A, Suzuki K, et al. Red, white, and processed meat consumption related to inflammatory and metabolic biomarkers among overweight and obese women. *Front Nutr* [Internet]. 2022 [cited 2023 Apr 6];9:1015566.

Sluijs I, Beulens JWJ, van der A DL, Spijkerman AMW, Grobbee DE, van der Schouw YT. Dietary intake of total, animal, and vegetable protein and risk of type 2 diabetes in the european prospective investigation into cancer and nutrition (EPIC)-NL study. *Diabetes Care.* 2009 Oct 13;33(1):43–48.

Struijk EA, Fung TT, Rodríguez-Artalejo F, Bischoff-Ferrari HA, Hu FB, Willett WC, Lopez-Garcia E. Protein intake and risk of frailty among older women in the Nurses' Health Study. *J Cachexia Sarcopenia Muscle.* 2022 Jun;13(3):1752–1761.

Sun L, Yuan J, Chen QC, Xiao WK, Ma GP, Liang JH, et al. Red meat consumption and risk for dyslipidaemia and inflammation: A systematic review and meta-analysis. *Front Cardiovasc Med* [Internet] [cited 2023 May 2]. 2022;9:996467.

Tabela TACO Online – Tabela Brasileira de Composição de Alimentos [Internet]. Available from: www.tabelatacoonline.com.br. https://www.tabelatacoonline.com.br/

Tian S, Xu Q, Jiang R, Han T, Sun C, Na L. Dietary protein consumption and the risk of type 2 diabetes: a systematic review and meta-analysis of cohort studies. *Nutrients.* 2017 Sep 6;9(9):982.

Tremblay F, Lavigne C, Jacques H, Marette A. Role of dietary proteins and amino acids in the pathogenesis of insulin resistance. *Annu Rev Nutr.* 2007;27:293–310.

Tong M, Neusner A, Longato L, Lawton M, Wands JR, de la Monte SM. Nitrosamine exposure causes insulin resistance diseases: relevance to type 2 diabetes mellitus, non-alcoholic steatohepatitis, and Alzheimer's disease. *J Alzheimers Dis.* JAD [Internet]. 2009;17(4):827–844.

Wang TJ, Larson MG, Vasan RS, Cheng S, Rhee EP, McCabe E, et al. Metabolite profiles and the risk of developing diabetes. *Nat Med.* 2011 Mar 20;17(4):448–53.

White PJ, McGarrah RW, Herman MA, Bain JR, Shah SH, Newgard CB. Insulin action, type 2 diabetes, and branched-chain amino acids: a two-way street. *Mol Metab.* 2021 May;101261.

Wittenbecher C, Mühlenbruch K, Kröger J, Jacobs S, Kuxhaus O, Floegel A, et al. Amino acids, lipid metabolites, and ferritin as potential mediators linking red meat consumption to type 2 diabetes. *Am J Clin Nutr* [Internet]. 2015 May 6;101(6):1241–1250.

Ye Z, Wang S, Zhang C, Zhao Y. Coordinated modulation of energy metabolism and inflammation by branched-chain amino acids and fatty acids. *Front Endocrinol.* 2020;11:617.

Zheng J, Zhu T, Yang G, Zhao L, Li F, Park YM, Tabung FK, Steck SE, Li X, Wang H. The isocaloric substitution of plant-based and animal-based protein in relation to aging-related health outcomes: a systematic review. *Nutrients.* 2022 Jan 9;14(2):272.

Zhenyukh O, González-Amor M, Rodrigues-Diez RR, Esteban V, Ruiz-Ortega M, Salaices M, et al. Branched-chain amino acids promote endothelial dysfunction through increased reactive oxygen species generation and inflammation. *J Cell Mol Med.* 2018 Jul 31;22(10):4948–4962.

Zhou M, Shao J, Wu CY, Shu L, Dong W, Liu Y, et al. Targeting BCAA catabolism to treat obesity-associated insulin resistance. *Diabetes* [Internet] [cited 2020 May 4]. 2019 Sep 1;68(9):1730–1746.

9 Animal Protein Intake and Cancer Risk

Adina Bianca Boşca, Carmen Mihaela Mihu, Anida Maria Băbţan, and Aranka Ilea

ABBREVIATIONS

AFB1	Aflatoxin B1
AFM1	Aflatoxin M1
CLA	Conjugated linoleic acid
CYP450	Cytochrome P450
DNA	Deoxyribonucleic acid
HAAs	Heterocyclic aromatic amines
IGF-1	Insulin-like growth factor-1
Neu5Gc	Nonhuman sialic acid N-glycolylneuraminic acid
NOCs	N-nitroso compounds
PAHs	Polycyclic aromatic hydrocarbons
PhIP	2-Amino-1-methyl-6-phenylimidazo[4,5-b]pyridine
PUFAs	Polyunsaturated fatty acids
TMAO	Trimethylamine N-oxide
TNF-α	Tumour necrosis factor-α
UHT	Ultra-high temperature

INTRODUCTION

In nutrition research, the effects of high-protein diet patterns on overall health have gained significant focus during the last decades. According to numerous population-based studies, the positive effects of high-quality protein diets include: (i) improved metabolism by delivering essential amino acids necessary for vital body functions; (ii) optimization of body weight through increased fat loss; and (iii) reduction in metabolic syndrome risk factors such as circulating glycaemic, lipid, and lipoprotein profiles. However, the type of dietary proteins is essential, since animal and plant sources vary significantly in terms of nutritional profiles – macronutrients, micronutrients, amino acid contents, and polyphenols – with different health outcomes. Numerous studies have demonstrated an association between long-term high animal protein intake and the risk of type 2 diabetes, cardiovascular diseases, and cancer (Budhathoki et al. 2019; Chen et al. 2020; Huang et al. 2020). Moreover, high protein intake leads to changes in dietary patterns, with subsequent influence on other macronutrients and micronutrients. Lower amounts of other dietary macronutrients, mainly carbohydrates, could have negative effects due to the lack of fibre (Budhathoki et al. 2019).

SOURCES AND CHARACTERISTICS OF DIFFERENT ANIMAL PROTEINS

Animal proteins encompass several categories: (i) unprocessed red meat; (ii) processed meats; (iii) poultry; (iv) fish; (v) dairy; and (vi) eggs (Table 9.1).

DOI: 10.1201/9781003597926-9

TABLE 9.1
Animal Protein Sources, Characteristics, and Constituents

Source	Characteristics	Macronutrients	Micronutrients	Constituents with Beneficial Effects	Constituents with Potential Negative Effects
Red meat (e.g., pork, beef, veal and lamb)	Lean red meat provides essential nutrients	Complete proteins and all essential amino acids, lipids	Vitamins: B3, B6, B12; Minerals: Fe, Zn, Se, P	Endogenous antioxidants and bioactive substances: taurine, L-carnitine, choline, glutathione, creatine, coenzyme Q10	Heme-iron, cholesterol, and saturated fatty acids
Processed meats (e.g., ham, salami, and bacon)	Prepared by drying, smoking, and/or curing the meat	Mainly proteins and lipids	Depending on the processing methods	Depending on the processing methods	Heme-iron and additives such as salt, preservatives based on nitrite and/or nitrate, artificial flavourings, and colourants
Poultry (e.g., chicken, turkey, ducks, or geese)	Lean meat, lower in saturated fat (if without skin)	Proteins, lipids	Vitamins: B2, B3, B6; Minerals: Se, K	Cationic antimicrobial peptides, cathelicidins	Cholesterol in skin; antibiotics; hormones
Fish and seafood	Fat fish contains more PUFAs	Proteins, lipids	Vitamins: A, D; Minerals: Se, Fe, Zn, Fe, Ca	PUFAs	Hg and environmental pollutants
Milk and dairy (e.g., yoghurt, kefir, cheese, and butter)	Contain growth factors, enzymes, and probiotics in milk derivates	Complete proteins, lipids, carbohydrates	Vitamins: D, B2, B12; Minerals: Ca, P, Mg, K, Zn	Antioxidants, caseins, PUFAs, CLA	Hormones, including IGF-1; aflatoxins; saturated fats
Eggs	Provide complex nutrients and contain growth factors	Proteins, lipids, carbohydrates	Vitamins: A, D, E, K, and almost all B vitamins; Minerals: S, K, Na, Ca, P, Mg, Fe	Egg peptides and phospholipids	Choline, cholesterol

CLA – conjugated linoleic acid; IGF-1 – insulin-like growth factor-1; PUFAs – polyunsaturated fatty acids.

Red meat, including pork, beef, veal, and lamb, is an important source of complete proteins containing all the amino acids and micronutrients, such as vitamins B3, B6, and B12, and minerals like iron, zinc, selenium, and phosphorus (Geiker et al. 2021). Lean red meat provides essential nutrients that are scarce or absent in other foods and also contains endogenous antioxidants and bioactive substances, such as taurine, L-carnitine, choline, glutathione, creatine, and coenzyme Q10. Depending on the source, meat can contain high amounts of cholesterol and saturated fatty acids, with potential negative health effects (Kulczyński et al. 2019).

Processed meats, such as ham, salami, and bacon, are prepared using various methods for preservation purposes for a longer period. Preparation methods involve drying, smoking, and/or curing the meat by adding ingredients such as salt, sugar, nitrite- and/or nitrate, flavourings and colourants. The body of evidence indicates that consumption of processed meat products is associated with an increased risk of different types of cancer (Chan et al. 2011; Guo J et al. 2015).

Dietary poultry meat is represented mainly by chicken and turkey, and less by other fowl such as ducks or geese. Evidence regarding the link between poultry consumption and the risk of cancer is controversial (Daniel et al. 2011).

Fish is a source of vitamin D and selenium, and high amounts of marine omega-3 polyunsaturated fatty acids (PUFAs) are abundant in fish fat (Zheng JS et al. 2013).

Milk and dairy products play an essential role in the diet due to their complex composition (Lu et al. 2016). Milk is rich in caseins and whey proteins, regarded as complete proteins due to the presence of all nine essential amino acids. Moreover, milk derivatives, like yoghurt and kefir, contain probiotic bacteria with beneficial effects (Guo Y et al. 2015). All dairy products also contain other macronutrients – lipids and carbohydrates – growth factors, enzymes, probiotics, and micronutrients, including minerals such as calcium, phosphorus, magnesium, zinc, potassium, and vitamins such as vitamin D, and some B vitamins, including B2 (riboflavin) and B12 (cobalamin) (Davoodi et al. 2016). Caseins and whey have numerous health benefits, including anticarcinogenic activity and immunomodulation (Davoodi et al. 2016). Some components, including insulin-like growth factor-1 (IGF-1), are associated with increased cancer risk, whereas others, such as conjugated linoleic acid (CLA), magnesium, and potassium, have anti-cancer properties (Alzahrani et al. 2022). A positive association between whole milk intake and prostate cancer risk has been reported in the meta-analysis conducted by Lu et al. (2016).

Eggs contain all the macronutrients necessary to support the developing embryo, especially proteins, as well as lipids, carbohydrates, growth factors, and micronutrients: vitamins and minerals (Lee and Paik 2019). Egg white and yolk contain proteins with high nutritional value; egg white contains mainly proteins like ovalbumin, ovotransferrin, ovomucoid, ovoglobulin, ovomucin, lysozyme, ovomacroglobulin, and others. Yolk proteins are represented by low-density lipoproteins and high-density lipoproteins, and smaller amounts of phosvitin, livetin, and riboflavin-binding proteins. Choline is present in all animal foods; in eggs, high amounts of choline are found in the structure of phospholipids, as different chemical compounds: phosphatidylcholine, lysophosphatidylcholine, and glycerophosphocholine (Awwad et al. 2012; Richman et al. 2012). Lipids are mainly present in the yolk and consist of triglycerides, phospholipids, cholesterol, and cerebroside (Richman et al. 2012). Carbohydrates are primarily represented by glucose in the egg white. Minerals such as sulphur, potassium, sodium, calcium, phosphorus, magnesium, and iron are found mainly in the egg white, whereas phosphorus is present in the yolk phospholipids. Egg peptides exert various biological effects, including anti-cancer, immunomodulatory, antioxidant, and antimicrobial activity (Lee and Paik 2019). Egg components with detrimental health effects include choline and cholesterol (Awwad et al. 2012; Richman et al. 2012; Keum et al. 2015).

An important aspect is that animal protein sources could also contain components and substances with carcinogenic effects or other negative impacts on health. These components include heme-iron found in red meat, liver, and processed meats; choline present in large amounts in dairy products, eggs, and liver; and cholesterol in eggs (Awwad et al. 2012). Some fish and seafood may contain mercury or other potential carcinogenic substances and environmental pollutants (Daniel et al. 2011).

The animal's diet has a major impact on the quality of meat and dairy products, with significant differences between grass or grain-fed cows, and the contents of potentially harmful compounds such as pesticides, antibiotics, and hormones. Grass-fed cows provide beef and dairy products with higher contents of antioxidants, omega-3 PUFAs, and CLA (Daley et al. 2010). Cow feedstuffs can be contaminated with mycotoxins, such as aflatoxin B1 (AFB1), which is metabolized and excreted in milk as aflatoxin M1, the hydroxylated metabolite of AFB1; both aflatoxins exert carcinogenic, toxic, mutagenic, and teratogenic effects on humans (Marchese et al. 2018). Moreover, dairy products may have different qualities depending on the production method and the hormones used for increasing milk production, such as recombinant bovine growth hormone, which could be responsible for increased cancer risk (Alzahrani et al. 2022).

IMPACT OF PREPARATION AND PROCESSING ON ANIMAL PROTEINS

Animal proteins can be altered during cooking, and the type and amounts of carcinogenic compounds produced in meats are related to temperature and cooking time. Direct exposure of meats to intense heat, such as in grilling, barbecuing, or frying, is more detrimental than indirect methods, such as boiling, poaching, or steaming. The reaction between amino acids and creatines occurs at temperatures higher than 100°C, resulting in the formation of heterocyclic aromatic amines (HAAs), whereas incomplete burning of organic substances at temperatures above 200°C gives rise to polycyclic aromatic hydrocarbons (PAHs). Particularly, one of the prominent HAAs generated in meat during cooking, 2-Amino-1-methyl-6-phenylimidazo[4,5-b]pyridine (PhIP), has been demonstrated to have carcinogenic potential (Farvid et al. 2021). Moreover, various chemicals may induce carcinogen formation; for example, N-nitroso compounds (NOCs) such as nitrosamines and nitrosamides can result due to nitrate and nitrite used as food additives during meat processing to improve colour and flavour (Farvid et al. 2021; Inoue-Choi et al. 2016). PAHs are combustion products occurring in charred meat and fish, which can promote cancer in different tissues (Pratt et al. 2011).

Thermal treatments of milk at temperatures between 90°C and 100°C change the quality and composition of dairy products. During normal ultra-high temperature (UHT) processing and in-container sterilization, milk proteins, mainly caseins, undergo cross-linking, whey proteins are denatured, vitamins are destroyed, and enzymes become inactivated. All these consequences alter the nutritive value of dairy products and negatively influence their beneficial health effects (Deeth 2021).

Similar to meat, preparing eggs and fish at high temperatures generates by-products such as HAAs and promotes lipid peroxidation, resulting in the formation of lipid radicals and reactive aldehydes, which have been associated with increased cancer risk. Moreover, these compounds can interact with proteins, carbohydrates, and vitamins in foods and alter their properties (Yu et al. 2014).

ASSOCIATION BETWEEN VARIOUS ANIMAL PROTEINS AND DIFFERENT TYPES OF CANCER

There is reliable evidence suggesting that diets rich in red and processed meats are linked to an increased risk of developing cancer. According to data published by several cohort and case-control studies, red meat and processed meats increase the risk of cancer in a dose-dependent manner (Zheng and Lee 2009; Wang et al. 2016). Consumption of more than 100 g of red meat daily, and more than three days a week, has been associated with the presence of tumours in different organs: oesophagus (Salehi et al. 2013), stomach (Song et al. 2014), colon (Bastide et al. 2011, Chan et al. 2011; Xu et al. 2013), pancreas (Larsson and Wolk 2012), breast (Guo J et al. 2015), prostate (Lauber and Goodherman 2011), and lung (Yang et al. 2012).

Current evidence indicates that the intake of dairy products is positively associated with prostate and ovarian cancer, possibly due to the high levels of hormones in milk (Herby et al. 2023). Men who ate dairy proteins in amounts higher than 30 g/day showed a significant increase in prostate cancer, and the risk was 10% higher with the supplementation of 20 g/day dairy protein (Alzahrani et al. 2022). Contrarily, earlier studies did not find a significant association between dairy product consumption and prostate cancer. (Huncharek et al. 2008). A case-control study on an extended population of Danish women reported a positive association between dairy product intake and ovarian cancer; interestingly, milk had a stronger association compared to other products, such as cheese (Faber et al. 2012).

Studies on breast cancer showed conflicting results: in populations with a high intake of dairy products, there was an increased breast cancer risk (Herby et al. 2023), even though CLA, calcium, and vitamin D are hypothesized to provide anti-cancer protection (Dong et al. 2011).

Furthermore, dairy products seem to have a protective effect on the gastrointestinal tract due to probiotics, vitamin D, and calcium content (Herby et al. 2023). However, some studies suggest a non-significant increase in the risk of gastric cancer due to dairy products (Tian et al. 2014).

The association between egg consumption and cancer risk has been presented depending on the number of eggs eaten per week. Intake of more than 2.5 eggs per week significantly increased the risk of prostate cancer (Richman et al. 2011). Consumption of more than five eggs per week was related to a higher risk of ovarian cancer and breast cancer (Keum et al. 2015). Egg intake was also linked to gastrointestinal cancers, mainly colon cancer (Tse and Eslick 2014).

Even though fish has a protective role against cancer, a case-control study showed that fried fish was associated with an increased risk of pancreatic cancer (Yu et al. 2014). The prospective investigation of Daniel et al. (2011) showed a positive association of canned tuna with ovarian cancer and melanoma.

MECHANISMS UNDERLYING THE CANCER RISK

According to existing evidence, various pathogenic mechanisms have been described linking animal proteins to cancer initiation and progression.

Mechanisms Induced by Red Meat and Processed Meat

The cancer risk related to the consumption of red meat seems to be caused by the high levels of heme-iron found in meat and the HAAs and PAHs generated during cooking meat at increased temperatures (Table 9.2).

Heme-iron derives from the dietary haemoglobin found in high amounts in red and processed meats. Several mechanisms have been described involving the association between heme-iron and increased cancer risk: (i) cytotoxicity on epithelial cells, induction of hyperplasia and apoptosis (Farvid et al. 2021); (ii) promoting growth of *Helicobacter pylori*, a known risk factor for gastric cancer (Song et al. 2014); (iii) catalyzation of endogenous NOC formation, which exerts carcinogenic effect (Inoue-Choi et al. 2016; Larsson and Wolk 2012); (iv) lipid peroxidation leading to the formation of aldehydes with cytotoxic and genotoxic activity (Bastide et al. 2011).

Animal proteins contain branched-chain and aromatic amino acids, which are linked to insulin resistance, one of the pathogenic mechanisms implicated in various cancers, including breast, prostate, and colorectal cancer (Farvid et al. 2021; Chen et al. 2020).

Among the HAAs derived from meat cooked at high temperatures, PhIP has been shown to exert genotoxic carcinogenic effects. Experimental animal studies conducted by Lauber and Goodherman (2011) demonstrated that PhIP increases the risk of colon, prostate, and mammary gland cancer and metastasis by potent oestrogenic activity and subsequent induction of cell proliferation, migration, and invasion.

TABLE 9.2
Carcinogens and Other Components with Potentially Negative Effects in Red Meat and Processed Meats; Types of Cancer and Pathogenic Mechanisms Associated with Meat Consumption

Components	Types of Cancer	Pathogenic Mechanisms
Heme-iron	Oesophageal, stomach, colorectal, pancreas, breast, prostate, and lung cancer	• Exerts cytotoxicity on epithelial cells • Promotes growth of *Helicobacter pylori* • Catalyzes endogenous NOC formation • Induces lipid peroxidation
Branched-chain and aromatic amino acids	Breast, prostate, and colorectal cancer	• Linked to insulin resistance
HAAs and PhIP	Colon, prostate, and breast cancer	• Exert potent oestrogenic activity • Induce cell proliferation, migration, and invasion
PAHs	Oesophageal, cervical, and prostate cancer	• Form DNA adducts
Neu5Gc	Colorectal cancer	• Induces chronic inflammation • Promotes growth and proliferation of cancer cells
NOCs	Colorectal cancer	• Form mutagenic agents • Exert genotoxicity
TMAO	Colorectal cancer	• Increases systemic inflammation and oxidative stress • Induces DNA damage, cell proliferation, and angiogenesis

IGF-1 – insulin-like growth factor-1; HAAs – heterocyclic aromatic amines; Neu5Gc – N-glycolylneuraminic acid; NOCs – N-nitroso compounds; PAHs – polycyclic aromatic hydrocarbons; PhIP – 2-amino-1-methyl-6-phenylimidazo[4, 5-b]pyridine; PUFAs – polyunsaturated fatty acids; TMAO – trimethylamine N-oxide.

Ingested PAHs can become bioactivated to form bindings with different cellular macromolecules, such as deoxyribonucleic acid (DNA), to form DNA adducts, one of the initial steps in carcinogenesis. Pratt et al. (2011) revealed the accumulation of PAH-DNA adducts within specific cell types in the oesophageal, cervical, prostatic, and trophoblastic epithelia and demonstrated the association with higher cancer risk in these organs.

The nitrate ingested with various processed meats is reduced to nitrite by microbiota in the oral cavity. Then, in the gastrointestinal tract, nitrite reacts with amines and amides and generates NOCs, responsible for DNA damage. Nitrosamines undergo metabolic activation by the cytochrome P450 (CYP450) monooxygenases to become alkylating species with genotoxic and carcinogenic potential. Nitrosamides decompose without enzymatic activation to form mutagenic agents (Inoue-Choi et al. 2016; Fahrer and Christmann 2023).

Red meat contains methionine, an essential amino acid, and a glycan, the non-human sialic acid N-glycolylneuraminic acid (Neu5Gc), both implicated in carcinogenesis. Methionine is essential for cancer progression because the growth of numerous types of tumour cells is dependent on this amino acid (Cellarier et al. 2003). Neu5Gc absorbed from animal products and accumulated in human tissues is responsible for chronic inflammation and the initiation of carcinoma development (Guo J et al. 2015; Samraj et al. 2015). Trimethylamine, a metabolite generated by the intestinal microbiota from L-carnitine and choline in animal-based diets, is further oxidated in the liver to trimethylamine N-oxide (TMAO). TMAO increases systemic inflammation and oxidative stress and plays a role in the oncogenesis of colorectal cancer by inducing DNA damage, cell proliferation, and angiogenesis (Yang et al. 2022).

TABLE 9.3
Carcinogens and Other Components with Potentially Negative Effects in Milk and Dairy Products; Types of Cancer and Pathogenic Mechanisms Associated with Dairy Consumption

Components	Types of Cancer	Pathogenic Mechanisms
Hormones – IGF-1	Prostate, breast, and ovarian cancer	• Induces cell proliferation and angiogenesis
Aflatoxins – AFB1 and AFM1	Hepatocellular carcinoma	• Form DNA adducts • Induce inflammation and oxidative stress

AFB1 – aflatoxin B1; AFM1 – aflatoxin M1; CLA – conjugated linoleic acid; IGF-1 – insulin-like growth factor-1.

Deleterious effects are also due to various factors associated with animal protein intake, including saturated fats, added salt, smoked meat, alcohol consumption, and cigarette smoking (Lin et al. 2015). Processed meats with high salt content may cause damage to the gastric mucosa and facilitate *Helicobacter pylori* colonization, further increasing the risk of gastric cancer (Zhu et al. 2013). Moreover, smoked meats have been significantly associated with an increased risk of breast cancer in both pre- and post-menopausal women (Lee et al. 2012).

Antibiotics in animal products alter the constituents and activity of intestinal microbiota, impacting the local and general immune response and increasing the risk of colorectal cancer (Becattini et al. 2016).

Mechanisms Induced by Milk and Dairy Products

The main mechanism linking high-protein dairy products to an increased risk of prostate and breast cancer is the IGF-1 content (Watling et al. 2023). Intake of dairy proteins in high dosages (more than 30 g/day) significantly elevates plasma levels of IGF-1, which promotes cell proliferation and cancer progression (Alzahrani et al. 2022; Sun et al. 2014).

Other components of dairy products could also influence cancer risk (Table 9.3).

The high amounts of calcium and phosphate interfere with the synthesis of 1,25-dihydroxy vitamin D, which has a protective role against prostate cancer (Aune et al. 2015; Newmark and Haeney 2010). Aflatoxins are associated with the development and progression of various tumours, especially hepatocellular carcinoma. Pathogenic mechanisms involve biotransformation reactions mediated by CYP450 enzymes, leading to the formation of hydroxylated and demethylated metabolites and 8,9-epoxide. The main hydroxylated metabolite of AFB1 is AFM1, excreted in the milk of mammals and found in dairy products. The reactive 8,9-epoxide has a high affinity for DNA and forms adducts, leading to DNA mutations. Other pathogenic pathways involve inflammation and oxidative stress, which are responsible for DNA damage and their carcinogenic effect (Marchese et al. 2018).

Mechanisms Induced by Eggs

The mechanisms underlying the association between egg consumption and prostate, ovarian, and breast cancer seem to be due to the increased cholesterol and choline contents (Table 9.4).

Choline, concentrated at 250 mg/egg, is converted to phospholipids that compose tumour cell membranes, thus promoting cell proliferation and tumour growth (Richman et al. 2012; Keum et al. 2015; Zeng et al. 2015). Another pathogenic pathway involves choline metabolization in the liver to generate TMAO, which is responsible for increasing systemic inflammation (Awwad et al. 2012). Cholesterol is a precursor for sex steroids, and androgens stimulate prostate tumour growth.

TABLE 9.4
Carcinogens and Other Components with Potentially Negative Effects in Eggs; Types of Cancer and Pathogenic Mechanisms Associated with Egg Consumption

Components	Types of Cancer	Pathogenic Mechanisms
Choline	Prostate, ovarian, breast, and gastrointestinal cancers	• Promotes cell proliferation and tumour growth
Cholesterol	Prostate and breast cancer	• Promotes proliferation and growth of malignant cells
TMAO	Colorectal cancer	• Increases systemic inflammation and oxidative stress • Induces DNA damage, cell proliferation and angiogenesis

TMAO – trimethylamine N-oxide.

Moreover, high levels of cholesterol enable the proliferation and growth of malignant cells since it is a structural component of the cell membrane. In breast cancer pathogenesis, circulating cholesterol is metabolized to 27-hydroxycholesterol, which binds to oestrogen receptors in tumour cells, stimulating cancer progression (Keum et al. 2015; Baek and Nelson 2016).

ANIMAL PROTEINS WITH PROTECTING AND ANTI-CANCER EFFECTS

According to recent data, poultry and fish – "white meat" – consumption is associated with lower cancer risk, which seems to be due to both the low amount of heme-iron and saturated fat and the overall healthier diet of the patients (Shi et al. 2015).

Daniel et al. reported an inverse association with digestive and lung cancers in patients who substituted red meat with white meat; moreover, even when red meat intake remained constant, poultry intake was still associated with a lower risk of gastrointestinal cancer, but fish intake showed mixed associations. These results suggest a protective effect of white meat, which is independent of the intake of red meat (Daniel et al. 2011).

Chicken meat contains antimicrobial cationic peptides, such as cathelicidins, which exert antimicrobial and immunomodulatory activities by activating toll-like receptor-2 and neutralizing lipopolysaccharides. The anti-cancer activity has been demonstrated by induced in vitro apoptosis on gastric cancer, colon cancer, and hematologic malignancies. Mahmoud et al. demonstrated the antitumourigenic activity of chicken cathelicidin peptides by inducing apoptosis on breast cancer cells in vitro and necrosis on solid tumours in mice (Mahmoud et al. 2022) (Figure 9.1).

Fish is regarded as a healthy choice due to its anti-inflammatory and anticarcinogenic effects (Daniel et al. 2011). According to several studies, the consumption of more than 50 g of fish daily could lower the risk of gastrointestinal, hepatic, ovarian, and breast cancer (Salehi et al. 2013). The most prominent constituents of fish foods with beneficial effects are the omega-3 PUFAs, which are associated with eicosanoid biosynthesis and play essential roles in immunomodulation and prevention of general diseases by reducing the systemic inflammatory burden and activity (Zheng et al. 2013). Moreover, omega-3 PUFAs interfere with tumour development by regulating multiple intracellular signalling pathways responsible for cell proliferation and angiogenesis (Yu et al. 2014). Jiang et al. make an important distinction between dietary marine omega-3 PUFAs and plant-based omega-3 PUFAs, as well as the type of fish consumed. Thus, plant-derived omega-3 PUFAs did not exert a significant protective effect in breast cancer. Furthermore, only fish intake with higher amounts of fatty acids significantly decreased the risk of ovarian cancer (Jiang et al. 2014).

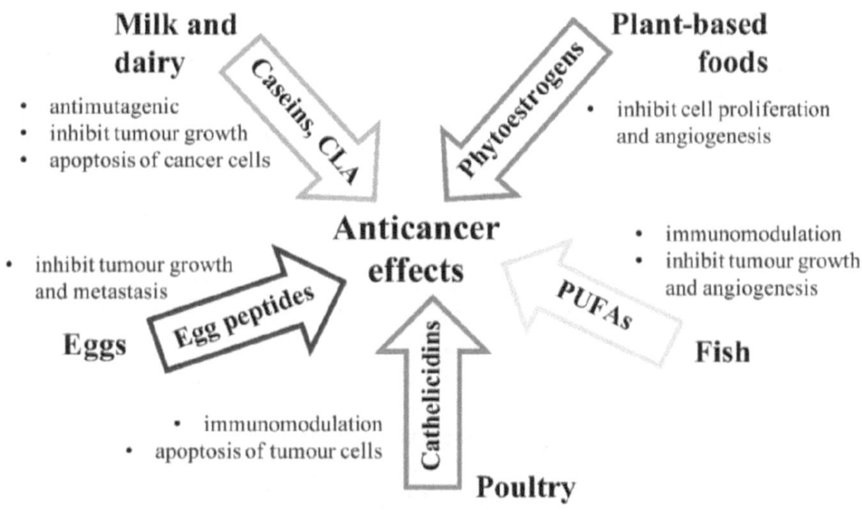

FIGURE 9.1 Protective anti-cancer effects of some animal proteins and plant-based foods.

Dairy components with protective anti-cancer effects include caseins, whey proteins, probiotics, CLA, and vitamin D (Herby et al. 2023). Whey proteins inhibit cell proliferation and tumour growth and exert anti-inflammatory and antioxidant effects; casein has anti-mutagenic activity and induces cytotoxicity and apoptosis in tumour cells (Davoodi et al. 2016). The probiotics in milk derivatives such as yoghurt and kefir exert a protective role against gastric cancer by inhibiting *Helicobacter pylori* colonization (Guo Y et al. 2015). A meta-analysis demonstrated that the risk of colorectal cancer was significantly reduced in people consuming high amounts of milk (more than 200 g/day) and other dairy products (more than 400 g/day), except for cheese; the protective effect seems to be due to calcium content (Aune et al. 2012).

Numerous studies describe several mechanisms implicating the egg proteins and peptides in anti-cancer activities: cystatin inhibits the activity of cysteine proteases, limiting tumour invasion and metastasis; avidin promotes binding of tumour necrosis factor-α (TNF-α) to tumour cells, with a significant increase in the anti-tumour effect of TNF-α; lysozyme and phosvitin inhibit tumour growth and metastasis (Lee and Paik 2019)

GUIDELINES REGARDING ANIMAL PROTEIN INTAKE TO REDUCE CANCER RISK

Red meat, poultry, fish, dairy, and eggs provide higher amounts and more balanced proteins compared to plant-derived foods (Wu 2016). In order to prevent cancer, it is not mandatory to eliminate red meat from the diet, but it is important to eat high-quality meat, consider individual dietary protein requirements, and improve eating patterns (Table 9.5).

Depending on age, intensity of physical activity, and health status, animal protein intake may be higher. For instance, in ill patients, animal proteins are necessary to support recovery, while in elderly people, meat consumption prevents sarcopenia. Red lean meat can be consumed in small servings of about 100 g raw weight or 65 g cooked meat 3–4 times a week. However, processed meats should be consumed in limited amounts or completely eliminated (Chen et al. 2020; Farvid et al. 2021).

Since overcooking animal foods may give rise to potentially carcinogenic substances, it is recommended to use healthier cooking methods. Direct and prolonged exposure of animal proteins to temperatures higher than 200°C should be avoided, and cooking by boiling or poaching is preferred to grilling or pan-frying (Yu et al. 2014). Moreover, marinating meat preserves moisture and

TABLE 9.5
Guidelines for Animal Protein Intake and Vegetarian Alternatives to Reduce Cancer Risk

Animal Proteins			Plant Protein Alternatives	
Red meat	Lean meat intake:	100 g raw weight or 65 g cooked meat 3–4 times a week	Cereals, pulses, fungi, or soy-based imitations	Higher in protein but lower in saturated fatty acids and salt compared to animal products
	Cooking methods:	Boiling or poaching		
	Recommendations:	Organic, grass-fed animal meat combined with vegetables		
Processed meats	Should be limited or avoided			
Poultry	Intake:	100 g raw weight or 85 g cooked meat	Soy-based imitations	Contain more carbohydrates than chicken
	Cooking methods:	Steaming, poaching or stewing		
	Recommendations:	Consumed without the skin		
Fish and seafood	Intake:	115 g raw weight or 100 g cooked fillet	Soy, pea protein, and wheat	Lower amounts of vitamin D and marine PUFAs
	Cooking methods:	Steaming or poaching		
	Recommendations:	Fattier fish is better		
Milk and dairy products	Intake:	2.5 servings of milk or equivalent of dairy products daily	Nuts, grains, and soy-based imitations	Lower in sugar, protein, calcium, and vitamin D content compared to milk; contain unsaturated fatty acids and fibre
	Preparation methods:	Avoid ultra-high temperatures		
	Recommendations:	Yoghurt and kefir contain probiotics; organic, grass-fed animal dairy		
Eggs	Intake:	2 eggs, 1–2 times per week	Various plant proteins and soybean protein isolates	Less cholesterol
	Cooking methods:	Boiling or poaching		
	Recommendations:	Should be avoided by patients with reproductive cancers		

prevents charring, and also adds flavour and beneficial ingredients. Consumption of organic, grass-fed, or pasture-raised animal products could prevent exposure to environmental toxic substances, carcinogenic agents, antibiotics, or hormones.

The combination of meat and vegetables provides fibre and antioxidants, which could counteract the pathogenic effects of heme-iron (Bastide et al. 2011).

Animal protein intake can also be supplemented by including poultry, eggs, and fish in other meals. Poultry, such as chicken or turkey, without the skin and prepared by steaming, poaching, or stewing, can be consumed in servings of about 100 g of raw weight or 85 g cooked meat. Fish can be included in the diet two or more times per week, as 115 g of raw weight or 100 g cooked fillet or canned in brine, without preservatives. Fattier fish is a better option due to the naturally occurring omega-3 PUFAs, with multiple health benefits (Jiang et al. 2014).

Recommendations referring to dairy intake vary depending on age, gender and health status. Adults can consume 2.5 servings of milk daily (a serving is equivalent to a cup, i.e., 250 ml) or milk products such as cheese, yoghurt, and kefir.

Depending on the amount of other dietary animal proteins, eggs should be limited to two eggs, 1–2 times per week. However, eggs should be avoided by patients at high risk or suffering from reproductive cancers, such as ovarian, breast, or prostate cancer. The best option is to prepare eggs by boiling or poaching instead of frying or scrambling (Keum et al. 2015).

Vegetarian alternatives to animal proteins could also be considered. Colourful fruits and vegetables are rich in vitamins and antioxidants and should be added to the diet on a regular basis (Farvid et al. 2014).

THE EFFECTS OF OTHER PROTEINS: PLANT PROTEIN INTAKE AND CANCER RISK

Plant-derived foods are regarded as a sustainable and high-quality protein source with the potential to supplement or substitute animal proteins (Xiao et al. 2023).

Plant foods based on whole grains, fruits, vegetables, legumes, and nuts are a rich source of proteins and bioactive substances. Among these, polyphenols with antioxidant activity, vitamins, and phytoestrogens have beneficial health effects and can reduce the risk of overall and cause-specific mortality, including cardiovascular diseases and cancer (Satija and Hu 2018; Farvid et al. 2014; Huang et al. 2020). Phytoestrogens seem to limit tumour growth by inhibiting cell proliferation and angiogenesis, whereas natural antioxidants counteract oxidative stress (Alzahrani et al. 2022).

A recent prospective cohort study conducted by Huang et al. over 16 years of observation reported that substitution of 3% of animal proteins in the diet with plant proteins resulted in a 10% lower risk of all-cause mortality in both men and women; the most protective effect was seen in the replacement of red meat and eggs with plant-derived foods (Huang et al. 2020).

A Rotterdam study conducted by Chen et al. reported that diets based on grains, which represent the main source of plant protein, were not associated with increased risk of all-cause mortality; instead, plant protein from other sources, such as legumes, fruits, and nuts showed inverse association with all-cause mortality (Chen et al. 2020; Satija and Hu 2018).

Recently, meat and dairy imitation products have become more and more popular, promoting sustainable dietary practices and supporting the transition from animal proteins to plant-derived daily diets. These are plant-based products with different main ingredients, e.g., cereals, pulses, and fungi in red meat, cold cuts, and sausage imitations; soy for poultry and red meat imitation; soy, pea protein, and wheat for fish imitations; nuts, grains, and soy for milk and yoghurt imitations; and soybean protein isolates and various plant proteins for analogue eggs (Xiao et al. 2023; Katidi et al. 2023). Depending on the ingredients, different protein content and nutritional composition have been reported in plant-based imitations compared with animal-based foods (Table 9.5). Katidi et al. reported that sausage imitations were higher in protein but lower in saturated fatty acids and salt; poultry imitations contained more carbohydrates; milk imitation was lower in sugar but contained unsaturated fatty acids and dietary fibres; and egg analogues contained less cholesterol compared with their animal-derived counterparts (Katidi et al. 2023).

Current trends in nutrition promote products based on plant proteins due to their similar nutritional value to animal proteins and for the advantage of being more healthful. However, plant proteins lack several essential amino acids; therefore, a healthy diet should be based on a diversification of protein sources to prevent nutritional deficiencies (Xiao et al. 2023).

MINI DICTIONARY OF TERMS

- **Carcinogen:** Any substance capable of inducing onset and promoting the growth of a malignant tumour, mainly by damaging the genome or by disrupting cellular metabolic processes.
- **Cathelicidins:** Positively charged antimicrobial peptides that are effective against bacteria, fungi, and parasites, and can also induce apoptosis in tumour cells to exert anti-cancer properties.
- **Conjugated linoleic acids:** Dietary omega-6 polyunsaturated fatty acids, isomers of linoleic acid, that are found in meat and dairy products and are beneficial for weight management, immunomodulation, and anti-cancer activity.
- **Deoxyribonucleic acid (DNA) adducts:** Compounds that are formed by a covalent bond between DNA and a chemical substance, inducing critical mutagenic changes and that are implicated in human carcinogenesis in a dose-dependent manner.
- **Heme-iron:** The complex form of iron derived from haemoglobin and present in red meat, poultry, and fish, which has increased bioavailability compared with non-heme-iron found in plant-based foods, including fruits, vegetables, and nuts.
- **Insulin-like growth factor 1:** A hormone with a molecular structure similar to insulin is produced in different tissues, mainly in the liver, which promotes body growth and regulates DNA synthesis and cell proliferation.
- **Long-chain omega-3 polyunsaturated fatty acids:** Essential fatty acids, present in both animal and plant-based diets, that are necessary for the production of proinflammatory prostaglandins.
- **Macronutrients:** Nutritive components included in large quantities in the diet that are represented by proteins, lipids, and carbohydrates, which provide essential amino acids, fatty acids, and saccharides to support the body's energy demands and vital functions.
- **Micronutrients:** Essential elements represented by vitamins and minerals that are required in varying amounts in the diet and are implicated in a range of physiological processes.
- **Nutrients:** Elements or compounds that are essential for an organism to ensure survival, normal growth, and maintenance of health.

SUMMARY POINTS

- This chapter focuses on the effects of animal protein intake on cancer risk.
- Animal proteins are a source of complete proteins, vitamins, and minerals, which cannot be obtained in sufficient amounts from other sources.
- In recent years, the association between long-term high animal protein intake and the risk of cancer has been well documented.
- Carcinogens in meat induce deoxyribonucleic acid (DNA) damage and the formation of DNA adducts, promoting tumour cell proliferation and angiogenesis.
- High intake of red meat and processed meats is associated with an increased risk of different types of cancer, including gastrointestinal, pancreatic, breast, and lung cancer.
- Poultry and fish can be regarded as healthful substitutes for red meat due to the lower amount of heme-iron and the content of chicken cathelicidins and marine omega-3 polyunsaturated fatty acids abundant in fish fat.
- Preparation by direct and prolonged exposure of animal proteins to high temperatures results in the formation of carcinogenic compounds.
- Some components from dairy products, including insulin-like growth factor 1, were associated with increased prostate cancer risk, whereas others, such as conjugated linoleic acid, magnesium, and potassium, have anti-cancer properties.

- Egg peptides seem to have a protective role, but high amounts of cholesterol and choline in eggs are related to an increased risk of ovarian, breast, and gastrointestinal cancer, mainly colon cancer.
- Vegetarian alternatives to animal proteins include a wide variety of whole grains, fruits, vegetables, legumes, nuts, and seeds.
- Plant protein-rich foods are associated with lower cancer risk due to fibre, phytoestrogens, and antioxidant substances.

REFERENCES

Alzahrani MA, Shakil Ahmad M, Alkhamees M, Aljuhayman A, Binsaleh S, Tiwari R, Almannie R. Dietary protein intake and prostate cancer risk in adults: a systematic review and dose-response meta-analysis of prospective cohort studies. *Complement Ther Med.* 2022 Nov;70:102851.

Aune D, Lau R, Chan DSM, Vieira R, Greenwood DC, Kampman E, Norat T. Dairy products and colorectal cancer risk: a systematic review and meta-analysis of cohort studies. *Ann Oncol.* 2012 Jan;23(1):37–45.

Aune D, Navarro Rosenblatt DA, Chan DS, Vieira AR, Vieira R, Greenwood DC, Vatten LJ, Norat T. Dairy products, calcium, and prostate cancer risk: a systematic review and meta-analysis of cohort studies. *Am J Clin Nutr.* 2015 Jan;101(1):87–117.

Awwad HM, Geisel J, Obeid R. The role of choline in prostate cancer. *Clin Biochem.* 2012;45:1548–53.

Baek AE, Nelson ER. The contribution of cholesterol and its metabolites to the pathophysiology of breast cancer. *Horm Cancer.* 2016 Aug;7(4):219–28.

Bastide NM, Pierre FH, Corpet DE. Heme iron from meat and risk of colorectal cancer: a meta-analysis and a review of the mechanisms involved. *Cancer Prev Res* (Philadelphia, Pa) 2011;4:177–84.

Becattini S, Taur Y, Pamer EG. Antibiotic-induced changes in the intestinal microbiota and disease. *Trends Mol Med.* 2016;22(6):458–78.

Budhathoki S, Sawada N, Iwasaki M, Yamaji T, Goto A, Kotemori A, Ishihara J, Takachi R, Charvat H, Mizoue T, Iso H, Tsugane S; Japan Public health center–based prospective study group. Association of animal and plant protein intake with all-cause and cause-specific mortality in a Japanese Cohort. *JAMA Intern Med.* 2019 Nov 1;179(11):1509–18.

Cellarier E, Durando X, Vasson MP, Farges MC, Demiden A, Maurizis JC, Madelmont JC, Chollet P. Methionine dependency and cancer treatment. *Cancer Treat Rev.* 2003 Dec;29(6):489–99.

Chan DS, Lau R, Aune D, Vieira R, Greenwood DC, Kampman E, Norat T. Red and processed meat and colorectal cancer incidence: meta-analysis of prospective studies. *PLoS One.* 2011;6(6):e20456.

Chen Z, Glisic M, Song M, Aliahmad HA, Zhang X, Moumdjian AC, Gonzalez-Jaramillo V, van der Schaft N, Bramer WM, Ikram MA, Voortman T. Dietary protein intake and all-cause and cause-specific mortality: results from the Rotterdam Study and a meta-analysis of prospective cohort studies. *Eur J Epidemiol.* 2020 May;35(5):411–29.

Daley CA, Abbott A, Doyle PS, Nader GA, Larson S. A review of fatty acid profiles and antioxidant content in grass-fed and grain-fed beef. *Nutr J.* 2010;9:10.

Daniel CR, Cross AJ, Graubard BI, Hollenbeck AR, Park Y, Sinha R. Prospective investigation of poultry and fish intake in relation to cancer risk. *Cancer Prev Res* (Phila). 2011 Nov;4(11):1903–11.

Davoodi SH, Shahbazi R, Esmaeili S, Sohrabvandi S, Mortazavian A, Jazayeri S, Taslimi A. Health-related aspects of milk proteins. *Iran J Pharm Res.* 2016 Summer;15(3):573–91.

Deeth HC. Effects of high-temperature milk processing. *Encyclopedia.* 2021;1(4):1312–21.

Dong JY, Zhang L, He K, Qin LQ. Dairy consumption and risk of breast cancer: a meta-analysis of prospective cohort studies. *Breast Cancer Res Treat.* 2011;127:23–31.

Faber MT, Jensen A, Sogaard M, et al. Use of dairy products, lactose, and calcium and risk of ovarian cancer – results from a Danish case-control study. *Acta Oncol.* 2012;51:454–64.

Fahrer J, Christmann M. DNA Alkylation damage by nitrosamines and relevant DNA repair pathways. *Int J Mol Sci.* 2023 Feb 28;24(5):4684.

Farvid MS, Cho E, Chen WY, Eliassen AH, Willett WC. Dietary protein sources in early adulthood and breast cancer incidence: prospective cohort study. *BMJ* (Clinical research ed) 2014;348:g3437.

Farvid MS, Sidahmed E, Spence ND, Mante Angua K, Rosner BA, Barnett JB. Consumption of red meat and processed meat and cancer incidence: a systematic review and meta-analysis of prospective studies. *Eur J Epidemiol.* 2021 Sep;36(9):937–51.

Geiker NRW, Bertram HC, Mejborn H, Dragsted LO, Kristensen L, Carrascal JR, Bügel S, Astrup A. Meat and human health-current knowledge and research gaps. *Foods*. 2021 Jul 5;10(7):1556.

Guo J, Wei W, Zhan L. Red and processed meat intake and risk of breast cancer: a meta-analysis of prospective studies. *Breast Cancer Res Treat*. 2015;151:191–8.

Guo Y, Shan Z, Ren H, Chen W. Dairy consumption and gastric cancer risk: a meta-analysis of epidemiological studies. *Nutr Cancer* 2015;67:555–68.

Herby AR, Cullimore JP, Paul-Quinn JL, Crosby LM. Dairy intake and incidence of common cancers in prospective studies: a narrative review. *IJDRP* [Internet]. 2023 Feb 28;5(1):14.

Huang J, Liao LM, Weinstein SJ, Sinha R, Graubard BI, Albanes D. Association between plant and animal protein intake and overall and cause-specific mortality. *JAMA Intern Med*. 2020 Sep 1;180(9):1173–84.

Huncharek M, Muscat J, Kupelnick B. Dairy products, dietary calcium and vitamin D intake as risk factors for prostate cancer: a meta-analysis of 26,769 cases from 45 observational studies. *Nutr Cancer*. 2008 Apr 1;138(7):1609–18.

Inoue-Choi M, Sinha R, Gierach GL, Ward MH. Red and processed meat, nitrite, and heme iron intakes and postmenopausal breast cancer risk in the NIH-AARP Diet and Health Study. *Int J Cancer*. 2016;60(4):421–41.

Jiang PY, Jiang ZB, Shen KX, Yue Y. Fish intake and ovarian cancer risk: a meta-analysis of 15 case-control and cohort studies. *PLoS One* 2014;9:e94601.

Katidi A, Xypolitaki K, Vlassopoulos A, Kapsokefalou M. Nutritional quality of plant-based meat and dairy imitation products and comparison with animal-based counterparts. *Nutrients*. 2023 Jan 12;15(2):401.

Keum N, Lee DH, Marchand N, Oh H, Liu H, Aune D, Greenwood DC, Giovannucci EL. Egg intake and cancers of the breast, ovary and prostate: a dose-response meta-analysis of prospective observational studies. *Br J Nutr*. 2015 Oct 14;114(7):1099–107.

Kulczyński B, Sidor A, Gramza-Michałowska A. Characteristics of selected antioxidative and bioactive compounds in meat and animal origin products. *Antioxidants* (Basel). 2019 Aug 22;8(9):335.

Larsson SC, Wolk A. Red and processed meat consumption and risk of pancreatic cancer: meta-analysis of prospective studies. *Br J Cancer*. 2012;106:603–7.

Lauber SN, Gooderham NJ. The cooked meat-derived mammary carcinogen 2-amino-1-methyl-6-phenyl imidazo[4,5-b]pyridine promotes invasive behaviour of breast cancer cells. *Toxicology*. 2011 Jan 11;279(1–3):139–45.

Lee JH, Paik HD. Anticancer and immunomodulatory activity of egg proteins and peptides: a review. *Poult Sci*. 2019 Dec 1;98(12):6505–16.

Lee JH, Wang Q, Yang F, Tao P, Li H, Huang Y, Li JY. SULT1A1 Arg213His polymorphism, smoked meat, and breast cancer risk: a case-control study and meta-analysis. *DNA Cell Biol*. 2012 May;31(5):688–99.

Lin S, Wang X, Huang C, Liu X, Zhao J, Yu IT, Christiani DC. Consumption of salted meat and its interactions with alcohol drinking and tobacco smoking on esophageal squamous-cell carcinoma. *Int J Cancer*. 2015 Aug 1;137(3):582–9.

Lu W, Chen H, Niu Y, Wu H, Xia D, Wu Y. Dairy products intake and cancer mortality risk: a meta-analysis of 11 population-based cohort studies. *Nutr J*. 2016 Oct 21;15(1):91.

Mahmoud MM, Alenezi M, Al-Hejin AM, Abujamel TS, Aljoud F, Noorwali A, Awad IA, Alkhaled M, Yacoub HA. Anticancer activity of chicken cathelicidin peptides against different types of cancer. *Mol Biol Rep*. 2022 Jun;49(6):4321–39.

Marchese S, Polo A, Ariano A, Velotto S, Costantini S, Severino L. Aflatoxin B1 and M1: Biological properties and their involvement in cancer development. *Toxins* (Basel). 2018 May 24;10(6):214.

Newmark HL, Heaney RP. Dairy products and prostate cancer risk. *Nutr Cancer* 2010;62:297–9.

Pratt MM, John K, MacLean AB, Afework S, Phillips DH, Poirier MC. Polycyclic aromatic hydrocarbon (PAH) exposure and DNA adduct semi-quantitation in archived human tissues. *Int J Environ Res Public Health*. 2011 Jul;8(7):2675–91.

Richman EL, Kenfield SA, Stampfer MJ, Giovannucci EL, Chan JM. Egg, red meat, and poultry intake and risk of lethal prostate cancer in the prostate-specific antigen-era: incidence and survival. *Cancer Prev Res* (Philadelphia, Pa) 2011;4:2110–21.

Richman EL, Kenfield SA, Stampfer MJ, Giovannucci EL, Zeisel SH, Willett WC, Chan JM. Choline intake and risk of lethal prostate cancer: incidence and survival. *Am J Clin Nutr*. 2012 Oct;96(4):855–63.

Salehi M, Moradi-Lakeh M, Salehi MH, Nojomi M, Kolahdooz F. Meat, fish, and esophageal cancer risk: a systematic review and dose-response meta-analysis. *Nutr Rev*. 2013;71:257–67.

Samraj AN, Pearce OM, Laubli H, Crittenden AN, Berg- feld AK, Banda K, et al. A red meat-derived glycan promotes inflammation and cancer progression. *Proc Natl Acad Sci USA*. 2015;112(2):542–7.

Satija A, Hu FB. Plant-based diets and cardiovascular health. *Trends Cardiovasc Med*. 2018;28(7):437–41.

Shi Y, Yu PW, Zeng DZ. Dose-response meta-analysis of poultry intake and colorectal cancer incidence and mortality. *Eur J Nutr.* 2015;54:243–50.

Song P, Lu M, Yin Q, Wu L, Zhang D, Fu B, Wang B, Zhao Q. Red meat consumption and stomach cancer risk: a meta-analysis. *J Cancer Res Clin Oncol.* 2014 Jun;140(6):979–92.

Sun Y, Lin LJ, Sang LX, Dai C, Jiang M, Zheng CQ. Dairy product consumption and gastric cancer risk: a meta-analysis. *World J Gastroenterol.* 2014;20:15879–98.

Tian SB, Yu JC, Kang WM, Ma ZQ, Ye X, Cao ZJ. Association between dairy intake and gastric cancer: a meta-analysis of observational studies. *PLoS One* 2014;9:e101728.

Tse G, Eslick GD. Egg consumption and risk of GI neoplasms: dose-response meta-analysis and systematic review. *Eur J Nutr.* 2014;53:1581–90.

Wang X, Lin X, Ouyang YY, Liu J, Zhao G, Pan A, Hu FB. Red and processed meat consumption and mortality: dose-response meta-analysis of prospective cohort studies. *Public Health Nutr.* 2016 Apr;19(5):893–905.

Watling CZ, Kelly RK, Dunneram Y, Knuppel A, Piernas C, Schmidt JA, Travis RC, Key TJ, Perez-Cornago A. Associations of intakes of total protein, protein from dairy sources, and dietary calcium with risks of colorectal, breast, and prostate cancer: a prospective analysis in UK Biobank. *Br J Cancer.* 2023 Sep;129(4):636–47.

Wu G. Dietary protein intake and human health. *Food Funct.* 2016 Mar;7(3):1251–65.

Xiao X, Zou PR, Hu F, Zhu W, Wei ZJ. Updates on plant-based protein products as an alternative to animal protein: technology, properties, and their health benefits. *Molecules.* 2023 May 11;28(10):4016.

Xu X, Yu E, Gao X, Song N, Liu L, Wei X, Zhang W, Fu C. Red and processed meat intake and risk of colorectal adenomas: a meta-analysis of observational studies. *Int J Cancer.* 2013 Jan 15;132(2):437–48.

Yang WS, Dai H, Lu Y, Li R, Gao C, Pan S. Trimethylamine N-oxide promotes cell proliferation and angiogenesis in colorectal cancer. *J Immunol Res.* 2022 Jul 4;2022:7043856.

Yang WS, Wong MY, Vogtmann E, Tang RQ, Xie L, Yang YS, Wu QJ, Zhang W, Xiang YB. Meat consumption and risk of lung cancer: evidence from observational studies. *Ann Oncol.* 2012 Dec;23(12):3163–70.

Yu XF, Zou J, Dong J. Fish consumption and risk of gastrointestinal cancers: a meta-analysis of cohort studies. *World J Gastroenterol.* 2014;20:15398–412.

Zeng ST, Guo L, Liu SK, Wang DH, Xi J, Huang P, Liu DT, Gao JF, Feng J, Zhang L. Egg consumption is associated with increased risk of ovarian cancer: Evidence from a meta-analysis of observational studies. *Clin Nutr.* 2015 Aug;34(4):635–41.

Zheng JS, Hu XJ, Zhao YM, Yang J, Li D. Intake of fish and marine n-3 polyunsaturated fatty acids and risk of breast cancer: meta-analysis of data from 21 independent prospective cohort studies. *BMJ* (Clinical research ed) 2013;346:f3706.

Zheng W, Lee SA. Well-done meat intake, heterocyclic amine exposure, and cancer risk. *Nutr Cancer.* 2009;61:437–46.

Zhu H, Yang X, Zhang C, Zhu C, Tao G, Zhao L, Tang S, Shu Z, Cai J, Dai S, Qin Q, Xu L, Cheng H, Sun X. Red and processed meat intake is associated with higher gastric cancer risk: a meta-analysis of epidemiological observational studies. *PLoS One.* 2013 Aug 14;8(8):e70955.

10 Bovine Milk Proteins
A Compositional Profile

Arpita Das, Ayushi Kapoor, Aparna Verma, and Kiran Ambatipudi

ABBREVIATIONS

ACE	Angiotensin-converting enzyme
BLAST	Basic local alignment search tool
BoMiProt	Bovine milk protein database
CAP1	Adenylyl cyclase-associated protein 1
CMT	California Mastitis Test
ESI-MS	Electrospray ionisation-mass spectrometry
FASTA	Fast-All
$GABA_A$	Gamma-aminobutyric acid A type
IVD	In vitro digestion
LC-MS/MS	Liquid chromatography with tandem mass spectrometry
MFG	Milk fat globules
MFGM	Milk fat globule membrane
NEB	Negative energy balance
PTM	Post-translational modification

INTRODUCTION

Bovine milk has long been considered a rich source of proteins, fats, sugars, vitamins, ions, milk fat globules (MFG), and beneficial microbes, providing nutritional needs for infants and adults. Milk proteins are considered promising food ingredients in various nutritional industries due to their structural flexibility and emulsifying and foaming properties (Dickinson 2001). Milk proteins are enriched in dairy products such as ice cream, cheese, yogurt, and chocolates to improve their nutritional value and importance (Smithers 2008). In addition, bovine milk proteins have many health-promoting effects, such as (i) lactoferrin possessing antimicrobial activities for protection against *Escherichia coli* and *Staphylococcus aureus* (Pino et al. 2022), (ii) maintaining a healthy gut microflora by regulating the growth of beneficial microbes in the gut microbiome (Sprong, Schonewille, and van der Meer 2010), (iii) antihypertensive and antioxidative activity (Nurminen et al. 2000), (iv) phosphoproteins providing essential nutrients for infant development as an important component of infant formula (Han et al. 2023).

Milk collection is non-invasive and inexpensive, making it a good indicator of nutritional characteristics. Various biochemical tests, such as the California Mastitis Test (CMT), somatic cell count, and pH test, help ensure safe milk consumption (Viguier et al. 2009). As a diagnostic fluid, milk proteomics is increasingly used to assess bovine animals' health and disease status by analysing the expression of proteins based on different variables. Recently, liquid chromatography-mass spectrometry (LC-MS/MS)-based milk proteomics have reported differential abundances of proteins as potential markers associated with bovine diseases such as mastitis, brucellosis, and immune-related diseases (Li et al. 2019; Elbehiry et al. 2022; Maity et al. 2020a). Notably, MS-based techniques

DOI: 10.1201/9781003597926-10

TABLE 10.1
Different Proteomic Studies Carried Out in the Field of Bovine Milk Proteins Concerning Human Health

S.No.	Proteomics Studies in Bovine Milk	Techniques Used	Milk Fraction	Reference
1.	Quantitative changes in milk proteins during *S. aureus* infection	ESI-MS/MS	MFGM, exosomes, whey	Reinhardt et al. (2013)
2.	Discovery of potential markers in SCM	ESI-MS/MS	Whey	Maity, Das, and Ambatipudi (2020b)
3.	Sleep-enhancing peptides in milk	ESI-MS/MS	Casein	Qian et al. (2021)
4.	Neuroprotective action of milk proteins for brain health	Behavioural tests on mice model	Casein	Joung et al. (2021)
5.	Antihypertensive peptides	ESI-LC/MS	Casein	Rutella et al. (2016)
6.	Hypocholesterolemic peptide from β-lactoglobulin	RP- HPLC	Whey	Nagaoka et al. (2001)
7.	Whey proteins to cure colitis in rat model	Biochemical assays, mucosal and faecal analysis	Whey	Sprong, Schonewille, and van der Meer 2010)
8.	Breed and season-specific variation in bovine milk proteins	ESI-LC/MS	Whey	Maity and Ambatipudi (2019a)
9.	Phosphoproteome analysis for infant formula	ESI-LC/MS	Whey, MFGM	Han et al. (2023)
10.	Proteomics of commercial infant formula	ESI-LC/MS	MFGM	Brink et al. (2020)

have unveiled the biological significance of highly complex bovine milk by identifying bioactive peptides and post-translational modifications (PTMs) of proteins (Table 10.1).

Many recent proteomics studies have focused on physiological factors (e.g., diet, breed, lactational stage, and seasonal variation) that affect the composition of bovine milk (Delosière et al. 2019; Maity and Ambatipudi 2019). Due to the necessity and consequential growing interest in bovine milk, comprehensive databases cataloguing milk proteins are essential for dairy researchers. A protein database is an organised collection of experimentally identified proteins with other data, such as their functionality, bioactivity, and structural and hierarchical information. Examples of proteomic databases include the Milk Bioactive Peptide database (Nielsen et al. 2017), the Bovine Milk Protein database (BoMiProt) (Maity, Das, and Ambatipudi 2020b), and the Milk Composition database (Foroutan et al. 2019). These databases provide a broad perspective of the ongoing research on bovine milk and possible information gaps that need attention to maximise its health-promoting effects.

Due to the advantages of MS-based proteomics in bovine milk research, and its ability to reveal thousands of proteins with potential benefits for human health, this chapter explores the health-promoting properties of bovine milk proteins alongside their potential industrial applications. Furthermore, this chapter reviews how advances in milk proteomics can be used to assess animal health status while discussing the recent increase in milk proteomics data compilation into databases, and the ways scientific communities and industry can maximise this data.

THE HISTORICAL ASPECT OF BOVINE MILK PROTEINS

Early History

Milk is the first form of nourishment for neonates and has long been recognised for its incredible biological significance. It has also been used extensively as a dietary component catering to the nutritional needs of growing children and adults since it is an unmatched source of high-quality protein. For a long time, bovine milk proteins have been recognised as potential biomolecules for supporting neonatal development and providing nutritional and immunological benefits for human health (Figure 10.1). In ancient times, Hippocrates, the father of modern medicine, prescribed whey proteins to boost the immune system (Hoffmann 1961). The chemical and biological properties of these proteins were first described by G.J. Mulder and J.J. Berzelius (Hartley 1951); Berzelius coined the term 'proteins' as an essential component of living beings. Milk proteins are of significant biological relevance, have been studied extensively, and are characterised as the superior protein system among food sources.

The exploration of milk proteins dates back to when casein proteins were analysed for the first time by Berzelius (Berzelius 1814). Casein is usually prepared by acid-mediated isoelectric precipitation at pH 4.6. The liquid remaining after coagulation is whey, a dilute solution of proteins, salts, and vitamins. Whey has become the primary source of research attention because of its immense health benefits. Whey proteins (e.g., serum amyloid A, immunoglobulins) are generally similar to blood proteins and are considered to have transferred directly from blood to milk. Whey contains a variety of functional proteins and bioactive peptides with anti-inflammatory and antimicrobial properties, drawing researchers' attention during the 1990s (Hoffmann 1961).

Whey constituents, namely lactalbumins, lactoferrin, and lactoglobulin, were discovered through isoelectric precipitation of the casein (Sebelien 1885). Using the techniques available then, protein preparation from bovine milk seemed to be a difficult task. The existence of lactoferrin in bovine milk was reported in 1940, and later on, B.D. Polis and H.W. Shmukler purified a red protein from bovine milk that was found to be associated with an iron-containing fraction of milk whey (Polis and Shmukler 1953). Similarly, Zweig and Block (1954) attempted to segregate the proteins with ferric chloride precipitation but achieved partial separation of α-lactalbumin with a much lower yield (Zweig and Block 1954). After several attempts, α-lactalbumin was isolated with ammonium sulphate fractionation, and later on, a more purified form was achieved utilising ion exchange chromatography (Groves 1960). Lactalbumin serves as a component of infant formula and has a central role in the synthesis of lactose in the udder, which is essential for milk production and, ultimately, milk volume. Similarly, it was frequently observed that lactoglobulin is incompletely segregated from other proteins due to interference from lactalbumin. However, with different fractionation methods, researchers could isolate β-lactoglobulin from α-lactalbumin using an improved precipitation (Aschaffenburg and Drewry 1957).

Modern History

In addition to the caseins and whey proteins, specific amino acid sequences of proteins, known as bioactive peptides, attracted the attention of researchers in the 1960s due to their numerous modulatory properties. For example, a glyco-macropeptide formed from the hydrolysis of κ-casein was later found to have antithrombotic activity and became well recognised in scientific research for its health benefits (Delfour et al. 1965). Subsequently, another group derived the primary structure of κ-casein B-I macropeptide (Mercier et al. 1972). Bioactive peptides such as casochemotide, exorphin, and lactorphines have since been demonstrated to play therapeutic roles, such as opioid-like features, immunomodulation, antihypertensive properties, and antimicrobial activity (Table 10.2). In another example of a bioactive peptide, proteomic analysis of glycoprotein PAS-6/7 purified from bovine MFGM has been reported to inhibit viral infection (Hvarregaard et al. 1996). Additionally, novel peptides from bovine milk proteins have been characterised as functional formulations with hypocholesterolemic, antihypertensive, and antidiabetic properties (Nurminen et al. 2000; Nagaoka et al. 2001; Mudgil et al. 2021).

Researchers have made significant advancements in the proteome annotation of bovine milk, which could render considerable economic and social benefits. For example, using LC/MS, a group identified essential proteins necessary for membrane trafficking and their role in mammary infection

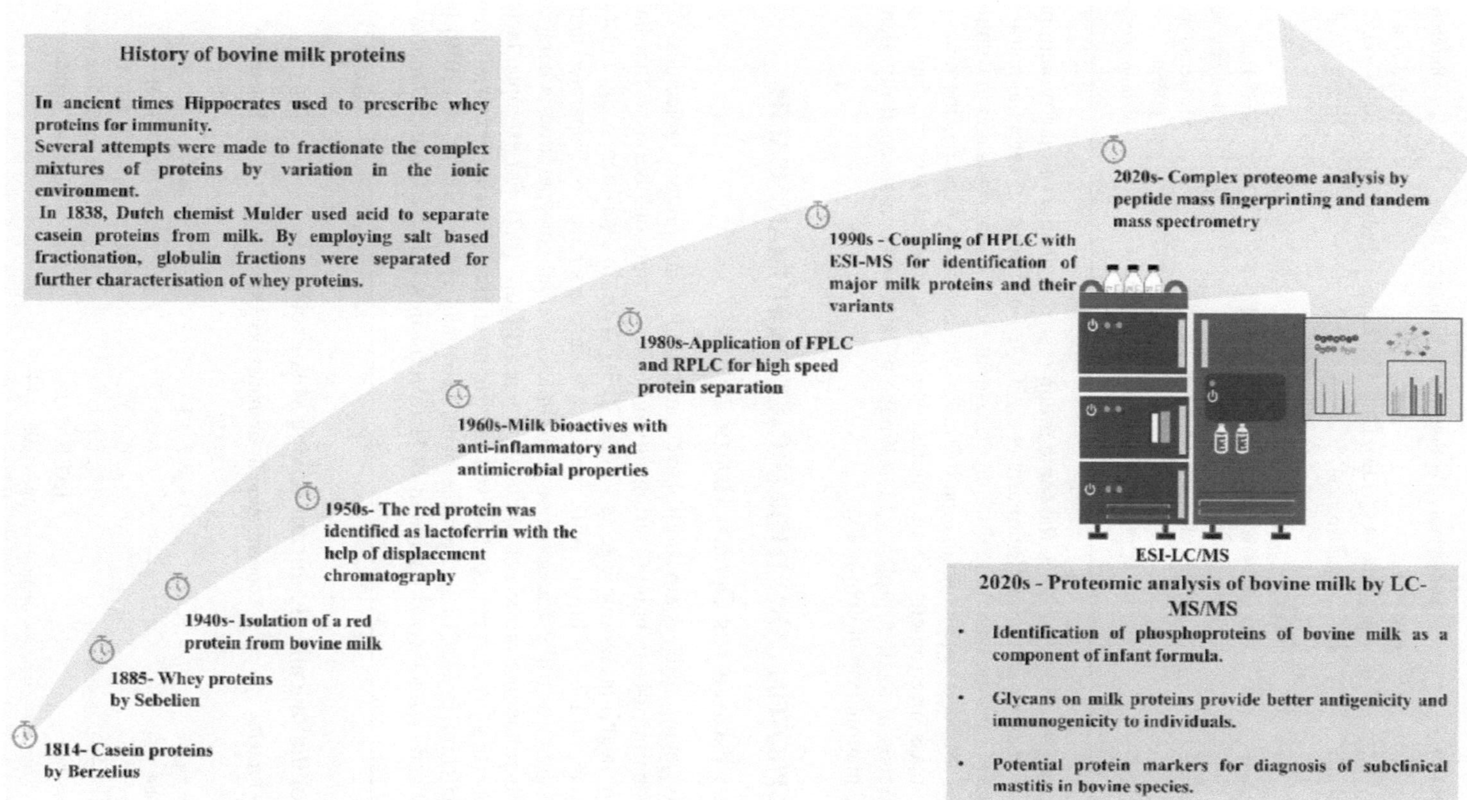

FIGURE 10.1 The timeline of major milestones associated with bovine milk proteins and proteomics. HPLC – high-performance liquid chromatography; FPLC – fast protein liquid chromatography; RPLC – reversed-phase liquid chromatography; ESI-MS – electrospray ionisation-mass spectrometry.

TABLE 10.2
Bioactive Peptides in Bovine Milk Proteins and Their Biological Roles

S.No.	Protein	Endogenous Peptide and Its Biological Role	References
1.	Casein	FLWPEYGA – antidiabetic YLGYLEQLLR – sleep-enhancing effect	Mudgil et al. (2021); Qian et al. (2021)
2.	β-lactoglobulin	HIRL – antihypertensive IIAEK – hypocholesterolemic	Nagaoka et al. (2001)
3.	Lactotransferrin	FKCRRWQWRMKKLGAPSICURRAF/A – antimicrobial	Meisel and Bockelmann (1999)
4.	Serum albumin	ALKAWSVAR – ACE inhibition	FitzGerald and Meisel (1999)
5.	α-lactalbumin	YGLF – ACE inhibition	Nurminen et al. (2000)

(Reinhardt and Lippolis 2006). In 2013, the same group reported changes in the protein profile of milk resulting from mastitis infection (Reinhardt et al. 2013). Furthermore, potential markers of the earliest onset stage of mastitis (subclinical stage) were identified for diagnosis and prevention at the preliminary stages (Maity, Das, and Ambatipudi 2020a). Proteomics is experiencing rapid progress due to continuous mass spectrometry advancements, which have enabled extensive data acquisition. As a result, thousands of distinct proteins from bovine milk have been successfully identified to better understand mammary pathophysiology.

BOVINE MILK PROTEINS AND THEIR IMPACT ON HUMAN HEALTH

Casein and Whey Proteins for Optimal Health

Explorations into bovine milk composition have elucidated many protein molecules – such as casein, β-lactoglobulin, α-lactalbumin, serum albumin, and immunoglobulins – that have been linked with many health-promoting effects (Table 10.3). With an ever-increasing understanding of the nutritional importance of bovine milk proteins, researchers have now separated and quantified thousands of proteins using fractionation techniques. Special consideration is being directed towards the health-enhancing properties of dairy proteins (Figure 10.2). For example, lactoferrin's iron-binding properties create an iron-deprived environment that prevents bacterial growth and biofilm formation (Pino et al. 2022). Because of its beneficial effects, Jin et al. (2019) heterologously expressed and characterised bovine milk lactoferrin in a safe bacterium, *Bacillus subtilis*,

TABLE 10.3
Concentration of Biologically Significant Bovine Milk Proteins

S.No.	Milk Proteins	Concentration in Grammes per Litre	Reference
1.	Casein	24–29	Sarode et al. (2016)
2.	β-lactoglobulin	3.2–3.3	Claeys et al. (2014)
3.	α-lactalbumin	0.7–1.5	Han et al. (2023)
5.	Lactoferrin	0.02–0.5	Claeys et al. (2014)
6.	Milk bovine serum albumin	0.1–0.4	Poutrel, Caffin, and Rainard (1983)
7.	Immunoglobulins	IgG: 0.15–0.8 IgA: 0.05–0.14 IgM: 0.04–1.0	Marnila and Korhonen (2011)
8.	Lysozyme	$(70–600) \times 10^{-6}$	Claeys et al. (2014)

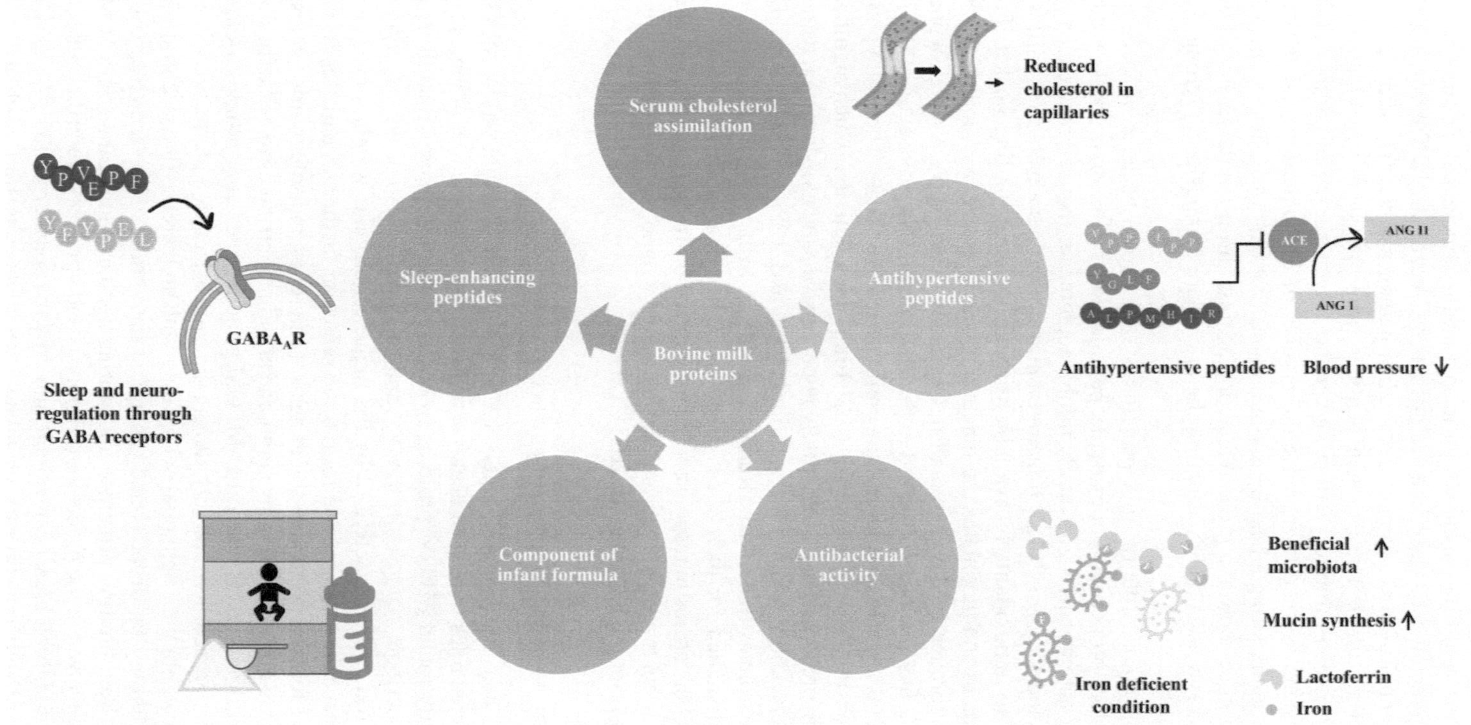

FIGURE 10.2 Potential health-promoting effects of bovine milk proteins include antihypertensive characteristics of multiple bioactive peptides, cholesterol-lowering properties of whey proteins, antibiofilm properties of lactoferrin, sleep-enhancing effects of casein hydrolysates, and use as infant formula. ACE – angiotensin-converting enzyme; ANG I and II – angiotensin I and II; GABA$_A$ – gamma-aminobutyric acid A type.

improving its antibacterial activity – a development that opens new avenues in the biomedical and nutraceutical industries (Jin et al. 2019).

In addition, much research has focused on antimicrobial proteins of bovine milk, such as lactoperoxidase, lysozyme, and β-defensin, which inactivate the adherence of pathogens and further colonisation of gut epithelial cells (Bielecka, Cichosz, and Czeczot 2022). Notably, a study reported the antibacterial potential of κ-casein peptides against pathogenic bacteria such as *E. coli* and *S. aureus* (Sedaghati et al. 2014). These casein peptides have also been investigated on probiotic strains, suggesting their non-inhibitory effect on beneficial bacteria in the gut microbiota. Bovine milk proteins have been observed to increase the number of *Lactobacillus* and *Bifidobacterium*, which are crucial for maintaining a healthy gut in humans. For example, dietary cheese whey protein supplemented in mice showed a protective action against chronic inflammatory bowel disease by increasing mucosa synthesis and modulating the microflora composition (Sprong, Schonewille, and van der Meer 2010).

In addition, the functional role of milk proteins is well known because of their antioxidative and immune-stimulatory properties. For example, peptides, such as casomorphins, exhibit superoxide anion scavenging activity and significantly inhibit angiotensin-induced reactive oxygen species (Bielecka, Cichosz, and Czeczot 2022). β-lactoglobulin is also responsible for milk's antioxidative nature by making antioxidants bioavailable through a ligand-binding pocket. Furthermore, β-lactoglobulin enhances and modulates the innate immune response by stimulating the proliferation of immune cells through IgM receptors (Tai, Chen, and Chen 2016). A novel hypocholesterolemic peptide 'IIAEK' has also been observed in β-lactoglobulin (Nagaoka et al. 2001).

Bovine milk proteins are also up-and-coming antihypertensive agents. The antihypertensive proteins possess angiotensin-converting enzyme (ACE) inhibition activity, which significantly regulates blood pressure in prehypertensive and mildly hypertensive patients. Moreover, using an in vitro digestion (IVD) system, antihypertensive tripeptides 'VPP' and 'IPP' were discovered from bovine casein during oro-gastrointestinal transit (Rutella et al. 2016). Milk proteins' association with brain health has been well studied for their stress-reducing effects. For example, a study reported the neuroprotective effect of caseins in response to stress-induced brain dysfunction (Joung et al. 2021). In addition, a novel casein tryptic hydrolysate was identified as a potential agent for stress-relieving and sleep-enhancing responses (Qian et al. 2021).

Beneficial Effects of Milk Fat Globule Proteins

The MFGM proteins constitute approximately 1% of the globule's weight on the MFG membrane and exhibit multifaceted roles in human health and disease by stabilising fat globules significantly. Among the commonly found MFGM proteins in bovine milk are mucin-1, xanthine dehydrogenase, butyrophilin, periodic acid-Schiff (PAS), and adipophilin (Smoczyński, Staniewski, and Kiełczewska 2012). Mucin-1, characterised by the highest molecular weight, emerges as a potential indicator for breast cancer. Its soluble form upon secretion further accentuates its significance. For instance, mucin-1 forms a protective shield against microbes and safeguards against chemical-related harm. PAS III, a glycosylated transmembrane protein, contributes to cell adhesion (Pallesen et al. 2007). Butyrophilin interacts with other MFGM proteins, such as xanthine oxidase, playing a crucial role in fat globule secretion. Notably, during the cattle's lactation phase, there is a substantial increase in secretion within their epithelial cells, along with an increase in concentration within the contractual regions linking fat droplets and the apical membrane of the secreting cell (Heid and Keenan 2005). Fatty acid-binding proteins, constituting another significant group of MFGM proteins, are intricately involved in the processes of lipolysis and lipogenesis. Furthermore, they appear to have the potential to inhibit breast cancer cell line growth (Spitsberg 2005).

Notably, MFGM protein constituents correlate with diverse factors, such as animal breed, health status, environment, nutrition, age, and physiological state (Maity and Ambatipudi 2019a). Importantly, the MFGM proteome profile changes along with the change in milk composition in different lactation stages. Such differences have been reported from colostrum through late-stage milk, highlighting their importance in cattle reproduction, udder health, and milk production.

BOVINE MILK PROTEOMICS: A DIAGNOSTIC APPROACH FOR ANIMAL DISEASES

The increasing demand for dairy products has led to the intensive commercialisation of the dairy industry, resulting in various animal health problems. Metabolic and management-prone diseases, such as mastitis, ketosis, and milk fever in dairy animals, are responsible for substantial economic losses to the dairy industry (Barkema et al. 2015). Poor health management and illness diagnosis are significant challenges for veterinarians, especially with the emergence of new pathogens every year. The dairy industry's future depends on early disease prediction, physiological wellness, and cost-effective diagnosis with technological precision to attain sustainable production of milk products. The discovery of physiological and behavioural indicators of disease in dairy ruminants has evolved through milk proteomics, enabling the development and establishment of biomarkers for better diagnostic approaches (Figure 10.3).

Brucellosis and Negative Energy Balance

Animals often undergo rigorous herd management in infectious environments, resulting in zoonotic infections due to several *Brucella* species, collectively known as brucellosis. Spontaneous antibiotic resistance has been observed in *Brucella* species due to the incorrect routine application of antibiotics, which affects animal health by reducing milk yield and causing reproduction and fertility problems. In this context, Elbehiry et al. (2022) employed proteomic-based analysis to screen both clinical and subclinical stages of brucellosis (Elbehiry et al. 2022). This MS-based approach aimed to discover the multi-drug-resistant bacterium early before its transmission to other animals and humans. Milk samples have also been utilised as a diagnostic medium to identify foot-and-mouth disease virus (serotype O) through enzyme-linked immunosorbent assay (Das et al. 2022)

Metabolic changes during the periparturient period in milking animals create a negative energy balance (NEB). Dairy animals in early lactation experience NEB due to low feed intake and high energy requirements for milk production. Mammary glands undergo metabolic changes impacting the health status of animals. Poor feeding conditions increase the risk of postpartum diseases like infertility, fatty liver, and ketosis (Barkema et al. 2015). Recently, a study by Delosière et al. (2019) detected 59 proteins in milk from early lactating cows. Interestingly, six of these proteins were associated with metabolic pathways such as ketogenesis, oxidative metabolism, and gluconeogenesis. These proteins may serve as putative biomarkers for detecting low-energy deficits in high milk-producing cows.

Clinical and Subclinical Mastitis

The proportions of bovine milk proteins appear to be affected by several factors, such as pathogens, environmental stressors, or mammary inflammation (Maity, Das, and Ambatipudi 2020). For example, clinical mastitis (CM) – an infectious cattle disease that results in severe mammary inflammation – causes substantial reductions in milk yield and quality. Mastitis is primarily caused by infectious pathogens such as *S. aureus* and *E. coli*, especially during milking processes, which can potentially infect other animals. More importantly, subclinical mastitis (SCM) – the asymptomatic early stage of mastitis – causes substantial economic losses to the dairy industry. Several diagnostic tests, such as CMT, pH, and culture tests, are currently used to detect disease pathogenesis in animals; however, these tests are limited in sensitivity and challenging to interpret (Viguier et al. 2009). In this context, several reports on the bovine milk proteome have revealed dynamic changes in the

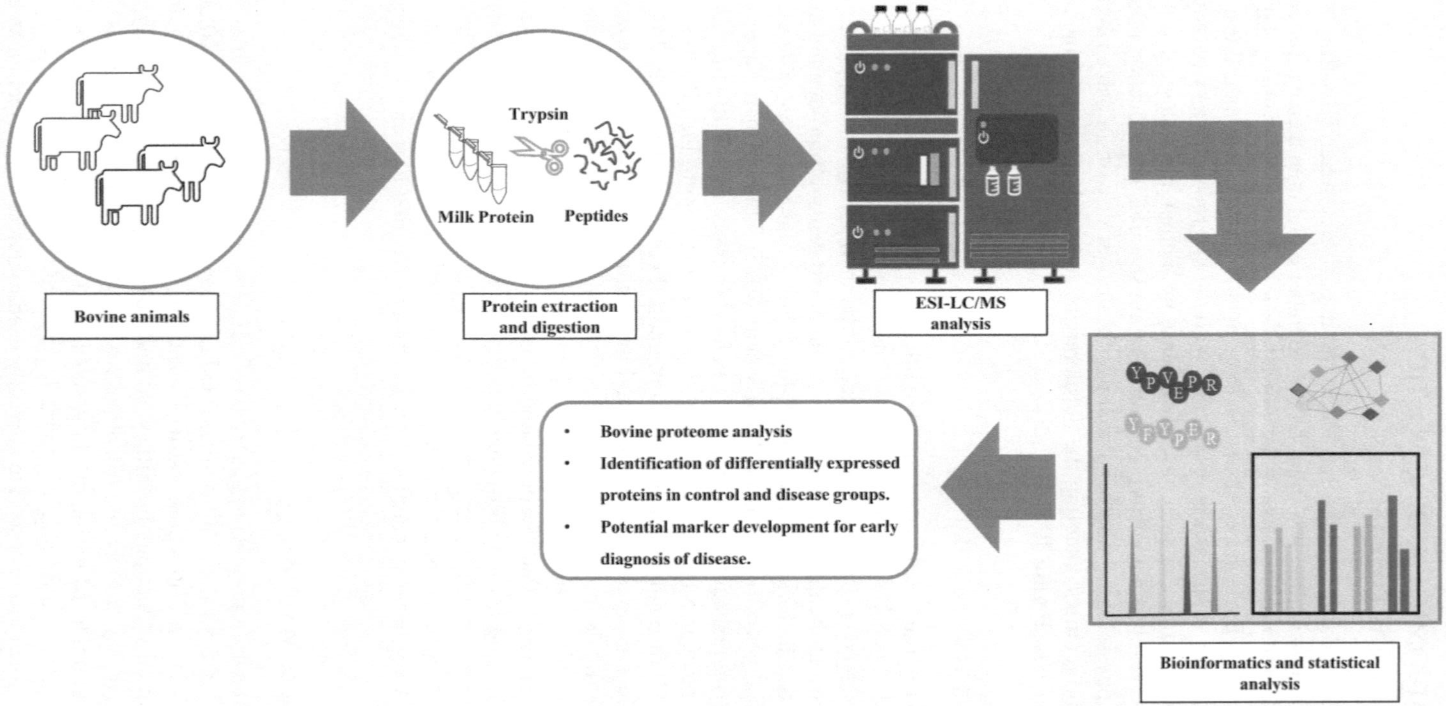

FIGURE 10.3 Schematic workflow of bovine milk proteomics. In the process of sample preparation, proteins are extracted from bovine milk and digested into peptides. The complex peptide mixture is separated in the nano-LC, followed by mass analysis in ESI-MS. Protein abundance across samples is quantified by comparing elution profiles across runs. Subsequently, bovine proteome analysis is carried out across the groups using several bioinformatics and statistical software for biomarker discovery.

expression of milk proteins across healthy, subclinical, and clinical mastitis. For example, Maity et al. (2020) identified signature patterns of adenylyl cyclase-associated protein 1 (CAP1), haptoglobin, and serum amyloid A (SAA) indicative of disease progression (Maity, Das, and Ambatipudi 2020). Although host defence proteins are naturally present in bovine milk, a differential change in their expression will serve in designing potential marker proteins for early mastitis detection. The findings from this proteomic investigation have established a deeper comprehension of the complexity of mastitis and other bacterial infections that will ultimately help facilitate early therapeutic and husbandry-based interventions to improve animal health and milk quality.

BOMIPROT: AN INTEGRATED DATABASE FOR BOVINE MILK PROTEINS

Mass spectrometry has revolutionised proteomic data generation by elucidating a vast expanse of proteins from various sources. Bovine milk research has garnered significant attention due to its nutritional value and immunological benefits. So far, over 500 research articles have reported changes in bovine milk protein abundances based on factors such as lactation, breed differences, health status, and milk fractions. For decades, there has been extensive research in bovine milk proteomics defining the significance of proteins for human health. However, there was a lack of a single database where the scientific community could avail of all the information. Therefore, to integrate the past and ongoing proteomic research on bovine milk into a single platform, BoMiProt (www.bomiprot.org) was created in 2019 as the first database dedicated explicitly to data derived from bovine milk samples (Maity, Das, and Ambatipudi 2020).

BoMiProt compiles data from 41 bovine milk proteome publications up to 2022 (Das et al. 2022). It provides detailed information on the significance of each protein, biochemical properties, bioactive peptides, three-dimensional structures, and disordered regions. Users can access the proteome data in BoMiProt through search parameters such as protein name, accession ID, and FASTA sequence. Multiple features allow the exploration of protein abundance values across milk fractions such as whey, exosome, and MFGM. The database includes over 1,392 defined proteins with secondary information such as function, biochemical properties, PTMs, hierarchical structures, and domains. In addition, a complete non-redundant bovine milk proteome in FASTA format provided by the BoMiProt database will be available for researchers to search for protein identity in MS-based protein identification. It is worth noting that the BLAST tool in the database facilitates identifying unknown milk protein sequences based on homologous sequence similarity and percentage identity. Recent developments in BoMiProt 2.0 have allowed extensive compilation and annotation of over 10,000 bovine milk proteins from newly peer-reviewed publications with updated primary and secondary information.

In conclusion, the vast amount of unorganised data available in the public domain has remained broadly scattered, neglected, and unaddressed. This data has been compiled together and curated to save the time and efforts of researchers working in the field of dairy science. In addition, aspects of health, nutrition, and disease related to bovine milk proteins have also been integrated into this database to diversify its applications.

INDUSTRIAL AND ECONOMIC ASPECTS OF BOVINE PROTEINS

Bovine milk contains two main classes of proteins: casein and whey. While casein constitutes approximately 80% of the total milk protein, whey protein has gained broader industrial application. Whey proteins, which make up 20% of the proteins in bovine milk, are present in the aqueous phase of milk and include ß-lactoglobulin, α-lactalbumin, immunoglobulins, bovine serum albumin, and other enzymes (Lin et al. 2021). Whey is commonly acquired as a co-product from cheese production, known as sweet whey, or during the production of acidified products like cottage cheese, yogurt, or casein whey, referred to as acid whey. Emerging sources include native whey from skim milk microfiltration or Greek whey produced during the straining and separation process used for the traditional production of Greek yogurt (Lagrange, Whitsett, and Burris 2015). Initially considered a co-product of cheese production, whey protein has evolved into a valuable supplement widely employed in various industries, such as food and beverage, cosmetics, and biotechnology, owing to its nutritional and functional benefits (Smithers 2008).

Technological advancements, such as ultrafiltration, microfiltration, nanofiltration, and reverse osmosis, have enabled industrial-scale processing and production of whey proteins (Figure 10.4). These membrane processes are highly efficient and cost-effective for whey protein production. Among these processes, ultrafiltration is the most commonly used for recovering whey protein concentrate, a popular form of whey protein. Moreover, the subsequent application of microfiltration in the processing yields whey protein isolates. Additionally, nanofiltration has emerged as a potential technique for concentrating whey up to 20–24% independently or alongside ultrafiltration to achieve a high retentate concentration (Khaire and Gogate 2019).

In 2013 alone, the United States produced approximately 39,501 metric tons of whey protein isolate, 108,060 metric tons of whey protein concentrate (50–89.9%), and 471,365 metric tons of whey lactose. Global exports of all whey ingredients amounted to 1.5 million metric tons, with the European Union leading exports at 530,772 metric tons, followed by the United States at 494,157 metric tons and Belarus at 115,451 metric tons (Lagrange, Whitsett, and Burris 2015). Asia has emerged as the leading permeate powder market, surpassing North America's market size. Despite India being the global leader in milk production, its bovine milk protein market is not experiencing significant growth on a global scale. At the same time, China maintains its dominant position as an importer of whey ingredients (Khaire and Gogate 2019).

The current emphasis on research to develop cost-efficient and highly effective technological advancements for the separation, purification, and production of whey proteins will continue to propel the growth and advancement of this sector. Due to their well-established presence and recognition, the market sector has already embraced the inclusion of high-value whey protein fractions, such as alpha-lactalbumin, glycomacropeptide, and lactoferrin (Lagrange, Whitsett, and Burris 2015). The presence of bovine milk proteins in the market sector will be further driven by their significant nutritional benefits, supported by research advancements and increasing consumer demands.

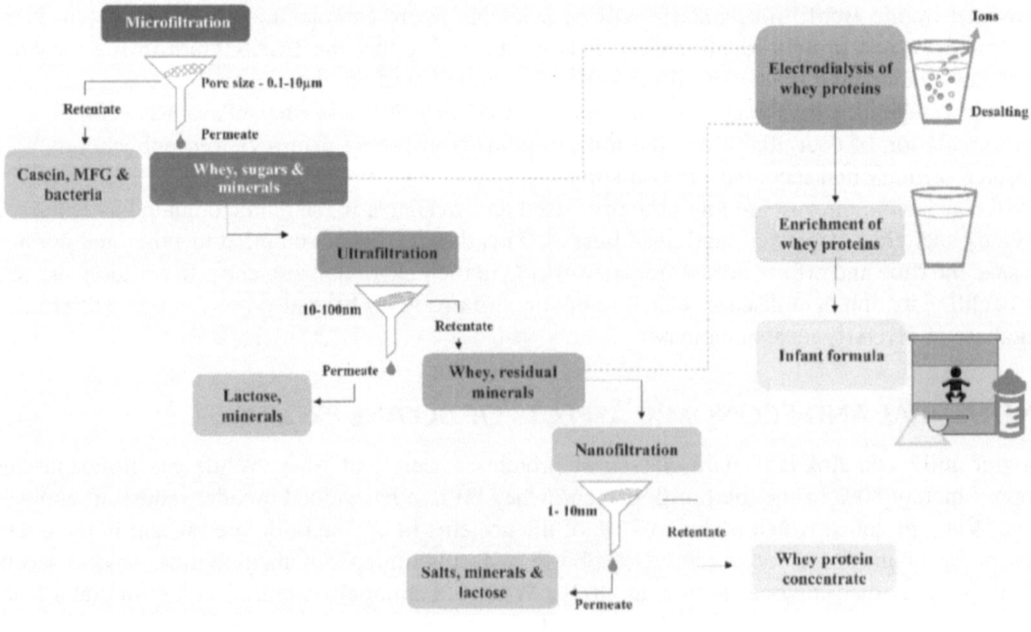

FIGURE 10.4 Schematic representation of different membrane-based filtration technologies for enriching whey proteins.

CONCLUSION

In summary, the advent of different methodologies of fractionation has made it possible to isolate even low-abundant whey proteins from caseins, which has advanced the current understanding of whey proteins (e.g., α-lactalbumin, β-lactoglobulin, and immunoglobulins). Furthermore, various enrichment methods such as ultrafiltration, microfiltration, precipitation, and reverse osmosis have enhanced the industrial production of whey proteins and their applications. Robust LC-MS/MS technologies have enabled researchers to analyse and quantify thousands of proteins from milk samples and address the biological significance of bioactives and PTMs important for human health. These inventions have made remarkable contributions to enhancing our understanding of the diverse roles of bovine milk proteins in human health and nutrition.

From an experimental perspective, understanding the comprehensive bovine milk proteome holds great importance, as it can improve milk's nutritional value and facilitate the identification of biomarkers for assessing animal health and production indicators. Analysing multiplexed samples through different labelling techniques enables the identification and quantification of protein abundances across milk fractions, seasons, and lactation stages, providing an in-depth picture of the bovine milk proteome. This has helped dairy nutritionists by offering insights into different parameters influencing milk quality and production. However, while many proteomic studies have reported potential markers for disease diagnosis, high-throughput targeted quantitation is needed to validate these potential biomarkers. Advancements in bovine milk proteomics have endowed researchers with a wealth of information on an array of milk proteins, enabling them to establish functionality and interrelationships within the milk proteome for the betterment of human and animal health.

The Effects of Other Proteins

In this chapter, the importance of bovine milk proteins for human health is discussed. Besides studies in milk proteins, the proteomic profiles of plasma, blood, and serum have been explored to study differentially expressed proteins for the early diagnosis of endometriosis in dairy cows (Ghaffari et al. 2020; Miller et al. 2019). However, proteomic analysis from blood or serum samples collected via invasive means is considered harmful to animal health. On the other hand, saliva is easy to obtain non-invasively and is enriched with a wide variety of constituents, including hormones, metabolites, and proteins that may serve as reliable biomarkers for health and disease. For example, some reports have shown the importance of bovine salivary proteomics in developing biomarkers for mastitis, disease resistance, productivity traits, and feed conversion efficiency in bovine groups (Franco-Martínez et al. 2021).

MINI DICTIONARY OF TERMS

- **Bioactive peptide:** A short protein peptide that displays various biomodulatory properties when subjected to enzymatic digestion.
- **Gut microbiome**: The collective community of microbes in the intestine that interact and provide various health benefits (e.g., digestion).
- **Infant formula:** A protein-based food supplement in liquid or powder form designed to meet infants' nutritional needs and support their growth and development.
- **Milk biomarker:** A biological molecule in milk that signifies a particular health or disease condition through differential expression.
- **Milk proteomics:** The study of the entire set of proteins in a milk sample in terms of their composition, function, structure, and interactions.

SUMMARY POINTS

- Milk proteins contain a vast array of bioactives with biomodulatory properties.
- Membrane-based filtration techniques aid in the enrichment of whey proteins, further enhancing the nutritional value of dairy products.
- High-throughput liquid chromatography with tandem mass spectrometry (LC-MS/MS) methods have enabled the comprehensive identification of proteins in the milk sample.
- The anti-biofilm properties of bovine milk proteins (such as lactoferrin) maintain a healthy gut microbiome.
- A vast amount of unorganised data on the bovine milk proteome up to 2022 has been compiled into BoMiProt to provide an in-depth outlook on the ongoing research in bovine milk proteins.

REFERENCES

Aschaffenburg, R., and J. Drewry. 1957. "Improved Method for the Preparation of Crystalline β-Lactoglobulin and α-Lactalbumin from Cow's Milk." *Biochemical Journal* 65 (2): 273–77. doi:10.1042/bj0650273.

Barkema, H.W., M.A.G. von Keyserlingk, J.P. Kastelic, T.J.G.M. Lam, C. Luby, J.-P. Roy, S.J. LeBlanc, G.P. Keefe, and D.F. Kelton. 2015. "Invited Review: Changes in the Dairy Industry Affecting Dairy Cattle Health and Welfare." *Journal of Dairy Science* 98 (11): 7426–45. doi:10.3168/jds.2015-9377.

Berzelius, J. J. 1814. "Über Thierische Chemie." *Schweiggers Journal für Chemie Physik* 11: 261–80. https://scholar.google.com/scholar?hl=en&as_sdt=0%2C5&q=Berzelius%2C+J.+J.+%281814%29.+Über+Thierische+Chemie.+Schweiggers+Journal+für+Chemie+Physik%2C+11%2C+261-280&btnG=.

Bielecka, Marika, Grażyna Cichosz, and Hanna Czeczot. 2022. "Antioxidant, Antimicrobial and Anticarcinogenic Activities of Bovine Milk Proteins and Their Hydrolysates – A Review." *International Dairy Journal* 127 (April): 105208. doi:10.1016/j.idairyj.2021.105208.

Brink, Lauren R., Anthony W. Herren, Shasta McMillen, Karl Fraser, Michael Agnew, Nicole Roy, and Bo Lönnerdal. 2020. "Omics Analysis Reveals Variations among Commercial Sources of Bovine Milk Fat Globule Membrane." *Journal of Dairy Science* 103 (4): 3002–16. doi:10.3168/jds.2019-17179.

Claeys, W.L., C. Verraes, S. Cardoen, J. De Block, A. Huyghebaert, K. Raes, K. Dewettinck, and L. Herman. 2014. "Consumption of Raw or Heated Milk from Different Species: An Evaluation of the Nutritional and Potential Health Benefits." *Food Control* 42 (August): 188–201. doi:10.1016/j.foodcont.2014.01.045.

Das, Arpita, Kuldeep Giri, Rama N. Behera, Sudipa Maity, and Kiran Ambatipudi. 2022. "BoMiProt 2.0: An Update of the Bovine Milk Protein Database." *Journal of Proteomics* 267 (September). Elsevier B.V. doi:10.1016/j.jprot.2022.104696.

Das, Leena, Krishna Sharma, Probodh Borah, and Md. Iftikar Hussain. 2022. "Detection of Foot-and-Mouth Disease Virus Serotype 'O' in Milk Samples of Cattle Using Rt-Pcr and Detection of Antibody Against Non-Structural Protein Using Diva Elisa." *Asian Journal of Microbiology, Biotechnology and Environmental Sciences*, no. March: 192–97. doi:10.53550/ajmbes.2022.v24i01.030.

Delfour, A., J. Jollès, C. Alais, and P. Jollès. 1965. "Caseino-Glycopeptides: Characterization of a Methionine Residue and of the N-Terminal Sequence." *Biochemical and Biophysical Research Communications* 19 (4): 452–55. doi:10.1016/0006-291X(65)90145-2.

Delosière, Mylène, José Pires, Laurence Bernard, Isabelle Cassar-Malek, and Muriel Bonnet. 2019. "Milk Proteome from in Silico Data Aggregation Allows the Identification of Putative Biomarkers of Negative Energy Balance in Dairy Cows." *Scientific Reports* 9 (1): 9718. doi:10.1038/s41598-019-46142-7.

Dickinson, Eric. 2001. "Milk Protein Interfacial Layers and the Relationship to Emulsion Stability and Rheology." *Colloids and Surfaces B: Biointerfaces* 20 (3): 197–210. doi:10.1016/S0927-7765(00)00204-6.

Elbehiry, Ayman, Musaad Aldubaib, Osamah Al Rugaie, Eman Marzouk, Marwan Abaalkhail, Ihab Moussa, Mohamed H. El-Husseiny, Adil Abalkhail, and Mohammed Rawway. 2022. "Proteomics-Based Screening and Antibiotic Resistance Assessment of Clinical and Sub-Clinical Brucella Species: An Evolution of Brucellosis Infection Control." Edited by Abdelazeem Mohamed Algammal. *PLoS One* 17 (1): e0262551. doi:10.1371/journal.pone.0262551.

FitzGerald, R. J., and H. Meisel. 1999. "Lactokinins: Whey Protein-Derived ACE Inhibitory Peptides." *Nahrung/Food* 43 (3): 165–67. doi:10.1002/(SICI)1521-3803(19990601)43:3<165::AID-FOOD165>3.0.CO;2-2.

Foroutan, Aidin, An Chi Guo, Rosa Vazquez-Fresno, Matthias Lipfert, Lun Zhang, Jiamin Zheng, Hasan Badran, et al. 2019. "Chemical Composition of Commercial Cow's Milk." *Journal of Agricultural and Food Chemistry* 67 (17): 4897–4914. doi:10.1021/acs.jafc.9b00204.

Franco-Martínez, L., A. Muñoz-Prieto, M.D. Contreras-Aguilar, R. Želvytė, I. Monkevičienė, A. Horvatić, J. Kuleš, V. Mrljak, J.J. Cerón, and D. Escribano. 2021. "Changes in Saliva Proteins in Cows with Mastitis: A Proteomic Approach." *Research in Veterinary Science* 140 (November): 91–99. doi:10.1016/j.rvsc.2021.08.008.

Ghaffari, Morteza H., Katharina Schuh, Josipa Kuleš, Nicolas Guillemin, Anita Horvatić, Vladimir Mrljak, Peter David Eckersall, et al. 2020. "Plasma Proteomic Profiling and Pathway Analysis of Normal and Overconditioned Dairy Cows during the Transition from Late Pregnancy to Early Lactation." *Journal of Dairy Science* 103 (5): 4806–21. doi:10.3168/jds.2019-17897.

Groves, L. 1960. "Red Protein from Milk2" 529 (7).

Han, Binsong, Lina Zhang, Ying Ma, Yanmei Hou, Kui Xie, Jinjing Zhong, and Peng Zhou. 2023. "Quantitative Phosphoproteome of Infant Formula: New Insights into the Difference of Phosphorylation in Milk Proteins between Bovine and Goat Species." *Journal of Agricultural and Food Chemistry* 71 (7): 3531–40. doi:10.1021/acs.jafc.2c07326.

Hartley, Harold. 1951. "Origin of the Word 'Protein.'" *Nature* 168 (4267): 244–44. doi:10.1038/168244a0.

Heid, Hans W., and Thomas W. Keenan. 2005. "Intracellular Origin and Secretion of Milk Fat Globules." *European Journal of Cell Biology* 84 (2–3): 245–58. doi:10.1016/j.ejcb.2004.12.002.

Hoffmann, K F. 1961. "[On the History of Whey Cures, Especially in the 17th, 18th, and 19th Centuries]." *Medizinische Monatsschrift* 15 (June): 411–14. http://www.ncbi.nlm.nih.gov/pubmed/13715057.

Hvarregaard, Jane, Mikkel H. Andersen, Lars Berglund, Jan T. Rasmussen, and Torben E. Petersen. 1996. "Characterization of Glycoprotein PAS-6/7 from Membranes of Bovine Milk Fat Globules." *European Journal of Biochemistry* 240 (3): 628–36. doi:10.1111/j.1432-1033.1996.0628h.x.

Jin, Liang, Lihong Li, Lixian Zhou, Rongzhen Zhang, Yan Xu, and Jiming Li. 2019. "Improving Expression of Bovine Lactoferrin N-Lobe by Promoter Optimization and Codon Engineering in Bacillus Subtilis and Its Antibacterial Activity." *Journal of Agricultural and Food Chemistry* 67 (35): 9749–56. doi:10.1021/acs.jafc.9b02350.

Joung, Jae Yeon, Jae Gwang Song, Hyung Wook Kim, and Nam Su Oh. 2021. "Protective Effects of Milk Casein on the Brain Function and Behavior in a Mouse Model of Chronic Stress." *Journal of Agricultural and Food Chemistry* 69 (6): 1936–41. doi:10.1021/acs.jafc.0c07292.

Khaire, Rajeshree A., and Parag R. Gogate. 2019. "Whey Proteins." In *Proteins: Sustainable Source, Processing and Applications*, 193–223. Elsevier. doi:10.1016/B978-0-12-816695-6.00007-6.

Lagrange, Veronique, Dacia Whitsett, and Cameron Burris. 2015. "Global Market for Dairy Proteins." *Journal of Food Science* 80 (S1): A16–22. doi:10.1111/1750-3841.12801.

Li, Lingling, John P. Bannantine, Joseph J. Campo, Arlo Randall, Yrjo T. Grohn, Megan A. Schilling, Robab Katani, Jessica Radzio-Basu, Laurel Easterling, and Vivek Kapur. 2019. "Identification of Sero-Diagnostic Antigens for the Early Diagnosis of Johne's Disease Using MAP Protein Microarrays." *Scientific Reports* 9 (1): 17573. doi:10.1038/s41598-019-53973-x.

Lin, Tiantian, Gopinathan Meletharayil, Rohit Kapoor, and Alireza Abbaspourrad. 2021. "Bioactives in Bovine Milk: Chemistry, Technology, and Applications." *Nutrition Reviews* 79 (Supplement_2): 48–69. doi:10.1093/nutrit/nuab099.

Maity, Sudipa, and Kiran Ambatipudi. 2019. "Quantitative Proteomics of Milk Whey Reveals Breed and Season Specific Variation in Protein Abundance in Holstein Friesian Cow and Murrah Buffalo." *Research in Veterinary Science* 125 (August): 244–52. doi:10.1016/j.rvsc.2019.07.001.

Maity, Sudipa, Aadil Hussain Bhat, Kuldeep Giri, and Kiran Ambatipudi. 2020. "BoMiProt: A Database of Bovine Milk Proteins." *Journal of Proteomics* 215 (March). J Proteomics. doi:10.1016/J.JPROT.2020.103648.

Maity, Sudipa, Debiprasanna Das, and Kiran Ambatipudi. 2020. "Quantitative Alterations in Bovine Milk Proteome from Healthy, Subclinical and Clinical Mastitis during S. Aureus Infection." *Journal of Proteomics* 223 (February). Elsevier: 103815. doi:10.1016/j.jprot.2020.103815.

Marnila, P., and H. Korhonen. 2011. "Milk Proteins: Immunoglobulins." *Encyclopedia of Dairy Sciences: Second Edition*, 807–15. doi:10.1016/B978-0-12-374407-4.00436-2.

Meisel, Hans, and Wilhelm Bockelmann. 1999. "Bioactive Peptides Encrypted in Milk Proteins: Proteolytic Activation and Thropho-Functional Properties." *Antonie van Leeuwenhoek, International Journal of General and Molecular Microbiology* 76 (1–4): 207–15. doi:10.1023/A:1002063805780.

Mercier, Jean-Claude, Joel URO, Bruno RIBADEAU-Dumas, and Francois GROSCLAUDE. 1972. "Structure Primaire Du Caseinomacropeptide de La Caseine KappaB1 Bovine." *European Journal of Biochemistry* 27 (3): 535–47. doi:10.1111/j.1432-1033.1972.tb01870.x.

Miller, Blake A., Amy Brewer, Paolo Nanni, Joseph J. Lim, John J. Callanan, Jonas Grossmann, Laura Kunz, André M. de Almeida, Kieran G. Meade, and Aspinas Chapwanya. 2019. "Characterization of Circulating Plasma Proteins in Dairy Cows with Cytological Endometritis." *Journal of Proteomics* 205 (August): 103421. doi:10.1016/j.jprot.2019.103421.

Mudgil, Priti, Hina Kamal, Bhanu Priya Kilari, Mohd Adam Salim Mohd Salim, Chee-Yuen Gan, and Sajid Maqsood. 2021. "Simulated Gastrointestinal Digestion of Camel and Bovine Casein Hydrolysates: Identification and Characterization of Novel Anti-Diabetic Bioactive Peptides." *Food Chemistry* 353 (August): 129374. doi:10.1016/j.foodchem.2021.129374.

Nagaoka, Satoshi, Yu Futamura, Keiji Miwa, Takako Awano, Kouhei Yamauchi, Yoshihiro Kanamaru, Kojima Tadashi, and Tamotsu Kuwata. 2001. "Identification of Novel Hypocholesterolemic Peptides Derived from Bovine Milk β-Lactoglobulin." *Biochemical and Biophysical Research Communications* 281 (1): 11–17. doi:10.1006/bbrc.2001.4298.

Nielsen, Søren Drud, Robert L. Beverly, Yunyao Qu, and David C. Dallas. 2017. "Milk Bioactive Peptide Database: A Comprehensive Database of Milk Protein-Derived Bioactive Peptides and Novel Visualization." *Food Chemistry* 232 (October): 673–82. doi:10.1016/j.foodchem.2017.04.056.

Nurminen, Marja-Leena, Marika Sipola, Hanna Kaarto, Anne Pihlanto-Leppälä, Kati Piilola, Riitta Korpela, Olli Tossavainen, Hannu Korhonen, and Heikki Vapaatalo. 2000. "α-Lactorphin Lowers Blood Pressure Measured by Radiotelemetry in Normotensive and Spontaneously Hypertensive Rats." *Life Sciences* 66 (16): 1535–43. doi:10.1016/S0024-3205(00)00471-9.

Pallesen, L.T., L.R.L. Pedersen, T.E. Petersen, and J.T. Rasmussen. 2007. "Characterization of Carbohydrate Structures of Bovine MUC15 and Distribution of the Mucin in Bovine Milk." *Journal of Dairy Science* 90 (7): 3143–52. doi:10.3168/jds.2007-0082.

Pino, Alessandra, Tommaso Mazza, Maura-Ann H. Matthews, Stefano Castellana, Cinzia Caggia, Cinzia L. Randazzo, and Gary A. Gelbfish. 2022. "Antimicrobial Activity of Bovine Lactoferrin against Gardnerella Species Clinical Isolates." *Frontiers in Microbiology* 13 (September). doi:10.3389/fmicb.2022.1000822.

Polis, B.D., and H.W. Shmukler. 1953. "Crystalline Lactoperoxidase. I. Isolation by Displacement Chromatography. II. Physicochemical and Enzymatic Properties." *The Journal of Biological Chemistry* 201 (1): 475–500. http://www.ncbi.nlm.nih.gov/pubmed/13044816.

Poutrel, B., J. P. Caffin, and P. Rainard. 1983. "Physiological and Pathological Factors Influencing Bovine Serum Albumin Content of Milk." *Journal of Dairy Science* 66 (3): 535–41. doi:10.3168/jds.S0022-0302(83)81822-0.

Qian, Jingjing, Lin Zheng, Guowan Su, Mingtao Huang, Donghui Luo, and Mouming Zhao. 2021. "Identification and Screening of Potential Bioactive Peptides with Sleep-Enhancing Effects in Bovine Milk Casein Hydrolysate." *Journal of Agricultural and Food Chemistry* 69 (38): 11246–58. doi:10.1021/acs.jafc.1c03937.

Reinhardt, Timothy A., and John D. Lippolis. 2006. "Bovine Milk Fat Globule Membrane Proteome." *Journal of Dairy Research* 73 (4): 406–16. doi:10.1017/S0022029906001889.

Reinhardt, Timothy A., Randy E. Sacco, Brian J. Nonnecke, and John D. Lippolis. 2013. "Bovine Milk Proteome: Quantitative Changes in Normal Milk Exosomes, Milk Fat Globule Membranes and Whey Proteomes Resulting from Staphylococcus Aureus Mastitis." *Journal of Proteomics* 82 (April): 141–54. doi:10.1016/j.jprot.2013.02.013.

Rutella, Giuseppina Sefora, Lisa Solieri, Serena Martini, and Davide Tagliazucchi. 2016. "Release of the Antihypertensive Tripeptides Valine-Proline-Proline and Isoleucine-Proline-Proline from Bovine Milk Caseins during in Vitro Gastrointestinal Digestion." *Journal of Agricultural and Food Chemistry* 64 (45): 8509–15. doi:10.1021/acs.jafc.6b03271.

Sarode, A.R., P.D. Sawale, C.D. Khedkar, S.D. Kalyankar, and R.D. Pawshe. 2016. "Casein and Caseinate: Methods of Manufacture." In *Encyclopedia of Food and Health*, 676–82. Elsevier. doi:10.1016/B978-0-12-384947-2.00122-7.

Sebelien, John. 1885. "Beitrag Zur Kenntniss Der Eiweisskörper Der Kuhmilch." *Bchm* 9 (4–5): 445–64. doi:10.1515/bchm1.1885.9.4-5.445.

Sedaghati, Marjaneh, Hamid Ezzatpanah, Masoud Mashhadi Akbar Boojar, Maryam Tajabadi Ebrahimi, and Mehdi Aminafshar. 2014. "Plasmin Digest of κ-Casein as a Source of Antibacterial Peptides." *Journal of Dairy Research* 81 (2): 245–51. doi:10.1017/S0022029914000120.

Smithers, Geoffrey W. 2008. "Whey and Whey Proteins—From 'Gutter-to-Gold.'" *International Dairy Journal* 18 (7): 695–704. doi:10.1016/j.idairyj.2008.03.008.

Smoczyński, Michał, Bogusław Staniewski, and Katarzyna Kiełczewska. 2012. "Composition and Structure of the Bovine Milk Fat Globule Membrane—Some Nutritional and Technological Implications." *Food Reviews International* 28 (2): 188–202. doi:10.1080/87559129.2011.595024.
Spitsberg, V.L. 2005. "Invited Review: Bovine Milk Fat Globule Membrane as a Potential Nutraceutical." *Journal of Dairy Science* 88 (7): 2289–94. doi:10.3168/jds.S0022-0302(05)72906-4.
Sprong, R.C., A.J. Schonewille, and R. van der Meer. 2010. "Dietary Cheese Whey Protein Protects Rats against Mild Dextran Sulfate Sodium–Induced Colitis: Role of Mucin and Microbiota." *Journal of Dairy Science* 93 (4): 1364–71. doi:10.3168/jds.2009-2397.
Tai, Chun San, Yi Yun Chen, and Wen Liang Chen. 2016. "β -Lactoglobulin Influences Human Immunity and Promotes Cell Proliferation." *BioMed Research International* 2016: 1–12. doi:10.1155/2016/7123587.
Viguier, Caroline, Sushrut Arora, Niamh Gilmartin, Katherine Welbeck, and Richard O'Kennedy. 2009. "Mastitis Detection: Current Trends and Future Perspectives." *Trends in Biotechnology* 27 (8): 486–93. doi:10.1016/j.tibtech.2009.05.004.
Zweig, Gunter, and Richard J. Block. 1954. "Studies on Bovine Whey Proteins. III. The Preparation of Crystalline Alpha-Lactalbumin and Beta-Lactoglobulin Ferrilactin." *Archives of Biochemistry and Biophysics* 51 (1). Arch Biochem Biophys: 200–7. doi:10.1016/0003-9861(54)90467-1.

11 Dairy Protein and the Risk of Non-Alcoholic Fatty Liver Disease

Jun-Hyuk Lee, Jihyun Yoon, and Yu-Jin Kwon

ABBREVIATIONS

CD36	Cluster of differentiation 36
CETP	Cholesteryl ester transfer protein
ChREBP	Carbohydrate-responsive element-binding protein
CLA	Conjugated linoleic acid
FFAs	Free fatty acids
Foxa2	Forkhead Box A2
GLUT4	Glucose transporter type 4
HOMA-IR	Homeostatic model assessment for insulin resistance
Ig	Immunoglobulins
IRS	Insulin receptor substrates
LXR	Liver X receptor
mTOR	(Mammalian Target of Rapamycin)
NAFLD	Non-alcoholic fatty liver disease
PI3K	Phosphoinositide 3-kinase
ROS	Reactive oxygen species
SREBP-1c	Sterol regulatory element-binding protein 1c
STAT	Signal transducers and activators of transcription
TNF-α	Tumor necrosis factor-α

INTRODUCTION

Milk and dairy products like yogurt, cheese, cream, and butter are highly regarded for their rich nutrient profile, providing essential proteins, fats, vitamins, and minerals. They have been proposed to be beneficial in preventing various health conditions, including obesity, cardiovascular disease, and type 2 diabetes. However, while these dairy products are endorsed by various governmental and healthcare professional organizations due to their high nutritional value (Carey and Whelton 2018), they may not be universally tolerated due to lactose intolerance and other dietary restrictions prevalent in certain populations (Bhatnagar and Aggarwal 2007). Moreover, the nutritional composition of dairy products can be quite variable due to differing production processes – such as lactic acid fermentation – and product types. These variations lead to differences in protein, fat, and carbohydrate contents.

Despite the potential benefits of dairy consumption, these foods are often calorie-dense and could contribute to weight gain if consumed in excess. It is important to moderate the intake of these foods to balance the potential health benefits with the risk of overconsumption. Additionally, further research is needed to fully understand and validate the proposed health benefits of dairy products,

DOI: 10.1201/9781003597926-11

especially in relation to chronic conditions like non-alcoholic fatty liver disease (NAFLD). NAFLD is the most prevalent chronic liver condition, and it is strongly linked to metabolic dysfunctions such as insulin resistance, obesity, and metabolic syndrome. Despite advances in pharmacological treatments targeting specific aspects of the disease, there is no universal treatment strategy for NAFLD. This chapter explores the nutritional characteristics and potential health benefits of dairy products related to NAFLD.

THE NUTRITIONAL CHARACTERISTICS OF DAIRY PRODUCTS

Dairy products, especially milk, contain specific proteins, fats, and carbohydrates alongside a variety of biologically active elements (Table 11.1). These include immunoglobulins, enzymes, antimicrobial peptides, oligosaccharides, hormones, cytokines, and growth factors, all of which play diverse biological roles.

PROTEINS

In bovine milk, the typical concentration of protein ranges between 3% and 4%, with the majority being casein (80%) and the remainder constituted by whey protein (20%) (Séverin and Wenshui 2005). Casein, representing 78–85% of the total protein content in milk, or 2.6–3.2% in terms of

TABLE 11.1
The Amount of Nutrients and Bioactive Components in a Serving of Selected Dairy Products

	Milk (Low Fat)	Milk (Whole)	Yogurt (Plain)	Cheese (Cheddar)	Butter
Serving size (g)	100	100	100	100	100
Energy (kcal)	42	65	89	298	761
Protein (g)	3.43	3.08	5.18	18.76	0.59
Total fat (g)	0.86	3.15	3.84	21.3	82.04
SFA (g)	0.29	2.17	2.46	14.46	48.05
MUFA (g)	0.2	0.74	0.9	3.97	15.96
PUFA (g)	0.03	0.1	0.11	0.45	1.84
Carbohydrates (g)	4.86	5.53	8.37	6.17	1.81
Lactose (g)	3.59	4.12	0.66	0	0
Cholesterol (mg)	9.1	9.69	13.64	64.62	232.12
Calcium (mg)	116	113	141	626	16
Phosphorus (mg)	87	84	105	857	19
Sodium (mg)	37	36	46	928	10
Magnesium (mg)	11	10	13	22	0
Potassium (mg)	149	143	174	62	29
Zinc (mg)	0.38	0.36	0.43	2.37	0.07
Iodine (μg)	11.89	6.08	4.2	11.28	4.19
Thiamin (mg)	0.017	0.021	0.021	0.059	0
Riboflavin (mg)	0.127	0.162	0.145	0.17	0.046
Vitamin A (RAE)	13	55	59	80	524

Abbreviations: MUFA, monounsaturated fatty acid; PUFA, polyunsaturated fatty acid; RAE, retinol activity equivalent; SFA, saturated fatty acid. Data from: The National Standard Food Composition Table published by the Rural Development Administration (https://koreanfood.rda.go.kr).

protein, is typically categorized into α-, β-, and κ-casein variants (Holt, Carver et al. 2013). Its nutritional superiority is underscored by its exceptional digestibility and optimal essential amino acid composition. Casein primarily functions as a mineral binder, serving as a transport medium for calcium and phosphorus. Additionally, it serves as a source for various physiologically active peptides that are beneficial to human health, encompassing antioxidants and immunoregulatory substances associated with cell regulation (Politis and Chronopoulou 2008). Whey protein, on the other hand, comprises heat-unstable α-lactalbumin and β-lactalbumin, as well as immunoglobulins, lactoferrin, proteoses, and certain enzymes, among others (Zapata et al. 2017). Immunoglobulins constitute 1.2–3.3% of milk protein and include types such as IgG2, IgA, and IgM. Notably, lactoferrin, a glycoprotein, exhibits potent antiviral and antibacterial properties and is inherently present solely in bovine and human colostrum (Shimazaki 2000). Milk proteins contain all nine essential amino acids, making them a source of complete protein. The presence of threonine, lysine, isoleucine, and tryptophan, which are essential amino acids vital for growth and somatic development in children, underscores the nutritive significance of milk proteins (Table 11.2).

FATS

The fat content in bovine milk ranges from 3 to 5%, predominantly made up of triglycerides of fatty acids, accounting for 95–96% of total milk fat (Lindmark Månsson 2008). The typical fat in milk consists of approximately 65% saturated fatty acids, 23% monounsaturated fatty acids, and 10% polyunsaturated fatty acids, of which approximately one-tenth are short-chain saturated fatty acids

TABLE 11.2
The Amino Acid Composition in Dairy Products

	Milk (Low Fat)	Milk (Whole)	Yogurt (Plain)	Cheese (Cheddar)	Butter
Serving size (g)	100	100	100	100	100
Total amino acids (mg)	3,079	3,033	4,070	18,519	517
Essential amino acid (mg)	1,398	1,381	1,698	8,821	242
Isoleucine (mg)	122	120	184	1,239	23
Leucine (mg)	333	333	367	1,513	51
Lysine (mg)	237	232	238	863	40
Methionine (mg)	69	72	78	803	18
Phenylalanine (mg)	135	135	21	1,060	24
Threonine (mg)	130	129	177	839	24
Tryptophan (mg)	35	31	31	306	2
Valine (mg)	165	158	226	1,042	28
Histidine (mg)	74	73	86	500	15
Arginine (mg)	98	98	100	656	17
Tyrosine (mg)	135	136	165	1,111	21
Cysteine (mg)	43	35	0	176	8
Alanine (mg)	97	96	147	696	16
Aspartic acid (mg)	227	224	307	1,133	38
Glutamic acid (mg)	637	628	932	4,192	99
Glycine (mg)	55	55	116	318	11
Proline (mg)	319	310	483	1,051	49
Serine (mg)	168	168	222	1,021	33

Source: Data from The National Standard Food Composition Table published by the Rural Development Administration.

with 4, 6, 8, or 10 carbon atoms. A notable proportion of these short-chain fatty acids is butyric acid (Marangoni et al. 2019). The unsaturated fatty acid component includes oleic acid, linoleic acid, and α-linolenic acid. Oleic acid (18:1, monounsaturated) comprises 25–30%. Essential fatty acids such as linoleic acid (18:2, n-6 series) and α-linolenic acid (18:3, n-3) are also present in milk.

Traditionally, all forms of saturated fatty acids were believed to elevate serum cholesterol levels. Current evidence, however, indicates that serum cholesterol levels are modulated by the unique properties of individual saturated fatty acids (Chowdhury et al. 2014). The atherogenic potential is ostensibly influenced by both the chain length and the physical state of these fatty acids. Free fatty acids (FFAs), including lauric, palmitic, and myristic acids, have been primarily implicated in inducing a surge in serum cholesterol (Bhat and Bhat 2011). Milk fat is notable for its short- and medium-chain fatty acids (C4–C12) – which constitute 11–12% of total fatty acids – and exhibits cardioprotective effects by reducing low-density lipoprotein (LDL) cholesterol levels (German and Dillard 2006). Additionally, milk fat promotes the absorption of fat-soluble vitamins such as A, D, E, and K. The overall cholesterol content in milk is relatively low at approximately 0.25–0.4% of total milk fat (3–4 mg/g) (Marangoni et al. 2019).

CARBOHYDRATES

Lactose, the primary carbohydrate in milk, is present at concentrations of approximately 4.6–4.9 g/100 mL of milk (Antunes et al. 2022). Lactic acid is derived from lactose through lactic fermentation and is cleaved into glucose and galactose by the enzyme lactase (β-galactosidase). These molecules play critical roles in maintaining blood glucose levels. Lactose significantly enhances the absorption of minerals like calcium, which is abundant in milk. However, its slow absorption rate can cause intestinal peristalsis and occasionally mild diarrhea. Lactose remains largely unhydrolyzed in the stomach and primarily descends into the small intestine, where it undergoes decomposition by lactase, an enzyme located in the epithelial cells of the intestinal mucosa. These breakdown products serve as nutrients for gut microbiota (Lomer et al. 2008).

MINERALS AND VITAMINS

Milk contains approximately 0.7% minerals, primarily in ionic and salt forms (Kaufmann and Hagemeister 1987). It is an optimal source of calcium due to its digestibility. Other constituents in milk, including lactose, vitamin D, and citric acid, have been observed to promote calcium absorption. Calcium and phosphorus are integral for the formation and maintenance of bones and teeth; their recommended ratio (1:1) can be achieved through sufficient milk intake. Milk also provides significant amounts of essential minerals such as potassium, magnesium, and sodium, alongside more than ten trace elements, including copper, iron, and zinc, all of which are crucial for metabolic functions within the human body (Stocco et al. 2021). Additionally, dairy products supply vitamins A, B2, and B6 but have relatively low levels of vitamin C and iron (Woźniak et al. 2022).

PHYSICAL PROPERTIES OF DAIRY PRODUCTS

The physical characteristics of dairy products can be divided into two main categories: physical state and composition. The physical state refers to appearance, texture, and consistency. Milk is an opaque white heterogeneous fluid where various components exist as emulsions, colloidal dispersions, or solutions. The state of milk components influences the nutritional and physiological characteristics of milk. Notably, the fat components of milk exist in the form of an emulsion that assists in the metabolism and absorption of milk fats.

Furthermore, the composition of dairy products indicates their chemical constitution. The composition of dairy products varies depending on the product type or processing method.

- Fresh milk is composed of water (87%), milk fat (3.5%), protein (3.3%), lactose (4.8%), and minerals (1%).
- Yogurt consists of water (88%), milk fat (3%), protein (4.2%), lactose (4.6%), and inorganic matter (0.4%).
- Cheese is composed of water (50–80%), milk fat (20–30%), protein (20–30%), and minerals (5–10%).
- Butter is made up of milk fat (80–90%), water (10–15%), and milk solids (1–5%).
- Ice cream is composed of water (55%), milk fat (10.5%), protein (3%), lactose (10%), and sugar (12%) (Chandan 2011).

The physical properties of dairy products are important for nutritional supply. For example, the high water content in fresh milk makes it a good source of hydration. The high protein content in yogurt provides a good source of satiety. And due to the high fat content in cheese, it becomes a good source of calories.

HEALTH BENEFITS OF DAIRY PRODUCTS

The nutritional role of milk is related to supplying essential and non-essential nutrients for optimizing human growth, development, and maintenance. With the shifting focus towards preventing chronic diseases through dietary and lifestyle modifications, certain constituents of dairy have been underscored for their potential health-boosting attributes. However, these claims need more support from a broader base of research evidence.

REDUCED RISK OF CARDIOVASCULAR DISEASE

Dairy products may help reduce the risk of heart disease by lowering blood pressure and cholesterol levels. Milk proteins, including casein, β-lactoglobulin, α-lactalbumin, immunoglobulin, lactoferrin, and serum albumin, break down into various peptides that show diverse biological effects such as immune regulation, antimicrobial activity, antithrombotic activity, blood pressure regulation, and mineral or vitamin binding (Meisel 1998). β-lactoglobulin, which constitutes about 50% of whey protein, plays a role in transporting lipophilic substances and lowering cholesterol. Conjugated linoleic acid (CLA) has various functionalities, including anti-cancer effects, cholesterol-lowering effects, and obesity-suppression effects (Akalin and Gonc 2006). Additionally, high plasma levels of saturated fatty acid C17:0 due to milk intake have been associated with a reduced risk of coronary heart disease (Chowdhury et al. 2014). According to a study in Europe, the typical short-chain saturated fatty acids of milk (with C4–C10) also provide a moderate protective effect against coronary artery risk (Warensjö et al. 2010).

MANAGEMENT OF TYPE 2 DIABETES, WEIGHT, AND METABOLIC SYNDROME

Previous studies indicate a potential correlation between milk consumption and a decreased risk of type 2 diabetes, as demonstrated in the longest cohort study and confirmed by recent meta-analyses (Elwood et al. 2007). This protective effect could be attributed to the high levels of calcium and magnesium in milk, minerals that are vital for insulin sensitivity and glucose tolerance. Additionally, dairy products may help manage weight by providing satiety and fullness. The protein in milk and dairy products helps to reduce body fat storage by preventing excessive energy consumption and is important for weight loss and subsequent weight maintenance due to its high satiety effect. Moreover, dairy protein is a good source of essential amino acids for muscle protein synthesis, thus helping to maintain metabolically active muscle mass during weight loss (Abargouei et al. 2012; Booth et al. 2015). Some meta-analyses report that dairy intake in adults helps to reduce body fat and preserve muscle mass by aiding in weight loss (Abargouei et al. 2012; Booth et al. 2015).

PREVALENCE OF NAFLD

NAFLD is defined as the presence of hepatic steatosis, characterized by the accumulation of fat in the liver exceeding 5% of its total weight, in the absence of other causative factors such as alcohol consumption, viral hepatitis, or medications known to induce hepatic lipid accumulation. The current global prevalence of NAFLD is steadily increasing, rising from 25.5% in or before 2005 to 37.8% in 2016 or later (Riazi et al. 2022). Furthermore, it is predicted that by 2040, 55.7% of all adults will be affected by NAFLD (Younossi et al. 2023).

The regional prevalence of NAFLD is highest in Latin America (44.4%), followed by the Middle East and North Africa (36.5%), South Asia (33.8%), Southeast Asia (33.1%), North America (31.2%), East Asia (29.7%), Asia Pacific (28.0%), and finally Western Europe (25.1%) (Younossi et al. 2023). As individuals age, the incidence of metabolic disorders tends to increase, leading to a rise in NAFLD prevalence. The peak prevalence of NAFLD was noted in men in their 50s (29.3%) and women in their 60s or over (25.4%) (Lazo et al. 2013). However, a recent shift in trends over several decades indicates a rapid surge in NAFLD cases predominantly affecting young adults (Allen et al. 2018). Over the last two decades, the prevalence of NAFLD among individuals aged 19–39 has increased sevenfold (Allen et al. 2018). These changes have been most prominent in low-to-middle sociodemographic regions such as the Middle East and North Africa. This increase seems to be associated with the rising trend of obesity prevalence among young adults in this area (Chen et al. 2022). The prevalence of NAFLD varies between genders as well. Men have a higher prevalence of NAFLD (40%) compared to women (26%) (Teng et al. 2023). Additionally, compared with premenopausal women, postmenopausal women are at a 2.37 times higher risk of NAFLD (Jaroenlapnopparat et al. 2023).

PATHOPHYSIOLOGY OF NAFLD

The pathophysiology of NAFLD is remarkably complex and involves a multitude of intertwined mechanisms (Figure 11.1). Traditionally, the pathophysiology of NAFLD was believed to follow a two-hit theory. The first hit is the accumulation of fat in the liver due to insulin resistance, followed by the second hit, which involves oxidative stress, lipid peroxidation, mitochondrial dysfunction, and pro-inflammatory cytokines, leading to hepatocyte damage, steatohepatitis, and liver fibrosis. Although these two-hit components are still considered to play the most critical role in the onset of NAFLD, they are inadequate in explaining the several molecular and metabolic changes that take place in NAFLD. Recent research suggests that NAFLD onset and progression occur through interactions of various factors, such as insulin resistance, cytokines/adipokines, changes in the gut microbiota, and genetic predispositions, leading to the emergence of multiple-hit theory.

INSULIN RESISTANCE

The first "hit" in the progression of NAFLD is characterized by the accumulation of lipids in the liver, primarily in the form of triacylglycerols. Excessive lipolysis in adipose tissues, coupled with a high-fat diet, leads to an increased influx of FFAs into the liver. Proteins such as cluster of differentiation 36 (CD36) and cholesteryl ester transfer protein (CETP) facilitate this influx, augmenting de novo lipogenesis and promoting the storage of triacylglycerols. This process alone accounts for about 26.1% of the total lipid content in the liver (Lambert et al. 2014). Insulin resistance exacerbates this process. The reduced effectiveness of insulin in suppressing adipose tissue lipolysis leads to increased circulation of FFAs, which triggers an inflammatory response and accounts for approximately 59% of the total hepatic lipid content. Furthermore, high-fat diets stimulate the transcription factor known as sterol regulatory element-binding protein 1c (SREBP-1c), which promotes lipid synthesis and contributes to an estimated 14.9% of the total hepatic lipid content (Donnelly et al. 2005).

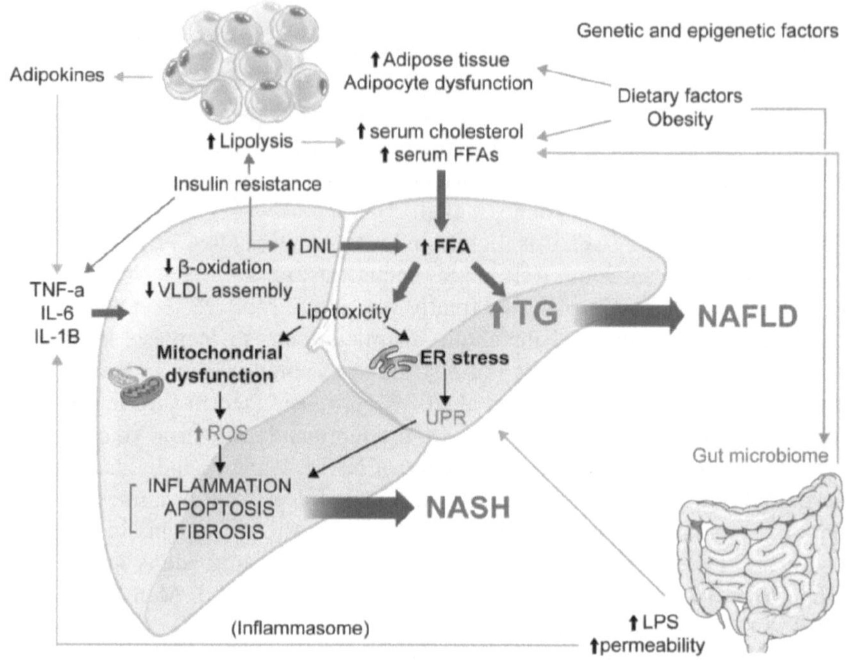

FIGURE 11.1 The pathophysiology of non-alcoholic fatty liver disease.

In normal insulin signaling, insulin binding to its receptor triggers phosphorylation of the receptor and two insulin receptor substrates (IRS)-1 and IRS-2. This initiates metabolic actions through various intracellular signaling pathways. First, through the phosphoinositide 3-kinase (PI3K)-AKT/protein kinase B (PKB) pathway, IRS-1 binds with PI3K, which activates AKT/PKB. This, in turn, phosphorylates and deactivates glycogen-synthase kinase-3, an inhibitory enzyme of glycogen activating enzyme, thereby increasing glycogen synthesis. At the same time, it translocates glucose transporter type 4 (GLUT4), which is in the cell, to the cell membrane, absorbing glucose from the blood into the cell. It also enhances the expression of SREBP-1c, inducing the synthesis of neutral fat, and by inhibiting cell death, it promotes cell survival. Second, after IRS-2 activation, the mitogen-activated protein kinases (MAPK)/extracellular signal-regulated kinases (ERK) pathway mainly affects cell growth and differentiation. It induces SREBP-1c, an important transcription factor for fat synthesis, playing a key role in new fat synthesis in hepatocytes.

Carbohydrate-responsive element-binding protein (ChREBP) is another crucial transcription factor for the expression of liver enzymes required for glucose metabolism, fatty acid, and neutral fat synthesis. Glucose regulates ChREBP by dictating its entry from the cytosol into the nucleus, promoting its binding to carbohydrate-responsive elements in the promoter regions of genes involved in glycolysis and lipogenesis. When intrahepatic glucose concentration increases, ChREBP is activated, promoting processes within the cell, stimulating fat formation, and converting excess glucose into fatty acids (Benhamed et al. 2012). Therefore, when consuming a high-carbohydrate diet, ChREBP activation can be promoted, leading to intrahepatic fat accumulation.

In a state of insulin resistance, de novo fat synthesis in the liver increases, fat breakdown in adipose tissue is stimulated, and the release of FFAs increases, leading to an increase in fatty acids flowing into the liver. This increases insulin resistance in the liver and simultaneously induces fatty acid oxidation in the mitochondria, peroxisomes, and microsomes. This process increases the generation of reactive oxygen species and lipid peroxidation products, damaging the liver cell membrane. This oxidative stress and inflammatory cytokines activate nuclear factor κ-B (NF-κB) kinase subunit-β (IKK-β) inhibitors and C-Jun N-terminal kinase (JNK), inhibiting insulin signal transmission, leading to further insulin resistance. This vicious cycle exacerbates NAFLD.

OXIDATIVE STRESS

After the first "hit," the liver becomes vulnerable to a second "hit" involving oxidative stress, lipid peroxidation, mitochondrial dysfunction, and the release of pro-inflammatory cytokines. The capacity of the liver to process and eliminate excessive lipids becomes overwhelmed, resulting in oxidative stress. This heightened state of stress prompts the production of reactive oxygen species (ROS), which promote lipid peroxidation and ultimately precipitate mitochondrial dysfunction (Gambino et al. 2011). In response to the cellular damage, hepatocytes release pro-inflammatory cytokines, heightening inflammation and starting a cycle of liver cell injury and inflammation. This vicious cycle can drive the progression to more severe stages of NAFLD, including non-alcoholic steatohepatitis (NASH), fibrosis, and cirrhosis. Research indicates that oxidative stress is a principal mechanism leading to liver injury in NAFLD (Gandhi 2012). The heightened production of ROS can incite lipid peroxidation, sparking inflammation and fibrogenesis by activating hepatic stellate cells (Gandhi 2012). This disruption of the oxidant/antioxidant balance further impacts metabolic processes within cellular organelles, propelling lipid peroxidation, mitochondrial dysfunction, and endoplasmic reticulum stress (Gambino et al. 2011).

CYTOKINES/ADIPOKINES

The involvement of leptin, an adipose-derived hormone, in NAFLD is well established, with leptin resistance being a common feature (Jiménez-Cortegana et al. 2021). Research has suggested a role for leptin in the activation of STAT3, which regulates energy balance and may also interact with other cytokines. Animal models have shown that leptin differentially regulates the activation of STAT3 in mice (Zhou et al. 2012). Furthermore, leptin receptor protein levels and basal hypothalamic phosphorylated STAT3 levels were similar in control and high-fructose diets, impacting weight gain and appetite (Chávez-Tapia et al. 2009).

Tumor necrosis factor (TNF)-α is secreted by Kupffer cells and adipocytes (Kakino et al. 2018). TNF-α induces insulin resistance by disrupting the insulin signaling pathway (Kakino et al. 2018). This is accomplished by inhibiting the function of IRS-1 through the activation of IKK-β/NFκB and JNK. Simultaneously, TNF-α enhances the expression of pro-inflammatory substances like interleukin (IL)-6 and IL-8 by activating the inflammatory pathway. This creates a vicious cycle between the inflammation and insulin resistance. Additionally, TNF-α induces mitochondrial permeability transition through death domains on the cell membrane, promoting cell apoptosis (Tiegs and Horst 2022). This process produces cytokeratin-18 breakdown products in the blood, serving as markers distinguishing steatohepatitis from simple steatosis.

IL-6, when binding to its receptor, activates the JAK/STAT3 signaling pathway similarly to leptin through glycoprotein 130 (Kroy et al. 2010). On the other hand, IL-6 induces the expression of suppressor of cytokine signaling 3, which is involved in leptin resistance and insulin resistance through the inhibition of IRS-1, contributing to the development of NAFLD.

GUT MICROBIOTA

The gut microbiota plays an integral role in the pathophysiology of NAFLD, and its complex and extensive influence on the development of NAFLD is commonly referred to as the "gut-liver axis." Connections between the gut and the liver are facilitated by the portal vein, which delivers products derived from the gut straight to the liver, and by the liver's feedback mechanism that returns bile and antibodies to the gut. Gut microbiota dysbiosis is characterized by decreased microbiota diversity, an increase in gram-negative bacteria (mainly *Proteobacteria*), and a decrease in gram-positive bacteria (primarily *Firmicutes*) (Di Ciaula et al. 2022). Studies report that increased levels of *Proteobacteria*, *Enterobacteriaceae*, *Escherichia*, *Bacteroides*, *Dorea*, and *Peptoniphilus*, alongside reduced levels of *Rikenellaceae*, *Ruminococcaceae*, *Faecalibacterium*, *Coprococcus*, *Anaerosporobacter*, and *Eubacterium* in patients with NAFLD (Iino et al. 2019). There is increasing evidence highlighting the pathological role of microbial metabolites, including trimethylamine, secondary bile acids, and short-chain fatty acids, in the development of NAFLD. Gut microbiota dysbiosis also induces inflammation in the gut, which results in the disruption of physical elements of the intestinal barriers, such as the epithelial layer and the gut-vascular barriers. Subsequently, inflammatory microbial metabolites or microbes translocate to systemic sites, including the liver, where they induce local inflammation and promote the development of NAFLD.

GENETIC PREDISPOSITIONS

The most extensively studied genes related to NAFLD to date are the patatin-like phospholipase domain-containing 3 (*PNPLA3*) gene, the Transmembrane 6 Superfamily Member 2 (*TM6SF2*) gene, and the membrane-bound O-acyltransferase domain-containing 7 (*MBOAT7*) gene (Longo et al. 2022). The rs738409 (C>G) single nucleotide polymorphism (SNP) in the *PNPLA3* gene (I148M), identified in 2008 genome-wide association studies, is common in Asians and Hispanics (Romeo et al. 2008). *PNPLA3* is a multifunctional enzyme believed to affect insulin signaling and fat metabolism, regulating the expression of lipase that controls the metabolism of neutral fats and retinoids. The *PNPLA3* 148M variant reduces enzyme activity, leading to fat accumulation in hepatocytes and stellate cells, thereby progressing liver damage. This mutation also reduces the secretion of very low-density lipoprotein, contributing to hepatic steatosis by promoting fat secretion disorder and fat accumulation within hepatocytes (Jiang et al. 2018). While wild-type carriers maintain a balance between fat creation and fat breakdown, those with the G allele mutation experience reduced fat breakdown due to the loss of lipase activity, leading to fat accumulation in the hepatocytes (Pirazzi et al. 2014). Thus, the G allele (rs738409) correlates with an increase in fatty liver, indicating that the role of *PNPLA3* I148M is associated with the pathogenesis of hepatic steatosis.

THE MECHANISMS UNDERLYING THE ASSOCIATION BETWEEN DAIRY PRODUCTS AND NAFLD RISK

Several clinical studies have established the association between dairy protein and NAFLD. Lee et al. (2021) found an inverse relationship between dairy protein intake and NAFLD development in a large population-based cohort study with a 10-year follow-up period. Zhang, Fu et al. (2020) reported that higher yogurt consumption inversely correlated with the prevalence of newly diagnosed NAFLD. Several possible mechanisms may explain the association between dairy protein intake and incident NAFLD (Figure 11.2).

Inflammation stands as a pivotal contributor to the progression of NAFLD to more severe stages. Certain dairy products, particularly those containing probiotics and bioactive peptides, have shown potential anti-inflammatory effects. Probiotics, abundantly present in fermented dairy items, possess the capability to influence the gut microbiota and modulate the body's inflammatory response, which might indirectly impact liver inflammation. NAFLD can involve an escalated generation of reactive oxygen species coupled with diminished levels of essential antioxidants like glutathione, vitamin E, β-carotene, and vitamin C. The conceivable anti-inflammatory and antioxidant properties inherent in dairy products could contribute to mitigating the oxidative stress and inflammation that fuel the progression of fibrosis. A study conducted by Hamad et al. (2011) demonstrated heightened levels of glutathione in rats that were fed whey protein isolates, hydrolysates, and β-lactoglobulin.

The intake of dairy proteins holds significance in fostering muscle synthesis and function. A previous study (Lee et al. 2020) reported that consuming more than one glass of milk per day was

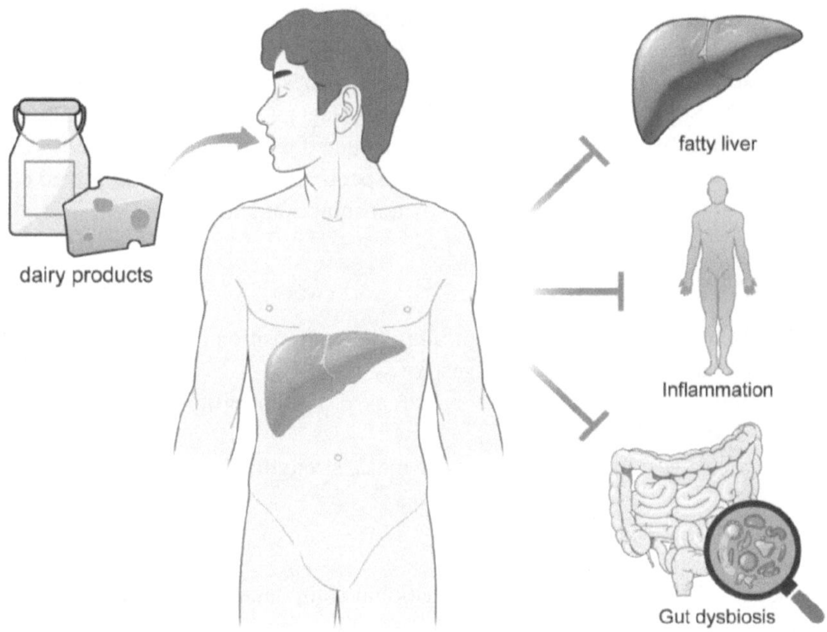

FIGURE 11.2 The mechanisms underlying the relationship between dairy products and non-alcoholic fatty liver disease.

associated with higher muscle mass index and muscle strength compared to consuming less than one glass. Dairy protein consumption might work in synergy with physical exercise to combat NAFLD and potentially forestall conditions such as sarcopenia, which poses a risk for NAFLD development. Adequate muscle mass can contribute to improved insulin sensitivity, which is beneficial for reducing the risk of insulin resistance and related metabolic conditions like NAFLD. Insulin resistance emerges as a crucial factor in the pathogenesis of NAFLD. The "Coronary Artery Risk Development in Young Adults" study unveiled an inverse correlation between the frequency of dairy consumption and the onset of insulin resistance syndrome (Pereira et al. 2002). A meta-analysis encompassing 30 randomized clinical trials demonstrated the potential benefits of dairy intake, particularly low-fat dairy products, on parameters like the homeostatic model assessment for insulin resistance (HOMA-IR), waist circumference, and body weight (Sochol et al. 2019).

THE EFFECTS OF OTHER PROTEINS

Soy foods have a long history of consumption in Asian countries. Soy protein is a significant contributor to plant-based protein sources in the human diet and contains all essential amino acids. Soybeans contain a wide range of nutrients, including proteins (primarily β-conglycinin and 11S glycinin), fats, carbohydrates, dietary fiber, vitamins, and isoflavones. Isoflavones are among the most extensively studied bioactive compounds found in soybeans. A previous study (Xiao and Hendry 2022) discovered that dietary soy proteins and their associated isoflavones can inhibit the formation and accumulation of lipid droplets in the liver. In non-obese animal models, soy protein and isoflavones accelerate hepatic lipolysis by activating SREBP-2 and increasing the expression of downstream genes (HMGC-R and LDLR). Meanwhile, soy protein inhibits hepatic lipogenesis by reducing the activity of SREBP-1 and its target genes (Xiao and Hendry 2022). This inhibition contributes to an improvement in NAFLD.

In a cohort study involving 4,622 participants aged 20–90 years, researchers found that a higher intake of soy food was linked to a reduced prevalence of NAFLD in Chinese adults (Zhang, Kumari et al. 2020). A systematic review and meta-analysis of randomized controlled clinical trials found that soybean and isoflavone may have varying effects on obesity-related anthropometric measures (Akhlaghi et al. 2017). Soy did not exhibit a significant effect on weight, waist circumference, or fat mass. In contrast, isoflavone studies, which were conducted exclusively in women, suggested that isoflavones may reduce body mass index. Further prospective studies and randomized clinical trials are needed to confirm the association between soy consumption and NAFLD.

MINI DICTIONARY OF TERMS

- **Gut dysbiosis:** An imbalance or disruption in the composition and function of the microorganisms that naturally inhabit the digestive system.
- **Predisposition:** A person's inherent or increased susceptibility to develop a particular condition or disease.
- **Sarcopenia:** The age-related loss of muscle mass, strength, and function.

SUMMARY POINTS

- Dairy products offer a diverse range of nutritional components and potential health advantages due to their varying proportions of proteins, fats, carbohydrates, minerals, and vitamins.
- Milk contains proteins, primarily casein (80%) and whey protein (20%), with casein providing essential amino acids.
- The global prevalence of non-alcoholic fatty liver disease (NAFLD), characterized by hepatic steatosis without other causative factors like alcohol consumption or viral hepatitis, has steadily risen.
- The underlying mechanisms of NAFLD involve insulin resistance, oxidative stress, cytokines, gut microbiota imbalances, and genetic factors.
- Dairy products have been found to mitigate NAFLD by addressing issues related to insulin resistance, inflammation, and oxidative stress.

REFERENCES

Abargouei, A. S., M. Janghorbani, M. Salehi-Marzijarani and A. Esmaillzadeh (2012). "Effect of dairy consumption on weight and body composition in adults: a systematic review and meta-analysis of randomized controlled clinical trials." *Int J Obes* **36**(12): 1485–1493.

Akalin, S. and S. Gonc (2006). "Functional properties of bioactive components of milk fat in metabolism." *Pak J Nutr.* **5**(3): 194–197

Akhlaghi, M., M. Zare and F. Nouripour (2017). "Effect of soy and soy isoflavones on obesity-related anthropometric measures: a systematic review and meta-analysis of randomized controlled clinical trials." *Adv Nutr* **8**(5): 705–717.

Allen, A. M., T. M. Therneau, J. J. Larson, A. Coward, V. K. Somers and P. S. Kamath (2018). "Nonalcoholic fatty liver disease incidence and impact on metabolic burden and death: A 20 year-community study." *Hepatology* **67**(5): 1726–1736.

Antunes, I., R. Bexiga, C. Pinto, L. Roseiro and M. Quaresma (2022). "Cow's milk in human nutrition and the emergence of plant-based milk alternatives." *Foods* **12**(1): 99.

Benhamed, F., P. D. Denechaud, M. Lemoine, C. Robichon, M. Moldes, J. Bertrand-Michel, V. Ratziu, L. Serfaty, C. Housset, J. Capeau, J. Girard, H. Guillou and C. Postic (2012). "The lipogenic transcription factor ChREBP dissociates hepatic steatosis from insulin resistance in mice and humans." *J Clin Invest* **122**(6): 2176–2194.

Bhat, Z. and H. Bhat (2011). "Milk and dairy products as functional foods: a review." *Int J Dairy Sci* **6**(1): 1–12.

Bhatnagar, S. and R. Aggarwal (2007). "Lactose intolerance." *BMJ* **334:** 1331–1332.

Booth, A. O., C. E. Huggins, N. Wattanapenpaiboon and C. A. Nowson (2015). "Effect of increasing dietary calcium through supplements and dairy food on body weight and body composition: a meta-analysis of randomised controlled trials." *Br J Nutr* **114**(7): 1013–1025.

Carey, R. M. and P. K. Whelton (2018). "Prevention, detection, evaluation, and management of high blood pressure in adults: synopsis of the 2017 American college of cardiology/American heart association hypertension guideline." *Ann Intern Med* **168**(5): 351–358.

Chandan, R. C. (2011). "Dairy ingredients for food processing: an overview." In: Chandan, R. C. and Kilara, A. (eds). *Dairy Ingredients for Food Processing.* Blackwell Publishing, Hoboken.

Chávez-Tapia, N. N., M. Uribe, G. Ponciano-Rodríguez, R. Medina-Santillán and N. Méndez-Sánchez (2009). "New insights into the pathophysiology of nonalcoholic fatty liver disease." *Ann Hepatol* **8**(Suppl 1): S9–17.

Chen, H., Y. Zhan, J. Zhang, S. Cheng, Y. Zhou, L. Chen and Z. Zeng (2022). "The global, regional, and national burden and trends of NAFLD in 204 countries and territories: an analysis from global burden of disease 2019." *JMIR Public Health Surveill* **8**(12): e34809.

Chowdhury, R., S. Warnakula, S. Kunutsor, F. Crowe, H. A. Ward, L. Johnson, O. H. Franco, A. S. Butterworth, N. G. Forouhi and S. G. Thompson (2014). "Association of dietary, circulating, and supplement fatty acids with coronary risk: a systematic review and meta-analysis." *Ann Intern Med* **160**(6): 398–406.

Chowdhury, R., S. Warnakula, S. Kunutsor, F. Crowe, H. A. Ward, L. Johnson, O. H. Franco, A. S. Butterworth, N. G. Forouhi, S. G. Thompson, K. T. Khaw, D. Mozaffarian, J. Danesh and E. Di Angelantonio (2014). "Association of dietary, circulating, and supplement fatty acids with coronary risk: a systematic review and meta-analysis." *Ann Intern Med* **160**(6): 398–406.

Di Ciaula, A., L. Bonfrate and P. Portincasa (2022). "The role of microbiota in nonalcoholic fatty liver disease." *Eur J Clin Invest* **52**(7): e13768.

Donnelly, K. L., C. I. Smith, S. J. Schwarzenberg, J. Jessurun, M. D. Boldt and E. J. Parks (2005). "Sources of fatty acids stored in liver and secreted via lipoproteins in patients with nonalcoholic fatty liver disease." *J Clin Invest* **115**(5): 1343–1351.

Elwood, P. C., J. E. Pickering and A. M. Fehily (2007). "Milk and dairy consumption, diabetes and the metabolic syndrome: the Caerphilly prospective study." *J Epidemiol Community Health* **61**(8): 695–698.

Gambino, R., G. Musso and M. Cassader (2011). "Redox balance in the pathogenesis of nonalcoholic fatty liver disease: mechanisms and therapeutic opportunities." *Antioxid Redox Signal* **15**(5): 1325–1365.

Gandhi, C. R. (2012). "Oxidative stress and hepatic stellate cells: a paradoxical relationship." *Trends Cell Mol Biol* **7**: 1–10.

German, J. B. and C. J. Dillard (2006). "Composition, structure and absorption of milk lipids: a source of energy, fat-soluble nutrients and bioactive molecules." *Crit Rev Food Sci Nutr* **46**(1): 57–92.

Hamad, E. M., S. H. Taha, A. G. Abou Dawood, M. Z. Sitohy and M. Abdel-Hamid (2011). "Protective effect of whey proteins against nonalcoholic fatty liver in rats." *Lipids Health Dis* **10**: 57.

Holt, C., J. Carver, H. Ecroyd and D. Thorn (2013). "Invited review: Caseins and the casein micelle: Their biological functions, structures, and behavior in foods." *J Dairy Sci* **96**(10): 6127–6146.

Iino, C., T. Endo, K. Mikami, T. Hasegawa, M. Kimura, N. Sawada, S. Nakaji and S. Fukuda (2019). "Significant decrease in Faecalibacterium among gut microbiota in nonalcoholic fatty liver disease: a large BMI- and sex-matched population study." *Hepatol Int* **13**(6): 748–756.

Jaroenlapnopparat, A., N. Charoenngam, B. Ponvilawan, M. Mariano, J. Thongpiya and P. Yingchoncharoen (2023). "Menopause is associated with increased prevalence of nonalcoholic fatty liver disease: a systematic review and meta-analysis." *Menopause* **30**(3): 348–354.

Jiang, Z. G., E. B. Tapper, M. Kim, M. A. Connelly, S. A. Krawczyk, E. U. Yee, M. A. Herman, K. J. Mukamal and M. Lai (2018). "Genetic determinants of circulating lipoproteins in nonalcoholic fatty liver disease." *J Clin Gastroenterol* **52**(5): 444–451.

Jiménez-Cortegana, C., A. García-Galey, M. Tami, P. Del Pino, I. Carmona, S. López, G. Alba and V. Sánchez-Margalet (2021). "Role of leptin in non-alcoholic fatty liver disease." *Biomedicines* **9**(7): 762.

Kakino, S., T. Ohki, H. Nakayama, X. Yuan, S. Otabe, T. Hashinaga, N. Wada, Y. Kurita, K. Tanaka, K. Hara, E. Soejima, Y. Tajiri and K. Yamada (2018). "Pivotal role of TNF-α in the development and progression of nonalcoholic fatty liver disease in a murine model." *Horm Metab Res* **50**(1): 80–87.

Kaufmann, W. and H. Hagemeister (1987). "Composition of milk." In: Grovert, H. O. (ed.). *Dairy-cattle Production. World Animal Science.* Elsevier Science Publishers, New York.

Kroy, D. C., N. Beraza, D. F. Tschaharganeh, L. E. Sander, S. Erschfeld, A. Giebeler, C. Liedtke, H. E. Wasmuth, C. Trautwein and K. L. Streetz (2010). "Lack of interleukin-6/glycoprotein 130/signal transducers and activators of transcription-3 signaling in hepatocytes predisposes to liver steatosis and injury in mice." *Hepatology* **51**(2): 463–473.

Lambert, J. E., M. A. Ramos-Roman, J. D. Browning and E. J. Parks (2014). "Increased de novo lipogenesis is a distinct characteristic of individuals with nonalcoholic fatty liver disease." *Gastroenterology* **146**(3): 726–735.

Lazo, M., R. Hernaez, M. S. Eberhardt, S. Bonekamp, I. Kamel, E. Guallar, A. Koteish, F. L. Brancati and J. M. Clark (2013). "Prevalence of nonalcoholic fatty liver disease in the United States: the third national health and nutrition examination survey, 1988–1994." *Am J Epidemiol* **178**(1): 38–45.

Lee, J. H., H. S. Lee, S. B. Ahn and Y. J. Kwon (2021). "Dairy protein intake is inversely related to development of non-alcoholic fatty liver disease." *Clin Nutr* **40**(10): 5252–5260.

Lee, J. H., H. S. Lee, H. Kim, Y. J. Kwon and J. W. Lee (2020). "Association of milk consumption frequency on muscle mass and strength: an analysis of three representative Korean population studies." *Eur J Nutr* **59**(7): 3257–3267.

Lindmark Månsson, H. (2008). "Fatty acids in bovine milk fat." *Food Nutr Res* **52**(1): 1821.

Lomer, M. C., G. Parkes and J. Sanderson (2008). "lactose intolerance in clinical practice–myths and realities." *Aliment Pharmacol Ther* **27**(2): 93–103.

Longo, M., M. Meroni, E. Paolini, V. Erconi, F. Carli, F. Fortunato, D. Ronchi, R. Piciotti, S. Sabatini, C. Macchi, A. Alisi, L. Miele, G. Soardo, G. P. Comi, L. Valenti, M. Ruscica, A. L. Fracanzani, A. Gastaldelli and P. Dongiovanni (2022). "TM6SF2/PNPLA3/MBOAT7 loss-of-function genetic variants impact on NAFLD development and progression both in patients and in in vitro models." *Cell Mol Gastroenterol Hepatol* **13**(3): 759–788.

Marangoni, F., L. Pellegrino, E. Verduci, A. Ghiselli, R. Bernabei, R. Calvani, I. Cetin, M. Giampietro, F. Perticone and L. Piretta (2019). "Cow's milk consumption and health: a health professional's guide." *J Am Coll Nutr* **38**(3): 197–208.

Meisel, H. (1998). "Overview on milk protein-derived peptides." *Int Dairy J* **8**(5–6): 363–373.

Pereira, M. A., D. R. Jacobs, Jr., L. Van Horn, M. L. Slattery, A. I. Kartashov and D. S. Ludwig (2002). "Dairy consumption, obesity, and the insulin resistance syndrome in young adults: the CARDIA Study." *JAMA* **287**(16): 2081–2089.

Pirazzi, C., L. Valenti, B. M. Motta, P. Pingitore, K. Hedfalk, R. M. Mancina, M. A. Burza, C. Indiveri, Y. Ferro, T. Montalcini, C. Maglio, P. Dongiovanni, S. Fargion, R. Rametta, A. Pujia, L. Andersson, S. Ghosal, M. Levin, O. Wiklund, M. Iacovino, J. Borén and S. Romeo (2014). "PNPLA3 has retinyl-palmitate lipase activity in human hepatic stellate cells." *Hum Mol Genet* **23**(15): 4077–4085.

Politis, I. and R. Chronopoulou (2008). "Milk peptides and immune response in the neonate." *Adv Exp Med Biol* **606**: 253.

Riazi, K., H. Azhari, J. H. Charette, F. E. Underwood, J. A. King, E. E. Afshar, M. G. Swain, S. E. Congly, G. G. Kaplan and A. A. Shaheen (2022). "The prevalence and incidence of NAFLD worldwide: a systematic review and meta-analysis." *Lancet Gastroenterol Hepatol* **7**(9): 851–861.

Romeo, S., J. Kozlitina, C. Xing, A. Pertsemlidis, D. Cox, L. A. Pennacchio, E. Boerwinkle, J. C. Cohen and H. H. Hobbs (2008). "Genetic variation in PNPLA3 confers susceptibility to nonalcoholic fatty liver disease." *Nat Genet* **40**(12): 1461–1465.

Séverin, S. and X. Wenshui (2005). "Milk biologically active components as nutraceuticals: review." *Crit Rev Food Sci Nutr* **45**(7–8): 645–656.

Shimazaki, K.-i. (2000). "Lactoferrin: A marvelous protein in milk." *Nihon Chikusan Gakkaiho* **71**(4): 329–347.

Sochol, K. M., T. S. Johns, R. S. Buttar, L. Randhawa, E. Sanchez, M. Gal, K. Lestrade, M. Merzkani, M. K. Abramowitz, Y. Mossavar-Rahmani and M. L. Melamed (2019). "The effects of dairy intake on insulin resistance: a systematic review and meta-analysis of randomized clinical trials." *Nutrients* **11**(9): 2237.

Stocco, G., A. Summer, C. Cipolat-Gotet, M. Malacarne, A. Cecchinato, N. Amalfitano and G. Bittante (2021). "The mineral profile affects the coagulation pattern and cheese-making efficiency of bovine milk." *J Dairy Sci* **104**(8): 8439–8453.

Teng, M. L., C. H. Ng, D. Q. Huang, K. E. Chan, D. J. Tan, W. H. Lim, J. D. Yang, E. Tan and M. D. Muthiah (2023). "Global incidence and prevalence of nonalcoholic fatty liver disease." *Clin Mol Hepatol* **29**(Suppl): S32–s42.

Tiegs, G. and A. K. Horst (2022). "TNF in the liver: targeting a central player in inflammation." *Semin Immunopathol* **44**(4): 445–459.

Warensjö, E., J.-H. Jansson, T. Cederholm, K. Boman, M. Eliasson, G. Hallmans, I. Johansson and P. Sjögren (2010). "Biomarkers of milk fat and the risk of myocardial infarction in men and women: a prospective, matched case-control study." *Am J Clin Nutr* **92**(1): 194–202.

Woźniak, D., W. Cichy, M. Dobrzyńska, J. Przysławski and S. Drzymała-Czyż (2022). "Reasonableness of enriching cow's cilk with vitamins and minerals." *Foods* **11**(8): 1079.

Xiao, C. W. and A. Hendry (2022). "Hypolipidemic effects of soy protein and isoflavones in the prevention of non-alcoholic fatty liver disease – a review." *Plant Foods Hum Nutr* **77**(3): 319–328.

Younossi, Z. M., P. Golabi, J. M. Paik, A. Henry, C. Van Dongen and L. Henry (2023). "The global epidemiology of nonalcoholic fatty liver disease (NAFLD) and nonalcoholic steatohepatitis (NASH): a systematic review." *Hepatology* **77**(4): 1335–1347.

Zapata, R. C., A. Singh, A. Pezeshki, T. Nibber and P. K. Chelikani (2017). "Whey protein components-lactalbumin and lactoferrin-improve energy balance and metabolism." *Sci Rep* **7**(1): 9917.

Zhang, S., J. Fu, Q. Zhang, L. Liu, M. Lu, G. Meng, Z. Yao, H. Wu, Y. Xia, X. Bao, Y. Gu, S. Sun, X. Wang, M. Zhou, Q. Jia, K. Song, Y. Wu, H. Xiang and K. Niu (2020). "Association between habitual yogurt consumption and newly diagnosed non-alcoholic fatty liver disease." *Eur J Clin Nutr* **74**(3): 491–499.

Zhang, S., S. Kumari, Y. Gu, X. Wu, X. Li, G. Meng, Q. Zhang, L. Liu, H. Wu, Y. Wang, T. Zhang, X. Wang, X. Cao, H. Li, Y. Liu, X. Wang, S. Sun, X. Wang, M. Zhou, Q. Jia, K. Song, Z. Sun and K. Niu (2020). "Soy food intake is inversely associated with newly diagnosed nonalcoholic fatty liver disease in the TCLSIH cohort study." *J Nutr* **150**(12): 3280–3287.

Zhou, Z., M. Neupane, H. R. Zhou, D. Wu, C. C. Chang, N. Moustaid-Moussa and K. J. Claycombe (2012). "Leptin differentially regulate STAT3 activation in ob/ob mouse adipose mesenchymal stem cells." *Nutr Metab (Lond)* **9**(1): 109.

12 Dairy Proteins and Metabolic Health

A Focus on Bioactive Peptides

Giovanni Tulipano

ABBREVIATIONS

ACE	angiotensin-converting enzyme
α-LA	α-lactalbumin
AMP	adenosine monophosphate
AMPK	AMP-activated protein kinase
BCAA	branched-chain amino acids
β-LG	β-lactoglobulin
CaSR	Calcium-sensing receptor
CCK	Cholecystokinin
DPP-IV	Dipeptidyl peptidase-4
GCPR	G-coupled protein receptor
GI	Gastrointestinal
GIP	Glucose-dependent insulinotropic peptide
GLP-1	Glucagon-like peptide-1
IC_{50}	Half-maximal inhibitory concentration
mTORC1	Mammalian target of rapamycin complex 1
PPARα	Peroxisome proliferator-activated receptor-alpha

INTRODUCTION

Milk is a whole food with a complex structural matrix, important for growth and development. In fact, milk and dairy products are also recommended as an essential component of a healthy diet in adulthood as sources of calcium, vitamin D, and proteins with high nutritional quality, as expressed by their digestible indispensable amino acid score (DIAAS) (Leksrisompong and Layman 2014).

In the coming decades, the global demand for protein to meet the needs of an increasing population is expected to face the challenge of sustainability. Dietary recommendations and consumer food habits will play an important role. In this regard, it has been suggested that the goal could be achieved by limiting the ongoing increase in animal product consumption and encouraging plant-based protein consumption. Indeed, while an increase in animal protein consumption is expected, the related growth in plant protein production demand to sustain it, is approximately seven times higher, requiring significant amounts of water and soil (Bruno 2015).

On the other hand, regarding the valorization of specific dietary proteins, there has been a growing interest in harnessing potential health-promoting benefits linked to biologically active components, in addition to considering their nutritional quality.

Milk and dairy products are currently the most extensively investigated source of proteins and peptides, with various purported health benefits. Apart from milk, dairy products include fresh and

DOI: 10.1201/9781003597926-12

ripened cheeses, yoghurt, and other fermented milk products produced using bacterial cultures. Moreover, advancements in fractionation and purification methods have led to the isolation of protein fractions and the preparation of concentrated forms of milk proteins for use as ingredients or dietary supplements, such as protein-fortified beverages.

DAIRY PROTEINS AS A SOURCE OF BIOACTIVE COMPOUNDS

Various components of dairy protein fractions are believed to produce a wide range of health benefits, spanning mood and sleep regulation, gastrointestinal function, cardiovascular health, immune response, mineral absorption and trafficking, neuroendocrine control of energy homeostasis, and skeletal muscle anabolism (Table 12.1).

Bioactive compounds may include full proteins, products of bacterial fermentation and ripening of dairy foods, or products of protein digestion in the gut. In this regard, it has long been accepted that dairy proteins can be disassembled into small peptides with biological functions distinct from those of the parent protein, including antimicrobial, immunomodulatory, antioxidative, and antiatherogenic functions, as well as mineral-binding, opioid-like, and enzyme-inhibitory activities (Table 12.2). More recently, new classes of peptides impacting energy balance and plasma glucose homeostasis have been identified (Tulipano 2020; Auestad and Layman 2021; Koirala et al. 2023).

Free amino acids derived from protein digestion also play functional roles beyond being metabolic substrates. Some amino acids act as precursors for signalling molecules; others directly interact with cell-surface receptors involved in secretory activity or cell bioenergetics.

In this chapter, "bioactivity" refers to a positive influence on physiological or metabolic functions based on scientific evidence derived largely from laboratory investigations. While beneficial effects on human health are expected, they have not necessarily been demonstrated through clinical trials.

TABLE 12.1
Milk Protein Fractions and Their Biochemical and Functional Properties

The Main Proteins in Milk	Biochemistry and Bioactivities
Casein fractions: αS1-casein, αS2-casein, β-casein, and κ-casein	Carry clusters of phosphorylated amino acids; exhibit mineral carrier activity (calcium binding); "slow" proteins associated with a lower and more prolonged amino acid absorption profile after a meal; rich in proline; form micellar structures in native milk to maintain water solubility.
Whey proteins: α-lactalbumin, β-lactoglobulin, lactoferrin, and glycomacropeptide	Water-soluble "fast" proteins that are rapidly digested, leading to a quick rise in plasma amino acid concentrations after a meal; they are rich in leucine.
α-lactalbumin	Contribute to effects on sleep quality, mood, gastrointestinal function, mineral absorption, and immunity.
β-lactoglobulin	Transport hydrophobic ligands; regulate enzyme activity; support the development of passive immunity in neonates; provide a rich source of essential amino acids.
Lactoferrin	Facilitate iron delivery; exhibit antibacterial and antiviral functions; enhance normal cell development; reduce inflammation in the gut mucosa.
Glycomacropeptide	Exhibit antibacterial and prebiotic activities; feature a unique amino acid composition (devoid of aromatic amino acids).

Amino acid composition, post-translational modifications (i.e., phosphorylation of serine/threonine clusters), and chain folding may confer specific bioactivities to the distinct milk proteins.

TABLE 12.2
Health-Related Activities of Peptides Derived from Dairy Proteins (Based on Preclinical Evidence)

Antihypertensive (ACE-inhibitory peptides)
Antioxidative
Antithrombotic
Anti-inflammatory
Antidiabetic (type 2 diabetes)
Opioid-like
Regulation of calcium and iron transport and tissue calcification (casein phosphopeptides)

Over time, an increasing number of small peptides (2–20 amino acids long) endowed with specific biological functions have been isolated from hydrolyzed dairy proteins. The bioactivities listed in Table 12.2 are largely based on preclinical evidence and do not necessarily indicate that health benefits have been convincingly demonstrated in humans.

Finally, characterizing functional properties within diets – and identifying bioactive compounds underlying these properties – may follow two approaches: (1) drawing inspiration from nutritional epidemiology studies investigating relationships between diet and health indices; (2) investigating specific nutrient functions within tissues or organs to "design diet from the bottom up" (Ryann and Seeley 2013; Kondrashina et al. 2020; Auestad and Layman 2021). In both cases, isolating bioactive compounds can support claims for functional food or dietary supplements with health-related benefits.

WHEY PROTEIN FRACTION AND METABOLIC HEALTH

For years, whey proteins have been extensively used in dietary supplements for anabolic recovery (Auestad and Layman 2021). Their potential role in controlling food intake, body weight gain, and postprandial glycemic excursions under pathological conditions has also been investigated in clinical trials (Rigamonti et al. 2020; Smedegaard et al. 2021; Sridonpai et al. 2021; Smith et al. 2022; Oberoi et al. 2023). Mealtime whey protein intake impacts metabolic health by slowing gastric emptying while increasing incretin peptide secretion and insulin release. These actions stem from whey's high content of specific amino acids combined with fast amino acid absorption into circulation upon digestion by gut proteases (Kondrashina et al. 2020; Tulipano 2020). This results in a satiating effect, supporting the use of mealtime whey protein supplements during body weight reduction programs and enhancing mechanisms that mitigate hyperglycemic excursions in type 2 diabetic patients (Jakubowicz et al. 2014; Rigamonti et al. 2020; Smith et al. 2022). However, despite promising results from acute studies in small cohorts of healthy subjects or patients, there are insufficient studies supporting long-term efficacy in larger populations. Thus, the clinical applicability remains unclear (Smith et al. 2020; Giglio et al. 2023). Unexplored areas that require further research include: timing of supplementation relative to meals, optimal whey protein dose, long-term efficacy, effects of combination therapy with antidiabetic drugs, potential adverse effects, and variability in patient responses based on clinical features.

Nevertheless, some recent proceedings from clinical research are worth mentioning. In 2022, Smith et al. assessed the timing and dose of daily whey protein supplements and suggested their efficacy in increasing time spent in euglycemic conditions over seven days in individuals with type

2 diabetes. In 2023, a novel hypothesis suggested that pre-meal whey protein shots significantly decrease postprandial insulin clearance compared to placebo in humans (Smith et al. 2023).

WHEY PROTEINS AS HIGH-QUALITY PROTEINS

Whey – the serum or water-soluble fraction of milk remaining after curd separation – is produced during the coagulation of caseins, triggered by acidic environments or proteolytic cleavage during cheese-making. Advances in scientific knowledge and processing technologies have transformed whey from a by-product of cheese manufacturing into a valuable dairy material with expanded applications in health care and pharmacy (Smithers 2008). Whey proteins are high-quality proteins due to their amino acid composition, bioavailability, and bioactivity. They also show physicochemical properties (e.g., emulsion and foam stabilization, high water retention capacity) that are widely exploited in the food industry (Auestad and Layman 2021).

Whey proteins contain substantial amounts of all essential amino acids and are remarkably rich in lysine, methionine, tryptophan, and leucine – amino acids often limiting in plant proteins.

The digestion of food protein in the gut lumen releases free amino acids that enhance hormone secretion from enteroendocrine cells in the gut mucosa (Ezcurra et al. 2013; Wauson et al. 2013; Tulipano 2020). These hormones help regulate food consumption and postprandial glycemia (Table 12.3).

After transport across the intestinal mucosa, circulating amino acids regulate anabolic hormones like insulin and growth hormone. L-arginine, L-lysine, L-leucine, and L-phenylalanine are potent insulin secretagogues. Free amino acids also directly affect cell metabolism across tissues like skeletal muscle. Branched-chain amino acids (BCAAs) – L-leucine, L-valine, and L-isoleucine – are particularly well-studied for their metabolic impact both in vitro and in vivo (Valerio et al. 2011; Auestad and Layman 2021).

In summary, the rapid rise in plasma amino acid concentrations following whey protein digestion contributes to satiety by reducing food intake. Whey proteins support anabolic recovery and weight management during illness or aging, and aid post-exercise recovery for athletes (Gilmartin et al. 2020; Auestad and Layman 2021). However, concerns remain about the effect of high BCAA intake on glucose tolerance due to conflicting evidence on positive versus negative effects (Tulipano 2020).

THE UNIQUE FATE OF WHEY PROTEINS IN THE GASTROINTESTINAL TRACT

The differential fate of whey proteins in the GI tract compared with other proteins like caseins is believed to contribute to their distinct effects. Whey proteins are so-called "fast" proteins, based on the rate of amino acid absorption and protein synthesis. After being ingested, whey proteins reach

TABLE 12.3
Gastroenteric Hormones Involved in Dairy Protein Intake Effects

Gastroenteric Hormones	Functions
Cholecystokynin (CCK)	Stimulates gallbladder contraction and pancreatic enzyme secretion; decreases gastric motility, emptying rate, appetite, and food intake.
Incretin hormones (glucagon-like peptide-1 [GLP-1] and glucose-dependent insulinotropic peptide [GIP])	Enhance glucose homeostasis by increasing insulin secretion and decreasing glucagon secretion post-meal; reduce gastric emptying rate and food intake.
Ghrelin	An orexigenic peptide released during fasting or reduced calorie intake; stimulates appetite.

the jejunum rapidly as intact polypeptides but are digested slowly in the small intestine. Despite longer digestion in the intestine, the amino acid absorption is still faster than for proteins like caseins (so-called "slow" proteins), producing a faster and higher, but short-lasting, rise in plasma amino acids, which is essential for stimulating protein synthesis through mammalian target of rapamycin (mTOR) pathway activation in skeletal muscle (Figure 12.1). On the other hand, caseins are prone to clot in the stomach, delaying their release to the intestine. The slow digestion results in a lower and more prolonged amino acid absorption profile. As a result, whey proteins can provide a maximum response with the least amount of protein and calorie intake and may be useful when food intake has to be restricted. Casein can be used to enhance and prolong post-meal anabolic responses, i.e., during sleep, when the total amount of protein is not restricted (Gilmartin et al. 2020; Tulipano 2020; Auestad and Layman 2021).

The characterization of the differential properties between whey proteins and caseins has significant implications for designing specific milk formulas (Tulipano 2020; Auestad and Layman 2021). Some whey protein-fortified milk formulations with a reversed whey-to-casein ratio have been investigated in rodents and humans for their effects compared to regular milk. The fortified milk was shown to improve muscle strength and exercise capacity without lean mass accretion in rats. In humans, reversing the whey-to-casein ratio enhanced incretin and insulin responses compared to regular cow milk with identical lactose and total protein content. Similarly, a comparable

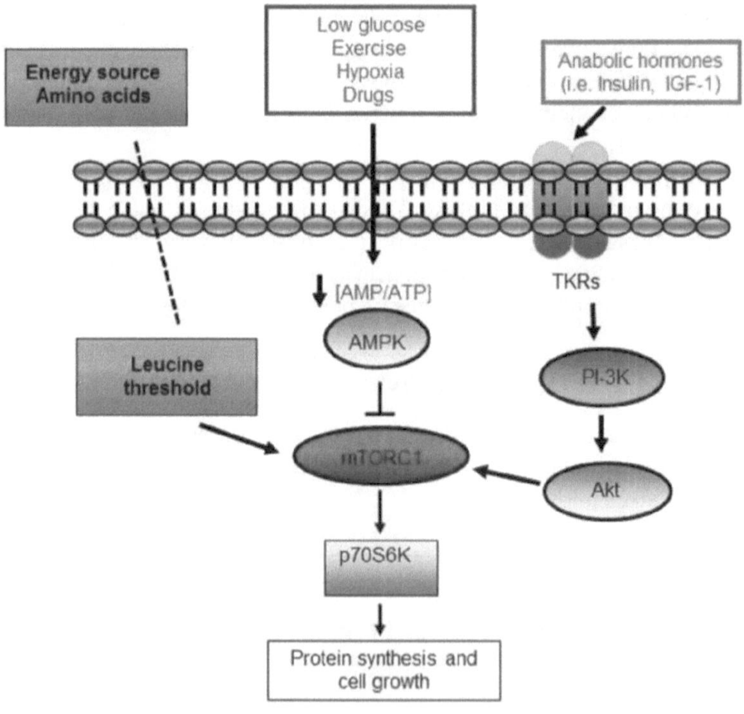

FIGURE 12.1 Role of mTORC1 in the intracellular signalling that regulates post-meal anabolic response in skeletal muscle fibers. mTOR is an intracellular complex which integrates multiple signals to determine whether an anabolic response in skeletal muscle tissue is sustainable. During fasting or calorie restriction, mTOR signalling is turned off in skeletal muscle, thereby shifting cells to net protein breakdown. When physical activity and nutrient availability are correctly balanced, mTOR signalling is activated and triggers the anabolic phase with protein synthesis. Among nutrients, BCAAs, especially leucine, play a main role. AMPK is an intracellular sensor of energy status activated in response to an increase in the AMP/ATP ratio, which limits the cell anabolic response and triggers catabolic pathways. mTORC1: mammalian target of rapamycin complex 1; BCAA: branched-chain amino acids; AMPK: AMP-activated kinase.

milk formula served with breakfast cereals in healthy adults was associated with a reduction in postprandial glycemia (El Khoury et al. 2019; Toffolon et al. 2021; Jeong et al. 2022).

ISOLATION AND CHARACTERIZATION OF BIOACTIVE PEPTIDES FROM FOOD PROTEINS

Bioactive peptides are defined as specific peptides (approximately 2–20 amino acids long) encrypted within the native amino acid sequence of food proteins. These peptides are released by proteolysis and exert positive effects on biochemical and cellular functions. They may ultimately benefit human health, by reducing or preventing chronic diseases during adulthood and aging. However, "bioactivity" does not necessarily mean that related health benefits have been convincingly demonstrated in humans through clinical trials.

Bioactive peptides can be released in three ways:

- Hydrolysis by digestive enzymes in the GI tract
- Hydrolysis by microbial fermentation
- The action of proteolytic enzymes isolated from microorganisms or plants

Bioinformatics (also known as in silico analysis) plays a key role in identifying food protein-derived peptides with biological functionality. Large databanks of full protein and peptide sequences, sequence alignment software, molecular docking simulations (to examine interactions between peptidic ligands and macromolecular targets), and quantitative structure-activity relationship (QSAR) modelling are all tools used to detect potential bioactive fragments encoded within a food protein's amino acid sequence. Computer software can also simulate proteolytic cleavage of food proteins by specific proteases (Minkiewicz et al. 2019; Nongonierma and FitzGerald 2016; Agyei et al. 2018; Chakrabarti et al. 2018).

A second strategy involves biochemical analysis and peptidomics, which include fractionation and separation of peptides via chromatographic methods and peptide identification using mass spectrometry combined with bioinformatics. These approaches have led to published lists of peptides released during gastrointestinal digestion of dairy proteins (in vivo or simulated in vitro) or during food processing (e.g., ripened cheeses or fermented milk products). Biochemical or biological assays allow researchers to isolate peptides exhibiting specific bioactivities from fractions of starting materials (Robinson et al. 2021; Baptista and Gigante 2021; Helal et al. 2023).

These investigations also improve methods for generating bioactive peptides from traditional foods or by-products of food processing, enabling the development of bioactive ingredients for dietary supplements or pharmaceuticals. Microbial fermentation or preliminary treatment of food proteins with specific proteases from plants or microbes may significantly alter substrates undergoing gastrointestinal digestion, thereby affecting the final products' patterns in the gut and their potential bioactivity. This consideration is appropriate for milk proteins in a variety of dairy products (Chakrabarti et al. 2018; Murtaza et al. 2022; Shukla et al. 2022).

LIMITED ORAL BIOAVAILABILITY CHALLENGES THE EFFECTIVENESS OF BIOACTIVE PEPTIDES IN VIVO

To reach their target tissues in active form, bioactive peptides must resist degradation in the gastrointestinal tract and cross the intestinal barrier into the bloodstream. For this reason, their effectiveness in humans has long been disputed due to limited evidence. Some peptides derived from food protein hydrolysis may be active directly within the gut lumen, skipping the need to reach the systemic circulation. In this context, gut microbiota and intestinal epithelial barriers – including dispersed enteroendocrine cells involved in the management of digestive functions and, ultimately, energy balance – represent easy targets for functional peptides (Figure 12.2).

Focussing on potential metabolic health benefits, a number of dairy protein-derived peptides with the ability to modulate food intake, body weight gain, and glucose homeostasis have been isolated and characterized (Tulipano 2020; Auestad and Layman 2021). The role played by bioactive peptides versus free amino acids needs to be discussed.

According to preclinical evidence, intact protein and partially hydrolyzed proteins can be more effective at inducing enteric hormone secretion than the products of their extensive hydrolysis. These data support the hypothesis that not only the relative content of specific amino acids (i.e., BCAAs) but also the spatial proximity between amino acid residues within a short sequence contributes to conferring functional activities to the products of food protein digestion. This means they are able to interact with specific biological systems. For example, a chymosin hydrolysate of sodium caseinate endowed with secretagogue activity in vitro was shown to reduce food intake after intraperitoneal administration in rodents. On the other hand, its effects on food intake and postprandial hormone levels were blunted after oral administration (Kondrashina et al. 2018; Kondrashina et al. 2020; Tulipano 2020). These data suggest that the bioactive component released after digestion with chymosin was not resistant to gastric acid and gastric proteases.

Moreover, the peptide ALPMH is an ACE-inhibitory peptide isolated from β-LG hydrolysates obtained using pepsin and trypsin. More recently, it was found to stimulate CCK secretion from

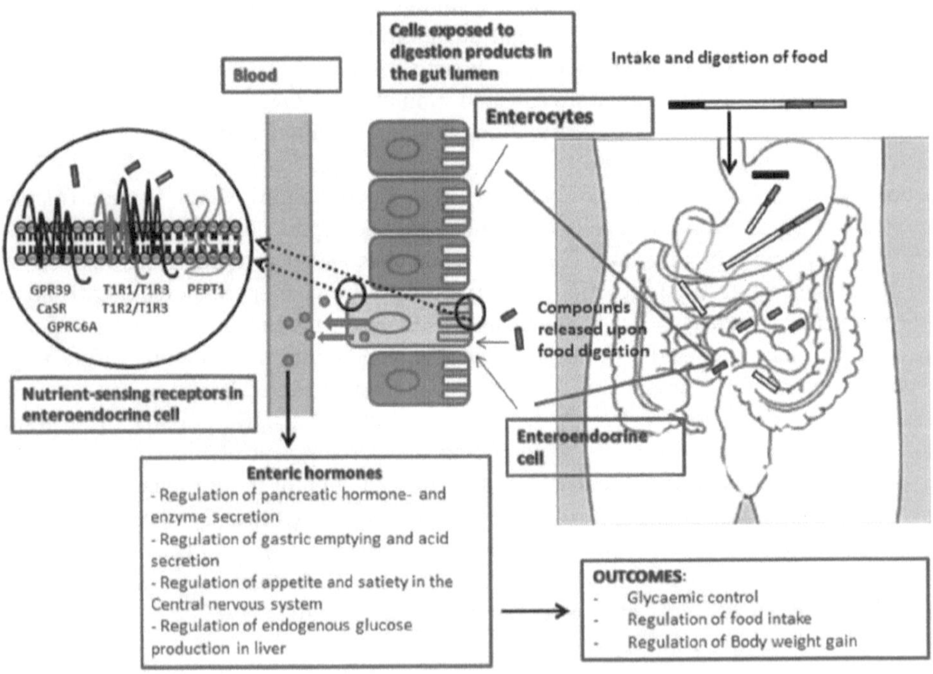

FIGURE 12.2 Interplay between nutrients and the neuroendocrine network is involved in the homeostatic control of food intake, body weight gain, and plasma glucose levels. The GI mucosa plays a crucial role in managing energy balance through dispersed enteroendocrine cells that release signals, mainly peptidic hormones and serotonin. Most enteroendocrine cells sense nutrients (carbohydrates, lipids, proteins) at their apical pole facing the gut lumen and their basolateral surface, and are induced to release hormones from their basal pole into circulation (i.e. GLP-1, GIP, and CCK). Receptors belonging to the class of GPCRs (GPR39, GPRC6A, CaSR, T1R1/T1R3 and T1R2/T1R3 heterodimers) and membrane transporters (PEPT1) have been implicated in peptide and free amino acid sensing in enteroendocrine cells. GLP-1: glucagon-like-peptide-1; GIP: glucose-dependent insulinotropic peptide; CCK: cholecystokinin; GPCR: G protein-coupled receptor.

enteroendocrine cells in vitro. In the same experimental settings, some di- and tripeptides with aliphatic side chains were ineffective, whereas the scrambled peptide PHLMA and two distinct peptides (six and eight amino acids long, respectively) were as effective as ALPMH. In summary, peptide length appears to be more relevant to their activity on enteroendocrine cells than specific amino acid sequences (Tulipano 2020).

PROTEOLYTIC CLEAVAGE OF DAIRY PROTEINS RELEASES BIOACTIVE PEPTIDES FOR METABOLIC HEALTH

Peptide YPFPGPI derives from β-casein (A1 genetic variant) and is resistant to degradation in the gastrointestinal tract. It has been called β-casomorphin-7 (β-CM7), meaning a heptapeptide from β-casein with μ-opioid receptor agonist activity. The activation of the μ-opioid receptors in the gut can increase gastrointestinal transit time and gut inflammation. Actually, β-CM7 also exerts non-opioid effects in the gut mucosa. It has been shown to stimulate CCK secretion and somatostatin release, which contribute to reducing gastric acid secretion, gastric motility, and the secretion of gastroenteric and pancreatic hormones.

There is evidence that β-CM7 and its fragment FPGPI are released in the jejunum after dairy product ingestion, and that FPGPI can move across the intestinal epithelial barrier. This peptide retains its ability to stimulate CCK secretion (Pupovac et al. 2002; Kondrashina et al. 2020).

β-CM7 bioactivity has significant implications for breeding and dairy production. Most bovine milk contains two genetic variants of β-casein: A1 and A2. β-CM7 is released upon digestion of A1 casein only; hence, it is absent in milk from animals expressing the A2 variant (so-called A2 milk). In conclusion, β-CM7 bioactivity has been associated with claims about differential functional properties between A1/A2 milk and A2 milk. A2 milk is claimed to be better tolerated by some consumers (Dantas et al. 2023).

Glycomacropeptide (GMP) is a large glycosylated peptide derived from κ-casein and released by the action of chymosin during cheese-making. It is a component of whey protein fractions. In animals and humans, evidence suggests that GMP can be effective after oral administration and may contribute to appetite-suppressant effects caused by whey protein intake. Its carbohydrate chains play a role in its bioactivity. Its effects on the release of satiety hormones like peptide YY, GLP-1, and CCK are at least partially indirect, mediated by alterations in gut microbiota composition (Veldhorst et al. 2009; Wernlund et al. 2021; Tulipano 2020).

Chymosin's action on sodium caseinate causes the release of the dipeptide RF, which has the potential to induce satiety. Specifically, it stimulates CCK secretion from enteroendocrine cells in vitro and is active in vivo after oral or intraperitoneal administration in mice, causing a delay in the gut transit of food and a short-lasting decrease in food intake (Kagebayashi et al. 2012; O'Halloran et al. 2018; Kondrashina et al. 2020).

MORE PEPTIDES DERIVED FROM DAIRY PROTEINS WERE SHOWN TO BE ACTIVE IN VIVO IN MICE

Peptide LIVTQTMKG and dipeptide MH (wheylin-1) were both isolated from the thermolysin digest of β-LG. LIVTQTMKG exerts an anorectic effect in fasted animals, mediated by antighrelinergic activity. This peptide also partially reversed the pancreatic β-cell damage in alloxan-induced diabetic mice with hyperglycemia. The peptide administration increased the expression of glucose transporter-2 (GLUT2) and suppressed apoptosis in β-cells, thus improving the insulin response and causing a reduction in plasma glucose and glycated serum protein levels (Aoki et al. 2017; Kondrashina et al. 2020; Koirala et al. 2023). Wheylin-1 is an anxiolytic-like dipeptide that also improves insulin sensitivity in mice by enhancing the activation of intracellular signalling pathways downstream of the insulin receptor. In summary, both peptides may contribute to the effects of whey protein intake on appetite and glucose control (Ogiwara et al. 2018; Tulipano 2020).

Peptide HIRL (β-lactotensin), isolated from the products of β-LG digestion with chymotrypsin, functions as a neurotensin receptor agonist (NT1 and NT2). However, its anorectic effect in fasted mice appears more closely linked to the activation of the corticotropin-releasing factor (CRF) system in the central nervous system, independently of the activation of NT1 or NT2 (Hou et al. 2009).

The tripeptide DQW from α-LA hydrolysates was administered by intragastric injection in mice fed a high-fat diet and was found to attenuate hepatic steatosis and insulin resistance. Its beneficial effects were related to an increase in the production of short-chain fatty acids, activation of the PPARα receptor in the liver, and partial reversal of gut microbiota dysbiosis (Chen et al. 2022; Koirala et al. 2023).

Finally, VPYPQ – a peptide derived from bovine β-casein – exerts antidiabetic effects in mice after oral administration by reducing postprandial plasma glucose levels in a dose-dependent manner and was effective in an oral glucose tolerance test at the highest dose tested (Koirala et al. 2023).

The search for bioactive compounds associated with appetite-suppressant or plasma glucose-lowering effects has garnered significant attention for their therapeutic implications. Notably, some products derived from dairy protein enzymatic digestion may also induce a reverse response. In this regard, a peptide mixture obtained by fractionation of casein hydrolysates was found to induce a short-term increase in food intake after administration by oral gavage to rats. A ghrelin receptor (GHSR-1a) agonist activity was proposed, although a specific bioactive peptide sequence was not isolated and identified (Howick et al. 2018; Tulipano 2020).

ENZYMES INVOLVED IN GLUCOSE HOMEOSTASIS AS TARGETS OF BIOACTIVE PEPTIDES

DPP-IV

CD26/dipeptidyl peptidase-4 (DPP-IV) is expressed by various cell types, including endothelial cells, immune cells, skeletal muscle cells, and enterocytes (Figure 12.3). DPP-IV inhibitors reduce the clearance of enteric hormones GIP and GLP-1 (incretins), thus enhancing their postprandial glycemic control activities. Indeed, some synthetic DPP-IV inhibitors are currently approved as oral drugs for treating type 2 diabetes.

Numerous short peptides encrypted in dairy protein sequences have been characterized as DPP-IV inhibitors in vitro. These include:

- Sequences released upon in silico digestion with gastrointestinal proteases
- Peptides isolated from hydrolysates prepared in vitro
- Peptides isolated from fermented milk products (Kondrashina et al. 2020; Tulipano 2020; Fleury et al. 2022)

However, conclusive evidence of the efficacy of food-derived DPP-IV inhibitors in vivo is lacking. While low bioavailability is expected for orally administered peptides or those released in the gut, transport across the intestinal mucosa to systemic circulation remains possible, especially when factors temporarily increase the permeability of the intestinal epithelial barrier (Drucker and Holst 2023).

The most potent dairy-derived DPP-IV inhibitors include some tryptophan-containing dipeptides (WR, WL, WK). Since peptide transporters at intestinal and renal epithelial cells mediate the transport of di- and tripeptides across lipid bilayers, these small inhibitors may reach the systemic circulation intact and remain active in vivo. Indeed, the peptide WR and longer peptides such as LKPTPEGDL, LPYPY, IPIQY, and IPI crossed Caco-2 cell monolayers in vitro, suggesting good intestinal absorption (Nongonierma and Fitzgerald 2013; Lacroix et al. 2017).

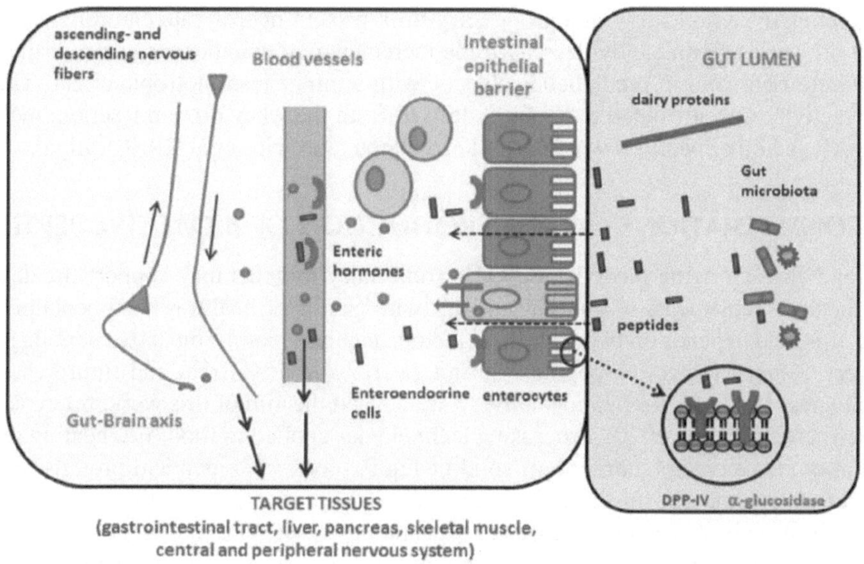

FIGURE 12.3 Schematic overview of the fate of bioactive components that are released in the gastrointestinal tract after dairy protein digestion, and their local and systemic targets. Local targets of bioactive peptides in the gut lumen include microbiota, enteroendocrine cells, and enzymatic activities expressed at the brush border of enterocytes. Some peptides may alter microbiota composition, inhibit α-glucosidase or DPP-IV enzymatic activities, or enhance enteric hormone secretion (GLP-1, GIP, peptide YY, CCK, somatostatin) from enteroendocrine cells. CD26/DPP-IV, a membrane protein with a releasable proteolytic domain, clears enteric hormones GIP and GLP-1. Potential systemic targets and effects include insulin sensitization in skeletal muscle cells, insulin secretion in the pancreas, ghrelin receptor (GHSR1a) agonism, and opioid receptor agonism. However, evidence of their in vivo activity remains limited. Systemic responses to bioactive peptides are often indirect, mediated by endocrine factors (i.e., enteric hormones) affecting pancreas, liver, and central nervous system activity. These factors can also affect communication between the central nervous system and the peripheral nervous systems, impacting visceral activity, appetite, food intake and metabolic functions. GLP-1: glucagon-like peptide-1; GIP: glucose-dependent insulinotropic peptide; CCK: cholecystokinin; DPP-IV: dipeptidyl peptidase-4.

Two in vivo rodent studies indirectly support the potential activity of some DPP-IV peptidic inhibitors. First, the peptide LPQNIPPL, isolated from a water-soluble Gouda cheese extract, inhibited DPP-IV in vitro and reduced postprandial plasma glucose levels during a glucose tolerance test in rats. Second, GLP-1 secretion triggered by carbohydrate, lipid, or casein intake was blunted in both DPP-IV-deficient rats and normal rats treated with the synthetic inhibitor sitagliptin compared to controls. Interestingly, whey protein intake did not significantly affect GLP-1 responses under these conditions. The authors concluded that whey protein intake itself significantly downregulated DPP-IV activity (Uenishi et al. 2012; Shimizu et al. 2021).

A-Glucosidase

The enzyme α-glucosidase converts complex carbohydrates to absorbable monosaccharides. Its pharmacological inhibition slows the absorption of simple carbohydrates in the small intestine, decreasing postprandial hyperglycemia in type 2 diabetes. Food can be a source of α-glucosidase inhibitors with saccharidic or non-saccharidic structures, including bioactive peptides isolated from the hydrolysates of various food proteins. While most peptides show low affinity for the enzyme, with the lowest IC_{50} values in the micromolar range, a clinical study supports the hypothesis that effects on glucose absorption can contribute to improved postprandial glucose control from dairy protein intake. Specifically, a preload with a proprietary milk protein hydrolysate claiming α-glucosidase inhibitory properties significantly decreased the incremental area under the curve of glucose after a carbohydrate-rich meal in prediabetic subjects, with a minor insulinotropic effect. The enzyme inhibitory activity was attributed to peptides derived from the whey protein fraction, including the dipeptide AP and other peptides which were not isolated (Sartorius et al. 2019; Tulipano 2020).

MORE CONSIDERATIONS ON THE PRODUCTION OF BIOACTIVE PEPTIDES

Isolation and characterizing bioactive peptides from dairy proteins may support the development of novel dietary supplements or pharmaceuticals with claims of health-related benefits. However, success in this field depends on two additional factors: technologies for bioactive peptide production and delivery systems protecting peptides during gastric transit. Current and future chemical and biotechnological strategies for peptide delivery are beyond the aim of this work; references may be found elsewhere (Tulipano 2020). Processing technologies applied to food (i.e., heating techniques, preparation of emulsions, preparation of solid or liquid foods with identical protein composition) and innovative technologies in the dairy industry can significantly alter the release of bioactive compounds from a given protein compared to expectations based on its native structure. This occurs by changing digestion rates, the protein's susceptibility to proteases, or inducing reactions involving amino acid side chains.

Ultrasound-assisted processing (UAP), microwave-assisted processing (MAP), and high-pressure processing (HPP) may be used as pretreatments combined with conventional methods (enzymatic hydrolysis and microbial fermentation) to improve the yields and modify the peptide profiles in the production of bioactive peptides from dairy proteins. These technologies do not break peptide bonds but can alter protein conformation and increase enzyme accessibility to the peptide bonds of food proteins (Murtaza et al. 2022).

THE EFFECTS OF OTHER PROTEINS

Research on bioactive peptides from traditional or alternative dietary proteins has grown steadily for two decades, making comprehensive reviews challenging.

Given this context, it is worth focussing on some vegetable proteins already featured in dietary recommendations (Bruno 2015; Duranti and Scarafoni 2015; Leksrisompong and Layman 2014). Legume seeds are protein-rich foods suggested to offer various dietary benefits due to their nutritional properties and positive effects on metabolic health. Specifically, lupin seeds have gained attention for their hypocholesterolemic, anti-inflammatory, and hypoglycemic properties. Researchers have attributed the postprandial glucose-lowering property of lupin seeds to a specific seed protein component, γ-conglutin, and to multiple mechanisms, including insulin-mimetic action in peripheral tissues, insulin-secretagogue activity, and DPP-IV and α-glucosidase inhibitory activities (Heinzl et al. 2022).

In conclusion, understanding the bioactivities of specific food protein fractions, in addition to their nutritional quality, may help develop new dietary recommendations using distinct sources of proteins as complements in a diet with more health benefits.

MINI DICTIONARY OF TERMS

- **Caco-2 cells:** An in vitro model using Caco-2 cell monolayers to simulate transport across the intestinal epithelial cell barrier.
- **DIAAS (digestible indispensable amino acid score):** The preferred method of protein quality measurement, as recommended by the FAO in 2013.

- **Essential amino acids:** Nine amino acids that human beings cannot produce de novo and must obtain from their diet: histidine, isoleucine, leucine, valine, phenylalanine, methionine, tryptophan, threonine, and lysine.
- **Incretins:** Enteric hormones (glucagon-like peptide-1 and glucose-dependent insulinotropic peptide) that are released in response to nutrients, enhancing the insulin response to postprandial increases in blood glucose.
- **Oral bioavailability:** The proportion of a substance that enters the systemic circulation in active form, expressed as a percentage of the total amount administered orally.

SUMMARY POINTS

- This chapter focuses on health benefits related to dairy protein intake in terms of controlling food intake, body weight gain, and glucose homeostasis.
- The chapter discusses evidence supporting the role of specific bioactive peptides derived from dairy protein digestion.
- It also considers the role played by free amino acids as functional compounds in metabolic control.
- The gastrointestinal mucosa contributes significantly to the interaction between foods and the signalling networks underlying energy and glucose homeostasis.
- Most peptide-related bioactivities discussed in the chapter are based on preclinical evidence.

REFERENCES

Agyei, D. et al. (2018). Bioinformatics and peptidomics approaches to the discovery and analysis of food-derived bioactive peptides. *Analytical and Bioanalytical Chemistry* 410: 3463–3472.

Aoki, H. et al. (2017). Lacto-ghrestatin, a novel bovine milk-derived peptide, suppresses ghrelin secretion. *FEBS Letters* 591: 2121–2130.

Auestad, N, and D.K. Layman. (2021). Dairy bioactive proteins and peptides: a narrative review. *Nutrition Reviews* 79(Suppl 2): 36–47.

Baptista, D.P. and M.L. Gigante. (2021). Bioactive peptides in ripened cheeses: release during technological processes and resistance to the gastrointestinal tract. *Journal of the Science of Food and Agriculture* 101(10): 4010–4017.

Bruno, G. (2015). The world needs proteins. *Agro FOOD Industry High Tech* 26(2): 4–7.

Chakrabarti, S. et al. (2018). Food derived bioactive peptides in human health: challenges and opportunities. *Nutrients* 10: 1738. https://www.mdpi.com/2072-6643/10/11/1738

Chen, H. et al. (2022). α-Lactalbumin peptide Asp-Gln-Trp alleviates hepatic insulin resistance and modulates gut microbiota dysbiosis in high-fat diet-induced NAFLD mice. *Food and Function* 13(19): 9878–9892.

Dantas, A. et al. (2023). An approach on detection, quantification, technological properties, and trends market of A2 cow milk. *Food Research International* 167:112690. https://www.sciencedirect.com/science/article/pii/S0963996923002351

Drucker D.J. and J.J. Holst. (2023). The expanding incretin universe: from basic biology to clinical translation. *Diabetologia*. https://link.springer.com/article/10.1007/s00125-023-05906-7

Duranti, M. and A. Scarafoni. (2015). An open window onto the food of the near future. *Agro FOOD Industry High Tech* 26(2): 8–10.

El Khoury, D. et al. (2019). Increased milk protein content and whey-to-casein ratio in milk served with breakfast cereal reduce postprandial glycemia in healthy adults: An examination of mechanisms of action. *Journal of Dairy Science* 102: 6766–6780.

Ezcurra, M. et al. (2013). Molecular mechanisms of incretin hormone secretion. *Current Opinion in Pharmacology* 13: 922–927.

Fleury, L. et al. (2022). In Vivo and in vitro comparison of the DPP-IV inhibitory potential of food proteins from different origins after gastrointestinal digestion. *International Journal of Molecular Sciences* 23: 8365. *https://www.mdpi.com/1422-0067/23/15/8365*

Giglio, B.M. et al. (2023). Effects of whey protein supplementation on adiposity, body weight, and glycemic parameters: A synthesis of evidence. *Nutrition, Metabolism & Cardiovascular Diseases* 33: 258–274.

Gilmartin, S. et al. (2020). Whey for Sarcopenia; Can whey peptides, hydrolysates or proteins play a beneficial role? *Foods* 9: 750. https://www.mdpi.com/2304-8158/9/6/750

Helal, A. and D. Tagliazucchi. (2023). Peptidomics profile, bioactive peptides identification and biological activities of six different cheese varieties. *Biology* (Basel) 12(1):78. https://www.mdpi.com/2079-7737/12/1/78

Heinzl, G.C. et al. (2022). Lupinus albus gamma-conglutin: new findings about its action at the intestinal barrier and a critical analysis of the state of the art on its postprandial glycaemic regulating activity. *Nutrients* 14: 3666. https://www.mdpi.com/2072-6643/14/17/3666

Hou, I.-C. et al. (2009). β-Lactotensin derived from bovine β-lactoglobulin suppresses food intake via the CRF system followed by the CGRP system in mice. *Peptides* 30: 2228–2232.

Howick, K. et al. (2018). A dairy-derived ghrelinergic hydrolysate modulates food intake in Vivo. *International Journal of Molecular Sciences* 19: 2780. https://www.mdpi.com/1422-0067/19/9/2780

Jakubowicz, D. et al. (2014). Incretin, insulinotropic and glucose-lowering effects of whey protein pre-load in type 2 diabetes: a randomised clinical trial. *Diabetologia* 57: 1807–1811.

Jeong, E.W. et al. (2022). Whey proteins-fortified milk with adjusted casein to whey proteins ratio improved muscle strength and endurance exercise capacity without lean mass accretion in rats. *Foods* 11: 574. *https://www.mdpi.com/2304-8158/11/4/574*

Kagebayashi, T. et al. (2012). Novel CCK-dependent vasorelaxing dipeptide, Arg-Phe, decreases blood pressure and food intake in rodents. *Molecular Nutrition & Food Research* 56: 1456–1463.

Koirala, P. et al. (2023). Dairy milk protein-derived bioactive peptides: avengers against metabolic syndrome. *Current Nutrition Reports* 12(2):308–326.

Kondrashina, A. et al. (2018). Satiating effect of a sodium caseinate hydrolysate and its fate in the upper gastrointestinal tract. *Journal of Functional Foods* 49: 306–313.

Kondrashina, A. et al. (2020). Dairy-derived peptides for satiety. *Journal of Functional Foods* 66: 103801. https://www.sciencedirect.com/science/article/pii/S1756464620300256

Lacroix, I.M.E. et al. (2017). Investigation into the bioavailability of milk protein-derived peptides with dipeptidyl-peptidase IV inhibitory activity using Caco-2 cell monolayers. *Food and Function* 8: 701–709.

Leksrisompong, P. and D.K. Layman. (2014). Whey protein isolate: the ideal ingredient for sports nutrition. *Agro FOOD Industry High Tech* 25(2): 19–23.

Minkiewicz, P. et al. (2019). BIOPEP-UWM database of bioactive peptides: current opportunities. *International Journal of Molecular Sciences* 20: 5978. https://www.mdpi.com/1422-0067/20/23/5978

Murtaza, M.A. et al. (2022). Conventional and novel technologies in the production of dairy bioactive peptides. *Frontiers in Nutrition* 9:780151. https://www.frontiersin.org/articles/10.3389/fnut.2022.780151/full

Nongonierma, A.B. and R.J. Fitzgerald. (2013). Inhibition of dipeptidyl peptidase IV (DPP-IV) by tryptophan containing dipeptides. *Food and Function* 4: 1843–1849.

Nongonierma, A.B. and R.J. FitzGerald. (2016). Learnings from quantitative structure-activity relationship (QSAR) studies with respect to food-protein-derived bioactive peptides: a review. *RSC Advances* 6: 75400–75413.

Oberoi, A. et al. (2023). Effects of co-ingesting glucose and whey protein on blood glucose, plasma insulin and glucagon concentrations, and gastric emptying, in older men with and without type 2 diabetes. *Diabetes, Obesity and Metabolism* 25(5):1321–1330.

Ogiwara, M. et al. (2018). Enzymatic digest of whey protein and wheylin-1, a dipeptide released in the digest, increase insulin sensitivity in an Akt phosphorylation-dependent manner. *Food and Function* 9: 4635–4641.

O'Halloran, F. et al. (2018). A casein hydrolysate increases GLP-1 secretion and reduces food intake. *Food Chemistry* 252: 303–310.

Pupovac, J. and G.H. Anderson. (2002). Dietary peptides induce satiety via cholecystokinin-A and peripheral opioid receptors in rats. *Journal of Nutrition* 132: 2775–2780.

Rigamonti, A.E. et al. (2020). The Appetite-suppressant and GLP-1-Stimulating effects of whey proteins in obese subjects are associated with increasing circulating levels of specific amino acids. *Nutrients* 12: 775. https://www.mdpi.com/2072-6643/12/3/775

Robinson, R.C. et al. (2021). Can cheese mites, maggots and molds enhance bioactivity? Peptidomic investigation of functional peptides in four traditional cheeses. *Food and Function* 12(2):633–645.

Ryann, K.K. and R.M. Seeley. (2013). Food as a hormone. *Science* 339: 918–919.

Sartorius, T. et al. (2019). Postprandial effects of a proprietary milk protein hydrolysate containing bioactive peptides in prediabetic subjects. *Nutrients 11: 1700. Erratum in: Nutrients 2020* 12(5). https://www.mdpi.com/2072-6643/11/7/1700

Shimizu, Y. et al. (2021). Glucagon-like peptide-1 response to whey protein is less diminished by dipeptidyl peptidase-4 in comparison with responses to dextrin, a lipid and casein in rats. *British Journal of Nutrition* 125: 398–407.

Shukla, P. et al. (2022). Exploring the potential of Lacticaseibacillus paracasei M11 on antidiabetic, anti-inflammatory, and ACE inhibitory effects of fermented dromedary camel milk (Camelus dromedaries) and the release of antidiabetic and anti-hypertensive peptides. *Journal of Food Biochemistry* 46(12): e14449. https://onlinelibrary.wiley.com/doi/full/10.1111/jfbc.14449

Smedegaard, S.B. et al. (2021). β-Lactoglobulin elevates insulin and glucagon concentrations compared with whey protein-a randomized double-blinded crossover trial in patients with type two diabetes mellitus. *Nutrients* 13(2): 308. *https://www.mdpi.com/2072-6643/13/2/308*

Smith, K. et al. (2020). The clinical application of mealtime whey protein for the treatment of postprandial hyperglycaemia for people with type 2 diabetes: a long whey to go. *Frontiers in Nutrion* 7:587843. https://www.frontiersin.org/articles/10.3389/fnut.2020.587843/full

Smith, K. et al. (2022). Thrice daily consumption of a novel, premeal shot containing a low dose of whey protein increases time in euglycemia during 7 days of free-living in individuals with type 2 diabetes. *BMJ Open Diabetes Research Care* 10(3): e002820. https://drc.bmj.com/content/10/3/e002820

Smith, K. et al. (2023). Pre-meal whey protein alters postprandial insulinemia by enhancing β-cell function and reducing insulin clearance in T2D. *Journal of Clinical Endocrinology and Metabolism* 108(8): e603–e612. https://academic.oup.com/jcem/article/108/8/e603/7025377

Smithers, G.W. (2008). Whey and whey proteins – from gutter-to-gold. *International Dairy Journal* 18: 695–704.

Sridonpai, P. et al. (2021). Postprandial effects of a whey protein-based multi-ingredient nutritional drink compared with a normal breakfast on glucose, insulin, and active GLP-1 response among type 2 diabetic subjects: a crossover randomised controlled trial. *Journal of Nutritional Science* 10: e49. https://doi.org/10.1017/jns.2021.41

Toffolon, A. et al. (2021). Effect of reversal of whey-protein to casein ratio of cow milk, on insulin, incretin, and amino acid responses in humans. *Molecular Nutrition and Food Reserach* 65(24): e2100069. *https://onlinelibrary.wiley.com/doi/10.1002/mnfr.202100069*

Tulipano, G. (2020). Role of bioactive peptide sequences in the potential impact of dairy protein intake on metabolic health. *International Journal of Molecular Sciences* 21: 8881. https://www.mdpi.com/1422-0067/21/22/8881

Uenishi, H. et al. (2012). Isolation and identification of casein-derived dipeptidyl-peptidase 4 (DPP-4)-inhibitory peptide LPQNIPPL from gouda-type cheese and its effect on plasma glucose in rats. *International Dairy Journal* 22: 24–30.

Valerio, A. et al. (2011). Branched-chain amino acids, mitochondrial biogenesis and healthspan: an evolutionary perspective. *Aging* 3: 464–478.

Veldhorst, M.A.B. et al. (2009). Effects of complete whey-protein breakfasts versus whey without GMP-breakfasts on energy intake and satiety. *Appetite* 52: 388–395.

Wauson, E.M. et al. (2013). Minireview: Nutrient sensing by G protein-coupled receptors. *Molecular Endocrinology* 27: 1188–97.

Wernlund, P.G. et al. (2021). Casein glycomacropeptide is well tolerated in healthy adults and changes neither high-sensitive C-reactive protein, gut microbiota nor faecal butyrate: a restricted randomised trial. *British Journal of Nutrition* 125:1374–1385.

13 Dairy Protein and Gut Microbiota

Burcu Ateş Özcan, Kübra Şahin, and Ayşe Betül Demirbaş

ABBREVIATIONS

CVD	Cardiovascular disease
DPD-KH	A low-protein diet supplemented with casein hydrolysate
DPD-SA	A low-protein diet supplemented with free amino acids
IBS	Inflammatory bowel disease
IGF	Insulin-like growth factor
MetS	Metabolic syndrome
NF-κB	Nuclear factor kappa B
NOD	Nucleotide-binding oligomerization domain protein
TLR4	Toll-like receptor 4
TMAO	Trimethylamine N-oxide
Treg	Foxp3+ T-regulatory

INTRODUCTION

Dairy products consist of milk obtained from mammals such as cows, sheep, and goats, as well as food products with high nutritional value, such as cheese, butter, and yogurt produced from this milk (Koushalya et al. 2022). Milk and dairy products, which have significant effects on physiological functions, constitute a common component of many dietary patterns. They are an important source not only of protein and calcium but also of some B-group vitamins, phosphorus, magnesium, zinc, and potassium. Therefore, in addition to strengthening immunity and protection from diseases, dairy products may also be related to some health conditions. With the recent popularity of research on gut microbiota, attention has turned to the effects of milk and dairy products on microbiota, and studies on the subject are gaining momentum (Aslam et al. 2020; Koushalya et al. 2022).

GUT MICROBIOTA

The entire collection of indigenous microorganisms inhabiting the gastrointestinal tract is referred to as the intestinal microbiota. The microbiota consists of anaerobic microorganisms that have adapted to living within the mucosal surface of the intestine. These microorganisms have undergone adaptations for survival within this microbial environment. Scientists discovered evidence of microorganisms associated with the human body, which they referred to as "beasts," toward the end of the 17th century and observed that microorganisms were associated with the mouth and feces of both healthy and sick individuals (Liu 2016; Ateş Özcan 2020). It is established that the cumulative weight of microorganisms within the body is approximately 2 kg, exceeding the weight of all its cells. The intestinal microbiota undergoes maturation during the early years of life and then maintains stability (Sun and Kato 2016; Sommer and Bäckhed 2016).

 DOI: 10.1201/9781003597926-13

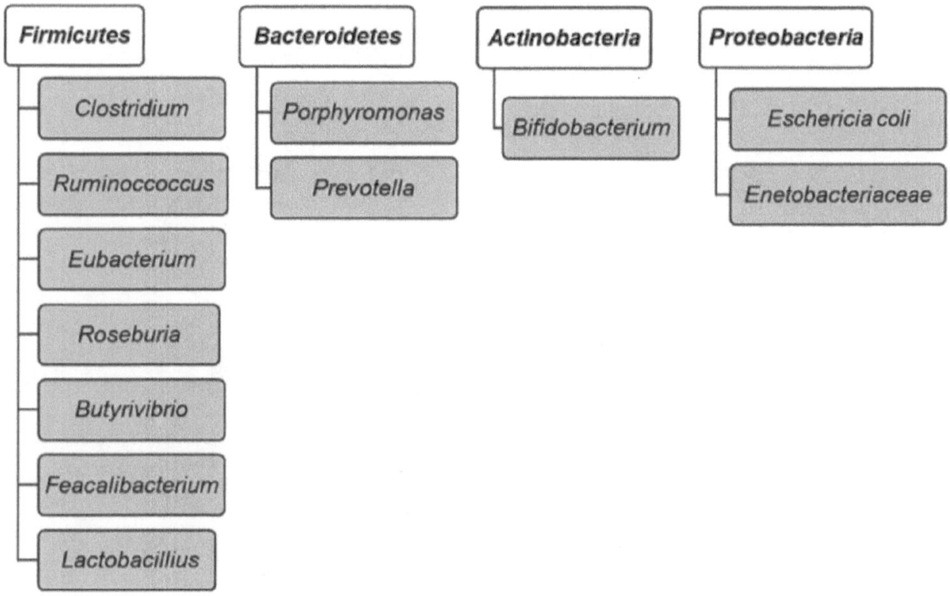

FIGURE 13.1 Four major phyla in the adult gut microbiota.

The gut microbiota is considered a hidden organ due to its impact on the physiological development and defense of the host (Liu 2016). It is a dynamic system consisting of tens of trillions of microorganisms that fulfills essential functions for the human host (Dominguez-Bello et al. 2010). In the microbiota of healthy individuals, there is a balanced distribution between symbionts and pathobionts. Dysbiosis, conversely, signifies the disruption of this equilibrium, resulting in the proliferation of pathogenic microorganisms (Özsoy 2019).

In an adult, 99% of the intestinal microbiota belongs to four major phyla: *Bacteroidetes*, *Firmicutes*, *Actinobacteria*, and *Proteobacteria*. *Firmicutes* and *Bacteroides* make up 95% of the intestinal microbiota. The microbiota consists primarily of gram-negative *Bacteroidetes* (mostly *Bacteroides* or *Prevotella* spp.) or gram-positive *Firmicutes* (mostly *Clostridium* and *Lactobacillus* spp.) bacteria, 97% of which are strict anaerobes. Less than 1% of the total intestinal microbiota consists of fungi and archaea (Adak and Khan 2019; Ateş Özcan 2020) (Figure 13.1).

FACTORS AFFECTING GUT MICROBIOTA

The gut microbial pattern is host-specific. The development of the intestinal microbiota begins during the intrauterine period, is influenced by the mode of delivery and dietary intake, and undergoes maturation over time (Herrema et al. 2017). It is associated with the physiological environment of the host throughout life and varies depending on environmental and non-environmental factors (Ateş Özcan 2020; Sommer and Bäckhed 2016) (Figure 13.2).

Adverse changes in the microbiota composition are referred to as "dysbiosis." The balance of gut microbiota is critical for maintaining cell proliferation, metabolism, inflammation, immunity, and the brain-gut relationship (Espín et al. 2017). When dysbiosis occurs, it can reduce beneficial symbiotic relationships in the gut, cause a decline in the diversity of microbiota composition, and lead to the emergence of undesirable pathogens (Krishnan et al. 2015).

The initial composition of the microbiota is acquired during birth, whether through a caesarean section or vaginal delivery, as microorganisms from both the mother and the surrounding environment colonize the gastrointestinal tract of the newborn. Hence, the mode of delivery constitutes a significant factor. The presence of bacteria in the placenta, umbilical cord, and amniotic fluid suggests that the fetus is exposed to various microorganisms. The establishment of the fetal

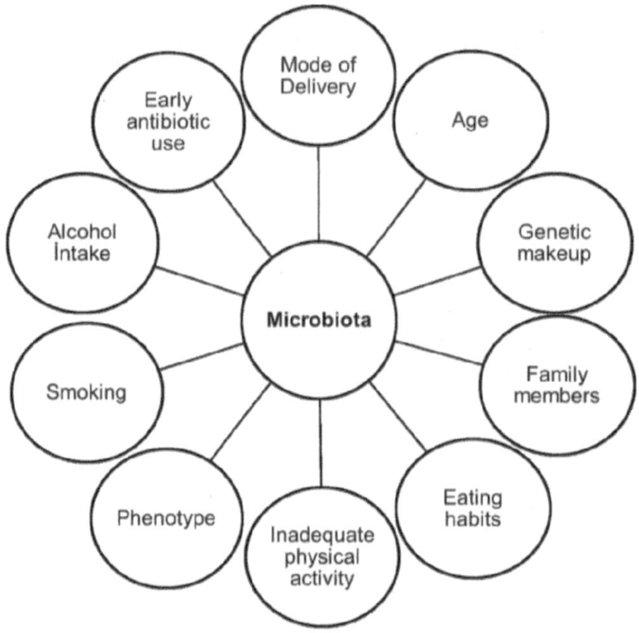

FIGURE 13.2 Important factors affecting the microbiota.

intestinal microbiota begins at birth and evolves through exposure to the vaginal, anal, and skin microbiota of the mother (Nagpal et al. 2016). The mode of delivery results in colonization either by *Lactobacillus*, *Prevotella*, or *Sneathia* spp. from the birth canal or by *Staphylococcus* spp. and *Propionibacterium* spp. in the case of a caesarean section. (Dominguez-Bello et al. 2010; Falony et al. 2016). The microbial composition differs on the first day of life for those born through vaginal delivery compared to those born via caesarean section. This affects the physiologic, metabolic, and immunologic development of the newborn (Nagpal et al. 2016).

The infant diet impacts the gut microbiota and is a major player in microbiota regulation (Power et al. 2014; Mayer et al. 2015). The intestinal microbiota resembles colostrum microbiota and is similar to amniotic fluid and placenta prenatally (Liu 2016). Breastfed infants are colonized first by *Streptococci* and *Staphylococci*, but lactic acid bacteria are also prevalent. The gut microbiota then shifts toward *Proteobacteria*, *Actinobacteria*, *Firmicutes*, and *Bacteroidetes*. In formula-fed infants, the enrichment of species such as *Staphylococcus aureus* and *Bacteroides* spp. is promoted (Liu 2016; Power et al. 2014). The relationship between the microbiota and the mother, with the transmission of bacteria from the birth canal and maternal feces during childbirth, persists postnatally through interactions like skin-to-skin contact, breastfeeding, and environmental exposure during the first year of life (Liu 2016). The infant microbiota is influenced by nutrition and diseases during the first three years of life, gradually maturing to resemble that of adults (Power et al. 2014). Geographical location, climate, cultural practices, gender, antibiotic usage, and a country's level of development all play significant roles in shaping the diversity of the gut microbiota (Liu 2016).

One of the most important factors affecting gut microbiota is diet. Variations in the composition and abundance of bacterial species, including *Bacteroidetes*, *Firmicutes*, *Actinobacteria*, *Verrucomicrobia*, and *Proteobacteria*, within the intestinal microbiota can occur, particularly in response to environmental factors like diet (Del Chierico et al. 2014). Metabolites formed by the digestion of food can impact the host's metabolism. Nevertheless, this composition typically reverts to its baseline within 48 hours after the diet is discontinued (David et al. 2014). Dietary changes may cause short-term changes in the gut microbiota. Yet, habitual diet has long-term consequences (Ayyıldız and Yıldıran 2019).

Antibiotic use has a negative impact on the composition of the gut microbiota. The diversity and stability of the microbiota decrease with advancing age. In particular, *Bifidobacterium* and *Bacteroides* show a decrease in species diversity and total number (Moon et al. 2015).

THE ROLE OF GUT MICROBIOTA

Research suggests that the gut microbiota may act as an "organ" that interacts with the human host and carries out numerous essential functions to protect human health. The gut microbiota includes at least a thousand bacterial species. It performs several vital functions, such as carbohydrate digestion, suppression of harmful microorganisms, vitamin synthesis, immune system activity, and drug metabolism (Table 13.1). The gut microbiota helps develop a functional immune system by protecting the gut from pathogenic microorganisms (Lepage et al. 2013). Foxp3+ T-regulatory (Treg) cells play an indispensable role in establishing this balance. Additionally, Treg cell differentiation and function can be regulated by the gut microbiota. The intestinal microbiota enables the proliferation of Treg cells in the intestinal cavity through short-chain fatty acids (SCFAs) (Bollrath and Powrie 2013).

The gut microbiota ferments complex, indigestible dietary fibers to produce SCFAs such as acetate, propionate, and butyrate. SCFAs positively affect intestinal epithelial cell development and differentiation. By reducing the pH of the intestine, SCFA production prevents the growth of pathogenic bacteria such as *Escherichia coli* (Lepage et al. 2013).

Within the human body, 'various microenvironments exist, each possessing its own distinct and finely-tuned "immunosurveillance" system (Belkaid and Naik 2013). The dense microbiota embedded in the gut strengthens the intestinal epithelial barrier and aids nutrient uptake. Both human hosts and microorganisms benefit from the abundant food supply in the small intestine. Pathogen-promoting (pathobiont) and inhibitory (symbiont) bacteria regulate the gut microbiota. The small intestine contains mostly *Proteobacteria* (*Enterobacteria*), *Lactobacillales*, and *Erysipelotrichales* (*Turicibacter*). In contrast, the large intestine harbors fewer bacteria because of its lower nutrient content. These bacteria are replaced by species like *Bacteroidetes* and *Clostridia*, which utilize indigestible host fibers as an energy source (Kamada et al. 2013).

The microbiota maintains the integrity of the epithelial barrier by protecting the "zonula occludens" (tight junction), "zonula adherens," and "desmosome" connections between intestinal epithelial cells. Some microbiota members contribute to producing antimicrobial peptides from intestinal mucus, thereby preventing pathogens from colonizing the intestine (Chung et al. 2012).

TABLE 13.1
Key Roles of Gut Microbiota in Health and Body Function

Mode of Action	
Carbohydrate digestion	Ferment complex, indigestible dietary fibers to produce SCFAs
Intestinal permeability	• Strengthens the intestinal epithelial barrier and aids nutrient uptake • Maintains the integrity of the epithelial barrier by protecting the tight junctions, zonula adherens, and desmosome connections between intestinal epithelial cells
Vitamin synthesis	Produces some B-group vitamins and vitamin K
Immune system regulation	Protects the gut from pathogenic microorganisms
Lipid metabolism	Suppresses lipoprotein lipase inhibition
Amino acid metabolism	Catabolizes aromatic amino acids such as phenylalanine and tyrosine

SCFAs: short-chain fatty acids.

In the colon, bacterial peptidases and proteases metabolize undigested proteins from the small intestine to produce neuroactive compounds such as gamma-aminobutyric acid, norepinephrine, dopamine, histamine, and serotonin (Adak and Khan 2019). The gut microbiota positively affects lipid metabolism by suppressing lipoprotein lipase inhibition. It synthesizes some B-group vitamins (thiamine, riboflavin, nicotinic acid, biotin, folate, pyridoxine, and cobalamin) and vitamin K. Additionally, the gut microbiota participates in amino acid metabolism by catabolizing aromatic amino acids such as phenylalanine and tyrosine (Rowland et al. 2018).

EUBIOSIS AND DYSBIOSIS

The gut microbiome is a dynamic ecosystem that can form its unique structure in response to various internal and external stimuli such as aging, diet, lifestyle, and disease. "Eubiosis" describes the balance between bacteria in the gut microbiota ecosystem. The eubiotic gut microbiota predominantly comprises *Firmicutes* and *Bacteroides*, with fewer pathogenic species such as *Proteobacteria*. "Dysbiosis" refers to the disruption of this eubiosis in the microbiota, where pathogenic bacteria become more dominant and biodiversity decreases (Lebba et al. 2016). As our understanding of the vital role of the intestinal microbiota in human health and disease development has grown, the concepts of a healthy microbiota (eubiosis) and dysbiosis, defined as the disruption of the microbiota structure that predisposes to diseases, have gained importance (Precup and Vodnar 2019). A eubiotic gut microbiota ensures optimal functioning of the microbiota and functions as an anti-inflammatory structure (Riccio and Rossano 2020). During dysbiosis, the microbial influence within the gut becomes progressively proinflammatory and adversely affects health. Dysbiosis is characterized by an increase in toxic components, including bile acid derivatives that can be detrimental to certain beneficial bacteria and trimethylamine N-oxide (TMO), which is harmful to the host (Velasquez et al. 2016). Moreover, intestinal permeability tends to rise in dysbiosis, leading to increased inflammation that may contribute to the development of various diseases, including cancer, cardiovascular diseases, obesity, metabolic syndrome, inflammatory bowel disease (IBS), rheumatoid arthritis, and allergies (Ateş Özcan 2020; Precup and Vodnar 2019) (Table 13.2). One study reported that a long-term high-fat, high-energy Western diet may lead to the development of dysbiosis in the gut microbiota (Litvak et al. 2018).

TABLE 13.2
Bacterial Composition and Effects of Eubiosis and Dysbiosis

Condition	Predominant Bacteria	Effects on the Organism
Eubiosis	Firmicutes ↑ Bacteroides ↑ Proteobacteria ↓ Actinobacteria ↓	• Optimal functioning of the microbiota • Anti-inflammatory effect
Dysbiosis	Firmicutes ↓ Bacteroides ↓ Proteobacteria ↑ Actinobacteria ↑	• Deterioration of microbiota health • Proinflammatory effect • Increase in toxic compounds (TMAO increase) • Increased permeability • Development of many diseases (IBS, obesity, MetS, CVD, etc.)

IBS: inflammatory bowel disease; MetS: metabolic syndrome; CVD: cardiovascular disease.

DAIRY PROTEINS

Dairy products include milk obtained from mammals such as cows, sheep, and goats, as well as food products with high nutritional value, such as cheese, butter, and yogurt produced from this milk (Koushalya et al. 2022). Codex Alimentarius defines dairy products as those "obtained by any form of milk processing, which may contain food additives and other ingredients functionally necessary for processing." Dairy products vary significantly between countries depending on social and cultural conditions, market demand, available milk processing technologies, and dietary habits (FAO 2022). Global milk production (81% cow milk, 15% buffalo milk, and 4% goat, sheep, and camel milk) increased by 1.6% in 2018 and is expected to increase by 1.7% annually until 2028 (OECD/FAO 2022). More than 6 billion people worldwide, especially in developing countries, consume milk and dairy products (FAO 2022).

Various factors, such as the species, breed, age, physical environment, season, and diet of dairy animals, influence the composition, flavor, and color of milk. Cow milk contains 5% lactose, 3.5% protein, and 3-4% fat. The composition of goat milk is similar to that of cow milk. Sheep milk has higher lactose, fat, and protein concentrations than cow and goat milk. Buffalo milk contains about twice as much fat as cow milk and has a fat:protein ratio of 2:1. Generally, milk and dairy products are rich in nutrients, including calcium, magnesium, riboflavin, vitamin B12, vitamin A, selenium, and pantothenic acid (FAO 2022; OECD/FAO 2022).

Milk, a highly significant component of human nutrition that is rich in nine essential amino acids, typically contains around 3.3%–3.5% protein. Total milk protein comprises casein and whey proteins. Casein has four different fractions: αs1-, αs2-, β-, and κ-casein. Whey protein comprises beta-lactoglobulin, alpha-lactalbumin, serum albumin, small amounts of immunoglobulins, lactoferrin, insulin-like growth factor, and the lactoperoxidase system (Muehlhoff et al. 2013) (Table 13.3). The ratios of αs1-, αs2-, β- and κ-casein in bovine milk are 38%, 10%, 35%, and 12%, respectively. β-lactoglobulin is found in 12% of bovine milk and accounts for approximately half of all whey proteins. Milk also contains small proteins such as metal-binding proteins, vitamin-binding proteins, β2-microglobulin, angiogenin, kininogen, osteopontin, glycoproteins, and milk fat globule membrane proteins (Boland and Singh 2019). In cow's milk, the casein ratio is higher, with a whey:casein ratio of 20:80. The amino acid profiles of whey and casein differ. Whey protein contains higher levels of branched-chain amino acids (BCAAs), including isoleucine, leucine, and valine, compared to casein. Casein contains higher levels of essential amino acids, including methionine, histidine (semi-essential), valine, and phenylalanine than whey protein. Casein also contains various nonessential amino acids such as proline, serine, glutamic acid, arginine, and tyrosine (McGregor and Poppitt 2013). Due to its essential amino acid content, milk protein has a high "protein-digestibility-corrected amino acid score" and "digestible indispensable amino acid score" (Michaelsen et al. 2011). Hence, incorporating milk and dairy products into the human diet enhances overall dietary quality (Muehlhoff et al. 2013).

Recently, plant-based milks such as coconut, almond, hazelnut, oat, soy, and rice milk have gained popularity as milk substitutes. Nevertheless, these alternatives are not categorized as dairy products due to variations in nutrient composition compared to animal milk. They also exhibit lower amino acid profiles and protein quality than animal milk, primarily due to their plant-based origin. However, soy milk and products enriched in protein content are included in the milk and dairy products group in the Turkish Dietary Guidelines (TUBER 2022).

THE IMPACT OF MILK AND DAIRY PRODUCTS ON GUT MICROBIOTA

Milk and dairy products can affect the intestinal microbiota through five main phyla, including *Firmicutes*, *Bacteroidetes*, *Fusobacteria*, *Proteobacteria*, and *Actinobacteria* via various mechanisms (Rinninella et al. 2019). Researchers believe that multiple nutrients in dairy products, such as carbohydrates, proteins, amino acids, lipids, vitamins, and minerals, may affect the gut microbiota

TABLE 13.3
Types of Dairy Proteins

Casein	Whey
αs1-casein	β-lactoglobulin
αs2- casein	α-lactalbumin
β- casein	Serum albumin
κ- casein	Immunoglobulins
	Lactoferrin
	Insulin-like growth factor (IGF)
	Lactoperoxidase

(Burton et al. 2017). Studies have also shown that dairy products may positively affect the intestinal microbiota through mechanical processes, including promoting beneficial bacteria growth, inhibiting pathogenic bacteria growth, and altering the gastrointestinal (GI) environment (Aslam et al. 2020) (Table 13.4). In a randomized controlled trial conducted over 24 weeks, obese participants were divided into two groups: one group received milk and a hypocaloric diet equivalent to 600 mg/day calcium, and the other group received milk and a hypocaloric diet equivalent to 1500 mg/day calcium intake. The two groups showed no significant difference in the composition and diversity of gut microbiota. However, the *Veillonella* genus decreased in the group with low milk intake at the end of 24 weeks (Bendtsen et al. 2018). *Lactobacillus* and *Bifidobacterium* species are considered probiotics because they positively affect host health, including metabolic homeostasis, immune system regulation, and anti-inflammatory effects. Milk components such as lactose and protein found in milk and dairy products promote the growth of these bacterial species (Turroni et al. 2014).

Live microorganisms that positively affect the gut microbiota are known as probiotics. Probiotics have beneficial effects, including suppressing the growth of pathogenic microorganisms by lowering intestinal pH, maintaining balance in the intestinal flora, increasing mucus secretion, strengthening the intestinal barrier and enterocytes by producing short-chain fatty acids, enhancing immune response, and preventing antibiotic-associated diarrhea. Probiotics also play a role in mitigating the risk of obesity and inflammatory bowel diseases, particularly colon cancer. Milk and dairy products, particularly kefir and yogurt, have probiotic properties (Demirören 2020). Kefir forms a mucosal structure in the gastrointestinal tract and increases the resistance of the intestines by cleansing the intestinal lumen. This increased resistance protects against *Escherichia coli* and other parasites. The bacteria and yeasts found in kefir also help digest incompletely digested nutrients, reducing nutrient loss. Due to its non-bloating nature in the stomach and intestines, individuals with digestive system issues can consume it more comfortably than other dairy products (Ozmen and Aydinli 2020).

Several studies (Fernandez-Raudales et al. 2012; Yılmaz et al. 2019) have demonstrated that milk and fermented dairy products can increase the growth of beneficial bacteria. In a study conducted by Fernandez-Raudales et al. (Fernandez-Raudales et al. 2012), bovine milk and two types of soy milk were given to participants with obesity. As a result, there was a significant increase in *Lactobacillus* in the bovine milk group compared to the soy milk groups. The researchers also observed a non-significant increase in the copy numbers of *Bifidobacterium*. Additionally, in the bovine milk group, the ratio of *Firmicutes/Bacteroidetes* remained unchanged, while *Roseburia* species tended to increase and *Prevotella* species tended to decrease (Fernandez-Raudales et al. 2012). In a study conducted on patients with inflammatory bowel syndrome, researchers observed that kefir consumption modulated the intestinal microbiota, and regular kefir consumption improved the patient's quality of life in the short term (Yılmaz et al. 2019). In an animal study conducted by Liu et al. (Liu et al. 2017), researchers showed that yogurt consumption improved constipation

TABLE 13.4
Potential Beneficial Effects of Dairy Products on Microbiota

- Facilitating the growth of beneficial bacteria
- Preventing the growth of pathogenic bacteria
- Positively affecting microbiota by changing the gastrointestinal (GI) environment

in mice with slow-transit constipation. Another study found that fermented milk protein products reduced cardiometabolic risk factors in mice with diet-induced obesity, possibly by modulating gut microbiota (Perazza et al. 2020). In a study conducted by Madsen et al. (Madsen et al. 2017), which evaluated the effects of varying amounts of amino acids found in dairy products on the intestinal microbiota and obesity, the authors stated that casein and other milk proteins are some of the most effective protein sources in preventing obesity due to their high BCAA content.

In a comprehensive meta-analysis study, researchers analyzed the potential alterations in the gut microbiota resulting from the biological characteristics of dairy products and varying milk consumption levels. They considered the distinct biological profiles of each dairy product category (nonfermented dairy products, fermented dairy products, and milk derivatives) and the diverse mechanisms through which they might impact the intestinal microbiota. The results showed that while certain dairy products such as yogurt, kefir, and milk have demonstrated similarities in promoting the growth of specific bacterial groups (e.g., *Bifidobacterium, Lactobacillus*), different dairy products have been associated with distinct impacts on the gut microbiota. Moreover, bacterial diversity decreased in individuals consuming bovine milk and in the control group. The study also found that *Prevotella* decreased in the bovine milk group. Some studies have reported that certain specific strains of *Prevotella*, which is considered a common type, may be associated with an inflammatory state. However, according to the study, dairy product derivatives such as casein and whey isolates and the amount of dairy products consumed do not appear to significantly affect the human intestinal microbiota composition. Therefore, the effect of milk consumption on gut microbiota remains uncertain (Aslam et al. 2020).

THE RELATIONSHIP BETWEEN CASEIN AND WHEY PROTEINS AND MICROBIOTA

Proteins are essential nutrients for the human body, and milk and its derivatives serve as a significant protein source. The total milk protein of milk and dairy products, which can provide nine essential amino acids, is divided into casein and whey proteins (Muehlhoff et al. 2013). Studies have indicated that both casein and whey proteins may affect microbiota (Boscaini et al. 2023; Guo et al. 2021).

Casein, rich in essential amino acids, is hydrolyzed by appropriate proteases to produce various bioactive peptides. Some of these peptides can rearrange the composition of the intestinal microbiota (Guo et al. 2021). Whey protein appears to provide complete protection, especially in infants, by stimulating beneficial bacteria such as *Bifidobacterium* and *Lactobacillus* and inhibiting the growth of pathogens. While studies show that whey protein may have similar properties in adult individuals (Sprong et al. 2010; McAllan et al. 2015), the effect of whey protein on adult gut microbiota is not fully understood. In most cases, whey protein supplementation to a normal diet or a high-fat diet has been shown to positively regulate the gut microbiota by increasing the growth of *Bifidobacterium* and *Lactobacillus* species, as well as beneficial taxa such as *Allobaculum*, *Akkermansia muciniphila*, and *Bacteroides*. In this context, alpha-lactalbumin (the second most prevalent protein in whey protein, constituting approximately 20%–25% of the total) and lactoferrin (a member of the transferrin protein family, making up about 1% of whey protein) are believed to be the key components responsible for this positive effect (Boscaini et al. 2023).

Whey protein contains various bioactive proteins such as lactoferrin, peptides, and glycomacropeptides that may be useful in preventing colitis. Whey is also a source of threonine, cysteine, serine, and, to a lesser extent, proline. These amino acids are the main constituents of gastrointestinal secretory mucins, and one study has shown that whey protein protects against diarrhea and reduces fecal blood loss by reducing inflammatory gene expression in dextran sulfate sodium-induced colitis in rats (Sprong et al. 2010).

Casein and whey proteins, which are thought to have several health impacts, may also be related to microbiota-related obesity. For instance, mice fed with whey protein isolate have a lower length of intestinal and stomach mucus. According to a study in which mice were fed a high-fat diet containing different doses of casein or whey protein isolate enriched with lactoferrin and lactoperoxidase, whey protein isolate specifically increased *Lactobacillaceae/Lactobacillus* and decreased *Clostridiaceae/Clostridium* in mice fed a high-fat diet (McAllan et al. 2015). Furthermore, another study (Shi et al. 2011) reported that replacing 5%, 50%, or 100% of the energy content derived from dietary casein with whey protein isolate resulted in proportional suppression of body weight gain in mice fed a high-fat diet. In a mouse colitis model, whey protein intake increased *Bifidobacteria* and *Lactobacilli* levels compared to casein (Sprong et al. 2010). Despite these findings, it remains unexplored whether the alterations detected in the gut microbiota are related to the anti-obesity effects of casein and whey proteins and the variations in these effects (Li et al. 2016).

Researchers have suggested that casein and whey proteins may also affect microbiota-related mucosal immunity. A study examining the effect of a low-protein diet supplemented with free amino acids (DPD-SA) and a low-protein diet supplemented with casein hydrolysate (DPD-KH) on colonic microbiota and mucosal immunity in pigs showed that compared to the DPD-SA diet, the DPD-KH diet potentially reduced the concentration of nitrogenous metabolites, the abundance of pathogenic bacteria, and the expression of proinflammatory Th1-cytokines. Reduced expression of Th1-cytokines resulted from the inhibition of the Toll-like receptor 4 (TLR4)/nucleotide-binding oligomerization domain (NOD) proteins-nuclear factor kappa B (NF-κB) (TLR4/NOD1-NF-κB) pathway. The DPD-KH diet was observed to enhance the abundance of *Lactobacillus* and increase total short-chain fatty acid concentrations to a greater extent than the DPD-SA diet. Additionally, it was found to enhance mucosal potential defense capabilities by stimulating humoral immunity. As a result, casein hydrolysate supplementation in a low-protein diet compared to free amino acid supplementation in a low-protein diet positively affected colonic microbiota and mucosal immunity in pigs (Wang et al. 2019).

Milk and dairy products could potentially influence the gut microbiota through their various nutrients, encompassing macro and micronutrients. Additionally, milk proteins are considered to be among the most potent protein sources for obesity prevention due to their rich BCAA content, which may potentially influence the gut microbiota and obesity. The potential impacts of milk proteins on obesity, the immune system, and other aspects suggest the need for more comprehensive research on their relationship with the microbiota and associated diseases.

THE EFFECTS OF OTHER PROTEINS

Proteins, which are extremely important for growth and development, sustaining life, and improving health, are of interest in terms of their relationships with the microbiota and their mechanisms of action. While studies show that dietary proteins may affect the microbiota, knowledge about how different dietary protein sources affect the intestinal microbiota is very limited. Nevertheless, in recent years, studies on red meat, chicken and fish proteins, soy, casein, and whey proteins have come to the fore. In a study examining the bacterial composition in the cecum of rats fed these proteins, researchers observed that the intestinal microbiota composition differed in rats fed meat-based and non-meat-based protein feeds, and that strict microbiota aggregation was higher in rats fed with non-meat proteins such as casein and soy protein. They found that the number of *Lactobacillus* species increased in young rats fed with chicken protein for 14 days (Zhu et al. 2015).

Regarding meat sources, researchers believe that L-carnitine and phosphatidylcholine (which can be converted into trimethylamine and trimethylamine oxide (TMAO)) contained in red meat and eggs may be associated with the development of cardiovascular diseases and obesity through their effects on the microbiota (Madsen et al. 2017). On the other hand, studies show the positive intestinal-related effects of protein sources and dairy products obtained through a vegetarian diet. In studies on the effect of soy on the microbiota, researchers observed that soy increases the levels of *Bifidobacteria* and *Lactobacilli* and can change the ratio of *Firmicutes* and *Bacteroidetes* (Huang et al. 2016).

MINI DICTIONARY OF TERMS

- **Codex Alimentarius:** Internationally recognized food standards and guidelines.
- **Host:** A cell or organism that supports the vitality of a virus or parasite by meeting its needs.
- **Lipoprotein lipase:** Enzyme involved in the entry of triglycerides from chylomicrons into adipose cells.
- **Pathobionts:** Pathogenic organisms that cause infectious diseases.
- **Proliferation:** Increase in the number of cells by division.
- **Symbiosis:** A relationship in which two different organisms benefit from each other as they continue their lives.

SUMMARY POINTS

- This chapter focuses on dairy protein and its effect on gut microbiota.
- Dairy products may positively affect the intestinal microbiota through mechanical processes, including promoting beneficial bacteria growth, inhibiting pathogenic bacteria growth, and altering the gastrointestinal environment.
- Some of the various bioactive peptides formed by the hydrolysis of casein with appropriate proteases can modulate the composition of the intestinal microbiota.
- Whey protein appears to provide complete protection, especially in infants, by stimulating beneficial bacteria such as Bifidobacterium and Lactobacillus and preventing the proliferation of pathogens.
- Milk and dairy products could potentially influence the gut microbiota.
- More comprehensive studies are needed on the effects of milk proteins on microbiota and related diseases.

REFERENCES

Adak, A., Khan, M.R. 2019. An insight into gut microbiota and its functionalities. *Cellular and Molecular Life Sciences* 76: 473–493.

Aslam, H., Marx, W., Rocks, T., Loughman, A., Chandrasekaran, V., Ruusunen, A., Dawson, S.L., West, M., Mullarkey, E., Pasco, J.A., Jacka, F.N. 2020. The effects of dairy and dairy derivatives on the gut microbiota: a systematic literature review. *Gut Microbes* 12(1): 1799533.

Ateş Özcan, B. 2020. Mikrobiyota ve obezite ilişkisi. In *Obezite, Nedenleri ve Sonuçları*, ed. M.E. Alphan, 137–157. Ankara: Hatiboğlu Yayıncılık.

Ayyıldız, F., Yıldıran, H. 2019. Farklı diyet modellerinin bağırsak mikrobiyotası üzerine etkisi. *Beslenme ve Diyet Dergisi* 47(2): 77–86.

Belkaid, Y., Naik, S. 2013. Compartmentalized and systemic control of tissue immunity by commensals. *Nature Immunology* 14(7): 646–653.

Bendtsen, L.Q., Blædel, T., Holm, J.B., Lorenzen, J.K., Mark, A.B., Kiilerich, P., Kristiansen, K., Astrup, A., Larsen, L.H. 2018. High intake of dairy during energy restriction does not affect energy balance or the intestinal microflora compared with low dairy intake in overweight individuals in a randomized controlled trial. *Applied Physiology, Nutrition, and Metabolism* 43(1): 1–10.

Boland, M., Singh, H. 2019. *Milk Proteins: From Expression to Food*. New Zealand: Academic Press.

Bollrath, J., Powrie, F.M. 2013. Controlling the frontier: regulatory t-cells and intestinal homeostasis. *Semin Immun* 25(5): 352–357.

Boscaini, S., Skuse, P., Nilaweera, K.N., Cryan, J.F., Cotter, P.D. 2023. The 'whey' to good health: whey protein and its beneficial effect on metabolism, gut microbiota and mental health. *Trends in Food Science & Technology* 133: 1–14.

Boulangé, C.L., Neves, A.L., Chilloux, J., Nicholson, J.K., Dumas, M.E. 2016. Impact of the gut microbiota on inflammation, obesity, and metabolic disease. *Genome Medicine* 8: 1–12.

Burton, K.J., Rosikiewicz, M., Pimentel, G., Bütikofer, U., Von Ah, U., Voirol, M.-J., Croxatto, A., Aeby, S., Drai, J., McTernan, P.G., Greub, G., Pralong, F.P., Vergères, G., Vionnet, N. 2017. Probiotic yogurt and acidified milk similarly reduce postprandial inflammation and both alter the gut microbiota of healthy, young men. *British Journal of Nutrition* 117(9): 1312–1322.

Chung, H., Pamp, S.J., Hill, J.A., Surana, N.K., Edelman, S.M., Troy, E.B., ... Kasper, D.L. 2012. Gut immune maturation depends on colonization with a host-specific microbiota. *Cell* 149(7): 1578–1593.

David, L.A., Maurice, C.F., Carmody, R.N., Gootenberg, D.B., Button, J.E., Wolfe, B.E., ... Turnbaugh, P.J. 2014. Diet rapidly and reproducibly alters the human gut microbiome. *Nature* 505(7484): 559–563.

Del Chierico, F., Vernocchi, P., Dallapiccola, B., Putignani, L. 2014. Mediterranean diet and health: food effects on gut microbiota and disease control. *International Journal of Molecular Sciences* 15(7): 11678–11699.

Demirören, K. 2020. Biyoaktif peptitler. In *Fonksiyonel Gıdalar*, ed. G. Baysoy, 209–221. Ankara: Nobel Tıp Kitabevleri.

Dominguez-Bello, M.G., Costello, E.K., Contreras, M., Magris, M., Hidalgo, G., Fierer, N., Knight, R. 2010. Delivery mode shapes the acquisition and structure of the initial microbiota across multiple body habitats in newborns. *Proceedings of the National Academy of Sciences* 107(26): 11971–11975.

Espín, J.C., González-Sarrías, A., Tomás-Barberán, F.A. 2017. The gut microbiota: a key factor in the therapeutic effects of (poly) phenols. *Biochemical Pharmacology* 139: 82–93.

Falony, G., Joossens, M., Vieira-Silva, S., Wang, J., Darzi, Y., Faust, K., ... Raes, J. 2016. Population-level analysis of gut microbiome variation. *Science* 352(6285): 560–564.

FAO. 2022. Gateway to dairy production and products. https://www.fao.org/dairy-production-products/products/en/ (accessed August 28, 2023).

Fernandez-Raudales, D., Hoeflinger, J.L., Bringe, N.A., Cox, S.B., Dowd, S.E., Miller, M.J., Gonzalez de Mejia, E. 2012. Consumption of different soymilk formulations differentially affects the gut microbiomes of overweight and obese men. *Gut Microbes* 3(6): 490–500.

Guo, Z., Yi, D., Hu, B., Shi, Y., Xin, Y., Gu, Z., ... Zhang, L. 2021. The alteration of gut microbiota by bioactive peptides: a review. Systems *Microbiology and Biomanufacturing* 1: 363–377.

Herrema, H., IJzerman, R.G., Nieuwdorp, M. 2017. Emerging role of intestinal microbiota and microbial metabolites in metabolic control. *Diabetologia* 60(4): 613–617.

Huang, H., Krishnan, H.B., Pham, Q., Yu, L.L., and Wang, T.T. 2016. Soy and gut microbiota: interaction and implication for human health. *Journal of Agricultural and Food Chemistry* 64(46): 8695–8709.

Kamada, N., Chen, G.Y., Inohara, N., Núñez, G. 2013. Control of pathogens and pathobionts by the gut microbiota. *Nature Immunology* 14(7): 685–690.

Koushalya, S., Vasantharaja, R., Hariprasad, P., Ariyadasa, T.U., Malik, A. 2022. Recent advances in the production of nutritional products from algal biomass. In *Algae and Aquatic Macrophytes in Cities: Bioremediation, Biomass, Biofuels and Bioproducts*, ed. V.C. Pandey, 235–260. Amsterdam: Elsevier.

Krishnan, S., Alden, N., Lee, K. 2015. Pathways and functions of gut microbiota metabolism impacting host physiology. *Current Opinion in Biotechnology* 36: 137–145.

Lebba, V., Totino, V., Gagliardi, A., Santangelo, F., Cacciotti, F., Trancassini, M., Mancini, C., Cicerone, C., Corazziari, E., Pantanella, F., Schippa, S. 2016. Eubiosis and dysbiosis: The two sides of the microbiota. *New Microbiology* 39(1): 1–12.

Lepage, P., Leclerc, M.C., Joossens, M., Mondot, S., Blottière, H.M., Raes, J., ... Doré, J. 2013. A metagenomic insight into our gut's microbiome. *Gut* 62(1): 146–158.

Li, Z., Jin, H., Oh, S.Y., Ji, G.E. 2016. Anti-obese effects of two lactobacilli and two bifidobacteria on ıcr mice fed on a high fat diet. *Biochemical and Biophysical Research Communications* 480: 222–227.

Litvak, Y., Byndloss, M.X., Bäumler, A.J. 2018. Colonocyte metabolism shapes the gut microbiota. *Science* 362(6418): eaat9076.

Liu, C.J., Tang, X.D., Yu, J., Zhang, H.Y., Li, X.R. 2017. Gut microbiota alterations from different lactobacillus probiotic-fermented yoghurt treatments in slow-transit constipation. *Journal of Functional Foods* 38: 110–118.

Liu, S. 2016. The development of our organ of other kinds- the gut microbiota. *Frontiers In Microbiology* 7: 2107.

Madsen, L., Myrmel, L.S., Fjære, E., Liaset, B., Kristiansen, K. 2017. Links between dietary protein sources, the gut microbiota, and obesity. *Frontiers in Physiology* 8: 1047.

Martin, F.P.J., Montoliu, I., Kussmann, M. 2017. Metabonomics of ageing–towards understanding metabolism of a long and healthy life. *Mechanisms of Ageing and Development* 165: 00171–179.

Mayer, E.A., Tillisch, K., Gupta, A. 2015. Gut/brain axis and the microbiota. *The Journal of Clinical Investigation* 125(3): 926–938.

McAllan, L., Speakman, J.R., Cryan, J.F., and Nilaweera, K.N. 2015. Whey protein isolate decreases murine stomach weight and intestinal length and alters the expression of Wnt signalling-associated genes. *British Journal of Nutrition* 113: 372–379.

McGregor, R.A., Poppitt, S.D. 2013. Milk protein for improved metabolic health: a review of the evidence. *Nutrition & Metabolism* 10(1): 46.

Michaelsen, K.F., Nielsen, A.L.H., Roos, N., Friis, H., Mølgaard, C. 2011. Cow's milk in treatment of moderate and severe undernutrition in low-income countries. *Nestle Nutr Workshop Ser Pediatr Program* 67: 99–111.

Moon, C., Baldridge, M.T., Wallace, M.A., Burnham, C.A.D., Virgin, H.W., Stappenbeck, T.S. 2015. Vertically transmitted faecal IgA levels determine extra-chromosomal phenotypic variation. *Nature* 521(7550): 90–93.

Muehlhoff, E., Bennett, A., MacMahon, D. 2013. Milk and dairy products in human nutrition. *International Journal of Diary Technology* 67(2): 303–304.

Nagpal, R., Tsuji, H., Takahashi, T., Kawashima, K., Nagata, S., Nomoto, K., Yamashiro, Y. (2016). Sensitive quantitative analysis of the meconium bacterial microbiota in healthy term infants born vaginally or by cesarean section. *Frontiers in Microbiology* 7, 1997.

OECD/FAO. 2022. Dairy and dairy products. In *OECD- FAO Agricultural Outlook 2022–2031*, ed. W. Legg, 212–223. Paris: OECD Publishing.

Ozmen, H., Aydinli, B. 2020. Bir probiyotik olarak kefir'in günlük besin desteğinden yoğun bakımda kullanımına uzanan öyküsü. *Mersin Üniversitesi Tıp Fakültesi Lokman Hekim Tıp Tarihi ve Folklorik Tıp Dergisi* 10(3): 295–301.

Özsoy, S. 2019. Polifenoller, mikrobiyota ve diyabet. *Beslenme ve Diyet Dergisi* 47: 102–109.

Perazza, L.R., Daniel, N., Dubois, M.-J., Pilon, G., Varin, T.V., Blais, M., Martinez Gonzales, J.L., Bouchard, M., Asselin, C., Lessard, M., Pouliot, Y., Roy, D., Marette, A. 2020. Distinct effects of milk-derived and fermented dairy protein on gut microbiota and cardiometabolic markers in diet-ınduced obese mice. *The Journal of Nutrition* 150(10): 2673–2686.

Power, S.E., O'Toole, P.W., Stanton, C., Ross, R.P., Fitzgerald, G.F. 2014. Intestinal microbiota, diet and health. *British Journal of Nutrition* 111(3): 387–402.

Precup, G., Vodnar, D.C. 2019. Gut prevotella as a possible biomarker of diet and its eubiotic versus dysbiotic roles: A comprehensive literature review. *British Journal of Nutrition* 122(2): 131–140.

Riccio, P., Rossano, R. 2020. The human gut microbiota is neither an organ nor a commensal. *FEBS Letters* 594(20): 3262–3271.

Rinninella, E., Cintoni, M., Raoul, P., Lopetuso, L.R., Scaldaferri, F., Pulcini, G., Miggiano, G.A.D., Gasbarrini, A., Mele, M.C. 2019. Food components and dietary habits: keys for a healthy gut microbiota composition. *Nutrients* 11(10): 2393.

Rowland, I., Gibson, G., Heinken, A., Scott, K., Swann, J., Thiele, I., Tuohy, K. 2018. Gut microbiota functions: metabolism of nutrients and other food components. *European Journal of Nutrition* 57: 1–24.

Shi, J., Tauriainen, E., Martonen, E., Finckenberg, P., Ahlroos-Lehmus, A., Tuomainen, A., Pilvi, T.K., Korpela, R., Mevaala, E.M. 2011. Whey protein isolate protects against dietinduced obesity and fatty liver formation. *International Dairy Journal* 21: 513–522.

Sommer, F., Bäckhed, F. 2016. Know your neighbor: microbiota and host epithelial cells interact locally to control intestinal function and physiology. *BioEssays* 38(5): 455–464.

Sprong, R.C., Schonewille, A.J., Van DerMeer, R. 2010. Dietary cheese whey protein protects rats against mild dextran sulfate sodium-induced colitis: role of mucin and microbiota. *Journal of Dairy Science* 93: 1364–1371.

Sun, J., Kato, I. 2016. Gut microbiota, inflammation and colorectal cancer. *Genes & Diseases* 3(2): 130–143.

T.C. Ministry of Health, General Directorate of Public Health. 2022. Türkiye Nutrition Guide (TUBER) 2022. https://hsgmdestek.saglik.gov.tr/depo/birimler/saglikli-beslenme-hareketli-hayat-db/Rehberler/T%C3%BCrkiye%20Beslenme%20Rehber%20(T%C3%9CBER)%202022.pdf (accessed August 28,2023).

Turroni, F., Ventura, M., Buttó, L.F., Duranti, S., O'Toole, P.W., Motherway, M.O., van Sinderen, D. 2014. Molecular dialogue between the human gut microbiota and the host: A lactobacillus and bifidobacterium perspective. *Cellular and Molecular Life Sciences* 71(2): 183–203.

Velasquez, M.T., Ramezani, A., Manal, A., Raj, D.S. 2016. Trimethylamine n-oxide: the good, the bad and the unknown. *Toxins* 8(11): 326.

Wang, H., Shen, J., Pi, Y., Gao, K., Zhu, W. 2019. Low-protein diets supplemented with casein hydrolysate favor the microbiota and enhance the mucosal humoral immunity in the colon of pigs. *Journal of Animal Science and Biotechnology* 10(1): 1–13.

Yılmaz, İ., Dolar, M.E., Özpınar, H. 2019. Effect of administering kefir on the changes in fecal microbiota and symptoms of inflammatory bowel disease: A randomized controlled trial. *The Turkish Journal of Gastroenterology* 30(3): 242–253.

Zhu, Y., Lin, X., Zhao, F., Shi, X., Li, H., Li, Y., Zhu, W., Xu, X., Li, C., Zhou, G. 2015. Meat, dairy and plant proteins alter bacterial composition of rat gut bacteria. *Scientific Reports* 5: 15220.

14 Dairy Proteins in the Diet and Skeletal Muscle Metabolism in Adults

Maria Spanoudaki, Sousana K. Papadopoulou, Stavros Pellios, and Constantinos Giagkinis

ABBREVIATIONS

Akt	Protein kinase B
BCAAs	Branched-chain amino acids
DIAAS	Digestible indispensable amino acid score
EAAs	Essential amino acids
IAAs	Irreplaceable amino acids
MPS	Muscle protein synthesis
mWPC	Microparticulated whey protein concentrate
NO	Nitrogen oxide
Thr	Threonine

INTRODUCTION

Adequate nutrition is crucial for survival and optimal growth at every phase of the human life cycle. Milk is the first fundamental food that the human body digests, absorbs and utilizes for growth and maintenance. It is clearly a complete nutrient source (Davoodi et al., 2016). Milk is intrinsically associated with the development of every cell in every system, supporting their proper function, optimal growth and health. Specifically, the digestion, absorption, distribution and utilization of milk components promote the growth and maintenance of human tissues from the earliest stages of life, providing adequate amounts of calories, protein, vitamins, minerals, trace elements and growth stimuli.

Dairy proteins are highly nutritious dried ingredients with several functional and nutritional properties (Huth et al., 2006; Fontecha et al., 2023). This category includes a variety of components, such as whey proteins and milk proteins with different protein and amino acid (AA) content. Dried caseins and caseinates, as well as serum proteins (whey protein), are also included in this group. Dairy proteins are widely used to promote lean mass by providing muscle protein synthesis (MPS). In addition, milk protein-derived peptides have been linked to various bioactivities, such as immune-protective, anticancer, metal-binding, antibacterial, anti-lipidemic, satiating, insulinotropic and anti-inflammatory properties in humans (Nongonierma and FitzGerald, 2015a).

Although the protein content of milk differs among mammals, with sheep's milk containing the highest amount of protein per 100 g, followed by buffalo's, camel's and goat's milk, the high content of whey and essential amino acids (leucine and arginine) forms a protein complex providing a high-quality profile. Several fermented dairy products, such as yoghurt and cheese, also retain the aforementioned compounds. Camel yoghurt has been found to be richer in terms of essential

DOI: 10.1201/9781003597926-14

amino acids (arginine, valine, lysine, tryptophan, phenylalanine) compared to bovine, sheep and goat yoghurts (Terzioğlu et al., 2023).

Research based on the chemical analysis of milk and dairy products has documented that whey and casein are the two predominant proteins (Nongonierma and FitzGerald, 2015b). The term "dairy proteins" includes whey and caseins derived from milk and other dairy products, while the term "milk" usually refers to bovine milk, which is a rich source of proteins and essential amino acids (EAAs), (Davoodi et al., 2016). Proteins derived from fermented dairy products also demonstrate enhanced absorption and increased postprandial MPS.

Casein proteins form complexes and are responsible for milk's white colour. The biological actions of caseins are based on the concentration of amino acids and mineral transport activity, which contribute to the secondary assimilation of minerals (Bär et al., 2019; Nongonierma and FitzGerald, 2015a; Trommelen et al., 2020).

Whey is the liquid byproduct of cheese production and concentrates a number of high-quality proteins (Auestad and Layman, 2021). Whey proteins are particularly dense in leucine, methionine, tryptophan and lysine, which are the limiting amino acids in plant food sources (Krissansen, 2007). The digestible indispensable amino acid score (DIAAS) protein quality scores for each of these amino acids have been found to be between 2.3 and 3.3 for whey, while DIAAS scores are below 0.8 for proteins derived from wheat and between 0.9 and 1.0 for proteins found in soy (Horstman et al., 2019; Rutherfurd et al., 2015).

Milk and dairy proteins, especially whey, have been linked to muscle tissue homeostasis (Alcantara et al., 2019). Proteins derived from milk and fermented milk have been associated with anabolic function, confirming the endogenous communication between gut microbiota and muscle tissue. Fermentation enhances amino acid uptake, which increases absorption and postprandial protein synthesis in muscles through Akt-independent pathways (Sumi et al., 2021; Vidal-Casariego et al., 2015).

The development of the muscular system from the neonatal period to its completion in adulthood requires energy substrates and growth stimulants. Muscle protein synthesis is critical for preserving the structural and functional integrity of skeletal muscle. Skeletal muscles are responsible for all movement and mobilization (Morgan et al., 2021). Thus, muscles are mechanically strained, being a large source of components necessary to maintain movement at any intensity performed daily. An assessment of the recommended dairy product intake in Europe found heterogeneity in compliance between countries, with lower than recommended intakes in adults of both genders. In 2019, the total prevalence of dairy consumption in Europe was 66.95% (63.35% and 69.8% in men and women, respectively) (Ribeiro et al., 2019).

Ageing exerts a negative effect on muscle strength and function. Muscle mass declines particularly after the fifth decade of life (or even earlier), leading to a condition known as sarcopenia, which has a great impact on the quality of life of older adults and elderly individuals. Although MPS and muscle protein breakdown are part of a remodelling cycle to maintain a net nitrogen balance that promotes muscle tissue reconstruction, muscle anabolic resistance is observed in the fifth decade of life or even earlier, leading to an imbalance between anabolic and catabolic rhythms in skeletal muscles (Mitchell et al., 2017). People with sarcopenia or with evidence of sarcopenia are prone to falls, fractures, inability to perform daily activities and frailty due to dysregulation within muscle tissue (Cuesta-Triana et al., 2019).

The type and role of proteins and amino acids in muscle fibre regeneration in health and disease have attracted the interest of the scientific community for at least the last two decades. Initially, the role of dairy proteins, particularly whey, in muscle growth and recovery was studied more extensively in athletes in the field of performance and injury rehabilitation. The low adherence to dairy intake recommendations, combined with the continuing increase in the population over 60 years of age, makes it necessary to investigate the importance of dairy protein intake and supplementation on muscle mass metabolism, particularly in middle-aged and older adults (Morgan et al., 2021).

The aim of this chapter is to highlight the effect of dairy proteins on skeletal MPS and function in adults. This study explores whether dairy proteins are the magic key to muscle remodelling.

SKELETAL MPS

As the main actor in protein synthesis, skeletal muscle is the body's largest source of protein. Energy, high-quality protein intake and exercise are the predominant stimulators for MPS. Skeletal muscle protein synthesis is essential for preserving functional and structural proteins. Protein and amino acid uptake promote muscle protein synthesis via the activation of the mechanical target of rapamycin complex 1 (mTORC1), a serine/threonine protein kinase that elevates muscle protein synthesis via translational regulation (Millward, 2021). Phosphorylation sites of mTORC1 involve S6 kinase 1 (S6K1) and the 4 eukaryotic binding protein 1 (4EBP1). After their phosphorylation, S6K1 stimulates cell development and proliferation, while 4EBP1 plays an indispensable role in the onset of eukaryotic translation. The activation of mTORC1 targets is mainly responsible for the anabolic response to exogenous amino acid uptake by muscles (Dideriksen et al., 2013; Thalacker-Mercer et al., 2020a).

Leucine, regardless of the presence of other EAAs, provides the stimuli for mTORC1 action and promotes the onset of MPS. Evidence-based studies have shown that the required dose of leucine for protein synthesis is age-dependent. Interestingly, the stimulation of MPS by leucine differs between young and older adults, with the latter requiring a higher dose when administered as a bolus (2 g vs. 3 g of leucine per day, respectively) (Thalacker-Mercer et al., 2020b). Leucine supplementation is beneficial in preventing age-related muscle mass impairment in older individuals, as it increases the fractional synthetic rate of muscle proteins (Thalacker-Mercer et al., 2020b; Xu et al., 2015).

Several amino acids, not only EAAs, play a crucial role in MPS, such as arginine. Arginine stimulates MPS via the mTORC1 pathway and through an NO-dependent vasodilation mechanism, thus increasing nutrient supply to the muscles. In addition, arginine induces the secretion of growth factors such as growth hormone and insulin and is a precursor of creatine. Remarkably, these pathways are only activated if arginine is depleted under critical conditions, such as anabolic resistance due to ageing or disease. Furthermore, arginine could be protective in muscle stress catabolism by acting directly on muscles (Argilés et al., 2016). However, arginine metabolism increases urea content, which limits its use (De Bandt, 2019) (Figure 14.1). Studies in healthy subjects have also revealed

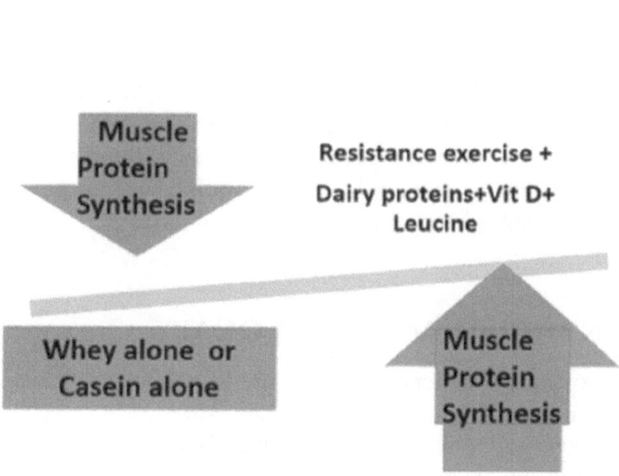

FIGURE 14.1 Dairy proteins' effect on muscle protein synthesis.

that arginine supplementation had limited results, demonstrating that the human body effectively synthesizes or recycles this AA via citrulline (De Bandt, 2019).

DAIRY PROTEINS

Whey and Casein Profile

Whey consists of many proteins such as α-lactalbumin, β-lactoglobulin, bovine glycomacropeptide, lactoferrin, α-lactalbumin, β-lactoglobulin and serum albumin (Bär et al., 2019) (Figure 14.1).

Whey has been extensively proposed to support or stimulate MPS. Its high amino acid profile, high solubility, bioavailability, rapid absorption and increased content of BCAA (particularly leucine) contribute to whey protein's great popularity in the athletic world and the sports nutrition market as well (Naclerio and Larumbe-Zabala, 2016a).

Several types of whey protein supplements are currently available on the market. The most widely used are whey protein isolate, hydrolyzed whey protein and whey protein concentrate. Milk protein concentrates are formed by the coagulation of milk with the enzyme rennet or acid, which results in separating the curd and whey. Additional drying and ultrafiltration produce whey protein concentrate with a content of more than 90% pure protein. Further processes such as selective elution or ion exchange chromatography can be used to achieve the production of purer and higher fractionated whey isolate containing more than 90% pure protein with traces of lipids and lactose. Both whey protein isolate and whey protein concentrate provide a blend of native intact proteins.

A new dairy protein is native whey protein produced by filtration of unprocessed raw milk, containing a higher content of leucine without glycolmacropeptides compared to whey protein concentrate and whey protein isolate (Dissanayake et al., 2012). Another form of dairy protein is a microparticulated form of whey protein concentrate (mWPC) produced by acidic precipitation and thermal agglomeration combined with a high-shear environment. Regarding the effect of mWPC on the stimulation of protein synthesis in human skeletal muscle compared to the common whey protein concentrate, no significant difference was found (Davoodi et al., 2016).

Caseins, a group of phospho-proteins, show high heterogeneity due to the existence of different isoforms with various amino acid combinations. Casein comprises the majority of milk proteins and includes a heterogeneous family of κ-casein, αs1-casein, αs2-casein and β-casein. It is characterized as a slow-digesting protein because of gradual digestion as it curdles in a low-pH environment (Horstman et al., 2019). Many studies have shown that casein can support MPS by reducing the rate of muscle protein breakdown and prolonging muscle anabolism (Bär et al., 2019; Hall et al., 2003). In terms of its amino acid profile, casein shows an optimal balance not only in BCAA content (leucine, isoleucine and valine) but also in non-BCAAs, such as arginine, a high proline content, traces of cysteine and glutamic acid (Auestad and Layman, 2021). Moreover, casein contains higher amounts of methionine, valine, phenylalanine, histidine, tyrosine and serine, while whey protein contains higher amounts of leucine and glycine. There is substantial scientific evidence for the effect of leucine on MPS, but not enough in the case of glycine. Glycine plays a key role in muscle recovery after injury and promotes MPS, thus making it a semi-essential amino acid for humans as well (Wang et al., 2013).

DAIRY PROTEINS IN THE DIET AND EFFECT ON MPS

Dairy products, milk protein supplements and milk are affordable worldwide, promoting muscle anabolism due to their content of EAAs and BCAAs.

EAAs or IAAs are those amino acids whose carbon skeleton cannot be synthesized or those that are not adequately produced de novo by the body in relation to its needs and must be provided by nutrition to best meet requirements. According to DIAAS (Wolfe et al., 2016), protein quality assessment of animal proteins, which includes whey and casein, among others, shows they have higher content and are complete in E A As compared to plant proteins such as potato, pea, brown rice and wheat (Kalman, 2014; Liu et al., 2019). For example, grain proteins are deficient in IAAs, such as threonine, tryptophan and lysine, while others derived from legumes are depleted in cysteine and methionine (Pinckaers et al., 2022). Hence, while DIAAS for dairy proteins is much higher than 100%, proteins of plants are scored below 80%. However, some protein extracts derived from soy, rice or peas have demonstrated scores close to or higher than 100% (Van Vliet et al., 2015). In contrast, the leucine content remains higher in whey isolate than in all other plant and animal proteins (Kalman, 2014), allowing whey protein to exert a larger effect on MPS stimuli (Witard et al., 2014a).

Moreover, dairy proteins are good sources of non-EAAs like cysteine. Cysteine plays a major role in the synthesis of glutathione, which in turn affects muscle tissue by increasing muscle cell apoptosis not only in older adults but in middle-aged adults as well (Sekhar et al., 2011). Meal patterns include animal and plant protein sources, and thus, older adults and the elderly consume a matrix of macro and micronutrients in daily life. The meal matrix changes the AA kinetics compared to dairy proteins in the form of supplements, such as whey, casein or a blend of whey and casein. Research has significantly supported that the consumption of full-fat milk after resistance exercise can induce a greater rate of MPS compared to fat-free milk (Elliot et al., 2006; Moore et al., 2014). Interestingly, the digestion of whey alone or combined with casein also stimulates MPS, but absorption and uptake in skeletal muscles were better preserved for casein in young adults (Du et al., 2019; Soop et al., 2012). Furthermore, the anabolic muscle response following ingestion of a combination of free EAAs and whey was found to be more than double the response to the administration of a similar dose of whey isolate in young adults (Park et al., 2020), as the rate of muscle protein synthesis was found to be significantly greater.

There is limited scientific evidence on the impact of dairy proteins on sarcopenia. The meta-analysis by Hanach and colleagues (2019) showed that consumption of dairy proteins as supplements enriched with vitamin D3 and/or leucine or in their native form in dairy products, such as ricotta cheese, can exert a positive effect on MPS but in middle-aged and older adults, the optimal intake was 14–40 g/day. However, the effect on muscle function assessed by the Short Physical Performance Battery was not significant (Hanach et al., 2019; Naclerio and Larumbe-Zabala, 2016b). In middle-aged men, it was also found that ingestion of 20 g of milk protein concentrate similarly affected resting myofibril fractional synthesis rates compared to equal amounts of whey protein (Mitchell et al., 2017).

Previous research has additionally indicated that a protein intake of 20 g of whole protein or 10 g of EAAs is sufficient for MPS stimuli before and after resistance exercise, while a larger dose may lead to EAA oxidation and urea genesis in rested and trained muscles in young men (Dideriksen et al., 2013; Witard et al., 2014b).

Alterations in amino acid and protein metabolism in response to a stimulus may be relevant to the observed changes in skeletal muscle mass and strength that follow ageing (Wolfe, 2015). The reaction to postprandial aminoacidemia and the switching of the stimuli for the protein synthesis pathway are likely to be influenced by age and dietary protein adequacy (Mitchell et al., 2017). Older adults, compared to younger ones, present a reduced anabolic response to dietary protein, even though the mechanism of muscle protein synthesis remains unchanged (Dideriksen et al., 2013; Thalacker-Mercer et al., 2020b). Focusing on sarcopenia as an outcome of ageing, the effect of dairy proteins and the dairy food matrix on MPS is still under consideration. Dairy protein supplementation, in combination with leucine or vitamin D, can exert a significant impact on MPS in the elderly (McGlory et al., 2019). It is worth noting that, apart from protein intake, muscle loading is the second stimulus for protein synthesis in the muscles. Combined with the loss of muscle strength, which occurs more rapidly than the loss of muscle mass, older people are prone to frailty (Goodpaster et al., 2006).

Older adults have demonstrated dairy and high-quality protein under-consumption (Ribeiro et al., 2019; Smeuninx et al., 2020), while higher consumption of low-fat yoghurt or low-fat milk, more than seven servings per week, was correlated to a decreased risk of frailty and an improvement in gait speed improvement (Hanach et al., 2019). Older women who reported higher consumption of dairy products (milk, cheese, yoghurt) also showed a reduced risk for fractures and an enhancement of appendicular muscle mass, hand grip strength and bone mass(Phillips and Martinson, 2018).

A recent meta-analysis revealed that long-term supplementation with 10–35 g/day of milk protein and resistance training helps maintain muscle mass or delays muscle loss in older adults, especially those with medical conditions such as obesity (Hidayat et al., 2018; Liao et al., 2017). In contrast, supplementation of 40 g/day of whey protein combined with 20 μg/day of vitamin D and low-intensity home exercise did not mitigate the decrease in muscle and physical capacity in sarcopenic older adults living in the community (Björkman et al., 2020). However, in non-regularly exercising older adults, muscle protein accumulation was greater after ingestion of 15 g of whey protein than after ingestion of 7 g of whey EAA content, revealing that the EAA content of whey is not entirely responsible for its anabolic effect (Katsanos et al., 2008). Additionally, the consumption of nine grams of milk protein concentrate with a single session of resistance exercise increased the positive effect on muscle anabolism in middle-aged men through the activation of the p70 S6 kinase phosphorylation metabolic pathway (Mitchell et al., 2017) (Figure 14.1).

The diet-related anabolic requirement for protein is higher in the elderly than in younger people. Thus, the recommendations for protein intake are 1.0–1.2 g/kg/day in older adults, compared to 0.8 g/kg/day for young adults (Zanini et al., 2020). Dairy proteins, easily found in food sources or as leucine-rich supplements, are effective for promoting myofibrillar synthesis. Notably, the response to leucine appears to be reduced in the elderly. Thus, higher leucine intake is necessary to induce muscle anabolism. The age dependence of protein synthesis and the magnitude of dairy protein intake are evident, and studies recommend more than 1.2 g/kg for the elderly population (Moore et al., 2014; Traylor et al., 2018; Cuesta-Triana et al., 2019; Zanini et al., 2020).

Studies in young and older adults have shown that digestion of dairy "fast protein" (whey), combined with dairy "slow protein" (casein), had the same effect on MPS or net nitrogen balance when taken after exercise. Some studies report no differences between casein and whey in terms of their effect on MPS in young adults with long-term training (Witard et al., 2014b).

Whole dairy proteins are widely used dietary supplements for gaining muscle mass through the stimulation of protein synthesis. Dairy protein supplementation is usually obtained as prepared protein-fortified foods, intact proteins or free AAs. Whey is the most widely used isolate protein supplement, and EAAs are the main active components of protein in the diet (Witard et al., 2016).

EFFECT OF DAIRY PROTEINS VERSUS PLANT PROTEINS ON MPS

Animal proteins have an AA profile that corresponds to body requirements and can trigger enhanced stimulation of MPS compared to plant proteins. As vegetarianism trends expand globally, a plant-based dietary pattern becomes favourable and reduces environmental strain. However, proteins of plant origin have a lower-quality AA profile than animal ones as they do not contain all essential AAs and have lower concentrations of methionine and lysine (Van Vliet et al., 2015). Consequently, it is essential to combine different plant-based protein sources to meet the full complement of EAAs (Smeuninx et al., 2020).

Soy is the most commonly studied plant protein, with a high concentration of BCAAs. Moreover, brown rice is a good source of protein, containing almost 40% of EAAs and 18% of BCAAs relative to its total protein content. When brown rice protein isolate was compared to soy protein and whey protein isolate, it had an equal AA profile; however, whey protein had higher EAA and BCAA content overall. Additionally, whey protein isolate exhibits higher digestibility than soy or brown rice protein isolate (Kalman, 2014). A study on AA bioavailability after ingestion of a mixture of dairy proteins (whey, casein) and vegetable proteins (soy, pea) revealed higher bioavailability for the blend compared to single proteins (Liu et al., 2019; Phillips et al., 2009).

A recent systematic review and meta-analysis demonstrated key differences between plant proteins (mostly soy) and animal proteins (whey and casein) regarding their effects on MPS, muscle mass maintenance and strength. In terms of body composition, significantly increased lean mass was observed in favour of animal proteins among adults under 50 years old when resistance training was not considered. However, when resistance training was analyzed, no difference was found between plant and animal proteins regarding absolute muscle mass, lean mass or lean mass percentage across trained and untrained subjects. Further analysis showed no statistically significant differences between animal and plant proteins regarding their effect on muscle strength (e.g., handgrip strength or leg extension/flexion).

Although animal proteins appear more beneficial for muscle gain and strength, especially in younger subjects, the source of protein does not seem to affect overall muscle strength outcomes (Lim et al., 2021).

CONCLUSIONS

A large body of scientific research confirms that dairy proteins are high-quality sources for promoting MPS.

Older adults and patients, especially those who are bedridden, are at great risk for energy-protein waste, muscle tissue loss and malnutrition. Providing adequate protein intake (1.2–1.5 g/kg body weight/day) and sufficient leucine supplementation may help limit these risks. Among older adults with chronic low protein intakes, whey or whey and casein supplementation may offer an optimal choice to enhance dairy protein intake and promote MPS.

MPS and muscle protein breakdown are part of a rebuilding cycle that promotes muscle tissue anabolism. Dairy proteins consumed through dietary intake play a key role in promoting MPS before and after exercise across all ages.

Maintaining a net nitrogen balance, combining exercise and dairy intake – or adding dairy-based supplements alongside resistance exercise tailored to each life stage – appears to have an optimal positive effect on gaining or maintaining muscle mass in both health and disease contexts.

Further research is required to investigate the optimal dose and the effect of dairy proteins as stimuli on MPS by exploring their mechanisms and efficacy in regulating anabolic resistance during ageing.

MINI DICTIONARY OF TERMS

- **Anabolic resistance:** The reduced stimulation of muscle protein synthesis at a given amount of protein/amino acids, which is associated with a reduction in skeletal muscle mass.
- **Dairy proteins:** Proteins derived from milk and dairy products.
- **DIAAS:** Score indicating EAA concentration and the digestion profile of any given protein source.
- **mTOR:** Mechanistic target of rapamycin (mTOR) is a type of serine-threonine protein kinase. The mTOR pathway is sensitive to muscle contraction and protein consumption stimuli.
- **Muscle protein breakdown:** The metabolic process of hydrolyzing protein into peptides and/or amino acids.
- **Muscle protein metabolism:** Muscle synthesis and muscle breakdown processes.
- **Muscle protein synthesis:** The metabolic process of binding amino acids to skeletal muscle proteins.
- **Older adults:** Adults aged over 60 years.
- **P70S6K:** A serine/threonine kinase with two different catalytic kinase sites that phosphorylate various ribosomal protein S6 residues.
- **Sarcopenia:** The loss of muscle mass and function.
- **Skeletal muscle:** The appendicular muscle.

SUMMARY POINTS

- Milk and dairy products promote muscle anabolism and growth.
- Whey and casein are the two predominant dairy proteins.
- Whey is rich in leucine, and leucine stimulates MPS.
- Whey is characterized as a "fast protein," while casein is characterized as a "slow protein."
- Older adults have greater protein and dairy protein requirements than younger ones.
- Whey protein and vegetable protein blends appear to be effective in MPS in older adults.
- Combining whey and casein intake with resistance exercise seems to have an optimal effect on aged muscles' protein synthesis.

REFERENCES

Alcantara, J.M.A., Sanchez-Delgado, G., Martinez-Tellez, B., Labayen, I., Ruiz, J.R., 2019. Impact of cow's milk intake on exercise performance and recovery of muscle function: a systematic review. *J. Int. Soc. Sports Nutr.* 16, 22. https://doi.org/10.1186/s12970-019-0288-5

Argilés, J.M., Campos, N., Lopez-Pedrosa, J.M., Rueda, R., Rodriguez-Mañas, L., 2016. Skeletal muscle regulates metabolism via interorgan crosstalk: roles in health and disease. *J. Am. Med. Dir. Assoc.* 17, 789–796. https://doi.org/10.1016/j.jamda.2016.04.019

Auestad, N., Layman, D.K., 2021. Dairy bioactive proteins and peptides: a narrative review. *Nutr. Rev.* 79, 36–47. https://doi.org/10.1093/nutrit/nuab097

Bär, C., Mathis, D., Neuhaus, P., Dürr, D., Bisig, W., Egger, L., Portmann, R., 2019. Protein profile of dairy products: Simultaneous quantification of twenty bovine milk proteins. *Int. Dairy J.* 97, 167–175. https://doi.org/10.1016/j.idairyj.2019.01.001

Björkman, M.P., Suominen, M.H., Kautiainen, H., Jyväkorpi, S.K., Finne-Soveri, H.U., Strandberg, T.E., Pitkälä, K.H., Tilvis, R.S., 2020. Effect of protein supplementation on physical performance in older people with sarcopenia–a randomized controlled trial. *J. Am. Med. Dir. Assoc.* 21, 226–232.e1. https://doi.org/10.1016/j.jamda.2019.09.006

Cuesta-Triana, F., Verdejo-Bravo, C., Fernández-Pérez, C., Martín-Sánchez, F.J., 2019. Effect of milk and other dairy products on the risk of frailty, sarcopenia, and cognitive performance decline in the elderly: a systematic review. *Adv. Nutr.* 10, S105–S119. https://doi.org/10.1093/advances/nmy105

Davoodi, S.H., Shahbazi, R., Esmaeili, S., Sohrabvandi, S., Mortazavian, A., Jazayeri, S., Taslimi, A., 2016. Health-related aspects of milk proteins. *Iran. J. Pharm. Res.* 2016, 15, 3, 573–559.

De Bandt, J.-P., 2019. Arginine and skeletal muscle. In: *Nutrition and Skeletal Muscle.* Elsevier, pp. 315–327. https://doi.org/10.1016/B978-0-12-810422-4.00018-X

Dideriksen, K., Reitelseder, S., Holm, L., 2013. Influence of amino acids, dietary protein, and physical activity on muscle mass development in humans. *Nutrients* 5, 852–876. https://doi.org/10.3390/nu5030852

Dissanayake, M., Liyanaarachchi, S., Vasiljevic, T., 2012. Functional properties of whey proteins microparticulated at low pH. *J. Dairy Sci.* 95, 1667–1679. https://doi.org/10.3168/jds.2011-4823

Du, Y., Oh, C., No, J., 2019. Advantage of dairy for improving aging muscle. *J. Obes. Metab. Syndr.* 28, 167–174. https://doi.org/10.7570/jomes.2019.28.3.167

Elliot, T.A., Cree, M.G., Sanford, A.P., Wolfe, R.R., Tipton, K.D., 2006. Milk ingestion stimulates net muscle protein synthesis following resistance exercise. *Med. Sci. Sports Exerc.* 38, 667–674. https://doi.org/10.1249/01.mss.0000210190.64458.25

Fontecha, J., Juárez, M., Gil, Á. 2023. Milk and dairy products. In: *Encyclopedia of Human Nutrition (Fourth Edition).* Academic Press, pp. 479–491. https://doi.org/10.1016/B978-0-12-821848-8.00144-X

Goodpaster, B.H., Park, S.W., Harris, T.B., Kritchevsky, S.B., Nevitt, M., Schwartz, A.V., Simonsick, E.M., Tylavsky, F.A., Visser, M., Newman, A.B., for the Health ABC Study, 2006. The loss of skeletal muscle strength, mass, and quality in older adults: the health, aging and body composition study. *J. Gerontol. A. Biol. Sci. Med. Sci.* 61, 1059–1064. https://doi.org/10.1093/gerona/61.10.1059

Hall, W.L., Millward, D.J., Long, S.J., Morgan, L.M., 2003. Casein and whey exert different effects on plasma amino acid profiles, gastrointestinal hormone secretion and appetite. *Br. J. Nutr.* 89, 239–248. https://doi.org/10.1079/BJN2002760

Hanach, N.I., McCullough, F., Avery, A., 2019. The impact of dairy protein intake on muscle mass, muscle strength, and physical performance in middle-aged to older adults with or without existing sarcopenia: a systematic review and meta-analysis. *Adv. Nutr.* 10, 59–69. https://doi.org/10.1093/advances/nmy065

Hidayat, K., Chen, G.-C., Wang, Y., Zhang, Z., Dai, X., Szeto, I.M.Y., Qin, L.-Q., 2018. Effects of milk proteins supplementation in older adults undergoing resistance training: A meta-analysis of randomized control trials. *J. Nutr. Health Aging*. 22, 237–245. https://doi.org/10.1007/s12603-017-0899-y

Horstman, A.M.H., Kouw, I.W.K., Van Dijk, J.-W., Hamer, H.M., Groen, B.B.L., Van Kranenburg, J., Gorissen, S.H.M., Van Loon, L.J.C., 2019. The muscle protein synthetic response to whey protein ingestion is greater in middle-aged women compared with men. *J. Clin. Endocrinol. Metab*. 104, 994–1004. https://doi.org/10.1210/jc.2018-01734

Huth, P.J., DiRienzo, D.B., Miller, G.D., 2006. Major scientific advances with dairy foods in nutrition and health, *J. Dairy Sci*., 89, 1207–1221. https://doi.org/10.3168/jds.S0022-0302(06)72190-7nce

Kalman, D., 2014. Amino acid composition of an organic brown rice protein concentrate and isolate compared to soy and whey concentrates and Isolates. *Foods* 3, 394–402. https://doi.org/10.3390/foods3030394

Katsanos, C.S., Chinkes, D.L., Paddon-Jones, D., Zhang, X., Aarsland, A., Wolfe, R.R., 2008. Whey protein ingestion in elderly persons results in greater muscle protein accrual than ingestion of its constituent essential amino acid content. *Nutr. Res*. 28, 651–658. https://doi.org/10.1016/j.nutres.2008.06.007

Krissansen, G.W., 2007. Emerging health properties of whey proteins and their clinical implications. *J. Am. Coll. Nutr.* 26, 713S–723S. https://doi.org/10.1080/07315724.2007.10719652

Liao, C.-D., Tsauo, J.-Y., Wu, Y.-T., Cheng, C.-P., Chen, Hui-Chuen, Huang, Y.-C., Chen, Hung-Chou, Liou, T.-H., 2017. Effects of protein supplementation combined with resistance exercise on body composition and physical function in older adults: a systematic review and meta-analysis. *Am. J. Clin. Nutr.* 106, 1078–1091. https://doi.org/10.3945/ajcn.116.143594

Lim, M.T., Pan, B.J., Toh, D.W.K., Sutanto, C.N., Kim, J.E., 2021. Animal protein versus plant protein in supporting lean mass and muscle strength: a systematic review and meta-analysis of randomized controlled trials. *Nutrients* 13, 661. https://doi.org/10.3390/nu13020661

Liu, J., Klebach, M., Visser, M., Hofman, Z., 2019. Amino acid availability of a dairy and vegetable protein blend compared to single casein, whey, soy, and pea proteins: a double-blind, cross-over trial. *Nutrients* 11, 2613. https://doi.org/10.3390/nu11112613

McGlory, C., Van Vliet, S., Stokes, T., Mittendorfer, B., Phillips, S.M., 2019. The impact of exercise and nutrition on the regulation of skeletal muscle mass. *J. Physiol.* 597, 1251–1258. https://doi.org/10.1113/JP275443

Millward, D.J., 2021. Interactions between growth of muscle and stature: mechanisms involved and their nutritional sensitivity to dietary protein: the protein-stat revisited. *Nutrients* 13, 729. https://doi.org/10.3390/nu13030729

Mitchell, C.J., Zeng, N., D'Souza, R.F., Mitchell, S.M., Aasen, K., Fanning, A.C., Poppitt, S.D., Cameron-Smith, D., 2017. Minimal dose of milk protein concentrate to enhance the anabolic signalling response to a single bout of resistance exercise; a randomised controlled trial. *J. Int. Soc. Sports Nutr.* 14, 17. https://doi.org/10.1186/s12970-017-0175-x

Moore, A.Z., Caturegli, G., Metter, E.J., Makrogiannis, S., Resnick, S.M., Harris, T.B., Ferrucci, L., 2014. Difference in muscle quality over the adult life span and biological correlates in the baltimore longitudinal study of aging. *J. Am. Geriatr. Soc.* 62, 230–236. https://doi.org/10.1111/jgs.12653

Morgan, P.T., Harris, D.O., Marshall, R.N., Quinlan, J.I., Edwards, S.J., Allen, S.L., Breen, L., 2021. Protein source and quality for skeletal muscle anabolism in young and older adults: a systematic review and meta-analysis. *J. Nutr.* 151, 1901–1920. https://doi.org/10.1093/jn/nxab055

Naclerio, F., Larumbe-Zabala, E., 2016a. Effects of whey protein alone or as part of a multi-ingredient formulation on strength, fat-free mass, or lean body mass in resistance-trained individuals: a meta-analysis. *Sports Med.* 46, 125–137. https://doi.org/10.1007/s40279-015-0403-y

Naclerio, F., Larumbe-Zabala, E., 2016b. Effects of whey protein alone or as part of a multi-ingredient formulation on strength, fat-free mass, or lean body mass in resistance-trained individuals: a meta-analysis. *Sports Med.* 46, 125–137. https://doi.org/10.1007/s40279-015-0403-y

Nongonierma, A.B., FitzGerald, R.J., 2015a. The scientific evidence for the role of milk protein-derived bioactive peptides in humans: A review. *J. Funct. Foods* 17, 640–656. https://doi.org/10.1016/j.jff.2015.06.021

Nongonierma, A.B., FitzGerald, R.J., 2015b. Bioactive properties of milk proteins in humans: A review. *Peptides* 73, 20–34. https://doi.org/10.1016/j.peptides.2015.08.009

Park, S., Church, D.D., Azhar, G., Schutzler, S.E., Ferrando, A.A., Wolfe, R.R., 2020. Anabolic response to essential amino acid plus whey protein composition is greater than whey protein alone in young healthy adults. *J. Int. Soc. Sports Nutr.* 17, 9. https://doi.org/10.1186/s12970-020-0340-5

Phillips, S.M., Martinson, W., 2018. Nutrient-rich, high-quality, protein-containing dairy foods in combination with exercise in aging persons to mitigate sarcopenia. *Nutr. Rev.* https://doi.org/10.1093/nutrit/nuy062

Phillips, S.M., Tang, J.E., Moore, D.R., 2009. The role of milk- and soy-based protein in support of muscle protein synthesis and muscle protein accretion in young and elderly persons. *J. Am. Coll. Nutr.* 28, 343–354. https://doi.org/10.1080/07315724.2009.10718096

Pinckaers, P.J., Kouw, I.W., Gorissen, S.H., Houben, L.H., Senden, J.M., Wodzig, W.K., De Groot, L.C., Verdijk, L.B., Snijders, T., Van Loon, L.J., 2022. The muscle protein synthetic response to the ingestion of a plant-derived protein blend does not differ from an equivalent amount of milk protein in healthy young males. *J. Nutr.* 152, 2734–2743. https://doi.org/10.1093/jn/nxac222

Ribeiro, I., Gomes, M., Figueiredo, D., Lourenço, J., Paúl, C., Costa, E., 2019. Dairy product intake in older adults across Europe based On the SHARE database. *J. Nutr. Gerontol. Geriatr.* 38, 297–306. https://doi.org/10.1080/21551197.2019.1627972

Rutherfurd, S.M., Fanning, A.C., Miller, B.J., Moughan, P.J., 2015. Protein digestibility-corrected amino acid scores and digestible indispensable amino acid scores differentially describe protein quality in growing male rats. *J. Nutr.* 145, 372–379. https://doi.org/10.3945/jn.114.195438

Sekhar, R.V., McKay, S.V., Patel, S.G., Guthikonda, A.P., Reddy, V.T., Balasubramanyam, A., Jahoor, F., 2011. Glutathione synthesis is diminished in patients with uncontrolled diabetes and restored by dietary supplementation with cysteine and glycine. *Diabetes Care* 34, 162–167. https://doi.org/10.2337/dc10-1006

Smeuninx, B., Greig, C.A., Breen, L., 2020. Amount, source and pattern of dietary protein intake across the adult lifespan: a cross-sectional study. *Front. Nutr.* 7, 25. https://doi.org/10.3389/fnut.2020.00025

Soop, M., Nehra, V., Henderson, G.C., Boirie, Y., Ford, G.C., Nair, K.S., 2012. Coingestion of whey protein and casein in a mixed meal: demonstration of a more sustained anabolic effect of casein. *Am. J. Physiol.-Endocrinol. Metab.* 303, E152–E162. https://doi.org/10.1152/ajpendo.00106.2012

Sumi, K., Osada, K., Sakuda, M., Ashida, K., Nakazato, K., 2021. Fermented milk retains beneficial effects on skeletal muscle protein anabolism after processing by centrifugation and supernatant removal. *J. Dairy Sci.* 104, 1336–1350. https://doi.org/10.3168/jds.2020-18780

Terzioğlu, M.E., Bakırcı, İ., Oz, E., Brennan, C.S., Huppertz, T., Amarowicz, R., Khan, M.R., Elobeid, T., Aadil, R.M., Oz, F., 2023. Comparison of camel, buffalo, cow, goat, and sheep yoghurts in terms of various physicochemical, biochemical, textural and rheological properties. *Int. Dairy J.* 146, 105749. https://doi.org/10.1016/j.idairyj.2023.105749

Thalacker-Mercer, A., Riddle, E., Barre, L., 2020a. Protein and amino acids for skeletal muscle health in aging. In: *Advances in Food and Nutrition Research*. Elsevier, pp. 29–64. https://doi.org/10.1016/bs.afnr.2019.08.002

Thalacker-Mercer, A., Riddle, E., Barre, L., 2020b. Protein and amino acids for skeletal muscle health in aging. In: *Advances in Food and Nutrition Research*. Elsevier, pp. 29–64. https://doi.org/10.1016/bs.afnr.2019.08.002

Traylor, D.A., Gorissen, S.H.M., Phillips, S.M., 2018. Perspective: protein requirements and optimal intakes in aging: are we ready to recommend more than the recommended daily allowance? *Adv. Nutr.* 9, 171–182. https://doi.org/10.1093/advances/nmy003

Trommelen, J., Weijzen, M.E.G., Van Kranenburg, J., Ganzevles, R.A., Beelen, M., Verdijk, L.B., Van Loon, L.J.C., 2020. Casein protein processing strongly modulates post-prandial plasma amino acid responses in vivo in humans. *Nutrients* 12, 2299. https://doi.org/10.3390/nu12082299

Van Vliet, S., Burd, N.A., Van Loon, L.J., 2015. The skeletal muscle anabolic response to plant- versus animal-based protein consumption. *J. Nutr.* 145, 1981–1991. https://doi.org/10.3945/jn.114.204305

Vidal-Casariego, A., Pintor-de La Maza, B., Calleja-Fernández, A., Villar-Taibo, R., Cano-Rodríguez, I., Ballesteros-Pomar, M.D., 2015. Consumption of low-fat dairy products and energy and protein intake in cancer patients at risk of malnutrition. *Nutr. Cancer* 67, 191–195. https://doi.org/10.1080/01635581.2015.967874

Wang, W., Wu, Z., Dai, Z., Yang, Y., Wang, J., Wu, G., 2013. Glycine metabolism in animals and humans: implications for nutrition and health. *Amino Acids* 45, 463–477. https://doi.org/10.1007/s00726-013-1493-1

Witard, O.C., Jackman, S.R., Breen, L., Smith, K., Selby, A., Tipton, K.D., 2014a. Myofibrillar muscle protein synthesis rates subsequent to a meal in response to increasing doses of whey protein at rest and after resistance exercise. *Am. J. Clin. Nutr.* 99, 86–95. https://doi.org/10.3945/ajcn.112.055517

Witard, O.C., Jackman, S.R., Breen, L., Smith, K., Selby, A., Tipton, K.D., 2014b. Myofibrillar muscle protein synthesis rates subsequent to a meal in response to increasing doses of whey protein at rest and after resistance exercise. *Am. J. Clin. Nutr.* 99, 86–95. https://doi.org/10.3945/ajcn.112.055517

Witard, O.C., Wardle, S., Macnaughton, L., Hodgson, A., Tipton, K., 2016. Protein considerations for optimising skeletal muscle mass in healthy young and older adults. *Nutrients* 8, 181. https://doi.org/10.3390/nu8040181

Wolfe, R.R., 2015. Update on protein intake: importance of milk proteins for health status of the elderly. *Nutr. Rev.* 73, 41–47. https://doi.org/10.1093/nutrit/nuv021

Wolfe, R.R., Rutherfurd, S.M., Kim, I.-Y., Moughan, P.J., 2016. Protein quality as determined by the Digestible Indispensable Amino Acid Score: evaluation of factors underlying the calculation: Table 1. *Nutr. Rev.* 74, 584–599. https://doi.org/10.1093/nutrit/nuw022

Xu, Z., Tan, Z., Zhang, Q., Gui, Q., Yang, Y., 2015. The effectiveness of leucine on muscle protein synthesis, lean body mass and leg lean mass accretion in older people: a systematic review and meta-analysis. *Br. J. Nutr.* 113, 25–34. https://doi.org/10.1017/S0007114514002475

Zanini, B., Simonetto, A., Zubani, M., Castellano, M., Gilioli, G., 2020. The effects of cow-milk protein supplementation in elderly population: systematic review and narrative synthesis. *Nutrients* 12, 2548. https://doi.org/10.3390/nu12092548

15 Antioxidant Peptides from Hydrolysis of Whey Protein

Ana Paula Vico, Marina del Rosario Bettiol, Yanina Estefanía Rossi, and Mariana Angélica Montenegro

ABBREVIATIONS

ABTS	2,2′-azino-bis-3-ethylbenzothiazoline-6-sulfonic acid
BSA	Bovine serum albumin
CPPs	Casein phosphopeptides
DPPH	2,2-diphenyl-1-picrylhydrazyl
FRAP	Ferric-reducing antioxidant power
GID	Gastrointestinal digestion
GMP	Glycomacropeptide
HHP	High hydrostatic pressure
ORAC	Oxygen radical absorbance capacity
ROS	Reactive oxygen species
SGID	Simulated gastrointestinal digestion

INTRODUCTION

Whey is the liquid by-product produced during cheesemaking or the coagulation of casein from milk. It represents approximately 85–95% of the milk volume used in cheesemaking and retains around 55% of the nutrients from milk (Eberhardt et al. 2019).

Whey is an important source of nutrients, including soluble proteins, lactose, vitamins, minerals, and fat (Zhao et al. 2022). Whey proteins possess high nutritional quality and biological value and are rich in essential amino acids for humans (Dullius et al. 2018). The main components of bovine whey proteins are β-lactoglobulin, α-lactalbumin, bovine serum albumin (BSA), lactoferrin, immunoglobulins, and glycomacropeptide (GMP) (Corrochano et al. 2018). The biological activity of whey proteins, including their beneficial effects on the cardiovascular, digestive, endocrine, immune, and nervous systems, makes them excellent food additives. However, much of this bioactivity stems from bioactive peptides encrypted within their native protein sequences. These peptides can be released during gastrointestinal digestion (GID), microbial fermentation, and *in vitro* enzymatic hydrolysis. Bioactive peptides can exert various physiological effects, such as antihypertensive, antioxidant, opioid, antimicrobial, and immunomodulatory activities (León-López et al. 2022). Among the wide range of reported bioactive peptides, those with antioxidant activity are of great interest because they can interact with reactive oxygen species (ROS), thereby reducing damage caused by oxidative stress, such as diabetes mellitus, atherosclerosis, cancer, and coronary heart disease (Pizzino et al. 2017). However, bioactive peptides have low bioavailability and biostability under gastrointestinal conditions, a bitter taste that reduces sensory acceptability, and high hygroscopicity, leading to physicochemical instability, loss of functional properties, and microbial degradation. Considering these factors, microencapsulation is extremely promising for improving

DOI: 10.1201/9781003597926-15

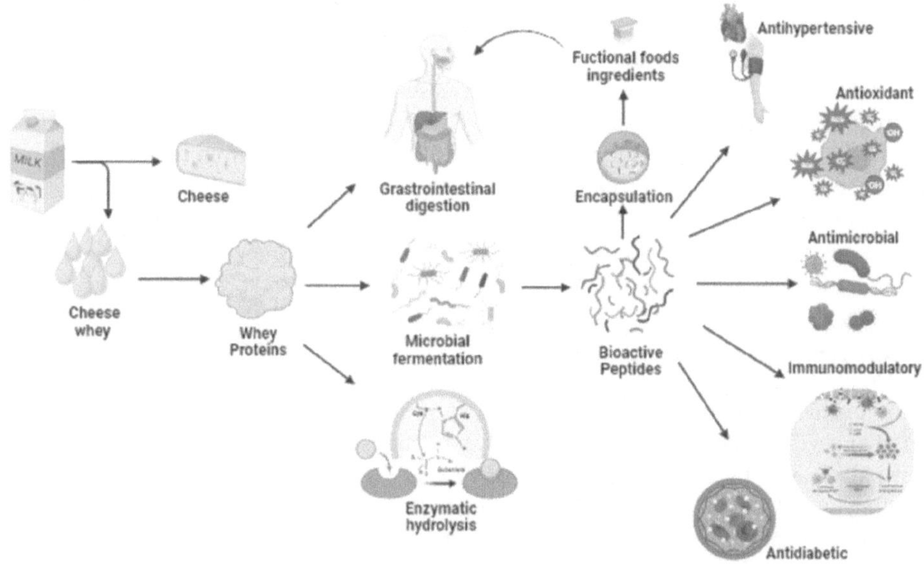

FIGURE 15.1 Whey protein antioxidant peptides, generation, mechanisms of action, and encapsulation as a strategy for the development of bioactive ingredients (created with BioRender.com).

delivery, protection, biocompatibility, and bioavailability, masking bitter taste, and enabling controlled release of bioactive peptides.

In this chapter, we review recent advances in the use of whey proteins as a source of antioxidant peptides, their mechanisms of action in cells, generation methods, and encapsulation strategies for developing bioactive ingredients for functional foods (Figure 15.1).

WHEY PROTEINS AND WHEY PROTEIN DERIVATIVES

Whey proteins are a group of soluble proteins that comprise approximately 20% of the total protein content in cow's milk. The protein fraction of whey consists of β-lactoglobulin (40–50%), α-lactalbumin (20–25%), BSA (5–10%), immunoglobulins (10–15%), GMP (10–15%), and lactoferrin (1–2%), which have a high nutritional value and a wide variety of biological and technological properties (Corrochano et al. 2018). However, the composition of proteins varies according to the type of whey; that is, sweet whey (pH 5.6, produced by coagulation with rennet during the cheesemaking process) or acid whey (pH 5, produced by direct acidification), milk type, cattle feed, lactation stage, and processing (León-López et al. 2022).

Whey proteins are recognized as potential sources of nutrients and have been exploited for their bioactive ingredients. Owing to their high nutritional value, they are used in several commercial food product applications.

Whey proteins have important biological functions. β-Lactoglobulin helps bind minerals like zinc and calcium. It also shows partial sequence homology with retinol-binding proteins. α-Lactalbumin is added to infant formulas or foods to enhance protein-rich dietary intakes. BSA can bind fatty acids and immunoglobulins, which helps develop passive immunity in consumers. Other protein fractions, such as lactoferrin, are iron-binding proteins that increase iron absorption in the digestive tract, inhibit enteric microorganisms, and promote beneficial microorganisms. Lactoferrin also modulates the immune system and is considered a major factor in resistance to nonspecific diseases in the mammary gland. GMP is a whey-derived casein peptide that has many health benefits, including promoting satiety and aiding in the management of phenylketonuria. Whey proteins are a rich source of essential amino acids, such as cysteine, and branched-chain amino acids, such as leucine, isoleucine, and valine. They are also high in sulfur-containing amino acids such as cysteine, which is a precursor of glutathione. Glutathione is a non-enzymatic thiol obtained from the diet that acts as an antioxidant. It helps to protect against diseases by reducing oxidative stress and regulating cellular processes (Deeth and Bansal 2018).

Various whey protein products are available on the market, made from different types of whey using processes such as ultrafiltration, diafiltration, and ion-exchange chromatography, accompanied by evaporation and drying. These include whey powders with 12–14% protein, whey protein concentrates with 35–80% protein, and whey protein isolates, with ≥90% protein. These products differ in protein, lipid, lactose, and mineral contents (Corrochano et al. 2018).

WHEY PROTEIN BIOACTIVE PEPTIDES

Within the primary amino acid sequence of whey proteins, encrypted peptides obtain biological activity when hydrolyzed, resulting in bioactive peptides (Cruz-Casas et al. 2021). These peptides can be released by enzymatic hydrolysis during GID; fermentation of milk by proteolytic starter cultures; or hydrolysis by proteolytic enzymes derived from microorganisms, animals, or plants. Bioactive peptides are protein fragments containing 2–20 amino acids, the composition and sequence of which define their functionality. Among these, antimicrobial, antihypertensive, antioxidant, and immunomodulatory effects are prominent, increasing their potential use for nutraceutical and therapeutic purposes (Bhandari et al. 2020). Some bioactive peptides may have multifunctional activities, and specific peptide sequences may have more than one biological activity. Bioactive peptides can modulate physiological functions by binding to specific receptors or by acting at specific sites in various body systems, such as the immune, nervous, cardiovascular, and gastrointestinal systems (Akbarian et al. 2022). Specifically, bioactive peptides derived from whey proteins exert beneficial health effects through various biological functions such as antioxidant, antihypertensive (generally evaluated as angiotensin-converting enzyme-inhibitor), anti-inflammatory, immunomodulatory, antimicrobial, and antidiabetic activities (Mann et al. 2015; Zhao and Ashaolu 2020; Dineshbhai et al. 2022). Table 15.1 shows some of the biological activities of peptides produced by the enzymatic hydrolysis of whey proteins. The biological functionality of bioactive whey protein peptides makes them excellent ingredients for functional foods. The enzymatic hydrolysis of whey proteins is the most widely used strategy to produce bioactive peptides as functional ingredients. However, recent studies have demonstrated an increasing use of microbial fermentation to produce bioactive peptides (Solieri et al. 2022; Rosa et al. 2023).

ANTIOXIDANT PEPTIDES

Recently, several researchers have focused on studying the mechanisms and characteristics of antioxidant peptides. The mechanisms by which peptides exert their antioxidant properties are not yet completely understood (Akbarian et al. 2022). However, it is well known that antioxidant peptides act as free radical and reactive species scavengers and metal ion chelators (Bhandari et al. 2020; Zhao et al. 2022; Lv et al. 2022).

The antioxidant activity of peptides is highly dependent on their structural properties, such as size, amino acid composition and sequence, and hydrophobicity (Lv et al. 2022; Akbarian et al. 2022). Peptides with a molecular weight below 3 kDa have shown strong antioxidant activity (Tadesse and Emire 2020). Small peptides may access free radicals and remove them more easily than large peptides (Akbarian et al. 2022). Ballatore et al. (2020) reported that a peptide fraction <3 kDa produced by the hydrolysis of whey proteins with trypsin showed the strongest scavenging activity of $O_2^{\bullet -}$ and $HO^{\bullet}$. Additionally, the presence of hydrophobic and aromatic amino acids, such as tyrosine, tryptophan, phenylalanine, histidine, and methionine, correlates with the antioxidant activity of peptides (Bhandari et al. 2020). The position of amino acids in the peptide sequence

TABLE 15.1
Biological Activity of Peptides Produced by the Enzymatic Hydrolysis and Microbial Fermentation of Whey Proteins and Whey-Milk Beverages

Peptide Production Process	Substrate	Enzyme/ Microorganism	Peptide	Protein Fragment Sequence	Bioactivity	Reference
Enzymatic hydrolysis	β-lactoglobulin	Trypsin	ALPMHIR	β-lactoglobulin *f*(142–148)	ACE-inhibitor	Power et al. 2014
			VAGTWY		Antioxidant	
		Pepsin	IPAVFK	β-lactoglobulin *f*(15–20)	Antidiabetic	Théolier et al. 2013
		Alcalase	KV AGT	β-lactoglobulin *f*(78–83)	Antimicrobial	
			HIRLS	β-lactoglobulin *f*(14-18) β–lactoglobulin *f*(146-150)	Antioxidant	Mann et al. 2015
	α-lactalbumin	Pepsin and pancreatin	VSLPEW		ACE-inhibitor	Xie et al. 2022
		Flavourzyme	VGINYWLAHK	α-lactalbumin *f*(99–108)	Antioxidant	Mann et al. 2015
		Pepsin	KVGIN	α-lactalbumin *f*(117–121)	Antimicrobial	Théolier et al. 2013

(*Continued*)

TABLE 15.1 (CONTINUED)
Biological Activity of Peptides Produced by the Enzymatic Hydrolysis and Microbial Fermentation of Whey Proteins and Whey-Milk Beverages

Peptide Production Process	Substrate	Enzyme/ Microorganism	Peptide	Protein Fragment Sequence	Bioactivity	Reference
Microbial fermentation	WPC80	*Streptococcus thermophilus* RBN16	LIVTQTMK	β-lactoglobulin *f*(17–24)	Cytotoxic	Solieri et al. 2022
			IDALNENK	β-lactoglobulin *f*(100–107)	Antimicrobial	
		Streptococcus thermophilus RBC06	HIR		ACE inhibition	
			ALPMH	β-lactoglobulin *f*(162–164) β-lactoglobulin *f*(158–162)	Hypocholesterolemic, ACE-inhibitor	
	WPC80	*Lactobacillus paracasei* and *Propionibacterium freudenreichii*	GGGPGPMGLMGPR YPFPGPI FVAPFPEVFGK	Collagen α-2(I) chain β-casein α-S1-casein	Antifungal	
	Whey-milk beverages	La-05, Bb-12, *L. casei*-01	LLYQEPVLGPVRGPFP WMHQPHQPLPPTVMFPPQ	β-casein f(189–204) β-casein f(143–160)	Antioxidant and ACE- inhibitor	Rosa et al. 2023
		CTL; La-03; La-05; *L. casei*-01 and Bb-12			Immunomodulatory	
			MHQPHQPLPPT	β-casein f(144–154)		
			HIQKEDVPSER	α-casein-S1 f(80–90)	Antirotaviral activity	
		CTL; La-05 and Bb-12	FVAPFPEVFGKE	α-casein-S1 f(24–35)	Antioxidative	
		Bb-12			ACE-inhibitor	
		La-03 and La-05				

ACE = angiotensin converting enzyme; WPC80 = whey protein concentrate with 80% protein; La-05 = *Lactobacillus acidophilus* 05; La-03 = *Lactobacillus acidophilus 03*; Bb-12 = *Bifidobacterium*-12; *L. casie*-01 = *Lacticaseibacillus casei*-01; *CTL* = *Lactococcus lactis* R-704.

also impacts their antioxidant activity; for example, the presence of a hydrophobic amino acid at the N-terminus (Akbarian et al. 2022). Recently, Bustamante et al. (2021) identified antioxidant peptides with these structural properties from hydrolysates of whey proteins treated with alcalase, chymotrypsin, and flavourzyme.

MECHANISM OF ACTION OF ANTIOXIDANT PEPTIDES AT THE CELL LEVEL

The antioxidant mechanism and cytoprotective effects of whey peptides in cell models resemble modifiers for many oxidative processes in the body. The most important effects include the regulation of the production of ROS, intracellular antioxidants, enzyme content, and activity interacting with redox-related signaling pathways. These functions relate to health benefits and reduced risk of chronic diseases, such as cancer, cardiovascular diseases, hypertension, and diabetes (Bhandari et al. 2020; Lv et al. 2022). When an organism is exposed to an external environment resulting in an imbalance of ROS in the biological system, various cellular processes, such as membrane lipid peroxidation and the degradation of enzymes, proteins, and nucleic acids, increase the possibility of many chronic pathologies (Lv et al. 2022).

Many authors have studied whey peptides' antioxidant activity at the cell level. Ballatore et al. (2020) compared the cell viability of peptide pre-treatment in IEC-18 cells induced by the stressor menadione. The cell viability increased significantly, showing an important cytoprotective effect. Similar studies showed that whey protein hydrolysate cytoprotects human lung fibroblast MRC-5 cells. Cell death decreased significantly when exposed to 24-hour pre-treatment with peptides (0.1–2.8 kDa) obtained from gel filtration of alcalase hydrolysate compared to the H_2O_2-damaged model control. Additionally, the authors observed an increase in the activity of cell superoxide dismutase, glutathione peroxidase, and catalase, and a decrease in the levels of malondialdehyde, indicating that peptides provided significant cell protection against H_2O_2-induced cytotoxicity. Studies in rat pheochromocytoma cell lines showed that pre-treated for 2 hours with peptides hydrolyzed by pepsin and trypsin and purified by macrospore absorption resins increased cell viability by 20–30% when incubated with H_2O_2 (Zhao et al. 2022). Other researchers demonstrated that whey peptides could modulate inflammatory cytokine production, for example, by inhibiting pro-inflammatory cytokine IL-8 secretion in intestinal cells (Bao and Wu 2021). Regarding enzyme activity, several studies reveal that direct cell exposure to whey peptides increases intracellular antioxidant enzymes such as glutathione peroxidase and superoxide dismutase (Corrochano et al. 2018; Zhao et al. 2022).

Chemical modification of the original polypeptide structure, including the Maillard reaction, can significantly improve the antioxidant activity of whey peptides. As shown by Zhang et al. (2018), glycosylated whey peptides exhibited higher antioxidant and proliferative activity in Caco-2 cell viability tests compared to vitamin C as a positive control (Lv et al. 2022).

Figure 15.2 summarizes the mechanisms of action and properties of whey antioxidant peptides.

WHEY PROTEIN BIOACTIVE PEPTIDES GENERATION

Fermentation

Bioactive peptides must be released from the polypeptide chains of whey proteins to exert their biological effects. This can be carried out using fermentation, enzymatic hydrolysis, *in vitro* GID, and novel processing technologies. In the last decade, researchers have made considerable efforts to develop new strategies for obtaining peptides with high antioxidant activity, focusing on optimizing resources, reducing costs, and finding biotechnological approaches. This section highlights some of the latest studies on whey antioxidant peptide generation. Previous noteworthy studies have been summarized by Corrochano et al. (2018).

Fermentation uses microorganisms to produce peptides, whereby proteins are hydrolyzed by peptidases secreted during microbial activity (Tadesse and Emire 2020). Therefore, the type of

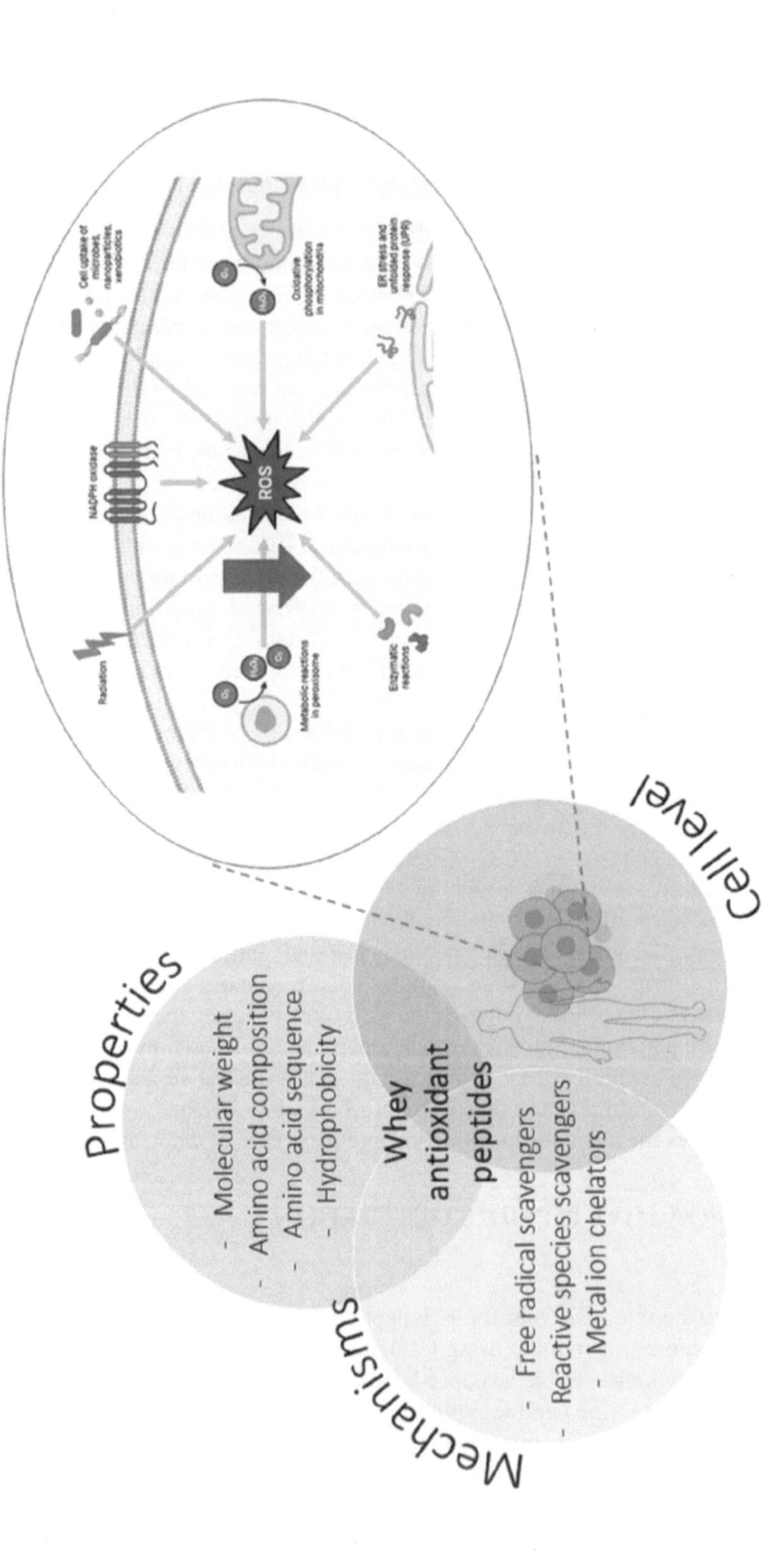

FIGURE 15.2 Whey antioxidant peptides mechanism and properties. (Adapted from "Sources of Reactive Oxygen Species (ROS) with Cell Background," by BioRender.com (2023). Retrieved from https://app.biorender.com/biorender-templates.)

microorganism is a key factor in obtaining peptides with high bioactivity (Cruz-Casas et al. 2021). Bacteria, fungi, and yeasts have been studied; however, lactic acid bacteria have been most frequently reported (Tadesse and Emire 2020; Cruz-Casas et al. 2021). Recently, Guo et al. (2023) purified a peptide fraction from whey proteins fermented by *Lactobacillus rhamnosus* B2-1, which showed high *in vitro* antioxidant activity (ORAC, ABTS, and HO• radical scavenging activity). Additionally, Cui et al. (2022) identified antioxidant peptides from casein and whey proteins fermented by three *Lactobacillus* strains (*brevis*, *reuteri*, and *plantarum*). Solieri et al. (2022) evaluated fermentation of whey proteins with strains isolated from natural whey starter, specifically two *Lactobacillus helveticus* strains and five *Streptococcus thermophilus* strains. The authors found that one of these *Streptococcus thermophilus* strains released peptides with the highest biological activities, adding value to this type of lactic acid bacterium. Simultaneous fermentation with different types of microorganisms is also possible, potentially enhancing the biological activities of the produced peptides (Cruz-Casas et al. 2021). For example, Dineshbhai et al. (2022) obtained and identified antioxidant peptides from whey proteins fermented with *Lactobacillus fermentum* and *Saccharomyces cerevisiae* strains.

Enzymatic Hydrolysis

Enzymatic hydrolysis is one of the most reported methods for producing bioactive peptides, which mainly depends on the specificity of the enzyme used (Tadesse and Emire 2020). Currently, there is a wide variety of enzymes from different sources due to the growing demand from industry, especially from the functional food sector (Kheroufi et al. 2022b). Thus, commercial enzymes from animal, microbial, and plant sources have been tested. Some of the latest studies carried out using commercial and new enzymes under their hydrolysis conditions to obtain antioxidant peptides are shown in Table 15.2. The most studied enzymes from animal sources have been gastrointestinal enzymes, such as pepsin, chymotrypsin, and trypsin. Recently, Kheroufi et al. (2022b) reported a whey protein hydrolysate produced by hydrolysis with chicken pepsin extract from chicken proventriculus (*Gallus gallus*) and compared it with commercial porcine pepsin. The authors found that the ORAC and ABTS antioxidant capacity of non-hydrolyzed whey proteins was enhanced by both enzymes, suggesting that chicken pepsin extract from chicken proventriculus is a way to take advantage of slaughter by-product. Additionally, a considerable number of proteases from microbial sources are commercially available, and one of the most extensively studied has been alcalase. Millan et al. (2022) reported a whey protein hydrolysate with increased antioxidant activity (ABTS and DPPH) produced by a protease from *Lysobacter* sp. A03, a cold-adapted bacterium isolated from Antarctica. The authors highlighted that *Lysobacter* sp. A03 protease can be used at low temperatures, which may represent a biotechnological advantage. In contrast, enzymatic hydrolysis with plant proteases to obtain antioxidant peptides has been less investigated (Kheroufi et al. 2022a). Only well-known proteases from vegetables, such as papain from papaya (*Carica papaya*) and bromelain from pineapple (*Ananas comosus*), have been studied. In this context, Kheroufi et al. (2022a) reported, for the first time, whey protein hydrolysis using a ficin crude extract obtained from fig latex (*Ficus carica*).

The resulting bioactive peptides depend not only on the specificity of the protease used but also on several processing factors, such as pre-treatment, reaction conditions (protein concentration, enzyme/substrate ratio, temperature, pH, time, etc.), and downstream processes (Dullius et al. 2018). Consequently, different conditions have been studied to find those that show high antioxidant activity. One strategy to evaluate several hydrolysis variables and their independent or synergistic effect on antioxidant activity is through response surface methodology (Ballatore et al. 2020; Hussein et al. 2020).

TABLE 15.2
Enzymatic Hydrolysis of Whey Proteins and Its Reaction Conditions Using Commercial and Novel Enzymes to Obtain Antioxidant Peptides

Source	Enzyme	Hydrolysis Conditions	Substrate	Antioxidant Assay	Reference
Animal	Trypsin (bovine)	pH 7.6, 41.1°C, 4.31 h, E/S = 1.7%	WPC35	ABTS HO• scavenging activity $O_2^{\bullet-}$ scavenging activity	Ballatore et al. 2020
	α-chymotrypsin (porcine)	pH 8, 45°C, 2 h, E/S = 5%	WPC	ABTS	Bustamante et al. 2021
	Pepsin (porcine)	pH 2, 37°C, 0–6 h, E/S = 0.5 and 1%	WPC80	ABTS ORAC	Kheroufi et al. 2022b
	Pepsin (chicken)	pH 2, 50°C, 0–6 h, E/S = 0.5 and 1%			
Microbial	Alcalase 2.4L (*Bacillus licheniformis*)	pH 8, 45°C, 7 h, E/S = 5%	WPC	ABTS	Bustamante et al. 2021
	Flavourzyme 1000L (*Aspergillus oryzae*)	pH 7, 45°C, 6 h, E/S = 5%			
	Alcalase 2.4L (*Bacillus licheniformis*)	pH 8, 50°C, 2.5 h, E/S = 1%	WPI	ABTS FRAP ORAC	Corrochano et al. 2019
	Neutrase 0.8L (*Bacillus amyloliquefaciens*)	pH 7, 50°C, 2.5 h, E/S = 1%			
	Alcalase (*Bacillus licheniformis*)	pH 7.5, 58.2°C, 6.03 h, E/S = 2.5%,	WPC	DPPH Iron(II) chelating activity	Hussein et al. 2020
	Protease from *Lysobacter* sp. A03	pH 8, 30°C, 0–4 h, E/S = 2% v/v	lyophilized bovine whey	ABTS DPPH Iron(II) chelating activity	Millan et al. 2022
Plant	Bromelain (pineapple)	pH 7, 50°C, 2.5 h, E/S = 5%	Sweet whey	ABTS	Abadía-García et al. 2016
	Papain (papaya)	pH 7, 60°C, 2.5 h, E/S = 5%			
	Bromelain (pineapple)	pH 7, 50°C, 2.5 h, E/S = 1%	WPI	ABTS FRAP ORAC	Corrochano et al. 2019
	Ficin (fig latex)	pH 7.5, 80°C, 0–6 h, E/S = 0.5 and 1%	WPC80	ABTS ORAC	Kheroufi et al. 2022a

E/S = enzyme/substrate ratio; WPC 35 = whey protein concentrate with 35% protein; WPC80 = whey protein concentrate with 80% protein; WPI = whey protein isolate with ≥90% protein; ABTS = 2,2′-azinobis-(3-ethylbenzothiazoline-6-sulfonic acid) radical scavenging method; ORAC = Oxygen Radical Absorbance Capacity Assay; FRAP = Ferric-Reducing Antioxidant Power Assay; DPPH = 2,2-diphenyl-1-picrylhydrazyl radical scavenging method.

In Vitro Gastrointestinal Digestion

Peptides and amino acids are produced during *in vivo* GID of dietary proteins, and to understand this process, several models of *in vitro* simulated gastrointestinal digestion (SGID) have been developed (Miralles et al. 2018). Currently, different static and dynamic models are available; however, for static models, the INFOGEST protocol is recommended (Brodkorb et al. 2019; Cruz-Casas et al. 2021). For example, (Corrochano et al. 2019) investigated the antioxidant activity of whey proteins before and after *in vitro* SGID under the INFOGEST protocol conditions. They found that post-SGID whey proteins had significantly higher ABTS, ORAC, and FRAP values. Similarly, Bustamante et al. (2021) found that whey protein concentrate obtained from Colombian traditional cheese whey, after *in vitro* SGID, had significantly higher ABTS values. Furthermore, *in vitro* SGID can be used to evaluate the bioaccessibility and bioactivity of peptides after gastrointestinal transit (Cruz-Casas et al. 2021). Bustamante et al. (2021) evaluated the peptide profile and bioactivity of whey protein hydrolysates with alcalase, chymotrypsin, and flavourzyme after *in vitro* SGID under the INFOGEST protocol conditions. They reported that 65% of the peptides identified in the hydrolysates with alcalase were resistant to the gastrointestinal tract, whereas 21% and 29% of the peptides in the hydrolysates with chymotrypsin and flavourzyme, respectively, were resistant to gastrointestinal conditions. They also found that the ABTS values of hydrolysates with alcalase and chymotrypsin increased after GID. Corrochano et al. (2019) reported that after GID, ABTS values of all hydrolysates decreased; ORAC values of all hydrolysates increased; and FRAP values of hydrolysates with alcalase and bromelain decreased, whereas those with neutrase increased.

Novel Processing Technologies

Biotechnological processes are the most commonly used ways to produce antioxidant peptides; however, they have some disadvantages at the industrial scale, such as high cost and low yield (Ulug et al. 2021). Accordingly, novel technologies based on physical methods such as high hydrostatic pressure (HHP), ultrasound, pulsed electric field, and microwaves have been studied to improve the hydrolytic process (Ulug et al. 2021). Some studies have reported the use of novel technologies in combination with enzymatic hydrolysis as pre-treatment or simultaneously (Abadía-García et al. 2016; Ma et al. 2018; Bamdad et al. 2017). Briefly, novel technologies enhance proteolysis and antioxidant activity because they induce structural changes in proteins and expose new cleavage sites for proteases (Tadesse and Emire 2020). The application of these new strategies for the pre-treatment of fermentation and *in vitro* SGID could be interesting. To the best of our knowledge, the use of novel technologies in combination with the microbial fermentation of whey proteins has not yet been reported. Recently, Ma et al. (2023) investigated the effect of HHP treatments on the digestibility and antioxidant activity of whey protein isolate after *in vitro* SGID model for the elderly. The authors found that HHP enhanced the digestibility and antioxidant activity of GID products. More recent studies, however, have focused on the use of novel technologies independently. Sarabandi et al. (2022) and Meng et al. (2021) have reported that sonication enhanced the ABTS and DPPH scavenging activities of whey proteins. The increase in antioxidant activity of whey proteins after sonication could be attributed to structural changes in proteins that produce larger amounts of exposed antioxidant amino acids (Meng et al. 2021).

APPLICATION OF BIOACTIVE PEPTIDES IN FUNCTIONAL FOODS

Encapsulation

The growing interest in the effect of diet on the prevention of nutritional deficiencies and diseases has driven the development of functional foods that can benefit the nutritional status and health of consumers. The beneficial effects of functional foods are associated with the presence of bioactive agents such as bioactive peptides, probiotics, prebiotics, postbiotics, antioxidants, polyunsaturated fatty acids, and fibers (Alongi and Anese 2021). Among these, bioactive peptides derived from whey proteins are of great interest because of their various physiological functions, as well as their contribution to sustainability, as they come from a by-product of the dairy industry. However, the bioactivity and bioavailability of peptides in functional foods remain a challenge because of their low resistance to technological processes, their instability under storage conditions and in the gastrointestinal tract, as well as their bitter taste and possible interactions with other components in the food matrix. For this reason, encapsulation has been proposed as an efficient technological alternative for the functionalization of foods with bioactive peptides (Rivero-Pino 2023). The ultimate goal of encapsulation is to transport bioactive compounds to the site of action through controlled release and improved bioavailability (Rossi et al. 2021).

There are two types of encapsulation: microencapsulation and nanoencapsulation. These can be achieved using various methods, such as double emulsion, freeze drying, emulsification-gelation, ionic gelation, or spray drying (used for both microencapsulation and nanoencapsulation). Other approaches include colloidal particles, such as microemulsions, nanoemulsions, emulsions, solid lipid nanoparticles, liposomes, nanoliposomes, niosomes, biopolymer nanoparticles, and hydrogel beads (Mohan et al. 2016; Aguilar-Toala et al. 2022). Table 15.3 outlines some methods used for encapsulating whey peptides along with their characteristics.

Liposomes and spray drying are among the most commonly used techniques for encapsulating peptides derived from whey proteins. Microencapsulation efficiently preserves the characteristics of the encapsulated material and facilitates uniform mixing and handling of bioactive compounds. Nanoencapsulation generates small particles with a large specific surface area that allows stable and uniform colloidal solutions to form effectively. Smaller particle sizes increase cell adhesion and improve delivery efficiency for bioactive ingredients, enhancing their bioavailability in food products (Alu'datt et al. 2022; Wang and Selomulya 2020).

Numerous biopolymers have been employed as wall materials for the microencapsulation of peptides; polysaccharides, lipids, and, to a lesser extent, proteins are among the most widely used (Aguilar-Toala et al. 2022). Polysaccharides are cost-effective, exhibit low viscosity at high solid ratios, and are biodegradable, making them suitable for encapsulating bioactive peptides. On the other hand, lipids are adequate for delivering bioactive compounds because of their similarity to cell membranes; however, their low stability in thermally processed foods and their susceptibility to oxidation limit their use. Some proteins have been utilized as encapsulating materials due to their nutritional benefits, as well as their emulsification and gelling properties. In general, selecting a wall material for encapsulating bioactive peptides intended for food use is based on properties such as biodegradability, non-toxicity, low cost, and suitability for the encapsulation method employed.

CHALLENGES AND FUTURE APPROACHES

The biological activities of peptides from whey proteins have raised interest in their utilization as functional food ingredients, given their ability to exert beneficial effects on various physiological functions. Therefore, it is important to consider the digestion, absorption, and metabolic processes of peptides. Some peptides can enter the bloodstream directly, whereas others may act on intestinal mucosa cells or affect the gut microbiota to exert their functions.

As a result, it is necessary to evaluate the toxicity and allergenicity of peptides obtained through enzymatic hydrolysis or microbial fermentation of whey. Recent clinical studies have found no toxic or adverse health effects from the intake of enzymatic whey protein hydrolysates. Additionally, a significant reduction in antigenicity has been demonstrated in whey peptides with molecular weights below 8 kDa (Zhao and Ashaolu 2020). However, more clinical studies are needed to assess the health effects of consuming foods supplemented with bioactive whey protein peptides and to understand how the food matrix and processing may modify the biological activity of these functional compounds.

Other challenges for utilizing bioactive whey protein peptides as functional food ingredients include cost-effective industrial-scale production, bitter taste, peptide stability, bioactivity within the food matrix, and the effects of thermal and non-thermal treatments on bioactivity.

TABLE 15.3
Some Methods Used to Develop Encapsulates with Whey Peptides

Encapsulation Type	Encapsulation Technique	Wall Material	Main Finding	Reference
Microencapsulation	Spray drying	Gelatin and chitosan	Chitosan yielded improved results compared to gelatin in terms of peptide protection during milk fermentation.	Gómez-Mascaraque et al. 2016
	Spray drying and freeze drying	Prebiotic gum arabic	Spray drying produced powders with better characteristics than freeze drying.	Correa et al. 2023
Nanoencapsulation	Nanocarriers (spray drying)	Omega-3 oils or starch	Nanocarrier-based encapsulation can increase the bioavailability of proteins and bioactive peptides.	Sarabandi et al. 2020
	Nanoliposomes	Soy lecithin-derived	Encapsulation efficiency ≥90%, the highest reported for food-derived peptides in liposome carriers.	Mohan et al. 2016
	Liposomes and niosomes	Ergosterol, β-sitosterol, mixed phytosterols, and stigmasterol	Niosomes could significantly improve the retention rate of peptides during gastrointestinal digestion, bioaccessibility, and hypoglycemic activity.	Du et al. 2022

To address these challenges, *in silico* and bioinformatic tools can be employed, such as molecular docking, structure-activity relationship studies, *in silico* digestion simulations, and food models, to understand peptide-nutrient interactions affecting bioactivity. Modeling studies can also be conducted to assess how different thermal or non-thermal treatments affect peptides (Rivero-Pino 2023). Figure 15.3 summarizes the challenges, tools, and solutions for incorporating bioactive peptides in functional foods.

THE EFFECTS OF OTHER PROTEINS

Antioxidant peptides can be obtained from various food-derived protein sources, such as animal, plant, insect, and marine products and by-products (Rossi et al. 2021). In this chapter, we focus on whey proteins as sources of bioactive peptides, particularly antioxidant peptides. However, other milk proteins, such as caseins, can also generate antioxidant peptides.

The hydrolysis of casein can cause an improvement in digestion, absorption, nutritional value, and antioxidant properties, as well as a reduction in allergenicity (Yin et al. 2021). The enzymatic hydrolysis of casein generates bioactive peptides such as β-casomorphins and casein phosphopeptides (CPPs), which have antioxidant effects due to their capacity to bind, transport, and increase the bioavailability of bivalent cations, in addition to eliminating ROS. It has been shown that CPPs minimize the damage caused by lipid peroxidation and exert protective effects against H_2O_2 in Caco-2 cells. Additionally, CPPs improve cell viability by increasing glutathione levels, inducing catalase activity, and regulating the cell cycle (Bielecka et al. 2022). Shazly et al. (2019) evaluated the release of antioxidant peptides from buffalo and bovine caseins and how proteases influence their antioxidant capacities. The enzymes used were alcalase, trypsin, pepsin, and papain. The authors concluded that the antioxidant capacity of the protein under study was linked to the type of enzyme used for enzymatic hydrolysis.

In addition, κ-casein and its released peptides can modulate the immune response by stimulating phagocytosis and macrophage proliferation, inhibiting the adhesion of bacteria that colonize the oral cavity, and preventing adhesion of *H. pylori* to the gastric mucosa (Bielecka et al. 2022).

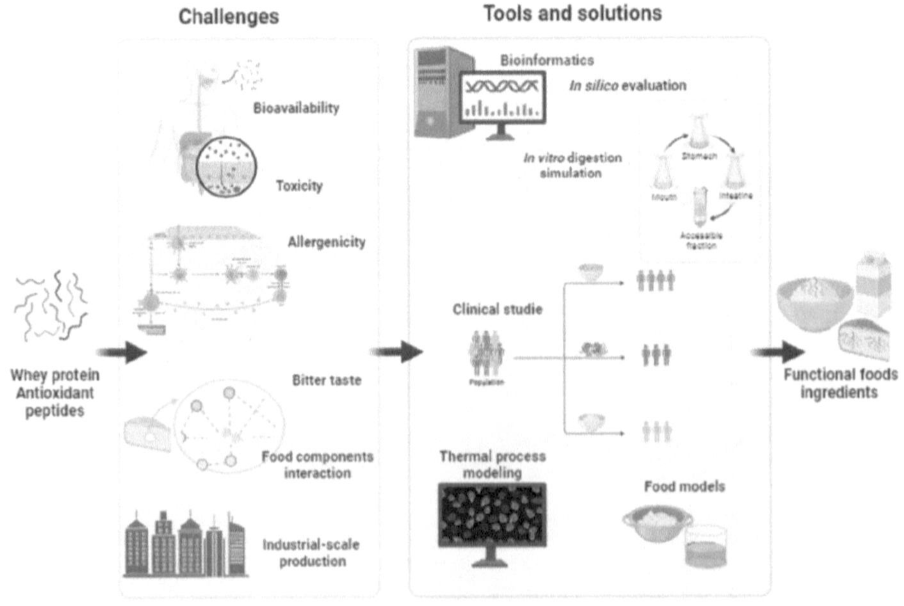

FIGURE 15.3 Challenges, tools, and solutions for incorporating whey protein antioxidant peptides in functional foods (created with BioRender.com).

MINI DICTIONARY OF TERMS

- **2,2′-azinobis-(3-ethylbenzothiazoline-6-sulfonic acid) (ABTS) radical scavenging method:** A spectrophotometric method used to evaluate the ability of antioxidant compounds (peptides) to scavenge ABTS radicals.
- **2,2-diphenyl-1-picrylhydrazyl (DPPH) radical scavenging assay:** A spectrophotometric method for evaluating antioxidant activity where the DPPH radical is reduced by an antioxidant compound (peptide).
- **Cytoprotection:** Protective effect on cell viability against an oxidative stressor agent.
- **Cytotoxicity:** Toxicity in cells; effects of bioactive compounds on general metabolism and/or enzymatic activity, resulting in a loss in viability cellular.
- **Ferric-Reducing Antioxidant Power (FRAP) Assay:** A method to evaluate antioxidant ability based on the electron transfer mechanism.
- **Oxygen Radical Absorbance Capacity (ORAC) Assay:** A method to evaluate antioxidant ability based on scavenging peroxyl radicals by donating hydrogen atom.

SUMMARY POINTS

- Whey proteins are of high nutritional quality and biological value.
- Whey proteins are a source of bioactive peptides.
- Bioactive peptides can be released during gastrointestinal digestion, microbial fermentation, and enzymatic hydrolysis.
- Peptides with antioxidant activity are of great interest because they can reduce the damage caused by oxidative stress.
- In this chapter, we present a review of recent advances in the use of whey proteins as a source of antioxidant peptides.

REFERENCES

Abadía-García, Lucía, Eduardo Castaño-Tostado, Lech Ozimek, Sergio Romero-Gómez, César Ozuna, and Silvia L. Amaya-Llano. 2016. Impact of ultrasound pretreatment on whey protein hydrolysis by vegetable proteases. *Innovative Food Science and Emerging Technologies* 37: 84–90.

Aguilar-Toala, J. E., D. Quintanar-Guerrero, A. M. Liceaga, and M. L. Zambrano- Zaragoza. 2022. Encapsulation of bioactive peptides: A strategy to improve the stability, protect the nutraceutical bioactivity and support their food applications. *RSC Advances* 12 (11): 6449–58.

Akbarian, Mohsen, Ali Khani, Sara Eghbalpour, and Vladimir N. Uversky. 2022. Bioactive peptides: Synthesis, sources, applications, and proposed mechanisms of action. *International Journal of Molecular Sciences* 23: 1445.

Alongi, Marilisa, and Monica Anese. 2021. Re-thinking functional food development through a holistic approach. *Journal of Functional Foods* 81: 104466.

Alu'datt, Muhammad H., Mohammad Alrosan, Sana Gammoh, Carole C. Tranchant, Mohammad N. Alhamad, Taha Rababah, Roa'a Zghoul, et al. 2022. Encapsulation-based technologies for bioactive compounds and their application in the food industry: A roadmap for food-derived functional and health-promoting ingredients. *Food Bioscience* 50: 101971.

Ballatore, María Belén, Marina del Rosario Bettiol, Noelia L. Vanden Braber, Carla Aylen Aminahuel, Yanina Estefanía Rossi, Gabriela Petroselli, Rosa Erra-Balsells, Lilia René Cavaglieri, and Mariana Angélica Montenegro. 2020. Antioxidant and cytoprotective effect of peptides produced by hydrolysis of whey protein concentrate with trypsin. *Food Chemistry* 319 126472.

Bamdad, Fatemeh, Seonghee Bark, Chul Hee Kwon, Joo Won Suh, and Hoon Sunwoo. 2017. Anti-inflammatory and antioxidant properties of peptides released from β-lactoglobulin by high hydrostatic pressure-assisted enzymatic hydrolysis. *Molecules* 22 (6).

Bao, Xiaoyu, and Jianping Wu. 2021. Impact of food-derived bioactive peptides on gut function and health. *Food Research International* 147 110485.

Bhandari, Divya, Shafiya Rafiq, Yogesh Gat, Punam Gat, Roji Waghmare, and Vikas Kumar. 2020. A review on bioactive peptides: Physiological functions, bioavailability and safety. *International Journal of Peptide Research and Therapeutics* 26 (1): 139–50.

Bielecka, Marika, Grażyna Cichosz, and Hanna Czeczot. 2022. Antioxidant, antimicrobial and anticarcinogenic activities of bovine milk proteins and their hydrolysates – A review. *International Dairy Journal* 127: 105208.

Brodkorb, André, Lotti Egger, Marie Alminger, Paula Alvito, Ricardo Assunção, Simon Ballance, Torsten Bohn, et al. 2019. INFOGEST static in vitro simulation of gastrointestinal food digestion. *Nature Protocols* 14 (4): 991–1014.

Bustamante, Sandra Zapata, Jesús Gil González, Stefano Sforza, and Tullia Tedeschi. 2021. Bioactivity and peptide profile of whey protein hydrolysates obtained from Colombian double-cream cheese production and their products after gastrointestinal digestion. *LWT* 145: 111334.

Corrêa, Ana Paula Folmer, Flávio Fonseca Veras, Camila Carvalho Lago, Caciano Pelayo Zapata Noreña, and Adriano Brandelli. 2023. Microencapsulation upholds biological activities of sheep whey hydrolysates and protects against in vitro gastrointestinal digestion. *International Dairy Journal* 138: 105554.

Corrochano, Alberto R., Vitaly Buckin, Phil M. Kelly, and Linda Giblin. 2018. Invited review: Whey proteins as antioxidants and promoters of cellular antioxidant pathways. *Journal of Dairy Science* 101 (6): 4747–61.

Corrochano, Alberto R., Yunus Sariçay, Elena Arranz, Phil M. Kelly, Vitaly Buckin, and Linda Giblin. 2019. Comparison of antioxidant activities of bovine whey proteins before and after simulated gastrointestinal digestion. *Journal of Dairy Science* 102 (1): 54–67.

Cruz-Casas, Dora Elisa, Cristóbal N. Aguilar, Juan A. Ascacio-Valdés, Raúl Rodríguez-Herrera, Mónica L. Chávez-González, and Adriana C. Flores-Gallegos. 2021. Enzymatic hydrolysis and microbial fermentation: The most favorable biotechnological methods for the release of bioactive peptides. *Food Chemistry: Molecular Sciences* 3: 100047.

Cui, Lei, Guo Yang, Shuyi Lu, Xiaoqun Zeng, Jun He, Yuxing Guo, Daodong Pan, and Zhen Wu. 2022. Antioxidant peptides derived from hydrolyzed milk proteins by Lactobacillus strains: A BIOPEP-UWM database-based analysis. *Food Research International* 156: 111339.

Deeth, Hilton, and Nidhi Bansal. 2018. Whey proteins: An overview. In *Whey Proteins: From Milk to Medicine*, ed. Hilton C. Deeth and Nidhi Bansal, 1–50. Elsevier Inc.

Dineshbhai, Chopada Kevalkumar, Bethsheba Basaiawmoit, Amar A. Sakure, Ruchika Maurya, Mahendra Bishnoi, Kanthi Kiran Kondepudi, G. B. Patil, Maunil Mankad, Zhenbin Liu, and Subrota Hati. 2022. Exploring the potential of Lactobacillus and Saccharomyces for biofunctionalities and the release of bioactive peptides from whey protein fermentate. *Food Bioscience* 48: 101758.

Du, Xiaojing, Xin Huang, Li Wang, Ling Mo, Huijuan Jing, Xinpeng Bai, and Hongxin Wang. 2022. Nanosized niosomes as effective delivery device to improve the stability and bioaccessibility of goat milk whey protein peptide. *Food Research International* 161: 111729.

Dullius, Anja, Márcia Inês Goettert, and Claucia Fernanda Volken de Souza. 2018. Whey protein hydrolysates as a source of bioactive peptides for functional foods – Biotechnological facilitation of industrial scale-up. *Journal of Functional Foods* 42: 58–74.

Eberhardt, Agustina, Emilse C. López, Roberto J. Ceruti, Fernanda Marino, Enrique J. Mammarella, Ricardo M. Manzo, and Guillermo A. Sihufe. 2019. Influence of the degree of hydrolysis on the bioactive properties of whey protein hydrolysates using Alcalase®. *International Journal of Dairy Technology* 72 (4): 573–84.

Gómez-Mascaraque, Laura G., Beatriz Miralles, Isidra Recio, and Amparo López-Rubio. 2016. Microencapsulation of a whey protein hydrolysate within micro-hydrogels: Impact on gastrointestinal stability and potential for functional yoghurt development. *Journal of Functional Foods* 26: 290–300.

Guo, Hao, Lei Fan, Lin Ding, Wenqin Yang, Chuangang Zang, and Hong Guan. 2023. Separation and purification of antioxidant peptide from fermented whey protein by lactobacillus rhamnosus B2-1. *Food Science of Animal Resources* 43 (1): 10–24.

Hussein, Fatima Abdelhameed, Shyan Yea Chay, Mohammad Zarei, Shehu Muhammad Auwal, Azizah Abdul Hamid, Wan Zunairah Wan Ibadullah, and Nazamid Saari. 2020. Whey protein concentrate as a novel source of bifunctional peptides with angiotensin-i converting enzyme inhibitory and antioxidant properties: RSM study. *Foods* 9 (1).

Kheroufi, Afaf, María E. Brassesco, Débora A. Campos, Halima Boughellout, and Manuela E. Pintado. 2022a. Functional properties of peptides obtained from whey proteins by ficin extract hydrolysis. *Food Bioscience* 47: 1–10.

Kheroufi, Afaf, María E. Brassesco, Débora A. Campos, Abdelghani Mouzai, Halima Boughellouta, and Manuela E. Pintado. 2022b. Whey protein-derived peptides: The impact of chicken pepsin hydrolysis upon whey proteins concentrate on their biological and technological properties. *International Dairy Journal* 134: 105442.

León-López, Arely, Xóchitl Alejandra Pérez-Marroquín, Ana Guadalupe Estrada-Fernández, Gieraldin Campos-Lozada, Alejandro Morales-Peñaloza, Rafael G. Campos-Montiel, and Gabriel Aguirre-álvarez. 2022. Milk whey hydrolysates as high value-added natural polymers: Functional properties and applications. *Polymers* 14: 1258.

Lv, Renzhi, Yifei Dong, Zhijie Bao, Simin Zhang, Songyi Lin, and Na Sun. 2022. Advances in the activity evaluation and cellular regulation pathways of food-derived antioxidant peptides. *Trends in Food Science and Technology* 122 (1): 171–86.

Ma, Shuang, Cuina Wang, and Mingruo Guo. 2018. Changes in structure and antioxidant activity of β-lactoglobulin by ultrasound and enzymatic treatment. *Ultrasonics Sonochemistry* 43: 227–36.

Ma, Yinlong, Jinzhao Xu, Ruibin Guo, Guoxin Teng, Yidan Chen, and Xiaoxi Xu. 2023. In vitro gastrointestinal model for the elderly: Effect of high hydrostatic pressure on protein structures and antioxidant activities of whey protein isolate. *Food Bioscience* 52: 102452.

Mann, Bimlesh, Anuradha Kumari, Rajesh Kumar, Rajan Sharma, Kishore Prajapati, Shaik Mahboob, and S. Athira. 2015. Antioxidant activity of whey protein hydrolysates in milk beverage system. *Journal of Food Science and Technology* 52 (6): 3235–41.

Meng, Yueyue, Zhiqiang Liang, Chenyi Zhang, Siqi Hao, Hongyang Han, Peng Du, Aili Li, Hong Shao, Chun Li, and Libo Liu. 2021. Ultrasonic modification of whey protein isolate: Implications for the structural and functional properties. *LWT* 152: 112272.

Millan, Gersi Cristina Lunar, Flávio Fonseca Veras, Paolo Stincone, Maria Elisa Paillië-Jiménez, and Adriano Brandelli. 2022. Biological activities of whey protein hydrolysate produced by protease from the Antarctic bacterium Lysobacter sp. A03. *Biocatalysis and Agricultural Biotechnology* 43: 102415.

Miralles, Beatriz, Roberto del Barrio, Carolina Cueva, Isidra Recio, and Lourdes Amigo. 2018. Dynamic gastric digestion of a commercial whey protein concentrate†. *Journal of the Science of Food and Agriculture* 98 (5): 1873–79.

Mohan, Aishwarya, David Julian McClements, and Chibuike C. Udenigwe. 2016. Encapsulation of bioactive whey peptides in soy lecithin-derived nanoliposomes: Influence of peptide molecular weight. *Food Chemistry* 213: 143–48.

Pizzino, Gabriele, Natasha Irrera, Mariapaola Cucinotta, Giovanni Pallio, Federica Mannino, Vincenzo Arcoraci, Francesco Squadrito, Domenica Altavilla, and Alessandra Bitto. 2017. *Oxidative Stress: Harms and Benefits for Human Health.* Oxidative Medicine and Cellular Longevity.

Power, O., A. Fernández, R. Norris, F. A. Riera, and R. J. FitzGerald. 2014. Selective enrichment of bioactive properties during ultrafiltration of a tryptic digest of β-lactoglobulin. *Journal of Functional Foods* 9 (1): 38–47.

Rivero-Pino, Fernando. 2023. Bioactive food-derived peptides for functional nutrition: Effect of fortification, processing and storage on peptide stability and bioactivity within food matrices. *Food Chemistry* 406: 135046.

Rosa, Lana S., Mariana L. Santos, Joel P. Abreu, Ramon S. Rocha, Erick A. Esmerino, Monica Q. Freitas, Eliane T. Mársico, et al. 2023. Probiotic fermented whey-milk beverages: Effect of different probiotic strains on the physicochemical characteristics, biological activity, and bioactive peptides. *Food Research International* 164: 112396.

Rossi, Yanina E., Noelia L. Vanden Braber, Ladislao I. Díaz Vergara, and Mariana A. Montenegro. 2021. Bioactive Ingredients Obtained from Agro-industrial Byproducts: Recent Advances and Innovation in Micro- And Nanoencapsulation. *Journal of Agricultural and Food Chemistry* 69 (50): 15066–75.

Sarabandi, Khashayar, Pouria Gharehbeglou, and Seid Mahdi Jafari. 2020. Spray-drying encapsulation of protein hydrolysates and bioactive peptides: Opportunities and challenges. *Drying Technology* 38 (5–6): 577–95.

Sarabandi, Khashayar, Fardin Tamjidi, Zahra Akbarbaglu, Katarzyna Samborska, Pouria Gharehbeglou, Mohammad Saeed Kharazmi, and Seid Mahdi Jafari. 2022. Modification of Whey Proteins by Sonication and Hydrolysis for the Emulsification and Spray Drying Encapsulation of Grape Seed Oil. *Pharmaceutics* 14 (11).

Shazly, Ahmed Behdal, Haibo Mu, Zhenmin Liu, Mahmoud Abd El-Aziz, Maomao Zeng, Fang Qin, Shuang Zhang, Zhiyong He, and Jie Chen. 2019. Release of antioxidant peptides from buffalo and bovine caseins: Influence of proteases on antioxidant capacities. *Food Chemistry* 274: 261–67.

Solieri, Lisa, Marta Valentini, Alice Cattivelli, Laura Sola, Ahmed Helal, Serena Martini, and Davide Tagliazucchi. 2022. Fermentation of whey protein concentrate by Streptococcus thermophilus strains releases peptides with biological activities. *Process Biochemistry* 121: 590–600.

Tadesse, Solomon Abebaw, and Shimelis Admassu Emire. 2020. Production and processing of antioxidant bioactive peptides: A driving force for the functional food market. *Heliyon* 6: e04765.

Théolier, Jérémie, Riadh Hammami, Philip Labelle, Ismail Fliss, and Julie Jean. 2013. Isolation and identification of antimicrobial peptides derived by peptic cleavage of whey protein isolate. *Journal of Functional Foods* 5 (2): 706–14.

Ulug, Sule Keskin, Forough Jahandideh, and Jianping Wu. 2021. Novel technologies for the production of bioactive peptides. *Trends in Food Science and Technology* 108: 27–39.

Wang, Yong, and Cordelia Selomulya. 2020. Spray drying strategy for encapsulation of bioactive peptide powders for food applications. *Advanced Powder Technology* 31 (1): 409–15.

Xie, Dewei, Lei Du, Haisheng Lin, Erzheng Su, Yaling Shen, Jingli Xie, and Dongzhi Wei. 2022. *In vitro-in silico* screening strategy and mechanism of angiotensin I-converting enzyme inhibitory peptides from α-lactalbumin. *LWT* 156: 112984.

Yin, Zhucheng, Yaru Wu, Yao Chen, Xuejiao Qie, Maomao Zeng, Zhaojun Wang, Fang Qin, Jie Chen, and Zhiyong He. 2021. Analysis of the interaction between cyanidin-3-O-glucoside and casein hydrolysates and its effect on the antioxidant ability of the complexes. *Food Chemistry* 340: 127915.

Zhang, Xinliu, Hao Gao, Chunyan Wang, Abdul Qayum, Zhishen Mu, Zengli Gao, and Zhanmei Jiang. 2018. Characterization and comparison of the structure and antioxidant activity of glycosylated whey peptides from two pathways. *Food Chemistry* 257: 279–88.

Zhao, Changhui, and Tolulope Joshua Ashaolu. 2020. Bioactivity and safety of whey peptides. *LWT* 134: 109935.

Zhao, Changhui, Nan Chen, and Tolulope Joshua Ashaolu. 2022. Whey proteins and peptides in health-promoting functions – A review. *International Dairy Journal* 126: 105269.

16 Using Whey Protein Concentrate and Curcumin as a Combinational Approach

Ceres Mattos Della Lucia, Kelly Aparecida Dias, Stephanie Michelin Santana Pereira, and Lívya Alves Oliveira

ABBREVIATIONS

ACE	Angiotensin-converting enzyme
AMPK	AMP-activated protein kinase
BCAAs	Branched-chain amino acids
cAMP	Cyclic AMP
CAT	Catalase
CCK	Cholecystokinin
CNS	Central nervous system
COX-2	Cyclooxygenase
CRP	C-reactive protein
GIP	Glucose-dependent insulinotropic polypeptide
GLP-1	Glucagon-like peptide 1
GLUT-4	Insulin-regulated glucose transporter
HbA1c	Glycosylated hemoglobin
HOMA-IR	Homeostatic model assessment of insulin resistance
HOMA-ß	Homeostatic model assessment of beta cell function
IgA	Immunoglobulin A
IL-1β	Interleukin 1β
iNOS	Inducible nitric oxide synthase
IPP	Isoleucine-proline-proline
IW	Isoleucine-tryptophan
LOX	Lipoxygenase
LPS	Lipopolysaccharide
NF-κB	Nuclear factor kappa B
NO	Nitric oxide
pI	Isoelectric pH
PI3K	Phosphatidylinositol 3-kinase
RCT	Renin-converting enzyme
ROS	Reactive oxygen species
SOD	Superoxide dismutase
TGF-β1	Transforming growth factor-beta
TNF-α	Tumour necrosis factor-alpha
VPP	Valine-proline-proline

DOI: 10.1201/9781003597926-16

INTRODUCTION

Whey protein has been extensively researched and is a popular dietary choice for athletes and individuals engaged in physical activity due to its rich composition of branched-chain amino acids (specifically leucine, isoleucine, and valine), bioactive peptides, vitamins, and minerals (Corrochano et al. 2018). It is recognised as a product with physiological and functional properties that enhance muscle growth (Stark et al. 2012). Furthermore, whey protein and its bioactive peptides offer numerous benefits for human health, with potential advantages in chronic diseases such as obesity, diabetes, and various other conditions (Alimoradi et al. 2016).

Whey proteins have also found applications as biopolymers, extending the shelf life of sensitive compounds and facilitating the controlled release of bioactive and nutritional substances within the body. They possess the unique ability to form gels and microcapsules through relatively moderate heating, without the need for chemical additives. This makes them a natural carrier for a wide range of bioactive components, both hydrophobic and hydrophilic, in both medical and food applications (Hu et al. 2019).

Turmeric, scientifically known as *Curcuma longa* L., belongs to the Zingiberaceae family. This medicinal plant is indigenous to India and Southeast Asia, where it is commonly referred to as turmeric, Indian saffron, and yellow ginger. Traditionally, turmeric's rhizome has been used as a colouring agent, flavour enhancer, and ingredient in the food industry for crafting seasonings, processed foods, and dairy products (Salehi et al. 2019). The health effects of turmeric generally focus on its main curcuminoid, curcumin [1,7-bis(4-hydroxy-3-methoxyphenyl)-1,6-heptadiene-3,5-dione] – a lipophilic polyphenol substance with a yellow-orange colour, acquired from the plant's rhizomes (Kocaadam and Şanlier 2017).

In the last decades, curcumin has gained attention in the field of sports medicine due to its potential as an antioxidant and anti-inflammatory agent (El-Saadony et al. 2023). It has also sparked great scientific interest due to its immunoregulatory, cardioprotective, antineoplastic, antimutagenic, anti-angiogenic, thrombosuppressive, and hepatoprotective effects, all associated with its antioxidant and anti-inflammatory potential (Liu et al. 2018). However, owing to curcumin's susceptibility to alkaline conditions, heat exposure, light, metal ions, enzymatic action, oxygen, and ascorbic acid, it is often encapsulated to enhance its solubility, stability, and bioavailability (Dar et al. 2017).

The primary aim of this chapter is to provide an overview of the potential benefits of whey protein and curcumin, both isolated and in combination, on various health conditions, metabolic control, physical exercise, inflammation, and oxidative stress.

WHEY PROTEIN AND ITS BIOACTIVE PEPTIDES

Whey is considered a rich source of biologically active components, mainly due to its protein fraction, exerting several health-promoting effects. Commercially available whey protein comes in three main forms: whey protein concentrate, isolate, or hydrolysed (Figure 16.1). Whey protein concentrate has a higher caloric value, contains all macro and micronutrients, and its protein percentage varies from 35% to 80%. Whey protein isolate is obtained through an additional purification step of whey, achieving a higher protein concentration (around 90%). Furthermore, whey protein concentrate and whey protein isolate can undergo a process involving treatment with acids, heat, or enzymes, breaking the protein into peptides and amino acids, resulting in whey protein hydrolysed (Mann et al. 2019).

The main proteins present in whey are β-lactoglobulin, α-lactalbumin, bovine serum albumin, and immunoglobulins. In lesser amounts, there are lactoferrin, lactoperoxidase, and proteosapeptone (Figure 16.2) (Olvera-Rosales et al. 2022). During the hydrolysis of proteins such as β-lactoglobulin, α-lactalbumin, bovine serum albumin, and lactoferrin, bioactive peptides are released, including α-lactotensin, β-lactotensin, serophin, albutensin A, lactoferricin B, and lactoferrampin (Madureira et al. 2010). Peptides can be released in several ways, either from precursor proteins or simpler

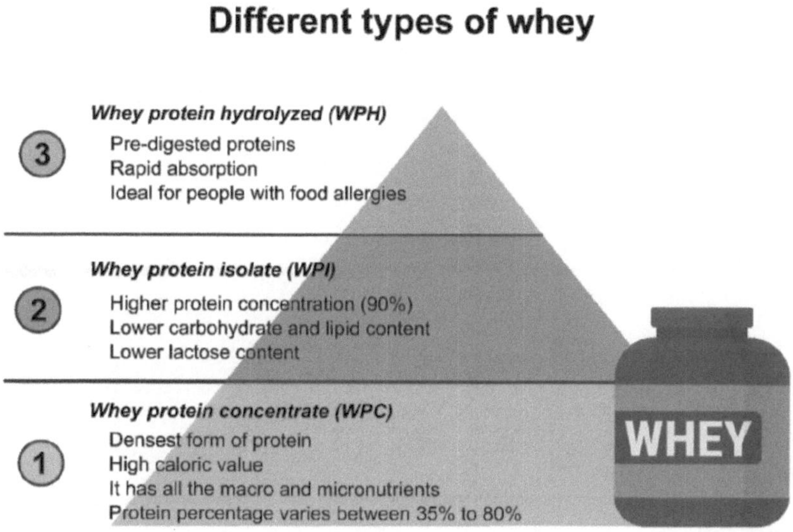

FIGURE 16.1 Different types of whey protein.

molecules, in addition to being hydrolysed through pancreatic, gastric, and microbial proteases (Madureira et al. 2010). The best-known way to obtain bioactive peptides is through enzymatic digestion by pancreatic enzymes, such as trypsin (Olvera-Rosales et al. 2022).

The physiological effects of bioactive peptides occur after they are released during intestinal digestion and reach their target sites in the brush border or after their absorption by peripheral organs (Madureira et al. 2010). This digestion occurs through the enzymatic hydrolysis of oligopeptides by peptidases, which cleaves them into free amino acids and dipeptides, favouring the passage of these compounds.

Peptides that are not cleaved by intestinal proteolysis are absorbed intact and enter the bloodstream, where serum peptidases subsequently hydrolyse the peptide bonds. Given this, resistance to peptidase degradation is an important factor in obtaining the physiological effect of bioactive peptides (Madureira et al. 2010).

The physiological effects of these peptides are associated with their antimicrobial, antioxidant, immunomodulatory, antihypertensive and opioid-like properties, which relate to health conditions (Madureira et al. 2010).

PEPTIDES WITH ANTIMICROBIAL ACTIVITY

Lactoferrin is the most studied component of whey regarding antimicrobial activity (Bruni et al. 2016), it is part of the innate immune system, showing activity against parasites, Gram-negative and Gram-positive bacteria, and fungi (Olvera-Rosales et al. 2022). The hydrolysis of lactoferrin, through gastric pepsin, produces lactoferricin, which has greater antimicrobial activity.

The antimicrobial mechanism of lactoferricin, as well as β-lactoglobulin and α-lactalbumin, involves the interactions of the electrons of its positively charged residues with those of the microbial surface, especially the negatively charged lipopolysaccharides (Sah et al. 2018). These residues will interact with the microbial lipid bilayer, causing a change in permeability, which allows cell lysis to occur (Olvera-Rosales et al. 2022).

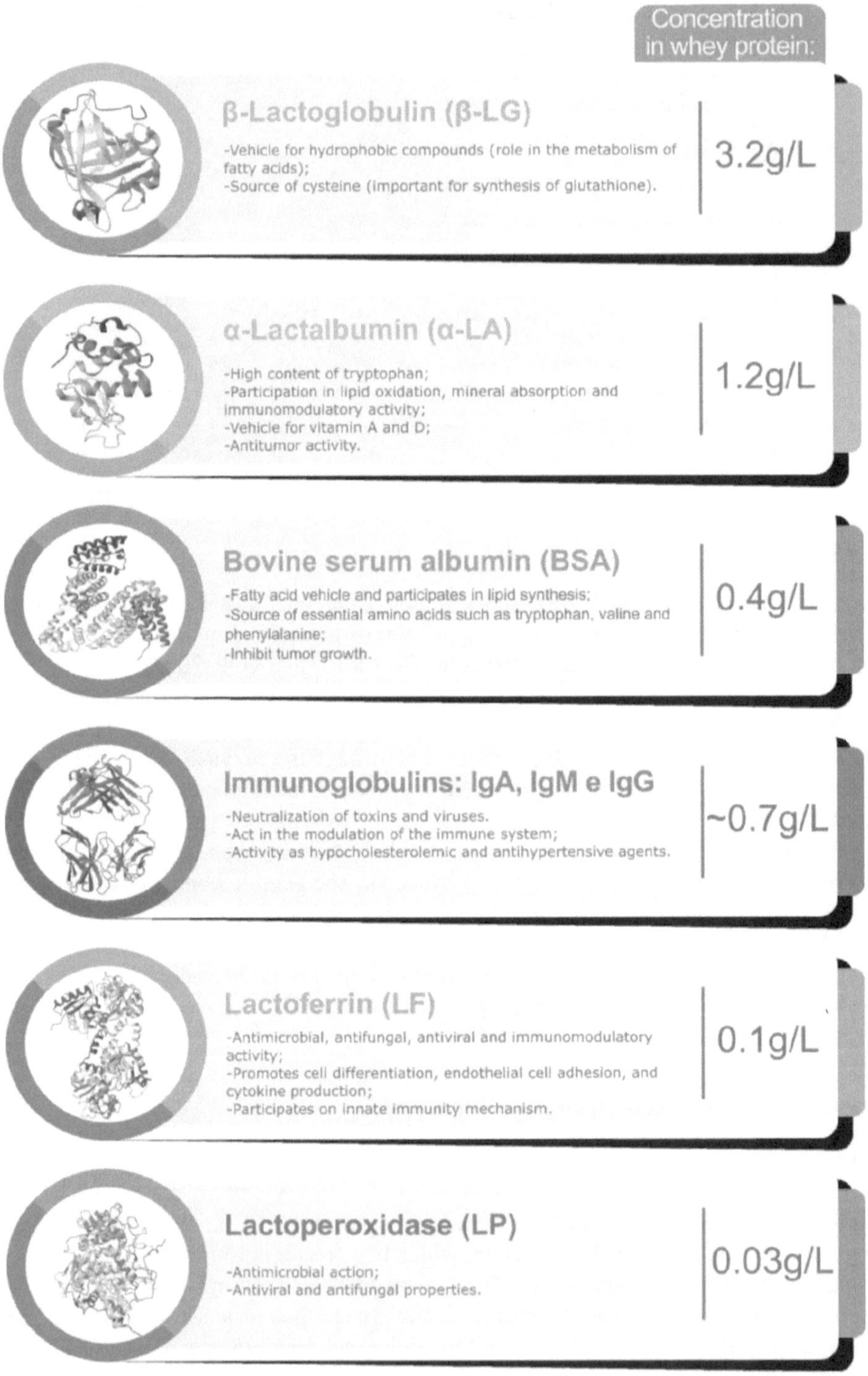

FIGURE 16.2 Main proteins present in whey protein.

ANTIOXIDANT PEPTIDES

The antioxidant activity of peptides relates to their structure, composition, and hydrophobicity. Amino acids with great antioxidant potential include aromatic ones, such as tyrosine, tryptophan, methionine, lysine, and histidine, and those with a sulphide group, such as cysteine, as they can donate protons to radicals that require electrons (Mann et al. 2019; Olvera-Rosales et al. 2022).

The functionality of antioxidant peptides may be related to the intracellular conversion of cysteine into glutathione, resulting in the protection of cells against damage from reactive oxygen species (ROS). These mechanisms include the inactivation of ROS and the elimination of free radicals; inhibition of lipid peroxidation; and chelation of metal ions that facilitate oxidation (Mann et al. 2019; Olvera-Rosales et al. 2022).

Furthermore, researchers have studied the role of antioxidant peptides in relation to the intestinal microbiota, as these peptides may reduce and even reverse the effects caused by dysbiosis by regulating the concentration of ROS (Dumitrescu et al. 2018). This type of bioactive peptide can modify the microbial community, as amino acid levels cause variations in the number of intestinal metabolites, reducing the abundance of bacteria involved in the production of ROS, such as *Escherichia coli* and *Clostridium perfringens* (Wang et al. 2019).

IMMUNOMODULATORY PEPTIDES

The immunomodulatory effect occurs through the hydrolysis of proteins, which releases peptides capable of affecting the immune system, improving the innate immunity of the intestinal mucosa (Brandelli et al. 2015; Olvera-Rosales et al. 2022). The modulation of the immune response by peptides can promote the proliferation of lymphocytes and the phagocytosis of macrophages, regulate the concentrations of cytokines, improve the synthesis of antibodies, and neutralise endotoxins of bacterial origin (LPS). The increase in lymphocytes, such as TGF-β1, correlates with the increase in IgA immunoglobulin after the consumption of whey protein; in addition, the production of lymphocytes can also be stimulated by the hydrolysis of β-lactoglobulin and α-lactalbumin (Kiewiet et al. 2018).

Furthermore, immunomodulatory peptides interfere with the interaction of LPS with toll-like receptors, affecting the production of inflammatory cytokines, such as C-reactive protein (CRP), interleukin 1β (IL-1β), interleukin 6, and tumour necrosis factor-alpha (TNF-α) (Adak and Khan, 2019).

PEPTIDES WITH ANTIHYPERTENSIVE ACTIVITY

The antihypertensive effect of peptides is related to their ability to inhibit the angiotensin-converting enzyme (ACE) in modulating the cardiovascular system. The decrease in blood pressure and the reduction in renin-converting enzyme (RCT) activity are linked to the peptides isoleucine-proline-proline (IPP), valine-proline-proline (VPP), and isoleucine-tryptophan (IW) (Martin et al. 2018).

These peptides have their inhibitory activity influenced by the amino acid sequence in the C-terminal position, and the amino acids phenylalanine, tryptophan, isoleucine, tyrosine, and proline have greater inhibitory potential on ACE (Olvera-Rosales et al. 2022). Additionally, ACE can be inhibited by peptides generated during the hydrolysis of β-lactoglobulin and α-lactalbumin by pepsin, pancreatin, trypsin, and chymotrypsin (Brandelli et al. 2015).

OPIOID-LIKE PEPTIDES

Opioid-like peptides, also known as enkephalins, demonstrate an affinity for opioid receptors such as μ, κ, and δ. When opioid receptors are activated, the enzyme adenylate cyclase is inhibited, resulting in a reduction in intracellular cyclic AMP (cAMP), and opening K^+ channels, which leads to hyperpolarisation at the postsynaptic level. Consequently, Ca^{++} channels are inhibited, reducing the release of neurotransmitters and neuronal excitability, causing an analgesic effect (Olvera-Rosales et al. 2022).

The most potent antinociceptive effects occur when peptide sequences derived from whey protein bind to μ receptors. Thus, the use of products that result in the production of opioid-like peptides is a good treatment alternative for neurological disorders, as their side effects are few and their production is not expensive (Olvera-Rosales et al. 2022).

HEALTH BENEFITS OF WHEY PROTEIN

As a high-quality protein, whey protein has gained increasing recognition for its numerous benefits for human health, and it is a popular choice among athletes. However, this versatile protein offers significant advantages for people of all ages and lifestyles due to its bioactive potential, which can act on the immune system and reduce the risk of chronic diseases such as type 2 diabetes and obesity, as reflected by metabolic syndrome (Alimoradi et al. 2016).

WHEY PROTEIN AND TYPE 2 DIABETES

The consumption of whey protein leads to a reduction in postprandial hyperglycemia, even when used in low doses. After consuming this protein source prior to a meal rich in macronutrients, there is a stimulus for the release of insulin, improving blood glucose and satiety (King et al. 2018).

The insulinotropic effect of whey protein relates to its composition, which is rich in branched-chain amino acids (BCAAs), which are digested quickly and easily, increasing BCAA levels in circulation and releasing insulin. Leucine, in particular, triggers the activation of the glutamate dehydrogenase enzyme in beta cells, stimulating an increase in Krebs cycle activity and oxygen consumption by these cells, resulting in an increase in insulin production. Isoleucine, on the other hand, influences the production of GLUT-4, essential for the transport of glucose in muscles, reducing insulin resistance in type 2 diabetics (Lesgards 2023).

Furthermore, bioactive peptides, when entering the digestive system, have the potential to stimulate the release of hormones such as glucose-dependent insulinotropic polypeptide (GIP) and glucagon-like peptide 1 (GLP-1), mainly in the colon wall. These hormones have the potential to increase insulin secretion and thus reduce blood sugar levels in diabetic patients, due to their ability to activate beta cells in the pancreas (Lesgards 2023).

WHEY PROTEIN AND OBESITY

An imbalance in protein, carbohydrate, and lipid intake can lead to overfeeding and increased energy intake, contributing to the development of obesity. Therefore, satiety plays a critical role in regulating food intake and in controlling obesity (Simonson et al. 2020).

Researchers have found that dietary proteins and specific amino acids exert significant influence in controlling gastric motility, pancreatic secretion, and, most importantly, inducing satiety. At the heart of this process are intestinal peptides that regulate digestion and signal to the central nervous system (CNS), influencing our hunger and satiety (Sousa et al. 2012).

Whey proteins are powerful stimulants of cholecystokinin (CCK) and GLP-1, which play a key role in promoting satiety. The glycomacropeptide, for example, stands out as an effective CCK secretagogue, which plays a crucial role in modulating satiety (Sousa et al. 2012).

Thus, the feeling of satiety associated with whey protein consumption is linked to the modulation of intestinal hormones, including increased release of anorectic hormones, such as CCK, leptin, and GLP-1, and decreased release of the orexigenic hormone, ghrelin. Additionally, there is a reduction in neuropeptide Y, which stimulates hunger, and an increase in pro-opiomelanocortin in the CNS, which inhibits appetite (Simonson et al. 2020).

WHEY PROTEIN AND ANTIOXIDANT ACTIVITY

The antioxidant effect of whey protein occurs due to the presence of powerful antioxidant components, through a series of mechanisms that help combat oxidative stress, a process linked to ageing and several chronic diseases (Corrochano et al. 2018). Whey is rich in cysteine, an amino acid that serves as a precursor to glutathione. Glutathione plays a crucial role in neutralising free radicals, reactive substances that damage our cells and DNA (Corrochano et al. 2018).

Furthermore, bioactive peptides from whey protein, such as lactoferrin, also have antioxidant properties, protecting cells from damage caused by free radicals (Olvera-Rosales et al. 2022). Whey protein is also a source of minerals, such as zinc and selenium, which are cofactors in antioxidant enzymes. Together with the natural antioxidants in whey, these minerals detoxify the body and reduce oxidative damage (Corrochano et al. 2018).

WHEY PROTEIN AND PHYSICAL PERFORMANCE

Whey protein has become common among athletes and physical activity practitioners who aim to gain lean mass and improve sports performance. The abundance of BCAAs in its composition, essential for the synthesis of muscle proteins and recovery after exercise, contributes to muscle growth and rapid repair, reducing post-workout pain and enabling more frequent and intense training. Additionally, whey protein's rapid digestion and absorption make it ideal as a post-workout supplement. Another benefit is its ability to reduce muscle catabolism, preventing the breakdown of muscle proteins, which is particularly relevant during intense training and periods of calorie restriction. This increase in sports performance, promotion of muscle growth, rapid recovery, and increased energy make this supplement valuable for a variety of sports (Atherton and Smith 2012).

CURCUMIN

Curcumin (1,7-bis(4-hydroxy-3-methoxyphenyl)-1,6-heptadiene-3,5-dione), the main polyphenol extracted from turmeric (*Curcuma longa* L.), was isolated for the first time by Vogel in 1815 and structurally characterised by Lampe and Milobedeska in 1910 (Hatcher et al. 2008). Also called diferuloylmethane, curcumin is a low-molecular-weight natural molecule comprising two 4-hydroxy-3-methoxyphenyl groups linked to an unsaturated carbon bridge with an α, β-diketone structure, and has the molecular formula $C_{21}H_{20}O_6$ (Figure 16.3) (Zhu et al. 2017).

This molecule has a hydrophobic nature, which makes it insoluble in water but soluble in substances such as dimethyl sulfoxide, acetone, ethanol, and oil (Beyene et al. 2021). The amount

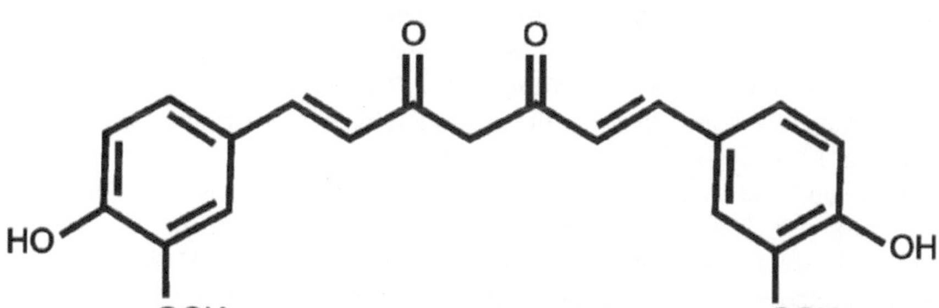

FIGURE 16.3 Chemical structure of curcumin. The chemical structure of curcumin is composed of two aromatic rings linked by a central chain.

of curcumin in turmeric varies from 3% to 8%, depending on the growing season. Therefore, a dessert spoon of turmeric powder, averaging 3 g, will typically contain between 30 mg and 90 mg of curcumin, although other plant species may also contain small amounts of this compound (Fabianowska-Majewska et al. 2021).

Numerous studies point to the benefits of curcumin due to its antioxidant, anti-inflammatory, immune-regulating, cardioprotective, antineoplastic, antimutagenic, antiangiogenic, thromboprotective, and hepatoprotective effects. Thus, curcumin is considered a nutraceutical compound because it not only nourishes but also provides therapeutic benefits to the body (Zheng et al. 2017).

ANTIOXIDANT ACTIVITY OF CURCUMIN

The oxidation of biomolecules manifests as oxidative damage to cells and, consequently, to tissues due to a tissue overload known as oxidative stress (Campbell et al. 2021). *In vitro* and *in vivo* studies have shown that curcumin's antioxidant action contributes to its therapeutic effects by reducing systemic markers of oxidative stress. Its chemical structure shows that electron-donating groups, especially the phenolic hydroxyl group, are the main contributors to its antioxidant activity (Sahebkar et al. 2015).

In this way, curcumin can reduce cellular oxidative stress by removing different forms of free radicals (Zheng et al. 2017). Curcumin can also increase the activity of antioxidant enzymes such as catalase (CAT), superoxide dismutase (SOD), and glutathione while inhibiting ROS-generating enzymes, such as lipoxygenase/cyclooxygenase and xanthine hydrogenase/oxidase (Lin et al. 2007; Sahebkar et al. 2015).

ANTI-INFLAMMATORY ACTIVITY OF CURCUMIN

Inflammation is a mediator for several diseases and can be caused by external or intrinsic factors, emerging as an immune system reaction associated with many diseases. In addition to reducing oxidative stress, curcumin can also protect against inflammation by modulating pro-inflammatory cytokines and signalling pathways, such as the nuclear factor kappa B (NF-κB) pathway (Zhang et al. 2018).

TNF-α is a mediator of inflammation in many diseases. Its effect is regulated by the activation of NF-κB. Once activated, TNF-α will activate downstream inflammatory pathways, such as cyclooxygenase (COX-2), lipoxygenase (LOX), and inducible nitric oxide synthase (iNOS). In addition to TNF-α, NF-κB is also activated by most inflammatory cytokines and by Gram-negative bacteria, viruses, chemical and physical stress, and other disease-causing factors. Curcumin has shown effectiveness in negatively regulating these downstream pathways, suppressing NF-κB (Sahin et al. 2016). Furthermore, it has shown the ability to inhibit the expression of pro-inflammatory cytokines, such as CXCL1, potentially reducing tumour metastasis (Killian et al. 2012).

Downregulation of pro-inflammatory cytokines, such as IL-6, IL-1β, and TNF-α, can reduce the incidence of inflammation (Wu and Wang 2014). Pretreatment with curcumin in human epithelial cells abrogated the upregulation of the pro-inflammatory cytokines TNF-α, IL-6, IL-8, and interferon-gamma 10 (IP-10)-induced proteins (Ferreira et al. 2015).

On the other hand, the upregulation of anti-inflammatory cytokines is essential to reduce the inflammatory response. The results of an experimental study showed that curcumin can inhibit inflammation and increase M2-type macrophages to the detriment of M1 macrophages in white adipose tissues, promoting the production of anti-inflammatory cytokines. Another study demonstrated in cultured macrophages that nanostructured carriers loaded with curcumin are taken up by these macrophages, which increase the release of anti-inflammatory cytokines, such as IL-10 and TGF-β (Song et al. 2018).

CURCUMIN IN HEALTH AND METABOLIC DISEASES

Curcumin has shown promising capabilities in preclinical and clinical studies. Recently, curcumin has been tested in humans for diseases such as metabolic syndrome, non-alcoholic fatty liver disease, atherosclerosis, and neurodegenerative conditions, among others (Akaberi et al. 2021). Its diverse beneficial effects may result from its ability to mediate many signalling pathways, decrease the inflammatory response, or indirectly maintain cellular homeostasis (Jabczyk et al. 2021).

Randomised clinical trials have shown that curcumin supplementation significantly reduces plasma TG levels, as well as the homeostasis model assessment of ß-cell dysfunction (HOMA-ß), insulin, HOMA-IR, and afamin – a glycoprotein associated with obesity, PCOS, type 2 diabetes, hypertension, and dyslipidemia (Bateni et al. 2021; Kheiripour et al. 2021).

Curcumin has been shown to reduce angiogenesis and adipogenesis by suppressing the expression of CCAAT/enhancer-binding protein alpha and PPAR, while also lowering cholesterol levels. Furthermore, curcumin can upregulate the gene expression of pancreatic glucose transporter 2 (GLUT2), GLUT3, and GLUT4, through the phosphatidylinositol 3-kinase (PI3K)/Akt pathway, thus stimulating insulin-mediated glucose uptake. (Shehzad et al. 2017; Chien et al. 2021). Another relevant aspect is its potential to inhibit hepatic gluconeogenesis through the modulation of 5′AMP-activated protein kinase (AMPK) (Heshmati et al. 2020).

Curcumin has also demonstrated potential in reducing lipids in the body, possibly through reducing levels of circulating lipid peroxides and total cholesterol (TC), as well as increasing levels of high-density lipoprotein (HDL). Several mechanisms may explain curcumin's beneficial influence on the lipid profile, such as its ability to suppress the expression of the Niemann-Pick C1-like protein (NPC1) in the intestine, which affects cholesterol absorption by hepatocytes (Panahi et al. 2018). Furthermore, curcumin improves dyslipidemia and activates the lipid metabolism pathway, increasing the activity of lipoprotein lipase and reducing triglyceride levels (Jamilian et al. 2020).

Curcumin limits the risk of lipid peroxidation, which contributes to the development of inflammatory responses associated with cardiovascular disease and atherosclerosis, due to its ability to neutralise and eliminate reactive forms of oxygen. Furthermore, curcumin and statins influence the same mediators of plasma lipid changes (Panahi et al. 2018).

CURCUMIN AND EXERCISE

Endogenous antioxidants protect the body against oxidative damage, mainly by activating the antioxidant response. However, in exhaustive physical exercises – especially acute, high-intensity, or long-duration activities with inadequate recovery – there may be a reduction in antioxidant activity (Radak and Taylor 2019). These exercises lead to muscle damage, delayed-onset muscle pain, impaired muscle regeneration, worsened protein catabolism, and immunological depression (Dias et al. 2021). Studies have shown that nutritional strategies that help regulate inflammation, immune function, and oxidative stress, such as the supply of exogenous antioxidants, can be beneficial. Thus, supplements such as curcumin have been identified as agents with significant therapeutic potential (El-Saadony et al. 2023).

A systematic review of clinical trials showed that curcumin supplementation at different doses was effective in improving sports performance, reducing exercise-induced muscle damage, and lowering fatigue by decreasing creatine kinase activity (Figure 16.4). Furthermore, curcumin has been shown to exert an anti-inflammatory effect by modulating pro-inflammatory cytokines, demonstrating its beneficial potential for sport and efficacy before and/or after acute physical exercise in sedentary individuals (Dias et al. 2021).

Other studies have shown the potential of curcumin in reducing post-exercise inflammation (Tanabe et al. 2019; Wang et al. 2019). The mechanisms that explain this potential are related to its ability to modulate pro-inflammatory cytokines and signalling pathways, in addition to its effectiveness in blocking the increase in NF-κB activation and regulating the expression of inflammatory

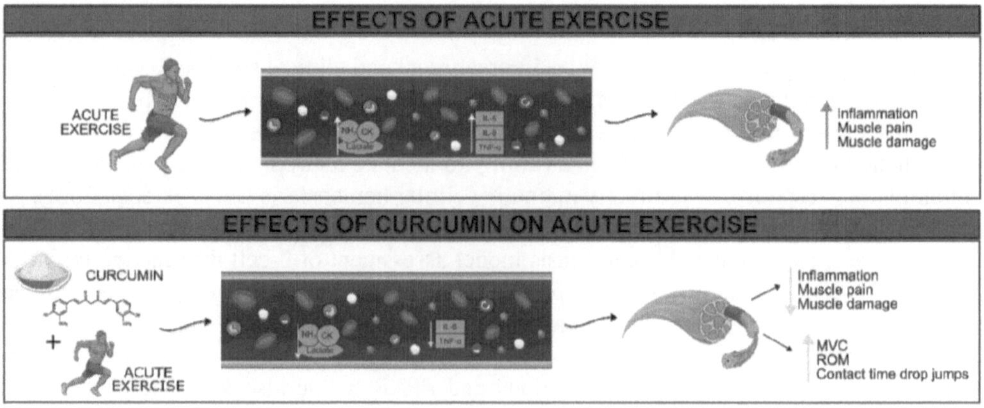

FIGURE 16.4 Effects of curcumin supplementation in acute physical exercises in sedentary individuals, based on a systematic review of clinical trials (adapted from Dias et al. 2021).

proteins (Zhang et al. 2018). Curcumin's inhibition of NF-κB may be directly related to the inhibition of ROS-generating enzymes, such as COX-2 (Dias et al. 2021).

BIOAVAILABILITY OF CURCUMIN

Despite the reported benefits of its anti-inflammatory and antioxidant mechanisms, curcumin's therapeutic results and clinical use are limited by its low bioavailability, poor intestinal absorption, and hydrophobic properties, leading to low solubility. Due to its tautomeric structure, high molecular weight, and aromatic groups, curcumin is extremely hydrophobic and therefore only partially absorbed through the gastrointestinal epithelium (El-Saadony et al. 2023). Furthermore, research related to the pharmacokinetics of curcumin revealed that its low absorption in plasma and tissues, rapid metabolism, and excretion considerably reduce its bioavailability (Salehi et al. 2019).

Several delivery strategies have been developed to overcome pharmacokinetic challenges that often result in low bioavailability when curcumin is ingested orally. These approaches include the use of adjuvants, nanoparticles, liposomes, and a drug self-emulsification system (El-Saadony et al. 2023). Thus, curcumin formulations have emerged as a result of research to improve bioavailability, permeability, circulation in the body, half-life, and resistance to metabolic processes. These formulations allow the incorporation of chemical compounds of curcumin and analogues with metabolic adjuvants, nanoparticles, liposomes, micelles, nanostructured lipid carriers, and phospholipid complexes (El-Saadony et al. 2023).

DEVELOPMENT OF A CURCUMIN-ADDED WHEY PROTEIN AS A STRATEGY TO PROMOTE HEALTH BENEFITS

Several studies have explored the health benefits of combining curcumin with whey protein, particularly regarding biochemical parameters, liver health, maintenance of muscle tissue integrity, improvement of oxidative balance, and attenuation of inflammatory responses. In addition, histopathological changes in the muscle and liver of rats during the strenuous exercise were also evaluated (Figure 16.5).

The first study aimed at producing curcumin-added whey protein and characterising its technological attributes was conducted by Gomes et al. (2020). Researchers prepared an ethanolic extract of turmeric before ultrafiltering the whey protein concentrate; turmeric extract was then added before spray drying the mixture. Morphological analyses included particle size distribution measurements, Raman spectroscopy assessments, sorption isotherms evaluations, and colourimetry

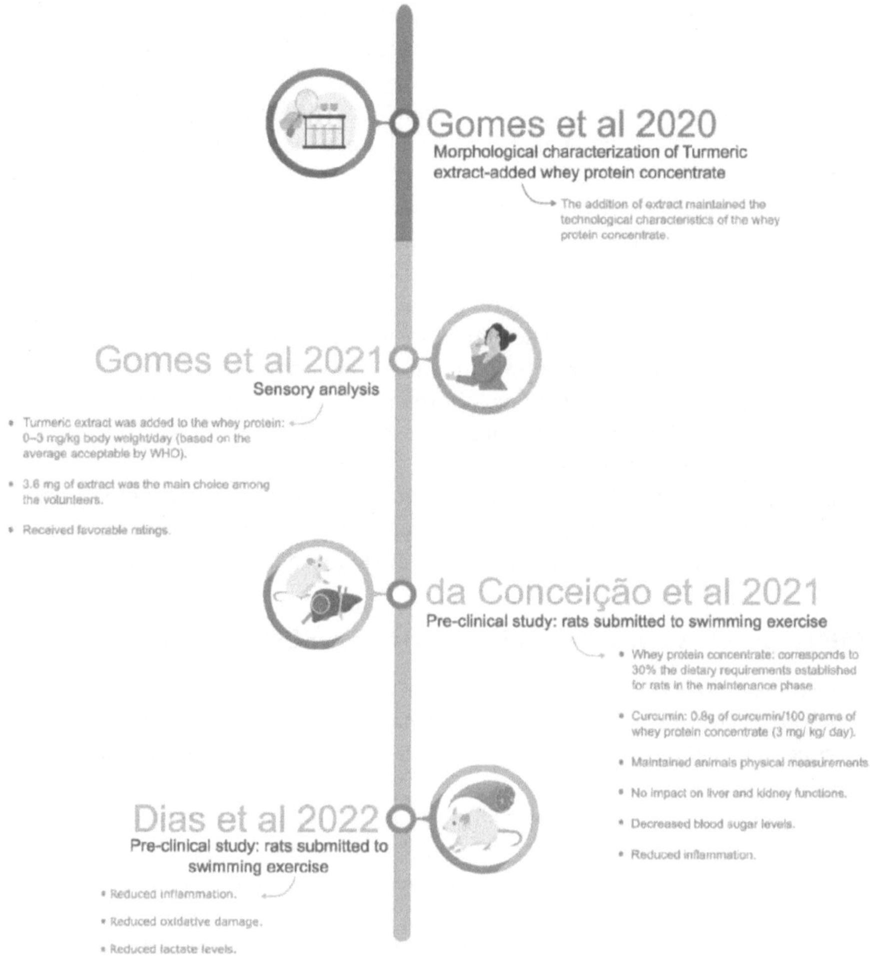
Gomes et al 2020
Morphological characterization of Turmeric extract-added whey protein concentrate
The addition of extract maintained the technological characteristics of the whey protein concentrate.
Gomes et al 2021
Sensory analysis
• Turmeric extract was added to the whey protein: 0–3 mg/kg body weight/day (based on the average acceptable by WHO).
• 3.6 mg of extract was the main choice among the volunteers.
• Received favorable ratings.
da Conceição et al 2021
Pre-clinical study: rats submitted to swimming exercise
• Whey protein concentrate: corresponds to 30% the dietary requirements established for rats in the maintenance phase
• Curcumin: 0.8g of curcumin/100 grams of whey protein concentrate (3 mg/ kg/ day).
• Maintained animals physical measurements
• No impact on liver and kidney functions.
• Decreased blood sugar levels.
• Reduced inflammation.
Dias et al 2022
Pre-clinical study: rats submitted to swimming exercise
• Reduced inflammation.
• Reduced oxidative damage.
• Reduced lactate levels.

FIGURE 16.5 Development and application of curcumin-added whey protein: phases of study design and observed results.

tests. The study also technologically compared whey concentrate formulations with and without turmeric extract, and results indicated that adding this extract did not change the technological characteristics of the whey protein concentrate.

The amount of turmeric extract added to the whey protein concentrate was based on the Food and Agriculture Organization's acceptable daily curcumin intake recommendation: 0–3 mg/kg body weight/day (FAO 2004). Two dosages were tested: 7.2 mg or 3.6 mg of curcumin per 30 g serving of whey protein. Based on the sensory analysis findings, the sample that included 3.6 mg of curcumin was the top choice among the volunteers and received favourable ratings (Gomes et al. 2021).

EFFECTS OF USING CURCUMIN-ADDED WHEY PROTEIN ON BIOCHEMICAL MARKERS AND LIVER FUNCTIONS

A preclinical study (da Conceição et al. 2021) was the first to use curcumin-added whey protein in a Wistar rat model to evaluate the impact of this combination on metabolic control, inflammation, and oxidative stress in animals subjected to an exhaustive exercise protocol. The curcumin was incorporated into whey protein concentrate at a concentration of 0.8 g of curcumin per 100 g of whey protein concentrate. This calculation was based on an assumed daily intake of 3 mg of curcumin per kg of body weight, which is the maximum acceptable daily intake for humans. The calculation accounted for an individual weighing 70 kg who replaces 0.3 g of protein per kg of body weight with whey protein concentrate, following the reference by Schoenfeld and Aragon (2018). Consequently, the protein substitution in animals using whey protein concentrate amounted to 30% of the dietary requirements established for rats in the maintenance phase, which is consistent with the substitution used for humans.

The curcumin used was Theracurmin®, a highly bioavailable curcumin developed using micronised technology, which can significantly increase bioavailability and water solubility compared to conventional curcumin. In preclinical and clinical studies, the absorption of Theracurmin® was shown to be 30 times greater than that of regular curcumin. Furthermore, its maximum plasma concentration increased by more than 50 times when Theracurmin® was used (da Conceição et al. 2021).

The intake of curcumin-added whey protein had no impact on the animals' physical measurements, food intake, liver or kidney functions, or protein balance. However, it did lead to a decrease in blood sugar levels and a decrease in the gene expression of TNF-α and IL-6, while increasing the expression of IL-10 (da Conceição et al. 2021).

To date, no studies have investigated this association in humans. Although preclinical studies on animals have demonstrated the benefits and safety of consuming curcumin combined with whey protein concentrate, further research is needed to confirm these effects in human populations.

CURCUMIN-ADDED WHEY PROTEIN IN THE MUSCLE TISSUE

Similarly, to evaluate the effect of curcumin-added whey protein on inflammatory and oxidative processes, as well as histopathological changes in muscle tissue, a study (Dias et al. 2022) under similar experimental conditions was conducted on Wistar rats subjected to an exhaustive swimming test (ET).

The results showed that curcumin-added whey protein reduced IL-6 and increased IL-10 expression in muscle tissue, thereby regulating inflammation. Additionally, higher nitric oxide (NO) concentrations were observed following the consumption of curcumin-added whey protein, along with reduced areas of inflammatory infiltrate and fibrotic tissue in muscle samples. These results show that curcumin-added whey protein contributes to the reduction in inflammation and oxidative damage caused by the exhaustive swimming test (Dias et al. 2022).

In addition to the results related to inflammatory cytokines, the findings on NO confirm that this combination may reduce inflammation. This is because NO suppresses inflammatory processes by decreasing lymphocyte activation and leukocyte adhesion, preventing cell rolling and migration, and, consequently, inhibiting tissue inflammation (Dias et al. 2022)

This study corroborates previous findings that consuming curcumin-added whey protein contributes to reducing inflammation and oxidative damage caused by exhaustive swimming tests at a dose of 3 mg/kg/day of curcumin. These markers do not directly reflect muscle damage; however, they can be used with other variables to infer muscle changes resulting from exhaustive physical exercise (Dias et al. 2022).

FUTURE PERSPECTIVES

In view of the beneficial results observed from combining whey protein with curcumin in preclinical studies – at safe doses and without risk of toxicity – future studies should focus on understanding how these findings can be extrapolated to humans.

Furthermore, both nutritional compounds individually have demonstrated positive effects in clinical trials for various health conditions, mainly due to their antioxidant and anti-inflammatory activities. Enhancing the beneficial effects of whey protein by combining it with curcumin, or vice versa, offers significant potential for disease prevention and global public health improvement, as well as applications in physical exercise contexts (Figure 16.6).

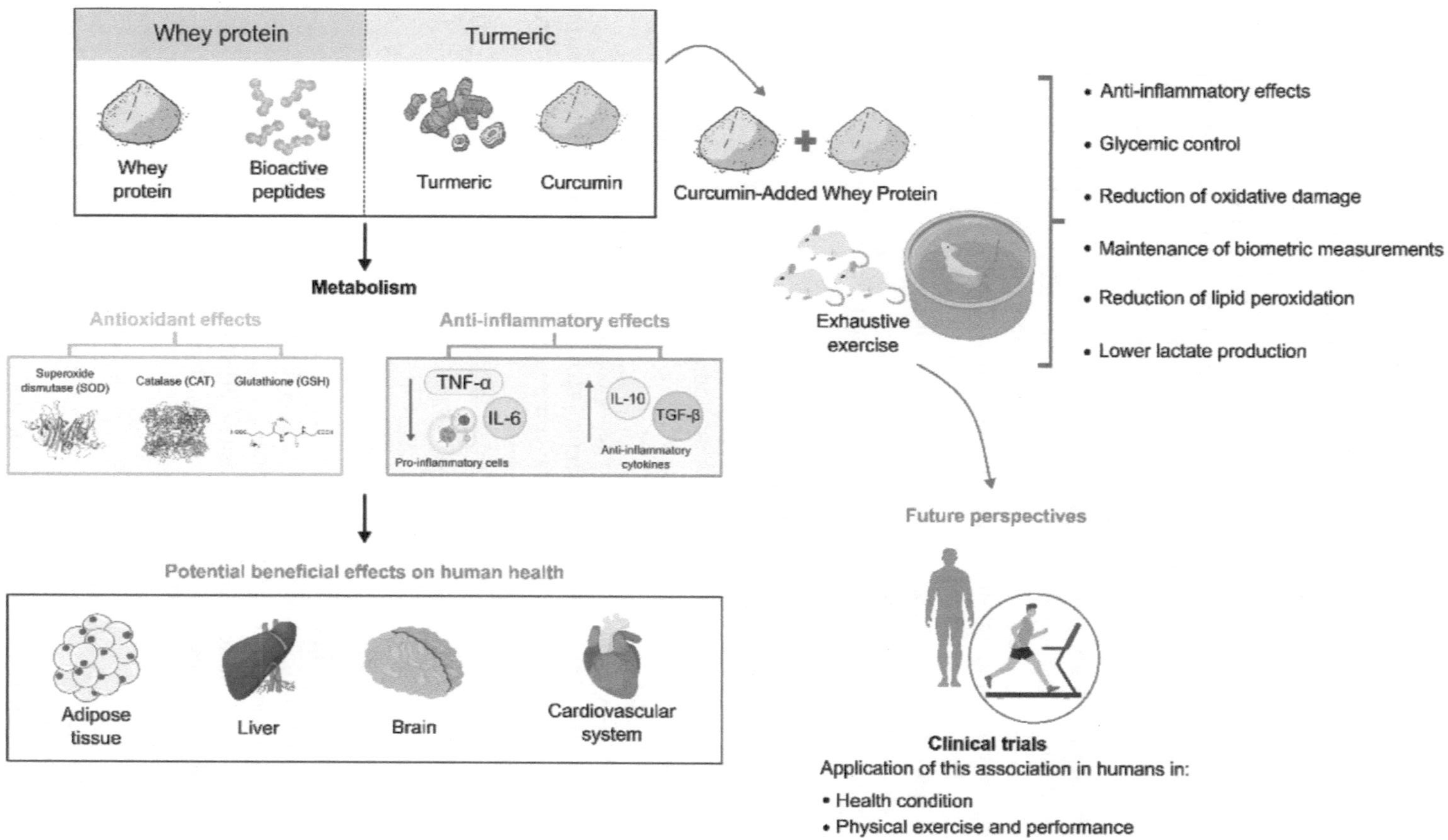

FIGURE 16.6 Effects of whey protein and its bioactive peptides and curcumin, isolated or combined, on different health conditions and exhaustive physical exercise. This figure summarises their antioxidant and anti-inflammatory effects across conditions such as obesity, liver disease, neurodegenerative disorders, cardiovascular diseases, and during exhaustive physical exercise based on preclinical studies. Future clinical trials are needed to evaluate this association further.

THE EFFECTS OF OTHER PROTEINS

This chapter summarises the potential benefits of whey protein and curcumin, used individually or combined, for regulating metabolism, reducing inflammation, and mitigating oxidative stress *in vivo*, with significant implications for general health and chronic diseases. However, it is also essential to consider the effects of other proteins, including casein, albumin, and vegetable proteins, taking into account factors like the timing of protein consumption, the form of protein (whole food vs. supplements), the type of exercise, and individual differences.

Casein is a slow-digesting protein that provides a sustained release of amino acids, which may help with muscle protein synthesis, potentially aiding in metabolic control and muscle recovery. Some studies suggest that casein may have anti-inflammatory properties due to its bioactive peptides, which may help reduce markers of inflammation, oxidative stress, and systolic and diastolic blood pressure (Fekete et al. 2015). In addition, casein peptides play a vital role in general health as they have antihypertensive, antithrombotic, and immunoregulatory properties (Petrotos et al. 2014).

Vegetable proteins, such as soy, pea, and rice protein, provide essential amino acids that support muscle protein synthesis, aiding in metabolic control and muscle recovery. However, their effects can vary depending on their specific source and composition. Some vegetable proteins contain bioactive compounds with potential anti-inflammatory properties (Gleeson et al. 2013). Additionally, including plant-based proteins in the diet is generally associated with a lower incidence of chronic diseases, such as heart disease, type 2 diabetes, cardiovascular disease, and the dysregulation of lipid metabolism (Nosworthy et al. 2023).

Research on the direct effects of dietary albumin on inflammation and oxidative stress during exercise is limited.

MINI DICTIONARY OF TERMS

- **Curcuminoids:** A group of chemical compounds found in turmeric.
- **Glycomacropeptide:** A protein derived from whey, with a low molecular weight and rich in glycomacromolecules.
- **Lipoxygenase/cyclooxygenase:** Reactive oxygen species-generating enzymes.
- **Opioid-like peptides:** Peptides that have chemical structures or bioactive properties similar to opioids, including natural and synthetic compounds that have the ability to interact with opioid receptors in the central nervous system.
- **Singlet oxygen:** A highly reactive form of molecular oxygen.
- **Xanthine hydrogenase/oxidase:** ROS-generating enzymes.

SUMMARY POINTS

- This chapter focuses on whey proteins and curcumin, isolated or combined.
- Whey protein is rich in bioactive peptides with beneficial effects on health.
- Curcumin has antioxidant and anti-inflammatory activity.
- Curcumin-added whey protein has shown positive effects in preclinical trials.
- Future studies should focus on investigating this combination in humans.

REFERENCES

Adak, A. and Khan, M.R. 2019. An insight into gut microbiota and its functionalities. *Cellular and Molecular Life Sciences* 76:473–493.

Akaberi, M. et al. 2021. Turmeric and curcumin: From traditional to modern medicine. In Guest, P.C. (Ed.) *Studies on Biomarkers and New Targets in Aging Research in Iran*. Springer, Cham. 1291:15–39.

Alimoradi, F.O.A.D. et al. 2016. Whey proteins: Health benefits and food applications. *Journal of International Research in Medical and Pharmaceutical Sciences* 9(2):63–73.

Atherton, P.J. and Smith, K. 2012. Muscle protein synthesis in response to nutrition and exercise. *The Journal of Physiology* 590(5):1049–1057.

Bateni, Z. et al. 2021. The effects of nano-curcumin supplementation on glycemic control, blood pressure, lipid profile, and insulin resistance in patients with the metabolic syndrome: A randomized, double-blind clinical trial. *Phytotherapy Research* 35(7):3945–3953.

Beyene, A.M. et al. 2021. Curcumin nanoformulations with metal oxide nanomaterials for biomedical applications. *Nanomaterials* 11(2):460.

Brandelli, A. et al. 2015. Whey as a source of peptides with remarkable biological activities. *Food Research International* 73:149–161

Bruni, N. et al. 2016. Antimicrobial activity of lactoferrin-related peptides and applications in human and veterinary medicine. *Molecules* 21(6):752.

Campbell, M.S.; et al. 2021. Influence of curcumin on performance na d post-exercise recovery. *Critical Reviews in Food Science and Nutrition* 61(7):1152–1162.

Chien, Y.J. et al. 2021. Effects of curcumin on glycemic control and lipid profile in polycystic ovary syndrome: systematic review with meta-analysis and trial sequential analysis. *Nutrients* 13(2):684.

Corrochano, A.R. et al. 2018. Invited review: Whey proteins as antioxidants and promoters of cellular antioxidant pathways. Journal of dairy science 101(6):4747–4761.

da Conceição, A.R. et al. 2021. Protective effects of whey protein concentrate admixtured of curcumin on metabolic control, inflammation and oxidative stress in Wistar rats submitted to exhaustive exercise. *British Journal of Nutrition* 127(4):526–539.

Dar, O.A. et al. 2017. Curcumin and its derivatives–Isolation, synthesis, and applications. In Shahid-ul-Islam (Ed.), *Plant-based Natural Products: Derivatives and Applications*, 145–174. John Wiley & Sons, Inc.

Deeth, H.C. and Mann, B. et al. 2019. Bioactive peptides from whey proteins. In Deeth, H.C. and Bansal, N. (Eds) *Whey Proteins*. Academic Press, 519–547.

Dias, K.A. et al. 2021. Effects of curcumin supplementation on inflammatory markers, muscle damage, and sports performance during acute physical exercise in sedentary individuals. *Oxidative Medicine and Cellular Longevity* 2021(1):9264639.

Dias, K.A. et al. 2022. Curcumin-added whey protein positively modulates skeletal muscle inflammation and oxidative damage after exhaustive exercise. *Nutrients* 14(22):4905.

Dumitrescu, L. et al. 2018. Oxidative stress and the microbiota-gut-brain axis. *Oxidative Medicine and Cellular Longevity* 2018:2406594.

El-Saadony et al. 2023. Impacts of turmeric and its principal bioactive curcumin on human health: Pharmaceutical, medicinal, and food applications: A comprehensive review. *Frontiers in Nutrition* 9:1040259.

Fabianowska-Majewska, K. et al. 2021. Curcumin from turmeric rhizome: A potential modulator of DNA methylation machinery in breast cancer inhibition. *Nutrients* 13(2):332.

Food and Agriculture Organization (FAO) 2004. Curcumin—Chemical and Technical Assessment. 61st JECFA, 1–8.

Fekete, Á.A. et al. 2015. Casein-derived lactotripeptides reduce systolic and diastolic blood pressure in a meta-analysis of randomised clinical trials. *Nutrients* 7(1):659–681.

Ferreira, V.H. et al. 2015. The anti-inflammatory activity of curcumin protects the genital mucosal epithelial barrier from disruption and blocks replication of HIV-1 and HSV-2. *PLoS One* 10(4):e0124903.

Gleeson et al. 2013. Dosing and efficacy of glutamine supplementation in human exercise and sport training. *The Journal of Nutrition* 138(10):2045S–2049S

Gomes, J.V.P. et al. 2020. Comparison of bioactive compounds and nutrient contents in whey protein concentrate admixture of turmeric extract produced by spray drying and foam mat drying. *Food Chemistry* 345:128772.

Gomes, J.V.P. et al. 2021. Morphological characterization of whey protein concentrate admixture of micro-encapsulated curcumin by spray drying. *Journal of Food Processing and Preservation* 45(2):e15141.

Hatcher, H. et al. 2008. Curcumin: From ancient medicine to current clinical trials. *Cellular and Molecular Life Sciences, Basel* 65(11):1631–1652.

Heshmati, J. et al. 2020. The effects of curcumin supplementation on óxidative stress, Sirtuin-1 and peroxisome proliferator activated receptor γ coactivator 1α gene expression in polycystic ovarian syndrome (PCOS) patients: A randomized placebo-controlled clinical trial. *Diabetes & Metabolic Syndrome: Clinical Research & Reviews* 14(2):77–82.

Hu, Y. et al. 2019. Protection and delivery of mandarin (Citrus reticulata Blanco) peel extracts by encapsulation of whey protein concentrate nanoparticles. *Food Science and Technology* 99:24–33.

Jabczyk, M. et al. 2021. Curcumin in metabolic health and disease. *Nutrients* 13(12):4440.

Jamilian, M. et al. 2020. Effects of curcumin on body weight, glycemic control and serum lipids in women with polycystic ovary syndrome: A randomized, double-blind, placebo-controlled trial. *Clinical Nutrition ESPEN* 36:128–133.

Kheiripour, N. et al. 2021. The positive effect of short-term nano-curcumin therapy on insulin resistance and serum levels of afamin in patients with metabolic syndrome. *Avicenna Journal of Phytomedicine* 11(2):146.

Kiewiet, M.B.G. et al. 2018. Immunomodulating protein aggregates in soy and whey hydrolysates and their resistance to digestion in an in vitro infant gastrointestinal model: New insights in the mechanism of immunomodulatory hydrolysates. *Food & Function* 9(1):604–613.

Killian, P.H. et al. 2012 Curcumin inhibits prostate cancer metastasis in vivo by targeting the inflammatory cytokines CXCL1 and-2. *Carcinogenesis* 33(12):2507–2519.

King, D.G. et al. 2018. A small dose of whey protein co-ingested with mixed-macronutrient breakfast and lunch meals improves postprandial glycemia and suppresses appetite in men with type 2 diabetes: A randomized controlled trial. *The American Journal of Clinical Nutrition* 107(4):550–557.

Kocaadam, B. and Şanlier, N. 2017. Curcumin, an active component of turmeric (Curcuma longa), and its effects on health. *Critical Reviews in Food Science and Nutrition* 57(13):2889–2895.

Lesgards, J.F. 2023. Benefits of whey proteins on type 2 diabetes mellitus parameters and prevention of cardiovascular diseases. *Nutrients* 15(5):1294.

Lin, Y.G. et al. 2007. Curcumin inhibits tumor growth and angiogenesis in ovarian carcinoma by targeting the nuclear factor-κB pathway. *Clinical Cancer Research* 13:3423–3430.

Liu, F. et al. 2018. Antitumor activity of curcumin by modulation of apoptosis and autophagy in human lung cancer A549 cells through inhibiting PI3K/Akt/mTOR pathway. *Oncology Reports* 39(3):1523–1531.

Madureira, A.R. et al. 2010 Invited review: Physiological properties of bioactive peptides obtained from whey proteins. *Journal of Dairy Science* 9(2):437–455.

Martin, M. et al. 2018. The angiotensin converting enzyme-inhibitory effects of the peptide isoleucine-tryptophan after oral intake via whey hydrolysate in men. *Journal of Hypertension* 36:e220.

Nosworthy, M.G. et al. 2023. Plant proteins: Methods of quality assessment and the human health benefits of pulses. *Foods* 2(15):2816.

Olvera-Rosales, L.B. et al. 2022. Bioactive peptides of whey: Obtaining, activity, mechanism of action, and further applications. *Critical Reviews in Food Science and Nutrition* 63(30):10351–10381.

Panahi, Y. et al. 2018. Curcumin as a potential candidate for treating hyperlipidemia: A review of cellular and metabolic mechanisms. *Journal of Cellular Physiology* 233(1):141–152.

Petrotos, K. et al. 2014. Casein and whey proteins in human health. In Kanekanian, A. (Ed.) *Milk and Dairy Products as Functional Foods.* John Wiley & Sons 1:94–146.

Radak, Z. and Taylor, A.W. 2019. Exercise and hormesis. In Rattan, S. and Kyriazi, M. (Eds) *The Science of Hormesis in Health and Longevity.* Academic Press 63–73.

Sah, B.N.P. et al. 2018. Antioxidative and antibacterial peptides derived from bovine milk proteins. *Critical Reviews in Food Science and Nutrition* 58(5):726–740.

Sahebkar, A. et al. 2015. Effect of curcuminoids on oxidative stress: A systematic review and meta-analysis of randomized controlled trials. *Journal of Functional Foods* 18:898–909.

Sahin, K. et al. 2016. Curcumin prevents muscle damage by regulating NF-κB and Nrf2 pathways and improves performance: an in vivo model. *Journal of Inflammation Research* 147–154.

Salehi, B. et al. 2019. The therapeutic potential of curcumin: A review of clinical trials. *European Journal of Medicinal Chemistry* 163:527–545.

Schoenfeld, B.J. and Aragon, A.A. 2018. How much protein can the body use in a single meal for muscle-building? Implications for daily protein distribution. *Journal of the International Society of Sports Nutrition* 15(1):10.

Shehzad, A. et al. 2017. Multifunctional curcumin mediate multitherapeutic effects. *Journal of Food Science* 82(9):2006–2015.

Simonson, M. et al. 2020. Protein, amino acids and obesity treatment. *Reviews in Endocrine and Metabolic Disorders* 21:341–353

Song, Z.L. et al. 2018 Dietary curcumin intervention targets mouse white adipose tissue inflammation and brown adipose tissue ucpl expression. *Obesity* 26:547–558

Sousa, G.T.D. et al. 2012. Dietary whey protein lessens several risk factors for metabolic diseases: a review. *Lipids in Health and Disease* 11:1–9.

Stark, M. et al. 2012. Protein timing and its effects on muscular hypertrophy and strength in individuals engaged in weight-training. *Journal of the International Society of Sports Nutrition* 9(1):54.

Tanabe, Y. et al. 2019. Effective timing of curcumin ingestion to attenuate eccentric exercise-induced muscle soreness in men. *Journal of Nutritional Science and Vitaminology* 65(1):82–89.

Wang, I.L. et al. 2019. Nanobubbles water curcumin extract reduces injury risks on drop jumps in women: a pilot study. *Evidence-Based Complementary and Alternative Medicine* 2019:8647587.

Wang, S. et al. 2019. Diet-induced remission in chronic enteropathy is associated with altered microbial community structure and synthesis of secondary bile acids. *Microbiome* (1):1–20.

Wu, N.C. and Wang, J.J. 2014. Curcumin attenuates liver warm ischemia and reperfusion-induced combined restrictive and obstructive lung disease by reducing matrix metalloprotease 9 activity. *Transplantation Proceedings* 46:1135–1138.

Zhang Y. et al. 2018. New MD2 inhibitors derived from curcumin with improved anti-inflammatory activity. *European Journal of Medicinal Chemistry* 148:291–305.

Zheng, Q.T. et al. 2017. Synthesis and antioxidant activity of curcumin analogs. *Journal of Asian Natural Products Research* 19:489–503.

Zhu J.K.Z. et al. 2017. Potential roles of chemical degradation in the biological activities of curcumin. *Food Function* 8:907–914.

17 Whey Protein and Impact on Obesity

Vahid Reza Askari, Ali Ebrahimi Dabagh, and Vafa Baradaran Rahimi

ABBREVIATIONS

BC	Body composition
BCAAs	Branched-chain amino acids
BLG	β-lactoglobulin
BMR	Basal metabolic rate
CCK	Cholecystokinin
CNS	Central nervous system
EAAs	Essential amino acids
GLP-1	Glucagon-like peptide-1
ISSN	International Society of Sports Nutrition
LBM	Lean body mass
MPS	Muscle protein synthesis
NEAA	Non-essential amino acid
NPY	Neuropeptide Y
NUCB2	Nucleobindin 2
POMC	Proopiomelanocortin
TEE	Total energy expenditure
TEF	Thermic energy of food
WPC	Whey protein concentrate
WPI	Whey protein isolate
WPH	Whey protein hydrolysate

INTRODUCTION

Obesity, a worldwide health issue, has escalated to widespread levels and is linked with a range of unfavorable health consequences. Dealing with this intricate problem demands a range of approaches, including changes in dietary patterns. Among the various elements of diet, whey protein has emerged as a promising candidate due to its potential to influence body composition (BC) and regulate metabolism. Understanding how whey protein affects obesity and the mechanisms involved could open the door for well-founded dietary measures to counteract this increasingly significant public health problem. As research progresses, leveraging the benefits of whey protein could become a valuable asset in the battle against obesity, consequently enhancing overall health and quality of life.

 DOI: 10.1201/9781003597926-17

WHEY PROTEIN

Whey protein is a well-recognized supplementary food source derived from cheese and other dairy items. It is abundant in components like lactoglobulin, lactalbumin, immunoglobulins, lactoferrin, lactose, minerals, vitamins, and lipids. Whey protein is widely used in the food and pharmaceutical industries (Andoyo et al. 2018). It accounts for roughly 20–30% of the complete protein composition in cow's milk (Devries and Phillips 2015). Its primary constituents include β-lactoglobulin (BLG) at 45–57%, α-lactoalbumin (ALA) at 15–25%, immunoglobulins at 10–15%, glycomacropeptide at 10–15%, bovine serum albumin at 10%, lactoferrin at around 1%, and lactoperoxidase at less than 1% (Bendtsen et al. 2013). In contrast to other types of proteins, whey protein is highly soluble in water, rapidly digested, and easily absorbed (Boirie et al. 1997). An investigation conducted among young individuals revealed that although whey protein digestion leads to a more pronounced initial increase in amino acids, casein proteins, which are digested at a slower rate, yield a greater leucine balance during the post-meal timeframe (Table 17.1). Curiously, a contrasting outcome has been witnessed in older individuals, wherein the consumption of whey protein results in a more significant increases in mixed muscle fractional synthesis rates compared to casein protein (Pennings et al. 2011).

Whey protein is available in diverse formats, encompassing whey protein concentrate (WPC), whey protein isolate (WPI), and whey protein hydrolysate (WPH). These variants can be found in powdered form or integrated into milk and specialized formulations containing elevated levels of specific amino acids (Sepandi et al. 2022). WPC comprises protein content ranging from about 25 to 89%, which may or may not include lactose (Table 17.1). WPI contains around 90–95% protein, generally devoid of carbohydrates. On the other hand, WPH features higher concentrations of peptide fractions (Keri Marshall 2004). Among athletes, WPH offers superior benefits compared to WPC and WPI because the process of hydrolyzing whey protein releases biologically active amino acids and peptides, resulting in enhanced physiological effects (Fassina et al. 2019).

Whey proteins are regarded highly for their quality, containing approximately 26% branched-chain amino acids (BCAAs) – specifically L-leucine, L-valine, and L-isoleucine (Walzem et al. 2002). These BCAAs are among the nine essential amino acids (isoleucine, leucine, lysine, methionine, phenylalanine, threonine, tryptophan, valine, and histidine) essential for facilitating muscle protein synthesis (MPS) (Burd et al. 2012), which supports muscle hypertrophy (Aoi et al. 2011). Notably, leucine plays a unique role in protein metabolism and is recognized as a pivotal signal in the initiation pathway for MPS (Anthony et al. 2001).

Whey protein is characterized as a biologically active protein, displaying a range of potential biological benefits. These encompass advantages for cardiovascular health, antioxidant attributes, heightened immune function, weight management, and reduced muscle mass breakdown during exercise. These attributes stem from the presence of numerous functional and nutritional

TABLE 17.1
Whey Protein Variants and Composition

Whey Protein Variant	Protein Content	Key Characteristics	Solubility	Digestibility
Whey protein concentrate	25–89%	Variable protein content may contain lactose	Good	Rapid
Whey protein isolate	90–95%	High protein content, low in carbohydrates	Excellent	Rapid
Whey protein hydrolysate	Variable	Rich in biologically active amino acids	Excellent	Rapid

constituents within whey protein. Particularly noteworthy are the essential and branched-chain amino acids, along with cysteine and immunoglobulin (Sousa et al. 2012). In theory, whey protein may contribute to weight loss by reducing appetite and enhancing the feeling of fullness through mechanisms involving the modulation of satiety hormones, changes in the production of glucose by the liver (hepatic gluconeogenesis), and diet-induced thermogenesis (Wirunsawanya et al. 2018).

EFFECTS OF WHEY PROTEIN ON APPETITE

Maintaining a reduced weight is particularly challenging due to an increased urge to eat and a decline in lean body mass (LBM), which results in a subsequent reduction of basal metabolic rate (BMR). These effects are common consequences of following a weight loss-focused diet (Gilbert et al. 2009). The nutritional composition of the diet, particularly its protein content, influences appetite perception, BC, and BMR (Martens and Westerterp-Plantenga 2014). Numerous studies have demonstrated that whey protein can mitigate various risk factors associated with metabolic disorders. These effects include a decrease in appetite sensation, reduced food intake, lowered blood pressure, improved insulin sensitivity, and diminished oxidative stress (Sousa et al. 2012). Whey protein has the potential to lower both short-term and long-term appetite. However, in terms of short-term appetite suppression, no discernible disparities have been observed between whey protein and carbohydrates (Mollahosseini et al. 2017). Distributing protein intake at approximately 25–30 g per meal may enhance appetite regulation, satiety, and weight management (Phillips et al. 2016). Consuming whey protein before meals reduces postprandial blood glucose levels, slows gastric emptying, and increases the peak insulin response. Furthermore, premeal whey protein consumption has the potential to raise plasma concentrations of glucagon-like peptide-1 (GLP-1) (Smedegaard et al. 2023).

One mechanism through which dietary proteins and amino acids might reduce appetite involves their influence on gut peptides, including cholecystokinin (CCK), GLP-1, glucose-dependent insulinotropic peptide (GIP), leptin, uroguanylin, and ghrelin (Table 17.2). These peptides are primarily synthesized and released from the gastrointestinal tract, impacting appetite regulation by modulating digestive processes and neural signaling within the central nervous system (CNS). Milk serum proteins, particularly whey protein, are highly effective in stimulating the secretion of CCK and GLP-1, both of which contribute to appetite suppression and satiety induction (Pimentel and Zemdegs 2010; Sousa et al. 2012).

In addition to their effects on gut peptides, whey protein amino acids also decrease the appetite-stimulating neuropeptide Y (NPY) and enhance the appetite-suppressing neuropeptide proopiomelanocortin (POMC) within the hypothalamus (Sousa et al. 2012). Conversely, whey protein

TABLE 17.2
Effects of Whey Protein on Hormones and Peptides

Hormones and Peptides	Mechanism and Effect	Effect of Whey Protein
Cholecystokinin (CCK)	Induces feelings of satiety and inhibits food intake	Increases satiety
Glucagon-like peptide-1 (GLP-1)	Enhances satiety, slows gastric emptying, reduces appetite	Increases satiety
Insulin	Influences appetite by affecting brain signals	Increases satiety, reduces appetite
Nesfatin	Enhances feelings of satiety and influences glucose levels	Increases satiety, influences glucose levels
Neuropeptide Y (NPY)	Stimulates appetite	Decreases appetite
Proopiomelanocortin (POMC)	Suppresses appetite	Increases suppression of appetite

is categorized as a soluble, rapidly digesting protein that demonstrates faster gastric emptying and absorption rates compared to other proteins like casein (Boirie et al. 1997). Moreover, whey protein's amino acid profile primarily consists of BCAAs, which are rapidly absorbed. This accelerated absorption may trigger an insulinotropic response, increasing insulin levels following digestion (Layman et al. 2003). Insulin acts as a satiety hormone capable of diminishing appetite through its impact on certain brain signals (Woods 2004).

An additional mechanism involves whey protein's impact on nesfatin. Following whey protein supplementation, nesfatin levels double despite no alterations to caloric intake (Giglio et al. 2019). Nesfatin influences glucose homeostasis, resulting in decreased glucose levels, although the underlying mechanisms remain incompletely understood (Ayada et al. 2015). Nesfatin is proposed as an anorectic hormone originating from the precursor peptide nucleobindin 2 (NUCB2), which enhances feelings of satiety (Table 17.2) (Shimizu et al. 2009). Furthermore, individuals carrying excess weight and displaying low nesfatin levels often exhibit an elevation in overall caloric consumption (Mirzaei et al. 2015).

Research indicates that whey protein's satiety outcomes may vary based on participants' body weight. For instance, a 50 g portion of whey protein could effectively reduce hunger in lean individuals but may not produce similar effects in overweight or obese individuals (Pal and Radavelli-Bagatini 2013).

EFFECTS OF WHEY PROTEIN ON BODY COMPOSITION

Body composition refers to the distribution of lean mass (comprising muscle, bones, and organs) and fat mass within the human body. Ensuring a healthy BC is crucial for overall well-being, optimizing athletic capabilities, and effective weight control (Table 17.3). Modifying BC and achieving weight loss typically involve two fundamental strategies: reducing calorie consumption and increasing calorie expenditure (Wycherley et al. 2012). High-protein diets represent an alternative strategy with significant catalytic potential for fat-burning attributes while curbing appetite, positively influencing both BC and weight loss outcomes (Wycherley et al. 2012).

Effects on Lean Body Mass (LBM)

Combining resistance training with whey protein supplementation has been shown to have a synergistic effect that promotes LBM gains. Therefore, it is recommended to add resistance training to one's lifestyle alongside whey protein supplementation.

Whey Protein Stimulates Muscle Protein Synthesis (MPS)

One of the central pathways by which whey protein enhances LBM is through its capacity to induce MPS. MPS denotes the mechanism through which muscle cells generate fresh proteins, ultimately fostering muscle growth and repair (Table 17.4). Maintaining elevated levels of amino acids in the bloodstream, known as plasma hyperaminoacidemia, is pivotal in triggering MPS (Bohé et al. 2003), but it is important to acknowledge that not all amino acids are equally potent in achieving

TABLE 17.3
Effects of Whey Protein on Body Composition and Weight Management

Aspects of Body Composition	Influences of Whey Protein
Lean body mass (LBM) enhancement	Stimulates muscle protein synthesis (MPS)
Body fat reduction	Increases thermic effect, aids weight loss
Energy expenditure and TEE	Elevates basal metabolic rate (BMR), TEF

TABLE 17.4
Whey Protein Dosage and Timing for Muscle Protein Synthesis (MPS)

Intervention	MPS Stimulation	Timing and Dosage
Whey protein isolate (20 g)	Rapid and significant	Immediately before/after exercise
EAAs enriched with leucine (1.5 g)	Maximum MPS activation	Resting periods (short-term boost)
EAAs (10 g)	Maximal MPS activation	Resting conditions
EAAs (20 g)	Maximal MPS activation	Resting conditions
Whey protein (40 g)	MPS peak stimulation	Resting conditions (elderly)

this. BCAAs and EAAs, with a specific emphasis on leucine, have demonstrated a heightened ability to stimulate MPS compared to non-essential amino acids (NEAAs).

Notably, studies have revealed that a mere 10 g of EAAs alone is sufficient to elicit maximal MPS activation in both younger and older individuals. Subsequent doses of 20 g and 40 g of EAAs do not exhibit further increases in MPS (Cuthbertson et al. 2005). In terms of the immediate stimulation of MPS, whey protein holds a notable advantage over other protein sources, such as soy (recognized for its rapid absorption) and casein (known for its slower release). Soy exhibits a higher capability to stimulate MPS compared to casein, although it still demonstrates lower effectiveness than whey protein, both during resting conditions and in response to the initiation of MPS prompted by acute resistance exercise (Tang et al. 2009). MPS rates are optimally stimulated with the consumption of 20 g of whey protein, and there are no additional increments in MPS observed with the intake of a 40 g portion (Witard et al. 2014a). The fact that a smaller quantity of EAAs is needed to achieve maximal stimulation of MPS compared to whey protein intake highlights the superior efficiency of EAAs compared to a protein source featuring a blend of amino acids.

Beyond the recognized advantages of EAAs alone, enhancing EAAs with leucine has been shown to intensify the effectiveness of these sources in triggering MPS. Notably, even a dose as low as 1.5 g of EAAs enriched with 0.6 g of leucine can induce maximum MPS rates during periods of rest (Wilkinson et al. 2018). The elevation in MPS subsequent to consuming 1.5 g of leucine-enriched EAAs demonstrates an equivalently robust response when compared to both 6 g of leucine-enriched EAAs and 40 g of whey protein. This implies that maximum MPS rates were effectively achieved through all three interventions without any significant differences observed among them at the two-hour and four-hour marks after feeding.

Given that LBM possesses higher metabolic activity than fat and plays a pivotal role in BMR, enhancing LBM increases BMR. Consequently, by increasing LBM through a combination of resistance training and increasing high-quality protein intake, body fat loss and maintaining the reduced weight will be guaranteed.

Whey Protein Dosage and Optimal Timing on LBM

The quantity of whey protein ingested can significantly affect its influence on LBM. The International Society of Sports Nutrition (ISSN) recommends a daily protein intake of approximately 1.4–2.0 g per kg of body weight for individuals engaging in consistent resistance exercise. This range supports muscle development and post-exercise recovery (Jäger et al. 2017). MPS rates peak 20 g intake of whey protein, with no additional increases in MPS observed at 40 g (Witard et al. 2014a). Elderly individuals require a dosage of 40 g of WPI to achieve maximal MPS rates (Yang et al. 2012).

The impact of insulin on MPS is linked to its ability to enhance amino acid availability, although this effect does not occur when insulin levels are raised systemically, such as after a meal (Trommelen et al. 2015). Insulin's ability to mitigate muscle protein breakdown is maximized at low-to-moderate levels (~15–30 μIU/mL) (Greenhaff et al. 2008). This range of insulin levels can be achieved through the consumption of 45 g of WPI alone (Power et al. 2009).

When whey protein is consumed near resistance exercise, it triggers an elevated activation (phosphorylation) of mTOR, a pivotal signaling protein present in myocytes that plays a role in MPS. Furthermore, this effect extends to its downstream mRNA translational signaling proteins, including p70s6 kinase and eIF4BP (Figure 17.1). This interaction strongly implies that a strategically timed intake of protein may enhance muscle hypertrophy (Farnfield et al. 2012). Elevated mTOR signaling has been shown to correlate with increased muscle hypertrophy over a 10-week training period (Hulmi et al. 2008). Elevated rates of MPS were attained through the consumption of a 20 g portion of WPI either immediately before or after resistance exercise (Tipton et al. 2004). A 40 g dose of whey protein resulted in a significant increase in MPS responses than a 20 g intake following an acute session of whole-body resistance exercise. This suggests that the absolute protein dosage may be more important than standardizing protein quantity relative to lean mass (Macnaughton et al. 2016).

MPS rates rise rapidly after whey protein ingestion, peaking within 30 minutes and remaining elevated for a up to three hours before gradually declining to basal levels. Interestingly, this decline occurs even though amino acids remain elevated in the bloodstream (Bohé et al. 2001). Employing an oral ingestion model involving 48 g of whey protein in healthy young men, MPS rates increased threefold within 45–90 minutes and then gradually declined to basal levels, despite sustained elevated plasma EAAs levels (Atherton et al. 2010).

A single dose of 25 g of whey protein induces a swift increase in amino acid levels in the bloodstream, stimulating MPS and anabolic signaling. Compared to dividing the same total amount into ten separate doses of 2.5 g each – designed to replicate the characteristics of a slower-digesting protein – the 25 g dose produces superior effects (West et al. 2011).

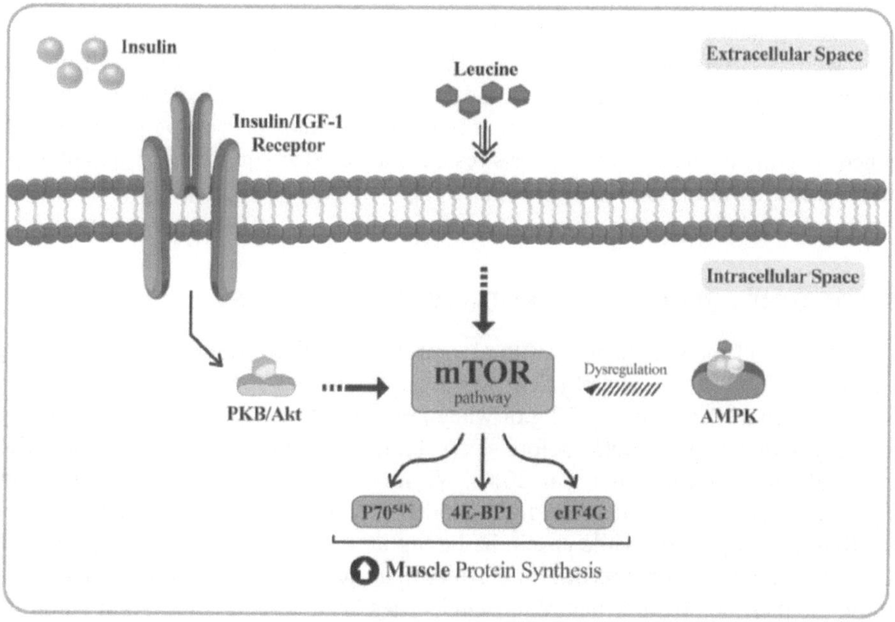

FIGURE 17.1 The mTOR pathway for muscle protein synthesis. Whey protein ingestion near resistance exercise boosts mTOR activation, a key protein in myocytes. This effect extends to downstream mRNA translational signaling proteins like p70s6 kinase and eIF4BP, suggesting strategic protein intake may enhance muscle hypertrophy.

In the morning following pre-sleep casein intake, the respiratory quotient remains unaltered. In contrast, both carbohydrate and whey protein can increase the respiratory quotient. This suggests that pre-sleep consumption of casein protein preserves the processes of overnight lipolysis and fat oxidation (Jäger et al. 2017).

Effects on Body Fat

Adopting a high-protein diet – approximately 1.2–1.6 g/kg/day – could yield advantages in terms of weight loss, fat mass reduction, and muscle mass preservation compared to a normoprotein diet with an intake of around 0.8 g/kg/day (Phillips et al. 2016). Supplementing with 40 g/day of whey protein for eight weeks without calorie restriction can reduce visceral fat in overweight and obese individuals (Giglio et al. 2019). Another study revealed that consuming a blend of WPI and additional peptides yielded greater potential for weight loss than glucose supplementation, with participants experiencing a substantial reduction in body fat (6.1%) and improved LBM preservation compared to the control group (Frestedt et al. 2008). Supplementing with 56 g/day of whey protein over 23 weeks reduced body weight and fat mass compared to carbohydrates in overweight individuals (Baer et al. 2011). It's crucial to emphasize that high-protein diets coupled with energy restriction lead to a more substantial decrease in body weight and fat mass while preserving LBM (Wycherley et al. 2013). Habitual consumption of supplementary protein may also contribute to long-term fat mass reduction and weight maintenance (Giglio et al. 2019).

HEALTH BENEFITS OF WHEY PROTEIN

Although athletes often regard whey protein as a prime source for repairing and sustaining skeletal muscle, it offers a range of additional health advantages. Notably, whey protein comprises various biologically active peptides, each possessing distinct signaling effects upon their release within the gastrointestinal tract due to their specific amino acid sequences. Whey protein contains high concentrations of β-lactoglobulin and α-lactalbumin, constituting around 75% of total bovine whey proteins, as well as EAAs, which account for approximately 50% of its weight. Moreover, whey protein seems to play a role in augmenting the responses of the lymphatic and immune systems (Staples et al. 2011). Its α-lactalbumin content is notably abundant in tryptophan, an amino acid that enhances cognitive performance under stress, enhances sleep quality, and potentially accelerates wound healing (Markus et al. 2002), benefits that can be especially relevant for recovery from contact sports or combat situations.

EFFECTS OF WHEY PROTEIN ON ENERGY EXPENDITURE

Under consistent food intake, changes in total energy expenditure (TEE) – encompassing BMR, thermic energy of food (TEF), and physical activity – can induce changes in body weight and BC. In a short-term scenario, consuming 30 g of whey protein, 30 g of casein protein, and 33 g of carbohydrate approximately 30 minutes before sleep can lead to an upsurge in morning BMR among young, physically fit men (Madzima et al. 2014). Within meals containing a blend of macronutrients (consisting of 50% protein, 40% carbohydrates, and 10% fat), whey protein exhibited a greater thermic effect than casein protein, while casein had a higher thermic effect than soy protein. Notably, all protein sources elicited a higher thermic effect than meals solely composed of carbohydrates. Importantly, the thermic effect of macronutrients varies between individuals and within the same individual over time (Hall et al. 2012). In various scenarios, protein consistently demonstrates a higher thermic effect than carbohydrates or fat. Therefore, increasing dietary protein intake, particularly whey protein, can elevate TEF and, consequently, TEE. If food consumption remains unchanged, this heightened TEE contributes to weight loss.

THE EFFECTS OF OTHER PROTEINS

In this chapter, we reviewed whey protein composition and its effects on weight and body composition, especially lean body mass. However, consideration should be given to other proteins such as egg or soy proteins and their effects on the discussed factors. Eggs, known for being an excellent source of high-quality protein with all essential amino acids, are acknowledged for their high biological value (Kovacs-Nolan et al. Mine 2005). The 2018 USDA National Nutrient Database reports that one large egg contains 6.3 g of protein, distributed between the egg white (3.6 g) and yolk (2.7 g) (Puglisi and Fernandez 2022). The advised leucine intake for maximizing muscle protein synthesis ranges from 700 mg to 3,000 mg per meal (Newman et al. 2006). A single egg provides around 500 mg of leucine, meeting the recommended "leucine threshold" with just 72 calories. (Newman et al. 2006). Though research on eggs and muscle protein synthesis is limited, Moore et al.'s study indicates promising results, highlighting the importance of protein quality (Moore et al. 2009). In this study, young men consumed varying doses of whole egg protein (0, 5, 10, 20, or 40 g) after leg resistance exercise. The results indicated that 20 g of egg protein maximized MPS, aligning with Witard et al.'s findings for whey protein (Witard et al. 2014b). This supports the International Society of Sports Nutrition's advice, suggesting 20–40 g of high-quality protein per serving. Norton et al.'s rat study further underscores eggs' anabolic potential (Norton et al. 2017). In this study, diets with egg or whey protein resulted in greater MPS than those with soy and/or wheat proteins. Rats consuming wheat protein had a 20% higher body fat percentage after 11 weeks compared to those on egg or whey diets (Norton et al. 2017).

CONCLUSION

Supplementing with whey protein in obese individuals primarily reduces body fat mass while improving metabolic syndrome indicators. When combined with caloric restriction and exercise, these positive outcomes are sustained, along with the preservation of fat-free mass. Whey protein also demonstrates age-specific advantages: it enhances feelings of fullness and regulates sugar levels in adolescents, while mitigating sarcopenia and ameliorating body composition when combined with resistance training in older individuals.

MINI DICTIONARY OF TERMS

- **Basal metabolic rate (BMR):** The energy expended by the body at rest to maintain basic physiological functions, excluding digestion and physical activity.
- **Branched-chain amino acids (BCAAs):** Essential amino acids – leucine, isoleucine, and valine – that support protein synthesis, muscle growth, and energy production.
- **Glucagon-like peptide-1 (GLP-1):** An incretin hormone released from the gut that enhances insulin secretion, inhibits glucagon, and promotes satiety, aiding in glucose homeostasis.
- **Glucose-dependent insulinotropic peptide (GIP):** An incretin hormone released from the gut that enhances insulin secretion in response to ingested glucose.
- **Lean body mass (LBM):** Total body weight minus the weight of body fat, including muscles, bones, organs, and other non-fat tissues.
- **mTOR (mammalian target of rapamycin):** A signaling pathway involved in cell growth, protein synthesis, and metabolism, responding to nutrient and energy availability.
- **Respiratory quotient (RQ):** The ratio of carbon dioxide produced to oxygen consumed during metabolism, reflecting the type of fuel (carbohydrates or fats) being utilized.
- **Thermic energy of food (TEF):** The energy expended during the digestion, absorption, and utilization of nutrients from food.

- **Total energy expenditure (TEE):** The total energy expended by the body, including basal metabolic rate, physical activity, and the thermic effect of food.

SUMMARY POINTS

- Constituting 20–30% of cow's milk protein, whey is primarily composed of β-lactoglobulin, α-lactalbumin, immunoglobulins, glycomacropeptide, bovine serum albumin, lactoferrin, and lactoperoxidase.
- Whey protein is renowned for its high-quality protein content, especially branched-chain amino acids (BCAAs), which promote muscle protein synthesis and hypertrophy.
- Biologically active, whey protein provides cardiovascular benefits, antioxidant properties, heightened immune function, weight management, and muscle mass preservation during exercise, influenced by gut peptides and amino acids' impact on appetite-regulating neuropeptides and insulin levels.
- Whey protein stimulates muscle protein synthesis (MPS), particularly through essential amino acids (EAAs) and leucine, showcasing its advantage over other protein sources in promoting lean body mass (LBM) growth.
- The International Society of Sports Nutrition recommends a protein intake range of 1.4–2.0 g/kg body weight/day for individuals engaged in regular resistance exercise, with 20 g of whey protein sufficient for optimal MPS stimulation.
- Whey protein's effects on body fat include reductions in visceral fat, potential weight loss, and preserving lean body mass in overweight and obese individuals.

REFERENCES

Andoyo, Robi, Vania Dianti Lestari, Efri Mardawati, and Bambang Nurhadi. 2018. "Fractal dimension analysis of texture formation of whey protein-based foods." *Int J Food Sci* 2018: 7673259. https://doi.org/10.1155/2018/7673259. https://doi.org/10.1155/2018/7673259.

Anthony, Joshua C., Tracy G. Anthony, Scot R. Kimball, and Leonard S. Jefferson. 2001. "Signaling pathways involved in translational control of protein synthesis in skeletal muscle by leucine." *J Nutr* 131 (3): 856S–60S.

Aoi, Wataru, Yoshikazu Takanami, Yukari Kawai, Masashi Morifuji, Jinichiro Koga, Minoru Kanegae, Kenichi Mihara, Taishi Yanohara, Jun Mukai, and Yuji Naito. 2011. "Dietary whey hydrolysate with exercise alters the plasma protein profile: a comprehensive protein analysis." *Nutrition* 27 (6): 687–92.

Atherton, P. J., T. Etheridge, P. W. Watt, D. Wilkinson, A. Selby, D. Rankin, K. Smith, and M. J. Rennie. 2010. "Muscle full effect after oral protein: time-dependent concordance and discordance between human muscle protein synthesis and mTORC1 signaling." *Am J Clin Nutr* 92 (5): 1080–8. https://doi.org/10.3945/ajcn.2010.29819.

Ayada, C., Ü Toru, and Y. Korkut. 2015. "Nesfatin-1 and its effects on different systems." *Hippokratia* 19 (1): 4–10.

Baer, D. J., K. S. Stote, D. R. Paul, G. Keith Harris, W. V. Rumpler, and B. A. Clevidence. 2011. "Whey protein but not soy protein supplementation alters body weight and composition in free-living overweight and obese adults." *J Nutr* 141 (8): 1489–94. https://doi.org/10.3945/jn.111.139840. https://www.scopus.com/inward/record.uri?eid=2-s2.0-79961107004&doi=10.3945%2fjn.111.139840&partnerID=40&md5=56b9a512da1fa8ac01bd86fdfd2cd887.

Bendtsen, Line Q, Janne K Lorenzen, Nathalie T Bendsen, Charlotte Rasmussen, and Arne Astrup. 2013. "Effect of dairy proteins on appetite, energy expenditure, body weight, and composition: a review of the evidence from controlled clinical trials." *Adv Nutr* 4 (4): 418–38.

Bohé, J., A. Low, R. R. Wolfe, and M. J. Rennie. 2003. "Human muscle protein synthesis is modulated by extracellular, not intramuscular amino acid availability: a dose-response study." *J Physiol* 552 (Pt 1): 315–24. https://doi.org/10.1113/jphysiol.2003.050674.

Bohé, J., J. F. Low, R. R. Wolfe, and M. J. Rennie. 2001. "Latency and duration of stimulation of human muscle protein synthesis during continuous infusion of amino acids." *J Physiol* 532 (Pt 2): 575–9. https://doi.org/10.1111/j.1469-7793.2001.0575f.x.

Boirie, Yves, Martial Dangin, Pierre Gachon, Marie-Paule Vasson, Jean-Louis Maubois, and Bernard Beaufrère. 1997. "Slow and fast dietary proteins differently modulate postprandial protein accretion." *Proc Natl Acad Sci* 94 (26): 14930–5.

Burd, Nicholas A, Yifan Yang, Daniel R Moore, Jason E Tang, Mark A Tarnopolsky, and Stuart M Phillips. 2012. "Greater stimulation of myofibrillar protein synthesis with ingestion of whey protein isolate v. micellar casein at rest and after resistance exercise in elderly men." *Br J Nutr* 108 (6): 958–62.

Cuthbertson, D., K. Smith, J. Babraj, G. Leese, T. Waddell, P. Atherton, H. Wackerhage, P. M. Taylor, and M. J. Rennie. 2005. "Anabolic signaling deficits underlie amino acid resistance of wasting, aging muscle." *Faseb J* 19 (3): 422–4. https://doi.org/10.1096/fj.04-2640fje.

Devries, Michaela C, and Stuart M Phillips. 2015. "Supplemental protein in support of muscle mass and health: advantage whey." *J Food Sci* 80 (S1): A8–A15.

Farnfield, M. M., L. Breen, K. A. Carey, A. Garnham, and D. Cameron-Smith. 2012. "Activation of mTOR signalling in young and old human skeletal muscle in response to combined resistance exercise and whey protein ingestion." *Appl Physiol Nutr Metab* 37 (1): 21–30. https://doi.org/10.1139/h11-132.

Fassina, P., G. Q. Nunes, F. S. Adami, M. I. Goettert, and C. F. V. De Souza. 2019. "Importance of cheese whey processing: Supplements for sports activities – A review." *Pol J Food Nutr Sci* 69 (1): 83–99. https://doi.org/10.31883/pjfns-2019-0008.

Frestedt, J. L., J. L. Zenk, M. A. Kuskowski, L. S. Ward, and E. D. Bastian. 2008. "A whey-protein supplement increases fat loss and spares lean muscle in obese subjects: a randomized human clinical study." *Nutr Metab (Lond)* 5: 8. https://doi.org/10.1186/1743-7075-5-8.

Giglio, B. M., R. M. Schincaglia, A. S. da Silva, I. C. S. Fazani, P. A. Monteiro, J. F. Mota, J. P. Cunha, C. Pichard, and G. D. Pimentel. 2019. "Whey protein supplementation compared to collagen increases blood nesfatin concentrations and decreases android fat in overweight women: a randomized double-blind study." *Nutrients* 11 (9). https://doi.org/10.3390/nu11092051.

Gilbert, Jo-Anne, Vicky Drapeau, Arne Astrup, and Angelo Tremblay. 2009. "Relationship between diet-induced changes in body fat and appetite sensations in women." *Appetite* 52 (3): 809–12.

Greenhaff, P. L., L. G. Karagounis, N. Peirce, E. J. Simpson, M. Hazell, R. Layfield, H. Wackerhage, K. Smith, P. Atherton, A. Selby, and M. J. Rennie. 2008. "Disassociation between the effects of amino acids and insulin on signaling, ubiquitin ligases, and protein turnover in human muscle." *Am J Physiol Endocrinol Metab* 295 (3): E595–604. https://doi.org/10.1152/ajpendo.90411.2008.

Hall, K. D., S. B. Heymsfield, J. W. Kemnitz, S. Klein, D. A. Schoeller, and J. R. Speakman. 2012. "Energy balance and its components: implications for body weight regulation." *Am J Clin Nutr* 95 (4): 989–94. https://doi.org/10.3945/ajcn.112.036350.

Hulmi, J. J., V. Kovanen, I. Lisko, H. Selänne, and A. A. Mero. 2008. "The effects of whey protein on myostatin and cell cycle-related gene expression responses to a single heavy resistance exercise bout in trained older men." *Eur J Appl Physiol* 102 (2): 205–13. https://doi.org/10.1007/s00421-007-0579-4.

Jäger, R., C. M. Kerksick, B. I. Campbell, P. J. Cribb, S. D. Wells, T. M. Skwiat, M. Purpura, T. N. Ziegenfuss, A. A. Ferrando, S. M. Arent, A. E. Smith-Ryan, J. R. Stout, P. J. Arciero, M. J. Ormsbee, L. W. Taylor, C. D. Wilborn, D. S. Kalman, R. B. Kreider, D. S. Willoughby, J. R. Hoffman, J. L. Krzykowski, and J. Antonio. 2017. "International society of sports nutrition position stand: protein and exercise." *J Int Soc Sports Nutr* 14: 20. https://doi.org/10.1186/s12970-017-0177-8.

Keri Marshall, N. 2004. "Therapeutic applications of whey protein." *Altern Med Rev* 9 (2): 136–56.

Kovacs-Nolan, Jennifer, Marshall Phillips, and Yoshinori Mine. 2005. "Advances in the value of eggs and egg components for human health." *J Agric Food Chem* 53 (22): 8421–31.

Layman, Donald K, Harn Shiue, Carl Sather, Donna J Erickson, and Jamie Baum. 2003. "Increased dietary protein modifies glucose and insulin homeostasis in adult women during weight loss." *J Nutr* 133 (2): 405–10.

Macnaughton, L. S., S. L. Wardle, O. C. Witard, C. McGlory, D. L. Hamilton, S. Jeromson, C. E. Lawrence, G. A. Wallis, and K. D. Tipton. 2016. "The response of muscle protein synthesis following whole-body resistance exercise is greater following 40 g than 20 g of ingested whey protein." *Physiol Rep* 4 (15). https://doi.org/10.14814/phy2.12893.

Madzima, T. A., L. B. Panton, S. K. Fretti, A. W. Kinsey, and M. J. Ormsbee. 2014. "Night-time consumption of protein or carbohydrate results in increased morning resting energy expenditure in active college-aged men." *Br J Nutr* 111 (1): 71–7. https://doi.org/10.1017/s000711451300192x.

Markus, C. R., B. Olivier, and E. H. de Haan. 2002. "Whey protein rich in alpha-lactalbumin increases the ratio of plasma tryptophan to the sum of the other large neutral amino acids and improves cognitive performance in stress-vulnerable subjects." *Am J Clin Nutr* 75 (6): 1051–6. https://doi.org/10.1093/ajcn/75.6.1051.

Martens, Eveline AP, and Margriet S Westerterp-Plantenga. 2014. "Protein diets, body weight loss and weight maintenance." *Curr Opin Clin Nutr Metab Care* 17 (1): 75–9.

Mirzaei, K., A. Hossein-nezhad, S. A. Keshavarz, F. Koohdani, M. R. Eshraghian, A. A. Saboor-Yaraghi, S. Hosseini, M. Chamari, M. Zareei, and M. Djalali. 2015. "Association of nesfatin-1 level with body composition, dietary intake and resting metabolic rate in obese and morbid obese subjects." *Diabetes Metab Syndr* 9 (4): 292–8. https://doi.org/10.1016/j.dsx.2014.04.010.

Mollahosseini, M., S. Shab-Bidar, M. H. Rahimi, and K. Djafarian. 2017. "Effect of whey protein supplementation on long and short term appetite: A meta-analysis of randomized controlled trials." *Clin Nutr ESPEN* 20: 34–40. https://doi.org/10.1016/j.clnesp.2017.04.002. https://www.scopus.com/inward/record.uri?eid=2-s2.0-85019036410&doi=10.1016%2fj.clnesp.2017.04.002&partnerID=40&md5=909fba62d5710849f739fcfdf9ff5b8d.

Moore, Daniel R., Meghann J. Robinson, Jessica L. Fry, Jason E. Tang, Elisa I. Glover, Sarah B. Wilkinson, Todd Prior, Mark A Tarnopolsky, and Stuart M Phillips. 2009. "Ingested protein dose response of muscle and albumin protein synthesis after resistance exercise in young men." *Am J Clin Nutr* 89 (1): 161–8.

Newman, Anne B., Varant Kupelian, Marjolein Visser, Eleanor M. Simonsick, Bret H. Goodpaster, Stephen B. Kritchevsky, Frances A. Tylavsky, Susan M. Rubin, and Tamara B. Harris. 2006. "Strength, but not muscle mass, is associated with mortality in the health, aging and body composition study cohort." *J Gerontol A Biol Sci Med Sci* 61 (1): 72–7.

Norton, Layne E., Gabriel J. Wilson, Christopher J. Moulton, and Donald K. Layman. 2017. "Meal distribution of dietary protein and leucine influences long-term muscle mass and body composition in adult rats." *J Nutr* 147 (2): 195–201.

Pal, Sebely, and Simone Radavelli-Bagatini. 2013. "The effects of whey protein on cardiometabolic risk factors." *Obes Rev* 14 (4): 324–43.

Pennings, B., Y. Boirie, J. M. Senden, A. P. Gijsen, H. Kuipers, and L. J. van Loon. 2011. "Whey protein stimulates postprandial muscle protein accretion more effectively than do casein and casein hydrolysate in older men." *Am J Clin Nutr* 93 (5): 997–1005. https://doi.org/10.3945/ajcn.110.008102.

Phillips, S. M., S. Chevalier, and H. J. Leidy. 2016. "Protein "requirements" beyond the RDA: implications for optimizing health." *Appl Physiol Nutr Metab* 41 (5): 565–72. https://doi.org/10.1139/apnm-2015-0550.

Pimentel, Gustavo D, and JC Zemdegs. 2010. "Foods and nutrients modulates the release of anorexigenic gastrointestinal hormones." *Acta Médica Portuguesa* 23 (5): 891–900.

Power, O., A. Hallihan, and P. Jakeman. 2009. "Human insulinotropic response to oral ingestion of native and hydrolysed whey protein." *Amino Acids* 37 (2): 333–9. https://doi.org/10.1007/s00726-008-0156-0.

Puglisi, Michael J., and Maria Luz Fernandez. 2022. "The health benefits of egg protein." *Nutrients* 14 (14): 2904.

Sepandi, M., M. Samadi, H. Shirvani, Y. Alimohamadi, M. Taghdir, F. Goudarzi, and I. Akbarzadeh. 2022. "Effect of whey protein supplementation on weight and body composition indicators: a meta-analysis of randomized clinical trials." *Clin Nutr ESPEN* 50: 74–83. https://doi.org/10.1016/j.clnesp.2022.05.020. https://www.scopus.com/inward/record.uri?eid=2-s2.0-85132540269&doi=10.1016%2fj.clnesp.2022.05.020&partnerID=40&md5=5a6bfba98c5dc5ef6d7c0d488267f913.

Shimizu, H., I. S. Oh, K. Hashimoto, M. Nakata, S. Yamamoto, N. Yoshida, H. Eguchi, I. Kato, K. Inoue, T. Satoh, S. Okada, M. Yamada, T. Yada, and M. Mori. 2009. "Peripheral administration of nesfatin-1 reduces food intake in mice: the leptin-independent mechanism." *Endocrinology* 150 (2): 662–71. https://doi.org/10.1210/en.2008-0598.

Smedegaard, S., U. Kampmann, P. G. Ovesen, H. Støvring, and N. Rittig. 2023. "Whey protein premeal lowers postprandial glucose concentrations in adults compared with water-the effect of timing, dose, and metabolic status: a systematic review and meta-analysis." *Am J Clin Nutr* 118 (2): 391–405. https://doi.org/10.1016/j.ajcnut.2023.05.012.

Sousa, Gabriela TD, Fábio S Lira, José C Rosa, Erick P de Oliveira, Lila M Oyama, Ronaldo V Santos, and Gustavo D Pimentel. 2012. "Dietary whey protein lessens several risk factors for metabolic diseases: a review." *Lipids Health Dis* 11: 1–9.

Staples, A. W., N. A. Burd, D. W. D. West, K. D. Currie, P. J. Atherton, D. R. Moore, M. J. Rennie, M. J. MacDonald, S. K. Baker, and S. M. Phillips. 2011. "Carbohydrate does not augment exercise-induced protein accretion versus protein alone." *Med Sci Sports Exerc* 43 (7): 1154–61. https://doi.org/10.1249/MSS.0b013e31820751cb. https://www.scopus.com/inward/record.uri?eid=2-s2.0-79959861066&doi=10.1249%2fMSS.0b013e31820751cb&partnerID=40&md5=8bb6941aff523ddca1e38d695a935f63.

Tang, J. E., D. R. Moore, G. W. Kujbida, M. A. Tarnopolsky, and S. M. Phillips. 2009. "Ingestion of whey hydrolysate, casein, or soy protein isolate: effects on mixed muscle protein synthesis at rest and following resistance exercise in young men." *J Appl Physiol (1985)* 107 (3): 987–92. https://doi.org/10.1152/japplphysiol.00076.2009.

Tipton, K. D., T. A. Elliott, M. G. Cree, S. E. Wolf, A. P. Sanford, and R. R. Wolfe. 2004. "Ingestion of casein and whey proteins result in muscle anabolism after resistance exercise." *Med Sci Sports Exerc* 36 (12): 2073–81. https://doi.org/10.1249/01.mss.0000147582.99810.c5.

Trommelen, J., B. B. Groen, H. M. Hamer, L. C. de Groot, and L. J. van Loon. 2015. "MECHANISMS IN ENDOCRINOLOGY: Exogenous insulin does not increase muscle protein synthesis rate when administered systemically: a systematic review." *Eur J Endocrinol* 173 (1): R25–34. https://doi.org/10.1530/eje-14-0902.

Walzem, RL, CJ Dillard, and J Bruce German. 2002. "Whey components: millennia of evolution create functionalities for mammalian nutrition: what we know and what we may be overlooking." *Crit Rev Food Sci Nutr* 42 (4): 353–75.

West, D. W., N. A. Burd, V. G. Coffey, S. K. Baker, L. M. Burke, J. A. Hawley, D. R. Moore, T. Stellingwerff, and S. M. Phillips. 2011. "Rapid aminoacidemia enhances myofibrillar protein synthesis and anabolic intramuscular signaling responses after resistance exercise." *Am J Clin Nutr* 94 (3): 795–803. https://doi.org/10.3945/ajcn.111.013722.

Wilkinson, D. J., S. S. I. Bukhari, B. E. Phillips, M. C. Limb, J. Cegielski, M. S. Brook, D. Rankin, W. K. Mitchell, H. Kobayashi, J. P. Williams, J. Lund, P. L. Greenhaff, K. Smith, and P. J. Atherton. 2018. "Effects of leucine-enriched essential amino acid and whey protein bolus dosing upon skeletal muscle protein synthesis at rest and after exercise in older women." *Clin Nutr* 37 (6 Pt A): 2011–21. https://doi.org/10.1016/j.clnu.2017.09.008.

Wirunsawanya, K., S. Upala, V. Jaruvongvanich, and A. Sanguankeo. 2018. "Whey protein supplementation improves body composition and cardiovascular risk factors in overweight and obese patients: a systematic review and meta-analysis." *J Am Coll Nutr* 37 (1): 60–70. https://doi.org/10.1080/07315724.2017.1344591. https://www.scopus.com/inward/record.uri?eid=2-s2.0-85032690652&doi=10.1080%2f07315724.2017.1344591&partnerID=40&md5=0c97d2a82dc0d39615917137ecfc342f.

Witard, O. C., S. R. Jackman, L. Breen, K. Smith, A. Selby, and K. D. Tipton. 2014a. "Myofibrillar muscle protein synthesis rates subsequent to a meal in response to increasing doses of whey protein at rest and after resistance exercise." *Am J Clin Nutr* 99 (1): 86–95. https://doi.org/10.3945/ajcn.112.055517.

Witard, Oliver C, Sarah R Jackman, Leigh Breen, Kenneth Smith, Anna Selby, and Kevin D Tipton. 2014b. "Myofibrillar muscle protein synthesis rates subsequent to a meal in response to increasing doses of whey protein at rest and after resistance exercise." *Am J Clin Nutr* 99 (1): 86–95.

Woods, Stephen C. 2004. "Gastrointestinal satiety signals I. An overview of gastrointestinal signals that influence food intake." *Am J Physiol Gastrointest Liver Physiol* 286 (1): G7–G13.

Wycherley, T. P., J. D. Buckley, M. Noakes, P. M. Clifton, and G. D. Brinkworth. 2013. "Comparison of the effects of weight loss from a high-protein versus standard-protein energy-restricted diet on strength and aerobic capacity in overweight and obese men." *Eur J Nutr* 52 (1): 317–25. https://doi.org/10.1007/s00394-012-0338-0.

Wycherley, Thomas P, Lisa J Moran, Peter M Clifton, Manny Noakes, and Grant D Brinkworth. 2012. "Effects of energy-restricted high-protein, low-fat compared with standard-protein, low-fat diets: a meta-analysis of randomized controlled trials." *Am J Clin Nutr* 96 (6): 1281–98.

Yang, Y., L. Breen, N. A. Burd, A. J. Hector, T. A. Churchward-Venne, A. R. Josse, M. A. Tarnopolsky, and S. M. Phillips. 2012. "Resistance exercise enhances myofibrillar protein synthesis with graded intakes of whey protein in older men." *Br J Nutr* 108 (10): 1780–8. https://doi.org/10.1017/s0007114511007422.

18 Use of Whey Protein in Children with Autism

Ana Maria Castejon, Jordan Ashley Spaw, Irina Rozenfeld, Nurit Sheinberg, Patrick Hardigan, Richard Deth, and Jimmy Gutman

ABBREVIATIONS

ABC	Aberrant Behavior Checklist
ADI-R	Autism Diagnostic Interview, Revised
ADOS	Autism Diagnostic Observation Schedule
ASD	Autism spectrum disorder
BCM7	Seven-amino acid peptide beta casomorphin-7
BV	Biological value
CARS	Childhood Autism Rating Scale
CBC	Complete blood count
CBCL	Child Behavior Checklist
CMP	Comprehensive metabolic panel
CRWP	Cysteine-rich whey protein
EAAT3	Excitatory amino acid transporter-3
GF/CF	Gluten-free/casein-free
GSH	Glutathione (active, reduced form)
GSSG	Glutathione (inactive, oxidized form)
MSEL	Mullen Scales of Early Learning
NAC	N-acetylcysteine
PLS-5	Preschool Language Scale, 5th edition
RBS-R	Repetitive behaviors using the Repetitive Behavior Scale, Revised
ROS	Reactive oxygen species
RRBI	Restricted and repetitive behaviors and interests
SAH	S-adenosylhomocysteine
SAM	S-adenosylmethionine
SCQ	Social Communication Questionnaire
SIDS	Sudden infant death syndrome
SNP	Single nucleotide polymorphism
SRS	Social Responsiveness Scale
tGSH	Total glutathione (reduced + oxidized)
VABS-II	Vineland Adaptive Behavior Scale, 2nd edition

AUTISM AND OXIDATIVE STRESS AND GLUTATHIONE

Autism is a complex neurodevelopmental disorder that affects 1 in 36 children in the United States, with four times as many males diagnosed as females (Maenner et al. 2023). The exact etiology remains undetermined. The spectrum of impairments noted in this disorder has led to the umbrella

DOI: 10.1201/9781003597926-18

term "autism spectrum disorder" (ASD). This condition is associated with "deficits in social interaction and communication together with restricted and repetitive behaviors and interests" (American Psychiatric Association 2013). A myriad of behavioral assessments are used for diagnosis, with the Autism Diagnostic Observation Schedule (ADOS) (Lord et al. 1989, 2000) considered the gold standard. Despite extensive research, researchers have not identified a definite biomarker for diagnosis or treatment (Loke, Hannan, and Craig 2015). Early intervention programs and special schooling are the most effective treatments for those with this neurodevelopmental disorder, and although outcomes of early intervention vary, all children benefit (Alabdali, Al-Ayadhi, and El-Ansary 2014).

The heterogeneity of ASD can be observed in the neurologic, metabolic, and immunologic systems, etc. (Ratajczak 2011; Zimmerman et al. 2005). Therefore, it is speculated to be a multifactorial disorder involving epigenetics, genetics, and environmental factors. Oxidative stress may serve as a link between the different systems affected by this condition (Zimmerman et al. 2005). Oxidative stress occurs when there is an imbalance between reactive oxygen species (ROS) and/or reactive nitrogen species and antioxidant capacity. Glutathione, the major endogenous antioxidant, is the body's primary defense against damage from ROS and is low in those with ASD (Chauhan, Audhya, and Chauhan 2012; Geier et al. 2010; Geier et al. 2009; Ghanizadeh et al. 2012; James et al. 2004, 2006, 2008; Kern and Jones 2006; Zoroglu et al. 2004).

Most importantly, children with ASD also have decreased levels of total glutathione and the reduced or active form of glutathione (James et al. 2004; James et al. 2006). Cysteine, the rate-limiting amino acid in glutathione synthesis, is significantly decreased in ASD relative to control children, suggesting that glutathione synthesis is insufficient to maintain redox homeostasis (James et al. 2004). These significant decreases in total and free plasma glutathione and the redox ratio (active reduced: inactive oxidized glutathione) in children with ASD are of particular concern due to the importance of this system for normal cell function.

Glutathione (GSH) is a ubiquitous intracellular peptide found in all mammalian tissues, performing many diverse functions, including detoxification, antioxidant defense, immune function regulation, and modulation of cell proliferation (Meister and Anderson 1983; Vašková et al. 2023; Lu 2013; Grimble 2006; Aw 2003).

Raising systemic glutathione levels in humans is poorly achieved through the ingestion of glutathione itself (Allen and Bradley 2011). Elevating GSH levels is most efficiently achieved through the use of glutathione precursors, notably containing the limiting amino acid for glutathione synthesis, cysteine (Forman, Zhang, and Rinna 2009). The most commonly used precursor is N-acetylcysteine (NAC) (Raghu et al. 2021). A lesser-known cysteine-delivery vehicle is the use of undenatured whey protein isolate (Ross et al. 2012).

NAC (N-acetylcysteine) is a synthetic derivative of the amino acid L-cysteine and a precursor of GSH. It has been used for several decades as a mucolytic and as an antidote to acetaminophen poisoning. Its toxicity depends on the route of administration and high dosages (Tenório et al. 2021). Arguably, it is the most widely used "antioxidant" in experimental cell and animal biology, as well as clinical studies (Pedre et al. 2021).

Cysteine-rich undenatured whey protein is a byproduct of cheese production (El-Sayed and Chase 2011), where the whey is handled at low temperatures and vigorous mechanical agitation is avoided, both of which can denature the three-dimensional configuration of the proteins (El-Sayed and Chase 2011). Loss of this native configuration negates the glutathione precursor effects of these proteins (Oka et al. 2022). The proteins predominantly acting as GSH precursors are lactoferrin, beta-lactoglobulin, alpha-lactalbumin, serum albumin, and immunoglobulin, all rich in cysteine and cystine moieties (Bounous and Gold 1991).

Unlike NAC, undenatured whey protein also delivers a rich source of protein nutrition. Containing all of the human essential amino acids, it carries the highest BV (Biological Value) of any known edible protein (Hoffman and Falvo 2004). Although a bovine milk protein, the isolate contains only negligible amounts of lactose or casein (Gangurde et al. 2011), both of which have been suspected of exacerbating autistic behavioral abnormalities (Quan et al. 2022; Kushak et al. 2011).

Immunocal® is a cysteine-rich non-denatured whey protein isolate (CRWP) that has been successfully used in several human clinical trials including cancer treatment (Tozer et al. 2008), sports performance (Lands, Grey, and Smountas 1999), lung disease (Grey et al. 2003), Parkinson's disease (Tosukhowong et al. 2016), and, notably, autistic spectrum disorder (Castejon et al. 2021). It appears in the American PDR (PDR.net 2023) and is described as a "glutathione precursor" (PDR .net 2023).

In a study examining the clinical and biochemical effects of Immunocal in Parkinson's disease patients, a statistically significant increase in both GSH and reduced/oxidized GSH levels was demonstrated after 6 months of ingesting 20 g protein/day (Tosukhowong et al. 2016). A McGill University team addressing oxidative stress in cystic fibrosis patients also used Immunocal 20 g/day vs. placebo for 3 months. After supplementation, they documented a 46.6% increase from baseline ($P < 0.05$) in lymphocytic GSH levels compared to placebo (Grey et al. 2003). Similar findings were observed in a trial looking at muscular performance in healthy young adults. Besides increases in peak power and work capacity, lymphocyte glutathione levels increased in the Immunocal-treated group (35.5%, $p = 0.02$) compared to the placebo group (Lands, Grey, and Smountas 1999). The use of whey protein as a functional food with many medical benefits continues to grow (Patel 2015).

CLINICAL STUDY EVALUATING THE EFFECTIVENESS OF CYSTEINE-RICH WHEY PROTEIN IN AUTISM

Although prior nutritional interventions addressing antioxidant capacity have successfully improved glutathione levels, the association between these changes and autistic behavior has been less compelling. Given that pharmacological alternatives targeting only specific comorbid conditions are limited and carry a significant burden of side effects, further studies utilizing complementary and alternative medicine for the treatment of ASD are justified.

A double-blind, placebo-controlled study was conducted to explore the effectiveness of a 90-day intervention with a nutritional supplement containing CRWP in treating ASD core behavioral symptoms and elevating glutathione levels in 3–5-year-old preschool children with ASD. The study also investigated whether improvements in intracellular glutathione correlated with behavioral changes. A comprehensive and age-specific behavioral assessment battery utilizing eight different tests was used to assess which core areas of ASD could be impacted by this intervention.

In brief, the effectiveness of a 90-day CRWP (Immunocal) intervention in children with ASD examined whether intracellular reduced and oxidized glutathione improvements correlated with behavioral changes. The study design was a double-blind, randomized, placebo-controlled trial in 3–5-year-old preschool children with confirmed ASD. The intervention group received daily CRWP (powder form: 0.5 g/kg for children <20 kg or a 10-g dose for those >20 kg), while the placebo group received rice protein, mimicking the protein load in the intervention group. White blood cell glutathione levels and ASD behaviors were assessed using different behavioral scales, such as the Childhood Autism Rating Scale, Preschool Language Scale, Social Communication Questionnaire, Child Behavior Checklist, and the parent-rated Vineland Adaptive Behavior Scale, 2nd edition (VABS-II) (Castejon et al. 2021).

A total of 40 participants completed the 90-day treatment period (CRWP, 21; placebo, 19). At baseline, the participants' demographic and diagnostic characteristics were similar across both groups. The average age of participants in both groups was 3.9 years. Most participants were male (placebo = 83% and CRWP = 90%), and a wide variety of races were represented in the study. There were no significant differences in the medications/supplements taken by the placebo or CRWP groups.

At baseline, average scores across groups were similar for most behavioral assessments; however, some differences were noted. In the VABS-II, the placebo group exhibited less severe clinical manifestations of ASD, and in the Child Behavior Checklist, the CRWP group had higher stress problem T-scores.

At baseline, the levels of total glutathione, oxidized glutathione, reduced glutathione, and the ratio of oxidized to reduced glutathione were measured in participants' leukocytes. There were no significant differences between groups in any of the glutathione measurements taken at baseline (Table 18.1).

BEHAVIORAL ASSESSMENTS AND GLUTATHIONE MEASUREMENTS

When comparing baseline to follow-up changes in the CRWP ($n = 21$) and placebo ($n = 19$) groups, behavioral improvements were seen in both groups; however, the CRWP group improved in more areas than the placebo group. No significant differences were observed after three months in the CARS, PLS, SCQ, or CBC behavioral scales between baseline and follow-up in the two groups (Δ vs. Δ). However, the parent-rated behavioral assessment VABS-II demonstrated significant improvements in the CRWP group compared to the placebo group in the composite score ($p = 0.03$). Further, significant changes were observed in multiple domains/sub-domains representing different aspects of adaptive behaviors associated with ASD symptoms in the intervention group.

Specifically, the socialization domain ($p = 0.04$), domestic daily living skills ($p = 0.05$), maladaptive behavior domain ($p = 0.04$), and internalizing subdomain ($p = 0.02$) all showed significant improvements with the CRWP supplementation after three months.

Higher increases in total and reduced glutathione were observed from baseline to follow-up in the CRWP group (Figure 18.1). In contrast, no significant changes in total, reduced, or oxidized glutathione levels were observed in the placebo group. After the 90-day supplementation, changes in both total ($p = 0.02$) and reduced glutathione ($p = 0.04$) in the CRWP group were significantly higher than changes in the placebo group (Figure 18.1). However, behavior improvements observed using the VABS-II were not significantly correlated with changes in glutathione levels.

SUB-ANALYSIS OF THE CRWP GROUP

Because a significant number of participants in the CRWP group showed significant improvements in adaptive behavior as measured by the VABS-II, researchers explored the common characteristics in this group of responders. Changes of >2 points or 1 SD in VABS-II composite scores were used to discriminate "responders." Out of 19 participants who completed behavioral assessments, 12 were identified as responders, compared to only 5 of the 21 who completed behavior assessments in the placebo group ($p = 0.03$). However, researchers found no difference between the two groups when comparing changes in total glutathione levels (responders $p = 0.05$, non-responders $p = 0.06$).

Further analysis of the VABS-II was used to compare the behavioral changes in the responders vs. the non-responders in the intervention group (Figure 18.2). The responders showed a much larger improvement in the given domains/sub-domains of the VABS-II, including the overall adaptive behavior composite score ($p<0.0001$ and $p = 0.0003$ compared to non-responders and placebo, respectively). In addition, researchers noted significant differences in the communication domain score, with differences in the receptive V-scale score and the expressive V-scale score, as well as in the daily living skills domain score, specifically in the personal V-scale score. Responder improvements were also noted in the socialization domain score, with significant differences in play and leisure time, coping skills, and the motor skills domain score, including the gross motor score. Moreover, the responders' group showed decreases in internalizing, externalizing, and maladaptive behavior scores (Table 18.2). It is important to highlight that no differences were found in baseline composite VABS-II scores between responders and non-responders ($p = 0.24$). These results show a favorable effect of CRWP on a range of behavior measures in those who responded to this intervention.

TABLE 18.1
Change in Glutathione Levels from Caseline to Follow-Up in Placebo and CRWP Groups

Glutathione Levels: (nM/10^5 WBC)	Placebo (Mean ± SEM)				CRWP (Mean ± SEM)				Baseline Placebo vs. Baseline Intervention	P-Value of Δ vs. Δ
	Baseline (n = 24)	12 Weeks (n = 16)	Δ	P-Value	Baseline (n = 20)	12 Weeks (n = 20)	Δ	P-Value		
tGSH	104.2 ± 15.8	88.0 ± 12.8	−16.22	0.50	113.1 ± 16.1	166.7 ± 37.2	53.6	0.17	0.77	0.02*
GSSG	10.9 ± 1.57	8.99 ± 1.36	−1.86	0.78	7.95 ± 1.34	12.88 ± 2.70	4.93	0.22	0.14	0.12
GSH	82.5 ± 13.9	66.3 ± 9.8	−16.16	0.53	97.2 ± 15.0	136.0 ± 34.4	38.8	0.47	0.13	0.04*

*$p < 0.05$.
CRWP: cysteine-rich whey protein; WBC: white blood cells; SEM: standard error of the mean; tGSH: total glutathione; GSSG: glutathione (inactive, oxidized form); GSH: glutathione (active, reduced form). Values are mean ± SEM.

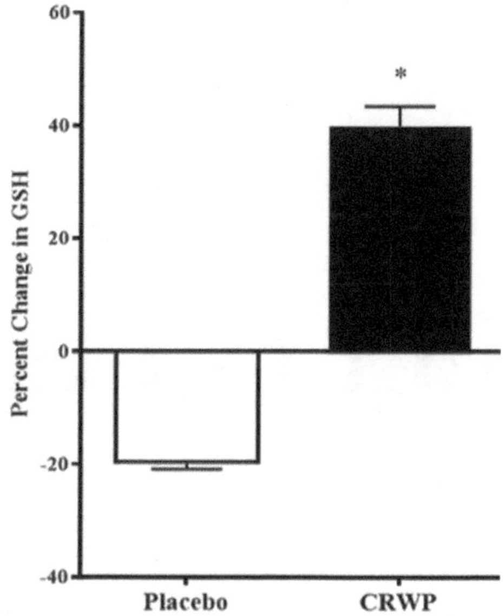

FIGURE 18.1 Percent change from baseline of reduced glutathione levels in placebo and CRWP groups. *p <0.05. CRWP = cysteine-rich whey protein.

It is important to highlight that no serious adverse events were reported in either treatment group. Compliance, assessed by the weight of the canisters before and after treatments, showed no significant differences between the groups (90.5% used in the placebo group vs. 89.9% in the CRWP group; p = 0.91).

Both groups showed significant improvements from baseline to follow-up behavioral score assessments in some tests. This was expected, as all children had access to high-standard care during the study, consisting of preschool centers and therapies providing special services to this population. However, when comparing the magnitude of changes between the two groups after the 3-month trial period (Δ vs. Δ), the CRWP group showed significant behavioral improvements with medium-large effect sizes in children's adaptive behavioral skills as measured by the VABS-II. This highlights the importance of randomized, double-blind, placebo-controlled studies in revealing accurate improvements with specific interventions. It is worth noting that children in the intervention group had to improve more than the placebo group for significant outcomes to be observed, as their baseline values indicated they were more severely affected by the disorder at the start of the trial.

Several behavioral improvements in children with ASD have been associated with nutritional interventions. NAC supplementation was associated with decreased irritability using the Aberrant Behavior Checklist (ABC) and reduced repetitive behaviors using the Repetitive Behavior Scale-Revised (RBS-R) and Social Responsiveness Scale (SRS) assessments in a pilot study (Hardan et al. 2012). In contrast, Wink et al. (2016) found no behavioral improvements with a similar study design. Vitamin B6 supplementation was associated with positive changes in sleep and gastrointestinal issues in a randomized, double-blind, placebo-controlled 3-month study in 20 children with ASD using a parent-rated scale (Adams and Holloway 2004). Additionally, this study mirrored the results of another study (Frye, Melnyk, et al. 2013), which showed significant increases in many of the same VABS-II scores after supplementation with methylcobalamin plus folinic acid. Each study used a clinician, parent, or a combination of scales to assess changes in behavior. The variety of scales and study designs used to assess behavioral changes makes it difficult to compare results with most previous studies using other nutritional interventions.

Twelve out of 20 children (60%) were identified as responders to the intervention due to a greater than two-point improvement in VABS-II overall adaptive composite score. Chatham et al. (2018)

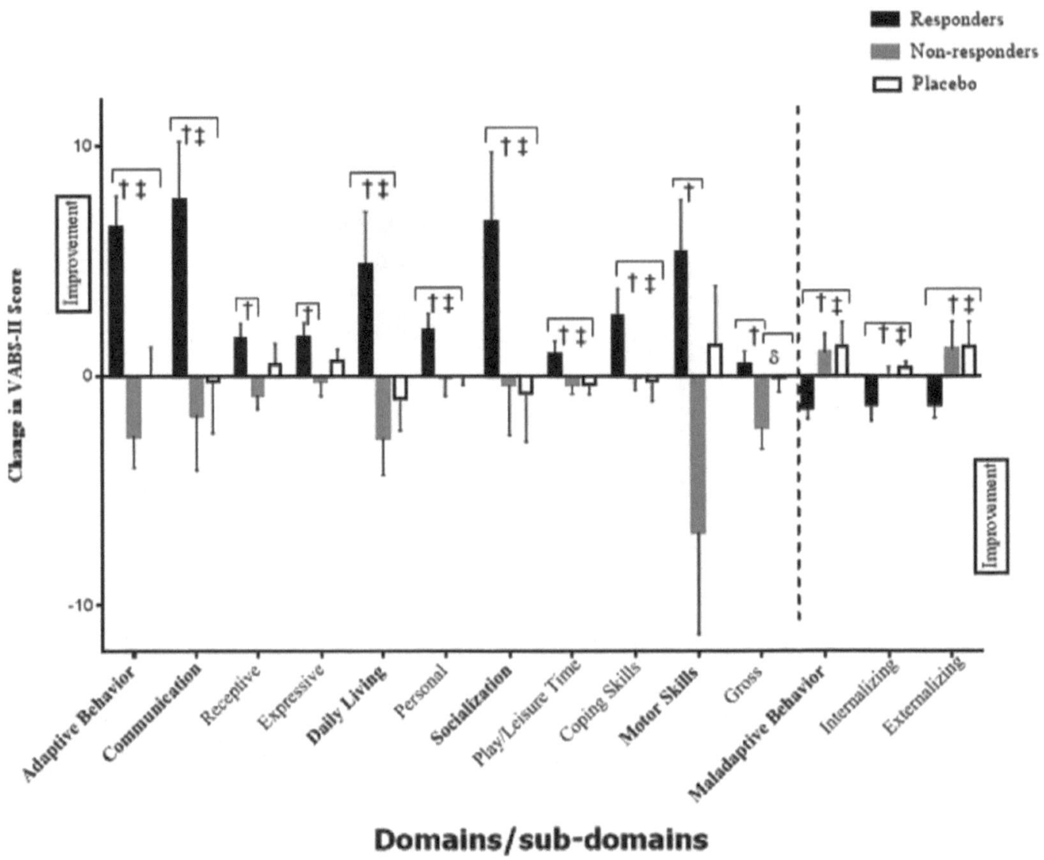

FIGURE 18.2 Significant differences in various domains/sub-domains of VABS-II in the responder, non-responder and placebo groups † significant difference between responder and non-responder groups. ‡ significant difference between responder and placebo groups. δ significant difference between non-responder and placebo groups. One-tail t-tests were utilized with significance reached at $p<0.05$. VABS-II = Vineland Adaptive Behavior Scale, 2nd edition.

showed that the minimal clinically significant difference in children with ASD ranged from 2 to 3.75 points, supporting our approach to identifying these children as responders.

The study also confirmed significant improvements in the glutathione levels of children with ASD using a nutritional approach known to increase glutathione biosynthesis. Children assigned to the supplement experienced a 40% increase in the reduced form of glutathione because this supplement provides a natural source of cysteine, the rate-limiting step in glutathione biosynthesis, leading to increased intracellular levels.

Other interventions have demonstrated comparable glutathione increases to those in our CRWP group. The combination of methylcobalamin and folinic acid induced increases of 15% in total glutathione and 20% in reduced glutathione (Frye, Melnyk, et al. 2013), while NAC treatment has demonstrated a 60% increase from baseline (Wink et al. 2016). Targeting glutathione levels is relevant because significant differences in glutathione and its related metabolites have been found in plasma (James et al. 2004, 2006), white blood cells (Ghanizadeh and Moghimi-Sarani 2013; Melnyk et al. 2012), and post-mortem brains (Chauhan, Audhya, and Chauhan 2012; Rose et al. 2012) of participants with ASD. This finding is supported by several genetic variations seen in ASD patients related to the transmethylation/transsulfuration pathway, where glutathione is one of the byproducts (James et al. 2004; James et al. 2006, 2008). The hypothesis that low glutathione levels are related to ASD symptoms has been partially validated, as several treatments targeting this deficiency have been

TABLE 18.2
Changes in VABS-II Scores in Responders, Non-Responders, and Placebo Groups

Vineland Adaptive Behavior Scale	Responders (n = 12)	Non-Responders (n = 7)	Placebo (n = 21)	P-Value Responders vs. Non-Responders	P-Value Responders vs. Placebo
Adaptive Behavior Composite Standard Score	6.5 ± 1.32	−2.86 ± 0.91	0.00 ± 1.25	<0.0001†	0.0003†
Communication Standard Total Score	7.67 ± 2.55	−1.71 ± 2.40	−0.29 ± 2.20	0.008†	0.01†
Receptive V-scale score	1.58 ± 0.69	−0.86 ± 0.59	0.48 ± 0.93	0.01†	0.21
Expressive V-scale score	1.67 ± 0.63	−0.29 ± 0.60	0.62 ± 0.54	0.03†	0.08
Written V-scale score	0.64 ± 0.47	0.29 ± 0.52	−0.29 ± 0.49	0.32	0.12
Daily Living Skills Standard Total Score	4.83 ± 2.31	−2.7 ± 1.6	−1.00 ± 1.39	0.008†	0.007†
Personal V-scale score	2 ± 0.71	−0.14 ± 0.77	−0.05 ± 0.36	0.03†	0.004†
Domestic V-scale score	−0.08 ± 0.57	−0.71 ± 0.60	0.05 ± 0.63	0.23	0.45
Community V-scale score	0.33 ± 0.45	−0.43 ± 0.62	−0.05 ± 0.51	0.19	0.20
Socialization Standard Total Score	6.67 ± 3.04	-0.43 ± 2.17	−0.81 ± 2.06	0.04†	0.02†
Interpersonal Relationships V-scale score	0.83 ± 0.82	0.29 ± 0.57	−0.38 ± 0.59	0.30	0.12
Play and Leisure Time V-scale score	0.92 ± 0.58	−0.43 ± 0.37	−0.38 ± 0.44	0.03†	0.04†
Coping Skills V-scale score	2.58 ± 1.18	−0.15 ± 0.51	−0.24 ± 0.89	0.03†	0.04†
Motor Skills Standard Total Score	5.33 ± 2.32	−6.86 ± 4.4	1.33 ± 2.56	0.02†	0.05
Gross V-scale score	0.5 ± 0.57	−2.29 ± 0.92	−0.14 ± 0.60δ	0.01†	0.09
Fine V-scale score	1.33 ± 0.54	0 ± 0.62	0.57 ± 0.39	0.07	0.13
Maladaptive Behavior Total V-Scale Score	−1.42 ± 0.47	1.0 ± 0.84	1.26 ± 1.05	0.01†	0.003†
Internalizing V-scale score	−1.33 ± 0.64	0 ± 0.37	0.37 ± 0.22	0.04†	0.0003†
Externalizing V-scale score	−1.33 ± 0.51	1.17 ± 1.20	1.26 ± 1.08	0.02†	0.008†

†p < 0.05, one-tail t-test.
δSignificant difference between placebo and non-responder subgroup where p < 0.05.
VABS-II, Vineland Adaptive Behavior Scale, 2nd edition. Values are mean ± SEM.

proven to be efficacious at modifying behavioral symptoms in children with this condition (Frye, Sequeira, et al. 2013).

Significant limitations of this study include the small sample size, narrow age sample, and short treatment intervention. Future studies, including a broader age group and using specific behavioral assessments and scales, are warranted. It would also be pertinent to include a cohort of neurotypical children in a similar study to compare any changes in glutathione levels and behaviors in that population with those of children with ASD.

INHIBITION OF CYSTEINE TRANSPORT BY CASEIN AND GLUTEN-DERIVED OPIOID PEPTIDES: IMPLICATIONS IN ASD

Cow milk-derived whey proteins are well known for their high content of the sulfur amino acid cysteine, but the absorption and systemic availability of this important nutrient are restricted by an opioid peptide released upon digestion of the milk curd protein beta casein. Specifically, the seven-amino-acid peptide beta casomorphin-7 (BCM7; Tyr-Pro-Phe-Pro-Gly-Pro-Ile) inhibits cellular cysteine uptake mediated by excitatory amino acid transporter-3 (EAAT3), also designated as EAAC1 in mice (Trivedi et al. 2014). While other members of the EAAT family transport glutamate and aspartate, EAAT3 preferentially transports cysteine and is expressed by gastrointestinal (GI) epithelial cells, especially in the distal ileum, as well as by neurons and immune cells. As a result, BCM7 can exert significant effects on antioxidant status, brain function, and inflammatory conditions.

Trivedi et al. (2014) demonstrated dose-dependent BCM7-mediated inhibition of cysteine uptake in GI-derived Caco-2 cells and SH-SY5Y neuronal cells, which paralleled inhibition by morphine and was blocked by a mu-opioid receptor antagonist. Inhibition of cysteine uptake was associated with decreased glutathione (GSH) and GSH/GSSG, as well as a lower ratio of S-adenosylmethionine (SAM) to S-adenosylhomocysteine (SAH), indicative of increased oxidative stress and impaired methylation, respectively. These actions were further accompanied by significant changes in the expression of redox-related genes as well as substantial effects on DNA methylation status, including gene pathways related to gastrointestinal disease and inflammation (Trivedi et al. 2015). Taken together, these actions of milk-derived BCM7 indicate an important potential influence on cellular metabolism and genomic regulation, with special importance for early infant development when milk is the sole or primary source of nutrition.

The discovery of BCM7-mediated inhibition of cysteine uptake can be traced back to the groundbreaking studies carried out in Norway by researchers who observed behavioral improvements in ASD subjects upon administration of a gluten/casein-free (GF/CF) diet accompanied by a decrease in urinary excretion of peptides (Knivsberg et al. 1990). Cessation of the GF/CF diet resulted in worsening behaviors and resumption of excessive urinary peptides. Reichelt and Knivsberg (2003) later reported that BCM7 and a similar opioid peptide released upon digestion of gluten, gliadinomorphin-7 (YPQPQPF; GM7), were among the elevated urinary peptides found in the ASD subjects. Since BCM7 and GM7 were food-derived, this prescient observation suggested that an ASD-associated "leaky gut" allowed systemic exposure to these opioid peptides (Reichelt and Knivsberg 2003). However, it should be noted that Dettmer et al. (2007) failed to identify BCM7 or GM7 in the urine of autistic subjects.

The amount of BCM7 released from bovine beta casein depends on the nature of the amino acid immediately following its sequence. A single nucleotide polymorphism (SNP) specifies either a histidine or a proline residue, denoted as A1 beta casein or A2 beta casein, respectively. Since the proline side chain is cyclic, it impairs protein cleavage at this locus, resulting in very little BCM7 being released from A2 beta casein compared to A1 beta casein. Consistent with this relationship, consumption of milk from homozygous A2/A2 cows results in an approximately twofold higher increase in plasma GSH compared to mixed A1/A2 (Deth et al. 2016), illustrating a crucial role for BCM7 in regulating GI absorption of whey protein-derived cysteine, whose availability is rate-limiting for GSH synthesis. Notably, the action of milk-derived BCM7 can also restrict cysteine absorption from other proteins consumed in the same meal.

The potential functional consequences of the inhibition of cysteine uptake by BCM7 and GM7 are broad and incompletely appreciated, reflecting the regulatory roles of redox status and methylation, including their influence on inflammation and immunity. Lower cysteine and GSH levels promote oxidative stress, and the folate and vitamin B12-dependent enzyme methionine synthase is highly sensitive to oxidative stress, which may account for BCM7/GM7 effects on DNA methylation and gene expression (Trivedi et al. 2014). Low GSH and oxidative stress increase the activity of the NLRP3 inflammasome (Bourgonje et al. 2021), while recent evidence indicates that cysteine-dependent persulfidation is crucial for terminating its cytokine-producing activity (Takeda et al. 2023). Thus, restriction of cysteine absorption could increase the risk of inflammation, not only in the GI tract but throughout the body.

Autoimmunity is associated with a Th2 pattern of CD4+ T-cell cytokine production, and autoimmune disorders have been linked to gluten and casein consumption and/or reversal by a GF/CF diet (Bangarusamy et al. 2021; Vojdani et al. 2003). Interleukin-1 (IL-4) is a key Th2 cytokine whose transcription is regulated by methylation of its promoter region, in an age-dependent manner reciprocal to that of interferon-gamma (IFN-γ), with IL-4/IFN-γ being normally higher in early development (Xia et al. 2016). Consumption of A1 milk was associated with higher IL-4 levels and inflammation in GI tissues (Ul Haq et al. 2014), while gluten-dependent celiac disease was associated with elevated IFN-γ in children (Björck et al. 2015), but elevated IL-4 in adults (Manavalan et al. 2010). Together, these findings indicate abnormal epigenetic regulation of cytokines, which might be related to redox and methylation consequences of BCM7/GM7.

THE EFFECT OF OTHER PROTEINS: CASEIN AND GLUTEN

This chapter has discussed the relationship between cysteine availability and its correlation with multiple physiological processes influencing cellular metabolism and genomic regulation, especially during early infant development.

Numerous studies have confirmed the benefits of a GF/CF diet, not only in autism but also in a variety of other conditions, as well as its widespread adoption as a health-promoting lifestyle choice (Poslt Königová et al. 2023; Whiteley et al. 2012). The link to cysteine transport arose because cysteine and GSH levels are markedly lower in ASD subjects (James et al. 2006), leading to the hypothesis that the GF/CF benefit might somehow improve cysteine availability. Thus, the health-promoting benefits of a GF/CF diet can, in large part, be attributed to an increased availability of cysteine due to avoidance of foods that release opioid peptides during their digestion and act to inhibit cysteine absorption. Moreover, low cysteine levels in ASD individuals may make them more sensitive to the inhibitory effects of BCM7 and GM7. Furthermore, since diet-derived urinary peptides decreased with a GF/CF diet, the ASD-associated "leaky gut" can tentatively be ascribed to a damaging effect of decreased cysteine on the barrier function of GI epithelial cells, most likely associated with inflammation.

Further research is needed to prove that GF/CF diets are effective in ASD and to determine if such dietary restrictions are more effective in those showing low cysteine and GSH levels.

MINI DICTIONARY OF TERMS

- **Aberrant Behavior Checklist:** A behavioral instrument that evaluates five domains: irritability, social withdrawal, stereotyped behavior, hyperactivity, and inappropriate speech. This scale is filled out by a caregiver.
- **Biological value:** Measures the proportion of absorbed protein from a given food and how much is incorporated into other proteins in the body.
- **Maladaptive behavior domain (Vineland):** Includes a child's problem behaviors in two forms: internalizing and externalizing behaviors. Internalizing behaviors are negative and focused inward, such as fearfulness, social withdrawal, and concentration problems. Externalizing behaviors are negative towards the environment, such as bullying, physical aggression, and disobeying rules.
- **Redox-related genes:** Genes that can regulate the expression of antioxidants under oxidative stress conditions.
- **Vineland Adaptive Behavior Scale:** A standardized test used to diagnose intellectual and developmental disabilities, autism, and developmental delays.

SUMMARY POINTS

- Lower antioxidant capacity, specifically lower GSH levels, is a common finding in ASD.
- Oxidative stress can be a major factor in many manifestations of ASD, such as abnormal methylation, inflammation, and immunity.
- GSH levels rely on cysteine availability, and dietary manipulations aimed at improving antioxidant capacity are centered on cysteine levels.
- A cysteine-rich whey protein supplement showed an effective increase in intracellular levels of GSH as well as some improvements in autistic behavior.
- Opioid peptide released upon digestion of the milk curd protein beta casein can decrease cysteine availability, providing a rationale for gluten- and casein-free diets in ASD.

The scientific evidence discussed in this chapter has been reported by Castejon et al. (2021).

ChatGPT was used to generate the abstract of this chapter.

REFERENCES

Adams, James B., and Charles Holloway. 2004. "Pilot study of a moderate dose multivitamin/mineral supplement for children with autistic spectrum disorder." *J Altern Complement Med* 10 (6): 1033–39.

Alabdali, Altaf, Laila Al-Ayadhi, and Afaf El-Ansary. 2014. "Association of social and cognitive impairment and biomarkers in autism spectrum disorders." *J Neuroinflammation* 11: 1–14.

Allen, J., and R. D. Bradley. 2011. "Effects of oral glutathione supplementation on systemic oxidative stress biomarkers in human volunteers." *J Altern Complement Med* 17 (9): 827–33. https://doi.org/10.1089/acm.2010.0716.

American Psychiatric Association, DSMTF, and American Psychiatric Association. 2013. *Diagnostic and Statistical Manual of Mental Disorders: DSM-5*. Vol. 5. Washington, DC: American Psychiatric Association.

Aw, T. Y. 2003. "Cellular redox: a modulator of intestinal epithelial cell proliferation." *News Physiol Sci* 18: 201–4. https://doi.org/10.1152/nips.01448.2003.

Bangarusamy, D. K., A. P. Lakshmanan, S. Al-Zaidan, S. Alabduljabbar, and A. Terranegra. 2021. "Nutriepigenetics: the effect of maternal diet and early nutrition on the pathogenesis of autoimmune diseases." *Minerva Pediatr (Torino)* 73 (2): 98–110. https://doi.org/10.23736/s2724-5276.20.06166-6.

Björck, S., S. R. Lindehammer, M. Fex, and D. Agardh. 2015. "Serum cytokine pattern in young children with screening detected coeliac disease." *Clin Exp Immunol* 179 (2): 230–5. https://doi.org/10.1111/cei.12454.

Bounous, G., and P. Gold. 1991. "The biological activity of undenatured dietary whey proteins: role of glutathione." *Clin Invest Med* 14 (4): 296–309.

Bourgonje, A. R., A. K. Offringa, L. E. van Eijk, A. E. Abdulle, J. L. Hillebrands, P. H. J. van der Voort, H. van Goor, and E. J. van Hezik. 2021. "N-Acetylcysteine and hydrogen sulfide in coronavirus disease 2019." *Antioxid Redox Signal* 35 (14): 1207–25. https://doi.org/10.1089/ars.2020.8247.

Castejon, A. M., J. A. Spaw, I. Rozenfeld, N. Sheinberg, S. Kabot, A. Shaw, P. Hardigan, R. Faillace, and E. E. Packer. 2021. "Improving antioxidant capacity in children with autism: a randomized, double-blind controlled study with cysteine-rich whey protein." *Front Psychiatry* 12: 669089. https://doi.org/10.3389/fpsyt.2021.669089.

Chatham, C. H., K. I. Taylor, Tony Charman, X. Liogier D'Ardhuy, E. Eule, Anegelina Fedele, A. Y. Hardan, E. Loth, L. Murtagh, and M. del Valle Rubido. 2018. "Adaptive behavior in autism: minimal clinically important differences on the Vineland-II." *Autism Res* 11 (2): 270–283.

Chauhan, Abha, Tapan Audhya, and Ved Chauhan. 2012. "Brain region-specific glutathione redox imbalance in autism." *Neurochem Res* 37: 1681–1689.

Deth, R., A. Clarke, J. Ni, and M. Trivedi. 2016. "Clinical evaluation of glutathione concentrations after consumption of milk containing different subtypes of β-casein: results from a randomized, cross-over clinical trial." *Nutr J* 15 (1): 82. https://doi.org/10.1186/s12937-016-0201-x.

Dettmer, K., D. Hanna, P. Whetstone, R. Hansen, and B. D. Hammock. 2007. "Autism and urinary exogenous neuropeptides: development of an on-line SPE-HPLC-tandem mass spectrometry method to test the opioid excess theory." *Anal Bioanal Chem* 388 (8): 1643–51. https://doi.org/10.1007/s00216-007-1301-4.

El-Sayed, M. M., and H. A. Chase. 2011. "Trends in whey protein fractionation." *Biotechnol Lett* 33 (8): 1501–11. https://doi.org/10.1007/s10529-011-0594-8.

Forman, H. J., H. Zhang, and A. Rinna. 2009. "Glutathione: overview of its protective roles, measurement, and biosynthesis." *Mol Aspects Med* 30 (1–2): 1–12. https://doi.org/10.1016/j.mam.2008.08.006.

Frye, Richard E., Stepan Melnyk, George Fuchs, Tyra Reid, Stefanie Jernigan, Oleksandra Pavliv, Amanda Hubanks, David W. Gaylor, Laura Walters, and S. Jill James. 2013. "Effectiveness of methylcobalamin and folinic acid treatment on adaptive behavior in children with autistic disorder is related to glutathione redox status." *Autism Res Treat* 609705: 9. https://doi.org/10.1155/2013/609705

Frye, Richard E., J. M. Sequeira, E. V. Quadros, S. J. James, and D. A. Rossignol. 2013. "Cerebral folate receptor autoantibodies in autism spectrum disorder." *Molecular Psychiatry* 18 (3): 369–381.

Gangurde, Hemant, Pooja S. Patil, Mayur Chordiya, and Nayana S. Baste. 2011. "Whey protein." *Sch Res J* 1: 69. https://doi.org/10.4103/2249-5975.99663.

Geier, David A., Tapan Audhya, Janet K. Kern, and Mark R. Geier. 2010. "Blood mercury levels in autism spectrum disorder: Is there a threshold level?" *Acta Neurobiol Exp* 70 (2): 177–186.

Geier, David A., Janet K. Kern, Carolyn R. Garver, James B. Adams, Tapan Audhya, and Mark R. Geier. 2009. "A prospective study of transsulfuration biomarkers in autistic disorders." *Neurochem Res* 34: 386–393.

Ghanizadeh, A., S. Akhondzadeh, M. Hormozi, A. Makarem, M. Abotorabi-Zarchi, and A. Firoozabadi. 2012. "Glutathione-related factors and oxidative stress in autism, a review." *Curr Med Chem* 19 (23): 4000–4005.

Ghanizadeh, Ahmad, and Ebrahim Moghimi-Sarani. 2013. "A randomized double blind placebo controlled clinical trial of N-Acetylcysteine added to risperidone for treating autistic disorders." *BMC Psychiatry* 13: 1–7.

Grey, Vijaylaxmi, Shawn R. Mohammed, Argyrios A. Smountas, Rasha Bahlool, and Larry C. Lands. 2003. "Improved glutathione status in young adult patients with cystic fibrosis supplemented with whey protein." *Journal of Cystic Fibrosis* 2 (4): 195–98.

Grimble, R. F. 2006. "The effects of sulfur amino acid intake on immune function in humans." *J Nutr* 136 (6 Suppl): 1660s–65s. https://doi.org/10.1093/jn/136.6.1660S.

Hardan, Antonio Y., Lawrence K. Fung, Robin A. Libove, Tetyana V. Obukhanych, Surekha Nair, Leonore A. Herzenberg, Thomas W. Frazier, and Rabindra Tirouvanziam. 2012. "A randomized controlled pilot trial of oral N-acetylcysteine in children with autism." *Biological Psychiatry* 71 (11): 956–61.

Hoffman, J. R., and M. J. Falvo. 2004. "Protein – which is best?" *J Sports Sci Med* 3 (3): 118–30.

James, S. Jill, Paul Cutler, Stepan Melnyk, Stefanie Jernigan, Laurette Janak, David W. Gaylor, and James A. Neubrander. 2004. "Metabolic biomarkers of increased oxidative stress and impaired methylation capacity in children with autism." *Am J Clin Nutr* 80 (6): 1611–17.

James, S. Jill, Stepan Melnyk, Stefanie Jernigan, Mario A. Cleves, Charles H. Halsted, Donna H. Wong, Paul Cutler, Kenneth Bock, Marvin Boris, and J. Jeffrey Bradstreet. 2006. "Metabolic endophenotype and related genotypes are associated with oxidative stress in children with autism." *Am J Med Genet B Neuropsychiatr Genet* 141 (8): 947–56.

Jill James, S., Stepan Melnyk, Stefanie Jernigan, Amanda Hubanks, Shannon Rose, and David W. Gaylor. 2008. "Abnormal transmethylation/transsulfuration metabolism and DNA hypomethylation among parents of children with autism." *J Autism Dev Disord* 38: 1966–75.

Kern, Janet K., and Anne M. Jones. 2006. "Evidence of toxicity, oxidative stress, and neuronal insult in autism." *J Toxicol Environ Health B* 9 (6): 485–99.

Knivsberg, Ann-Mari, Kirsti Wiig, Gunnar Lind, Magne Nødland, et al. 1990. "Dietary intervention in autistic syndromes." *Brain Dysfunction* 3 (5–6): 315–27.

Kushak, R. I., G. Y. Lauwers, H. S. Winter, and T. M. Buie. 2011. "Intestinal disaccharidase activity in patients with autism: effect of age, gender, and intestinal inflammation." *Autism* 15 (3): 285–94. https://doi.org/10.1177/1362361310369142.

Lands, L. C., V. L. Grey, and A. A. Smountas. 1999. "Effect of supplementation with a cysteine donor on muscular performance." *J Appl Physiol (1985)* 87 (4): 1381–5. https://doi.org/10.1152/jappl.1999.87.4.1381.

Loke, Yuk Jing, Anthony John Hannan, and Jeffrey Mark Craig. 2015. "The role of epigenetic change in autism spectrum disorders." *Front Neurol* 6: 107.

Lord, Catherine, Susan Risi, Linda Lambrecht, Edwin H. Cook, Bennett L. Leventhal, Pamela C. DiLavore, Andrew Pickles, and Michael Rutter. 2000. "The autism diagnostic observation schedule—Generic: a standard measure of social and communication deficits associated with the spectrum of autism." *J Autism Dev Disord* 30: 205–223.

Lord, Catherine, Michael Rutter, Susan Goode, Jacquelyn Heemsbergen, Heather Jordan, Lynn Mawhood, and Eric Schopler. 1989. "Austism diagnostic observation schedule: A standardized observation of communicative and social behavior." *J Autism Dev Disord* 19 (2): 185–212.

Lu, S. C. 2013. "Glutathione synthesis." *Biochim Biophys Acta* 1830 (5): 3143–53. https://doi.org/10.1016/j.bbagen.2012.09.008.

Maenner, M. J., Z. Warren, A. R. Williams, E. Amoakohene, A. V. Bakian, D. A. Bilder, M. S. Durkin, R. T. Fitzgerald, S. M. Furnier, M. M. Hughes, C. M. Ladd-Acosta, D. McArthur, E. T. Pas, A. Salinas, A. Vehorn, S. Williams, A. Esler, A. Grzybowski, J. Hall-Lande, R. H. N. Nguyen, K. Pierce, W. Zahorodny, A. Hudson, L. Hallas, K. C. Mancilla, M. Patrick, J. Shenouda, K. Sidwell, M. DiRienzo, J. Gutierrez, M. H. Spivey, M. Lopez, S. Pettygrove, Y. D. Schwenk, A. Washington, and K. A. Shaw. 2023. "Prevalence and characteristics of autism spectrum disorder among children aged 8 years – autism and developmental disabilities monitoring network, 11 sites, United States, 2020." *MMWR Surveill Summ* 72 (2): 1–14. https://doi.org/10.15585/mmwr.ss7202a1.

Manavalan, J. S., L. Hernandez, J. G. Shah, J. Konikkara, A. J. Naiyer, A. R. Lee, E. Ciaccio, M. T. Minaya, P. H. Green, and G. Bhagat. 2010. "Serum cytokine elevations in celiac disease: association with disease presentation." *Hum Immunol* 71 (1): 50–7. https://doi.org/10.1016/j.humimm.2009.09.351.

Meister, A., and M. E. Anderson. 1983. "Glutathione." *Annu Rev Biochem* 52: 711–60. https://doi.org/10.1146/annurev.bi.52.070183.003431.

Melnyk, Stepan, George J Fuchs, Eldon Schulz, Maya Lopez, Stephen G Kahler, Jill J Fussell, Jayne Bellando, Oleksandra Pavliv, Shannon Rose, and Lisa Seidel. 2012. "Metabolic imbalance associated with methylation dysregulation and oxidative damage in children with autism." *J Autism Dev Disord* 42: 367–377.

Oka, D., W. Ono, S. Tamaki, T. Noguchi, and K. Takano. 2022. "Effects of the thermal denaturation degree of a whey protein isolate on the strength of acid milk gels and the dissociation of κ-casein." *J Dairy Res*: 1–5. https://doi.org/10.1017/s0022029922000103.

Patel, Seema. 2015. "Functional food relevance of whey protein: A review of recent findings and scopes ahead." *J Funct Foods* 19: 308–19. https://doi.org/https://doi.org/10.1016/j.jff.2015.09.040. https://www.sciencedirect.com/science/article/pii/S1756464615004570.

Pedre, B., U. Barayeu, D. Ezeriņa, and T. P. Dick. 2021. "The mechanism of action of N-acetylcysteine (NAC): The emerging role of H(2)S and sulfane sulfur species." *Pharmacol Ther* 228: 107916. https://doi.org/10.1016/j.pharmthera.2021.107916.

PDR.net. "Immunocal." Last modified July 12, 2023. https://www.pdr.net/full-prescribing-information/hl/?druglabelid=257.

Poslt Königová, M., M. Sebalo Vňuková, P. Řehořková, M. Anders, and R. Ptáček. 2023. "The effectiveness of gluten-free dietary interventions: a systematic review." *Front Psychol* 14: 1107022. https://doi.org/10.3389/fpsyg.2023.1107022.

Quan, L., X. Xu, Y. Cui, H. Han, R. L. Hendren, L. Zhao, and X. You. 2022. "A systematic review and meta-analysis of the benefits of a gluten-free diet and/or casein-free diet for children with autism spectrum disorder." *Nutr Rev* 80 (5): 1237–46. https://doi.org/10.1093/nutrit/nuab073.

Raghu, G., M. Berk, P. A. Campochiaro, H. Jaeschke, G. Marenzi, L. Richeldi, F. Q. Wen, F. Nicoletti, and P. M. A. Calverley. 2021. "The multifaceted therapeutic role of N-Acetylcysteine (NAC) in disorders characterized by oxidative stress." *Curr Neuropharmacol* 19 (8): 1202–24. https://doi.org/10.2174/1570159x19666201230144109.

Ratajczak, Helen V. 2011. "Theoretical aspects of autism: biomarkers—a review." *J Immunotoxicol* 8 (1): 80–94.

Reichelt, K. L., and A. M. Knivsberg. 2003. "Can the pathophysiology of autism be explained by the nature of the discovered urine peptides?" *Nutr Neurosci* 6 (1): 19–28. https://doi.org/10.1080/1028415021000042839.

Rose, S., S. Melnyk, O. Pavliv, S. Bai, T. G. Nick, R. E. Frye, and S. J. James. 2012. "Evidence of oxidative damage and inflammation associated with low glutathione redox status in the autism brain." *Transl Psychiatry* 2 (7): e134.

Ross, E. K., J. J. Gray, A. N. Winter, and D. A. Linseman. 2012. "Immunocal® and preservation of glutathione as a novel neuroprotective strategy for degenerative disorders of the nervous system." *Recent Pat CNS Drug Discov* 7 (3): 230–5. https://doi.org/10.2174/157488912803252014.

Takeda, H., S. Murakami, Z. Liu, T. Sawa, M. Takahashi, Y. Izumi, T. Bamba, H. Sato, T. Akaike, H. Sekine, and H. Motohashi. 2023. "Sulfur metabolic response in macrophage limits excessive inflammatory response by creating a negative feedback loop." *Redox Biol* 65: 102834. https://doi.org/10.1016/j.redox.2023.102834.

Tenório, Mcds, N. G. Graciliano, F. A. Moura, A. C. M. Oliveira, and M. O. F. Goulart. 2021. "N-Acetylcysteine (NAC): impacts on human health." *Antioxidants (Basel)* 10 (6). https://doi.org/10.3390/antiox10060967.

Tosukhowong, P., C. Boonla, T. Dissayabutra, L. Kaewwilai, S. Muensri, C. Chotipanich, J. Joutsa, J. Rinne, and R. Bhidayasiri. 2016. "Biochemical and clinical effects of Whey protein supplementation in Parkinson's disease: A pilot study." *J Neurol Sci* 367: 162–70. https://doi.org/10.1016/j.jns.2016.05.056.

Tozer, R. G., P. Tai, W. Falconer, T. Ducruet, A. Karabadjian, G. Bounous, J. H. Molson, and W. Dröge. 2008. "Cysteine-rich protein reverses weight loss in lung cancer patients receiving chemotherapy or radiotherapy." *Antioxid Redox Signal* 10 (2): 395–402. https://doi.org/10.1089/ars.2007.1919.

Trivedi, M. S., Nathaniel W. Hodgson, Stephen J. Walker, Geert Trooskens, Vineeth Nair, and Richard C. Deth. 2015. "Epigenetic effects of casein-derived opioid peptides in SH-SY5Y human neuroblastoma cells." *Nutrition & Metabolism* 12 (1): 54. https://doi.org/10.1186/s12986-015-0050-1. https://doi.org/10.1186/s12986-015-0050-1.

Trivedi, M. S., J. S. Shah, S. Al-Mughairy, N. W. Hodgson, B. Simms, G. A. Trooskens, W. Van Criekinge, and R. C. Deth. 2014. "Food-derived opioid peptides inhibit cysteine uptake with redox and epigenetic consequences." *J Nutr Biochem* 25 (10): 1011–8. https://doi.org/10.1016/j.jnutbio.2014.05.004.

Ul Haq, M. R., R. Kapila, R. Sharma, V. Saliganti, and S. Kapila. 2014. "Comparative evaluation of cow β-casein variants (A1/A2) consumption on Th2-mediated inflammatory response in mouse gut." *Eur J Nutr* 53 (4): 1039–49. https://doi.org/10.1007/s00394-013-0606-7.

Vašková, J., L. Kočan, L. Vaško, and P. Perjési. 2023. "Glutathione-related enzymes and proteins: a review." *Molecules* 28 (3). https://doi.org/10.3390/molecules28031447.

Vojdani, A., J. B. Pangborn, E. Vojdani, and E. L. Cooper. 2003. "Infections, toxic chemicals and dietary peptides binding to lymphocyte receptors and tissue enzymes are major instigators of autoimmunity in autism." *Int J Immunopathol Pharmacol* 16 (3): 189–99. https://doi.org/10.1177/039463200301600302.

Whiteley, P., P. Shattock, A. M. Knivsberg, A. Seim, K. L. Reichelt, L. Todd, K. Carr, and M. Hooper. 2012. "Gluten- and casein-free dietary intervention for autism spectrum conditions." *Front Hum Neurosci* 6: 344. https://doi.org/10.3389/fnhum.2012.00344.

Wink, Logan K., Ryan Adams, Zemin Wang, James E. Klaunig, Martin H. Plawecki, David J. Posey, Christopher J. McDougle, and Craig A. Erickson. 2016. "A randomized placebo-controlled pilot study of N-acetylcysteine in youth with autism spectrum disorder." *Molecular Autism* 7: 1–9.

Xia, Y., J. Yang, G. Wang, C. Li, and Q. Li. 2016. "Age-related changes in DNA methylation associated with shifting Th1/Th2 balance." *Inflammation* 39 (6): 1892–903. https://doi.org/10.1007/s10753-016-0425-0.

Zimmerman, Andrew W., Harumi Jyonouchi, Anne M. Comi, Susan L. Connors, Sheldon Milstien, Angeliki Varsou, and Melvyn P. Heyes. 2005. "Cerebrospinal fluid and serum markers of inflammation in autism." *Pediatric Neurol* 33 (3): 195–201.

Zoroglu, S Salih, Ferah Armutcu, Sakir Ozen, Ahmet Gurel, Ercan Sivasli, Ozer Yetkin, and Iclal Meram. 2004. "Increased oxidative stress and altered activities of erythrocyte free radical scavenging enzymes in autism." *Eur Arch Psychiatry Clin Neurosci* 254: 143–147.

19 Fish Protein and Peptides
Impact on Health

Vahid Reza Askari, Ali Ebrahimi Dabagh, and Vafa Baradaran Rahimi

ABBREVIATIONS

ACE	Angiotensin-converting enzyme
ACEI	Angiotensin-converting enzyme inhibitor
BBI	Bowman–Birk inhibitor
BMD	Bone mineral density
CART	Cocaine and amphetamine-regulated transcript
CCK	Cholecystokinin
CHO	Carbohydrate
CRP	C-reactive protein
DHA	Docosahexaenoic acid
DPP-4	Dipeptidylpeptidase-4
DXA	Dual-energy X-ray absorptiometry
EPA	Eicosapentaenoic acid
FBP	Fish bone peptides
FPH	Fish protein hydrolysate
GIP	Gastric inhibitory polypeptide
GLP-1	Glucagon-like peptide-1
IgY	Immunoglobulin Y
MCP-1	Monocyte chemoattractant protein-1
NSAID	Nonsteroidal anti-inflammatory drug
POMC	Pro-opiomelanocortin
PRO	Protein
PYY	Peptide YY
RER	Respiratory exchange ratio
T2DM	Type 2 diabetes mellitus
TT	Time trial

INTRODUCTION

Lower-income countries generally have a higher proportion of protein intake derived from aquatic sources compared to wealthier nations. This discrepancy highlights the economic viability of aquatic foods as a readily available and cost-effective animal protein source, surpassing alternative sources in terms of affordability and accessibility. Moreover, these foods are held in high regard due to their strong desirability and integral role in local gastronomic customs.

DOI: 10.1201/9781003597926-19

Recent investigations have identified several bioactive peptides sourced from different types of fish. These peptides consist of short sequences spanning around 2 to 20 amino acids, which demonstrate positive physiological effects when ingested by living organisms. These beneficial compounds can be generated through proteolytic hydrolysis, achieved using commonly accessible enzymes like trypsin, chymotrypsin, alcalase, or proteolytic microorganisms, often employing fermentation techniques (Vercruysse, Van Camp, and Smagghe 2005). Numerous bioactive compounds have been extracted from residual fish muscle proteins, collagen, gelatin, fish oil, fish bones, and internal organs (Jeon and Kim 2002).

ANTIOXIDANT ACTIVITY

Peptides derived from fish proteins have demonstrated a remarkable capacity to exhibit robust antioxidative activities across various oxidative systems (Rajapakse et al. 2005). Antioxidants can help mitigate problems that occur when molecules in our bodies become oxidized. In one study, researchers isolated a helpful substance from the backbone of tuna. They called it VKAGFAWTANQQLS (Table 19.1). This finding is significant for developing foods that are beneficial for our bodies. The researchers found that these special substances can clean up harmful particles and act as antioxidants (Je et al. 2007).

Another research project discovered an antioxidant peptide in hoki fish frame protein through the process of digestion in the stomach and intestines (Kim, Je, and Kim 2007). Various enzymes were employed to break down the proteins, and the resulting peptides demonstrated powerful antioxidant effects in different experimental setups.

ANTIHYPERTENSIVE ACTIVITY

Peptides that inhibit ACE (angiotensin-converting enzyme) have been extracted from the skin of skate fish and act as noncompetitive inhibitors (J.K. Lee, Jeon, and Byun 2011). Seafood by-products from the fishing industry, such as tuna backbones, have yielded a range of isolated peptides (S.-H. Lee, Qian, and Kim 2010). To obtain an antioxidant peptide, tuna backbones were subjected to hydrolysis using a variety of proteases, including alcalase, α-chymotrypsin, neutrase, papain, pepsin, and trypsin (Je et al. 2007).

Gelatin peptides contain a distinctive repeating sequence of Gly-Pro-Ala in their structure (Table 19.1). The antihypertensive properties observed in gelatin peptides are believed to be linked to their special arrangement of amino acids.

ANTIMICROBIAL ACTIVITY

Antimicrobial peptides are found in many animals and have the potential to fight against microbes. There are three versions of a new type of peptide that have their ends modified, called chrysophsin-1, chrysophsin-2, and chrysophsin-3. These peptides have 25, 25, and 20 amino acids, respectively, and they are very positively charged. They have an uncommon sequence of amino acids at their ends, specifically RRRH. These peptides were discovered in the gills of red sea bream, scientifically known as *Chrysophrys* (*Pagrus*) *major* (Iijima et al. 2003). Pleurocidin is anticipated to adopt a structure shaped like an amphipathic α-helix, resembling various other linear antimicrobial peptides. It demonstrated the ability to combat *Escherichia coli* bacteria, as evident in a bacterial cell lysis plate experiment. Additionally, a research endeavor focused on skate skin involved both creating collagen and isolating an antimicrobial peptide (S.-h. Cho, Jahncke, and Eun 2004).

TABLE 19.1
Fish Peptides and Their Bioactive Effects, Mechanisms, and Potential Applications

Peptide	Source	Bioactive Effects	Mechanism of Action	Potential Applications
VKAGFAWTANQQLS	Tuna backbone	Antioxidant	Neutralizes harmful particles, acts as an antioxidant	Functional foods, health supplements
Gelatin peptides	Fish gelatin	Antioxidant	Specific arrangement of amino acids	Food additives, nutraceuticals
Met-Tyr	Sardine muscle	Antioxidant defense	Triggers antioxidant defense protein production	Antioxidant-rich products, supplements
ACE-inhibiting peptides	Skate fish skin	Antihypertensive	Inhibit angiotensin-converting enzyme	Hypertension management, supplements
Chrysophsin peptides	Red sea bream gills	Antimicrobial	Amphipathic secondary structures, combat bacteria	Food preservation, antimicrobial agents
Pleurocidin	Winter flounder skin	Antimicrobial	Amphipathic α-helix, combat *Escherichia coli*	Antibacterial agents, medical products
Fish muscle peptides	Fish muscle	Anticoagulant	Inhibit coagulation factors, hinder blood clotting	Thrombosis prevention, medical use

ANTICOAGULANT POTENTIAL

Peptides extracted from fish muscle through enzymatic processes have also exhibited anticoagulant and antiplatelet traits when tested in laboratory conditions. These findings imply that fish-derived peptides possess the ability to hinder coagulation factors in the intrinsic pathway of blood clotting (Rajapakse et al. 2005). From the yellowfin sole, a specific peptide was isolated and found to block the activity of activated coagulation factor XII. This peptide, with anticoagulant properties, also works against platelet membrane glycoprotein integrin, which helps prevent the aggregation of platelets.

ANTICANCER POTENTIAL

Some reports indicate that proteins, peptides, and amino acids might possess properties that counteract tumor growth or proliferation. However, research on the inhibitory effects on cell growth from peptides originating from fish protein is less common. The hydrolysates derived from three blue whiting, three cod, three plaice, and one salmon can inhibit the growth of two human breast cancer cell lines, namely MCF-7/6 and MDA-MB-231 (Picot et al. 2006). The hydrolysates consisted of a diverse blend of free amino acids, peptides, lipids, and sodium chloride (Table 19.1). Furthermore, from the dark muscle of tuna, two peptides with antiproliferative properties were isolated. This isolation was achieved through enzymatic breakdown using papain and protease on the MCF-7 human breast cancer cell line (Hsu, Li-Chan, and Jao 2011).

ANTIHYPERGLYCEMIC POTENTIAL

Diabetes is a serious metabolic condition projected to impact approximately 451 million individuals globally (N.H. Cho et al. 2018). Around 90% of diabetes cases are attributed to type 2 insulin-resistant diabetes mellitus (T2DM).

Certain enhancements in glycemic measurements due to fish hydrolysates have been linked to hormonal responses. These include the stimulation of insulin release, the inhibition of dipeptidyl-peptidase-4 (DPP-4) enzyme (which extends the lifespan of natural incretin hormones), and the secretion of incretin hormones like glucagon-like peptide-1 (GLP-1) and glucose-dependent insulinotropic polypeptide (GIP). While some *in vitro* studies suggest that fish protein hydrolysates (FPHs) might enhance insulin secretion (Sharkey et al. 2020), none of the human trials conducted with fish hydrolysates have demonstrated an elevation in plasma insulin levels. In fact, one study even indicated a reduction in plasma insulin (Dale et al. 2018). A portion of hydrolysate obtained from salmon frames showed a glucose uptake level equivalent to that induced by insulin in rat skeletal muscle (L6) cells (Zhu et al. 2010). Both salmon and blue whiting protein hydrolysates were found to increase glucose uptake in mouse adipose (3T3-L1) cells (Harnedy et al. 2018). Additionally, although diabetic patients showed no significant change in plasma insulin levels, there was an observed enhancement in insulin sensitivity following a six-week regimen of marine collagen peptides treatment (Ayabe et al. 2015).

BONE AND CARTILAGE HEALTH

Bones perform multiple vital functions within the body. They safeguard organs, offer structural support, facilitate movement, generate both red and white blood cells, and store minerals. Bone's primary components are collagen and calcium. Collagen is responsible for transmitting forces and upholding the structure of tissues (Daneault et al. 2017). With aging, the flexibility and strength of bones diminish, leading to the development of osteoporotic fractures. Osteoporosis is a chronic condition that typically lacks noticeable symptoms. It arises from low bone mineral density (BMD) and disrupted skeletal microarchitecture, leading to a heightened susceptibility to fractures (Zhang et al. 2018).

Fish peptides accelerate the process of calcium absorption (Jung et al. 2005). Scientists have discovered that FPHs contain peptides and growth factors that act similarly to hormones, enhancing the speed of calcium absorption (Fouchereau-Peron et al. 1999). These peptides can attach to receptors on the surface of osteoclasts and play a significant role in calcium metabolism by reducing the osteoclast count. As a result, these peptides hold potential for treating conditions like osteoporosis and Paget's disease.

Furthermore, gelatin peptides have demonstrated the ability to enhance the absorption of dietary calcium in animal models, thereby boosting the bioavailability of calcium. In a research study, it was found that fish bone peptide (FBP) II had the ability to prevent the creation of insoluble calcium salts under neutral pH conditions. During the course of the experiment, including FBP II in the diets of ovariectomized rats led to an increase in calcium retention and a reduction in the loss of bone mineral. Moreover, the levels of total calcium in the femur, BMD, and strength were markedly elevated by the FBP II diet, comparable to those observed in the group fed with a diet containing casein phosphopeptide (Jung, Lee, and Kim 2006).

ANOREXIGENIC POTENTIAL

Obesity, another chronic metabolic condition, impacts approximately 650 million individuals worldwide. This ailment is associated with various health issues, such as cardiovascular diseases, cancer, and T2DM. Notably, obesity accounts for around 80% of T2DM risk. Inflammation, adipokines, and excessive accumulation of lipids in pancreatic, liver, and muscle tissues are believed to contribute to the intricate connection between the development of obesity and T2DM.

Numerous hormones within the entero-insular axis, which have an impact on diabetes, also influence the regulation of appetite. Examples of such hormones include GLP-1, GIP, cholecystokinin (CCK), and peptide YY (PYY) (Holst 2013). Nonetheless, attempts to develop pharmaceutical treatments that target specific hormones like CCK and PYY have faced considerable challenges. As a consequence, functional foods have emerged as an appealing alternative. Unlike high-dose pharmacotherapies, functional foods administered at lower doses orally may circumvent adverse effects. While they may not fully resolve symptoms, they could serve as preventive measures or early-stage treatments when combined with lifestyle adjustments. Several FPHs have demonstrated the ability to reduce weight gain, as observed in both animal trials and human research. However, the precise mechanism underlying this effect remains inadequately understood. This conclusion is derived from a single study, and further investigation is necessary to gain a comprehensive understanding of these impacts. Some of the diminished food intake might also stem from the delayed emptying of the stomach, potentially facilitated by protein-carbohydrate binding (Geirsdottir et al. 2011).

EFFECTS ON BODY COMPOSITION

A study by Nobile et al. (2016) found that 90-day supplementation with FPHs (1.4 g or 2.8 g) combined with a 300 kcal daily caloric deficit led to a decrease in body weight, body mass index, fat mass measured through dual-energy X-ray absorptiometry (DXA), and waist, hip, and thigh circumference. These outcomes were comparable to those achieved with a control group using whey protein isolate. The study revealed no significant alterations in extracellular water and no notable differences between FPH doses and the whey protein isolate control across all endpoints. However, the study did not report DXA measurements of lean mass, fat-free mass, and bone mineral content. Therefore, the role of these tissues in overall body weight reductions, based on the three-compartment model, remains uncertain (Oldroyd, Treadgold, and Hind 2018). Given the available data, it's difficult to conclude that FPH had a discernible impact on body composition. The changes observed likely result from the caloric deficit achieved through dietary monitoring.

EFFECTS ON SKELETAL MUSCLE FUNCTION AND EXERCISE PERFORMANCE

Mjøs et al. (2019) investigated FPH's influence on short-term recovery between cycling sessions among healthy middle-aged cyclists. They found no differences in time to exhaustion, heart rate, RER, blood lactate levels, and glucose levels after adding FPH (20 mg) to a formulation containing whey protein and carbohydrates, compared to an isoenergetic and isonitrogenous supplement without FPH. The relatively low dosage of FPH may not have been potent enough to produce a significant impact. Additionally, the concurrent provision of whey protein and carbohydrates (contributing to 12% and 66% of the energy composition in each beverage, respectively) could have influenced the outcomes. All three exercise performance studies employed small FPH doses, and the potential effects of larger doses—taken acutely or chronically—on cycling-related fat oxidation rates remain unexplored. Currently, these findings appear to confirm that, for highly trained athletes, the availability of carbohydrates is the limiting factor affecting performance in events lasting up to three hours (Hawley and Leckey 2015). Given this information, the available performance data do not sufficiently support FPH use in this specific context.

A feasibility study involving nursing home residents aged over 80 years (Drotningsvik et al. 2019) showed no notable differences in body weight and handgrip strength between groups initially, and these parameters did not significantly change by the study's endpoint (although exact data were not provided). The amount of protein administered (5.2 g per day) and the duration of supplementation may have been insufficient to yield positive outcomes in this population. The potential benefits of FPH supplementation in conjunction with a resistance exercise program have yet to be investigated in older and/or frail populations (Figure 19.1).

Considering all findings, there is not yet enough evidence to endorse FPH use for the performance and functional outcomes examined in the aforementioned studies.

OTHER EFFECTS

Acidic peptide fractions from Atlantic cod hydrolysate have exhibited robust immunostimulatory effects. Treatment with these peptides has led to the activation of the oxidative burst in Atlantic salmon leucocytes (Gildberg et al. 1996). Immunomodulators stimulate macrophages to produce oxygen metabolites, triggering the oxidative burst, which is crucial for the bactericidal capability of phagocytes.

Certain peptides extracted from different fish sources and fermented fish products can inhibit prolyl endopeptidase (Sørensen et al. 2004). Peptides derived from salmon, trout, and cod muscles, along with those from Norwegian fermented trout muscle, have been examined for their potential to inhibit prolyl endopeptidase activity. Results indicate that these sources are indeed promising reservoirs of such inhibitory activity.

Research suggests that brief supplementation with FPH derived from Pacific whiting (administered through 1 g capsules of FPH three times daily for seven days) might help prevent intestinal injury caused by nonsteroidal anti-inflammatory drugs (NSAIDs) (Marchbank et al. 2008). However, evidence regarding the potential advantages of long-term or chronic supplementation remains limited.

In a study of nursing home residents, serum levels of the inflammatory marker monocyte chemoattractant protein-1 (MCP-1) notably decreased following six weeks of FPH supplementation. However, C-reactive protein (CRP) increased significantly in the FPH group compared to the control group (Figure 19.2) (Drotningsvik et al. 2019).

THE EFFECTS OF OTHER PROTEINS

In this chapter, we have reviewed fish proteins and their effects on health, particularly regarding oxidant status, blood pressure, infection, coagulation, glycemic measurement, bone and cartilage

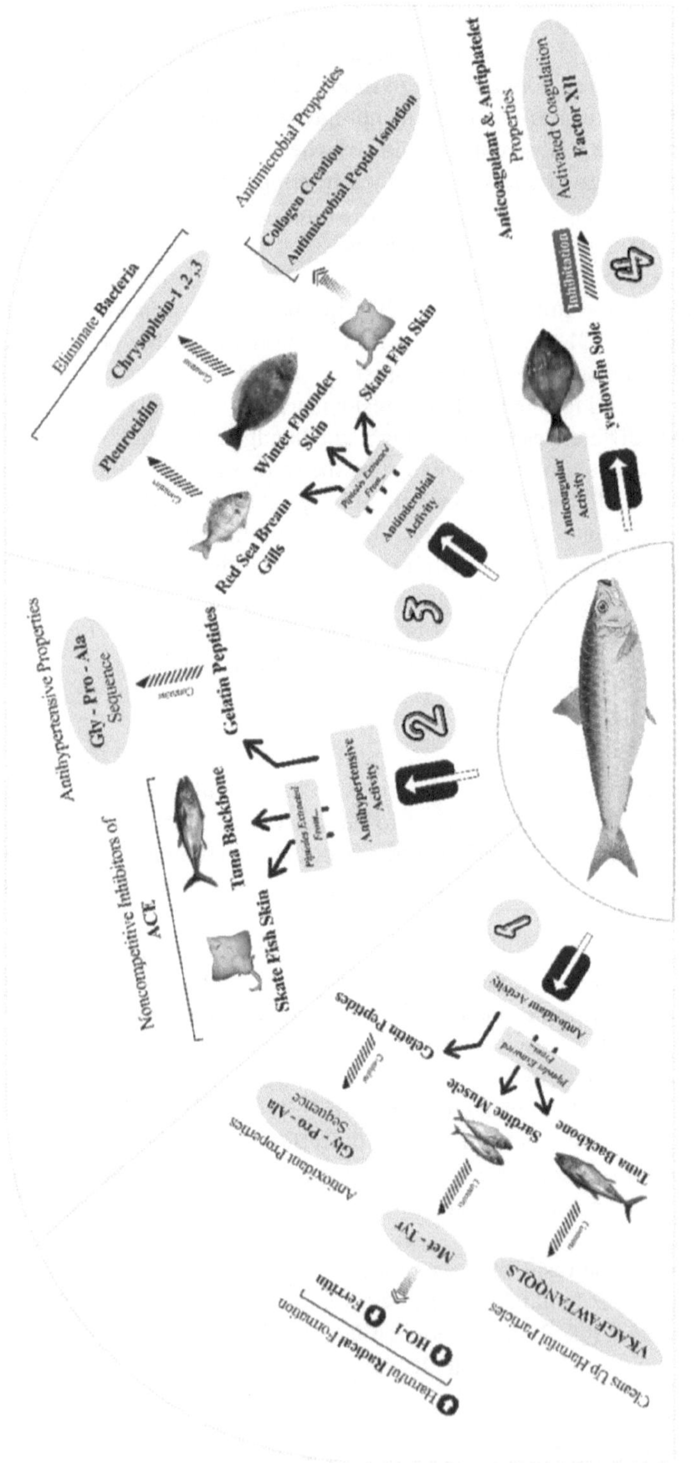

FIGURE 19.1 Summary of the effects of fish proteins on health. This figure illustrates the health benefits of peptides extracted from various fish types. ACE: angiotensin-converting enzyme.

health, and anthropometric factors. However, it's crucial to consider the effects of other proteins, such as those from eggs or soy, on health status. The properties of egg proteins, including their antimicrobial and immune-protective aspects, suggest promising therapeutic applications (Maria Luz Fernandez 2015). Immunoglobulin Y (IgY), equivalent to mammalian IgG, protects developing chickens similarly to how IgG safeguards human fetuses (Chucri et al. 2010). IgY is crucial for passive immunization, contributing valuable treatment and disease prevention in humans and animals (Kovacs-Nolan and Mine 2012). Notably, egg yolk IgY has proven its efficacy by diminishing intestinal inflammation in mice infected with *Salmonella typhimurium* (Li et al. 2016).

Egg proteins contain additional protective elements against infection, such as lysozyme, which hydrolyzes bacterial cell wall peptidoglycans (Ibrahim, Aoki, and Pellegrini 2002). Avidin, another component, binds biotin, hindering its use by bacteria (Banks, Board, and Sparks 1986). Phosvitin demonstrates protective effects against *Streptococcus* bacteria (Brady et al. 2002), and ovotransferrin's antimicrobial activity stems from trapping iron, inhibiting bacterial growth (Wu and Acero-Lopez 2012).

The protective influence of egg proteins extends to chronic diseases. Rats consuming albumin-derived peptides experienced hypotensive effects (Fujita, Sasaki, and Yoshikawa 1995), highlighting the significance of protein hydrolysis in releasing hypotensive peptides (Jahandideh et al. 2014). A study of young, healthy individuals indicated that daily egg consumption led to reduced blood pressure compared to abstaining from eggs (Barona and Fernandez 2012). Egg proteins also protect against colon cancer, possibly through cysteine peptidase inhibitors isolated from chicken eggs (Hap et al. 2011) or direct suppression of colon tumors by egg yolk proteins (Ishikawa et al. 2009). In summary, eggs contain proteins with biologically active components that may offer protection against hypertension, inflammatory bowel disease, and cancer.

Soybeans provide high-quality proteins with all essential amino acids found in animal proteins, without cholesterol, and with lower saturated fat (Chatterjee, Gleddie, and Xiao 2018). Soy peptides' primary bioactivity is their hypolipidemic effect. Many soy peptides, including LPYPR from the glycinin subunit, have demonstrated the ability to lower cholesterol and triglycerides, inhibiting fat synthesis and storage in various experimental settings. Yoshikawa et al. (2000) first identified LPYPR, administering it at 50 mg/kg for two days without isoflavones, resulting in ~25% reductions in both serum total and low-density lipoprotein (LDL) cholesterol in rats (Yoshikawa et al. 2000). Further investigations highlighted LPYP as a hypocholesterolemic peptide, operating as a competitive inhibitor of 3-hydroxy-3-methylglutaryl CoA reductase (HMGR), a key enzyme in cholesterol biosynthesis (Pak et al. 2012). This peptide enhanced LDL uptake in cultured liver cells by activating the LDL receptor (LDLR)–sterol regulatory element-binding protein 2 (SREBP2) pathway (Lammi, Zanoni, and Arnoldi 2015).

Several soy peptides known for their hypolipidemic effects also exhibit antidiabetic properties across various experimental models. For instance, soy peptides like LPYP, IAVPGEVA, and IAVPTGVA, recognized for their hypocholesterolemic action, demonstrated improved glucose metabolism. They achieved this by enhancing glucose uptake in cultured hepatic cells through glucose transporters (GLUT) 1 and 4 (Lammi, Zanoni, and Arnoldi 2015). High blood pressure is a risk factor for coronary heart disease. Antihypertensive peptides in Asian fermented soybean foods block ACE to regulate blood pressure(de Mejia and Ben 2006). These peptides, like HHL in Korean soybean paste treated with chymotrypsin (Singh, Vij, and Hati 2014), inhibit ACE. Peptides SY and GY in soybean seasoning reduce hypertension in rats (Nakahara et al. 2011). Various soy peptides, e.g., FFYY and LHPGDAQR from soy milk, show enhanced ACE inhibition (Tomatsu et al. 2013). Certain structural features, such as Pro or hydroxyl-Pro at the C-terminus, make peptides resistant to degradation, while Tyr at the C-terminus enhances antihypertensive effects (Figure 19.2) (Wang and de Mejia 2005).

Soy isoflavones have been extensively studied for their dual role in cancer promotion and prevention (He and Chen 2013). Notably, soy peptides, particularly lunasin and Bowman–Birk inhibitor (BBI) from the minor 2S fraction of soy proteins, exhibit anticancer properties (Chatterjee,

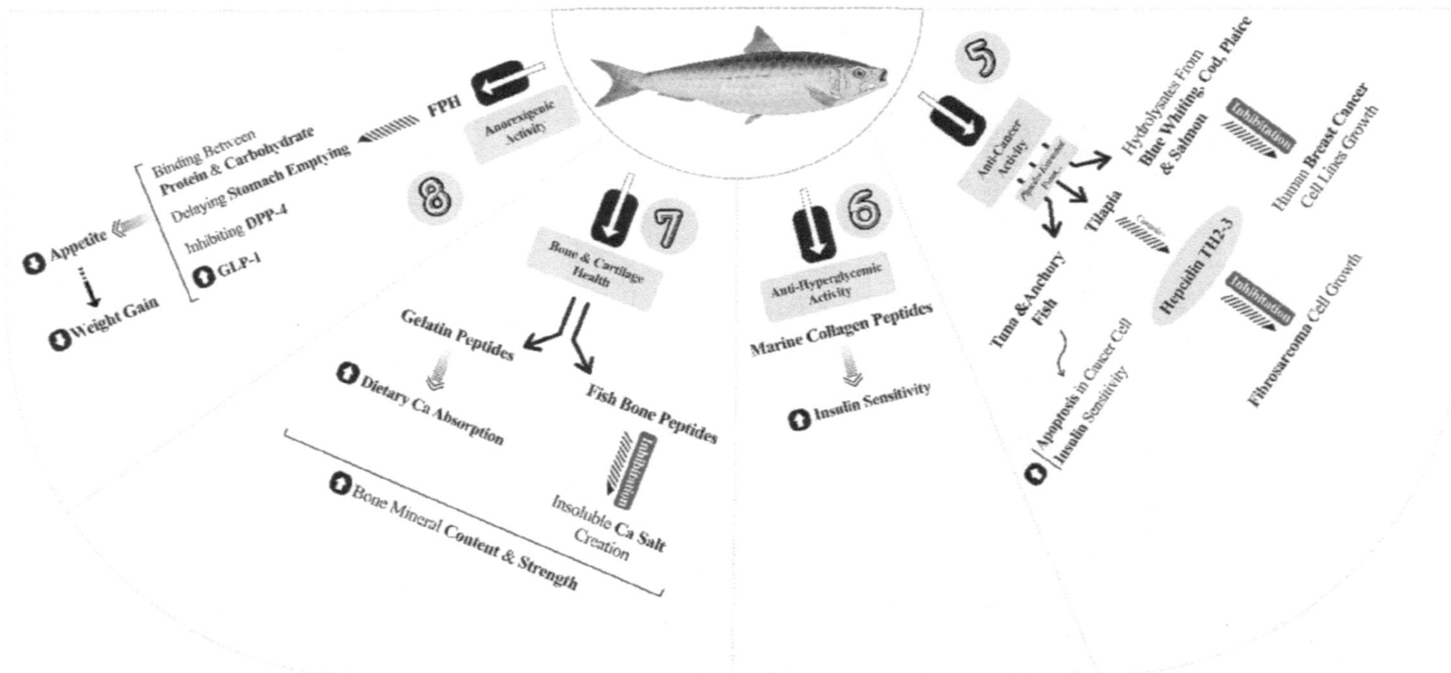

FIGURE 19.2 Summary of the effects of fish proteins on health. This figure illustrates the health benefits of peptides extracted from various fish types. DPP-4: dipeptidylpeptidase-4; GLP-1: glucagon-like peptide-1; FPH: fish protein hydrolysate; Ca: calcium.

Gleddie, and Xiao 2018). BBI, initially considered an antinutrient, demonstrated anticarcinogenic effects across various tissues and species, even undergoing FDA Investigational Drug evaluation (Losso 2008). In human trials, BBI proved to be a safe cancer chemopreventive agent at doses ranging from 800 to 2000 chymotrypsin inhibitor units (Lin et al. 2014). Its anticancer mechanism involves apoptosis, reactive oxygen species-induced mitochondrial damage, proteasomal inhibition, and antiangiogenesis.

The interplay between soy peptides and cancer presents promising avenues for cancer prevention and treatment. Carcinogenesis involves pro-inflammatory, pro-oxidant, and immunosuppressive mechanisms, contributing to abnormal tissue growth. Proteins and peptides with anticancer properties often exhibit anti-inflammatory and antioxidant effects (Lule et al. 2015). Soy protein, with or without isoflavones, reduces oxidative stress and inflammation by inhibiting NF-κB and pro-inflammatory cytokines in various models and human subjects (Draganidis et al. 2016).

Soy milk hydrolysates produce peptides, like RQRK and VIK, which demonstrate anti-inflammatory effects in murine macrophages (Dia, Bringe, and de Mejia 2014). Lunasin, known for its anticancer potential, acts as an antioxidant by inhibiting radical scavengers and reducing pro-inflammatory cytokine secretion (Hernández-Ledesma, Hsieh, and de Lumen 2009; Lule et al. 2015). Its RGD motif blocks inflammation in human macrophages by interacting with αVβ3 integrin through an Akt-mediated NF-κB pathway (Figure 19.1) (Cam and de Mejia 2012). In one trial, soy protein ingestion resulted in the absorption of ~4.5% of the total ingested lunasin (Dia et al. 2009).

MINI DICTIONARY OF TERMS

- **Cholecystokinin (CCK):** A peptide hormone crucial in the digestive system. It is released in response to the presence of food, especially fats and proteins, in the duodenum and jejunum of the small intestine. CCK stimulates gallbladder contraction and digestive enzyme secretion and contributes to satiety.
- **Dipeptidylpeptidase-4 (DPP-4) enzyme:** Also known as CD26, this enzyme regulates glucose metabolism. DPP-4 inhibitors, also known as gliptins, are used in the treatment of type 2 diabetes by increasing circulating levels of active incretin hormones, leading to improved glucose regulation.
- **Glucagon-like peptide-1 (GLP-1):** A hormone released by the L cells in the intestine, primarily in the ileum and colon, in response to food intake, especially carbohydrates. It plays a crucial role in the regulation of glucose metabolism and is an important target in the treatment of type 2 diabetes.
- **Glucose-dependent insulinotropic polypeptide (GIP):** A hormone released by the K cells (or L cells) in the duodenum and jejunum of the small intestine in response to the ingestion of food, especially glucose and fatty acids.
- **Peptide YY (PYY):** A peptide hormone produced by cells in the lining of the gastrointestinal tract, particularly in the ileum and colon, in response to the presence of fatty acids and amino acids. PYY acts as an appetite suppressant and slows gastric emptying.
- **Respiratory exchange ratio (RER):** A measure of the ratio between carbon dioxide produced and oxygen consumed during metabolism, providing insights into the primary energy substrate used during physical activity or metabolic processes.
- **Seafood by-products:** Parts of marine animals not typically consumed as primary food but repurposed or utilized in various ways. These by-products often result from seafood processing for human consumption.

SUMMARY POINTS

- The skin of skate fish yields peptides that inhibit angiotensin-converting enzyme (ACE), serving as noncompetitive inhibitors. Tuna backbones subjected to hydrolysis produce antioxidant peptides through various proteases.
- Antimicrobial peptides, such as chrysophsin-1, chrysophsin-2, and chrysophsin-3, found in red sea bream gills, display positive charges and unique amino acid sequences, demonstrating efficacy against both Gram-negative and Gram-positive bacteria.
- Peptides from fish muscle exhibit anticoagulant and antiplatelet properties, blocking the activity of coagulation factor XII and inhibiting platelet membrane glycoprotein integrin.
- Functional foods with fish hydrolysates demonstrate anorexigenic potential by reducing weight gain and suppressing appetite-stimulating factors in the brain.
- Short-term supplementation with Pacific whiting-derived fish hydrolysates may protect against intestinal injury caused by nonsteroidal anti-inflammatory drugs (NSAIDs).
- Supplementation with fish hydrolysates in nursing home residents results in decreased serum levels of the inflammatory marker MCP-1 but increased CRP, suggesting potential anti-inflammatory effects.

REFERENCES

Ayabe, Tatsuhiro, Takafumi Mizushige, Wakana Ota, Fuminori Kawabata, Kohsuke Hayamizu, Li Han, Tomoko Tsuji, Ryuhei Kanamoto, and Kousaku Ohinata. 2015. "A novel Alaska pollack-derived peptide, which increases glucose uptake in skeletal muscle cells, lowers the blood glucose level in diabetic mice." *Food & Function* 6 (8): 2749–2757.

Banks, JG, Ronald George Board, and NH Sparks. 1986. "Natural antimicrobial systems and their potential in food preservation of the future." *Biotechnology and Applied Biochemistry* 8 (2–3): 103–147.

Barona, Jacqueline, and Maria Luz Fernandez. 2012. "Dietary cholesterol affects plasma lipid levels, the intravascular processing of lipoproteins and reverse cholesterol transport without increasing the risk for heart disease." *Nutrients* 4 (8): 1015–1025.

Brady, D, S Gaines, L Fenelon, J McPartlin, and C O'farrelly. 2002. "A lipoprotein-derived antimicrobial factor from hen-egg yolk is active against Streptococcus species." *Journal of Food science* 67 (8): 3096–3103.

Cam, Anthony, and Elvira Gonzalez de Mejia. 2012. "RGD-peptide lunasin inhibits Akt-mediated NF- κB activation in human macrophages through interaction with the αVβ3 integrin." *Molecular Nutrition & Food Research* 56 (10): 1569–1581.

Chatterjee, Cynthia, Stephen Gleddie, and Chao-Wu Xiao. 2018. "Soybean bioactive peptides and their functional properties." *Nutrients* 10 (9): 1211.

Cho, Nam H, JE Shaw, Suvi Karuranga, Yafang Huang, JD da Rocha Fernandes, AW Ohlrogge, and BIDF Malanda. 2018. "IDF diabetes atlas: global estimates of diabetes prevalence for 2017 and projections for 2045." *Diabetes Research and Clinical Practice* 138: 271–281.

Cho, Soung-hun, Michael L Jahncke, and Jong-bang Eun. 2004. "Nutritional composition and microflora of the fresh and fermented skate (Raja Kenojei) skins." *International Journal of Food Sciences and Nutrition* 55 (1): 45–51.

Chucri, Thaís Martins, JM Monteiro, AR Lima, MLB Salvadori, JR Kfoury Junior, and Maria Angélica Miglino. 2010. "A review of immune transfer by the placenta." *Journal of Reproductive Immunology* 87 (1–2): 14–20.

Dale, Hanna Fjeldheim, Caroline Jensen, Trygve Hausken, Einar Lied, Jan Gunnar Hatlebakk, Ingeborg Brønstad, Dag Arne Lihaug Hoff, and Gülen Arslan Lied. 2018. "Effect of a cod protein hydrolysate on postprandial glucose metabolism in healthy subjects: A double-blind cross-over trial." *Journal of Nutritional Science* 7: e33.

Daneault, Audrey, Janne Prawitt, Véronique Fabien Soulé, Véronique Coxam, and Yohann Wittrant. 2017. "Biological effect of hydrolyzed collagen on bone metabolism." *Critical Reviews in Food Science and Nutrition* 57 (9): 1922–1937.

De Mejia, Elvira, and O Ben. 2006. "Soybean bioactive peptides: a new horizon in preventing chronic diseases." *Sexuality, Reproduction and Menopause* 4 (2): 91–95.

Dia, Vermont P, Neal A Bringe, and Elvira G De Mejia. 2014. "Peptides in pepsin–pancreatin hydrolysates from commercially available soy products that inhibit lipopolysaccharide-induced inflammation in macrophages." *Food Chemistry* 152: 423–431.

Dia, Vermont P, Sofia Torres, Ben O De Lumen, John W Erdman Jr, and Elvira Gonzalez De Mejia. 2009. "Presence of lunasin in plasma of men after soy protein consumption." *Journal of Agricultural and Food Chemistry* 57 (4): 1260–1266.

Draganidis, Dimitrios, Leonidas G Karagounis, Ioannis Athanailidis, Athanasios Chatzinikolaou, Athanasios Z Jamurtas, and Ioannis G Fatouros. 2016. "Inflammaging and skeletal muscle: can protein intake make a difference?" *The Journal of Nutrition* 146 (10): 1940–1952.

Drotningsvik, Aslaug, Åge Oterhals, Ola Flesland, Ottar Nygård, and Oddrun A Gudbrandsen. 2019. "Fish protein supplementation in older nursing home residents: A randomised, double-blind, pilot study." *Pilot and Feasibility Studies* 5: 1–8.

Fouchereau-Peron, M, L Duvail, C Michel, A Gildberg, I Batista, and Y Le Gal. 1999. "Isolation of an acid fraction from a fish protein hydrolysate with a calcitonin-gene-related-peptide-like biological activity." *Biotechnology and Applied Biochemistry* 29 (1): 87–92.

Fujita, Hiroyuki, Ryuzo Sasaki, and Masaaki Yoshikawa. 1995. "Potentiation of the antihypertensive activity of orally administered ovokinin, a vasorelaxing peptide derived from ovalbumin, by emulsification in egg phosphatidylcholine." *Bioscience, Biotechnology, and Biochemistry* 59 (12): 2344–2345.

Geirsdottir, Margret, Sjofn Sigurgisladottir, Patricia Y Hamaguchi, Gudjon Thorkelsson, Ragnar Johannsson, Hordur G Kristinsson, and Magnus M Kristjansson. 2011. "Enzymatic hydrolysis of blue whiting (Micromesistius poutassou); functional and bioactive properties." *Journal of Food Science* 76 (1): C14–C20.

Gildberg, Asbjorn, Jarl Bøgwald, Audny Johansen, and Even Stenberg. 1996. "Isolation of acid peptide fractions from a fish protein hydrolysate with strong stimulatory effect on Atlantic salmon (Salmo salar) head kidney leucocytes." *Comparative Biochemistry and Physiology Part B: Biochemistry and Molecular Biology* 114 (1): 97–101.

Hap, Andrzej, Wojciech Kielan, Zygmunt Grzebieniak, Maciej Siewinski, Jerzy Rudnicki, Robert Tarnawa, Julia Rudno-Rudzinska, and Anil Kumar Agrawal. 2011. "Control of active B and L cathepsins in tissues of colorectal cancer using cystatins isolated from chicken egg proteins: in vitro studies." *Folia Histochemica et Cytobiologica* 49 (4): 670–676.

Harnedy, Pádraigín A, Vadivel Parthsarathy, Chris M McLaughlin, Martina B O'Keeffe, Philip J Allsopp, Emeir M McSorley, Finbarr PM O'Harte, and Richard J FitzGerald. 2018. "Atlantic salmon (Salmo salar) co-product-derived protein hydrolysates: a source of antidiabetic peptides." *Food Research International* 106: 598–606.

Hawley, John A, and Jill J Leckey. 2015. "Carbohydrate dependence during prolonged, intense endurance exercise." *Sports Medicine* 45: 5–12.

He, Fen-Jin, and Jin-Qiang Chen. 2013. "Consumption of soybean, soy foods, soy isoflavones and breast cancer incidence: differences between Chinese women and women in Western countries and possible mechanisms." *Food science and Human Wellness* 2 (3–4): 146–161.

Hernández-Ledesma, Blanca, Chia-Chien Hsieh, and Ben O de Lumen. 2009. "Antioxidant and anti-inflammatory properties of cancer preventive peptide lunasin in RAW 264.7 macrophages." *Biochemical and Biophysical Research Communications* 390 (3): 803–808.

Holst, Jens Juul. 2013. "Enteroendocrine secretion of gut hormones in diabetes, obesity and after bariatric surgery." *Current Opinion in Pharmacology* 13 (6): 983–988.

Hsu, Kuo-Chiang, Eunice CY Li-Chan, and Chia-Ling Jao. 2011. "Antiproliferative activity of peptides prepared from enzymatic hydrolysates of tuna dark muscle on human breast cancer cell line MCF 7." *Food Chemistry* 126 (2): 617–622.

Ibrahim, Hisham R, Takayoshi Aoki, and Antonio Pellegrini. 2002. "Strategies for new antimicrobial proteins and peptides: lysozyme and aprotinin as model molecules." *Current Pharmaceutical Design* 8 (9): 671–693.

Iijima, Noriaki, Norio Tanimoto, Yohko Emoto, Yohko Morita, Kazumasa Uematsu, Tomoya Murakami, and Toshihiro Nakai. 2003. "Purification and characterization of three isoforms of chrysophsin, a novel antimicrobial peptide in the gills of the red sea bream, Chrysophrys major." *European Journal of Biochemistry* 270 (4): 675–686.

Ishikawa, Shin-ichi, Takayuki Asano, Shingo Takenoshita, Yuuya Nozawa, Keizo Arihara, and Makoto Itoh. 2009. "Egg yolk proteins suppress azoxymethane-induced aberrant crypt foci formation and cell proliferation in the colon of rats." *Nutrition Research* 29 (1): 64–69.

Jahandideh, Forough, Kaustav Majumder, Subhadeep Chakrabarti, Jude S Morton, Sareh Panahi, Susan Kaufman, Sandra T Davidge, and Jianping Wu. 2014. "Beneficial effects of simulated gastro-intestinal digests of fried egg and its fractions on blood pressure, plasma lipids and oxidative stress in spontaneously hypertensive rats." *PLoS One* 9 (12): e115006.

Je, Jae-Young, Zhong-Ji Qian, Hee-Guk Byun, and Se-Kwon Kim. 2007. "Purification and characterization of an antioxidant peptide obtained from tuna backbone protein by enzymatic hydrolysis." *Process Biochemistry* 42 (5): 840–846.

Jeon, You-Jin, and Se-Kwon Kim. 2002. "Antitumor activity of chitosan oligosaccharides produced in ultrafiltration membrane reactor system." *Journal of Microbiology and Biotechnology* 12 (3): 503–507.

Jung, Won-Kyo, Bae-Jin Lee, and Se-Kwon Kim. 2006. "Fish-bone peptide increases calcium solubility and bioavailability in ovariectomised rats." *British Journal of Nutrition* 95 (1): 124–128.

Jung, Won-Kyo, Pyo-Jam Park, Hee-Guk Byun, Sung-Hoon Moon, and Se-Kwon Kim. 2005. "Preparation of hoki (Johnius belengerii) bone oligophosphopeptide with a high affinity to calcium by carnivorous intestine crude proteinase." *Food Chemistry* 91 (2): 333–340.

Kim, Soo-Yong, Jae-Young Je, and Se-Kwon Kim. 2007. "Purification and characterization of antioxidant peptide from hoki (Johnius belengerii) frame protein by gastrointestinal digestion." *The Journal of Nutritional Biochemistry* 18 (1): 31–38.

Kovacs-Nolan, Jennifer, and Yoshinori Mine. 2012. "Egg yolk antibodies for passive immunity." *Annual Review of Food Science and Technology* 3: 163–182.

Lammi, Carmen, Chiara Zanoni, and Anna Arnoldi. 2015. "IAVPGEVA, IAVPTGVA, and LPYP, three peptides from soy glycinin, modulate cholesterol metabolism in HepG2 cells through the activation of the LDLR-SREBP2 pathway." *Journal of Functional Foods* 14: 469–478.

Lee, Jung Kwon, Joong-Kyun Jeon, and Hee-Guk Byun. 2011. "Effect of angiotensin I converting enzyme inhibitory peptide purified from skate skin hydrolysate." *Food Chemistry* 125 (2): 495–499.

Lee, Sang-Hoon, Zhong-Ji Qian, and Se-Kwon Kim. 2010. "A novel angiotensin I converting enzyme inhibitory peptide from tuna frame protein hydrolysate and its antihypertensive effect in spontaneously hypertensive rats." *Food Chemistry* 118 (1): 96–102.

Li Xiaoyu, Ying Yao, Xitao Wang, Yuhong Zhen, Philip A Thacker, Lili Wang, Ming Shi, Junjun Zhao, Ying Zong, and Ni Wang. 2016. "Chicken egg yolk antibodies (IgY) modulate the intestinal mucosal immune response in a mouse model of Salmonella typhimurium infection." *International Immunopharmacology* 36: 305–314.

Lin, Lilie L, Rosemarie Mick, Jeffrey Ware, James Metz, Robert Lustig, Neha Vapiwala, Ramesh Rengan, and Ann R Kennedy. 2014. "Phase I randomized double-blind placebo-controlled single-dose safety studies of Bowman-Birk inhibitor concentrate." *Oncology Letters* 7 (4): 1151–1158.

Losso, Jack N. 2008. "The biochemical and functional food properties of the Bowman–Birk inhibitor." *Critical Reviews in Food Science and Nutrition* 48 (1): 94–118.

Lule, Vaibhao Kisanrao, Sheenam Garg, Sarang Dilip Pophaly, Hitesh, and Sudhir Kumar Tomar. 2015. "Potential health benefits of lunasin: a multifaceted soy-derived bioactive peptide." *Journal of Food Science* 80 (3): R485–R494.

Marchbank, T, JK Limdi, A Mahmood, G Elia, and RJ Playford. 2008. "Clinical trial: protective effect of a commercial fish protein hydrolysate against indomethacin (NSAID)-induced small intestinal injury." *Alimentary Pharmacology & Therapeutics* 28 (6): 799–804.

Maria Luz Fernandez, Catherine J Andersen. 2015. "Eggs, composition and health." In *Encyclopedia of food and health*, edited by Benjamin Caballero, Paul Finglas and Fidel Toldrá, 470–475. Amsterdam, The Netherlands: Elsevier.

Mjøs, Ingunn, Einar Thorsen, Trygve Hausken, Einar Lied, Roy M Nilsen, Ingeborg Brønstad, Elisabeth Edvardsen, and Bente Frisk. 2019. "The effect of low dose marine protein hydrolysates on short-term recovery after high intensity performance cycling: a double-blinded crossover study." *Journal of the International Society of Sports Nutrition* 16 (1): 48.

Nakahara, Takeharu, Katsutoshi Sugimoto, Atsushi Sano, Hitomi Yamaguchi, Hiroshi Katayama, and Riichiro Uchida. 2011. "Antihypertensive mechanism of a peptide-enriched soy sauce-like seasoning: The active constituents and its suppressive effect on renin–angiotensin–aldosterone system." *Journal of Food Science* 76 (8): H201–H206.

Nobile, Vincenzo, Elisa Duclos, Angela Michelotti, Gioia Bizzaro, Massimo Negro, and Florian Soisson. 2016. "Supplementation with a fish protein hydrolysate (Micromesistius poutassou): effects on body weight, body composition, and CCK/GLP-1 secretion." *Food & Nutrition Research* 60 (1): 29857.

Oldroyd, Brian, Laura Treadgold, and Karen Hind. 2018. "Cross calibration of the GE prodigy and iDXA for the measurement of total and regional body composition in adults." *Journal of Clinical Densitometry* 21 (3): 383–393.

Pak, Valeriy V, Minseon Koo, Dae Young Kwon, and Lyubov Yun. 2012. "Design of a highly potent inhibitory peptide acting as a competitive inhibitor of HMG-CoA reductase." *Amino Acids* 43: 2015–2025.

Picot, L, S Bordenave, S Didelot, I Fruitier-Arnaudin, F Sannier, G Thorkelsson, JP Bergé, Fabienne Guérard, A Chabeaud, and JM Piot. 2006. "Antiproliferative activity of fish protein hydrolysates on human breast cancer cell lines." *Process Biochemistry* 41 (5): 1217–1222.

Rajapakse, Niranjan, Won-Kyo Jung, Eresha Mendis, Sung-Hoon Moon, and Se-Kwon Kim. 2005. "A novel anticoagulant purified from fish protein hydrolysate inhibits factor XIIa and platelet aggregation." *Life Sciences* 76 (22): 2607–2619.

Sharkey, Shaun J, Pádraigín A Harnedy-Rothwell, Philip J Allsopp, Lynsey E Hollywood, Richard J FitzGerald, and Finbarr PM O'Harte. 2020. "A narrative review of the anti-hyperglycemic and satiating effects of fish protein hydrolysates and their bioactive peptides." *Molecular Nutrition & Food Research* 64 (21): 2000403.

Singh, Brij Pal, Shilpa Vij, and Subrota Hati. 2014. "Functional significance of bioactive peptides derived from soybean." *Peptides* 54: 171–179.

Sørensen, Raymond, Elisabeth Kildal, Leszek Stepaniak, Are Hugo Pripp, and Terje Sørhaug. 2004. "Screening for peptides from fish and cheese inhibitory to prolyl endopeptidase." *Food/Nahrung* 48 (1): 53–56.

Tomatsu, Makoto, Atsushi Shimakage, Mamoru Shinbo, Seihan Yamada, and Saori Takahashi. 2013. "Novel angiotensin I-converting enzyme inhibitory peptides derived from soya milk." *Food Chemistry* 136 (2): 612–616.

Vercruysse, Lieselot, John Van Camp, and Guy Smagghe. 2005. "ACE inhibitory peptides derived from enzymatic hydrolysates of animal muscle protein: a review." *Journal of Agricultural and Food Chemistry* 53 (21): 8106–8115.

Wang, Wenyi, and Elvira Gonzalez De Mejia. 2005. "A new frontier in soy bioactive peptides that may prevent age-related chronic diseases." *Comprehensive Reviews in Food Science and Food Safety* 4 (4): 63–78.

Wu, Jianping, and Alexandra Acero-Lopez. 2012. "Ovotransferrin: Structure, bioactivities, and preparation." *Food Research International* 46 (2): 480–487.

Yoshikawa, Masaaki, Hiroyuki Fujita, Nobuyuki Matoba, Yasuyuki Takenaka, Taichi Yamamoto, Rena Yamauchi, Hirotaka Tsuruki, and Kyoya Takahata. 2000. "Bioactive peptides derived from food proteins preventing lifestyle-related diseases." *Biofactors* 12 (1–4): 143–146.

Zhang, Ling, Siqi Zhang, Hongdong Song, and Bo Li. 2018. "Effect of collagen hydrolysates from silver carp skin (Hypophthalmichthys molitrix) on osteoporosis in chronologically aged mice: increasing bone remodeling." *Nutrients* 10 (10): 1434.

Zhu, Cui-Feng, Guan-Zhi Li, Hong-Bin Peng, Fan Zhang, Yun Chen, and Yong Li. 2010. "Treatment with marine collagen peptides modulates glucose and lipid metabolism in Chinese patients with type 2 diabetes mellitus." *Applied Physiology, Nutrition, and Metabolism* 35 (6): 797–804.

20 Amino Acid Score, Nitrogen-to-Protein Conversion Factor, and Digestibility of Edible Insect Proteins

Masaru Ochiai

ABBREVIATIONS

AA	Amino acid
AAS	Amino acid score
EFSA	The European Food Safety Authority
ELISA	Enzyme-linked immunosorbent assay
FAO	Food and Agriculture Organization
IgE	Immunoglobulin E
NPF	Nitrogen-to-protein conversion factor
PDCAAS	Protein digestibility-corrected amino acid score
SDGs	Sustainable development goals
SDS-PAGE	Sodium dodecylsulfate polyacrylamide gel electrophoresis

INTRODUCTION

Why are Edible Insect Proteins Recommended?

The global population is estimated to reach 9.7 billion by 2050 (United Nations 2022). This population expansion necessitates adequate resources to satisfy human health and nutritional requirements (United Nations 2022). Currently, livestock meat, chicken eggs, and soybeans—with high protein contents, adequate amino acid (AA) profiles, gut-intestinal digestibility, and palatability—are widely utilized as major food protein resources; however, their use can result in severe environmental problems. According to the dairy report from the Food and Agriculture Organization of the United Nations (FAO), global meat production and the demand for crops to sustain livestock production will increase by more than 50% by 2050 to ensure food security for the increasing global population (van Huis et al. 2013). However, the low feed-to-meat conversion efficiency of livestock necessitates the exploration of alternative and sustainable food resources. The development of alternative food protein resources is crucial, particularly for low-middle-income countries and certain countries that rely heavily on imports of numerous food protein sources.

Recently, increasing concerns regarding food security have prompted the exploration of new sustainable protein resources (Figure 20.1). Among them, edible insects are recommended for consumption because of their high nutritional, environmental, and feeding efficiency benefits (van Huis et al. 2013; Hawkey et al. 2021). In 2018, the EU authorized insects raised and processed in an appropriate environment as novel foods. In 2021, the FAO published a book regarding edible insects and food safety perspectives (FAO 2021). Additionally, in 2015, in line with the global

 DOI: 10.1201/9781003597926-20

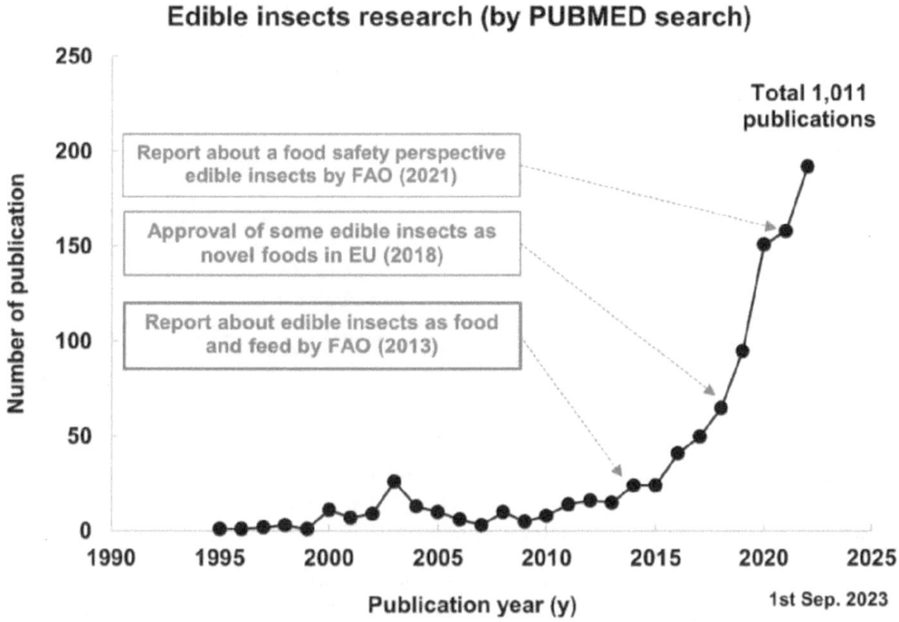

FIGURE 20.1 The number of publications about edible insects to date. The search was conducted on September 1, 2023, using PubMed (https://pubmed.ncbi.nlm.nih.gov/) with the search term "edible insects." The total number is shown in the figure, along with significant events related to edible insects.

sustainable development agenda, the United Nations' "Transforming our World: The 2030 Agenda for Sustainable Development" adopted 17 Sustainable Development Goals (SDGs), which are intended to "stimulate action over the next 15 years in areas of critical importance for humanity and the planet." As demonstrated in a review (Moruzzo et al. 2021), utilizing edible insects in society can contribute to the SDGs through direct and indirect interactions.

HOW MANY EDIBLE INSECT SPECIES ARE OFFICIALLY RECOGNIZED?

Currently, data show that over 2,100 edible insect species were reported in 2017 (Jongema 2017), but the number of edible insects officially recognized as safe is limited to a few species: the migratory locust (*Locusta migratoria*, adult), house cricket (*Acheta domesticus*, adult), lesser mealworm (*Alphitobius diaperinus*, larva), and yellow mealworm (*Tenebrio molitor*, larva). The European Food Safety Authority (EFSA) has published some reviews in the *EFSA Journal* regarding the safety of edible insects as novel foods (EFSA Panel on Nutrition, Novel Foods and Food Allergens (NDA) 2021a, 2021b, 2021c, 2021d, 2022, 2023). Frozen and dried formulations of these edible insects are generally recommended for recognition as novel foods and can be utilized for processed foods such as stick bars, bread, cakes, biscuits, and powdered foods.

Food cultures differ from country to country, and attitudes towards edible insects and their acceptability as novel foods vary. It is necessary to adhere to methods of using edible insects that are appropriate for the food culture.

Are Edible Insect Macronutrients Well Balanced?

Edible insects are generally recognized as alternative protein sources, along with plant protein materials (soybeans, peas, etc.), seaweed, microalgae, and cultured meat (Liceaga et al. 2022). Macronutrient compositions and food functional components of edible insects are introduced in reviews by van Huis et al. (2021) and Tang et al. (2019). As shown in Figure 20.2, some edible insect

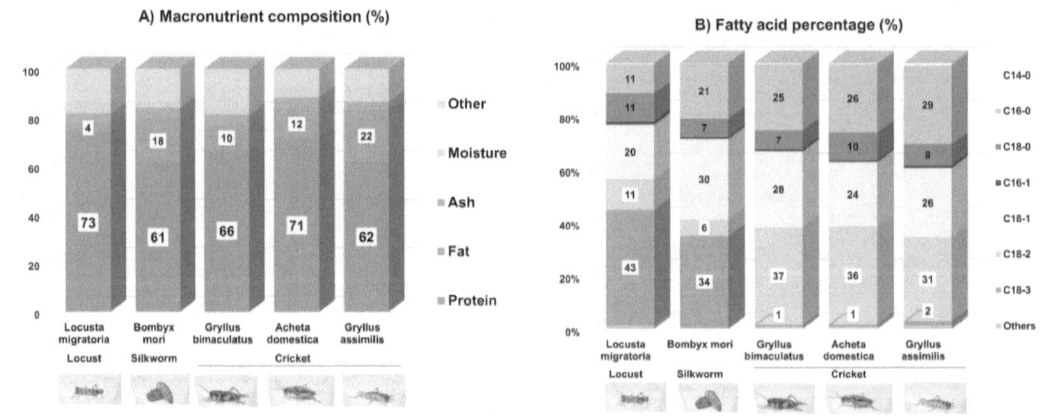

FIGURE 20.2 Macronutrient composition of selected edible insects. A) Composition of macronutrients (crude protein, crude fat, crude ash, moisture, others) of edible insects (migratory locusts, silkworms, two-spotted crickets, house crickets, Jamaican field crickets). B) Fatty acid composition of the edible insects. Images of each insect were provided by Takeo (Tokyo, Japan).

powders (migratory locusts, silkworms, and crickets) are mainly composed of macronutrients such as protein, fat, carbohydrates (including dietary fiber), and minerals, with well-balanced macronutrient compositions. Protein content, which is calculated by multiplying the nitrogen content by 6.25, a conventional nitrogen-to-protein conversion factor (NPF) value, is 73.4% (migratory locust), 61.2% (silkworm), and 61.5–71.0% (crickets). Ochiai and Komiya (2021) reported results comparable to those of several previous reports (Tang et al. 2019; Jantzen da Silva Lucas et al. 2020; Liceaga 2022).

The fat content in edible insects is high, particularly in silkworms and crickets, compared with conventional food protein materials such as milk casein, chicken egg white, and livestock meats. Regarding characteristics of fats and lipids in edible insects, Ochiai and Komiya (2021) reported that edible insects contained lipids not only in triacylglycerol form but also in several kinds of phospholipid forms at a similar level to soybean, chicken egg yolk, fish, and livestock meat (Ochiai and Komiya 2021). The fatty acid composition of the lipids also differs significantly by insect species: rich in α-linolenic acid (n-3) in the migratory locust and silkworm, but linoleic acid (n-6) in the cricket species. Therefore, it is characteristic that when whole edible insects are utilized as dietary protein sources, the nutritional properties of each unsaturated fatty acid are more pronounced compared to conventional dietary protein materials.

Important Issues Regarding Methods for Quantitative Analysis of Edible Insect Proteins

While edible insects represent protein abundance, some recent reviews have raised controversial points regarding the quantitative protein analysis of edible insects (Mariotti et al. 2008; Jonas-Levi and Martinez 2017; Janssen et al. 2017; Churchward-Venne et al. 2017; Boulos et al. 2020; Smets et al. 2021). For the quantitative determination of dietary protein materials, the Kjeldahl method is generally applied. The Kjeldahl method is the most frequently used approach and is still recognized as the official method by AOAC International. Hayes (2020) and Mæ̀hre et al. (2018) discussed the advantages and disadvantages of several protein determination methods that are frequently used in food science and by the food industry.

The Kjeldahl method involves the digestion of food with a strong acid to release nitrogen, which is subsequently quantified via titration. Protein quality is then calculated from the nitrogen concentration of the food using an NPF value (typically 6.25, which is often called the "Jones factor") (Mariotti et al. 2008). This value is based on the assumption that the general nitrogen content in food proteins is 16% and that all nitrogen in foods is protein-bound. However, this method does not consider the nitrogen content of a specific AAs, which depends on their molecular weight and the number of nitrogen atoms. This default factor value has also been applied to unknown proteins, such as insect proteins (Regulation (EU) No 1169/2011 (2011) on the provision of food information to consumers).

Mæ̀hre et al. (2018) and Mariotti et al. (2008) have suggested that the Kjeldahl method does not measure true protein and that the NPF value of 6.25 may not always be suitable for all protein types. In the case of edible insect proteins, many researchers have indicated that the amount of nitrogen from chitin, a nitrogen-rich polysaccharide, influences the total amount of nitrogen, and the protein content of insects in food is overestimated when an NPF value of 6.25 is used (Mariotti et al. 2008; Jonas-Levi and Martinez 2017; Janssen et al. 2017; Churchward-Venne et al. 2017; Boulos et al. 2020; Smets et al. 2021). Therefore, as the total nitrogen content calculated using the Kjeldahl method is derived from the sum of the true protein and dietary fiber chitin, using the NPF value of 6.25 is less suitable; however, this value has been commonly and incorrectly used in some reports, as suggested by Jonas-Levi and Martinez (2017). More accurate calculation of the species-specific NPF value necessitates the analysis and separation of the nitrogen source, followed by an accurate measurement of the chitin and true protein content in edible insects.

True Protein, Chitin Content, and Net Nitrogen-Protein Conversion Factor (NPF) of Edible Insects

For example, Boulos et al. (2020) investigated the chitin content of several insect species (mealworms, crickets, and migratory locusts), finding it to be 4.3–5.1% dry weight. Aguilera et al. (2021) also reported that the chitin contents of mealworms, beetles, caterpillars, ants, crickets, and locust flours ranged from 5.1 to 12.1%. Janssen et al. (2017), who highlighted the overestimation of the protein content of edible insects, also reported that chitin-derived (N-acetyl) glucosamine accounted for 4.4–9.1% of dry weight in mealworms, lesser mealworms, and black soldier flies, corresponding to approximately one-third of the total carbohydrate.

Ochiai et al. (2024) examined the distinction between protein-derived nitrogen and chitin-derived nitrogen in several edible insects using the method described by Aguilera et al. (2021) (Figure 20.3). Chitin-derived nitrogen content comprised 17%, 8%, 14%, 17%, and 21% of total nitrogen content in migratory locusts, silkworms, two-spotted crickets, house crickets, and Jamaican field crickets, respectively. Corresponding chitin content was 10.7%, 1.6%, 6.3%, 5.9%, and 7.2%. These findings demonstrate that chitin content in edible insects significantly affects true protein content and net NPF values.

The calculated true protein content for migratory locusts, silkworms, two-spotted crickets, house crickets, and Jamaican field crickets was 60.9%, 56.4%, 57.5%, 59.2%, and 48.5%, respectively, using true protein-derived nitrogen multiplied by 6.25. In contrast, using total nitrogen content multiplied by 6.25 yielded protein contents of 73.4%, 61.2%, 66.5%, 71.0%, and 61.5%, respectively. The discrepancies were significant: 12.5%, 4.8%, 9.0%, 11.8%, and 13.0%, respectively. These results underscore the need for caution in true protein quantification of edible insects due to their non-protein nitrogen content.

Net NPF values, calculated by dividing true protein content by total nitrogen content, were 5.19, 5.76, 5.40, 5.21, and 4.93 for the aforementioned insects, respectively. Other researchers have also recommended more precise NPF values for edible insects. For example, Janssen et al. (2017) reported NPF values of 4.75 and 4.86 for mealworms and lesser mealworms (larvae), respectively, with extracted protein yielding an NPF value of 5.59. Boulos et al. (2020) reported that the NPF values for mealworms, house crickets, and migratory locusts were 5.41, 5.25, and 5.33, respectively. These studies consistently show net NPF values below the conventional NPF value of 6.25.

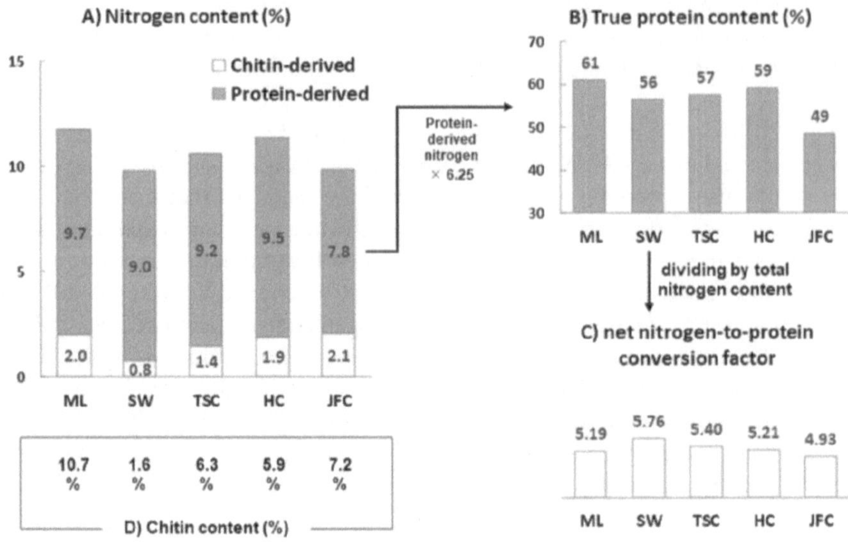

FIGURE 20.3 True protein and chitin contents and net NPF of edible insects. Edible insects contain dietary fiber chitin, which is composed of nitrogen atoms. Chitin content can affect the true protein content when the Kjeldahl method with a conventional NPF (6.25) is applied for protein content determination. Thus, (A) total nitrogen contents are divided into protein-derived and chitin-derived nitrogen contents. (B) True protein content is calculated by multiplying a protein-derived nitrogen content by a conventional NPF (6.25). (C) The net NPF of edible insects is calculated by dividing true protein content by total nitrogen content. (D) Chitin content was also quantified by an acid-base hydrolysis method.

Edible Insect Protein Amino Acid Scores

Beyond protein-derived AA abundance, the AA composition and AA scores (AAS) of food protein materials are crucial for determining protein quality. Our previous study (Ochiai et al. 2022; 2024) revealed AAS of 63, 94, 87, 84, and 85 for migratory locusts, silkworms, two-spotted crickets, house crickets, and Jamaican field crickets, respectively (Table 20.1). Edible insects typically show insufficient essential AA balance: limiting AAs were Trp, Met, and Lys for migratory locusts and crickets, and Leu and Lys for silkworms. Compared to the higher AAS of milk casein, beef, egg white, and soybean protein (Schaafsma 2000), these low AAS values indicate suboptimal AA composition despite high nitrogen and amino acid content. Other studies corroborate these findings: locusts and crickets are deficient in Trp, Met, and Lys (Højrup et al. 1986), many herbivorous edible insects lack Trp, Lys, and Met/Cys (Raheem et al. 2019), and silkworms are deficient in Leu (Longvah et al. 2011). Thus, edible insects may serve as supplementary, rather than completely alternative, protein sources for human foods.

Gut-Intestinal Digestibility of Edible Insect Proteins

Protein digestibility in gut-intestinal tracts is another important factor in determining protein quality. Some plant-based and edible insect proteins exhibit resistance to gut-intestinal digestion. Ochiai et al. (2022) demonstrated this resistance, potentially caused by structural alterations during sample production or the characteristics of edible insect proteins. Their study showed that migratory locust powder resisted digestion by gut pepsin (6 hours) but was digestible by intestinal trypsin and/or chymotrypsin (2 hours) *in vitro* (Figure 20.4). In a rat experiment, proteins with molecular weights between 30 and 44 kDa from migratory locusts also resisted gut digestion but were digested in lower

TABLE 20.1
AAS and Limiting AA of Edible Insect Proteins

	Migratory Locust (*Locusta migratoria*)	Silkworm (*Bombyx mori*)	Two-Spotted Cricket (*Gryllus bimaculatus*)	House Cricket (*Acheta domestica*)	Jamaican Field Cricket (*Gryllus assimilis*)	Casein
Essential Amino Acid (EAA)						
Isoleucine (Ile)	124	131	134	128	124	177
Leucine (Leu)	115	94	108	101	108	181
Lysine (Lys)	83	98	88	90	90	177
Methionine (Met)	71	152	92	90	98	133
Phenylalanine (Phe)	137	147	127	135	132	105
Threonine (The)	105	111	102	104	106	165
Tryptophan (Trp)	63	126	87	84	85	135
Valine (Val)	162	139	160	154	147	189
Histidine (His)	105	134	106	100	108	181
Restricted Amino Acid						
1	Trp 63	Leu 94	Trp 87	Trp 84	Trp 85	-
2	Met 71	Lys 98	Lys 88	Met 90	Lys 90	-
3	Lys 83	-	Met 92	Lys 90	Met 98	-
Reference	Ochiai et al. (2022)	-	-	-	-	Ochiai et al. (2022)

AAS of edible insects (migratory locusts, silkworms, two-spotted crickets, house crickets, Jamaican field crickets) were calculated based on the AA scoring pattern for preschool children (2–5 years old) (1985), as suggested by the FAO/WHO/UNU (1991). The limiting AA of the edible insect proteins are also described.

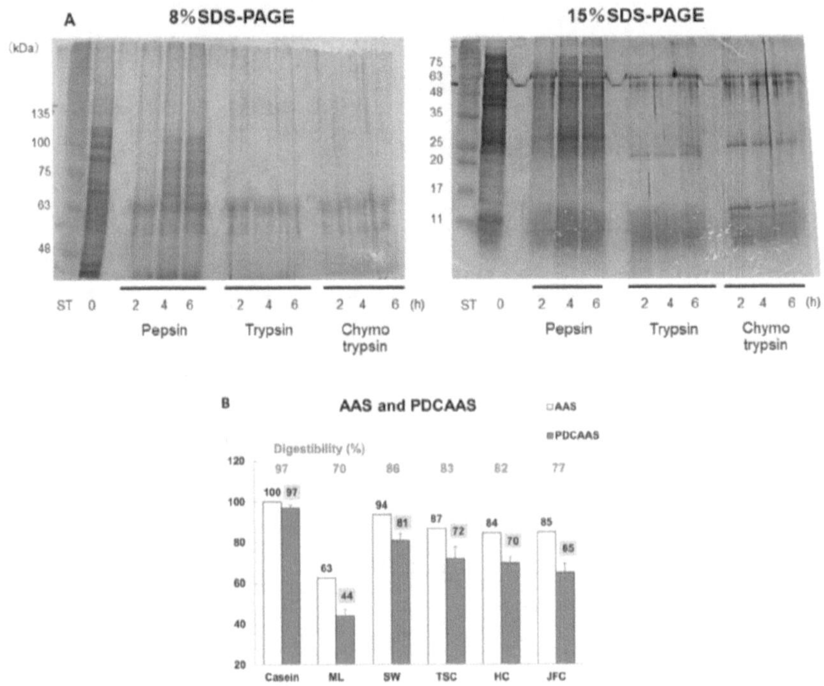

FIGURE 20.4 Evaluation of gut-intestinal digestibility of edible insect proteins *in vitro* and *in vivo*. (A) *In vitro* assessment involved treating proteins with pepsin, chymotrypsin, or trypsin for 6 hours, followed by SDS-PAGE and silver staining. (B) *In vivo* assessment involved feeding rats a diet containing edible insect proteins, then analyzing digestive tract contents using SDS-PAGE and silver straining after 3 hours. Apparent protein digestibility was determined by comparing dietary protein intake to fecal protein excretion over 9 days in rats fed a diet with 20% edible insect protein.

intestinal tracts (SDS-PAGE data in Ochiai et al. 2022). These findings suggest that migratory locust proteins may be slowly absorbed from the small intestine. Notably, rat plasma levels of individual AAs remained unchanged following dietary migratory locust consumption.

Several reports indicate that crustacean allergens like tropomyosin and tropomyosin-like compounds in edible insects remain undegraded in gut-intestinal tracts, which suggests that shellfish tropomyosin immunoglobulin E (IgE) displays cross-reactivity with edible insect species (Ribeiro et al. 2018; Kamemura et al. 2019; Palmer et al. 2020; De Marchi et al. 2021). Tropomyosin, a known insect allergen protein with 33–40 kDa molecular weight (De Marchi et al. 2021), was detected in migratory locusts (7.9 µg/g) using a commercial crustacean allergen ELISA kit (Ochiai et al. 2022). Consequently, some processed foods in Japan now carry warnings about shellfish allergy risks from insect-derived ingredients.

These findings suggest that edible insect proteins containing crustacean allergens have low intestinal digestibility. Our previous study investigated the apparent gut-intestinal digestibility (true protein digestibility) of edible insect proteins in growing rats fed various edible insect diets for 9 days. The true protein digestibility was calculated using the following formula from the FAO/WHO protocol (FAO/WHO 1991; Hughes et al. 2011). The protein digestibility of migratory locusts, silkworms, two-spotted crickets, house crickets, Jamaican field crickets, and casein was 70%, 86%, 83%, 82%, 77%, and 97%, respectively. These results indicate that low-protein digestibility and dietary fiber chitin could suppress and delay intestinal AA absorption and enhance fecal nutrient excretion.

However, other studies have found high protein digestibility in insect meals, supporting their suitability for food product formulation, while also noting large differences in protein digestibility between insect species and processing methods (Rodríguez-Rodríguez et al. 2022). For example, heat treatment of dietary protein materials can decrease digestibility and PDCAAS, as demonstrated in skim milk and soy protein isolates (Schaafsma 2005). Thus, food hygiene heat treatments of edible insects may alter gut-intestinal digestibility due to heat-induced protein structural modifications (Manditsera et al. 2019).

PDCAAS of Edible Insect Proteins and its Effect Rat Growth

The protein digestibility-corrected AA score (PDCAAS) is calculated by multiplying each AAS by true protein digestibility (%) and is utilized to determine protein quality (Boye et al. 2012). As shown in Figure 20.4, the PDCAAS of migratory locusts, silkworms, two-spotted crickets, house crickets, and Jamaican field crickets was 44, 81, 72, 70, and 65, respectively, compared to 97 for casein. Migratory locusts had the lowest PDCAAS (44) among edible insects. The PDCAAS of silkworms was similar to the result (86) reported by Longvah et al. (2011).

Previous studies have reported PDCAAS values for other food protein sources: milk or whey protein (99–100), pea protein concentrate (75), soy protein isolate (93), and wheat protein (50) (Mathai et al. 2017). Hughes et al. (2011) reported PDCAAS values for soy protein isolate (100), milk casein (100), egg white (100), beef (92), pea protein concentrate (73), kidney beans (68), rice (53), whole wheat (40), wheat gluten (25), and almonds (23). Rutherfurd et al. (2015) found high digestibility and PDCAAS for milk proteins (100) and soy proteins (94–97), but lower values for proteins from peas (86), wheat bran (48), and rice (38). These data show that animal-based proteins and soy proteins have high PDCAAS values, while edible insects and many plant-based proteins have lower values.

Ochiai et al. (2024) investigated the effect of dietary edible insect proteins on growth parameters in growing rats over 9 days. The dietary protein source was completely replaced with each edible insect powder (migratory locusts, silkworms, two-spotted crickets, house crickets, Jamaican field crickets) (20% in diet) or casein (20% in diet). As shown in Figure 20.5, rat growth was suppressed when fed edible insect proteins compared to casein, correlating with the AAS of edible insect proteins.

CONCLUSIONS AND FUTURE PERSPECTIVES

This chapter concludes that some edible insects can serve as additional protein sources when consumed with other nutrients; however, they cannot be considered high-quality protein resources due to their insufficient AAS and gut-intestinal digestibility. The PDCAAS of the edible insects was lower than their individual AAS, and rat growth was suppressed when each edible insect was fed as the sole protein source, which correlates with AAS. The NPF of edible insects was largely influenced by their dietary fiber chitin content and was lower than the conventional NPF value (6.25). This study also confirmed that more accurate net NPF values can be calculated by dividing the true nitrogen content by the total protein content.

Recently, there has been an increased focus on edible insects as alternative food protein resources and processed foods containing edible insects are expected to increase worldwide. Edible insects can be effective as additional protein sources. However, when using edible insects in processed foods, more attention should be paid to food ingredient labeling and the calculation of protein and dietary fiber content.

Regarding food functional properties, some edible insects contain bioactive components such as peptides, functional lipids, dietary fiber, polyphenols, and carotenoids that have anti-oxidative and anti-obesity effects (D'Antonio et al. 2021; Liceaga et al. 2022; Aguilar-Toalá et al. 2022; Aiello et al. 2023; Teixeira et al. 2023; Quah et al. 2023; Lange and Nakamura 2023). However, *in vivo* investigations are limited. Considering the metabolic characteristics of bioactive components, further animal studies are needed. These investigations are expected to advance edible insect food science, technology, and applications for functional human foods.

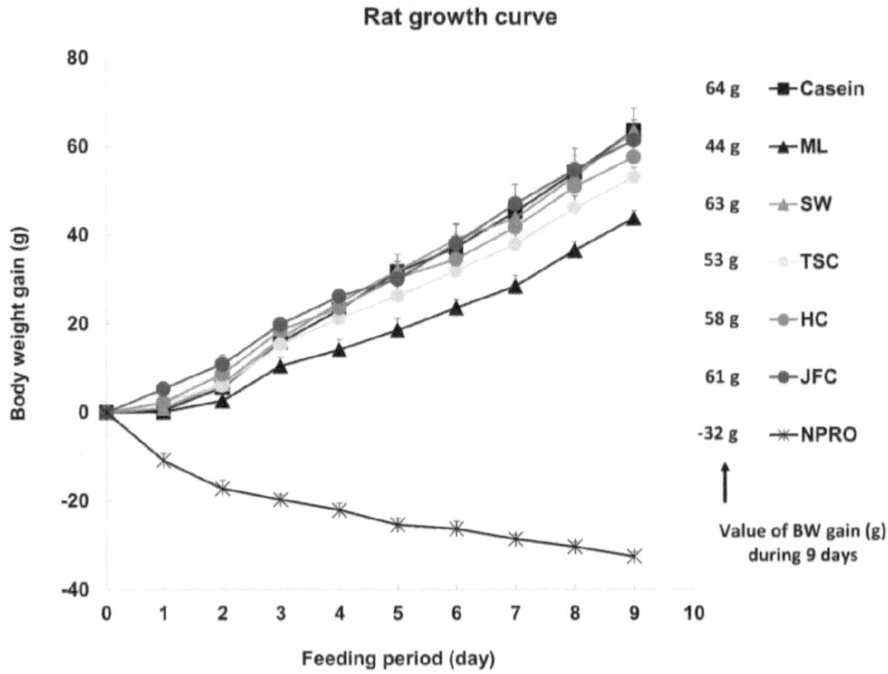

FIGURE 20.5 Effect of edible insect protein quality on rat growth. Body weight gain curves of rats (Means ± SE, n=5) fed diets containing 20% protein from various edible insects or a non-protein diet for 9 days. Values represent the average body weight gain during the treatment period. ML, migratory locust; SW, silkworm; TSC, two-spotted cricket; HC, house cricket; JFC, Jamaican field cricket; NPRO, non-protein.

More information and *in vivo* research on safety, nutrition, and food functional properties are needed to apply edible insects as alternative food protein resources and functional food materials.

THE EFFECTS OF OTHER PROTEINS

Conventional food protein resources primarily include animal products such as milk, eggs, meat, and fish, and plant resources such as soybeans and peas. As this chapter shows, conventional animal proteins have nutritionally sufficient amounts of each AA and an AAS of 100, based on AA composition. In addition, many studies have shown that animal proteins have excellent protein digestibility, with a PDCAAS close to 100. Therefore, milk casein, egg white, soybean meal, and fish meat are used as protein sources in animal experiments (rats and mice). Furthermore, functional food research has increased focus on the nutritional and physiological value of both soybean protein, a representative plant protein, and animal protein. For example, egg white proteins suppress food intake (appetite) and improve glucose and lipid metabolism in rats (Ochai and Matsuo 2014; Ochiai et al. 2014, 2017; Ochiai and Azuma 2017). Notably, egg white proteins strongly inhibit lipid synthesis in adipose tissues and liver and are considered protein sources for weight loss, similar to soybean proteins. The functionality of hydrolyzed peptides has also gained attention, with many studies revealing that specific peptides obtained enzymatically from milk casein and egg white proteins have nutritional and physiological functions.

While the effectiveness and safety of proteins and peptides derived from animal resources are clear, the recent rapid increase in global population has led to increased demand for food, especially food protein, and rising costs of food import and export. Due to factors including changes in the agricultural environment caused by global warming and livestock and poultry feeding management responding to increased awareness of animal welfare, securing food resources to meet population needs is becoming increasingly difficult worldwide. The imbalance between food resource demand and supply is expected to continue, making the development of alternative food resources a critical food issue.

DETAILS OF IMPORTANT AREAS RELATED TO EDIBLE INSECT PROTEINS

Kjeldahl method: An analytical chemistry method for the quantitative determination of nitrogen in organic substances and inorganic compounds such as ammonia and ammonium substances. It involves food digestion with a strong acid to release nitrogen (ammonium sulfate). The amount of nitrogen is then quantified via titration from the amount of ammonia generated by distillation. Crude protein content is calculated from the total nitrogen content of the food using a nitrogen-to-protein conversion factor value.

Nitrogen-protein conversion factor (NPF): For many years, the protein content of foods has been determined based on total nitrogen content, with the Kjeldahl method widely applied for this purpose. Nitrogen content is multiplied by a factor to calculate protein content. This approach is based on two assumptions: that dietary carbohydrates and fats do not contain nitrogen, and that nearly all dietary nitrogen is present as AA in proteins. Early determinations found the average nitrogen (N) content of proteins to be about 16%, which led to the use of the calculation N × 6.25 (1/0.16 = 6.25) to convert nitrogen content into protein content. However, this single factor (NPF) of 6.25 is complicated by two factors. First, not all nitrogen in foods is in proteins: it also exists in variable quantities of other compounds, such as free AA, nucleotides, creatine, and choline, referred to as non-protein nitrogen. Second, the nitrogen content of specific AA varies according to their molecular and number of nitrogen atoms. Consequently, the nitrogen content of proteins actually varies from about 13% to 19%, equating to NPF values ranging from 5.26 to 7.69. In response to these considerations, Jones (1941) suggested replacing N × 6.25 with N × a food-specific factor. These specific factors, now referred to as "Jones factors," have been widely adopted. Jones factors for commonly eaten foods range from 5.18 (nuts, seeds) to 6.38 (milk). However, most foods with a high proportion of non-protein nitrogen contain relatively small amounts of total nitrogen. As a result, the range of Jones factors for major dietary sources of protein is narrower. Jones factors for animal proteins such as meat, milk, and eggs are between 6.25 and 6.38; those for plant proteins that supply substantial quantities of protein in cereal- or legume-based diets generally range from 5.70 to 6.25.

Chitin: A linear nitrogen-containing polysaccharide polymer of poly-β1-4-N-acetylglucosamine. It is a main component of the cuticle that covers the body surface of many invertebrates, such as the exoskeletons of arthropods and crustaceans, the surface of mollusk shells, and the cell walls of fungi such as molds and mushrooms. Chitin contains not only N-acetylglucosamine but also glucosamine, in an approximate ratio of 9:1. Purification involves obtaining chitin from the shells of crustaceans such as crabs and shrimps, which are mainly caught as marine products. Purification includes demineralization using hydrochloric acid, deproteinization using alkali treatment, and depigmentation using alcohol extraction and bleaching methods to remove proteins, pigments such as carotenoids, and calcium salts. In the food sector, it is obtained from the shells of crabs and other crustaceans that are caught as seafood. Although its *in vivo* functionality has not been fully demonstrated, glucosamine obtained by acid hydrolysis of chitin is used in supplements.

Amino Acid Score (AAS): A numerical value evaluating the content ratio of essential AA in foods. It evaluates the amount of essential AA in a specific food per gram of nitrogen compared to standard values. AAS is calculated as mg of each essential AA per gram of nitrogen in protein and as a ratio to the AA scoring pattern based on the FAO/WHO joint committee. (Example: FAO/WHO/UNU (1985) AA Reference Values). On average, 1 g of nitrogen, which makes up protein, is equivalent to 6.25 g of protein. This is a method that compares the standard essential AA pattern with the ratio of essential AA in each food protein, using the value of the AA with the lowest value (first limiting AA) as the evaluation value, also called the chemical evaluation method.

Protein digestibility-corrected amino acid score (PDCAAS): Adopted by FAO/WHO (1991) as the preferred method for measuring the protein value in human nutrition. The method is based on a comparison of the concentration of the first limiting essential AA in the test protein with the concentration of that AA in a reference (scoring) pattern. This scoring pattern is derived from the essential AA requirements of preschool-age children (FAO/WHO/UNU 1985). The resulting chemical score is corrected for true fecal digestibility of the test protein. PDCAAS values higher than 100% are truncated to 100%. Although the PDCAAS method is widely accepted, critical questions have been raised in the scientific community about a number of issues. These questions relate to 1) the validity of the preschool-age child AA requirement values, 2) the validity of correction for fecal instead of ileal digestibility, and 3) the truncation of PDCAAS values to 100%. In recent years, new methods for qualitative evaluation of proteins have been proposed, such as DIAAS (digestible indispensable AA score), which address the above-mentioned issues.

MINI DICTIONARY OF TERMS

- **Cultured meat:** Cultured meat is edible meat obtained by tissue culturing cells from the edible parts of animals. It is attracting attention as an alternative to conventional meat.
- **Food allergens:** Food allergens are proteins, etc., contained in food that the body recognizes as foreign substances when ingested, causing the body to overprotect itself and causing harmful symptoms.
- **Insect:** Insects are pan-crustacean hexapod invertebrates of the class Insecta. They are the largest group within the arthropod phylum. Insects have a chitinous exoskeleton, a three-part body, three pairs of jointed legs, compound eyes, and one pair of antennae.
- **Microalgae:** Microalgae are unicellular species and microscopic algae invisible to the naked eye. They are phytoplankton typically found in freshwater and marine systems, living in both the water column and sediment.
- **Shellfish allergy:** Shellfish allergy is caused by ingesting crustaceans such as shrimp and crabs, which results in various systemic symptoms and sometimes symptoms of anaphylactic shock. Tropomyosin is known to be a major allergen in crustaceans.

SUMMARY POINTS

- Some species of edible insects have been authorized as novel foods in the EU and recommended to be utilized as food protein resources.
- Some edible insects show well-balanced nutrients and contain fat content more than conventional food protein resources.
- Edible insects contain nitrogen-containing dietary fiber chitin at a level of ~2%–11%, inducing the overestimation of protein content when the Kjeldahl method is applied for protein determination.
- The net NPF values of edible insects are lower those of conventional NPF (6.25).
- AAS of edible insect proteins was lower (~63–94) than that of conventional dietary protein resources (milk, soybean, meat, fish) (100).
- Proteins from the edible insect show resistance to gut-intestinal digestion, inducing a lower protein digestibility-corrected AA score (PDCAAS) (44–81) than each AAS and PDCAAS of casein (97).
- Low AAS and PDCAAS of edible insect proteins show the suppression of growth in rats.

- Some proteins and peptides derived from edible insects are expected to represent food functional properties mainly *in vitro* assays, but more investigations are needed *in vivo* considering the protein and AA metabolism.

REFERENCES

Aguilera, Y. et al. 2021. Investigating edible insects as a sustainable food source: nutritional value and techno-functional and physiological properties. *Food Funct* 12:6309–22.

Aguilar-Toalá, J. E. et al. 2022. Beyond human nutrition of edible insects: health benefits and safety aspects. *Insects* 13:1007.

Aiello, D. et al. 2023. Edible insects an alternative nutritional source of bioactive compounds: a review. *Molecules* 28:699.

Boulos, S. et al. 2020. Nitrogen-to-protein conversion factors for edible insects on the swiss market: *T. molitor, A. domesticus*, and *L. migratoria*. *Front Nutr* 7:89.

Boye, J. et al. 2012. Protein quality evaluation twenty years after the introduction of the protein digestibility corrected amino acid score method. *Br J Nutr* 108:S183–211.

Churchward-Venne, T. A. et al. 2017. Consideration of insects as a source of dietary protein for human consumption. *Nutr Rev* 75:1035–45.

D'Antonio, V. et al. 2021. Dietary modulation of oxidative stress from edible insects: a mini-review. *Front Nutr* 8:642551.

De Marchi et al. 2021. Allergens from edible insects: cross-reactivity and effects of processing. *Curr Allergy Asthma Rep* 21:35.

EFSA Panel on Nutrition, Novel Foods and Food Allergens (NDA). 2021a. Safety of dried yellow mealworm (*Tenebrio molitor* larva) as a novel food pursuant to Regulation (EU) 2015/2283. *EFSA J* 19:e06343.

EFSA Panel on Nutrition, Novel Foods and Food Allergens (NDA). 2021b. Safety of frozen and dried formulations from migratory locust (*Locusta migratoria*) as a Novel food pursuant to Regulation (EU) 2015/2283. *EFSA J* 19:e06667.

EFSA Panel on Nutrition, Novel Foods and Food Allergens (NDA). 2021c. Safety of frozen and dried formulations from whole yellow mealworm (*Tenebrio molitor larva*) as a novel food pursuant to Regulation (EU) 2015/2283. *EFSA J* 19:e06778.

EFSA Panel on Nutrition, Novel Foods and Food Allergens (NDA). 2021d. Safety of frozen and dried formulations from whole house crickets (*Acheta domesticus*) as a Novel food pursuant to Regulation (EU) 2015/2283. *EFSA J* 19:e06779.

EFSA Panel on Nutrition, Novel Foods and Food Allergens (NDA). 2022. Safety of frozen and freeze-dried formulations of the lesser mealworm (*Alphitobius diaperinus* larva) as a Novel food pursuant to Regulation (EU) 2015/2283. *EFSA J* 20:e07325.

EFSA Panel on Nutrition, Novel Foods and Food Allergens (NDA). 2023. Safety of UV-treated powder of whole yellow mealworm (*Tenebrio molitor larva*) as a novel food pursuant to Regulation (EU) 2015/2283. *EFSA J* 21:e08009.

Energy and protein requirements. Report of a joint FAO/WHO/UNU Expert Consultation. *World Health Organ Tech Rep Ser.* 1985;724:1–206.

FAO. 2021. Looking at edible insects from a food safety perspective. Challenges and opportunities for the sector. Rome, Italy. https://doi.org/10.4060/cb4094en.

FAO/WHO. 1991. Protein Quality Evaluation; Report of a Joint FAO/WHO Expert Consultation, United Nations; Rome, Italy. https://www.fao.org/ag/humannutrition/35978-02317b979a686a57aa4593304f-fc17f06.pdf.

Hawkey, K. J. et al. 2021. Insects: a potential source of protein and other nutrients for feed and food. *Annu Rev Anim Biosci* 9:333–54.

Hayes, M. 2020. Measuring protein content in food: an overview of methods. *Foods* 9:1340.

Højrup, P. et al. 1986. Isolation, characterization, and N-terminal sequence studies of cuticular proteins from the migratory locust, *Locusta migratoria*. *Eur J Biochem* 154:153–9.

Hughes, G. J. et al. 2011. Protein digestibility-corrected amino acid scores (PDCAAS) for soy protein isolates and concentrate: criteria for evaluation. *J Agri Food Chem* 59:12707–12.

Janssen, R. H. et al. 2017. Nitrogen-to-protein conversion factors for three edible insects: *Tenebrio molitor, Alphitobius diaperinus*, and *Hermetia illucens*. *J Agric Food Chem* 65:2275–8.

Jantzen da Silva Lucas A. et al. 2020. Edible insects: an alternative of nutritional, functional and bioactive compounds. *Food Chem* 311:126022.

Jonas-Levi, A. and Martinez, J. J. I. 2017. The high level of protein content reported in insects for food and feed is overestimated. *J Food Compos Anal* 62:184–8.

Jones, D. B. 1941. Factors for converting percentages of nitrogen in foods and feeds into percentages of protein. Washington, DC, US Department of Agriculture-circ. 183.

Jongema, Y. 2017. List of edible insects of the world, 2017. https://www.wur.nl/en/research-results/chair-groups/plant-sciences/laboratory-of-entomology/edible-insects/worldwide-species-list.htm. (accessed September 1, 2023).

Kamemura, N. et al. 2019. Cross-allergenicity of crustacean and the edible insect *Gryllus bimaculatus* in patients with shrimp allergy. *Mol Immunol* 106:127–34.

Lange, K. W. and Nakamura, Y. 2023. Edible insects and their potential anti-obesity effects: a review. *Food Sci Anim Prod* 1:9240008.

Liceaga, A. M. 2022. Edible insects, a valuable protein source from ancient to modern times. *Adv Food Nutr Res* 101:129–52.

Liceaga, A. M. et al. 2022. Insects as an alternative protein source. *Annu Rev Food Sci Technol* 13:19–34.

Longvah, T. et al. 2011. Nutrient profile and protein quality evaluation of eri silkworm (*Samia ricinii*) prepupae and pupae. *Food Chem* 128:400–3.

Manditsera, F. A. et al. 2019. Effect of domestic cooking methods on protein digestibility and mineral bioaccessibility of wild harvested adult edible insects. *Food Res Int* 121:404–11.

Mathai, J. K. et al. 2017. Values for digestible indispensable amino acid scores (DIAAS) for some dairy and plant proteins may better describe protein quality than values calculated using the concept for protein digestibility-corrected amino acid scores (PDCAAS). *Br J Nutr* 117:490–9.

Mæhre, H. K. et al. 2018. Protein determination-method matters. *Foods* 7:5.

Mariotti, F. et al. 2008. Converting nitrogen into protein-beyond 6.25 and Jones' factors. *Crit Rev Food Sci Nutr* 48:177–84.

Moruzzo, R. et al. 2021. Edible insects and sustainable development goals. *Insects* 12:557.

Ochiai, M. and Azuma, Y. 2017. Egg white hydrolysate improves glucose tolerance in type-2 diabetic NSY mice. *J Nutr Sci Vitaminol* 63:422–9.

Ochiai, M. and Komiya, Y. 2021. Detection of edible insect derived phospholipids with polyunsaturated fatty acids by thin-layer chromatography, gas chromatography, and enzymatic methods. *J Food Compos Anal* 99:103869.

Ochiai, M. and Matsuo, T. 2014. Effect of egg white and its hydrolysate on stearoyl-CoA desaturase index and fat accumulation in rat tissues. *Int J Food Sci Nutr* 65:948–52.

Ochiai, M. et al. 2014. Increased muscular triglyceride content and hyperglycemia in Goto-Kakizaki rat are decreased by egg white hydrolysate. *Int J Food Sci Nutr* 65:495–501.

Ochiai, M. et al. 2017. Egg white hydrolysate can be a low-allergenic food material to suppress ectopic fat accumulation in rats fed an equicaloric diet. *J Nutr Sci Vitaminol* 63:111–19.

Ochiai, M. et al. 2022. Edible insect *Locusta migratoria* shows intestinal protein digestibility and improves plasma and hepatic lipid metabolism in male rats. *Food Chem* 396:133701.

Ochiai, M. et al. 2024. Low protein digestibility-corrected amino acid score and net nitrogen-to-protein conversion factor value of edible insects. *Food Chem* 454:139781.

Palmer, L. K. et al. 2020. Shellfish tropomyosin IgE cross-reactivity differs among edible insect species. *Mol Nutr Food Res* 64:e1900923.

Quah, Y. et al. 2023. Bioactive peptide discovery from edible insects for potential applications in human health and agriculture. *Molecules* 28:1233.

Raheem, D. et al. 2019. Traditional consumption of and rearing edible insects in Africa, Asia and Europe. *Crit Rev Food Sci Nutr* 59:2169–88.

Ribeiro, J. C. et al. 2018. Allergic risks of consuming edible insects: a systematic review. *Mol Nutr Food Res* 62.

Rodríguez-Rodríguez, M. et al. 2022. In vitro crude protein digestibility of insects: a review. *Insects* 13:682.

Rutherfurd, S. M. et al. 2015. Protein digestibility-corrected amino acid scores and digestible indispensable amino acid scores differentially describe protein quality in growing male rats. *J Nutr* 145:372–9.

Schaafsma, G. 2000. The protein digestibility-corrected amino acid score. *J Nutr* 130:1865S–7S.

Schaafsma, G. 2005. The protein digestibility-corrected amino acid score (PDCAAS)—a concept for describing protein quality in foods and food ingredients: a critical review. *J AOAC Int* 88:988–94.

Smets, R. et al. 2021. On the nitrogen content and a robust nitrogen-to-protein conversion factor of black soldier fly larvae (Hermetia illucens). *Anal Bioanal Chem* 413:6365–77.

Tang, C. et al. 2019. Edible insects as a food source: a review. *Food Prod Process and Nutr* 1;8.

Teixeira, C. S. S. et al. 2023. Edible insects as a novel source of bioactive peptides: a systematic review. *Foods* 12:2026.

United Nations, Department of Economic and Social Affairs, 2022. *World Population Prospects 2022. Summary of Results*. New York: United Nations.

van Huis, A. et al. 2013. Edible insects: future prospects for food and feed security. *FAO Forestry Paper* no. 171, Rome, Italy. https://www.fao.org/3/i3253e/i3253e.pdf.

van Huis, A. et al. 2021. Nutritional qualities and enhancement of edible insects. *Annu Rev Nutr* 41:551–76.

21 Cultivated Meat as a New Source of Sustainable Alternative Protein

Samantha Robertson and Masatoshi Suzuki

ABBREVIATIONS

3D	Three-dimensional
ECM	Extracellular matrix
ESC	Embryonic stem cell
FAP	Fibro-adipogenic progenitor
GMO	Genetically modified organism
GRAS	Generally recognized as safe
iPSC	Induced pluripotent stem cell
SARS-CoV-2	Severe acute respiratory syndrome coronavirus 2
SMPC	Skeletal muscle progenitor/stem cell

INTRODUCTION

Cellular agriculture is quickly becoming a growing scientific field, supported by multidisciplinary concepts and knowledge in bioengineering, animal science, and cell biology (Eibl et al. 2021; Reiss et al. 2021; Chodkowska et al. 2022). Specifically, cultivated meat represents a new type of meat manufactured from cell and tissue cultures. It is also known as cell-based meat and is an artificial product produced through *in vitro* methods using animal cells. The fundamental strategy of cultivated meat production is supported by muscle tissue engineering (Samandari et al. 2023; Sugii et al. 2023).

This technology may become a game changer in resolving various concerns associated with conventional meat production. For instance, cellular agriculture is expected to address environmental concerns by reducing the carbon footprint associated with traditional livestock agriculture and being more eco-friendly (Gerber et al. 2013; Bellarby et al. 2013; Sinke and Odegard 2021). Cultivated meat can also potentially eliminate ethical concerns regarding animal welfare, which are inherent in the process of conventional meat production through livestock farming. Furthermore, it can address health concerns arising from animal-borne diseases and the use of antibiotics (Webster 2002; Zhao et al. 2010).

Cultivated meat can also offer an effective solution to meet future projections of an ever-increasing global population and overall demand for meat (Mcconnell et al. 2023; Food and Agriculture Organization of the United Nations 2017). The recent SARS-CoV-2 pandemic, which had incredible impacts on meat production and consumer needs, has also highlighted the importance of a more sustainable meat supply (Ijaz et al. 2021). All these factors motivating the creation of a cultivated meat food supply will be heightened by increasing consumer awareness and greater public knowledge about healthy eating habits, optimal conditions for keeping animals, and animal welfare.

DOI: 10.1201/9781003597926-21

The ultimate goal of cultivated meat manufacturing is to make a low-cost meat substitute with the organoleptic and nutritional properties of real meat.

One considerable impact of cellular agriculture is that it can offer sustainable products as a new protein alternative. Meat is animal flesh composed of skeletal muscle, fat, and connective tissue, representing one of the essential components of a balanced human diet (Klurfeld 2018). It is rich in nutrients such as proteins, iron, vitamins, and fatty acids. As cultivated meat is derived from animal cells, the product can serve as an animal protein-rich alternative to traditional meat. Current products in development target species including livestock such as cattle, pigs, chickens, crustaceans, and fish.

The production process of cultivated meat is supported by muscle tissue engineering, a strategy for generating *in vitro* muscle tissues using cell culture and tissue-engineering techniques (Pajcin et al. 2022). The technology has several attractive advantages, but cellular agriculture still faces many technical hurdles to achieving high-quality and high-quantity production at relatively reasonable costs and for wide-range commercialization (Reiss et al. 2021).

This chapter discusses the potential of cultivated meat as a new source of sustainable alternative protein. First, it examines the definition and background of cultivated meat as a type of artificial meat. Next, it overviews a typical manufacturing strategy for cultivated meat production. Additionally, the chapter discusses the potential and promises of cultivated meat as an animal protein alternative. Lastly, it addresses the current status and existing challenges associated with cultivated meat production. A main discussion point is how cultivated meat can sustainably contribute to society as an alternative protein source.

CULTIVATED MEAT AS AN EMERGING TYPE OF ARTIFICIAL MEAT

Cultivated meat is classified as one type of artificial meat. Artificial meat is broadly defined as meat replacements with three types: meat substitutes, cultured meat, and modified meat (Figure 21.1) (Bonny et al. 2015; Mateti et al. 2022). The first type comprises meat substitutes composed of non-animal materials from plants and fungi. Representative products of meat substitutes are fermentation-based meat substitutes manufactured from soybean (such as tofu) and fungal proteins (Quorn). These products are already accessible in the market and have gradually gained acceptance among consumers. However, they still constitute a small portion of the total market due to consumers' preferences regarding taste, texture, and price.

The second type of artificial meat is cultured meat, which is formulated with cells *in vitro* by tissue engineering. Recent advances in tissue engineering allow for the manufacture of *in vitro* products by large-scale expansion of seeding cells in culture and three-dimensional (3D) tissue formation. Lastly, modified meat is a product using materials or cells (partially or mainly) originating from genetically modified organisms (GMOs). Genetic engineering and biotechnology enable the development of GMOs such as transgenic pigs and cows. While GMOs offer attractive potential to improve the production of meat alternatives, consumers' general skepticism toward GMOs largely influences their acceptance of GMO-derived meat products. If genetically modified cells are used for production, these meat products may also be considered a type of cultivated meat (Bonny et al. 2015; Mateti et al. 2022). Meat derived from cloned animals, if available in the future, may be considered a fourth category of artificial meat because the cloning process is artificially manipulated (Bonny et al. 2015; Mateti et al. 2022).

There are many "synonyms" used as technical, lay, and media terms when referring to artificial meat and cultivated meat. Sometimes these terms are conceptually confused when used. For instance, cultivated meat is often misunderstood as a genetically modified food because both are associated with laboratory work and biotechnology. These words are available in Figure 21.1, although the list is not exhaustive.

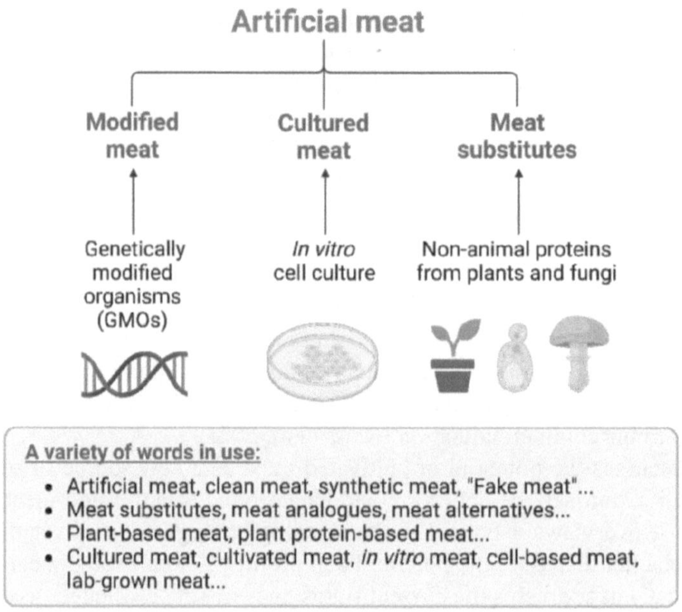

FIGURE 21.1 Classification of artificial meat. Artificial meat has three main types of meat replacements: meat substitutes, cultured meat, and modified meat. Meat substitutes are non-animal products containing plant- and/or myo-proteins. Cultured meat is produced from cells through tissue engineering. Modified meat is derived from genetically modified organisms (GMOs). This classification is based on previous publications (Bonny et al. 2015; Mateti et al. 2022). This figure was created using BioRender (http://biorender.com/).

SHIFTING CONCEPTS TOWARD CULTIVATED MEAT AND ITS OVERALL PRODUCTION WORKFLOW

The idea of meat replacement in food products is not new, but it has become the rationale for cultivated meat (Figure 21.2) (Ismail et al. 2020). Traditionally, soy protein-based products such as tofu (also known as bean curd) and tempeh (fermented soybean cake) have been consumed for centuries in Asia. Plant-based proteins are not limited to these traditional Asian products; they have been actively used for the production of meat alternatives. While the acceptance of plant-based foods has increased based on historical use, these products have potential concerns for some people in terms of flavor and allergies to soy proteins and gluten. Meanwhile, interest in healthy food and environmental sustainability has been highlighted in the public eye.

Along with technological developments in cell culture and tissue engineering, the current trend in meat alternative production has expanded toward cultivated meat production. Since the original concept was proposed in the early 1900s, several notable milestones have guided the history of cultivated meat (Figure 21.3) (Yap et al. 2023; Eibl et al. 2021; Kumar et al. 2021; Ye et al. 2022; Ramani et al. 2021). These milestones include significant advances in development, foundation, commercialization, and policy.

The production of cultivated meat requires three steps: 1) cell sourcing and line establishment, 2) large-scale cell expansion, and 3) tissue biomanufacturing as meat products (Figure 21.4) (Reiss et al. 2021). This production workflow has been formulated by a combination of relevant bioengineering approaches. Specific techniques and biomaterials include cell culture, small molecule-based signaling, bioreactors, and biocompatible scaffolds for tissue engineering.

The isolation and establishment of required cell types are the first steps of the production process. These cells are expanded to a large scale in a culture medium, which is supplemented with various small molecules for cell proliferation. The expanded cells are then seeded into biocompatible tissue scaffolds to prepare 3D tissue formation following proper cell differentiation and maturation. For

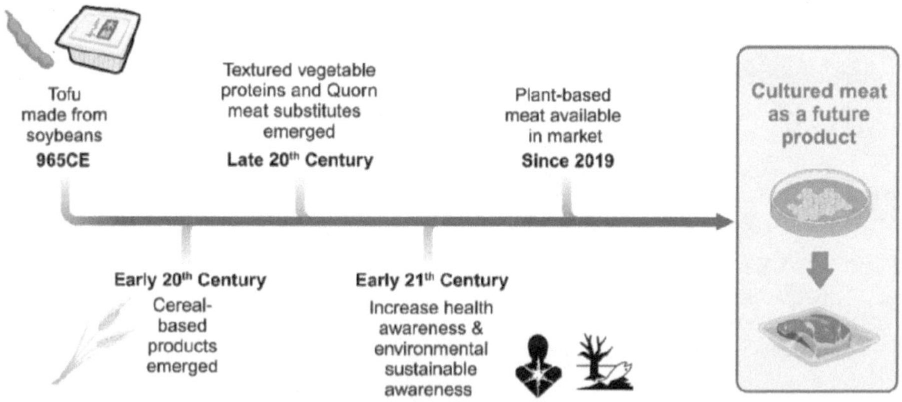

FIGURE 21.2 The history of meat alternatives and cultivated meat as a future prospect. The introduction of meat replacements in food products began with fermentation-based substitutes and soybean-based diets such as tofu and tempeh (fermented soybean cake developed in Indonesia). Following other significant milestones in history, cultivated meat shows great promise as an alternative type of artificial meat in the field. This figure was modified from Ismail et al. (2020). This figure was created using BioRender (http://biorender.com/).

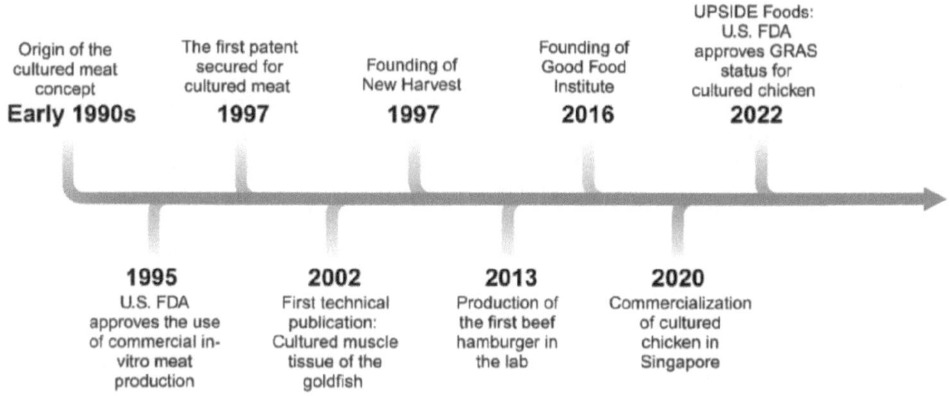

FIGURE 21.3 The major milestones in the development of cultivated meat. US FDA, US Food and Drug Administration; GRAS, generally recognized as safe. This figure was adapted from previous literature (Yap et al. 2023; Eibl et al. 2021; Kumar et al. 2021; Ye et al. 2022; Ramani et al. 2021) and was created using BioRender (http://biorender.com/).

manufacturing cells and tissues, different types of bioreactors are available for scaling up production to a commercially viable size.

CELL TYPES AND SOURCING FOR CULTIVATED MEAT PRODUCTION

The sourcing of specific cell types, such as skeletal myocytes and adipocytes, is the first step in the manufacturing workflow of cultivated meat production. Meat comprises approximately 90% muscle and 10% fat and connective tissue, although there are differences depending on species and muscle types (Warriss and Rhodes 1977; Listrat et al. 2016). Considering this initial composition of tissue types, the main cellular components present in meat are skeletal myocytes, adipocytes, and fibroblasts. Additional cell types, such as mesenchymal stromal cells, endothelial cells, chondrocytes, osteocytes, and hematopoietic cells, also play supporting roles in tissue formation during the production of cultivated meat. Due to these variations in cell and tissue types, the nutritive composition

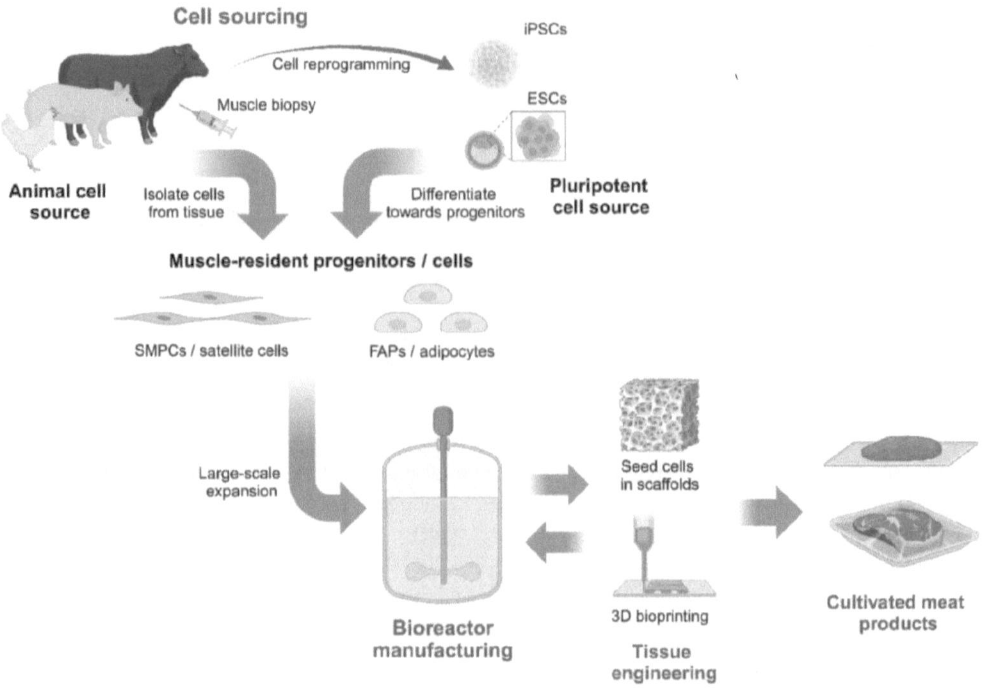

FIGURE 21.4 A typical workflow of cultivated meat production. Cell sourcing is the first step of the workflow. Available cells may be sourced from either an animal cell source or a pluripotent cell source. Muscle-resident progenitors, skeletal muscle progenitor stem cells (SMPCs) and fibro-adipogenic progenitors (FAPs), are prepared from the chosen cell source. These cells are expanded in a bioreactor to yield a large quantity of cells. Tissue-engineering approaches, such as biocompatible tissue scaffolds and 3D bioprinting, can facilitate tissue formation and provide the cultivated meat product with a specific structure. This figure was modified from Reiss et al. (2021) and created using BioRender (http://biorender.com/).

of protein, total fat, and fatty acids in skeletal muscle differs between species (Bomkamp et al. 2022).

Cell sourcing is the most critical step in achieving efficient production. It is ideal to have highly proliferative and immature cell lines to fulfill this requirement, as the quality of these cells ensures cell proliferation and differentiation at a scale appropriate for commercial production. To prepare a variety of highly proliferative cells, progenitor/stem cells are commonly used for cultivated meat production. These cells can differentiate into musculoskeletal tissues, such as skeletal muscle progenitor/stem cells (SMPCs, also known as myogenic progenitors) and fibro-adipogenic progenitors (FAPs). These cells can be differentiated into several critical cell types: skeletal myocytes, adipocytes, and fibroblasts (Samandari et al. 2023). Since cultivated meat is a type of bioengineered skeletal muscle tissue, SMPCs for cultivated meat production should have a high affinity for forming elongated myocytes, multinucleated myotubes, and myofibers. Various types of SMPCs are potentially available for muscle tissue engineering (Hosoyama et al. 2012).

There are two major sources of progenitor/stem cells for muscle tissue engineering (Reiss et al. 2021; Pajcin et al. 2022; Jara et al. 2023): 1) primary cells isolated from animal tissues, and 2) progenitor/stem cells prepared from pluripotent stem cells. Such cell types are identified in pre- or post-natal muscles as well as non-muscle somatic tissues (Figure 21.4). Furthermore, pluripotent stem cells can be used to derive SMPCs and other progenitor/stem cells using specific derivation protocols in culture.

SKELETAL MUSCLE SATELLITE CELLS AND FIBRO-ADIPOGENIC PROGENITORS

Primary cells are directly isolated from a biopsy or post-mortem tissue. While embryonic, postnatal, and adult tissues are available as primary cell sources, adult muscle tissues are often chosen to isolate primary cells for cultivated meat production. Cell sorting or extra cell plating procedures may be required to enrich specific cells of interest and obtain a good population of target cells. As a primary cell source of SMPCs, muscle-resident progenitors can be isolated from skeletal muscle tissues (Figure 21.5). These progenitors are known as satellite cells (or myosatellite cells), a type of adult stem cell with a high potential to differentiate into well-matured myotubes and myofibers. Satellite cells are found under the basement membrane of muscle fibers. These cells are normally quiescent in adult muscles but respond to stress, trauma, and other stimulations. These activated cells can then contribute to muscle repair and plasticity (Bischoff and Heintz 1994; Morgan and Partridge 2003; Kuang et al. 2007; Xu et al. 2015). Although current knowledge of satellite cell biology is mainly based on research in rodents and humans, the significance of these cells in livestock *in vivo* and *in vitro* has also been well explored (Ding et al. 2018; Li et al. 2015; Kolkmann et al. 2022).

Throughout different species, muscle satellite cells can be identified by specific markers (Tey et al. 2019) (Figure 21.5). Both quiescent and activated satellite cells express the transcription factor Pax7. With the expression of another transcription factor, MyoD, satellite cells are committed to becoming myoblasts or myogenic precursor cells, which then terminally differentiate into multinucleated myotubes positive for myosin heavy chain. Desmin, a major subunit of muscle-type intermediate filaments, is also known to be specific to postmitotic myoblasts and myotubes.

Other types of progenitor/stem cells are also necessary to add non-muscle cellular and nutritive components like fat. Among these cells, FAPs are considered a type of adipogenic cell. FAPs are multipotent mesenchymal stem cells that can preferentially differentiate into either adipocytes or fibroblasts. These cells normally reside in the interstitial space between myofibers (Low et al. 2017). FAPs are essential in supporting regeneration in skeletal muscle cells (Biferali et al. 2019) as the main source of excess extracellular matrix (ECM) in normal and pathological conditions. The two

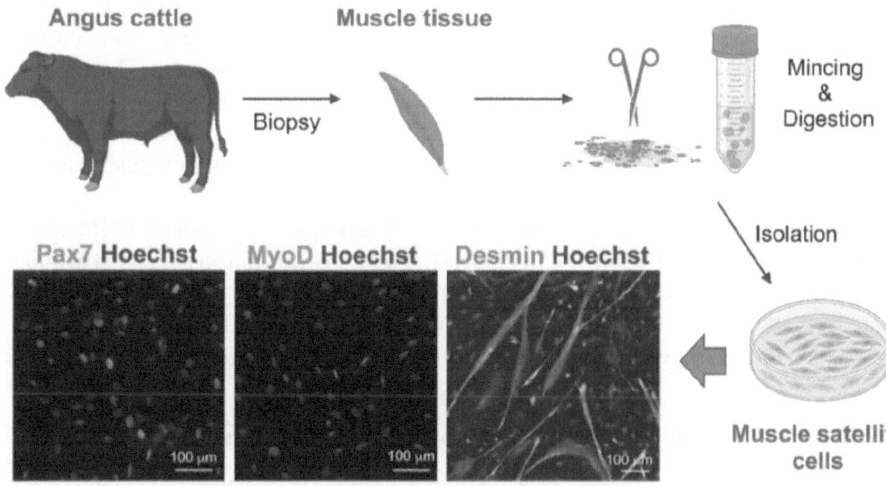

FIGURE 21.5 A representative process of muscle satellite cell isolation as a primary cell source is presented. This figure represents a recent workflow for isolating bovine satellite cells from Angus cattle. Muscle tissue samples were collected from different muscle types (neck, back, cheek, and hindlimb) in the body by biopsy. Tissues were minced with scissors and then enzymatically digested by collagenase. After isolating cell fractions by repeated centrifugation, primary satellite cells were isolated and expanded in culture. These satellite cells were plated on coverslips and differentiated for 2 weeks. After fixation, the cells were immunostained for specific markers (Pax7, MyoD, and Desmin) targeting satellite cells and myoblasts. This figure was created using BioRender (http://biorender.com/).

progenitor/stem cells, SMPCs and FAPs, can cover the creation of required tissue types that formulate meat products. These adult stem cells would be easily accessible for establishing cultivated meat production. In fact, current efforts in the field mainly focus on the potential use of SMPCs and FAPs derived from primary tissue sources. However, one disadvantage of adult stem cells is their limited capacity for proliferation (Redondo et al. 2017).

PLURIPOTENT STEM CELLS AS ANOTHER CELL SOURCE FOR CULTIVATED MEAT PRODUCTION

Another cell source for cultivated meat production is progenitor/stem cells derived from pluripotent stem cells. There are two types of pluripotent stem cells: embryonic stem cells (ESCs) and induced pluripotent stem cells (iPSCs). While ESCs are derived from the inner cell mass of the blastocyst, iPSCs are created from adult somatic cells by cell reprogramming back into an embryonic-like pluripotent state (Takahashi and Yamanaka 2006; Yu et al. 2007). Both ESCs and iPSCs have attractive potential for sourcing specific cell types such as SMPCs and FAPs. These pluripotent stem cells are highly proliferative in culture while maintaining their undifferentiated state. As their name implies, their pluripotency is a considerable advantage: the ability to differentiate into any cell type in the three germ layers – mesoderm, ectoderm, and endoderm. Livestock ESCs and iPSCs have already been established, although their availability is still limited compared to mouse or human cell lines.

When pluripotent stem cells are used for cultivated meat production, they need to be differentiated into specific cell types. Therefore, well-established differentiation protocols for livestock pluripotent stem cells must be available to secure high-quality progenitor/stem cells on a sufficient scale for production, which is an ongoing challenge in the field. Differentiation protocols for human and murine cells have already been reported to yield a significant number of progenitors and mature cells, such as SMPCs and skeletal myocytes (Jiwlawat et al. 2017; Jiwlawat et al. 2018), satellite cells (Al Tanoury et al. 2020), FAPs (Hynes et al. 2016), and adipocytes (Guénantin et al. 2017). Typically, the genetic modification of myogenic genes (such as Pax7 and MyoD) is quite effective in forcing specific cell differentiation into the skeletal muscle lineage. However, this approach may not be ideal for cultivated meat production because the end products are considered genetically modified foods, which are not always acceptable to a wide range of consumers. Therefore, potential risks and concerns associated with genetically modified organisms should be carefully considered when using these cells for cultivated meat production. Instead, it is important to focus on optimizing culture conditions that are efficient and provide a large scale of cells without genetic modifications for livestock ESCs and iPSCs.

Primary cells can be easily obtained from a biopsy of any species or muscle of interest, but they are limited in their proliferative capacity. In contrast, the highly proliferative capacity of pluripotent stem cells is an attractive feature of these immortalized cells. However, the expansion and differentiation procedures of pluripotent stem cells are often more complicated. The production cost may be more expensive to obtain progenitor/stem cells for cultivated meat production from pluripotent cells.

LARGE-SCALE CELL EXPANSION USING BIOREACTOR SYSTEMS

After the required cells are established, scaling up cell sources is the subsequent step for cultivated meat production. For large-scale production of cell culture biopharmaceuticals, bioreactor systems have commonly been used to provide the necessary stimuli and capacity in culture (Pajcin et al. 2022). A bioreactor is an engineered vessel that can manage the culture environment, supporting the growth and development of cells or tissues within its chamber. Bioreactors continuously aid in nutrient diffusion and cell development by stirring or stimulating the cells to support their proliferation and maturation. In the context of cultivated meat production, bioreactors can maintain cells and culture medium at the desired biological conditions from a lab-grown scale up to a manufacturing scale. At the initial stage of cultivated meat production, maintaining active cell proliferation is critical. Therefore, a bioreactor plays a key role in enabling large-scale cell culture. It can also simplify medium recycling and replacement throughout the proliferation stage, which helps with bioprocessing in the manufacturing workflow. Currently, different types of bioreactors are available, such as stirred-tank, hollow fiber, roller bottle, rocking bed, fluidized-bed, and fixed (packed) bed systems (Pajcin et al. 2022). In some workflows, a secondary step using a bioreactor is also included for the prepared tissues or cell aggregates with microcarriers that have already been seeded with myocytes or other cell types. This step is expected to maintain the culture long-term until tissue differentiation and maturation are fully achieved.

TISSUE ENGINEERING TO SUPPORT WELL-ORGANIZED TISSUE FORMATION

Many artificial meat products are currently available, such as ground beef, meatballs, and meat nuggets. These products do not need prominent scaffolding architecture. However, if the production of cultivated steak is considered, the organization of 3D tissue structure will be required. Multiple bioengineering approaches can create well-defined 3D cellular organization in the final product, including microcarriers, 3D bioprinting, ECMs, and biological scaffolds. Specifically, microcarriers can promote cell expansion and differentiation in culture. Recent advances in 3D bioprinting technology allow researchers to generate structurally organized tissues by design. Furthermore, a good choice of ECM types can sufficiently simulate the cellular microenvironment, which can facilitate the differentiation and maturation of seeded cells. Indeed, hydrogels have commonly been used commonly as a major choice of bioink for 3D bioprinting in the field of tissue engineering.

To date, different types of biological scaffolds have been developed and tested to achieve 3D muscle tissue formation, including cultivated meat production (Bomkamp et al. 2022). Unique types of biomaterials are also being explored, such as materials and scaffolds derived from plants and microalgae. For instance, decellularized plant materials have been proposed for use as 3D tissue scaffolds for cultivated meat production and muscle tissue engineering (Ben-Arye et al. 2020; Gershlak et al. 2017; Fontana et al. 2017; Yun et al. 2023). These scaffolds can provide the architecture of the cultivated meat product. A scaffold is a biocompatible material that can support the development and differentiation of cells that adhere to it. Many scaffolds also have specific porosity and degradability to help nutrient diffusion to seeded cells. Specifically, SMPCs and myoblasts are adherent and need a scaffold during their 3D tissue formation development to facilitate proliferation and differentiation into myocytes. As a result, a scaffold is often required during the stages of differentiation and tissue maturation in the production workflow of cultivated meat. Typically, for cultivated meat production, tissue scaffolds should be edible, nontoxic, and biodegradable. Although tissue-engineering approaches using different biomaterials and techniques are still in the process of development, the choice of bioengineering approaches will influence the quality of the final products.

PROMISES OF CULTIVATED MEAT AS A NEW SOURCE OF SUSTAINABLE PROTEIN ALTERNATIVES

The new movement for cultivated meat is supported by different stakeholders in academia, industry, and the economy. Several companies have already launched plant-based or insect products as meat substitutes. These products offer solutions to meet the demands and needs of both consumers and the environment. Likewise, cellular agriculture has many promising advantages in addressing these issues (Figure 21.6) (Sexton et al. 2019; Hocquette 2016).

When considering cultivated meat as an alternative protein, one strength is that the technology can secure safe and stable meat production because the products are fabricated in labs and factories. Cultivated meat production is based on a sequence of bioprocesses initially founded on cell biological and bioengineering approaches. Once the manufacturing workflow is established, production

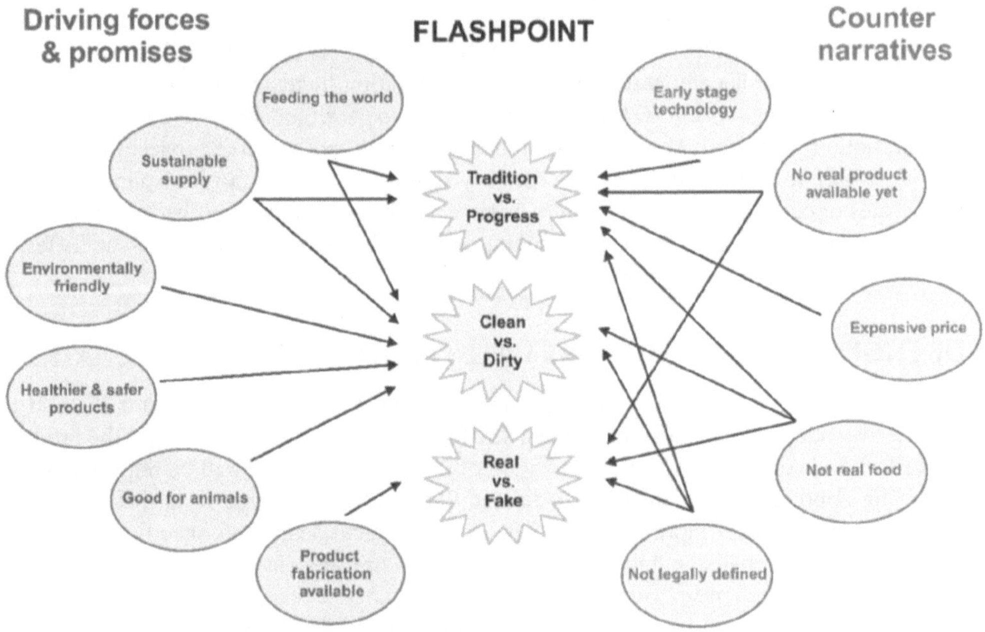

FIGURE 21.6 Narratives and flashpoints of cultivated meat as a source of alternative protein. Three flashpoints (middle column) are listed between the promises (left) and the counter-narratives (right). The concept of this figure was based on information from two papers (Sexton et al. 2019; Hocquette 2016). This figure was created using BioRender (http://biorender.com/).

can be managed to minimize potential influences from external factors such as climate, shortages of natural resources, and animal health conditions.

Furthermore, there are opportunities to modify the nutritive composition of the product during manufacturing. First, different proportions of cell types can alter the ratio of protein, acid, and fat in the final product. If different ratios of SMPCs and/or FAPs are applied for seeding, the composition of myocytes and adipocytes will change. It is also possible to add extra nutritive supplements to the product at a specific step of bioprocessing. For instance, vitamins, minerals, amino acids, and lipids can be supplemented when 3D tissue structure is organized. This means that cultivated meat has the potential to become a new type of health food. Additionally, the use of unique materials in the tissue engineering step can create a new product with different components. For instance, scaffolding with plant-based materials can add plant-derived proteins, ECM, and fibers (Ben-Arye et al. 2020; Gershlak et al. 2017; Fontana et al. 2017; Yun et al. 2023). This results in a final product that differs from conventional meat products. While the current direction of cellular agriculture is to develop products that completely resemble conventional meat, production can be altered to accommodate any type of modification, which is the most significant advantage of this technology compared to conventional meat production.

Another benefit of cultivated meat is that it can serve as a sustainable source of alternative proteins while maintaining sufficient quality, cleanliness, and safety in the resulting products. Conventional meat factories frequently experience supply recalls or shortages due to widespread disease outbreaks in livestock. The COVID-19 pandemic adversely affected production in the farming and meat industries (Ijaz et al. 2021). Also, there are continuous concerns regarding the contamination of hormones, antibiotics, and pesticides in conventionally produced meat and other dairy products (Welsh et al. 2019; Grzinic et al. 2023). All of these issues may pose potential risks of foodborne illness to consumers. Well-established manufacturing of cultivated meat could address these concerns in the near future.

REMAINING HURDLES FOR CULTIVATED MEAT PRODUCTION

While the potential of cultivated meat is attractive, it remains a fairly young field with many discoveries yet to be made. It is expected to achieve well-controlled and sustainable manufacturing of agricultural products using cells and tissues. To date, several technical hurdles remain (Figure 21.6) (Reiss et al. 2021; Chodkowska et al. 2022; Sexton et al. 2019; Hocquette 2016).

First, an ongoing challenge for cultivated meat production is the limited availability of high-quality progenitor/stem cell lines to fulfill the quality and quantity needed to obtain relevant immature cells and mature tissue types. Primary cells have a limited capacity for proliferation. More active use of pluripotent stem cells may resolve this limitation, but further studies of progenitor derivation methods using livestock ESCs and iPSCs are still needed.

Next, a well-designed protocol for cell and tissue culture should be established to address existing obstacles related to product quality and production cost. An ideal medium formulation should be pathogen-free, xeno-free, and chemically defined. Additional considerations are needed to secure the high quality of the final products. Furthermore, the current production costs are higher than conventional meat products, because cell and tissue culture require expensive materials such as culture media, growth factors, reagents, and plasticware. Without better cell lines showing a high capacity for cell proliferation and cost-effective culture protocols for manufacturing, it may be challenging to offer competitive pricing. Additionally, further applications of bioreactor systems may support cost-effective and efficient manufacturing.

As almost all cultivated meat industries are in the beginning stages of product development, they haven't yet demonstrated whether the technology can offer more attractive products than traditional meat. Not only must cultivated meat fulfill its role as an alternative source of protein and other nutrients, it would need a good balance of traditional meat characteristics as well. This includes taste, smell, and texture, which can make consumers satisfied with cultivated meat as a "good" product to eat with specific benefits. Ideally, cellular agriculture is expected to achieve a perfect balance to create better food with clean, safe, guilt-free, healthy, and pleasurable options, surpassing any existing animal-based products.

CONCLUDING REMARKS

The narrative landscape of cellular agriculture and cultivated meat technology is quite promising as the next movement in alternative proteins (Sexton et al. 2019; Hocquette 2016). Cultivated meat is a new, attractive field for both science and business because it has the potential to address both ethical and environmental concerns associated with conventional meat production. While the approach has many possibilities, several technological fronts need further advancements in research and optimization. Cell sourcing is critical in determining expansion potential and differentiation capacity for desired cells. Furthermore, any downstream steps in production should sufficiently meet all demands for both quality and quantity at the end. To achieve this goal, broader debates and considerations may be required from all aspects of academia, industries, consumers, and regulatory agencies. By applying this attractive technology, the ultimate goal will be to determine what constitutes safe and sustainable production and consumption as a better source of alternative nutrients.

ACKNOWLEDGMENTS

Research in the author's current laboratory was funded in part by a grant from the US National Institutes of Health (R01AR077191), the Good Food Institute, the UW Stem Cell & Regenerative Medicine Center, and the University of Wisconsin Foundation. All figures were created with BioRender.com.

CONFLICTS OF INTEREST

The authors declare no conflict of interest.

THE EFFECTS OF OTHER PROTEINS

In this chapter, we discussed the potential of cultivated meat and how it can sustainably contribute to the community as an alternative protein source. As a type of cellular agriculture, cultivated meat will be manufactured by tissue engineering using animal cells. While plant-based meat alternatives have historically been accepted by consumers, the development of cultivated meat is rapidly expanding as an emerging field. The technology has attractive benefits in resolving existing issues in food safety, the environment, forthcoming population growth, and animal ethics. To make cultivated meat comparable to traditional meat in the market, several technical challenges and complicated questions still remain for development. These technical hurdles include cell sourcing, the optimization of industrial-scale culture, and the novel use of bioengineering approaches to create 3D tissue. These challenges are critical because they significantly influence the quantity and quality of the product as a source of alternative proteins. Cultivated meat products are not yet widely available in the market, but based on current progress in the field, their availability may not be too far off. On the other hand, other meat alternatives, such as plant-based or insect products, are already available on the market and serve as protein substitutes. For cultivated meat, both the potential benefits and limitations of artificial meat production should be discussed more by different stakeholders in academia, industry, regulatory agencies, and consumers. By applying innovative and attractive technology, our ultimate goal will be to provide safe and sustainable products as a better source of alternative nutrients.

MINI DICTIONARY OF TERMS

- **Adipocytes:** Fat cells.
- **Artificial meat:** A broad term that encompasses three main types of meat replacements.
- **Biocompatible:** Materials that are not harmful to living organisms; in this case, they are safe not only for cells to grow but also for human consumption.
- **Biomaterials:** Components relating to the creation and manipulation of live cells or cell products like organoids, tissues, or (in this context) cell-based meat.
- **Bioreactor:** A cell culture device used to rapidly culture and expand cells.
- **Cellular agriculture:** The field of creating meat products through the use of cell culture techniques.
- **Cultivated meat/cell-based meat:** Products made of muscle/fat cells (meat) from animals to circumvent traditional farming; they are often made to resemble traditional meat products.
- **Differentiation/derivation:** Cells maturing into a specific cell type with a certain job (i.e., muscle or fat) rather than remaining as progenitor cells.
- **Multipotent:** Having the ability to mature into several types of different cells in the organism, but not any kind of cell.
- **Pluripotent:** Having the ability to mature into any type of cell in the organism.
- **Progenitor:** A cell that has not yet matured into a specific cell type.
- **Skeletal myocytes:** "Normal" muscle cells, as would be found in traditional meat products.
- **Xeno-free:** Not including products sourced from outside the species of interest, i.e., not using chicken growth factors in pig cell products, etc.

SUMMARY POINTS

- This chapter focuses on cultivated meat as a new source of alternative proteins.
- A typical manufacturing strategy for cultivated meat production is discussed.
- The production of cultivated meat requires three steps.
- Cell sourcing is the most critical step to achieving efficient production.
- There are two major sources of cells for cultivated meat production.
- Tissue engineering supports large-scale culture expansion and muscle tissue formation.
- Cultivated meat has significant potential as an alternative source of animal protein and nutrition.
- The current status of cultivated meat technology remains a fairly young field.

REFERENCES

Al Tanoury, Ziad, Jyoti Rao, Olivier Tassy, Bénédicte Gobert, Svetlana Gapon, Jean-Marie Garnier, Erica Wagner, Aurore Hick, Arielle Hall, Emanuela Gussoni, and Olivier Pourquié. 2020. "Differentiation of the human PAX7-positive myogenic precursors/satellite cell lineage *in vitro*." *Development* 147 (12):dev187344. doi: 10.1242/dev.187344.

Bellarby, J., R. Tirado, A. Leip, F. Weiss, J. P. Lesschen, and P. Smith. 2013. "Livestock greenhouse gas emissions and mitigation potential in Europe." *Glob Chang Biol* 19 (1):3–18. doi: 10.1111/j.1365-2486.2012.02786.x.

Ben-Arye, Tom, Yulia Shandalov, Shahar Ben-Shaul, Shira Landau, Yedidya Zagury, Iris Ianovici, Neta Lavon, and Shulamit Levenberg. 2020. "Textured soy protein scaffolds enable the generation of three-dimensional bovine skeletal muscle tissue for cell-based meat." *Nature Food* 1 (4):210–220. doi: 10.1038/s43016-020-0046-5.

Biferali, B., Proietti, D., Mozzetta, C., Madaro, L. 2019. Fibro-adipogenic progenitors cross-talk in skeletal muscle: The social network. *Front Physiol* 10:1074. doi: 10.3389/fphys.2019.01074.

Bischoff, R., and C. Heintz. 1994. "Enhancement of skeletal muscle regeneration." *Dev Dyn* 201 (1):41–54. doi: 10.1002/aja.1002010105.

Bomkamp, C., S. C. Skaalure, G. F. Fernando, T. Ben-Arye, E. W. Swartz, and E. A. Specht. 2022. "Scaffolding biomaterials for 3D cultivated meat: Prospects and challenges." *Adv Sci (Weinh)* 9 (3):e2102908. doi: 10.1002/advs.202102908.

Bonny, S. F. P., G. E. Gardner, D. W. Pethick, and J.-F. Hocquette. 2015. "What is artificial meat and what does it mean for the future of the meat industry?" *Journal of Integrative Agriculture* 14 (2):255–263. doi: 10.1016/S2095-3119(14)60888-1.

Chodkowska, K. A., K. Wodz, and J. Wojciechowski. 2022. "Sustainable future protein foods: The challenges and the future of cultivated meat." *Foods* 11 (24). doi: 10.3390/foods11244008.

Ding, Shijie, G. N. M. Swennen, Tobias Messmer, Mick Gagliardi, Daniël G. M. Molin, Chunbao Li, Guanghong Zhou, and Mark J. Post. 2018. "Maintaining bovine satellite cells stemness through p38 pathway." *Scientific Reports* 8 (1):10808. doi: 10.1038/s41598-018-28746-7.

Eibl, R., Y. Senn, G. Gubser, V. Jossen, C. van den Bos, and D. Eibl. 2021. "Cellular agriculture: Opportunities and challenges." *Annu Rev Food Sci Technol* 12:51–73. doi: 10.1146/annurev-food-063020-123940.

Fontana, G., J. Gershlak, M. Adamski, J. S. Lee, S. Matsumoto, H. D. Le, B. Binder, J. Wirth, G. Gaudette, and W. L. Murphy. 2017. "Biofunctionalized plants as diverse biomaterials for human cell culture." *Adv Healthc Mater* 6 (8). doi: 10.1002/adhm.201601225.

Food and Agriculture Organization of the United Nations. 2017. *The Future of Food and Agriculture: Trends and Challenges*. Rome: Food and Agriculture Organization of the United Nations.

Gerber, P. J., H. Steinfeld, B. Henderson, A. Mottet, C. Opio, J. Dijkman, A. Falcucci, and G. Tempio. 2013. *Tackling* Climate Change Through Livestock – *A* Global Assessment of Emissions and Mitigation *Opportunities*. Rome, Italy: FAO.

Gershlak, J. R., S. Hernandez, G. Fontana, L. R. Perreault, K. J. Hansen, S. A. Larson, B. Y. Binder, D. M. Dolivo, T. Yang, T. Dominko, M. W. Rolle, P. J. Weathers, F. Medina-Bolivar, C. L. Cramer, W. L. Murphy, and G. R. Gaudette. 2017. "Crossing kingdoms: Using decellularized plants as perfusable tissue engineering scaffolds." *Biomaterials* 125:13–22. doi: 10.1016/j.biomaterials.2017.02.011.

Grzinic, G., A. Piotrowicz-Cieslak, A. Klimkowicz-Pawlas, R. L. Gorny, A. Lawniczek-Walczyk, L. Piechowicz, E. Olkowska, M. Potrykus, M. Tankiewicz, M. Krupka, G. Siebielec, and L. Wolska. 2023. "Intensive poultry farming: A review of the impact on the environment and human health." *Sci Total Environ* 858 (Pt 3):160014. doi: 10.1016/j.scitotenv.2022.160014.

Guénantin, Anne-Claire, Nolwenn Briand, Emilie Capel, Florent Dumont, Romain Morichon, Claire Provost, Francesca Stillitano, Dorota Jeziorowska, Jean-Pierre Siffroi, Roger J. Hajjar, Bruno Fève, Jean-Sébastien Hulot, Philippe Collas, Jacqueline Capeau, and Corinne Vigouroux. 2017. "Functional human beige adipocytes from induced pluripotent stem cells." *Diabetes* 66 (6):1470. doi: 10.2337/db16-1107.

Hocquette, J. F. 2016. "Is in vitro meat the solution for the future?" *Meat Sci* 120:167–176. doi: 10.1016/j.meatsci.2016.04.036.

Hosoyama, T., J. Van Dyke, and M. Suzuki. 2012. "Applications of skeletal muscle progenitor cells for neuromuscular diseases." *Am J Stem Cells* 1 (3):253–263.

Hynes, Kim, Danijela Menicanin, Stan Gronthos, and Mark P. Bartold. 2016. "Differentiation of iPSC to mesenchymal stem-like cells and their characterization." In *Induced Pluripotent Stem (iPS) Cells: Methods and Protocols*, edited by Kursad Turksen and Andras Nagy, 353–374. New York, NY: Springer New York.

Ijaz, M., M. K. Yar, I. H. Badar, S. Ali, M. S. Islam, M. H. Jaspal, Z. Hayat, A. Sardar, S. Ullah, and D. Guevara-Ruiz. 2021. "Meat production and supply chain under COVID–19 scenario: Current trends and future prospects." *Front Vet Sci* 8:660736. doi: 10.3389/fvets.2021.660736.

Ismail, I., Y. H. Hwang, and S. T. Joo. 2020. "Meat analog as future food: A review." *J Anim Sci Technol* 62 (2):111–120. doi: 10.5187/jast.2020.62.2.111.

Jara, T. C., K. Park, P. Vahmani, A. L. Van Eenennaam, L. R. Smith, and A. C. Denicol. 2023. "Stem cell-based strategies and challenges for production of cultivated meat." *Nat Food* 4 (10):841–853. doi: 10.1038/s43016-023-00857-z.

Jiwlawat, N., E. Lynch, J. Jeffrey, J. M. Van Dyke, and M. Suzuki. 2018. "Current progress and challenges for skeletal muscle differentiation from human pluripotent stem cells using transgene-free approaches." *Stem Cells Int* 2018:6241681. doi: 10.1155/2018/6241681.

Jiwlawat, S., E. Lynch, J. Glaser, I. Smit-Oistad, J. Jeffrey, J. M. Van Dyke, and M. Suzuki. 2017. "Differentiation and sarcomere formation in skeletal myocytes directly prepared from human induced pluripotent stem cells using a sphere-based culture." *Differentiation* 96:70–81. doi: 10.1016/j.diff.2017.07.004.

Klurfeld, D. M. 2018. "What is the role of meat in a healthy diet?" *Anim Front* 8 (3):5–10. doi: 10.1093/af/vfy009.

Kolkmann, A. M., A. Van Essen, M. J. Post, and P. Moutsatsou. 2022. "Development of a chemically defined medium for in vitro expansion of primary bovine satellite cells." *Front Bioeng Biotechnol* 10:895289. doi: 10.3389/fbioe.2022.895289.

Kuang, S., K. Kuroda, F. Le Grand, and M. A. Rudnicki. 2007. "Asymmetric self-renewal and commitment of satellite stem cells in muscle." *Cell* 129 (5):999–1010. doi: 10.1016/j.cell.2007.03.044.

Kumar, P., N. Sharma, S. Sharma, N. Mehta, A. K. Verma, S. Chemmalar, and A. Q. Sazili. 2021. "In-vitro meat: A promising solution for sustainability of meat sector." *J Anim Sci Technol* 63 (4):693–724. doi: 10.5187/jast.2021.e85.

Li, B. J., P. H. Li, R. H. Huang, W. X. Sun, H. Wang, Q. F. Li, J. Chen, W. J. Wu, and H. L. Liu. 2015. "Isolation, culture and identification of porcine skeletal muscle satellite cells." *Asian-Australas J Anim Sci* 28 (8):1171–1177. doi: 10.5713/ajas.14.0848.

Listrat, Anne, Bénédicte Lebret, Isabelle Louveau, Thierry Astruc, Muriel Bonnet, Louis Lefaucheur, Brigitte Picard, and Jérôme Bugeon. 2016. "How muscle structure and composition influence meat and flesh quality." *Sci World J* 2016:3182746. doi: 10.1155/2016/3182746.

Low, M., Eisner, C., Rossi, F. 2017. "Fibro/adipogenic progenitors (FAPs): Isolation by FACS and culture." *Methods Mol Biol* 1556:179–189. doi: 10.1007/978-1-4939-6771-1_9.

Mateti, Tarun, Anindita Laha, and Pushpalatha Shenoy. 2022. "Artificial meat industry: Production methodology, challenges, and future." *JOM* 74 (9):3428–3444. doi: 10.1007/s11837-022-05316-x.

Mcconnell, L. L., C. Osorio, and T. Hofmann. 2023. "The future of agriculture and food: sustainable approaches to achieve zero hunger." *J Agric Food Chem* 71 (36):13165–13167. doi: 10.1021/acs.jafc.3c05433.

Morgan, J. E., and T. A. Partridge. 2003. "Muscle satellite cells." *Int J Biochem Cell Biol* 35 (8):1151–1156. doi: 10.1016/s1357-2725(03)00042-6.

Pajcin, I., T. Knezic, I. Savic Azoulay, V. Vlajkov, M. Djisalov, L. Janjusevic, J. Grahovac, and I. Gadjanski. 2022. "Bioengineering outlook on cultivated meat production." *Micromachines (Basel)* 13 (3). doi: 10.3390/mi13030402.

Ramani, S., D. Ko, B. Kim, C. Cho, W. Kim, C. Jo, C. K. Lee, J. Kang, S. Hur, and S. Park. 2021. "Technical requirements for cultured meat production: A review." *J Anim Sci Technol* 63 (4):681–692. doi: 10.5187/jast.2021.e45.

Redondo, P.A., Pavlou, M., Loizidou, M., Cheema, U. 2017. Elements of the niche for adult stem cell expansion. *J Tissue Eng* 8:2041731417725464. doi: 10.1177/2041731417725464.

Reiss, J., S. Robertson, and M. Suzuki. 2021. "Cell sources for cultivated meat: Applications and considerations throughout the production workflow." *Int J Mol Sci* 22 (14). doi: 10.3390/ijms22147513.

Samandari, M., F. Saeedinejad, J. Quint, S. X. Y. Chuah, R. Farzad, and A. Tamayol. 2023. "Repurposing biomedical muscle tissue engineering for cellular agriculture: Challenges and opportunities." *Trends Biotechnol* 41 (7):887–906. doi: 10.1016/j.tibtech.2023.02.002.

Sexton, A. E., T. Garnett, and J. Lorimer. 2019. "Framing the future of food: The contested promises of alternative proteins." *Environ Plan E Nat Space* 2 (1):47–72. doi: 10.1177/2514848619827009.

Sinke, Pelle, and Ingrid Odegard. 2021. "LCA of cultivated meat Future predictions for different scenarios." CE Delft. Accessed February 2021. https://cedelft.eu/publications/rapport-lca-of-cultivated-meat-future-projections-for-different-scenarios/.

Sugii, S., C. Y. Q. Wong, A. K. O. Lwin, and L. J. M. Chew. 2023. "Alternative fat: Redefining adipocytes for biomanufacturing cultivated meat." *Trends Biotechnol* 41 (5):686–700. doi: 10.1016/j.tibtech.2022.08.005.

Takahashi, K., and S. Yamanaka. 2006. "Induction of pluripotent stem cells from mouse embryonic and adult fibroblast cultures by defined factors." *Cell* 126 (4). http://www.ncbi.nlm.nih.gov/entrez/query.fcgi?cmd=Retrieve&db=PubMed&dopt=Citation&list_uids=16904174

Tey, S. R., S. Robertson, E. Lynch, and M. Suzuki. 2019. "Coding cell identity of human skeletal muscle progenitor cells using cell surface markers: Current status and remaining challenges for characterization and isolation." *Front Cell Dev Biol* 7:284. doi: 10.3389/fcell.2019.00284.

Warriss, P. D., and D. N. Rhodes. 1977. "Haemoglobin concentrations in beef." *J Sci Food Agric* 28 (10):931–934. doi: 10.1002/jsfa.2740281012.

Webster, R. G. 2002. "The importance of animal influenza for human disease." *Vaccine* 20 Suppl 2:S16–20. doi: 10.1016/s0264-410x(02)00123-8.

Welsh, J. A., H. Braun, N. Brown, C. Um, K. Ehret, J. Figueroa, and D. Boyd Barr. 2019. "Production-related contaminants (pesticides, antibiotics and hormones) in organic and conventionally produced milk samples sold in the USA." *Public Health Nutr* 22 (16):2972–2980. doi: 10.1017/S136898001900106X.

Xu, X., K. J. Wilschut, G. Kouklis, H. Tian, R. Hesse, C. Garland, H. Sbitany, S. Hansen, R. Seth, P. D. Knott, W. Y. Hoffman, and J. H. Pomerantz. 2015. "Human satellite cell transplantation and regeneration from diverse skeletal muscles." *Stem Cell Reports* 5 (3):419–434. doi: 10.1016/j.stemcr.2015.07.016.

Yap, Wee Swan, Deepak Choudhury, and Ratima Suntornnond. 2023. "Towards biomanufacturing of cultured meat." *Trends in Biotechnology* 41 (3):292–294. doi: 10.1016/j.tibtech.2023.01.014.

Ye, Yongli, Jingwen Zhou, Xin Guan, and Xiulan Sun. 2022. "Commercialization of cultured meat products: Current status, challenges, and strategic prospects." *Future Foods* 6:100177. doi: https://doi.org/10.1016/j.fufo.2022.100177.

Yu, J., M. A. Vodyanik, K. Smuga-Otto, J. Antosiewicz-Bourget, J. L. Frane, S. Tian, J. Nie, G. A. Jonsdottir, V. Ruotti, R. Stewart, Slukvin, II, and J. A. Thomson. 2007. "Induced pluripotent stem cell lines derived from human somatic cells." *Science* 318 (5858):1917–1920. doi: 10.1126/science.1151526.

Yun, J., S. Robertson, C. Kim, M. Suzuki, W. L. Murphy, and P. Gopalan. 2023. "Aligned skeletal muscle assembly on a biofunctionalized plant leaf scaffold." *Acta Biomater* 171:327–335. doi: 10.1016/j.actbio.2023.09.016.

Zhao, L., Y. H. Dong, and H. Wang. 2010. "Residues of veterinary antibiotics in manures from feedlot livestock in eight provinces of China." *Sci Total Environ* 408 (5):1069–1075. doi: 10.1016/j.scitotenv.2009.11.014.

22 Soy Protein and Its Influence on Hepatic Inflammation in Non-Alcoholic Fatty Liver Disease (NAFLD)

Wei Li and Reza Hakkak

ABBREVIATIONS

BMI	Body mass index
COVID-19	Coronavirus disease 2019
CRP	C-reactive protein
FFA	Free fatty acids
GI	Gastrointestinal
HCC	Hepatocellular carcinoma
IL-1β	Interleukin-1β
IL-6	Interleukin-6
IL-8	Interleukin-8
IL-12	Interleukin-12
IP-10	Interferon gamma-induced protein-10
LPS	Lipopolysaccharide
MCP-1	Monocyte chemoattractant protein-1
MIP-1α	Macrophage inflammatory protein-1α
MIP-1β	Macrophage inflammatory protein-1β
NAFLD	Non-alcoholic fatty liver disease
NASH	Non-alcoholic steatohepatitis
TNF-α	Tumor necrosis factor-α
VAT	Visceral adipose tissue
WHO	World Health Organization

INTRODUCTION

Non-alcoholic fatty liver disease (NAFLD) has become the most prevalent liver disease worldwide due to the increased rate of obesity in recent decades. Currently, there are no approved pharmaceutical drugs to prevent or treat NAFLD. Easing the NAFLD disease burden primarily relies on lifestyle changes such as dietary interventions. Soy protein intake is associated with reduced NAFLD risk in humans and has been shown to protect against NAFLD in animal models. The protection afforded by soy protein against NAFLD may be mediated by multiple mechanisms. This chapter focuses on the anti-inflammatory functions of soy protein and discusses how it may reduce NAFLD risk and severity by inhibiting systemic and tissue inflammation.

DOI: 10.1201/9781003597926-22

NON-ALCOHOLIC FATTY LIVER DISEASE

NAFLD is characterized by an excessive accumulation of lipids in the liver that is not caused by alcohol overconsumption (NIDDK 2021). NAFLD is the most common cause of chronic liver disease worldwide, affecting about 25% of the global population (Shetty and Syn 2019; Mitra, De, and Chowdhury 2019). NAFLD is also becoming increasingly common among children and adolescents. The prevalence rate of NAFLD is between 5% and 10% among all children and adolescents in the United States and can be greater than 30% in obese children and adolescents (Anderson et al. 2015; Yu and Schwimmer 2021). According to a 2022 meta-analysis, the global prevalence of pediatric NAFLD is 7.40% in the general population and 52.49% among those who are obese (Li et al. 2022). These children and adolescents are potentially at lifelong risk of developing NAFLD-related complications.

NAFLD has four main stages of progression: simple steatosis, non-alcoholic steatohepatitis (NASH), cirrhosis, and hepatocellular carcinoma (HCC). NAFLD starts with simple steatosis, a largely harmless stage characterized by the accumulation of fat in liver cells. Although simple steatosis is generally considered a benign condition, individuals with simple steatosis are more susceptible to other insults to the liver, such as the toxic effects of alcohol and drugs (Mazzolini et al. 2020). Because simple steatosis does not present symptoms, diagnosis is difficult without liver biopsies. About 25% of those with simple steatosis may progress to NASH, which is characterized by inflammation and hepatocyte ballooning (Mazzolini et al. 2020). NASH affects about 3–5% of the global population, and approximately 20% of NASH patients have advanced fibrosis or cirrhosis (Takahashi and Fukusato 2014; Estes et al. 2018). Eventually, some patients progress to the end-stage liver disease HCC, which leads to death or requires liver transplantation (Perumpail et al. 2017). NAFLD does not affect the liver alone. NAFLD is an independent risk factor for cardiovascular diseases (Lu et al. 2013; Francque, van der Graaff, and Kwanten 2016; Stahl et al. 2019). The risk of developing type 2 diabetes is more than twofold higher in individuals with NAFLD (Gastaldelli and Cusi 2019).

OBESITY IS A MAJOR RISK FACTOR FOR NAFLD DEVELOPMENT

The prevalence of obesity continues to rise globally and remains a major public health burden (Agha and Agha 2017). According to the World Health Organization (WHO), globally, 1.9 billion adults 18 years and older were overweight, including 650 million who were obese. Among children and adolescents, 39 million under the age of 5 years and over 340 million aged 5–19 years were overweight or obese (WHO 2021). Emerging data indicate that the COVID-19 pandemic has worsened obesity rates in countries such as the United States (Restrepo 2022; Lange et al. 2021). In a large, longitudinal cohort of 432,302 children and adolescents in the United States aged 2–19 years, body mass index (BMI) increased sharply during the COVID-19 pandemic, with the monthly rate of increase in BMI nearly doubling due to school closures, stress, improper nutrition, and loss of opportunities for structured exercise (Lange et al. 2021).

Obesity is a risk factor for many chronic diseases, including NAFLD (Sarwar, Pierce, and Koppe 2018). The prevalence rate of NAFLD may be as high as 50% in the obese population (Divella et al. 2019). NAFLD will likely remain the most prevalent liver disease in children and adolescents. Experts have proposed that NAFLD should be suspected in all overweight or obese children and adolescents older than 3 years of age with increased waist circumference, especially if there is a family history of NAFLD (Vajro et al. 2012). In a recent study, Park et al. analyzed 1,737 Korean families with two parents and adolescent children aged 12–18 and reported that adolescent children with one parent with NAFLD were at risk of NAFLD, and the risk was higher when both parents had NAFLD (Park et al. 2023).

LOW-GRADE SYSTEMIC INFLAMMATION IN OBESITY

While the etiology of obesity-associated chronic diseases is multifactorial, a common paradigm is chronic low-grade inflammation (Kawai, Autieri, and Scalia 2021; Iyengar et al. 2016; Saltiel and Olefsky 2017; Luo and Lin 2021; Gregor and Hotamisligil 2011). Adipose tissue acts as an endocrine organ to release adipokines, cytokines, chemokines, and lipids into the circulation (Zatterale et al. 2020; Skurk et al. 2007). The macrophage populations in adipose tissue play an important role in obesity-induced systemic inflammation and insulin resistance (Kunz et al. 2021). Macrophages are the main leukocyte population in adipose tissue. The presence of macrophages in adipose tissue was first reported in 2000 (Bornstein et al. 2000). Researchers subsequently discovered that macrophage infiltration into adipose tissue increases in obesity, and inflammatory cytokines secreted by adipose tissue, such as TNF-α and MIP-1α, are almost entirely of macrophage origin (Xu et al. 2003; Weisberg et al. 2003).

Macrophages are generally classified as M1 macrophages or M2 macrophages based on activation stimuli, subsequent function, and cytokine profile (Martinez and Gordon 2014). Also known as classically activated macrophages, M1 macrophages are pro-inflammatory and secrete cytokines, including TNF-α, IL-1β, IL-6, IL-12, and IL-23 (Goerdt et al. 1999; Hao et al. 2012). In contrast, M2 macrophages are alternatively activated macrophages that secrete anti-inflammatory cytokines and growth factors such as IL-10 and TGF-β (Fuentes, Roszer, and Ricote 2010; Bohlson et al. 2014). Macrophage polarization and the function of M1 vs. M2 macrophages have been reviewed in detail elsewhere (Martinez and Gordon 2014). In obese adipose tissue, M2 macrophages switch to the M1 phenotype, leading to increased secretion of pro-inflammatory cytokines and subsequent insulin resistance (Castoldi et al. 2015).

The size of adipocytes is another important determinant of adipose tissue inflammation. In cultured adipocytes isolated from patients who underwent elective plastic abdominal surgery, the secretion of inflammatory cytokines/chemokines positively correlates with adipocyte size. The larger cell fraction secretes more leptin, IL-6, IL-8, TNF-α, MCP-1, IP-10, and MIP-1β (Skurk et al. 2007).

In addition to adipose tissue, inflammatory signals may also originate from the gastrointestinal (GI) tract in obese individuals. GI tract commensal bacteria-associated molecules, such as lipopolysaccharides (LPS), traverse the portal vein to enter the circulation, a process known as LPS translocation (Ghosh et al. 2020). Elevated blood LPS levels are associated with obesity in humans and animals (Boutagy et al. 2016).

NAFLD AND INFLAMMATION

Like many other chronic diseases, NAFLD is linked to inflammation. Increased levels of C-reactive protein (CRP), IL-1β, IL-6, TNF-α, and ICAM-1 are associated with an increased risk of NAFLD (Duan et al. 2022). Inflammatory signals arising from dysfunctional adipose tissue in obesity promote the development and progression of NAFLD (Cordeiro et al. 2020). The pro-inflammatory cytokines released into the systemic circulation from obese adipose tissue induce liver insulin resistance and secretion of CRP from the liver, further promoting systemic inflammation (Cordeiro et al. 2020).

Inflammatory stimuli from the GI tract are particularly relevant to liver inflammation because the liver is exposed to bacterial molecules that enter the portal vein (Raetz and Whitfield 2002). These inflammatory stimuli, such as LPS, traverse the portal vein to the liver, leading to liver inflammation and dysregulation of liver metabolism (Casagrande et al. 2020; Item and Konrad 2012). Higher LPS concentrations have been reported in the blood of NAFLD patients (Nier et al. 2020).

Because NAFLD has no obvious symptoms, diagnosis mainly relies on imaging or histology. The observational nature of the human studies on the relationship between tissue LPS levels and NAFLD reveals only correlations. In contrast, animal studies have shown a potential causal relationship between LPS translocation and NAFLD. LPS injection in animals exacerbates liver steatosis (Fukunishi et al. 2014; He et al. 2020). The positive correlation between LPS and NAFLD in humans and the causal relationship between LPS and liver steatosis in animals suggest that LPS translocation and liver inflammation may contribute to NAFLD in humans.

SOYBEAN AND SOY PROTEIN

Soybean (*Glycine max*) is a legume of the pea family known for its edible seeds. Soybean likely originated from the domestication of wild soybeans in East Asia 6,000–9,000 years ago (Carter, Hymowitz, and Nelson 2004; Kim et al. 2012; Sedivy, Wu, and Hanzawa 2017). It has been a part of the East Asian diet for thousands of years in the form of traditional soy foods, such as tofu, soy sauce, tempeh, and edamame. Soybean is a highly valuable crop in modern agriculture, ranking among the most economically important crops worldwide. Soybeans are an excellent source of high-quality protein and contain higher oil content than most legumes. Every 100 g of mature raw soybean seeds contains approximately 36.5 g of protein, 19.9 g of lipids, 30.2 g of carbohydrates (including 9.3 g of fiber), 4.9 g of ash/minerals, and 8.5 g of water (Service 2018).

The total global soy production in 2023 is estimated at 403 million metric tons, with Brazil, the United States, and Argentina together contributing approximately 80% of global soy production (Service 2023). Despite this large production volume, soy is not an established ingredient in Western diets. For example, soy contributes less than 6% of total protein to the food supply in the United States (Promotion 2014).

Soy protein is considered a high-quality protein, with a protein digestibility-corrected amino acid score (PDCAAS) ranging from 0.92 to 1.00, which is comparable to proteins from meat and dairy, and much higher than most other plant proteins (Qin, Wang, and Luo 2022). Compared to animal proteins, soy protein is lower in sulfur-containing amino acids such as methionine and cysteine. Therefore, methionine and cysteine are often supplemented in soy protein diets in animal studies to allow fair comparisons between soy and animal proteins (Hakkak et al. 2022). Despite its slightly lower levels of sulfur-containing amino acids compared to animal proteins in general, soy protein is still considered a "complete protein" that contains adequate amounts of all essential amino acids to support normal human growth (Michelfelder 2009). In Western countries, soy protein products like soy protein concentrates (SPC) and soy protein isolates (SPI) have been developed as economical and high-quality vegetable protein sources for humans.

In addition to its protein content, soy protein products also contain isoflavones – plant secondary metabolites naturally found in high amounts in soybeans, mainly in the glycoside forms of daidzin and genistin, with smaller amounts in the aglycone forms of daidzein and genistein (Kalaiselvan et al. 2010; Miadoková 2009). Isoflavone concentrations are about 2 mg/g protein in textured soy protein and 0.6–1.0 mg/g protein in isolated soy proteins (Sacks et al. 2006).

In recent years, soy foods have gained more acceptance in Western societies. The increasing popularity of soy foods may be attributed to several reasons, including public interest in plant-based meat substitutes, food manufacturers' efforts to develop new varieties of foods with soy ingredients, and perhaps above all, increased awareness of soy's health benefits.

The health benefits of consuming soy foods have been extensively studied and well-documented. These benefits include reduced risks of coronary heart disease and some cancers, improved bone health, reduced systemic inflammation, and fewer menopausal symptoms. The health benefits of soy and soy protein have been reviewed in depth elsewhere (Messina 2016).

SOY PROTEIN AND NAFLD PROTECTION

Consuming soy protein has been associated with a decreased risk of NAFLD. A cross-sectional study involving 24,622 Chinese adults aged 20 to 90 found an association between high soy food intake and a lower prevalence of NAFLD after adjusting for potential confounding factors (Zhang et al. 2020). Because of the time required for humans to develop NAFLD, there is a lack of randomized controlled human trials for soy protein's protective effect against NAFLD. However, soy protein's protection against NAFLD has been demonstrated in animal experiments. In male Wistar rats, feeding soy protein decreases high-fat diet (HFD)-induced liver expression of SREBP-1 and FAS and prevents the development of fatty liver compared to a casein protein control diet (Ascencio et al. 2004). Feeding soy protein diets to male and female obese Zucker rats reduces liver steatosis compared to a casein control diet (Zhou et al. 2014; Hakkak et al. 2012, 2018, 2022).

Several studies have investigated the effect of specific soy protein components in preventing NAFLD. The soy protein β-conglycinin prevents the development of NAFLD in HFD-fed obese mice by down-regulating PPARγ (Li, Ikaga, and Yamazaki 2018). Because soy protein contains isoflavones, its protective effect against NAFLD may be partly mediated by these compounds. In both humans and animals, the soy isoflavone genistein has been shown to improve insulin sensitivity, decrease inflammation markers, optimize lipid profiles, and decrease serum AST and ALT levels (Xin et al. 2019). Genistein can reduce HFD-induced liver steatosis in some rat and mouse NAFLD models (Lee et al. 2006; Kim, Kang, and Lee 2010; Kim et al. 2005; Yalniz et al. 2007). In an experiment designed to investigate the contribution of soy protein isoflavone to the prevention of liver steatosis, Hakkak et al. reported that soy protein diets with both normal amounts of isoflavone (~2 mg/g) and negligible amounts of isoflavone (0.154 mg/g) reduced liver steatosis in obese Zucker rats compared to a casein control diet. The effect was more pronounced in rats fed the soy diet with normal amounts of isoflavone, suggesting the protective effect may be mediated by both the protein and the isoflavone components of the soy protein diet (Hakkak et al. 2022).

SOY PROTEIN AND NAFLD TREATMENT

Although studies in humans have only demonstrated an association between soy protein consumption and a decreased risk of developing NAFLD, randomized clinical trials have reported soy protein's benefits in treating patients with existing NAFLD. In a parallel randomized clinical trial involving 45 patients with NAFLD, participants consumed one of three diets: a low-calorie diet, a low-calorie, low-carbohydrate diet, or a low-calorie, low-carbohydrate soy-containing diet for 8 weeks. The latter diet incorporated 30 g of soy nuts containing 11.3 g protein and 103 mg of isoflavones to replace 30 g of red meat in the other diets. This soy-containing diet reduced serum ALT, AST, fibrinogen, and malondialdehyde levels more than the other diets (Kani et al. 2014). The same study also showed that the soy protein-containing diet reduced fasting blood glucose, serum insulin, serum hs-CRP, and both systolic and diastolic blood pressure levels compared to the other diets. At the end of the study, some patients either no longer had NAFLD or had reduced NAFLD severity (Kani et al. 2017). In a more recent clinical trial, 70 patients with NAFLD were assigned either to a low-calorie diet or to a low-calorie diet plus 240 ml of soy milk daily for 8 weeks. At the end of the trial, the soy milk group showed a significantly greater decrease in serum ALT and hs-CRP compared to the control group. Soy milk also led to greater improvements in insulin sensitivity markers and larger decreases in blood pressure compared to the diet without soy milk (Eslami et al. 2019). Taken together, these studies suggest that soy protein may provide additional benefits in protecting against NAFLD-associated liver stress and improving metabolic markers when combined with low-calorie diets.

THE ANTI-INFLAMMATORY EFFECT OF SOY PROTEIN

Soy's protective effect against chronic diseases such as NAFLD may be partly mediated by its anti-inflammatory properties. In a study of Chinese women, higher soy food consumption was associated with lower circulating levels of IL-6, TNF-α, and soluble TNF receptors 1 and 2 (Wu et al. 2012). In a randomized crossover clinical trial involving 42 postmenopausal women with metabolic syndrome, both soy nut and soy protein consumption reduced serum CRP compared to a control diet (Dietary Approach to Stop Hypertension [DASH] diet) (Azadbakht et al. 2007). In another randomized crossover trial, replacing 25 g of non-soy protein daily with protein from soy nuts for 8 weeks reduced soluble vascular cell adhesion molecule-1 compared to a therapeutic lifestyle change (TLC) diet in hypertensive postmenopausal women, suggesting soy may reduce endothelial cell inflammation (Nasca, Zhou, and Welty 2008).

Many ingredients in soy have anti-inflammatory properties. The ability of soy isoflavones to reduce inflammation has been reported (Yu et al. 2016; Goh et al. 2022). In addition to soy isoflavones, researchers have identified some soy protein-derived anti-inflammatory peptides. For example, a soy-derived angiotensin-converting enzyme (ACE)-inhibitory peptide inhibits inflammation in vascular smooth muscle cells (Lin et al. 2017). Several soy peptides protect against LPS-induced inflammation in cultured intestinal cells by reducing nitric oxide and inflammatory cytokine expression and in cultured macrophages by suppressing TLR4-mediated pathways such as NFκB activation (Wen et al. 2022; Yi et al. 2020). The soy-derived tripeptide Phe-Leu-Val reduces TNF-α-induced inflammation and insulin resistance in adipocytes (Kwak et al. 2016). Although most of the evidence for the anti-inflammatory properties of soy peptides has come from *in vitro* experiments, soy-derived peptides can be absorbed into the circulation from the GI tract (Erdmann, Cheung, and Schröder 2008). The soy peptide lunasin has been shown to have anticancer effects *in vivo* (Hsieh, Hernández-Ledesma, and de Lumen 2010). The functional properties of soy bioactive peptides in reducing the risk of chronic diseases have been reviewed in detail, and researchers attribute many of their health benefits to their anti-inflammatory functions (Hu, Liu, and Liu 2023; Chatterjee, Gleddie, and Xiao 2018).

Given soy protein's anti-inflammatory properties and the contribution of inflammation to NAFLD, soy protein's protection against NAFLD may be partly attributed to the inhibition of inflammation. Feeding obese Zucker rats a casein diet supplemented with soy protein enriched with isoflavones decreases liver inflammation and steatosis compared to the casein diet alone (Gudbrandsen, Wergedahl, and Berge 2009). In both human and animal studies, the reduction of NAFLD by soy protein is accompanied by decreased systemic inflammation (Li et al. 2023; Kani et al. 2017). Soy protein may reduce inflammation and NAFLD through multiple mechanisms. As discussed above, soy protein bioactive peptides and isoflavones may inhibit liver and adipose tissue inflammation. Soy protein may also reduce the inflammatory stimuli from the GI tract by modifying gut microbiota. Soy protein consumption has been shown to increase the levels of bifidobacteria and lactobacilli and alter the ratio between Firmicutes and Bacteroidetes in both animals and humans (Huang et al. 2016). Future studies should investigate whether the effect of soy protein on tissue inflammation and the composition of gut microbiota directly mediates its protection against NAFLD and identify the exact soy protein-derived bioactive compounds that exert the benefits.

THE EFFECTS OF OTHER PROTEINS

In this chapter, we review the compositional profile of soy protein and how dietary soy protein may protect against obesity-associated NAFLD. However, researchers must also consider other high-quality proteins of both animal and plant origins, such as whey protein, and proteins from beans, seeds, and nuts. For example, in a prospective study of patients with type 2 diabetes, diets high in protein from both animal and plant sources reduced liver steatosis and inflammation and improved insulin sensitivity (Markova et al. 2017). On the other hand, a recent report from a cohort study in North China suggested that replacing animal protein with plant protein in general is associated with a significant reduction in NAFLD risk (Zhang et al. 2023). Taken together, although incorporating more soy protein into the daily diet may offer promising protection against NAFLD, it is also important to emphasize the benefit of an overall healthy dietary pattern with a balanced intake of high-quality proteins from all sources in reducing the risk of not only NAFLD but also other chronic diseases.

MINI DICTIONARY OF TERMS

- **Casein:** An animal protein that contributes the majority of the protein content in cow's milk.
- **Cirrhosis:** The scarring of tissue due to chronic damage.
- **Cytokines:** Signaling proteins/peptides that are secreted primarily by cells of the immune system.
- **Isoflavones:** A family of phytochemicals found in plants, especially in beans. Some isoflavones have weak estrogen activity.
- **Lipopolysaccharide (LPS):** An outer membrane component of gram-negative bacteria, also commonly known as endotoxin.
- **LPS translocation:** The entry of LPS derived from intestinal bacteria into tissues that occurs through the hepatic portal vein or via lipoprotein transportation.
- **Steatosis:** The accumulation of lipids, especially triacylglycerols, in tissues.
- **Whey:** An animal protein of milk origin, whey is produced as a byproduct of casein or cheese manufacturing.

SUMMARY POINTS

- This chapter focuses on the effects of dietary soy protein on NAFLD.
- Obesity is a major risk factor for NAFLD.
- Inflammation contributes to the development of NAFLD.
- Soy protein consumption is associated with a lower NAFLD risk in humans.
- Soy protein protects against NAFLD in animal studies.
- Soy protein's anti-inflammatory properties may mediate its protection against NAFLD.

REFERENCES

Agha, M., and R. Agha. 2017. "The rising prevalence of obesity: part A: impact on public health." *Int J Surg Oncol (N Y)* 2 (7):e17. https://doi.org/10.1097/ij9.0000000000000017.

Anderson, E. L., L. D. Howe, H. E. Jones, J. P. Higgins, D. A. Lawlor, and A. Fraser. 2015. "The prevalence of non-alcoholic fatty liver disease in children and adolescents: A systematic review and meta-analysis." *PLoS One* 10 (10):e0140908. https://doi.org/10.1371/journal.pone.0140908.

Ascencio, Claudia, Nimbe Torres, Fernando Isoard-Acosta, Armando R. Tovar, Francisco J. Gómez-Pérez, and Rogelio Hernández-Pando. 2004. "Soy protein affects serum insulin and hepatic SREBP-1 mRNA and reduces fatty liver in rats." *J Nutr* 134 (3):522–529. https://doi.org/10.1093/jn/134.3.522.

Azadbakht, Leila, Masoud Kimiagar, Yadollah Mehrabi, Ahmad Esmaillzadeh, Frank B. Hu, and Walter C. Willett. 2007. "Soy consumption, markers of inflammation, and endothelial function: A cross-over study in postmenopausal women with the metabolic syndrome." *Diabetes Care* 30 (4):967–973. https://doi.org/10.2337/dc06-2126.

Bohlson, S. S., S. D. O'Conner, H. J. Hulsebus, M. M. Ho, and D. A. Fraser. 2014. "Complement, c1q, and c1q-related molecules regulate macrophage polarization." *Front Immunol* 5:402. https://doi.org/10.3389/fimmu.2014.00402.

Bornstein, S. R., M. Abu-Asab, A. Glasow, G. Päth, H. Hauner, M. Tsokos, G. P. Chrousos, and W. A. Scherbaum. 2000. "Immunohistochemical and ultrastructural localization of leptin and leptin receptor in human white adipose tissue and differentiating human adipose cells in primary culture." *Diabetes* 49 (4):532–538. https://doi.org/10.2337/diabetes.49.4.532.

Boutagy, N. E., R. P. McMillan, M. I. Frisard, and M. W. Hulver. 2016. "Metabolic endotoxemia with obesity: Is it real and is it relevant?" *Biochimie* 124:11–20. https://doi.org/10.1016/j.biochi.2015.06.020.

Carter, T. E., T. Hymowitz, and R. L. Nelson. 2004. *Biogeography, Local Adaptation, Vavilov, and Genetic Diversity in Soybean*. Berlin, Heidelberg: Biological Resources and Migration.

Casagrande, Breno Picin, Daniel Vitor de Souza, Daniel Araki Ribeiro, Alessandra Medeiros, Luciana Pellegrini Pisani, and Debora Estadella. 2020. "Hepatic inflammation precedes steatosis and is mediated by visceral fat accumulation." *J Endocrinol* 245 (3):369–380. https://doi.org/10.1530/joe-20-0073.

Castoldi, A., C. Naffah de Souza, N. O. Câmara, and P. M. Moraes-Vieira. 2015. "The macrophage switch in obesity development." *Front Immunol* 6:637. https://doi.org/10.3389/fimmu.2015.00637.

CDC. "Overweight and obesity." accessed September 15, 2023. https://www.cdc.gov/obesity/index.html.

Chatterjee, Cynthia, Stephen Gleddie, and Chao-Wu Xiao. 2018. "Soybean bioactive peptides and their functional properties." *Nutrients* 10 (9):1211.

Cordeiro, Adryana, Raquel Costa, Nelson Andrade, Cláudia Silva, Natalia Canabrava, Maria João Pena, Ilda Rodrigues, Sara Andrade, and Andrea Ramalho. 2020. "Does adipose tissue inflammation drive the development of non-alcoholic fatty liver disease in obesity?" *Clin Res Hepatol Gastroenterol* 44 (4):394–402. https://doi.org/10.1016/j.clinre.2019.10.001.

Divella, R., A. Mazzocca, A. Daniele, C. Sabbà, and A. Paradiso. 2019. "Obesity, nonalcoholic fatty liver disease and adipocytokines network in promotion of cancer." *Int J Biol Sci* 15 (3):610–616. https://doi.org/10.7150/ijbs.29599.

Duan, Y., X. Pan, J. Luo, X. Xiao, J. Li, P. L. Bestman, and M. Luo. 2022. "Association of inflammatory cytokines with non-alcoholic fatty liver disease." *Front Immunol* 13:880298. https://doi.org/10.3389/fimmu.2022.880298.

Erdmann, K., B. W. Cheung, and H. Schröder. 2008. "The possible roles of food-derived bioactive peptides in reducing the risk of cardiovascular disease." *J Nutr Biochem* 19 (10):643–654. https://doi.org/10.1016/j.jnutbio.2007.11.010.

Eslami, O., F. Shidfar, Z. Maleki, S. Jazayeri, A. F. Hosseini, S. Agah, and F. Ardiyani. 2019. "Effect of soy milk on metabolic status of patients with nonalcoholic fatty liver disease: A randomized clinical trial." *J Am Coll Nutr* 38 (1):51–58. https://doi.org/10.1080/07315724.2018.1479990.

Estes, C., H. Razavi, R. Loomba, Z. Younossi, and A. J. Sanyal. 2018. "Modeling the epidemic of nonalcoholic fatty liver disease demonstrates an exponential increase in burden of disease." *Hepatology* 67 (1):123–133. https://doi.org/10.1002/hep.29466.

Francque, S. M., D. van der Graaff, and W. J. Kwanten. 2016. "Non-alcoholic fatty liver disease and cardiovascular risk: Pathophysiological mechanisms and implications." *J Hepatol* 65 (2):425–43. https://doi.org/10.1016/j.jhep.2016.04.005.

Fuentes, L., T. Roszer, and M. Ricote. 2010. "Inflammatory mediators and insulin resistance in obesity: Role of nuclear receptor signaling in macrophages." *Mediators Inflamm* 2010:219583. https://doi.org/10.1155/2010/219583.

Fukunishi, Shinya, Tetsuya Sujishi, Atsushi Takeshita, Hideko Ohama, Yusuke Tsuchimoto, Akira Asai, Yasuhiro Tsuda, and Kazuhide Higuchi. 2014. "Lipopolysaccharides accelerate hepatic steatosis in the development of nonalcoholic fatty liver disease in Zucker rats." *J Clini Biochem Nutr* 54 (1):39–44. https://doi.org/10.3164/jcbn.13-49.

Gastaldelli, A., and K. Cusi. 2019. "From NASH to diabetes and from diabetes to NASH: Mechanisms and treatment options." *JHEP Rep* 1 (4):312–328. https://doi.org/10.1016/j.jhepr.2019.07.002.

Ghosh, Siddhartha, Jing Wang, Paul Yannie, and Shobha Ghosh. 2020. "Intestinal barrier dysfunction, LPS translocation, and disease development." *J Endocr Soc* 4. https://doi.org/10.1210/jendso/bvz039.

Goerdt, S., O. Politz, K. Schledzewski, R. Birk, A. Gratchev, P. Guillot, N. Hakiy, C. D. Klemke, E. Dippel, V. Kodelja, and C. E. Orfanos. 1999. "Alternative versus classical activation of macrophages." *Pathobiology* 67 (5–6):222–226. https://doi.org/10.1159/000028096.

Goh, Yu Xian, Juriyati Jalil, Kok Wai Lam, Khairana Husain, and Chandini Menon Premakumar. 2022. "Genistein: A review on its anti-inflammatory properties." *Frontiers in Pharmacology* 13:820969. https://doi.org/10.3389/fphar.2022.820969.

Gregor, M. F., and G. S. Hotamisligil. 2011. "Inflammatory mechanisms in obesity." *Annu Rev Immunol* 29:415–445. https://doi.org/10.1146/annurev-immunol-031210-101322.

Gudbrandsen, O. A., H. Wergedahl, and R. K. Berge. 2009. "A casein diet added isoflavone-enriched soy protein favorably affects biomarkers of steatohepatitis in obese Zucker rats." *Nutrition* 25 (5):574–580. https://doi.org/10.1016/j.nut.2008.10.020.

Hakkak, R., A. Al-Dwairi, G. J. Fuchs, S. Korourian, and F. A. Simmen. 2012. "Dietary soy protein induces hepatic lipogenic enzyme gene expression while suppressing hepatosteatosis in obese female Zucker rats bearing DMBA-initiated mammary tumors." *Genes Nutr* 7 (4):549–558. https://doi.org/10.1007/s12263-012-0294-6.

Hakkak, Reza, C. Heath Gauss, Andrea Bell, and Soheila Korourian. 2018. "Short-term soy protein isolate feeding prevents liver steatosis and reduces serum ALT and AST levels in obese female zucker rats." *Biomedicines* 6 (2):55.

Hakkak, Reza, Beverly Spray, Elisabet Børsheim, and Soheila Korourian. 2022. "Diet containing soy protein concentrate with low and high isoflavones for 9 weeks protects against non-alcoholic fatty liver steatosis using obese zucker rats." *Frontiers in Nutrition* 9. https://doi.org/10.3389/fnut.2022.913571.

Hao, N. B., M. H. Lü, Y. H. Fan, Y. L. Cao, Z. R. Zhang, and S. M. Yang. 2012. "Macrophages in tumor microenvironments and the progression of tumors." *Clin Dev Immunol* 2012:948098. https://doi.org/10.1155/2012/948098.

He, Qian, Jun Zeng, Kecheng Yao, Wei Wang, Qiong Wu, Renmin Tang, Xuan Xia, and Xiulan Zou. 2020. "Long-term subcutaneous injection of lipopolysaccharides and high-fat diet induced non-alcoholic fatty liver disease through IKKε/ NF-κB signaling." *Biochem Biophys Res Commun* 532 (3):362–369. https://doi.org/10.1016/j.bbrc.2020.08.036.

Hsieh, C. C., B. Hernández-Ledesma, and B. O. de Lumen. 2010. "Soybean peptide lunasin suppresses in vitro and in vivo 7,12-dimethylbenz[a]anthracene-induced tumorigenesis." *J Food Sci* 75 (9):H311–H316. https://doi.org/10.1111/j.1750-3841.2010.01861.x.

Hu, Sumei, Caiyu Liu, and Xinqi Liu. 2023. "The beneficial effects of soybean proteins and peptides on chronic diseases." *Nutrients* 15 (8):1811.

Huang, H., H. B. Krishnan, Q. Pham, L. L. Yu, and T. T. Wang. 2016. "Soy and gut microbiota: Interaction and implication for human health." *J Agric Food Chem* 64 (46):8695–8709. https://doi.org/10.1021/acs.jafc.6b03725.

Item, F., and D. Konrad. 2012. "Visceral fat and metabolic inflammation: the portal theory revisited." *Obes Rev* 13 Suppl 2:30–39. https://doi.org/10.1111/j.1467-789X.2012.01035.x.

Iyengar, N. M., A. Gucalp, A. J. Dannenberg, and C. A. Hudis. 2016. "Obesity and cancer mechanisms: Tumor microenvironment and inflammation." *J Clin Oncol* 34 (35):4270–4276. https://doi.org/10.1200/jco.2016.67.4283.

Kalaiselvan, V., M. Kalaivani, A. Vijayakumar, K. Sureshkumar, and K. Venkateskumar. 2010. "Current knowledge and future direction of research on soy isoflavones as a therapeutic agents." *Pharmacogn Rev* 4 (8):111–117. https://doi.org/10.4103/0973-7847.70900.

Kani, A. H., S. M. Alavian, A. Esmaillzadeh, P. Adibi, and L. Azadbakht. 2014. "Effects of a novel therapeutic diet on liver enzymes and coagulating factors in patients with non-alcoholic fatty liver disease: A parallel randomized trial." *Nutrition* 30 (7–8):814–821. https://doi.org/10.1016/j.nut.2013.11.008.

Kani, A. H., S. M. Alavian, A. Esmaillzadeh, P. Adibi, F. Haghighatdoost, and L. Azadbakht. 2017. "Effects of a low-calorie, low-carbohydrate soy containing diet on systemic inflammation among patients with nonalcoholic fatty liver disease: A parallel randomized clinical trial." *Horm Metab Res* 49 (9):687–692. https://doi.org/10.1055/s-0042-118707.

Kawai, T., M. V. Autieri, and R. Scalia. 2021. "Adipose tissue inflammation and metabolic dysfunction in obesity." *Am J Physiol Cell Physiol* 320 (3):C375–c391. https://doi.org/10.1152/ajpcell.00379.2020.

Kim, M. Y., K. Van, Y. J. Kang, K. H. Kim, and S. H. Lee. 2012. "Tracing soybean domestication history: From nucleotide to genome." *Breed Sci* 61 (5):445–452. https://doi.org/10.1270/jsbbs.61.445.

Kim, Mi-Hyun, Kyung-Sun Kang, and Yeon-Sook Lee. 2010. "The inhibitory effect of genistein on hepatic steatosis is linked to visceral adipocyte metabolism in mice with diet-induced non-alcoholic fatty liver disease." *British Journal of Nutrition* 104 (9):1333–1342. https://doi.org/10.1017/S0007114510002266.

Kim, Sujong, Insuk Sohn, Yeon Sook Lee, and Yong Sung Lee. 2005. "Hepatic gene expression profiles are altered by genistein supplementation in mice with diet-induced obesity." *J Nutr* 135 (1):33–41.

Kunz, Hawley E., Corey R. Hart, Kevin J. Gries, Mojtaba Parvizi, Marcello Laurenti, Chiara Dalla Man, Natalie Moore, Xiaoyan Zhang, Zachary Ryan, Eric C. Polley, Michael D. Jensen, Adrian Vella, and Ian R. Lanza. 2021. "Adipose tissue macrophage populations and inflammation are associated with systemic inflammation and insulin resistance in obesity." *Am J Physiol Endocrinol Metab* 321 (1):E105–E121. https://doi.org/10.1152/ajpendo.00070.2021.

Kwak, S. J., C. S. Kim, M. S. Choi, T. Park, M. K. Sung, J. W. Yun, H. Yoo, Y. Mine, and R. Yu. 2016. "The soy peptide phe-leu-val reduces TNFα-induced inflammatory response and insulin resistance in adipocytes." *J Med Food* 19 (7):678–685. https://doi.org/10.1089/jmf.2016.3685.

Lange, S. J., L. Kompaniyets, D. S. Freedman, E. M. Kraus, R. Porter, H. M. Blanck, and A. B. Goodman. 2021. "Longitudinal trends in body mass index before and during the COVID–19 pandemic among persons aged 2–19 years – United States, 2018–2020." *MMWR Morb Mortal Wkly Rep* 70 (37):1278–1283. https://doi.org/10.15585/mmwr.mm7037a3.

Lee, Young Min, Joo Sun Choi, Mi Hyun Kim, Myeong Ho Jung, Yeon Sook Lee, and Jihyun Song. 2006. "Effects of dietary genistein on hepatic lipid metabolism and mitochondrial function in mice fed high-fat diets." *Nutrition* 22 (9):956–964. https://doi.org/10.1016/j.nut.2005.12.014.

Li, D., R. Ikaga, and T. Yamazaki. 2018. "Soya protein β-conglycinin ameliorates fatty liver and obesity in diet-induced obese mice through the down-regulation of PPARγ." *Br J Nutr* 119 (11):1220–1232. https://doi.org/10.1017/s0007114518000739.

Li, J., A. Ha, F. Rui, B. Zou, H. Yang, Q. Xue, X. Hu, Y. Xu, L. Henry, M. Barakat, C. D. Stave, J. Shi, C. Wu, R. Cheung, and M. H. Nguyen. 2022. "Meta-analysis: Global prevalence, trend and forecasting of non-alcoholic fatty liver disease in children and adolescents, 2000–2021." *Aliment Pharmacol Ther* 56 (3):396–406. https://doi.org/10.1111/apt.17096.

Li, Wei, Nathan C. Twaddle, Beverly Spray, Bernice Nounamo, Behjatolah Monzavi-Karbassi, and Reza Hakkak. 2023. "Feeding soy protein concentrates with low and high isoflavones alters 9 and 18 weeks serum isoflavones and inflammatory protein levels in lean and obese zucker rats." *Journal of Medicinal Food* 26 (2):120–127. https://doi.org/10.1089/jmf.2022.0100.

Lin, Qinlu, Wang Liao, Jie Bai, Wei Wu, and Jianping Wu. 2017. "Soy protein-derived ACE-inhibitory peptide LSW (Leu-Ser-Trp) shows anti-inflammatory activity on vascular smooth muscle cells." *Journal of Functional Foods* 34:248–253. https://doi.org/10.1016/j.jff.2017.04.029.

Lu, Hongyun, Hong Liu, Fang Hu, Lingling Zou, Shunkui Luo, and Liao Sun. 2013. "Independent association between nonalcoholic fatty liver disease and cardiovascular disease: A systematic review and meta-analysis." *International Journal of Endocrinology* 2013:124958. https://doi.org/10.1155/2013/124958.

Luo, Y., and H. Lin. 2021. "Inflammation initiates a vicious cycle between obesity and nonalcoholic fatty liver disease." *Immun Inflamm Dis* 9 (1):59–73. https://doi.org/10.1002/iid3.391.

Markova, M., O. Pivovarova, S. Hornemann, S. Sucher, T. Frahnow, K. Wegner, J. Machann, K. J. Petzke, J. Hierholzer, R. Lichtinghagen, C. Herder, M. Carstensen-Kirberg, M. Roden, N. Rudovich, S. Klaus, R. Thomann, R. Schneeweiss, S. Rohn, and A. F. Pfeiffer. 2017. "Isocaloric diets high in animal or plant protein reduce liver fat and inflammation in individuals with type 2 diabetes." *Gastroenterology* 152 (3):571–585.e8. https://doi.org/10.1053/j.gastro.2016.10.007.

Martinez, F. O., and S. Gordon. 2014. "The M1 and M2 paradigm of macrophage activation: Time for reassessment." *F1000Prime Rep* 6:13. https://doi.org/10.12703/p6-13.

Mazzolini, G., J. P. Sowa, C. Atorrasagasti, Ö Kücükoglu, W. K. Syn, and A. Canbay. 2020. "Significance of simple steatosis: An update on the clinical and molecular evidence." *Cells* 9 (11). https://doi.org/10.3390/cells9112458.

Messina, M. 2016. "Soy and health update: Evaluation of the clinical and epidemiologic literature." *Nutrients* 8 (12). https://doi.org/10.3390/nu8120754.

Miadoková, E. 2009. "Isoflavonoids – an overview of their biological activities and potential health benefits." *Interdiscip Toxicol* 2 (4):211–218. https://doi.org/10.2478/v10102-009-0021-3.

Michelfelder, A. J. 2009. "Soy: A complete source of protein." *Am Fam Physician* 79 (1):43–47.

Mitra, Souveek, Arka De, and Abhijit Chowdhury. 2019. "Epidemiology of non-alcoholic and alcoholic fatty liver diseases." *Transl Gastroenterol Hepatol* 5. https://doi.org/10.21037/tgh.2019.09.08.

Nasca, Melita M., Jin-Rong Zhou, and Francine K. Welty. 2008. "Effect of soy nuts on adhesion molecules and markers of inflammation in hypertensive and normotensive postmenopausal women." *The American Journal of Cardiology* 102 (1):84–86. https://doi.org/10.1016/j.amjcard.2008.02.100.

NIDDK. 2021a. "Definition & Facts of NAFLD & NASH." accessed August 6, 2023. https://www.niddk.nih.gov/health-information/liver-disease/nafld-nash/definition-facts.

Nier, Anika, Yvonne Huber, Christian Labenz, Maurice Michel, Ina Bergheim, and Jörn M. Schattenberg. 2020. "Adipokines and endotoxemia correlate with hepatic steatosis in non-alcoholic fatty liver disease (NAFLD)." *Nutrients* 12 (3):699. https://doi.org/10.3390/nu12030699.

Park, Yewan, Dong Hyun Sinn, Kyunga Kim, and Geum-Youn Gwak. 2023. "The association of non-alcoholic fatty liver disease between parents and adolescent children." *Aliment Pharmacol Ther* 57 (2):245–252. https://doi.org/https://doi.org/10.1111/apt.17257.

Perumpail, B. J., M. A. Khan, E. R. Yoo, G. Cholankeril, D. Kim, and A. Ahmed. 2017. "Clinical epidemiology and disease burden of nonalcoholic fatty liver disease." *World J Gastroenterol* 23 (47):8263–8276. https://doi.org/10.3748/wjg.v23.i47.8263.

Promotion, US Department of Agriculture. Center for Nutrition Policy. 2014. "US department of agriculture. Center for nutrition policy and promotion." June.

Qin, Pingxu, Taoran Wang, and Yangchao Luo. 2022. "A review on plant-based proteins from soybean: Health benefits and soy product development." *J Agric Res* 7:100265. https://doi.org/10.1016/j.jafr.2021.100265.

Raetz, C. R., and C. Whitfield. 2002. "Lipopolysaccharide endotoxins." *Annu Rev Biochem* 71:635–700. https://doi.org/10.1146/annurev.biochem.71.110601.135414.

Restrepo, Brandon J. 2022. "Obesity prevalence among U.S. Adults during the COVID-19 pandemic." *Am J Prev Med* 63 (1):102–106. https://doi.org/10.1016/j.amepre.2022.01.012.

Sacks, Frank M., Alice Lichtenstein, Linda Van Horn, William Harris, Penny Kris-Etherton, and Mary Winston. 2006. "Soy protein, isoflavones, and cardiovascular health." *Circulation* 113 (7):1034–1044. https://doi.org/doi:10.1161/CIRCULATIONAHA.106.171052.

Saltiel, A. R., and J. M. Olefsky. 2017. "Inflammatory mechanisms linking obesity and metabolic disease." *J Clin Invest* 127 (1):1–4. https://doi.org/10.1172/jci92035.

Sarwar, R., N. Pierce, and S. Koppe. 2018. "Obesity and nonalcoholic fatty liver disease: current perspectives." *Diabetes Metab Syndr Obes* 11:533–542. https://doi.org/10.2147/dmso.S146339.

Sedivy, Eric J., Faqiang Wu, and Yoshie Hanzawa. 2017. "Soybean domestication: the origin, genetic architecture and molecular bases." *New Phytologist* 214 (2):539–553. https://doi.org/10.1111/nph.14418.

Service, USDA Agriculture Research. 2018. "FooodData central." accessed August 14. https://fdc.nal.usda.gov/fdc-app.html#/food-details/174270/nutrients.

Service, USDA Foreign Agriculture. 2023. "Soyben explorer." accessed August 14. https://ipad.fas.usda.gov/cropexplorer/cropview/commodityView.aspx?cropid=2222000.

Shetty, Akshay, and Wing-Kin Syn. 2019. "Health and economic burden of nonalcoholic fatty liver disease in the united states and its impact on veterans." *Federal Practitioner: For the Health Care Professionals of the VA, DoD, and PHS* 36 (1):14–19.

Skurk, Thomas, Catherine Alberti-Huber, Christian Herder, and Hans Hauner. 2007. "Relationship between adipocyte size and adipokine expression and secretion." *J Clin Endocrinol Metab* 92 (3):1023–1033. https://doi.org/10.1210/jc.2006-1055.

Stahl, E. P., D. S. Dhindsa, S. K. Lee, P. B. Sandesara, N. P. Chalasani, and L. S. Sperling. 2019. "Nonalcoholic fatty liver disease and the heart: JACC state-of-the-art review." *J Am Coll Cardiol* 73 (8):948–963. https://doi.org/10.1016/j.jacc.2018.11.050.

Takahashi, Y., and T. Fukusato. 2014. "Histopathology of nonalcoholic fatty liver disease/nonalcoholic steatohepatitis." *World J Gastroenterol* 20 (42):15539–48. https://doi.org/10.3748/wjg.v20.i42.15539.

Vajro, P., S. Lenta, P. Socha, A. Dhawan, P. McKiernan, U. Baumann, O. Durmaz, F. Lacaille, V. McLin, and V. Nobili. 2012. "Diagnosis of nonalcoholic fatty liver disease in children and adolescents: Position paper of the ESPGHAN hepatology committee." *J Pediatr Gastroenterol Nutr* 54 (5):700–713. https://doi.org/10.1097/MPG.0b013e318252a13f.

Weisberg, S. P., D. McCann, M. Desai, M. Rosenbaum, R. L. Leibel, and A. W. Ferrante, Jr. 2003. "Obesity is associated with macrophage accumulation in adipose tissue." *J Clin Invest* 112 (12):1796–1808. https://doi.org/10.1172/jci19246.

Wen, Lingrong, Huimin Bi, Xuesong Zhou, Yueming Jiang, Hong Zhu, Xiong Fu, and Bao Yang. 2022. "Structure characterization of soybean peptides and their protective activity against intestinal inflammation." *Food Chemistry* 387:132868. https://doi.org/10.1016/j.foodchem.2022.132868.

WHO. 2021. "Obesity and overweight." accessed September 15, 2023. https://www.who.int/news-room/fact-sheets/detail/obesity-and-overweight.

Wu, Sheng Hui, Xiao Ou Shu, Wong-Ho Chow, Yong-Bing Xiang, Xianglan Zhang, Hong-Lan Li, Qiuyin Cai, Bu-Tian Ji, Hui Cai, Nathaniel Rothman, Yu-Tang Gao, Wei Zheng, and Gong Yang. 2012. "Soy food intake and circulating levels of inflammatory markers in Chinese women." *J Acad Nutr Diet* 112 (7):996–1004.e4. https://doi.org/10.1016/j.jand.2012.04.001.

Xin, Xin, Cheng Chen, Yi-Yang Hu, and Qin Feng. 2019. "Protective effect of genistein on nonalcoholic fatty liver disease (NAFLD)." *Biomed Pharmacother* 117:109047. https://doi.org/10.1016/j.biopha.2019.109047.

Xu, H., G. T. Barnes, Q. Yang, G. Tan, D. Yang, C. J. Chou, J. Sole, A. Nichols, J. S. Ross, L. A. Tartaglia, and H. Chen. 2003. "Chronic inflammation in fat plays a crucial role in the development of obesity-related insulin resistance." *J Clin Invest* 112 (12):1821–30. https://doi.org/10.1172/jci19451.

Yalniz, Mehmet, Ibrahim Halil Bahcecioglu, Nalan Kuzu, Orhan Kursat Poyrazoglu, Ozgur Bulmus, Selman Celebi, Bilal Ustundag, Ibrahim Hanefi Ozercan, and Kazim Sahin. 2007. "Preventive role of genistein in an experimental non-alcoholic steatohepatitis model." *J Gastroenterol Hepatol* 22 (11):2009–2014.

Yi, Guofu, He Li, Menglan Liu, Zhiwei Ying, Jian Zhang, and Xinqi Liu. 2020. "Soybean protein-derived peptides inhibit inflammation in LPS-induced RAW264.7 macrophages via the suppression of TLR4-mediated MAPK-JNK and NF-kappa B activation." *J Food Biochem* 44 (8):e13289. https://doi.org/10.1111/jfbc.13289.

Yu, E. L., and J. B. Schwimmer. 2021. "Epidemiology of pediatric nonalcoholic fatty liver disease." *Clin Liver Dis (Hoboken)* 17 (3):196–199. https://doi.org/10.1002/cld.1027.

Yu, J., X. Bi, B. Yu, and D. Chen. 2016. "Isoflavones: Anti-inflammatory benefit and possible caveats." *Nutrients* 8 (6). https://doi.org/10.3390/nu8060361.

Zatterale, Federica, Michele Longo, Jamal Naderi, Gregory Alexander Raciti, Antonella Desiderio, Claudia Miele, and Francesco Beguinot. 2020. "Chronic adipose tissue inflammation linking obesity to insulin resistance and type 2 diabetes." *Frontiers in Physiology* 10. https://doi.org/10.3389/fphys.2019.01607.

Zhang, Shunming, Shubham Kumari, Yeqing Gu, Xiaohui Wu, Xiaoyue Li, Ge Meng, Qing Zhang, Li Liu, Hongmei Wu, Yawen Wang, Tingjing Zhang, Xuena Wang, Xingqi Cao, Huiping Li, Yunyun Liu, Xiaohe Wang, Shaomei Sun, Xing Wang, Ming Zhou, Qiyu Jia, Kun Song, Zhong Sun, and Kaijun Niu. 2020. "Soy food intake is inversely associated with newly diagnosed nonalcoholic fatty liver disease in the TCLSIH cohort study." *J Nutr* 150 (12):3280–3287. https://doi.org/10.1093/jn/nxaa297.

Zhang, Shunming, Yan Yan, Ge Meng, Qing Zhang, Li Liu, Hongmei Wu, Yeqing Gu, Xuena Wang, Juanjuan Zhang, Shaomei Sun, Xing Wang, Ming Zhou, Qiyu Jia, Kun Song, Yan Borné, Lu Qi, Yu-Ming Chen, and Kaijun Niu. 2023. "Protein foods from animal sources and risk of nonalcoholic fatty liver disease in representative cohorts from North and South China." *J Intern Med* 293 (3):340–353. https://doi.org/10.1111/joim.13586.

Zhou, Dan, Stephane Lezmi, Huan Wang, Jeremy Davis, William Banz, and Hong Chen. 2014. "Fat accumulation in the liver of obese rats is alleviated by soy protein isolate through β-catenin signaling." *Obesity* 22 (1):151–158. https://doi.org/10.1002/oby.20421.

23 Identifying the Anti-Cancer Components in Soy

Ingrid Elisia and Gerald Krystal

ABBREVIATIONS

BBIs	Bowman–Birk inhibitors
GI	Gastrointestinal
PSA	Prostate-specific antigen
SPI	Soy protein isolate

INTRODUCTION

Early population studies showing lower breast cancer incidence rates among women in regions consuming high levels of soy food led to the hypothesis that soy foods might lower cancer rates (Messina and Barnes 1991; Tominaga 1985). Subsequent animal studies confirmed that diets containing soy were indeed effective in preventing the formation of certain tumors (Hakkak et al. 2000; Appelt and Reicks 1999; Landstrom et al. 1998; Aronson et al. 1999). Specifically, when compared to casein, a milk protein commonly used in standard rodent diets, soy protein isolates (SPIs) – highly refined soy protein preparations depleted of most other ingredients in soybeans, with minimum protein contents of 90% (Messina et al. 2022) – were found to be superior in preventing mammary, prostate, liver, ovarian, colon, and cervical cancers (Mercer et al. 2017; Taha et al. 2018; Robles-Ramirez Mdel et al. 2012; Hakkak et al. 2001; Simmen et al. 2005; Zhou et al. 2002). Recently, results from the authors' laboratory, in which cigarette smoke carcinogen-induced lung cancer in A/J mice was monitored, have confirmed SPIs' superiority over casein in preventing lung cancer (Elisia et al. 2019). Countering these promising results, however, several reports published in the early 2000s suggested that isoflavones (phytoestrogens uniquely found in soy) might promote mammary and prostate cancers in rodents (Hsieh et al. 1998; Ju et al. 2001; Nakamura et al. 2011). This has led to ongoing controversy surrounding soy consumption, particularly among breast cancer patients, which we will address below.

Despite multiple decades of research, the active components in soy that are responsible for its anti-cancer activity have not been unequivocally identified. Several components have been reported to have anti-cancer activities. These include the isoflavones, a group of phytochemicals with weak estrogenic activity; Bowman–Birk inhibitors (BBIs), which are small polypeptides with protease inhibitor activity; soy proteins themselves; lunasin (a bioactive peptide); and the saponins (Figure 23.1)

The relative concentrations of these components in soy are shown in Table 23.1

This narrative review aims to highlight each component of soy thought to have anti-cancer activity and explore its merits.

DOI: 10.1201/9781003597926-23

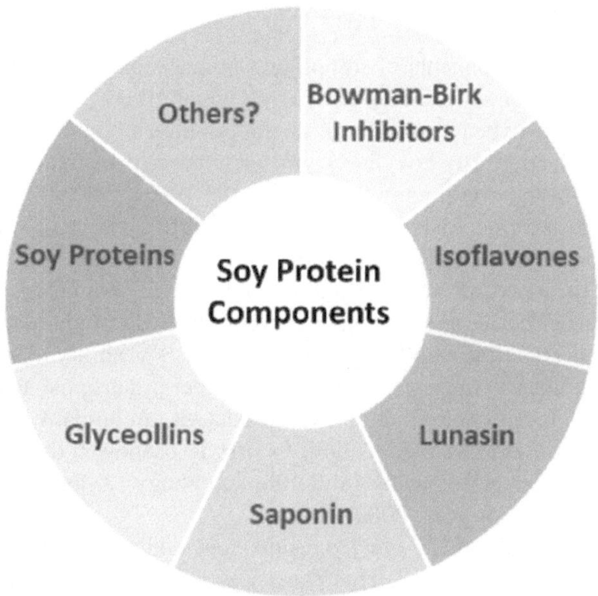

FIGURE 23.1 Soy protein components with purported cancer chemopreventive properties. Several soy protein components have been investigated for their potential chemopreventive properties, including the Bowman–Birk inhibitors, the isoflavones, and lunasin. There are other components in soy with promising anti-cancer effects that need further research, including saponins, glyceollins, gma-mIR159a, peptides, and hydrolysates derived from soy protein digestion. There may be others as well that have not yet been identified.

TABLE 23.1
Approximate Concentrations of Putative Chemopreventive Agents in Soy

Substance	Concentration	Reference
Saponin	0.62–6.16%[a]	Shiraiwa et al. (1991)
Lunasin	0.1–1.33 g/100 g flour[b]	de Mejia et al. (2004)
Soy protein/hydrolysates	35–40% dry weight[c]	Duan et al. (2022)
Isoflavones	~3.5 mg/g soy protein[d]	Messina (2016)
Bowman–Birk inhibitors	1.89–11.4 mg/g dry weight[e]	Mittal et al. (2020)

[a] Shiraiwa, Masakazu, Harada, Kyuya; Okubo, Kazuyoshi. 1991. "Composition and Content of Saponins in Soybean Seed According to Variety, Cultivation Year and Maturity." *Bioscience, Biotechnology & Biochemistry* 55 (2).

[b] Gonzalez de Mejia, E., M. Vasconez, B. O. de Lumen, and R. Nelson. 2004. "Lunasin concentration in different soybean genotypes, commercial soy protein, and isoflavone products." *J Agric Food Chem* 52 (19):5882–7. doi: 1021/jf0496752.

[c] Duan, Ying, Qi Qi, Zihao Liu, Min Zhang, and Huaqing Liu. 2022. "Soy consumption and serum uric acid levels: A systematic review and meta-analysis." *Frontiers in Nutrition* 9.

[d] Messina, M. 2016. "Soy and Health Update: Evaluation of the Clinical and Epidemiologic Literature." *Nutrients* 8 (12). doi: 10.3390/nu8120754.

[e] Mittal, P., V. Kumar, and A. Rani. 2020. *"Effect of Genotype, Seed Development Stages, and Processing Treatments on Bowman–Birk Inhibitor in Soybean and Its Level in Commercial Soy Products"* 49 (3).

BOWMAN–BIRK INHIBITORS

BBIs were among the first components of soy protein preparations investigated for potential anticarcinogenic activity. These small proteins (6–9 kDa), which likely play an important role in protecting storage proteins in soybean seeds from degradation, are potent serine protease inhibitors that bind and inactivate the digestive enzymes trypsin, chymotrypsin, and elastase (Cid-Gallegos et al. 2022). Early reports from several animal studies in the 1980s and 1990s, mainly from the Ann R. Kennedy Lab, suggested that BBIs have a chemopreventive effect in various chemically and genetically induced cancer models (Kennedy 1998). Dietary BBIs also decreased the tumor load of the prostate cancer line, LNCaP, xenografted onto nude mice (Wan et al. 1999). This suggested that, in addition to their effectiveness in cancer prevention, BBIs might also be useful in treating established prostate cancer. These results highlight dietary BBIs' ability to survive gastrointestinal (GI) digestion, allowing them to impact the GI tract and other organs post-absorption. In 1992, BBI concentrate, investigated for possible chemopreventive activity in humans, received Investigational New Drug status from the FDA (Kennedy 1998). *In vitro* tests showed that BBIs directly inhibited the growth of various cancer cell lines by inhibiting autophagy (Kyani et al. 2021) and inducing apoptosis (Olias et al. 2019; Tang et al. 2009).

Despite these promising animal and *in vitro* results, few studies currently evaluate the impact of BBIs on cancer development in humans. This paucity of research persists despite a phase 1 clinical trial involving 19 male participants with benign prostate hyperplasia, which showed that BBIs are not toxic at the dose tested and are effective at reducing serum prostate-specific antigen (PSA) and prostate volumes (Malkowicz et al. 2001). However, in a more recent randomized, placebo-controlled phase IIb trial involving 132 subjects with oral leukoplakia, BBI concentrate failed to decrease oral lesions more effectively than the placebo arm (Armstrong et al. 2013). The authors suggested that inadvertent refrigeration or freezing of the BBI might account for the negative results since storing at refrigerated or frozen temperatures has been shown to diminish BBIs' efficacy in preventing malignant transformation of cells *in vitro* (Kennedy 1998; Armstrong et al. 2013). To our knowledge, no subsequent clinical trials evaluating BBIs' impact on cancer have been carried out.

One possible reason for the lack of research or clinical interest in using BBIs as a chemopreventive agent could be their instability during processing or storage. The bioactive function of BBIs has been linked to their ability to act as serine protease inhibitors (Gitlin-Domagalska et al. 2020), suggesting that changes in BBI protein conformation might reduce their chemopreventive activity. While BBIs were reported to be resistant to GI digestion and pure BBIs were reported to be heat-resistant, the BBIs in soy extracts are not as heat-stable as originally thought (DiPietro and Liener 1989). Glycation, which is expected to occur in BBIs during food processing, was also found, *in vitro*, to reduce the antiproliferative activity of a specific form of BBI (Clemente et al. 2010). The suggestion that freezing or refrigerating BBIs may reduce their efficacy, potentially leading to the negative results in the phase IIb clinical trial described above, highlights another challenge related to the BBI stability during storage (Armstrong et al. 2013).

Since common soy processing may diminish BBI activity, it is reasonable to conclude that the BBIs in soy are unlikely to be responsible for the observed relationship between soy food intake and reduced cancer risk in countries that traditionally consume soy. This is because consumers typically eat most soy foods only after some heat processing, as raw soy contains heat-labile antinutritive factors that may inhibit growth and cause pancreatic enlargement (Messina and Barnes 1991). Whether purified BBIs can be developed into a nutraceutical product that helps to prevent cancer remains an open question.

ISOFLAVONES AND EQUOL

Soybeans contain high levels of isoflavones, a group of phytochemicals, some of which have been shown to bind estrogen receptors, potentially eliciting both estrogenic and/or anti-estrogenic activities (Messina and Wood 2008; Messina and Barnes 1991). The three most abundant isoflavones in soy are genistein, daidzein, and glycitein, which are the glycosylated forms of the aglycones genistin, daidzin, and glycetin, respectively (Figure 23.2).

Because soy is a rich source of isoflavones, it was originally hypothesized that these compounds were the bioactive components in soy that reduced the risk of hormone-sensitive cancers such as breast and prostate cancers. Additionally, the gut microbiome can metabolize daidzein to generate equol, which also has estrogenic activity (Setchell and Clerici 2010). Since the discovery that some people are "equol producers" while others are not, it was also hypothesized that only equol producers might benefit from isoflavone consumption (Setchell and Clerici 2010). Barnes et al., however, noticed that although inhibition of mammary tumorigenesis suggests an anti-estrogenic activity of isoflavones, the ability of SPIs to reduce mammary tumor burden in their animal studies was greater than the observed reduction in mammary tumor estrogen receptors (Messina and Barnes 1991). The authors concluded that the anti-cancer activity of isoflavones, if they were indeed responsible for the reduction in mammary tumors, may not related to their potential to bind with estrogen receptors and that isoflavones' efficacy may extend beyond tumors containing a functional steroid receptor system (Messina and Barnes 1991).

Most *in vitro* studies evaluating the ability of isoflavones and equol to inhibit cancer cell line proliferation suggest that they are indeed promising anti-cancer agents. Their ability to suppress cancer cell growth was shown in multiple cancer cell types, hormone-responsive or not (Itsumi et al. 2016; Anastasius et al. 2009; Kim et al. 2009; Zhang et al. 2019). However, several animal studies from the late 1990s and early 2000s reported that genistein, the major isoflavone in soy, promoted the growth of estrogen receptor-positive human breast cancer cells in ovariectomized athymic nude mice (Hsieh et al. 1998; Ju et al. 2001), creating controversy in the general public and casting doubt on the potential benefit of soy-containing diets for breast cancer patients (Messina et al. 2022). Subsequently published *in vitro* and animal studies suggested that both isoflavones and equol promoted mammary (Martinez-Montemayor et al. 2010) or prostate (Nakamura et al. 2011) tumor growth and stimulated metastatic tumor formation (Yang et al. 2015; Andrade et al. 2015). As a result, research interest in soy and isoflavones has tapered off, as can be seen by the declining number of publications when searching the words "soy" and "cancer" in PubMed.

Nevertheless, most observational or prospective case-control studies in humans do not support the idea that soy food consumption is harmful to cancer patients, and several studies confirm the

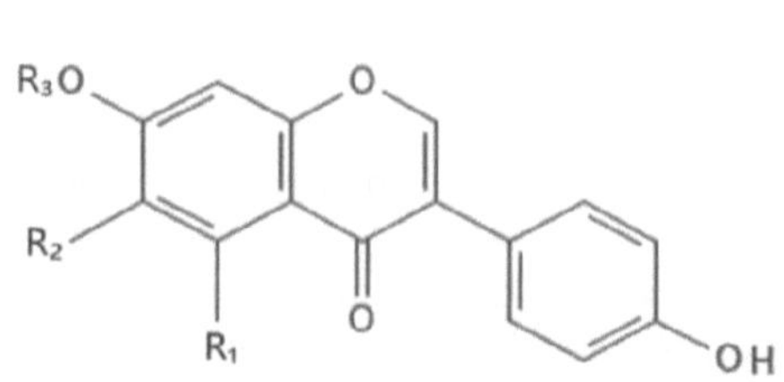

Isoflavone	R1	R2	R3
Aglycones:			
Genistein	OH	H	H
Daidzein	H	H	H
Glycitein	H	O-CH3	H
Glycosides:			
Genistin	OH	H	O-Glucoside
Daidzin	H	H	O-Glucoside
Glycitin	H	O-CH3	O-Glucoside

FIGURE 23.2 Chemical structure of the commonly found isoflavones in soy. The three isoflavones most commonly found in soy can exist either glycosylated or as aglycones.

positive relationship between soy consumption and a reduced risk of cancer (Sim et al. 2020; Tan et al. 2018; Baglia et al. 2016; Lee et al. 2009; Yang et al. 2009). One possible reason for this discrepancy is highlighted in a study evaluating the kinetics of genistein in mice vs. humans. Setchell et al. (2011) reported that rodents metabolize isoflavones differently than humans; while humans quickly metabolize isoflavones to their inactive forms, rodents are less efficient in conjugating them, leading to a high proportion of unconjugated, active isoflavones in mice. The plasma percentages of unconjugated genistein in mice, for example, were approximately 20–150 times higher than those found in humans in this study (Setchell et al. 2011). Thus, soy consumption in humans may not result in an isoflavone concentration that would be effective in preventing or promoting tumor growth in mice. While this brings into question the validity of research utilizing rodents to evaluate isoflavones' efficacy, it should alleviate concerns regarding the safety of soy foods for breast cancer patients. Unfortunately, this also means that isoflavones are unlikely to be the active components in soy that reduce the risk of cancer in humans.

Many randomized clinical trials performed on participants at high risk for breast or prostate cancer have led to the conclusion that isoflavones do not have beneficial or adverse effects, supporting the idea that isoflavones are likely not the chemopreventive agent in soy. Specifically, a double-blind, randomized clinical trial evaluating the impact of 6 months of soy isoflavone (150 mg genistein, 74 mg daidzein, and 11 mg glycitein/day) supplementation in women at increased risk of breast cancer suggested that the isoflavones had no impact on breast epithelial proliferation (Khan et al. 2012). In addition, a longer double-blind, placebo-controlled randomized trial with breast cancer patients or with high-risk women found that taking soy isoflavones (50 mg/day for 12 months) did not change breast tissue density (Wu et al. 2015). Similarly, long-term (6–12 months) supplementation with isoflavones (83–100 mg/day) did not reduce serum PSA in healthy older men (Adams et al. 2004) or impact prostate tumor markers when given to men with a high risk of prostate cancer or low-grade prostate cancer (Hamilton-Reeves et al. 2008). When given at a high dose (160 mg/day) to men with prostate cancer undergoing androgen deprivation therapy for 12 weeks, soy isoflavones also did not improve metabolic or inflammatory parameters in these men (Napora et al. 2011). Consequently, isoflavone supplementation does not appear to reduce the incidence or progression of breast or prostate cancer.

SOY PROTEINS, INCLUDING LUNASIN, PROTEIN HYDROLYSATES, AND PEPTIDES

In addition to the randomized clinical trials mentioned above, which suggested that isoflavones were unlikely to contribute to the anti-cancer effect of soy foods, multiple animal studies have reported that soy extracts or SPIs are superior to isoflavones in preventing cancer. For example, SPI, but not genistein, was found to reduce alcohol-induced tumor progression in diethylnitrosamine-treated mice (Mercer et al. 2018). In another study using a transgenic mouse (MMTV-neu) model of breast carcinoma, isoflavone-poor soy protein concentrate was more effective than isoflavone-containing soy protein concentrate in reducing mammary tumor weights (Chiesa et al. 2008). Since the body digests soy protein upon consumption, these findings led to the idea that protein hydrolysates or bioactive peptides derived from soy digestion might be chemopreventive.

In vitro tests show that soy peptides or soy protein hydrolysates, obtained from hydrolysis using digestive enzymes, suppressed the growth of multiple cancer cell lines, including human cervical cancer cells (HeLa) and human colon cancer cells (Caco-2, HT-29, HCT-116) (Gonzalez-Montoya et al. 2018; Robles-Ramirez Mdel et al. 2012). Of all the components within these hydrolysates, the most investigated bioactive peptide from soy has been lunasin, a 43-amino-acid polypeptide with a molecular mass of 5.5 kDa (Wan et al. 2017). The discovery of lunasin was reported in 1999 when mammalian cells transfected with the lunasin gene led to inhibition of mitosis and subsequent cell death (Galvez and de Lumen 1999). Later studies showed that lunasin inhibited the chemical carcinogen-induced transformation of cells by preventing histone acetylation. Importantly, it appeared to selectively induce apoptosis in cells undergoing transformation, not in non-transformed cells. Since then, studies have shown that lunasin inhibits the proliferation or induces the apoptosis of various cancer cell lines, such as breast, colon, non-small lung cancer, and leukemic cells (Pabona et al. 2013; Hsieh et al. 2010a; Dia and Mejia 2010; Dia and Gonzalez de Mejia 2011; McConnell et al. 2015; Inaba et al. 2014; de Mejia et al. 2010).

One of the earliest pieces of evidence that lunasin might be chemopreventive *in vivo* came from its dermal application to SENCAR mice (Galvez et al. 2001). In these studies, lunasin reduced skin tumor incidence following chemically induced skin cancer. However, a subsequent study evaluating the efficacy of dietary lunasin in DMBA-induced mammary tumors suggested only a non-significant trend towards reducing mammary tumor development (Hsieh et al. 2010b). When given to mice by subcutaneous injection or topical application, lunasin also did not prevent melanoma tumor development (Castaneda-Reyes et al. 2022). Pure lunasin only showed efficacy in suppressing the growth of MDA-MB-231 mammary tumors in athymic nude mice when it was given intraperitoneally (4–20 mg/kg) (Hsieh et al. 2010). This suggests that lunasin may indeed be chemopreventive with certain types of cancers if intact lunasin can be present at high enough concentrations after GI digestion.

While clinical trials evaluating the lunasin's effect on cancer prevention have not yet been conducted, Dia et al. (2009) showed that lunasin could be detected in the plasma of men who consumed 50 g of soy protein for 4 days. On average, 4.5% of the total lunasin was absorbed, reaching 71 ng/mL (33.5–122.7 ng/mL) in plasma 1 hour after ingestion on day 5. Whether this concentration is high enough to elicit chemopreventive activity still needs to be established. The cost associated with producing lunasin may be prohibitive for clinical trials. Moreover, based on the above study where 4 mg/kg lunasin effectively reduced mammary tumor burden (Hsieh et al. 2010), we estimate that the effective concentration in an 80 kg man is equivalent to 6.4 μg/mL (assuming a 5 L blood volume). This is almost 90 times higher than the concentration found in plasma by Dia et al., suggesting that lunasin may not be the likely component in soy that reduces the risk of cancer in humans. Several studies reporting that isoflavone-depleted soy protein had no impact on cancer formation further support the idea that lunasin is unlikely to contribute to the chemopreventive activity of soy (Cohen et al. 2000; Zhou et al. 2002).

It should also be mentioned that plant proteins in general differ from animal proteins in essential amino acid content, and this is especially true for methionine, which is significantly lower in soy proteins than in casein (Gorissen et al. 2018). This could be important, given that methionine promotes cancer cell growth and metabolism (Wanders, Hobson, and Ji 2020). However, unpublished results from the authors' laboratory, using cigarette smoke carcinogen-induced lung cancer in A/J mice, suggest that there is no difference in lung nodule numbers or size when comparing amino acid cocktails identical to soy proteins and casein.

OTHER SOY COMPONENTS

Several other components in soy with potential anti-cancer activity have not yet been thoroughly investigated, and we hypothesize that one or more of these components could be the major contributors to the chemopreventive effects of soy foods. For example, soy saponins, which comprise approximately 5% of soybeans (dry weight) (Messina and Barnes 1991), have been shown *in vitro* to reduce liver cell viability and the growth of breast and colon cancer cell lines (Huang et al. 2021; Rowlands et al. 2002; Zhang and Popovich 2008). *In vivo* tests show that soyasaponin Ag extracted from soy effectively represses MDA-MB-231 mammary tumor growth when xenografted into athymic nude Balb/C mice (Huang et al. 2021). As a crude extract, soy saponins have also been shown to reduce, *in vivo*, the number of carcinogen-induced aberrant crypt foci in rats (Guo et al. 2013), consistent with the *in vitro* chemopreventive activity of the saponins in colon cancer cells.

Another class of compounds of interest is glyceollins, which are soy phytoalexins that also exhibit anti-estrogenic activity (Bamji and Corbitt 2017). Few publications address soy glyceollins, but the limited available evidence suggests that they inhibit both the growth of the prostate (LNCaP) cancer cell line *in vitro* (Payton-Stewart et al. 2009) and subcutaneously implanted Lewis lung carcinoma cells in C57BL/6J mice (Lee et al. 2013).

One of the most recently identified potential anti-cancer components from soy is the plant-derived microRNA (miRNA), gma-miR159a. *In vitro,* gma-miR159a has been shown to suppress the expression of the Myc oncogene, and this, in turn, inhibits the growth of Caco-2 colon cancer cells (Liu et al. 2021). *In vivo* tests show that dietary gma-miR159a given through oral gavage significantly attenuates azoxymethane/dextran sodium sulfate-induced colitis and reduces the occurrence of colon cancer in C57BL/6 mice. Gma-miR159a also remains stable in cooked soybeans, although food processing into tofu or soy milk causes a significant loss of this miRNA (Liu et al. 2021). Whether the saponins, glyceollins, and gma-miR159a are bioavailable and capable of eliciting anti-cancer effects in humans remains to be determined.

CONCLUSIONS/FUTURE DIRECTIONS

This chapter highlighted several compounds found in soy foods that could contribute to the positive relationship between soy consumption and reduced cancer risk. Based on currently available evidence from the last few decades, it appears that the most commonly investigated compounds – the BBIs, isoflavones, and lunasin, or other peptides derived from GI hydrolysis – are unlikely to be the chemopreventive agents in soy. However, other promising components in soy have not been thoroughly investigated *in vitro* or *in vivo*, and these components could act independently or synergistically with other soy components to prevent cancer development. Future research should focus on exploring the potential independent or synergistic actions of these components and their role in reducing the risk of cancer.

MINI DICTIONARY OF TERMS

- **Aglycones:** Molecules lacking sugar residues.
- **Apoptosis:** Programmed cell death that does not trigger the immune system.
- **Autophagy:** An intracellular, self-devouring process for self-preservation.
- **Chemopreventive:** Cancer-preventing.
- **Hyperplasia:** Increase in cell number.
- **Leukoplakia:** White lesion in the oral cavity that may be an early sign of cancer.
- **Lewis lung carcinoma cells:** Lung tumor cell line derived from the lung of a C57BL mouse.
- **LNCaP cells:** Androgen-sensitive human prostate cancer cell line.
- **MicroRNA:** Small, conserved, non-coding RNA involved in regulating gene expression.
- **MMTV-neu:** Transgenic mice that spontaneously develop mammary tumors because they carry the activated c-neu oncogene under the control of the mouse mammary tumor virus (MMTV) long terminal repeat.
- **Phytochemicals:** Chemicals derived from plants.
- **Phytoestrogen:** Estrogen-mimicking compound from plants.
- **Nude mice:** Mice without a thymus, fur, or T cells.
- **Soyasaponin Ag:** An isomer of soysaponin A.
- **Xenograft:** Transplant of cells from one species to another.

SUMMARY POINTS

- This chapter reviews components of soy that may prevent cancer.
- Observational studies suggest that countries with high soy consumption have a low incidence of cancer.
- Several soy components may contribute to the chemopreventive effect of soy.

- Bowman–Birk inhibitors (BBIs), isoflavones, soy proteins, and lunasin have been extensively investigated both *in vitro* and in rodents.
- BBIs are likely destroyed during food processing, while the bioavailability of lunasin appears too low to elicit anti-cancer effects.
- Isoflavones are controversial because they were found to promote cancer in rodents.
- However, humans metabolize isoflavones more quickly, and these compounds are unlikely to reach concentrations in humans that elicit either harmful or chemopreventive effects.
- Other compounds in soy warrant further investigation.
- These include saponins, glyceollins, and gma-miR159a.

REFERENCES

Adams, K. F., C. Chen, K. M. Newton, J. D. Potter, and J. W. Lampe. 2004. "Soy isoflavones do not modulate prostate-specific antigen concentrations in older men in a randomized controlled trial." *Cancer Epidemiol Biomarkers Prev* 13 (4):644–8.

Anastasius, N., S. Boston, M. Lacey, N. Storing, and S. A. Whitehead. 2009. "Evidence that low-dose, long-term genistein treatment inhibits oestradiol-stimulated growth in MCF-7 cells by down-regulation of the PI3-kinase/Akt signalling pathway." *J Steroid Biochem Mol Biol* 116 (1–2):50–5. doi: 10.1016/j.jsbmb.2009.04.009.

Andrade, J. E., Y. H. Ju, C. Baker, D. R. Doerge, and W. G. Helferich. 2015. "Long-term exposure to dietary sources of genistein induces estrogen-independence in the human breast cancer (MCF-7) xenograft model." *Mol Nutr Food Res* 59 (3):413–23. doi: 10.1002/mnfr.201300780.

Appelt, L. C., and M. M. Reicks. 1999. "Soy induces phase II enzymes but does not inhibit dimethylbenz[a]anthracene-induced carcinogenesis in female rats." *J Nutr* 129 (10):1820–6. doi: 10.1093/jn/129.10.1820.

Armstrong, W. B., T. H. Taylor, A. R. Kennedy, R. J. Melrose, D. V. Messadi, M. Gu, A. D. Le, M. Perloff, F. Civantos, W. J. Goodwin, L. J. Wirth, A. R. Kerr, and F. L. Meyskens, Jr. 2013. "Bowman birk inhibitor concentrate and oral leukoplakia: a randomized phase IIb trial." *Cancer Prev Res (Phila)* 6 (5):410–8. doi: 10.1158/1940-6207.CAPR-13-0004.

Aronson, W. J., C. N. Tymchuk, R. M. Elashoff, W. H. McBride, C. McLean, H. Wang, and D. Heber. 1999. "Decreased growth of human prostate LNCaP tumors in SCID mice fed a low-fat, soy protein diet with isoflavones." *Nutr Cancer* 35 (2):130–6. doi: 10.1207/S15327914NC352_6.

Baglia, M. L., W. Zheng, H. Li, G. Yang, J. Gao, Y. T. Gao, and X. O. Shu. 2016. "The association of soy food consumption with the risk of subtype of breast cancers defined by hormone receptor and HER2 status." *Int J Cancer* 139 (4):742–8. doi: 10.1002/ijc.30117.

Bamji, Sanaya F., and Cynthia Corbitt. 2017. "Glyceollins: Soybean phytoalexins that exhibit a wide range of health-promoting effects." *J Funct Foods* 34:98–105. doi: https://doi.org/10.1016/j.jff.2017.04.020.

Castaneda-Reyes, E. D., M. J. Perea-Flores, G. Davila-Ortiz, and E. Gonzalez de Mejia. 2022. "Liposomes loaded with Amaranth unsaponifiable matter and Soybean Lunasin prevented melanoma tumor development overexpressing caspase-3 in an in Vivo model." *Pharmaceutics* 14 (10). doi: 10.3390/pharmaceutics14102214.

Chiesa, G., E. Rigamonti, M. R. Lovati, E. Disconzi, S. Soldati, M. G. Sacco, E. M. Cato, V. Patton, E. Scanziani, P. Vezzoni, A. Arnoldi, D. Locati, and C. R. Sirtori. 2008. "Reduced mammary tumor progression in a transgenic mouse model fed an isoflavone-poor soy protein concentrate." *Mol Nutr Food Res* 52 (10):1121–9. doi: 10.1002/mnfr.200700296.

Cid-Gallegos, M. S., L. J. Corzo-Rios, C. Jimenez-Martinez, and X. M. Sanchez-Chino. 2022. "Protease inhibitors from plants as therapeutic agents- a review." *Plant Foods Hum Nutr* 77 (1):20–9. doi: 10.1007/s11130-022-00949-4.

Clemente, A., F. J. Moreno, C. Marin-Manzano Mdel, E. Jimenez, and C. Domoney. 2010. "The cytotoxic effect of Bowman–Birk isoinhibitors, IBB1 and IBBD2, from soybean (Glycine max) on HT29 human colorectal cancer cells is related to their intrinsic ability to inhibit serine proteases." *Mol Nutr Food Res* 54 (3):396–405. doi: 10.1002/mnfr.200900122.

Cohen, L. A., Z. Zhao, B. Pittman, and J. A. Scimeca. 2000. "Effect of intact and isoflavone-depleted soy protein on NMU-induced rat mammary tumorigenesis." *Carcinogenesis* 21 (5):929–35. doi: 10.1093/carcin/21.5.929.

de Mejia, E. G., M. Vasconez, B. O. de Lumen, and R. Nelson. 2004. "Lunasin concentration in different soybean genotypes, commercial soy protein, and isoflavone products." *J Agric Food Chem* 52 (19):5882–7. doi: 10.1021/jf0496752.

de Mejia, E. G., W. Wang, and V. P. Dia. 2010. "Lunasin, with an arginine-glycine-aspartic acid motif, causes apoptosis to L1210 leukemia cells by activation of caspase-3." *Mol Nutr Food Res* 54 (3):406–14. doi: 10.1002/mnfr.200900073.

Dia, V. P., and E. G. Mejia. 2010. "Lunasin promotes apoptosis in human colon cancer cells by mitochondrial pathway activation and induction of nuclear clusterin expression." *Cancer Lett* 295 (1):44–53. doi: 10.1016/j.canlet.2010.02.010.

Dia, V. P., and E. Gonzalez de Mejia. 2011. "Lunasin induces apoptosis and modifies the expression of genes associated with extracellular matrix and cell adhesion in human metastatic colon cancer cells." *Mol Nutr Food Res* 55 (4):623–34. doi: 10.1002/mnfr.201000419.

Dia, V. P., S. Torres, B. O. De Lumen, J. W. Erdman, Jr. and E. G. De Mejia. 2009. "Presence of lunasin in plasma of men after soy protein consumption." *J Agric Food Chem* 57 (4):1260–6. doi: 10.1021/jf803303k.

DiPietro, Christina M., and Irvin E. Liener. 1989. "Heat inactivation of the Kunitz and Bowman–Birk soybean protease inhibitors." *J Agric Food Chem* 37 (1):39–44. doi: 10.1021/jf00085a010.

Duan, Ying, Qi Qi, Zihao Liu, Min Zhang, and Huaqing Liu. 2022. "Soy consumption and serum uric acid levels: A systematic review and meta-analysis." *Frontiers in Nutrition* 9.

Elisia, I., B. Cho, M. Hay, M. Y. Li, E. Hofs, V. Lam, R. A. Dyer, J. Lum, and G. Krystal. 2019. "The effect of diet and exercise on tobacco carcinogen-induced lung cancer." *Carcinogenesis* 40 (3):448–60. doi: 10.1093/carcin/bgz060.

Galvez, A. F., N. Chen, J. Macasieb, and B. O. de Lumen. 2001. "Chemopreventive property of a soybean peptide (lunasin) that binds to deacetylated histones and inhibits acetylation." *Cancer Res* 61 (20):7473–8.

Galvez, A. F., and B. O. de Lumen. 1999. "A soybean cDNA encoding a chromatin-binding peptide inhibits mitosis of mammalian cells." *Nat Biotechnol* 17 (5):495–500. doi: 10.1038/8676.

Gitlin-Domagalska, A., A. Maciejewska, and D. Debowski. 2020. "Bowman–birk inhibitors: insights into family of multifunctional proteins and peptides with potential therapeutical applications." *Pharmaceuticals (Basel)* 13 (12). doi: 10.3390/ph13120421.

Gonzalez-Montoya, M., B. Hernandez-Ledesma, J. M. Silvan, R. Mora-Escobedo, and C. Martinez-Villaluenga. 2018. "Peptides derived from in vitro gastrointestinal digestion of germinated soybean proteins inhibit human colon cancer cells proliferation and inflammation." *Food Chem* 242:75–82. doi: 10.1016/j.foodchem.2017.09.035.

Gorissen, S. H. M., J. J. R. Crombag, J. M. G. Senden, W. A. H. Waterval, J. Bierau, L. B. Verdijk, and L. J. C. van Loon. 2018. "Protein content and amino acid composition of commercially available plant-based protein isolates." *Amino Acids* 50 (12):1685–95. doi: 10.1007/s00726-018-2640-5.

Guo, Y. W., Y. H. Chen, W. C. Chiu, H. Liao, and S. H. Lin. 2013. "Soy saponins meditate the progression of colon cancer in rats by inhibiting the activity of beta -glucuronidase and the number of aberrant crypt foci but not cyclooxygenase-2 activity." *ISRN Oncol* 2013:645817. doi: 10.1155/2013/645817.

Hakkak, R., S. Korourian, M. J. Ronis, J. M. Johnston, and T. M. Badger. 2001. "Soy protein isolate consumption protects against azoxymethane-induced colon tumors in male rats." *Cancer Lett* 166 (1):27–32. doi: 10.1016/s0304-3835(01)00441-4.

Hakkak, R., S. Korourian, S. R. Shelnutt, S. Lensing, M. J. Ronis, and T. M. Badger. 2000. "Diets containing whey proteins or soy protein isolate protect against 7,12-dimethylbenz(a)anthracene-induced mammary tumors in female rats." *Cancer Epidemiol Biomarkers Prev* 9 (1):113–7.

Hamilton-Reeves, J. M., S. A. Rebello, W. Thomas, M. S. Kurzer, and J. W. Slaton. 2008. "Effects of soy protein isolate consumption on prostate cancer biomarkers in men with HGPIN, ASAP, and low-grade prostate cancer." *Nutr Cancer* 60 (1):7–13. doi: 10.1080/01635580701586770.

Hsieh, C. C., B. Hernandez-Ledesma, H. J. Jeong, J. H. Park, and B. O. de Lumen. 2010. "Complementary roles in cancer prevention: protease inhibitor makes the cancer preventive peptide lunasin bioavailable." *PLoS One* 5 (1):e8890. doi: 10.1371/journal.pone.0008890.

Hsieh, C. C., B. Hernandez-Ledesma, and B. O. de Lumen. 2010a. "Lunasin, a novel seed peptide, sensitizes human breast cancer MDA-MB-231 cells to aspirin-arrested cell cycle and induced apoptosis." *Chem Biol Interact* 186 (2):127–34. doi: 10.1016/j.cbi.2010.04.027.

Hsieh, C. C., B. Hernandez-Ledesma, and B. O. de Lumen. 2010b. "Soybean peptide lunasin suppresses in vitro and in vivo 7,12-dimethylbenz[a]anthracene-induced tumorigenesis." *J Food Sci* 75 (9):H311–6. doi: 10.1111/j.1750-3841.2010.01861.x.

Hsieh, C. Y., R. C. Santell, S. Z. Haslam, and W. G. Helferich. 1998. “Estrogenic effects of genistein on the growth of estrogen receptor-positive human breast cancer (MCF-7) cells in vitro and in vivo.” *Cancer Res* 58 (17):3833–8.

Huang, S., P. Huang, H. Wu, S. Wang, and G. Liu. 2021. “Soyasaponin Ag inhibits triple-negative breast cancer progression via targeting the DUSP6/MAPK signaling.” *Folia Histochem Cytobiol* 59 (4):291–301. doi: 10.5603/FHC.a2021.0029.

Inaba, J., E. J. McConnell, and K. R. Davis. 2014. “Lunasin sensitivity in non-small cell lung cancer cells is linked to suppression of integrin signaling and changes in histone acetylation.” *Int J Mol Sci* 15 (12):23705–24. doi: 10.3390/ijms151223705.

Itsumi, M., M. Shiota, A. Takeuchi, E. Kashiwagi, J. Inokuchi, K. Tatsugami, S. Kajioka, T. Uchiumi, S. Naito, M. Eto, and A. Yokomizo. 2016. “Equol inhibits prostate cancer growth through degradation of androgen receptor by S-phase kinase-associated protein 2.” *Cancer Sci* 107 (7):1022–8. doi: 10.1111/cas.12948.

Ju, Y. H., C. D. Allred, K. F. Allred, K. L. Karko, D. R. Doerge, and W. G. Helferich. 2001. “Physiological concentrations of dietary genistein dose-dependently stimulate growth of estrogen-dependent human breast cancer (MCF-7) tumors implanted in athymic nude mice.” *J Nutr* 131 (11):2957–62. doi: 10.1093/jn/131.11.2957.

Kennedy, A. R. 1998. “The Bowman–Birk inhibitor from soybeans as an anticarcinogenic agent.” *Am J Clin Nutr* 68 (6 Suppl):1406S–12S. doi: 10.1093/ajcn/68.6.1406S.

Khan, S. A., R. T. Chatterton, N. Michel, M. Bryk, O. Lee, D. Ivancic, R. Heinz, C. M. Zalles, I. B. Helenowski, B. D. Jovanovic, A. A. Franke, M. C. Bosland, J. Wang, N. M. Hansen, K. P. Bethke, A. Dew, M. Coomes, and R. C. Bergan. 2012. “Soy isoflavone supplementation for breast cancer risk reduction: a randomized phase II trial.” *Cancer Prev Res (Phila)* 5 (2):309–19. doi: 10.1158/1940-6207.CAPR-11-0251.

Kim, S. H., S. H. Kim, S. C. Lee, and Y. S. Song. 2009. “Involvement of both extrinsic and intrinsic apoptotic pathways in apoptosis induced by genistein in human cervical cancer cells.” *Ann N Y Acad Sci* 1171:196–201. doi: 10.1111/j.1749-6632.2009.04902.x.

Kyani, S., H. Akrami, A. Mostafaei, S. Akbari, and Z. Salehi. 2021. “Inhibitory effect of Bowman–Birk protease inhibitor on autophagy in MDAMB231 breast cancer cell line.” *J Cancer Res Ther* 17 (2):504–9. doi: 10.4103/jcrt.JCRT_622_18.

Landstrom, M., J. X. Zhang, G. Hallmans, P. Aman, A. Bergh, J. E. Damber, W. Mazur, K. Wahala, and H. Adlercreutz. 1998. “Inhibitory effects of soy and rye diets on the development of Dunning R3327 prostate adenocarcinoma in rats.” *Prostate* 36 (3):151–61. doi: 10.1002/(sici)1097-0045(19980801)36:3<151::aid-pros2>3.0.co;2-k.

Lee, S. A., X. O. Shu, H. Li, G. Yang, H. Cai, W. Wen, B. T. Ji, J. Gao, Y. T. Gao, and W. Zheng. 2009. “Adolescent and adult soy food intake and breast cancer risk: results from the Shanghai women's health study.” *Am J Clin Nutr* 89 (6):1920–6. doi: 10.3945/ajcn.2008.27361.

Lee, S. H., J. Lee, M. H. Jung, and Y. M. Lee. 2013. “Glyceollins, a novel class of soy phytoalexins, inhibit angiogenesis by blocking the VEGF and bFGF signaling pathways.” *Mol Nutr Food Res* 57 (2):225–34. doi: 10.1002/mnfr.201200489.

Liu, J., F. Wang, H. Song, Z. Weng, Y. Bao, Y. Fang, X. Tang, and X. Shen. 2021. “Soybean-derived gma-miR159a alleviates colon tumorigenesis by suppressing TCF7/MYC in mice.” *J Nutr Biochem* 92:108627. doi: 10.1016/j.jnutbio.2021.108627.

Malkowicz, S. B., W. G. McKenna, D. J. Vaughn, X. S. Wan, K. J. Propert, K. Rockwell, S. H. Marks, A. J. Wein, and A. R. Kennedy. 2001. “Effects of Bowman–Birk inhibitor concentrate (BBIC) in patients with benign prostatic hyperplasia.” *Prostate* 48 (1):16–28. doi: 10.1002/pros.1077.

Martinez-Montemayor, M. M., E. Otero-Franqui, J. Martinez, A. De La Mota-Peynado, L. A. Cubano, and S. Dharmawardhane. 2010. “Individual and combined soy isoflavones exert differential effects on metastatic cancer progression.” *Clin Exp Metastasis* 27 (7):465–80. doi: 10.1007/s10585-010-9336-x.

McConnell, E. J., B. Devapatla, K. Yaddanapudi, and K. R. Davis. 2015. “The soybean-derived peptide lunasin inhibits non-small cell lung cancer cell proliferation by suppressing phosphorylation of the retinoblastoma protein.” *Oncotarget* 6 (7):4649–62. doi: 10.18632/oncotarget.3080.

Mercer, K. E., C. F. Pulliam, L. Hennings, M. A. Cleves, E. E. Jones, R. R. Drake, and M. J. J. Ronis. 2018. “Diet supplementation with soy protein isolate, but not the isoflavone genistein, protects against alcohol-induced tumor progression in DEN-treated male mice.” *Adv Exp Med Biol* 1032:115–26. doi: 10.1007/978-3-319-98788-0_9.

Mercer, K. E., C. F. Pulliam, K. B. Pedersen, L. Hennings, and M. J. Ronis. 2017. “Soy protein isolate inhibits hepatic tumor promotion in mice fed a high-fat liquid diet.” *Exp Biol Med (Maywood)* 242 (6):635–44. doi: 10.1177/1535370216685436.

Messina, M. 2016. "Soy and Health Update: Evaluation of the Clinical and Epidemiologic Literature." *Nutrients* 8 (12). doi: 10.3390/nu8120754.

Messina, M. J., and S. Barnes. 1991. "The role of soy products in reducing risk of cancer." *J Natl Cancer Inst* 83 (8):541–6. doi: 10.1093/jnci/83.8.541.

Messina, M. J., A. Duncan, V. Messina, H. Lynch, J. Kiel, and J. W. Erdman, Jr. 2022. "The health effects of soy: A reference guide for health professionals." *Front Nutr* 9:970364. doi: 10.3389/fnut.2022.970364.

Messina, M. J., and C. E. Wood. 2008. "Soy isoflavones, estrogen therapy, and breast cancer risk: analysis and commentary." *Nutr J* 7:17. doi: 10.1186/1475-2891-7-17.

Mittal, P., V. Kumar, and A. Rani. 2020. *Effect of Genotype, Seed Development Stages, and Processing Treatments on Bowman–Birk Inhibitor in Soybean and Its Level in Commercial Soy Products* 49 (3).

Nakamura, H., Y. Wang, T. Kurita, H. Adomat, G. R. Cunha, and Y. Wang. 2011. "Genistein increases epidermal growth factor receptor signaling and promotes tumor progression in advanced human prostate cancer." *PLoS One* 6 (5):e20034. doi: 10.1371/journal.pone.0020034.

Napora, J. K., R. G. Short, D. C. Muller, O. D. Carlson, J. O. Odetunde, X. Xu, M. Carducci, T. G. Travison, M. Maggio, J. M. Egan, and S. Basaria. 2011. "High-dose isoflavones do not improve metabolic and inflammatory parameters in androgen-deprived men with prostate cancer." *J Androl* 32 (1):40–8. doi: 10.2164/jandrol.110.010983.

Olias, R., C. Becerra-Rodriguez, J. R. Soliz-Rueda, F. J. Moreno, C. Delgado-Andrade, and A. Clemente. 2019. "Glycation affects differently the main soybean Bowman–Birk isoinhibitors, IBB1 and IBBD2, altering their antiproliferative properties against HT29 colon cancer cells." *Food Funct* 10 (9):6193–202. doi: 10.1039/c9fo01421g.

Pabona, J. M., B. Dave, Y. Su, M. T. Montales, B. O. de Lumen, E. G. de Mejia, O. M. Rahal, and R. C. Simmen. 2013. "The soybean peptide lunasin promotes apoptosis of mammary epithelial cells via induction of tumor suppressor PTEN: similarities and distinct actions from soy isoflavone genistein." *Genes Nutr* 8 (1):79–90. doi: 10.1007/s12263-012-0307-5.

Payton-Stewart, F., N. W. Schoene, Y. S. Kim, M. E. Burow, T. E. Cleveland, S. M. Boue, and T. T. Wang. 2009. "Molecular effects of soy phytoalexin glyceollins in human prostate cancer cells LNCaP." *Mol Carcinog* 48 (9):862–71. doi: 10.1002/mc.20532.

Robles-Ramirez Mdel, C., E. Ramon-Gallegos, R. Mora-Escobedo, and N. Torres-Torres. 2012. "A peptide fraction from germinated soybean protein down-regulates PTTG1 and TOP2A mRNA expression, inducing apoptosis in cervical cancer cells." *J Exp Ther Oncol* 9 (4):255–63.

Rowlands, J. C., M. A. Berhow, and T. M. Badger. 2002. "Estrogenic and antiproliferative properties of soy sapogenols in human breast cancer cells in vitro." *Food Chem Toxicol* 40 (12):1767–74. doi: 10.1016/s0278-6915(02)00181-3.

Setchell, K. D., N. M. Brown, X. Zhao, S. L. Lindley, J. E. Heubi, E. C. King, and M. J. Messina. 2011. "Soy isoflavone phase II metabolism differs between rodents and humans: implications for the effect on breast cancer risk." *Am J Clin Nutr* 94 (5):1284–94. doi: 10.3945/ajcn.111.019638.

Setchell, K. D., and C. Clerici. 2010. "Equol: history, chemistry, and formation." *J Nutr* 140 (7):1355S–62S. doi: 10.3945/jn.109.119776.

Shiraiwa, Masakazu, Harada, Kyuya; Okubo, Kazuyoshi. 1991. "Composition and Content of Saponins in Soybean Seed According to Variety, Cultivation Year and Maturity." *Bioscience, Biotechnology & Biochemistry* 55 (2).

Sim, E. J., K. P. Ko, C. Ahn, S. M. Park, Y. J. Surh, S. An, S. W. Kim, M. H. Lee, J. W. Lee, J. E. Lee, K. S. Kim, C. K. Yom, H. A. Kim, and S. K. Park. 2020. "Isoflavone intake on the risk of overall breast cancer and molecular subtypes in women at high risk for hereditary breast cancer." *Breast Cancer Res Treat* 184 (2):615–26. doi: 10.1007/s10549-020-05875-0.

Simmen, R. C., R. R. Eason, S. R. Till, L. Chatman, Jr., M. C. Velarde, Y. Geng, S. Korourian, and T. M. Badger. 2005. "Inhibition of NMU-induced mammary tumorigenesis by dietary soy." *Cancer Lett* 224 (1):45–52. doi: 10.1016/j.canlet.2004.11.009.

Taha, A. A. A., M. Koshiyama, N. Matsumura, K. Abiko, K. Yamaguchi, J. Hamanishi, T. Baba, B. Kharma, I. H. Mohamed, M. M. Ameen, S. A. Ismail, I. Konishi, and M. Mandai. 2018. "The effect of the type of dietary protein on the development of ovarian cancer." *Oncotarget* 9 (35):23987–99. doi: 10.18632/oncotarget.25253.

Tan, M. M., W. K. Ho, S. Y. Yoon, S. Mariapun, S. N. Hasan, D. S. Lee, T. Hassan, S. Y. Lee, S. Y. Phuah, K. Sivanandan, P. P. Ng, N. Rajaram, M. Jaganathan, S. Jamaris, T. Islam, K. Rahmat, F. Fadzli, A. Vijayananthan, P. Rajadurai, M. H. See, M. K. Thong, N. A. Mohd Taib, C. H. Yip, and S. H. Teo. 2018. "A case-control study of breast cancer risk factors in 7,663 women in Malaysia." *PLoS One* 13 (9):e0203469. doi: 10.1371/journal.pone.0203469.

Tang, M., M. Asamoto, K. Ogawa, A. Naiki-Ito, S. Sato, S. Takahashi, and T. Shirai. 2009. "Induction of apoptosis in the LNCaP human prostate carcinoma cell line and prostate adenocarcinomas of SV40T antigen transgenic rats by the Bowman–Birk inhibitor." *Pathol Int* 59 (11):790–6. doi: 10.1111/j.1440-1827.2009.02445.x.

Tominaga, S. 1985. "Cancer incidence in Japanese in Japan, Hawaii, and western United States." *Natl Cancer Inst Monogr* 69:83–92.

Wan, X. S., H. Liu, Y. Sun, J. Zhang, X. Chen, and N. Chen. 2017. "Lunasin: A promising polypeptide for the prevention and treatment of cancer." *Oncol Lett* 13 (6):3997–4001. doi: 10.3892/ol.2017.6017.

Wan, X. S., J. H. Ware, L. Zhang, P. M. Newberne, S. M. Evans, L. C. Clark, and A. R. Kennedy. 1999. "Treatment with soybean-derived Bowman Birk inhibitor increases serum prostate-specific antigen concentration while suppressing growth of human prostate cancer xenografts in nude mice." *Prostate* 41 (4):243–52. doi: 10.1002/(sici)1097-0045(19991201)41:4<243::aid-pros4>3.0.co;2-f.

Wanders, D., K. Hobson, and X. Ji. 2020. "Methionine restriction and cancer biology." *Nutrients* 12 (3). doi: 10.3390/nu12030684.

Wu, A. H., D. Spicer, A. Garcia, C. C. Tseng, L. Hovanessian-Larsen, P. Sheth, S. E. Martin, D. Hawes, C. Russell, H. MacDonald, D. Tripathy, M. Y. Su, G. Ursin, and M. C. Pike. 2015. "Double-blind randomized 12-month soy intervention had no effects on breast MRI fibroglandular tissue density or mammographic density." *Cancer Prev Res (Phila)* 8 (10):942–51. doi: 10.1158/1940-6207.CAPR-15-0125.

Yang, G., X. O. Shu, H. Li, W. H. Chow, H. Cai, X. Zhang, Y. T. Gao, and W. Zheng. 2009. "Prospective cohort study of soy food intake and colorectal cancer risk in women." *Am J Clin Nutr* 89 (2):577–83. doi: 10.3945/ajcn.2008.26742.

Yang, X., A. Belosay, J. A. Hartman, H. Song, Y. Zhang, W. Wang, D. R. Doerge, and W. G. Helferich. 2015. "Dietary soy isoflavones increase metastasis to lungs in an experimental model of breast cancer with bone micro-tumors." *Clin Exp Metastasis* 32 (4):323–33. doi: 10.1007/s10585-015-9709-2.

Zhang, Q., W. S. Cao, X. Q. Wang, M. Zhang, X. M. Lu, J. Q. Chen, Y. Chen, M. M. Ge, C. Y. Zhong, and H. Y. Han. 2019. "Genistein inhibits nasopharyngeal cancer stem cells through sonic hedgehog signaling." *Phytother Res* 33 (10):2783–91. doi: 10.1002/ptr.6464.

Zhang, W., and D. G. Popovich. 2008. "Effect of soyasapogenol A and soyasapogenol B concentrated extracts on HEP-G2 cell proliferation and apoptosis." *J Agric Food Chem* 56 (8):2603–8. doi: 10.1021/jf0731550.

Zhou, J. R., L. Yu, Y. Zhong, R. L. Nassr, A. A. Franke, S. M. Gaston, and G. L. Blackburn. 2002. "Inhibition of orthotopic growth and metastasis of androgen-sensitive human prostate tumors in mice by bioactive soybean components." *Prostate* 53 (2):143–53. doi: 10.1002/pros.10141.

24 Soy Protein Supplementation

Effects on Prostate Cancer and Hormones in Males

Maarten C. Bosland

ABBREVIATIONS

BPH	Benign prostatic hypertrophy
CI	Confidence interval
DHEAS	Dehydroepiandrosterone
DHT	5α-dihydrotestosterone
EGF	Epidermal growth factor
FSH	Follicle-stimulating hormone
LH	Luteinizing hormone
NHANES	National Health and Nutrition Examination Survey
PCNA	Proliferating cell nuclear antigen
PSA	Prostate-specific antigen
SHBG	Sex hormone-binding globulin
T3	Triiodothyronine
T4	Thyroxine
TSH	Thyroid-stimulating hormone (also known as thyrotrophin or thyrotropic hormone)

INTRODUCTION

Prostate cancer is often the most common male malignancy in countries where people eat little soy and is less common in countries where soy intake is typically high, such as Japan and parts of China and Southeast Asia (Sung et al. 2021). Migrant studies of Japanese men who moved to the US have shown that they assume the much higher (5–10 times) risk of prostate cancer experienced by American men within one or two generations (summarized in Bosland 1988). (These migrant studies were conducted when prostate cancer was detected clinically and not by screening in both Japan and the US, allowing proper epidemiological comparisons.) These studies demonstrated that environment, particularly lifestyle and diet, are major determinants of prostate cancer risk. This notion led to the idea that soy consumption might have preventive activity against prostate cancer, first proposed about 30 years ago (Barnes et al. 1995; Wynder et al. 1994).

Soy contains estrogenic compounds associated with its protein fraction (Setchell 1998, 2002). Prostate cancer has historically been treated with estrogens, and this treatment is still used in some low-resource areas of the world (Ali et al. 2019; Turo et al. 2014; Okuku et al. 2016). Hence, there may be an inverse relation between prostate cancer risk and soy consumption, particularly soy protein and its estrogenic constituents, as this chapter addresses. These estrogenic constituents, particularly the isoflavone genistein, have inhibitory activity on prostate cancer cells *in vitro* (Mahmoud et al. 2014) and can inhibit prostate cancer development in animal models (McCormick et al. 2007). Researchers have also demonstrated this *in vivo* inhibitory effect for soy protein (Bylund et al. 2000;

 DOI: 10.1201/9781003597926-24

Pollard and Suckow 2006). Soy consumption has also been shown to affect hormones associated with prostate cancer, such as the androgen testosterone, as detailed in this review. Based on these and other observations, supplementation with soy protein has been proposed as an approach to prevent and possibly treat prostate cancer (Messina 2003; Perabo et al. 2008; van Die et al. 2016).

The objective of this chapter is to provide a review of the effects of soy protein supplementation on the risk of prostate cancer and its progression and recurrence after treatment, as well as on associated hormones.

One challenge is that soy contains, besides abundant protein, several micronutrients with considerable biological properties, such as the estrogenic compounds mentioned above, and most research has focused on those. Thus, it is difficult to disentangle the effects of soy protein itself and those of non-protein constituents in soy protein. Fortunately, several studies have compared whole soy protein with protein depleted of isoflavones, allowing conclusions about the effects of soy protein by itself. Because the effects of protein cannot be studied using *in vitro* systems, this review is limited to the *in vivo* effects of soy protein supplementation in humans and some animal models. The review will mention the effects of isolated isoflavones where relevant but will not address them in detail.

ASSOCIATION BETWEEN CONSUMPTION OF SOY AND ISOFLAVONES AND RISK OF PROSTATE CANCER

Many cohort and case-control studies have examined the epidemiology of soy consumption and the risk of prostate cancer. Rather than summarizing each study, Table 24.1 details five meta-analyses published between 2009 and 2022. This table demonstrates considerable consistency in the finding that the consumption of soy-containing foods and products is associated with a statistically significant 12–29% reduction in the risk of prostate cancer development. In addition, only non-fermented soy consumption is associated with this risk reduction (25–36% lower risk); fermented soy products such as miso and natto are not associated with reduced prostate cancer risk. Of note, these meta-analyses did not pertain to prostate cancer mortality.

The consistency among these meta-analyses is not surprising because they included partially overlapping epidemiological studies. However, these meta-analyses were published over more than 12 years, included both cohort and case-control studies over a wide geographical and soy consumption range (e.g., Japan, China, US, Europe), and varied in inclusion and exclusion criteria and statistical methods. Therefore, the consistency across these five meta-analyses provides a high degree of confidence that the association between soy consumption and reduced risk of prostate cancer is real and substantial. Notably, this type of study addresses long-term habitual dietary habits and cannot easily or conclusively separate dietary from other lifestyle factors. However, most of the epidemiological studies included in these meta-analyses applied extensive adjustments for other lifestyle factors and potential confounders such as body mass index.

Applegate et al. (2018) list five studies (three cohort and two case-control studies) that assessed the association between soy consumption and risk of advanced prostate cancer and found a non-significant ($P = 0.119$) relative risk of 0.87 (0.74, 1.04; 95% CI) for the association of risk and soy. Even though the number of studies that included advanced prostate cancer is small, this is an important observation because advanced prostate cancer is difficult to treat, while non-advanced (early-stage) prostate cancers are often treatable, resulting in nearly 100% 5-year survival in high-income countries.

The association between prostate cancer risk and isoflavone intake calculated from food frequency and food isoflavone concentrations in these meta-analyses is less substantial and consistent (0–33%) than for soy consumption. Nevertheless, Table 24.1 suggests that isoflavones are likely at least partly responsible for the risk reduction associated with soy consumption.

In conclusion, considerable and consistent evidence shows that the consumption of non-fermented soy food and products is associated with a reduced risk of prostate cancer in the range of 25–30%

TABLE 24.1
Meta-Analyses of Cohort and Case-Control Studies on Soy and Isoflavone Consumption and Prostate Cancer Risk

Study (Year of Publication)	Yan & Spitznagel (2009)	Hwang et al. (2009)	Zhang et al. (2016)	Applegate et al. (2018)	Fan et al. (2022)
All soy foods & products (non-fermented plus fermented)					
Relative risk or odds ratio	0.74 (0.63, 0.89)[a] P = 0.01	0.69 (057, 0.84)[a] P < 0.001	0.78 (0.66, 0.90)[a] P value N/P	0.71 (0.58, 0.85)[a] P < 0.001	0.88 (0.78, 0.99)[a] P value N/P
Number (type) of studies	14 (5 cohort; 9 case-control)	5 (2 cohort; 3 case-control)	12 (4 cohort; 8 case-control)	16 (7 cohort; 9 case-control)	7 (all cohort); 2 studies after 2017
Non-fermented soy foods (tofu and/or soy milk)					
Relative risk or odds ratio	0.70 (0.56, 0.88)[a] P = 0.01	0.75 (0.62, 0.89)[a] P < 0.01	0.64 (0.48, 0.80)[a] P value N/P	0.65 (0.56, 0.83)[a] P < 0.001	N/D
Number (type) of studies	8 (3 cohort; 5 case-control)	8 (4 cohort; 4 case-control)	6 (3 cohort; 3 case-control)	11 (5 cohort; 6 case-control)	
Fermented soy foods (miso, miso soup and/or natto)					
Relative risk or odds ratio	1.02 (0.73, 1.42)[a] P = 0.92	1.10 (0.76, 1.57)[a] P = 0.62	N/D	0.86 (0.66, 1.13)[a] P < 0.218	N/D
Number (type) of studies	8 (3 cohort; 5 case-control)	5 (3 cohort; 2 case-control)		11 (5 cohort; 6 case-control)	
Isoflavones (total isoflavones)					
Relative risk or odds ratio	0.88 (0.76, 1.02)[a] P = 0.09	0.67 (0.52, 0.86)[a] P = 0.002[b]	0.77 (0.66, 0.88)[a] P value N/P	1.03 (0.84, 1.10)[a] P = 0.313	0.99 (0.87, 1.13)[a] P value N/P
Number (type) of studies	14 (5 cohort; 9 case-control)	8 (4 cohort; 4 case-control)	21 (14 cohort; 9 case-control)	16 (7 cohort; 9 case-control)	4 (all cohort)

[a] 95% confidence interval.
[b] Calculated for genistein and daidzein, not total isoflavones.
N/P = not presented; N/D = not determined.

and that soy isoflavones are probably partly responsible for this reduced risk. Based on a limited number of studies, the risk reduction appears to be mostly limited to localized-early stage prostate cancer rather than advanced cancer, i.e., metastatic, extracapsular, and/or pathologically high-grade (Gleason score 8 and higher, or in some cases 7 or higher). By contrast, a meta-analysis of 12 reports found no significant association between the risk of prostate cancer and intake of total, animal, and vegetable protein (Mao et al. 2018). Thus, the association of soy consumption with prostate cancer risk is specific to soy protein.

EFFECT OF SOY PROTEIN SUPPLEMENTATION ON PSA

Prostate-specific antigen (PSA) is a serine protease produced by prostatic epithelial cells and secreted into the prostatic fluid to cleave proteins to maintain semen fluidity (Balk et al. 2003). Its expression is androgen-regulated via androgen receptors in the prostatic epithelium. If the structural integrity of the multilayered prostatic epithelium is compromised by diseases including inflammation (prostatitis), benign prostatic hyperplasia (BPH), or cancer, PSA leaks into the interstitial fluid around the prostatic acini and ducts and enters the bloodstream (Balk et al. 2003). A tiny amount of PSA can leak into the bloodstream even in the absence of these disease processes. Thus, the circulating level of PSA in the serum depends on the absence/presence of these diseases, the number of normal or cancerous prostatic cells, and androgenic stimuli to the prostatic cells.

Serum PSA levels below 4 ng/mL are unlikely to be associated with prostate cancer, except in African American men, where a lower cutoff value is often used clinically (Balk et al. 2003). PSA levels between 4 and 10 ng/mL occur in men with prostatitis, BPH, or cancer and require clinical follow-up, often using prostate biopsies, to determine which disease is present. If PSA levels exceed 10 ng/mL, cancer is likely to be present once prostatitis is ruled out. Following successful prostate cancer treatment with surgery (radical prostatectomy) or radiotherapy (using radioactive seeds implanted in the prostate or external beam radiation), PSA levels are either undetectable or very low (<1 ng/mL). If recurrence occurs, PSA levels start to rise (biochemical recurrence), and clinicians use PSA measurements for follow-up after treatment to detect recurrence and, when surgery or radiotherapy is not possible or in case of recurrence, to assess the effectiveness of further treatments.

Effect of Soy Protein Supplementation on Circulating PSA

Effects of soy consumption on circulating PSA levels have been examined in clinical trials with men without prostate disease, men with early-stage cancer under watchful waiting, men with cancer in the weeks prior to radical prostatectomy, and men who developed detectable and rising PSA after treatment.

Four randomized clinical trials have examined the effects of soy food or soy protein isolate consumption compared to a placebo milk-based product or a low-soy diet on PSA in men without prostate cancer, with untreated prostate cancer, or with biochemical recurrence (Table 24.2). These studies clearly demonstrate that soy protein supplementation for up to 6 months does not affect circulating levels of PSA in these three populations.

Three studies of men without prostate cancer or men with cancer on watchful waiting examined the effect of 6 weeks to 12 months of supplementation with soy stripped of its isoflavones on circulating PSA (Table 24.3). None of these studies found evidence of effects of soy protein consumption on serum PSA, regardless of the presence or absence of isoflavones in the protein isolate.

There are several reports of single-arm, non-randomized studies of men prior to radical prostatectomy or men with biochemical recurrence (Van Veldhuizen et al. 2006; Kwan et al. 2010; Pendleton et al. 2008) in which researchers observed inconsistent effects of soy supplementation for 3–4 weeks to 12 months on PSA. In addition, there are two randomized studies with more complex total diet changes, one of which, with men prior to radical prostatectomy, was too short in duration and too small to allow conclusions (Dalais et al. 2004). The other combined the results of three separate studies with healthy men and found no effect of soy supplementation for up to 3 months on PSA (Jenkins et al. 2003). This review does not discuss other studies that involved supplementation with soy in combination with other substances because it is impossible to unravel the specific effect of soy protein.

Several other studies addressed the effects of supplementation with 40–80 mg/day pure isoflavones, but not protein, ranging in duration from 2–6 weeks to 12 weeks or 12 months (Kumar et al. 2020; Miyanaga et al. 2012; Hamilton-Reeves et al. 2013). None of these studies observed a significant effect of the intervention on serum PSA. Two meta-analyses concurred with the absence of effects of oral isoflavone supplementation on circulating PSA (van Die et al. 2014; Ratha et al. 2021).

In summary, randomized clinical trials provide conclusive evidence that the consumption of soy protein, with or without isoflavones, does not affect serum PSA levels in men with and without prostate cancer.

TABLE 24.2
Studies of the Effects of Soy and Soy Protein on Circulating PSA

Study Characteristics	Maskarinec et al. (2006)	Kumar et al. (2004)	Hamilton-Reeves et al. (2008)	Bosland et al. (2022a)
Study Design	Randomized cross-over with a 1-month washout	Randomized to soy protein or placebo	Randomized to soy protein or milk protein placebo	Randomized to soy protein or casein
Study Duration	3 months-3 months	12 weeks	3 and 6 months	6 months
Study Subjects				
Number	23 total, 11-12 per arm	29 on soy; 30 on placebo	20 on soy and 18 on milk protein	8 on soy; 8 on placebo
Age	59 ± 7[a] (44-69) years	73 ± 5 and 71 ± 5 yrs,[a] respectively	68 ± 8 and 68 ± 7 yrs,[a] respectively	66 (60, 71) and 64 (59, 69) yrs,[b] respectively
Race	10 Asian; 13 white or other	≥ 94% white	100% white	10 white; 6 non-white
Clinical status	No evidence of prostate cancer (normal PSA)	Elevated PSA; prostate cancer on watchful waiting	Elevated PSA; 90% preneoplastic prostate lesions (2 and 1 subjects prostate cancer on biopsy), but no treatment	Elevated-rising PSA after radical prostatectomy
Intervention	Two daily soy servings (tofu, soy milk, protein and nuts) versus habitual low soy diet	Soy protein isolate or isocaloric placebo	Soy protein isolate or casein placebo	Soy protein isolate or casein placebo
Dose	soy providing 69 vs. 4 mg/day total isoflavones or (soy dose not provided) isoflavones	Soy providing 60 mg/day genistein vs. low isoflavones (soy dose not provided)	40 g protein supplement/day providing 107 or <6 mg/day	20 g/day soy protein or casein providing 41 or <1 mg/day
Source	Various including Solae	Protein Technologies (Solae)	Solae (St. Louis, MO, USA)	Solae
Change in total serum PSA	baseline → 3 months	baseline → 12 weeks	Baseline → 3 months → 6 months	baseline → 6 months
On soy food or soy protein	2.02 ± 1.45 → 1.74 ± 1.40 ng/ml[a]	7.38 ± 5.62 → 6.77 ± 4.96 ng/ml[a]	5.4 ± 1 → - 0.8 ± 0.5 → - 0.5 ± 0.6 ng/ml[c]	0.495 → 0.685 ng/ml; 34% change (7, 61%)[d]
On placebo or usual diet	1.83 ± 1.45 → 1.95 ± 1.60 ng/ml[a]	1.83 ± 1.45 → 1.95 ± 1.60 ng/ml[a]	5.1 ± 1 → - 0.6 ± 0.6 → - 0.2 ± 0.6 ng/ml[a]	0.205 → 0.240 ng/ml; 54% change (11, 118)[d]
Difference in change	- 0.28 (soy); + 0.12 ng/ml (placebo) P = 0.10	+ 8% (soy) versus + 6% (placebo) P = 0.96	*P* > 0.05 (no values presented)	PSA doubling time: 10.1 (soy); 6.1 months (placebo); P = 0.721

[a] Values are mean ± standard deviation.
[b] Values are median (95% confidence interval).
[c] Change from baseline.
[d] Percent change (95% confidence interval).
PSA = prostate-specific antigen.

TABLE 24.3
Studies of the Effects of Soy Protein And Soy Protein Depleted of Isoflavones on Circulating PSA

Study Characteristics	Urban et al. (2001)		Adams et al. (2004)	Hamilton-Reeves et al. (2008)
Study Design	Blinded cross-over randomized to soy protein or stripped soy protein without washout		Randomized to soy protein or stripped soy protein	Randomized to soy protein or stripped soy protein
Study Duration	6 weeks-6 weeks		12 months	6 months with 3 month interim time-point
Study Subjects				
Number	34 total, 17 per arm		35 on soy and 47 on stripped soy	20 on soy and 20 on stripped soy
Age	65 ± 2 yrs[a]		64 ± 7 and 65 ± 8 yrs, respectively[a]	68 ± 8 and 68 ± 5 yrs, respectively[a]
Race	74% white; 24% Black; 2% other		89% and 88% white, respectively	100% white
Clinical status	Elevated PSA, but no evidence of prostate cancer		Colon polyps, no prostate cancer, no elevated PSA	Elevated PSA; 90-95% had preneoplastic prostate lesions on biopsy; 2 and 1 subjects had prostate cancer but no treatment
Intervention	Soy protein isolate with or without isoflavones		Soy protein isolate with or without isoflavones	Soy protein isolate with or without isoflavones
Dose	2 x 18.8 (37.6) g protein/day providing 69 or 3.4 mg/day isoflavones		40 g protein supplement/day providing 107 mg or <6 mg/day isoflavones	40 g protein supplement/day providing 107 mg or <6 mg/ day isoflavones
Source	Protein Technologies (Solae)		Protein Technologies (Solae)	Solae (St. Louis, MO, USA)
Change in total serum PSA	First arm	Second arm	baseline → 12 months	baseline → 3 months → 6 months
On soy protein with isoflavones	8.7 → 8.7	7.6 → 7.8 ng/ml[a]	1.7 ± 2.9 → 2.0 ± 3.5 ng/ml[a]	5.4 ± 1 →- 0.8 ± 0.5 b → - 0.5 ± 0.6[a] ng/ml[b]
On soy protein stripped of isoflavones	9.1 → 8.7	7.8 → 8.2 ng/ml[a]	1.7 ± 3.1 → 2.0 ± 3.2 ng/ml[a]	5.0 ± 1 → - 0.8 ± 0.5 b → - 0.8 ± 0.6[a] ng/ml[b]
Difference in change between the two groups	- 0.4 ng/ml	+ 0.2 ng/ml P = 0.622	0.5% (-17.3, 22.2)[c]	P > 0.05

[a] Values are mean ± standard deviation.
[b] Change from baseline.
[c] 95% confidence interval.
PSA = prostate-specific antigen.

SOY SUPPLEMENTATION AND PROSTATE CANCER CLINICAL OUTCOME

Few studies have examined the effect of soy protein supplementation on prostate cancer clinical outcomes. Bosland et al. (2013) conducted a clinical trial with men at risk of recurrence after radical prostatectomy for prostate cancer, randomizing 81 to a soy protein beverage supplement (19.2 g protein/day providing 40.9 mg of aglycone isoflavone equivalents) and 78 to a casein-based supplement (19.8 g/day) for 2 years after surgery (the supplements were provided by Solae, St. Louis, MO, US). The primary endpoint was biochemical recurrence, defined as the development of a serum PSA level of 0.07 ng/mL or higher confirmed by two subsequent PSA values of 0.07 ng/mL or higher at least 1 month apart. Recurrence-free survival curves overlapped, showing no difference in recurrence (hazard ratio: 0.96; 95% CI: 0.53–1.72; P = 0.89 [log-rank test]) (Bosland et al. 2013).

Kumar et al. (2004) conducted a clinical trial with men with biopsy-confirmed prostate cancer under watchful waiting, randomized to soy protein or an isocaloric placebo for 12 weeks (see Table 24.2). Serum PSA in both groups decreased by 6-8%, suggesting no progression in either group. Bosland et al. (2022a) conducted a small clinical trial with men with prostate cancer recurrence after radical prostatectomy, randomized to soy protein or a casein placebo for 6 months (see Table 24.2). PSA doubling time increased by 34% in the soy group and 54% in men on placebo, a non-significant difference (P = 0.721; two-sided Mann-Whitney test), suggesting no difference in disease progression.

Hamilton-Reeves et al. (2008) randomized men with biopsy evidence of preneoplastic lesions but not cancer in their prostate to a 6-month intervention with a soy protein isolate (40 g/day providing 107 mg of aglycone isoflavone equivalents), the same supplement with >95% of the isoflavones chemically removed, or 40 g/day of a milk protein isolate (the supplements were provided by Solae) (see Tables 24.2 and 24.3). At the end of the study, 1 of 17 men on soy protein had developed prostate cancer, 1 of 16 men on isoflavone-depleted soy protein, and 6 of 16 men on milk protein. The incidence difference between men on milk protein and men on both soy protein groups combined was significant (P = 0.010; two-sided Fisher exact test), as was the difference between men on milk protein and men on depleted soy protein (P = 0.039; two-sided Fisher exact test); the difference between men on milk protein and those on isoflavone-rich soy protein was borderline significant (P = 0.083; two-sided Fisher exact test). There was no difference between the soy and depleted soy groups, suggesting that in this small study isoflavones were not responsible for the incidence difference with the milk protein group. However, the results of a randomized clinical trial by Miyanaga et al. (2012) do not support this conclusion.

Miyanaga et al. (2012) randomized 50–75-year-old Japanese men with biopsy-proven absence of prostate cancer to tablets containing isoflavones (60 mg/day) or placebo tablets for 12 months. The incidence of prostate cancer in men who underwent an end-of-study biopsy (n = 89) was 21.4% (9/42) in the isoflavone group and 34.0% (16/47) in the placebo group, a non-significant difference (P = 0.139; one-sided Fisher exact test). However, in men older than 64 years, the difference was significant: 28.0% (7/25) in the isoflavone group and 51.1% (16/28) in the placebo group (P = 0.031; one-sided Fisher exact test); the difference was borderline significant when a two-sided test was used (P = 0.052).

In conclusion, three small randomized clinical trials and one larger randomized clinical trial provide inconclusive evidence that soy protein or isoflavones inhibit the development of prostate cancer, while one large randomized trial provides conclusive evidence that soy protein supplementation for 2 years does not reduce the risk of prostate cancer recurrence after radical prostatectomy.

EFFECT OF SOY PROTEIN ON PROSTATE TISSUE BIOMARKERS

Only one study, with two reports, has examined the effects of soy protein supplementation on prostate tissue biomarkers relevant to cancer, comparing supplementation of soy protein, soy protein depleted of isoflavones, and milk protein (Hamilton-Reeves et al. 2007a, 2008; see also Tables 24.2

and 24.3). Prostate biopsy tissue was collected at baseline and after 6 months of supplementation, and immunohistochemical expression of the following proteins was semiquantitatively scored: androgen receptor, estrogen receptor-β, PCNA, Bax, Bcl-2, and EGF receptor, and the ratios of Bax:Bcl-2 and Bax:PCNA expression were calculated. In the tissue of subjects on isoflavone-depleted soy protein, expression of Bax (n = 16) and PCNA (n = 13) was reduced at the end of the study (P <0.05), but the Bax:PCNA ratio did not change (Hamilton-Reeves et al. 2008). Bax expression in the tissue of men on isoflavone-depleted soy protein was significantly lower than in men on non-depleted soy protein (n = 14) or milk protein (n = 14). In the tissue of subjects on milk protein (n = 14), expression of the androgen receptor (n = 14) increased at the end of the study compared to baseline and compared to tissue from men on non-isoflavone-depleted soy protein (n = 14) (*P* <0.05), but estrogen receptor expression was similar in all three groups at baseline and after 6 months of intervention (Hamilton-Reeves et al. 2007a). The biological significance of these findings is not clear, although isoflavones may play a role. Hamilton-Reeves et al. (2007a, 2008) provide a potential explanation.

Clinical trials with isoflavone intervention (not soy protein itself) have reported the effects of these compounds on prostate tissue biomarkers of cell proliferation. These studies involved intervention with isoflavones in the 3–6 weeks prior to radical prostatectomy to treat prostate cancer. Kumar et al. (2007, 2010, 2020) randomized men to 40–80 mg/day of aglycone isoflavone tablets or placebo pills and collected prostate tissue at the time of surgery. They did not find differences in the immunohistochemically scored expression of the proliferation marker Ki67. Hamilton-Reeves et al. (2013) found differences in prostate tissue expression of several genes involved in cell cycle control and apoptosis, comparing two men given isoflavone capsules (51 mg aglycone equivalent/day) and one man on placebo capsules. Given the small number of subjects involved, no conclusions can be drawn from this observation.

EFFECTS OF SOY ON HOEMONES IN MALES

The major hormones that affect the prostate and are or may be involved in prostate cancer development are androgens, particularly testosterone, and estrogens, specifically 17-β estradiol (Bosland, 2013; Liu et al. 2020). It is assumed that the free forms of these steroid hormones, unbound to sex hormone-binding globulin (SHBG) and, to a lesser degree, serum albumen, are bioavailable to cells, making it important to determine their concentration in addition to total testosterone and estradiol (Hammond 2016). Thus, this review focuses on the effects of soy consumption on these two hormones and SHBG, as these effects may mediate soy's effects on prostate cancer.

Table 24.4 summarizes two randomized studies of soy protein supplementation for 3–6 months versus a milk protein placebo and one 4-week single-arm study of soy protein supplementation. These studies found no effects of soy or differences between treatment groups on circulating free or total testosterone and estradiol, even though in one study, SHBG decreased in both the soy and the placebo groups and testosterone decreased in the placebo group in another study. One study measured LH and observed no effects of soy or placebo. By contrast, in a much longer duration randomized study (18 months), both serum total testosterone and SHBG decreased significantly in the soy protein supplementation group, but free testosterone and estradiol did not. This study observed no changes in the casein placebo group, while the difference between the treatment groups in these hormone changes over 18 months was not significant or, for SHBG, borderline significant.

In the 6-month randomized study by Hamilton-Reeves et al. (2007a, 2007b) comparing soy protein and milk protein supplementation, the researchers also measured androgen and estrogen precursors in the serum and estrogens and several estrogen metabolites in the urine. Soy protein supplementation increased the levels of estradiol and estrone in the urine but not in the serum, while in the milk protein placebo group, the estrogen metabolite 2-hydroxy-estradiol decreased in response to the intervention; the differences between treatment groups in these changes in urinary levels were significant. Neither intervention affected serum levels of androgen and estrogen

TABLE 24.4
Effects of Soy and Soy Protein Consumption on Hormone Levels In Males

Study Characteristic	Kumar et al. (2004)	Goodin et al. (2007)	Hamilton-Reeves et al. (2007a, 2007b)	Bosland et al. (2022b)
Study Design	Randomized to soy protein or isocaloric placebo	Single arm trial	Randomized to soy protein or placebo	Randomized to soy protein or placebo
Study Duration	12 weeks	4 weeks followed by 2 weeks recovery	6 months with 3 month interim time-point	18 months and interim time points at 2, 4, 8 months
Study Subjects				
Number	29 on soy; 30 on placebo	12	19 on soy and 19 on stripped soy	10-13; 18-21 for testosterone only
Age	73 ± 5 and 71 ± 5 yrs, respectively[a]	32 (25 - 47) years[b]	68 ± 8 and 68 ± 5 yrs, respectively[a]	58 - 59 yrs (soy); 60 - 61 (placebo)[b]
Race	≥ 94% white	Not provided	100% white	10-22 white, 0-2 Black
Clinical status	Elevated PSA; prostate cancer on watchful waiting	"Healthy"	Elevated PSA; 90-95% preneoplastic prostate lesions on biopsy; 2 or 1 subjects had prostate cancer	Biochemical recurrence-free after radical prostatectomy
Intervention	Soy protein isolate or isocaloric placebo	Soy protein ("pure soy protein powder")	Soy protein isolate with isoflavones or milk protein placebo	Soy protein isolate or casein placebo
Dose	Soy protein providing 60 mg/day genistein versus low isoflavones (protein dose not provided)	57 g protein supplement per day or usual diet	40 g protein supplement per day; soy providing 107 mg isoflavones	20 g/day soy protein or casein providing 41 or <1 mg/day total isoflavones
Source	Protein Technologies (Solae)	Puritan's Pride (Oakdale, NY, USA)	Solae (St. Louis, MO, USA)	Solae
Change in serum or urinary hormone levels from baseline				
On soy food or soy protein	No change in serum SHBG, (free) testosterone, or (free) estradiol	No significant change in serum testosterone and LH	Serum SHBG decreased ($P < 0.05$), but no change in serum (free) testosterone, DHT, estradiol, estrone, DHEAS, androstenedione, and androstanediol glucuronide; urinary estradiol and estrone increased ($P < 0.05$), but estrogen metabolites did not change	Serum testosterone and SHBG decreased 14% and 21% at 18 months ($P^{trend} = 0.004$ and < 0.001), but free testosterone and estradiol did not change

(*Continued*)

TABLE 24.4 (CONTINUED)
Effects of Soy and Soy Protein Consumption on Hormone Levels In Males

On placebo or usual diet	Significant decrease in total testosterone ($P = 0.01$); no change in SHBG, free testosterone, (free) estradiol	No significant change in testosterone or LH	Serum SHBG decreased ($P < 0.05$), but no change in serum (free) testosterone, DHT, estradiol, estrone, DHEAS, androstenedione, and androstanediol glucuronide; urinary estrogens and estrogen metabolites did not change, except 2-hydroxy-estradiol which decreased ($P < 0.05$)	(Free) testosterone, SHBG, and estradiol did not change significantly
Difference in change between the two groups	No significant differences ($P > 0.10$)	No significant differences ($P > 0.20$)	Significant ($P < 0.05$) between-group differences in changes were only found for urinary, but not serum, estradiol and estrone levels and for urinary 2-hydroxy-estradiol	Differences in serum hormone levels at 2-18 months were not significant or, for SHBG, borderline significant ($P = 0.064$; 2-way ANOVA)

[a] Values are mean ± standard deviation.
[b] Only range was provided.
DHEAS = dehydroepiandrosterone; DHT = 5α-dihydrotestosterone; LH = luteinizing hormone; PSA = prostate-specific antigen; SHBG = sex hormone-binding globulin.

precursors or other estradiol metabolites. The increases in urinary estradiol and estrone in the soy group were considerable, nearly doubling from baseline.

In the studies by Hamilton-Reeves et al. (2007a, 2007b) comparing the soy protein group and a group supplemented with soy protein from which isoflavones had been removed, urinary estradiol and estrone increased in both groups, but less in the group supplemented with isoflavone-depleted soy protein than in the undepleted group (Table 24.5). By contrast, serum estradiol and estrone increased only in the isoflavone-depleted group, as did androstenedione. The reason soy protein supplementation would increase urinary output of estrogens is probably partly associated with isoflavone intake, but it is unclear why isoflavone-depleted soy, but not undepleted soy, would increase serum estrogens. A decrease in serum SHBG occurred in both groups, while total and free testosterone levels remained unaffected. The level of DHEAS went down in the undepleted group and up in the isoflavone-depleted group, although not to a statistically significant degree. However, the difference in serum DHEAS change between groups was significant and related to the difference in serum estrogen levels between groups.

By contrast, Sathyapalan et al. (2017) did not find significant changes in serum levels of SHBG, (free) testosterone, estradiol, LH, and FSH in a 3-month study comparing soy protein (in soy bars) with or without isoflavones removed. The difference from the results of Hamilton-Reeves et al. (2007a) may be due to the difference in the amount of soy supplementation, 15 g of soy protein per day in the former study versus 40 g/day in the latter.

In conclusion, the effects of soy protein supplementation on sex steroids appear to be complex and may depend on the duration and dose of the intervention as well as the presence or absence of isoflavones in the supplements. Several studies found a decrease in serum SHBG in the soy-supplemented groups, but free testosterone levels were not affected by the interventions. Soy protein supplementation, regardless of the presence of isoflavones, resulted in an increase in urinary

TABLE 24.5
Effects of Soy Protein With and Without Isoflavones on Hormones in Males

Study Characteristic	Hamilton-Reeves et al. (2007a)	Hamilton-Reeves et al. (2007b)	Sathyapalan et al. (2017)
Study Design	Randomized to soy protein or stripped soy protein	Randomized to soy protein or stripped soy protein	Randomized to soy protein or low isoflavone soy protein
Study Duration	6 months with 3 month time-point	6 months with 3 month time-point	3 months
Study Subjects			
Number	20 on soy and 20 on stripped soy	19 on soy and 19 on stripped soy	100 on soy; 100 on low isoflavone soy
Age	68 ± 8 and 68 ± 5 yrs, respectively[a]	68 ± 8 and 68 ± 5 yrs, respectively[a]	52 (50, 55) and 52 (50, 55), respectively.[b]
Race	100% white	100% white	100% white
Clinical status	Elevated PSA; 90-95% preneoplastic prostate lesions on biopsy; 2 or 1 subjects had prostate cancer	Elevated PSA; 90-95% preneoplastic prostate lesions on biopsy; 2 or 1 subjects had prostate cancer	Treated type-2 diabetes and sub-clinical hypogonadism but no testosterone treatment
Intervention	Soy protein isolate with or without isoflavones	Soy protein isolate with or without isoflavones	Soy protein bars with or without isoflavones
Dose	40 g protein supplement/day providing 107 mg isoflavones	40 g protein supplement/day providing 107 mg isoflavones	2 x 7.5 (15) g protein/day providing 2 x 33 (66) mg isoflavones
Source	Solae (St. Louis, MO, USA)	Solae	Solbar (Ashdod, Israel)
Change in serum or urinary hormone levels from baseline			
On soy protein with isoflavones	Significant decrease in serum SHBG ($P < 0.05$); no changes in serum levels of (free) testosterone, DHT, estradiol, estrone, DHEAS, androstenedione, androstanediol	Significant ($P < 0.05$) increases in urinary levels of estradiol and estrone; no changes in urinary 2-methoxy-estradiol and -estrone, 2-hydroxy-estradiol and -estrone, 16α-hydroxy estrone, and estriol	No significant change in (free) testosterone, SHBG, estradiol, LH, and FSH
On soy protein stripped of isoflavones	Significant ($P < 0.05$) decrease in serum levels of SHBG and increases in estradiol, estrone, DHEAS, and androstenedione; no changes in serum (free) testosterone, DHT, androstanediol	Significant ($P < 0.05$) increases in urinary levels of estradiol and estrone; no changes in urinary 2-methoxy-estradiol and -estrone, 2-hydroxy-estradiol and -estrone, 16α-hydroxy estrone, and estriol	No significant change in (free) testosterone, SHBG, estradiol, LH, and FSH
Difference in change between the two groups	Significant differences in changes in serum estradiol, androstenedione, and DHEAS ($P < 0.05$)	Significant less increase in urinary estrone with isoflavone-depleted soy than undepleted soy ($P < 0.05$)	No significant differences between the two treatment groups for any hormone

[a] Values are mean ± standard deviation.
[b] Values are median (25th, 75th percentile).
DHEAS = dehydroepiandrosterone; DHT = 5α-dihydrotestosterone; FSH = follicle-stimulating hormone; LH = luteinizing hormone; PSA = prostate-specific antigen; SHBG = sex hormone-binding globulin.

estrogens in the only study examining this, and these increases were considerable and, therefore, likely real. Serum estrogen levels, by contrast, were not changed by soy protein supplementation in several studies. It should be noted that all but one of these studies had a duration of 6 months or less. Therefore, it is difficult to make inferences between the observed hormone changes and the reduction in risk of prostate cancer with long-term soy consumption. Reed et al. (2021) reported in a meta-analysis that supplementation with soy foods, soy protein, or isoflavones did not significantly modify serum levels of total and free testosterone, SHBG, estradiol, and estrone. Although their conclusions broadly concur with those drawn here, they combined a large number of quite diverse studies and combined studies with soy or soy protein with studies of isolated isoflavones, and they did not include soy's effects on urinary estrogens in their analysis.

CONCLUDING AND SUMMARIZING REMARKS

The published literature on soy and prostate cancer provides considerable and consistent evidence that long-term, perhaps life-long, consumption of non-fermented soy food and soy products reduces the risk of prostate cancer. The risk reduction is sizable, 25–30%, but probably requires decades of soy consumption, which is unlikely to be feasible as a general preventive approach. Soy isoflavones are probably partly responsible for the reduction in risk. The risk reduction appears, based on a limited number of studies, to be mostly limited to localized-early stage prostate cancer rather than advanced cancer. By contrast, a meta-analysis found no significant association between the risk of prostate cancer and the intake of total, animal, and vegetable protein (Mao et al. 2018). Thus, the association of soy consumption with reduced prostate cancer risk appears to be specific to soy protein.

Randomized clinical trials provide conclusive evidence that supplementation of soy protein, with or without isoflavones, for up to 12 months does not affect serum PSA levels in men with and without prostate cancer compared to men on a placebo supplement or low-soy diet. Furthermore, the evidence that supplementation of soy protein or isoflavones inhibits the development of prostate cancer from randomized clinical trials is overall inconclusive. However, one randomized trial provides conclusive evidence that soy protein supplementation for 2 years does not reduce the risk of recurrence of prostate cancer after surgical treatment.

The discrepancy between epidemiological evidence showing soy inhibits or prevents prostate cancer development and randomized studies showing a lack of such an effect from soy or isoflavone supplementation may relate to the short duration of the supplementation studies (at most 2 years) compared to the long-term habitual dietary soy exposure assessed in epidemiological studies. Unfortunately, longer-term randomized supplementation trials to resolve this issue are unlikely to ever be conducted.

Soy protein supplementation for up to 3, 6, or even 18 months reduced SHBG levels in several randomized trials but did not change the amount of bioavailable free testosterone or serum levels of estrogens in these studies. In one 6-month study, soy protein supplementation, with or without isoflavones, increased urinary estrogen output. The relation of this finding to the prostate cancer risk reduction identified in epidemiological studies is not clear, but this observation is intriguing and worthy of further investigation. The few short-term randomized trials of the effects of soy protein supplementation on cancer-related biomarkers in prostate tissue obtained from biopsies have not yielded information that helps explain why epidemiological studies have found the risk of prostate cancer to be reduced by soy consumption.

In conclusion, randomized clinical trials provide limited evidence that soy protein supplementation, with or without isoflavones, for up to 2 years does not appear to delay or prevent the development or recurrence of prostate cancer, while epidemiological studies consistently show that long-term consumption of soy is associated with an approximately 25–30% reduction in risk of prostate cancer. This reduction in risk is probably at least partly associated with the intake of soy isoflavones. Randomized studies of the effects of soy protein supplementation on sex steroid hormones or prostate tissue biomarkers related to prostate cancer provide no clear mechanistic explanations for this discrepancy.

THE EFFECTS OF OTHER PROTEINS

In randomized clinical trials studying the effects of soy protein supplementation, researchers have often used a milk protein (casein)-based placebo. The studies summarized in Tables 24.2 and 24.3 clearly show that casein supplementation does not affect serum PSA levels in men without or with prostate cancer or with recurrent prostate cancer. Tables 24.4 and 24.5 indicate that casein supplementation reduces circulating SHBG without affecting free testosterone, just like soy protein does. In addition, casein supplementation increased urinary estrogens, similar to soy protein, but, unlike soy protein, it also increased serum estrogen levels and some steroid hormone precursors (DHEAS and androstenedione).

There are no other studies of specific non-soy proteins and prostate cancer. However, as indicated earlier, a meta-analysis found no significant association between the risk of prostate cancer and intake of total, animal, and vegetable protein (Mao et al. 2018). Interestingly, using data from the US National Health and Nutrition Examination Survey (NHANES), researchers have reported a non-linear positive relationship between the intake of total dietary protein and serum PSA levels for protein intakes exceeding 182 g/day (Song et al. 2020). However, this threshold probably applied to less than 20–25% of the NHANES surveyed population, and no association was found between total protein intake and PSA.

MINI DICTIONARY OF TERMS

- **DHT (5α-dihydrotestosterone):** The active metabolite of testosterone that is produced by the enzyme 5α-reductase in prostate cells and binds with high affinity to the androgen receptor in these cells.
- **Estradiol (17β-estradiol):** The major female sex steroid (estrogen) that is produced by conversion from androgens by the enzyme aromatase in fat tissue and, in males, in the prostate.
- **Prostate:** A gland that surrounds the urethra at the base of the bladder, which produces prostatic fluid that is secreted into the seminal fluid during ejaculation.
- **Prostate cancer:** A malignancy arising from the epithelial cells of the prostate gland.
- **Prostate-specific antigen (PSA):** A serine protease produced by prostatic epithelial cells and secreted into the prostatic fluid that can leak into the bloodstream during injuries to the prostate, including cancer.
- **Sex hormone-binding globulin:** A serum protein produced by the liver that binds a high proportion of androgenic and estrogenic sex steroid hormones, leaving a small fraction of these hormones free and bioavailable in the blood.
- **Soy:** Products derived from soybeans, such as tofu, miso, and natto that all contain soy protein and soy sauce.
- **Soy isoflavones:** Naturally occurring compounds in soy that have biological activities, particularly estrogenic properties; major isoflavones are daidzein, which can be converted to equol in some people's intestinal tract, genistein, and glycitein.
- **Testosterone:** The major male sex steroid hormone (androgen) that is produced by the testes.

SUMMARY POINTS

- Long-term consumption of soy is associated with an approximately 25–30% reduction in the risk of prostate cancer in epidemiological studies.

- This reduction in risk is probably at least partly associated with the intake of soy isoflavones.
- Randomized clinical trials provide limited evidence that soy protein supplementation, with or without isoflavones, for up to 2 years does not delay or prevent the development or recurrence of prostate cancer.
- Soy protein supplementation, with or without isoflavones, for up to 12 months does not affect serum PSA levels in men with or without prostate cancer.
- Randomized trials have found some effects on sex steroids from soy protein supplementation for up to 6 or 18 months, but these observations do not clearly explain why epidemiological studies have associated long-term soy consumption with reduced risk of prostate cancer.

REFERENCES

Adams K F, Chen C, Newton K M, Potter J D and Lampe J W. 2004. Soy isoflavones do not modulate prostate-specific antigen concentrations in older men in a randomized controlled trial. *Cancer Epidemiology, Biomarkers & Prevention* 13: 644–648.

Ali A, Khalil M A I, Khan N, Abu Bakar M, Amjad A, Ahmed I and Mir K. 2019. Diethylstilbestrol in the treatment of castration-resistant prostate cancer: a lower-middle-income country experience. *Cureus* 11: e4470.

Applegate C C, Rowles J L, Ranard K M, Jeon S and Erdman J W. 2018. Soy consumption and the risk of prostate cancer: an updated systematic review and meta-analysis. *Nutrients* 10, no. 1 (January 4): 40. https://doi.org/10.3390/nu10010040.

Balk S P, Ko Y J and Bubley G J. 2003. Biology of prostate-specific antigen. *Journal of Clinical Oncology* 21: 383–391.

Barnes S, Peterson T G and Coward L. 1995. Rationale for the use of genistein-containing soy matrices in chemoprevention trials for breast and prostate cancer. *Journal of Cellular Biochemistry Supply* 22: 181–187.

Bosland M C. 1988. The etiopathogenesis of prostatic cancer with special reference to environmental factors. *Advances in Cancer Research* 51: 1–106.

Bosland M C. 2013. A perspective on the role of estrogen in hormone-induced prostate carcinogenesis. *Cancer Letters* 334: 28–33.

Bosland M C, Huang J, Schlicht M J, Enk E, Xie H and Kato I. 2022b. Impact of 18-month soy protein supplementation on steroid hormones and serum biomarkers of angiogenesis, apoptosis, and the growth Hormone/IGF-1 axis: results of a randomized, placebo-controlled trial in males following prostatectomy. *Nutrition and Cancer* 74: 110–121.

Bosland M C, Kato I, Zeleniuch-Jacquotte A, Schmoll J, Enk Rueter E, Melamed J, Kong M X, Macias V, Kajdacsy-Balla A, Lumey L H, Xie H, Gao W, Walden P, Lepor H, Taneja S S, Randolph C, Schlicht M J, Meserve-Watanabe H, Deaton RJ and Davies J A. 2013. Effect of soy protein isolate supplementation on biochemical recurrence of prostate cancer after radical prostatectomy: a randomized trial. *JAMA* 310: 170–178.

Bosland M C, Schmoll J, Watanabe H, Randolph C and Kato I. 2022a. Randomized, placebo-controlled six-month intervention study of soy protein isolate in men with biochemical recurrence after radical prostatectomy: a pilot study. *Nutrition and Cancer* 74: 555–564.

Bylund A, Zhang J X, Bergh A, Damber J E, Widmark A, Johansson A, Adlercreutz H, Aman P, Shepherd M J and Hallmans G. 2000. Rye bran and soy protein delay growth and increase apoptosis of human LNCaP prostate adenocarcinoma in nude mice. *Prostate* 42: 304–314.

Dalais FS, Meliala A, Wattanapenpaiboon N, Frydenberg M, Suter D A, Thomson W K and Wahlqvist M L. 2004. Effects of a diet rich in phytoestrogens on prostate-specific antigen and sex hormones in men diagnosed with prostate cancer. *Urology* 64: 510–515.

Fan Y, Wang M, Li Z, Jiang H, Shi J, Shi X, Liu S, Zhao J, Kong L, Zhang W and Ma L. 2022. Intake of soy, soy isoflavones and soy protein and risk of cancer incidence and mortality. *Frontiers in Nutrition* 9 (March 4): 847421. https://doi.org/10.3389/fnut.2022.847421.

Goodin S, Shen F, Shih W J, Dave N, Kane M P, Medina P, Lambert G H, Aisner J, Gallo M and DiPaola R S. 2007. Clinical and biological activity of soy protein powder supplementation in healthy male volunteers. *Cancer Epidemiology, Biomarkers & Prevention* 16: 829–833.

Hamilton-Reeves J M, Banerjee S, Banerjee S K, Holzbeierlein J M, Thrasher J B, Kambhampati S, Keighley J and Van Veldhuizen P. 2013. Short-term soy isoflavone intervention in patients with localized prostate cancer: a randomized, double-blind, placebo-controlled trial. *PLoS One* 8, no.7 (July): e68331. https://doi.org/10.1371/journal.pone.0068331.

Hamilton-Reeves J M, Rebello S A, Thomas W, Kurzer M S and Slaton J W. 2008. Effects of soy protein isolate consumption on prostate cancer biomarkers in men with HGPIN, ASAP, and low-grade prostate cancer. *Nutrition and Cancer* 60: 7–13.

Hamilton-Reeves J M, Rebello S A, Thomas W, Slaton J W and Kurzer M S. 2007a. Isoflavone-rich soy protein isolate suppresses androgen receptor expression without altering estrogen receptor-beta expression or serum hormonal profiles in men at high risk of prostate cancer. *Journal of Nutrition* 137: 1769–1775.

Hamilton-Reeves J M, Rebello S A, Thomas W, Slaton J W and Kurzer M S. 2007b. Soy protein isolate increases urinary estrogens and the ratio of 2:16alpha-hydroxyestrone in men at high risk of prostate cancer. *Journal of Nutrition* 137: 2258–2263.

Hammond G L. 2016. Plasma steroid-binding proteins: primary gatekeepers of steroid hormone action. *Journal of Endocrinology* 230: R13–R25.

Hwang Y W, Kim S Y, Jee S H, Kim Y N and Nam C M. 2009. Soy food consumption and risk of prostate cancer: a meta-analysis of observational studies. *Nutrition and Cancer* 61: 598–606.

Jenkins D J, Kendall C W, D'Costa M A, Jackson C J, Vidgen E, Singer W, Silverman J A, Koumbridis G, Honey J, Rao A V, Fleshner N and Klotz L. 2003. Soy consumption and phytoestrogens: effect on serum prostate specific antigen when blood lipids and oxidized low-density lipoprotein are reduced in hyperlipidemic men. *Journal of Urology* 169:507–511.

Kumar N B, Cantor A, Allen K, Riccardi D, Besterman-Dahan K, Seigne J, Helal M, Salup R and Pow-Sang J. 2004.The specific role of isoflavones in reducing prostate cancer risk. *Prostate* 59: 141–147.

Kumar N B, Kang L, Pow-Sang J, Xu P, Allen K, Riccardi D, Besterman-Dahan K and Krischer J P. 2010. Results of a randomized phase I dose-finding trial of several doses of isoflavones in men with localized prostate cancer: administration prior to radical prostatectomy. *Journal of the Society for Integrative Oncology* 8: 3–13.

Kumar N B, Krischer J P, Allen K, Riccardi D, Besterman-Dahan K, Salup R, Kang L, Xu P and Pow-Sang J. 2007. A Phase II randomized, placebo-controlled clinical trial of purified isoflavones in modulating steroid hormones in men diagnosed with localized prostate cancer. *Nutrition and Cancer* 59: 163–168.

Kumar N B, Pow-Sang J, Spiess P, Dickinson S and Schell M J. 2020. A phase II randomized clinical trial using aglycone isoflavones to treat patients with localized prostate cancer in the pre-surgical period prior to radical prostatectomy. *Oncotarget* 11: 1218–1234.

Kwan W, Duncan G, Van Patten C, Liu M and Lim J. 2010. A phase II trial of a soy beverage for subjects without clinical disease with rising prostate-specific antigen after radical radiation for prostate cancer. *Nutrition and Cancer* 62: 198–207.

Liu W J, Zhao G, Zhang C Y, Yang C Q, Zeng X B, Li J, Zhu K, Zhao S Q, Lu HM, Yin D C and Lin S X. 2020. Comparison of the roles of estrogens and androgens in breast cancer and prostate cancer. *Journal of Cellular Biochemistry* 121: 2756–2769.

Mahmoud A M, Yang W and Bosland M C. 2014. Soy isoflavones and prostate cancer: a review of molecular mechanisms. *Journal of Steroid Biochemistry and Molecular Biology* 140: 116–132.

Mao Y, Tie Y and Du J. 2018. Association between dietary protein intake and prostate cancer risk: evidence from a meta-analysis. *World Journal of Surgical Oncology* 16, no. 1: 152. https://doi.org/10.1186/s12957-018-1452-0.

Maskarinec G, Morimoto Y, Hebshi S, Sharma S, Franke A A and Stanczyk F Z. 2006. Serum prostate-specific antigen but not testosterone levels decrease in a randomized soy intervention among men. *European Journal of Clinical Nutrition* 60: 1423–1429.

Messina M J. 2003. Emerging evidence on the role of soy in reducing prostate cancer risk. *Nutrition Reviews* 61: 117–131.

Miyanaga N, Akaza H, Hinotsu S, Fujioka T, Naito S, Namiki M, Takahashi S, Hirao Y, Horie S, Tsukamoto T, Mori M and Tsuji H. 2012. Prostate cancer chemoprevention study: an investigative randomized control study using purified isoflavones in men with rising prostate-specific antigen. *Cancer Science* 103: 125–130.

McCormick D L, Johnson W D, Bosland M C, Lubet R A and Steele V E. 2007. Chemoprevention of rat prostate carcinogenesis by soy isoflavones and by Bowman–Birk inhibitor. *Nutrition and Cancer* 57: 184–193.

Okuku F, Orem J, Holoya G, De Boer C, Thompson C L and Cooney M M. 2016. Prostate cancer burden at the Uganda Cancer Institute. *Journal of Global Oncology* 2: 181–185.

Pendleton J M, Tan W W, Anai S, Chang M, Hou W, Shiverick K T and Rosser C J. 2008. Phase II trial of isoflavone in prostate-specific antigen recurrent prostate cancer after previous local therapy. *BMC Cancer* 8: 132.

Perabo F G, Von Löw E C, Ellinger J, von Rücker A, Müller S C and Bastian P J. 2008. Soy isoflavone genistein in prevention and treatment of prostate cancer. *Prostate Cancer and Prostatic Diseases* 11: 6–12.

Pollard M and Suckow M A. 2006. Dietary prevention of hormone refractory prostate cancer in Lobund-Wistar rats: a review of studies in a relevant animal model. *Comparative Medicine* 56: 461–467.

Ratha P, Neumann T, Schmidt C A and Schneidewind L. 2021. Can isoflavones influence prostate specific antigen serum levels in localized prostate cancer? A systematic review. *Nutrition and Cancer* 73: 361–368.

Reed K E, Camargo J, Hamilton-Reeves J, Kurzer M and Messina M. 2021. Neither soy nor isoflavone intake affects male reproductive hormones: An expanded and updated meta-analysis of clinical studies. *Reproductive Toxicology* 100: 60–67.

Sathyapalan T, Rigby A S, Bhasin S, Thatcher N J, Kilpatrick E S and Atkin S L. 2017. Effect of soy in men with Type 2 diabetes mellitus and subclinical hypogonadism: a randomized controlled study. *Journal of Clinical Endocrinology and Metabolism* 102: 425–433.

Setchell K D. 1998. Phytoestrogens: the biochemistry, physiology, and implications for human health of soy isoflavones. *American Journal of Clinical Nutrition* 68: 1333S–1346S.

Setchell K D, Brown N M and Lydeking-Olsen E. 2002. The clinical importance of the metabolite equol – a clue to the effectiveness of soy and its isoflavones. *Journal of Nutrition* 132: 3577–3584.

Song J, Chen C, He S, Chen W, Su J, Yuan D, Sun Fand Zhu J. 2020. Is there a non-linear relationship between dietary protein intake and prostate-specific antigen: proof from the national health and nutrition examination survey (2003–2010). *Lipids in Health and Disease* 19: 82. https://doi.org/10.1186/s12944-020-01234-6.

Sung H, Ferlay J, Siegel R L, Laversanne M, Soerjomataram I, Jemal A and Bray F. 2021. Global cancer statistics 2020: GLOBOCAN estimates of incidence and mortality worldwide for 36 cancers in 185 countries. *CA: A Cancer Journal for Clinicians* 71: 209–249.

Turo R, Smolski M, Esler R, Kujawa M L, Bromage S J, Oakley N, Adeyoju A, Brown S C, Brough R, Sinclair A and Collins G N. 2014. Diethylstilboestrol for the treatment of prostate cancer: past, present and future. *Scandinavian Journal of Urology* 48: 4–14.

Urban D, Irwin W, Kirk M, Markiewicz M A, Myers R, Smith M, Weiss H, Grizzle W E and Barnes S. 2001. The effect of isolated soy protein on plasma biomarkers in elderly men with elevated serum prostate specific antigen. *Journal of Urology* 165: 294–300.

van Die M D, Bone K M, Emery J, Williams S G, Pirotta M V and Paller C J. 2016. Phytotherapeutic interventions in the management of biochemically recurrent prostate cancer: a systematic review of randomised trials. *BJU International* 117 (Suppl 4): 17–34.

van Die M D, Bone K M, Williams S G and Pirotta M V. 2014. Soy and soy isoflavones in prostate cancer: a systematic review and meta-analysis of randomized controlled trials. *BJU International* 113: E119–130.

van Veldhuizen P J, Thrasher J B, Ray G, Cherian R, Ward J, Holzbeierlein J, Gutow S and Banerjee S K. 2006. Dose effect of soy supplementation in prostate cancer: a pilot study. *Oncology Reports* 16: 1221–1224.

Wynder E L, Rose D P and Cohen L A. 1994. Nutrition and prostate cancer: a proposal for dietary intervention. *Nutrition and Cancer* 22: 1–10.

Yan L and Spitznagel E L. 2009. Soy consumption and prostate cancer risk in men: a revisit of a meta-analysis. *American Journal of Clinical Nutrition* 89: 1155–1163.

Zhang M, Wang K, Chen L, Yin B and Song Y. 2016. Is phytoestrogen intake associated with decreased risk of prostate cancer? A systematic review of epidemiological studies based on 17,546 cases. *Andrology* 4: 745–756.

25 Effects of Soy Protein on Diabetes

Maria do Carmo de Carvalho e Martins, Joyce Lopes Macedo, Izabela Cristina Pereira de Araújo, and Vanessa Brito Lira de Carvalho

ABBREVIATIONS

AMPK	Adenosine monophosphate-activated protein kinase
CRP	C-reactive protein
DM	Diabetes mellitus
DM1	Type 1 diabetes mellitus
DM2	Type 2 diabetes mellitus
DPP-IV	Dipeptidyl peptidase IV enzyme
GI	Glycemic index
GIP	Glucose-dependent insulinotropic polypeptide
GLP-1	Glucagon-like peptide-1
GLUT4	Glucose transporter 4
HOMA-IR	Homeostatic Model Assessment of Insulin Resistance
IL-1β	Interleukin 1-beta
IL-6	Interleukin 6
LDL-c	Low-density lipoprotein cholesterol
MUFA	Monounsaturated fatty acids
PUFA	Polyunsaturated fatty acids
TNF-α	Tumor necrosis factor-alpha

INTRODUCTION

Diabetes mellitus (DM) is a public health problem on a global scale, as it is one of the fastest-growing chronic diseases worldwide and represents the seventh-leading cause of death in the world (Zheng et al 2018). It is a systemic metabolic disease characterized by hyperglycemia resulting from insufficient insulin secretion and/or action (Cole and Florez 2020).

Type 1 diabetes mellitus (DM1) is characterized by significant insulin deficiency due to the destruction of pancreatic ß-cells, often related to autoimmune processes, and is more common in children and adolescents. In contrast, type 2 (DM2) is characterized by insulin resistance and a partial deficiency in insulin secretion by pancreatic islet ß-cells, as well as alterations in the secretion of incretins. It is the most prevalent type of diabetes, accounting for approximately 90% of cases, and is correlated with high mortality rates, significant medical costs, and various complications, including retinopathy, kidney disease, microvascular complications, and neuropathies (World Health Organization 2019).

DM2 is commonly linked to obesity and aging, manifesting gradually and insidiously. Glucose intolerance is associated with a complex interaction of influences, including genetic predisposition, environmental factors, inadequate dietary choices, low levels of physical activity, and overweight,

 DOI: 10.1201/9781003597926-25

all of which play a substantial role in the evolution of insulin resistance and the onset of this type of diabetes (Petersmann et al 2019).

Treating DM requires both pharmacological and non-pharmacological approaches. The latter category includes interventions such as diet and body weight control, which have been highlighted as accessible and low-cost options. In this context, researchers have considered nutrients and bioactive compounds present in foods a promising strategy as an auxiliary resource in glycemic control (Hu et al 2023).

Bioactive peptides derived from food proteins could be an affordable option with few side effects. Researchers have identified different foods containing a variety of bioactive peptides with antidiabetic, antihypertensive, and anticancer properties (Cicero et al 2017; Tovar and Torres 2010). Soy-derived peptides, for example, are among the most popular bioactive components obtained from soy proteins and are widely used with functional claims to help promote health in various aspects, including preventing chronic non-communicable diseases and conditions, such as obesity, DM2, cardiovascular diseases, and cancer (Chatterjee et al 2018).

Soy is an excellent source of highly beneficial proteins and peptides. This legume contains all 20 amino acids, including the nine essential amino acids (Zhang et al, 2017). The nutritional value of soy protein is comparable to that of animal-origin proteins, which qualifies it as a protein of high biological value. Table 25.1 shows the essential amino acid content of soy protein and animal proteins such as meat, eggs, and cow's milk casein (Pires et al, 2006). In addition, soy is rich in bioactive compounds, such as various peptides derived from its proteins, as well as isoflavones and oligosaccharides, all of which contribute to promoting longevity and maintaining good health (Nagaoka et al 2021).

Soy peptides result from breaking down the proteins present in soybeans through the action of various proteolytic enzymes. They are oligopeptides containing three to six amino acids, with molecular weights ranging from 300 to 700 (Wen et al 2021). Their composition and proportion of amino acids are identical to those of the original soy proteins, but they have the advantage of being more readily absorbed and more stable. The biological functions of soy peptides relate to the size of the molecules and the particular amino acid sequences that make them up. Researchers have conducted few studies on peptides derived from soy proteins, which have mainly addressed the relationship between the structure and activities of these peptides, and this area of research remains little explored (Lin et al 2017; Singh and Vij 2018).

This chapter describes the effects of soy proteins/peptides in improving glycemic control and reducing insulin resistance and their potential role as an auxiliary resource in managing diabetes mellitus. It highlights the effects of soy proteins in improving glucose metabolism, aiming to contribute to preventing or delaying the onset of complications related to DM.

TABLE 25.1
Essential Amino Acid Content of Soy and Animal Proteins (mg/g Protein)

	Food/Protein			
Essential Amino Acids	**Soy**	**Beef**	**Egg Powder**	**Casein**
Leucine	81.34	92.24	83.9	93.05
Isoleucine	45.71	39.43	34.64	46.91
Valine	48.16	43.0	47.52	54.95
Lysine	82.69	95.28	91.44	78.66
Methionine	18.65	35.59	40.05	30.14
Phenylalanine	96.99	83.86	98.64	109.71
Threonine	51.34	48.23	53.5	43.22
Histidine	96.99	38.10	22.12	18.99

SOY PROTEIN'S EFFECTS ON GLYCEMIC CONTROL

Soy (*Glycine max*) contains high-quality proteins that can aid in managing various diseases, including DM and its metabolic complications (Das et al 2022).

Habitual soy protein consumption has been associated with a reduction in the risk of DM2, and encouraging the consumption of this protein may be extremely important, especially given the increase in the worldwide prevalence of diabetes. The beneficial effects of soy protein intake on glycemic control involve a reduction in glycemia, hemoglobin glycation, and insulin resistance (Tang et al 2020).

Konya et al (2019) described improved glycemic control resulting from soy protein supplementation in a randomized clinical trial with 60 people with DM2. Using intervention with isolated soy protein and casein protein as a comparator, they found reduced percentages of hemoglobin glycation in the group that received isolated soy protein.

Sedaghat et al (2015) also found benefits in glycemic control parameters in response to soy protein supplementation in a study of 69 patients with DM2. The intervention group received 60 grams of soy protein in their morning and afternoon snacks for eight weeks, while the control group maintained their usual diabetes diet (but without soy). As a result, soy protein consumption reduced fasting glycemia and the percentage of glycated hemoglobin while increasing plasma insulin concentrations and reducing insulin resistance.

In addition to protein, various peptides derived from soy can modulate physiological actions related to glucose homeostasis and insulin metabolism (Lecerf et al 2020), and researchers have demonstrated this antidiabetic activity using different experimental models *in vitro* and *in vivo* (Das et al 2022).

Lu et al (2012) used *in vivo* and *in vitro* experimental protocols to evaluate the pharmacological activity of aglycine (a natural bioactive peptide isolated from soy). They observed that *in vivo* treatment in an experimental model of DM2 in mice effectively controlled hyperglycemia and improved oral glucose tolerance. In an *in vitro* diabetes model using C2C12 muscle cells, they demonstrated increased glucose uptake and translocation of glucose transporter 4 (GLUT4) to the plasma membrane.

Finally, other studies using *in vivo* experimental protocols with diabetic rats and mice revealed that consuming soy protein peptides such as β-conglycinin, soymorphin-5, and aglycine promoted increased insulin sensitivity, improved glucose uptake by the muscle cell and GLUT4 translocation to the plasma membrane, reduced blood glucose concentrations, restored pancreatic function, increased plasma adiponectin concentration, and increased phosphorylated AMP-activated protein kinase (AMPK) activity (Figure 25.1) (Jiang et al 2014; Tachibana et al 2014).

MECHANISMS ASSOCIATED WITH SOY PROTEIN AND PEPTIDES' EFFECTS ON GLYCEMIC CONTROL

Evidence shows that soy protein and peptides can act on a variety of molecular targets, such as the enzymes alpha-amylase and alpha-glucosidases, digestive enzymes that hydrolyze glycosidic bonds in carbohydrates (Lecerf et al 2020). α-Amylase (1,4-α-D-glycan glycohydrolase) has endohydrolytic activity, initiating starch digestion by randomly hydrolyzing α 1,4-glycosidic bonds, which breaks down polysaccharides into a mixture of glucose, maltose, and dextrins (Tricarico et al 2008).

α-Glycosidases are enzymes that hydrolyze the α-1,4-glycosidic bond in short-chain glycans such as maltose or maltotriose, resulting from the action of other enzymes, as well as on amylopectin to release α-D-glucose from the non-reducing end of the glycosidic chain. Inhibiting these enzymes effectively reduces intestinal glucose absorption and postprandial hyperglycemia (Figure 25.2) (Telagari and Hullati 2015).

In addition, soy protein and peptides can inhibit the enzyme dipeptidyl peptidase IV (DPP-IV), which is considered a potential therapeutic target in treating diabetic hyperglycemia. DPP-IV

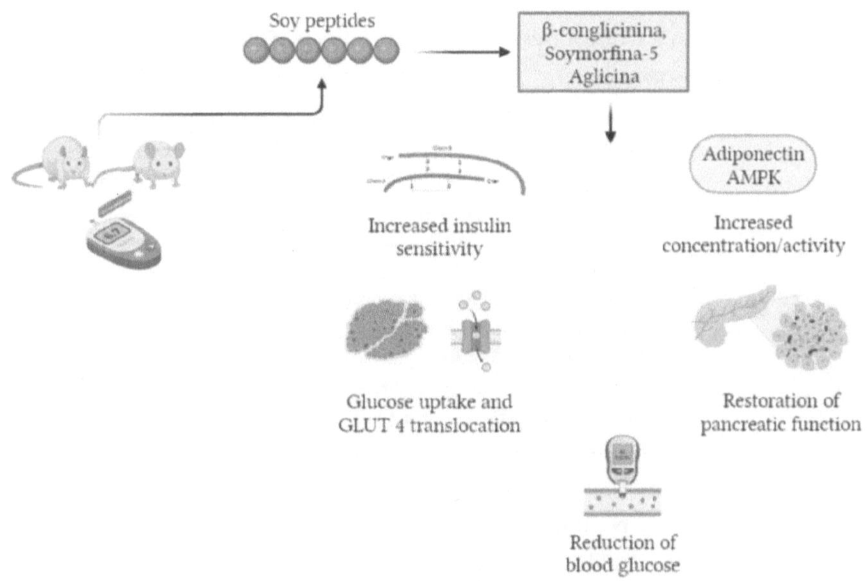

FIGURE 25.1 Effects of consuming soy peptides on glycaemic control in experimental models of diabetes. Legend: GLUT 4 = glucose transporter 4; AMPK = AMP-activated protein kinase.

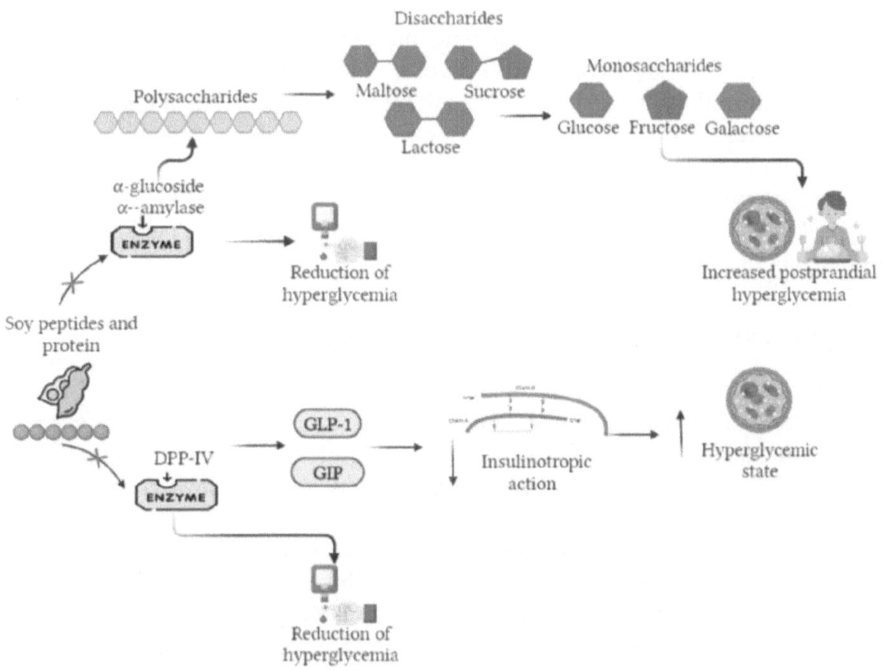

FIGURE 25.2 Mechanism of action of soy protein and peptides on the enzymes alpha-amylase, alpha-glucosidase and dipeptidyl peptidase IV in glycaemic control. Legend: GLP-1 = glucagon-like peptide-1; GIP = Glucose-dependent insulinotropic polypeptide; DPP-IV = dipeptidyl peptidase-4.

TABLE 25.2
Effects of Soy's Bioactive Components on Intermediary Metabolism

Bioactive Constituent	Action on Intermediary Metabolism
Aglycine	• *In vitro*: Increased glucose uptake and GLUT4 translocation to muscle cell plasma membrane. • *In vivo*: Hypoglycemic effect and improved oral glucose tolerance.
β-conglicinin, soymorphin-5	• Increased insulin sensitivity. • Increased glucose uptake by muscle cells and GLUT4 translocation to the plasma membrane. • Increased plasma adiponectin concentration and AMPK activity.
Isoflavones	• Inhibition of insulin release. • Inhibition of brush border α-glucosidases, reducing intestinal glucose absorption. • Increased number and affinity of insulin receptors and intracellular phosphorylation. • Inhibition of tyrosine kinase activity and changes in glucose transporters.

promotes the inactivation of peptides from the incretin family, which includes glucagon-like peptide-1 (GLP-1) and glucose-dependent insulinotropic polypeptide (GIP). As incretins exert an insulinotropic action, hyperactivity of the DPP-IV enzyme contributes to maintaining a hyperglycemic state (Figure 25.2) (Zani et al 2018).

Soy peptides can also improve insulin sensitivity and increase glucose uptake by muscle cells (Lecerf et al 2020), as well as modulate cell signaling pathways in multiple organs to maintain glucose homeostasis, energy balance, and regulate parameters associated with the pathophysiology of diabetes mellitus (Das et al 2022).

Other components present in soy, such as isoflavones, also have effects related to improved glycemic control (Zuo et al 2023). Isoflavones can inhibit insulin release and act as inhibitors of α-glucosidases linked to the brush border, reducing intestinal glucose absorption (Chen et al 2006). Other isoflavone actions in glycemic control involve changes in the number and affinity of the insulin receptor, intracellular phosphorylation, inhibitory action of tyrosine kinase, and changes in glucose transporters (Li et al 2020). The effects of soy's bioactive components on intermediary metabolism are shown in Table 25.2.

In summary, soy protein and its peptides can act in different ways to modulate various cell signaling pathways to ensure glucose homeostasis and regulate inflammatory parameters related to the pathophysiology of diabetes.

SOY PROTEIN'S EFFECTS ON INSULIN RESISTANCE

Soy is rich in proteins of high biological value, with essential amino acids found in animal proteins but without cholesterol or saturated fat (Chatterjee et al 2018). Evidence shows that soy protein is associated with reduced insulin resistance, lower fasting blood glucose, and improved glycemic control (Figure 25.3), which may contribute to fewer deaths from cardiovascular diseases and DM (Konya et al 2019; Yi et al 2023).

Reduced insulin resistance and lower blood glucose may result from the biochemical effects of soy proteins and peptides, as well as the action of soy's bioactive compounds (Costa et al 2020). Thus, consuming soy products may reduce the risk of developing DM2 (Li et al 2018).

Insulin resistance generally occurs when insulin-sensitive cells stop responding and/or due to a relative deficiency of this hormone in the body. Insulin, a peptide hormone, binds to receptors on target cell plasma membranes to activate an anabolic response to nutrient availability and control

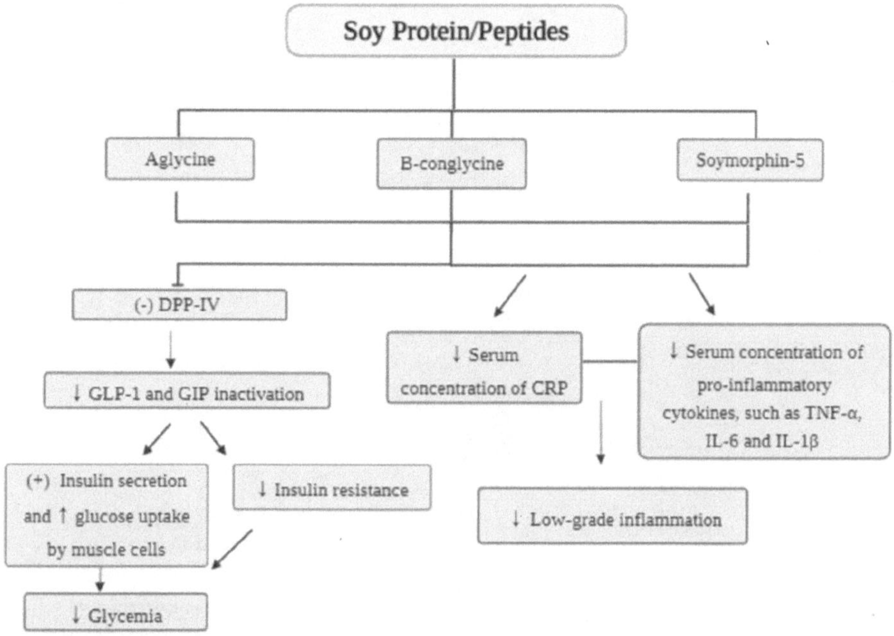

FIGURE 25.3 Effects of soy protein on insulin resistance and inflammation. Legend: DPP-IV dipeptidyl peptidase IV enzyme; GLP-1 glucagon-like peptide-1; GIP Glucose-dependent insulinotropic polypeptide; CRP C-reactive protein; TNF-α Tumor necrosis factor α ; IL-6 Interleukin 6; IL-1β interleukin 1-beta, (-) = inhibition; (+) stimulation.

metabolic flows. Thus, insulin plays an important role in energy metabolism and in cardiovascular and neurological processes (Petersen and Shulman 2018; Gutiérrez-Rodelo et al 2017).

Soy plays an important role in reducing insulin resistance and oxidative stress not only due to the action of its proteins and peptides (Figure 25.4) but also due to its high content of unsaturated fatty acids and dietary fiber (Bakhtiari et al 2019). With regard to the effects of soy and its constituents, Sedaghat et al (2015) evaluated soy's effectiveness on glycemic control, blood pressure, lipid profile, and insulin resistance in individuals with DM2 and showed that daily consumption of 60 g/day of soybeans for eight weeks resulted in decreased percentages of glycated hemoglobin and serum concentrations of fasting glucose, LDL-c (low-density lipoprotein cholesterol), and total cholesterol, as well as insulin resistance.

A study by Nakamoto et al (2015) with a cohort of 1148 Japanese participants showed that a higher frequency of soy-based food consumption was inversely associated with insulin resistance, especially in women. Higher soy consumption may be associated with a lower risk of developing diabetes.

Researchers have also studied soy as part of a dietary strategy to combat obesity, a condition associated with insulin resistance and DM2. This effect has been linked to its high protein content, which positively affects body weight and adiposity control, including central adiposity, thus reducing waist circumference (Akhlaghi et al 2017; Aguiar et al 2019).

THE RELATIONSHIP BETWEEN SOY PROTEIN CONSUMPTION AND INFLAMMATION MARKERS

Soy proteins and peptides may also reduce serum concentrations of pro-inflammatory substances (Figure 25.3). Obesity is marked by a chronic low-grade inflammatory state, and C-reactive protein (CRP), tumor necrosis factor-alpha (TNF-α), and other pro-inflammatory cytokines, such as

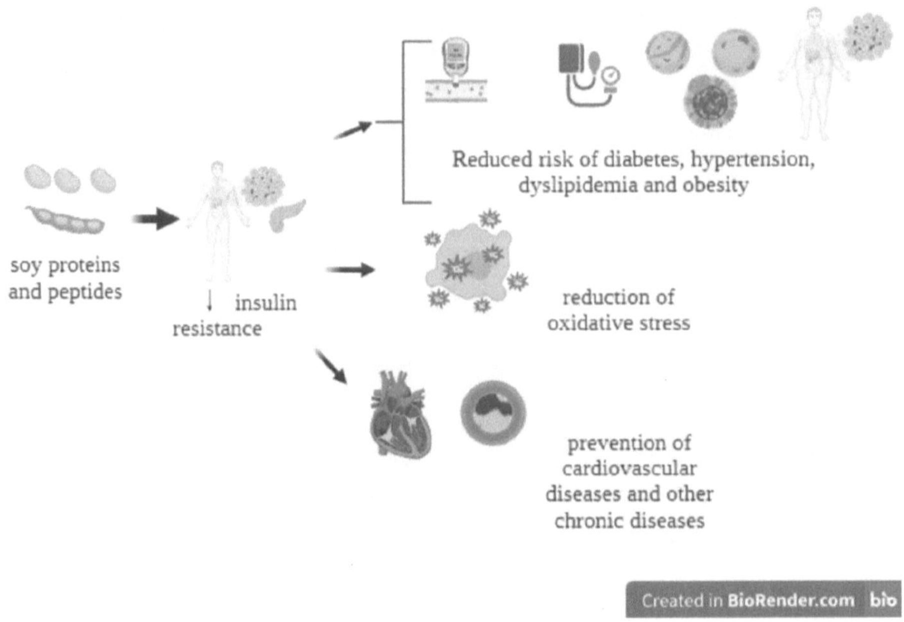

FIGURE 25.4 Functional effects of soy protein and peptides related to the reduction of insulin resistance.

interleukin 6 (IL-6) and interleukin 1-beta (IL-1β), directly relate to increased insulin resistance. This decreased sensitivity to insulin action can impair glucose homeostasis and increase the risk of developing DM2 (Liu et al 2016).

Regarding the relationship between the presence of chronic inflammation and T2DM, CRP, a systemic marker of inflammation, is a suitable biomarker for this type of diabetes (Luersen et al 2023). A meta-analysis of randomized clinical trials evaluating the potential effects of soy milk consumption on cardiometabolic risk factors in adults showed that soy milk intake, in addition to reducing systolic and diastolic blood pressure and serum concentrations of low-density lipoproteins and cholesterol, also had anti-inflammatory effects, evidenced by reduced serum concentrations of C-reactive protein and pro-inflammatory cytokines, such as IL-6 and TNF-α (Sohouli et al 2021). Similarly, in a systematic review of randomized clinical trials, Prokopidis et al (2023) also reported that soy protein has anti-inflammatory effects, decreasing circulating levels of IL-6 and TNF-α.

In addition, an experimental study on rats assessing the effects of soy protein on insulin resistance in the presence of hepatic steatosis over 10 weeks found reduced insulin resistance, improved lipid levels, and increased antioxidant capacity (Yang et al 2011).

Thus, soy consumption can, through its proteins and peptides, as well as other compounds, contribute to reducing insulin resistance and serve as an auxiliary resource in improving glycemic control. Soy or soy protein consumption can be highlighted as an accessible and low-cost strategy to promote metabolic health, aid in weight control and body composition, and reduce the inflammatory state in obesity. The combined effects of soy protein and peptides, among other components, can be exploited for preventing and treating DM, as well as preventing cardiovascular diseases and other chronic non-communicable diseases, constituting a health promotion approach and a promising adjunct therapy for the general well-being of the population (Figure 25.4).

OTHER PLANT PROTEINS' EFFECTS ON DIABETES

Besides soy protein, researchers have studied other plant proteins as potential adjuvant resources for treating DM. Antidiabetic action is one of the biological effects produced by plant proteins and peptides, mainly sourced from cereals and legumes (Chan-Zapata et al 2020).

In a systematic review by Pfeiffer et al (2020), diets rich in plant proteins improved fasting glycemia and total cholesterol levels in people with DM2 compared to diets rich in red meat proteins.

Plant protein sources, such as beans, dried peas, chickpeas, and lentils, can reduce insulin resistance, among other parameters associated with T2DM, including the Homeostatic Model Assessment for Insulin Resistance (HOMA-IR), with stronger evidence for chickpeas compared to the other protein sources mentioned (Mullins and Arjmandi 2021).

Improved glycemic control after consuming chickpeas, in terms of increased glucose tolerance and insulin secretion, can be explained by their high protein and fiber content, low simple carbohydrates content, slow digestibility, slow absorption rates, high content of monounsaturated fatty acids (MUFA) and polyunsaturated fatty acids (PUFA), and high content of resistant starch, which is digested and absorbed slowly, and increases secretion of GLP-1 and peptide YY due to the fermentation of amylose (Reister, Belote, and Leidy 2020).

Jenkins et al (2012) conducted a study with 121 participants with DM2, randomized to consume a diet rich in legumes with a low glycemic index (GI). Participants increased their legume intake by at least one cup a day for three months. The study showed that a low-GI diet containing 190 g (1 cup) of vegetable protein from legumes (baked beans, chickpeas, or lentils) per day for three months reduced hemoglobin glycation. In another study of 18 participants, consuming black bean pasta meals containing different protein concentrations reduced postprandial glycemia and insulinemia compared to the control group, which received white bread (Winham et al 2022).

In view of the above, consuming other plant proteins can help improve glucose metabolism and long-term glycemic control, reducing hemoglobin glycation, with benefits in various parameters related to DM. Therefore, this dietary strategy could be appropriate for treating and preventing diabetes (Pires 2023).

CONCLUSION

Consuming soy protein and its peptides may constitute a promising, accessible, and low-cost dietary strategy for health promotion and adjuvant therapy in preventing and managing diabetes mellitus through important metabolic health benefits related to improved glycemic control, reduced insulin resistance, and modulation of inflammation markers.

MINI DICTIONARY OF TERMS

- **Alpha-amylase:** An enzyme that initiates carbohydrate digestion by hydrolyzing α-1,4-glycosidic bonds of polysaccharides into oligosaccharides and disaccharides.
- **Alpha-glucosidase:** Enzymes that act in the hydrolysis of the α-1,4-glycosidic bonds in short-chain glycans, such as maltose or maltotriose, resulting from the action of other enzymes, as well as on amylopectin to release α-D-glucose from the non-reducing end of the glycosidic chain.
- **AMP-activated protein kinase (AMPK):** An enzyme that activates or inhibits different proteins in the cell cytoplasm and acts as an important sensor and regulator of energy metabolism.
- **Chronic low-grade inflammation:** A state of mild and persistent systemic inflammation associated with various chronic diseases, including DM2, heart disease, obesity, cancer, and autoimmune disorders. It can contribute to tissue damage over time and increase the risk of chronic diseases.

- **Dipeptidyl peptidase IV (DPP-IV):** An enzyme that inactivates various bioactive peptides, including glucagon-like peptide-1 (GLP-1) and glucose-dependent insulinotropic polypeptide (GIP); its inhibition may help maintain glycemic control.
- **Essential amino acids:** Amino acids that the human body cannot produce on its own and must, therefore, be obtained from the diet.
- **Glucose homeostasis:** The physiological balance of blood glucose concentrations maintained through the regulatory action of hormones such as insulin and glucagon, among others.
- **Insulin resistance:** A condition in which cells have difficulty responding to insulin, resulting in high concentrations of glucose in the blood.
- **Isoflavones:** Bioactive compounds found in soy that, among other effects, can inhibit insulin release and α-glucosidase activity, thus showing positive effects in improving glycemic control.

SUMMARY POINTS

- Soy protein and its peptides potentially benefit glycemic control by reducing glycemia and hemoglobin glycation.
- Soy protein and peptides improve glycemic control, as evidenced by a reduction in insulin resistance.
- Inhibiting digestive enzymes such as alpha-amylase and alpha-glucosidase, as well as the DPP-IV enzyme, contributes to maintaining glycemic control.
- Consuming soy protein and its peptides helps reduce serum concentrations of pro-inflammatory cytokines such as CRP, TNF-α, IL-6, and IL-1β.
- Soy, because it is rich in high-quality proteins, has a low glycemic index, and is rich in fiber, may offer additional benefits in preventing obesity, a risk factor for diabetes mellitus.

REFERENCES

Aguiar, C, Duarte, R and Carvalho, D. 2019. New approach to diabetes care: from blood glucose to cardiovascular disease. *Rev Port Cardiol (Engl Ed)* 38(1):53–63. https://doi.org/10.1016/j.repc.2018.03.013

Akhlaghi, M, Zare, M and Nouripour, F. 2017. Effect of soy and soy isoflavones on obesity-related anthropometric measures: a systematic review and meta-analysis of randomized controlled clinical trials. *Adv Nutr* 8(5):705–717. https://doi.org/10.3945/an.117.015370

Bakhtiari, A et al. 2019. Clinical and metabolic response to soy administration in older women with metabolic syndrome: a randomized controlled trial. *Diabetol Metab Syndr* 11(47). https://doi.org/10.1186/s13098-019-0441-y

Chan-Zapata, I, Sandoval-Castro, C and Segura-Campos, M. 2020. Proteins and peptides from vegetable food sources as therapeutic adjuvants for the type 2 diabetes mellitus. *Crit Rev Food Sci Nutr* 62(10):2673–2682. https://doi.org/10.1080/10408398.2020.1857331

Chatterjee, C, Gleddie, S and Xiao, CW. 2018. Soybean bioactive peptides and their functional properties. *Nutrients* 10(9):1211. https://doi.org/10.3390/nu10091211

Chen, SW, Zhang, HM, Zhang, LS, Feng, XF and Peng, X. 2006. Effects of soy isoflavone on gene expression of adiponectin in insulin-resistance rats induced by high-fat and high-sugar diet. *Wei Sheng Yan Jiu* 35(1):46–49.

Cicero, AF, Fogacci, F and Colletti, A. 2017. Potential role of bioactive peptides in prevention and treatment of chronic diseases: a narrative review. *Br J Pharmacol* 174(11):1378–1394. https://doi.org/10.1111/bph.13608

Cole, JB and Florez, JC. 2020. Genetics of diabetes mellitus and diabetes complications. *Nat Rev Nephrol* 16(7):377–390. https://doi.org/10.1038/s41581-020-0278-5

Costa, IS, Medeiros, AF, Piuvezam, G, Medeiros, GCBS, Maciel, BLL and Morais, AHA. 2020. Insulin-like proteins in plant sources: a systematic review. *Diabetes Metab Syndr Obes.* September 30(13):3421–3431. https://doi.org/10.2147/DMSO.S256883

Das, D, Kabir, ME, Sarkar, S, Wann, SB, Kalita, J and Manna, P. 2022. Antidiabetic potential of soy protein/peptide: A therapeutic insight. *Int J Biol Macromol* 1 (194):276–288. https://doi.org/10.1016/j.ijbiomac.2021.11.131

Gutiérrez-Rodelo, C, Roura-Guiberna, A and Olivares-Reyes, JA. 2017. Mecanismos Moleculares de la Resistencia a la Insulina: Una Actualización [Molecular Mechanisms of Insulin Resistance: An Update]. *Gac Med Mex* 153(2):214–228.

Hu, S, Liu, C and Liu, X. 2023. The beneficial effects of soybean proteins and peptides on chronic diseases. *Nutrients* 15(8):811. https://doi.org/10.3390/nu15081811

Jenkins, DJ, Kendall, CW, Agostinho, LS and Mitchell, S. 2012. Efeito das leguminosas como parte de uma dieta com baixo índice glicêmico no controle glicêmico e fatores de risco cardiovascular no diabetes mellitus tipo 2: um ensaio clínico randomizado. *Arco Estagiário Med* 172:1653–1660.

Jiang, H, Feng, J, Du, Z, Zhen, H, Lin, M, Jia, S, Li, T, Huang, X, Ostenson, CG and Chen, Z. 2014. taOral administration of soybean peptide Vglycin normalizes fasting glucose and restores impaired pancreatic function in Type 2 diabetic Wistar rats. *J Nutr Biochem* 25(9):954–963. https://doi.org/10.1016/j.jnutbio.2014.04.010

Konya, J, Sathyapalan, T, Kilpatrick, ES and Atkin, SL. 2019. The effects of soy protein and cocoa with or without isoflavones on glycemic control in type 2 diabetes. A double-blind, randomized, placebo-controlled study. *Front Endocrinol (Lausanne)* 9(10). https://doi.org/10.3389/fendo.2019.00296

Lecerf, JM, Arnoldi, A, Rowland, I, Trabal, J, Widhalm, K, Aiking, H and Messina, M. 2020. Soyfoods, glycemic control and diabetes. *Nutrition Clinique et Métabolisme* 34:141–148. https://doi.org/10.1016/j.nupar.2020.02.437

Li, N, Wu, X, Zhuang, W, Xia, L, Chen, Y, Zhao, R, Yi, M, Wan, Q, Du, L and Zhou, Y. 2020. Soy and Isoflavone consumption and multiple health outcomes: umbrella review of systematic reviews and meta-analyses of observational studies and randomized trials in humans. *Mol Nutr Food Res* 64(4). https://doi.org/10.1002/mnfr.201900751

Li, W, Ruan, W, Peng, Y and Wang, D. 2018. Soy and the risk of type 2 diabetes mellitus: a systematic review and meta-analysis of observational studies. *Diabetes Res Clin Pract* 137:190–199. https://doi.org/10.1016/j.diabres.2018.01.010

Lin, Q, Xu, Q, Bai, J, Wu, W, Hong, H and Wu, J. 2017. Transport of soybean protein-derived antihypertensive peptide LSW across Caco-2 monolayers. *J Funct Foods* 39:96–102. https://doi.org/10.1016/j.jff.2017.10.011

Liu, C, Feng, X, Li, Q, Wang, Y, Li, Q and Hua, M. 2016. Adiponectin, TNF-α and inflammatory cytokines and risk of type 2 diabetes: a systematic review and meta-analysis. *Cytokine* 86:100–109. https://doi.org/10.1016/j.cyto.2016.06.028

Lu, J, Zeng, Y, Hou, W, Zhang, S, Li L. Luo, X, Xi, W, Chen, Z and Xiang, M. 2012. The soybean peptide aglycin regulates glucose homeostasis in type 2 diabetic mice via IR/IRS1 pathway. *J Nutr Biochem* 23(11):1449–1457. https://doi.org/10.1016/j.jnutbio.2011.09.007

Lüersen, K, Fischer, A, Bauer, I, Huebbe, P, Uekaji, Y, Chikamoto, K, Nakata, D, Hiramatsu, N, Terao, K and Rimbach, G. 2023. Soy extract, rich in hydroxylated isoflavones, exhibits antidiabetic properties in vitro and in *Drosophila melanogaster* in Vivo. *Nutrients* 15(6):1392. https://doi.org/10.3390/nu15061392

Mullins, AP and Arjmandi, BH. 2021. Benefícios para a saúde da nutrição vegetal: foco no feijão nas doenças cardiometabólicas. *Nutrientes* 13:519.

Nagaoka, S, Takeuchi, A and Banno, A. 2021. Plant-derived peptides improving lipid and glucose metabolism. *Peptides* 142:170577. https://doi.org/10.1016/j.peptides.2021.170577

Nakamoto, M, Uemura, H, Sakai, T, Katsuura-Kamano, S, Yamaguchi, M. Hiyoshi, M and Arisawa, K. 2015 Inverse association between soya food consumption and insulin resistance in Japanese adults. *Public Health Nutr* 18(11):2031–2040. https://doi.org/10.1017/S136898001400247X

Petersmann, A, Müller-Wieland, D, Müller, UA, Landgraf, R, Nauck, M, Freckmann, G and Schleicher, E. 2019. Definition, classification and diagnosis of diabetes mellitus. *Exp Clin Endocrinol Diabetes* 127(S 01):S1–S7. https://doi.org/10.1055/a-1018-9078

Petersen, MC and Shulman, GI. 2018. Mechanisms of insulin action and insulin resistance. *Physiol Rev* 98(4):2133–2223. https://doi: 10.1152/physrev.00063.2017.

Pfeiffer, AFH, Pedersen, E, Schwab, U, Risérus, U, Aas, AM, Uusitupa, M, Thanopoulou, A, Kendall, C, Sievenpiper, JL, Kahleová, H, Rahélic, D, Salas-Salvadó, J, Gebauer, S, Hermansen, K. 2020. The effects of different quantities and qualities of protein intake in people with diabetes mellitus. *Nutrients* 12(2):365. https://doi: 10.3390/nu12020365.

Pires CV. 2023. Superfoods for type 2 diabetes: a narrative review and proposal for new international recommendations. *Medicina* 59(7):1184. https://doi.org/10.3390/medicina59071184

Pires, CV, Oliveira, MGDA, Rosa, JC and Costa, NMB. 2006. Qualidade nutricional e escore químico de aminoácidos de diferentes fontes protéicas. *Food Sci Technol* 26:179–187. https://doi.org/10.1590/S0101-20612006000100029

Prokopidis, K, Mazidi, M, Sankaranarayanan, R, Tajik, B, McArdle, A and Isanejad, M. 2023. Effects of whey and soy protein supplementation on inflammatory cytokines in older adults: a systematic review and meta-analysis. *Br J Nutr.* March 14 129(5):759–770. https://doi.org/10.1017/S0007114522001787

Reister, EJ, Belote, LN and Leidy, HJ. 2020. Os benefícios da inclusão de ingredientes de homus e homus na dieta americana para promover a qualidade e a saúde da dieta: uma revisão abrangente. *Nutrientes* 12(3678):1–12.

Sedaghat, A, Shahbazian, H. Haidari, F, Payami, S, Jahanshahi, A and Latifi, S. 2015. The effect of soy nuts on glycemic control, lipid profile and insulin-resistance in type 2 diabetic patients. *Open J Endocr Metab Dis* 5:1–7. https://doi.org/10.4236/ojemd.2015.51001

Singh, BP and Vij, S. 2018. In vitro stability of bioactive peptides derived from fermented soy milk against heat treatment, pH and gastrointestinal enzymes. *Lwt* 91:303–307. https://doi.org/10.1016/j.lwt.2018.01.066

Sohouli, MH et al. 2021. Impact of soy milk consumption on cardiometabolic risk factors: A systematic review and meta-analysis of randomized controlled trials. *J Funct Foods* 83. https://doi.org/10.1016/j.jff.2021.104499

Tachibana, N, Yamashita, Y, Nagata, M, Wanezaki, S, Ashida, H, Horio, F and Kohno, M. 2014. Soy β-conglycinin improves glucose uptake in skeletal muscle and ameliorates hepatic insulin resistance in Goto-Kakizaki rats. *Nutr Res* 34(2):160–167. https://doi.org10.1016/j.nutres.2013.12.001

Tang, J, Wan, Y, Zhao, M, Zhong, H, Zheng, JS and Feng, F. 2020. Legume and soy intake and risk of type 2 diabetes: a systematic review and meta-analysis of prospective cohort studies. *Am J Clin Nutr* 111(3):677–688. https://doi.org/10.1093/ajcn/nqz338

Telagari, M and Hullatti, K. 2015. In-vitro α-amylase and α-glucosidase inhibitory activity of Adiantum caudatum Linn. and Celosia argentea Linn. Extracts and fractions. *Indian J Pharmacol* 47(4):425–429. https://doi.org/10.4103/0253-7613.161270

Tovar, AR and Torres N. 2010. The role of dietary protein on lipotoxicity. *Biochimica et Biophysica Acta (BBA)-Molecular and Cell Biology of Lipids* 1801(3):367–371. https://doi.org/10.1016/j.bbalip.2009.09.007

Tricarico, JM, Johnston, JD and Dawson, KA. 2008. Dietary supplementation of ruminant diets with an Aspergillus oryzae α-amylase. *Anim Feed Sci Technol* 145(1–4):136–150. https://doi.org/10.3389/fnut.2022.847156

Yang, HY, Tzeng, YH, Chai, CY, Hsieh, AT, Chen, JR, Chang, LS and Yang, SS. 2011. Soy protein retards the progression of non-alcoholic steatohepatitis via improvement of insulin resistance and steatosis. *Nutrition* 27(9):943–948. https://doi.org/10.1016/j.nut.2010.09.004

Yi, G, Sang, X, Zhu, Y, Zhou, D, Yang, S, Huo, Y, Liu, Y, Safdar, B and Bu, X. 2023. The SWGEDWGEIW from soybean peptides reduces insulin resistance in 3T3-L1 adipocytes by activating p-Akt/GLUT4 signaling pathway. Molecules. March 28 28(7):3001. https://doi.org/10.3390/molecules28073001

Zani, SC, Wu, J and Chan, CB. 2018. Egg and soy-derived peptides and hydrolysates: a review of their physiological actions against diabetes and obesity. *Nutrients* 10(5):1–15. https://doi.org/10.3390/nu10050549

Zhang, Y, Zhou, F, Zhao, M, Ning, Z, Sun-Waterhouse, D and Sun, B. 2017. Soy peptide aggregates formed during hydrolysis reduced protein extraction without decreasing their nutritional value. *Food & Function* 8(12):4384–4395. https://doi.org/10.1039/C7FO00812K

Zheng, Y, Ley, SH and Hu, FB. 2018. Global etiology and epidemiology of type 2 diabetes mellitus and its complications. *Nat Rev Endocrinol* 14(2):88–98. https://doi.org/10.1038/nrendo.2017.151

Zuo, X, Zhao, R, Wu, M, Wan, Q and Li, T. 2023. Soy consumption and the risk of type 2 diabetes and cardiovascular diseases: a systematic review and meta-analysis. *Nutrients* 15(6):1–18. https://doi.org/10.3390/nu15061358

Wen, L, Jiang, Y, Zhou, X Bi, H and Yang, B. 2021. Structure identification of soybean peptides and their immunomodulatory activity. *Food Chem* 359:129970. https://doi.org/10.1016/j.foodchem.2021.129970

Winham, DM, Thompson, SV, Heer, MM, David, ED, Hooper, SD and Cichy, KA, 2022. Refeições de massa de feijão preto ST com concentrações variadas de proteínas reduzem a glicemia pós-prandial e a insulina da mesma forma em comparação com o controle de pão branco em adultos. *Alimentos* 11(1652):1–17.

World Health Organization. 2019. *Classification of Diabetes Mellitus*. Geneva: Licence: CC BY-NC-SA 3.0 IGO.

26 Soybean Proteins and Effects on Atherosclerosis

Modelling in ApoE Deficiency

Roberto Martínez-Beamonte, María Angeles Navarro, José M. Lou-Bonafonte, and Jesús Osada

ABBREVIATIONS

Apo	Apolipoprotein
ApoE	Apolipoprotein E
BCAA	Branched-chain amino acids
βCG	Beta-conglycinin
CETP	Cholesteryl ester transfer protein
CAS	Casein
ER	Oestrogen receptor
HDL	High-density lipoproteins
ICAM-1	Intercellular adhesion molecule-1
IFN-γ	Interferon-gamma
I-κB	Inhibitor of kappa B
IL-6	Interleukin 6
IL-1β	Interleukin 1β
IL-17A	Interleukin 17A
LDL	Low-density lipoprotein
LPS	Lipopolysaccharide
LSW	Tripeptide containing Leu-Ser-Trp
LY96	Restricting lymphocyte antigen 96
MCP-1	Monocyte chemoattractant protein
miRNA-145	Micro ribonucleic acid 145
NF-κB	Nuclear factor-kappa B
NO	Nitric oxide
OX40	Tumour necrosis factor receptor superfamily member 4
SPI	Soy protein isolate
TAG	Triacylglycerol
TNF-α	Tumour necrosis factor-alpha
VCAM-1	Vascular cell adhesion molecule-1
VLDL	Very-low-density lipoprotein

DOI: 10.1201/9781003597926-26

INTRODUCTION

Atherosclerosis

As a chronic disease, atherosclerosis serves as a common pathogenic basis for several cardiovascular diseases. In humans, it is a multifactorial, long-term process in which plasma lipoproteins and environmental factors such as cigarette smoking, diet, air pollution, and environmental stress play an important role in its development (Osada, Joven, and Maeda 2000). Inflammation has been added to the traditional risk factors, together with the properties of arterial wall cells and their interactions with the coagulation cascade through thrombotic events (Figure 26.1). These are all current hallmarks of atherosclerotic development (Libby 2021; Bonacina et al. 2023).

The period of atherogenesis in humans is very long, making it virtually impossible to test the influence of all diets and their components on the process in a timely manner. Accordingly, animal models exhibiting more rapid changes can be useful for studying this process, and their use in preclinical research remains essential for understanding this and other pathologies (Mukherjee, Roy, Ghosh, and Nandi 2022). The more criteria a model meets in terms of development time, characteristics of the pathological process, genetics of the species, size of offspring, cost, and handling, the more relevant it will be (Osada, Joven, and Maeda 2000).

Apolipoprotein E-Deficient Mice

Apolipoprotein E (ApoE) is a component of all plasma lipoproteins except low-density lipoproteins (LDLs). Its presence is critical for the clearance of chylomicron and very-low-density lipoprotein (VLDL) remnants. Therefore, defective binding or absence of ApoE has been associated with the development of atherosclerosis (Hofker, van Vlijmen, and Havekes 1998). For this reason, three independent research groups generated ApoE-deficient mice (Plump et al. 1992; Zhang, Reddick, Piedrahita, and Maeda 1992; van Ree et al. 1994). These mice show impaired clearance of remnant plasma lipoproteins and consequently have plasma cholesterol levels five times higher than those of wild-type mice when fed a chow diet of 4% fat and 0.01% (w/w) cholesterol (Plump et al. 1992; Zhang, Reddick, Piedrahita, and Maeda 1992; van Ree et al. 1994). On the same diet and as early as 3 months after birth, they also develop spontaneous atherosclerosis at the base of the aorta, which spreads along the aorta and preferentially at the origin of its branching vessels. The initial fatty streak lesions observed progress with age or diet to a fibro-proliferative intermediate lesion and the formation of a fibrous cap, similar to the human process (Nakashima et al. 1994; Reddick, Zhang, and Maeda 1994; Tamminen et al. 1999) (Table 26.1).

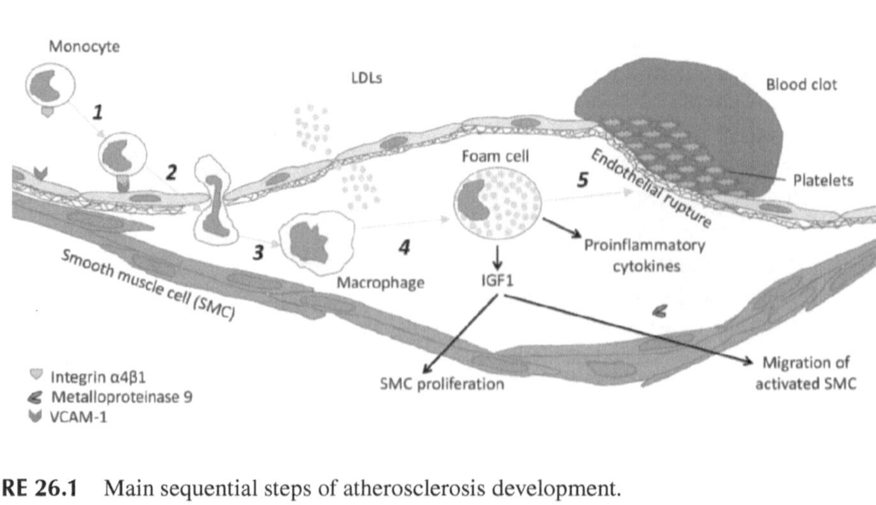

FIGURE 26.1 Main sequential steps of atherosclerosis development.

TABLE 26.1
Phenotype of ApoE-Deficient Mice

Diet	Plasma	Vascular Bed
Chow diet (4% fat, 0.01% w/w cholesterol)	Hypercholesterolaemia: 5× levels of wild-type mice	At 3 months: spontaneous atherosclerosis (fatty streak) at base of aorta, pulmonary and innominate arteries, and origin of branching vessels. After 8 months: lesions progress to a fibro-proliferative stage with fibrous cap formation.
Western diet (20% fat, 0.15% w/w cholesterol)	Hypercholesterolaemia: 13× levels of wild-type mice	Rapid development of atherosclerotic features in less than 5 months.

Adapted from Nakashima et al. (1994); Reddick, Zhang, and Maeda (1994); Tamminen et al. (1999).

All these features make this an excellent model for gaining insight into the human process, and its use has allowed researchers to scrutinise the effects of dietary components and the putative mechanisms by which they may act (Osada, Joven, and Maeda 2000; Imaizumi 2011).

Soy Protein Fraction

Soybean seeds are organically extracted to produce oil and soybean cake. Drying and grinding produces soybean flour (50% protein), which can be treated with alcohol or water to remove carbohydrates and produce soy protein concentrate (70% protein). Then, removing fibre and insoluble carbohydrates by a precipitation step produces soy protein isolate (90% protein) (Preece, Hooshyar, and Zuidam 2017).

Ultracentrifugation separates soy proteins into four major groups known as the 2S, 7S, 11S, and 15S fractions (Table 26.2).

The 2S fraction represents 20% of the soy protein and contains proteins such as albumin, 2S globulin, cytochrome C, and Kunitz and Bowman–Birk protease inhibitors. The 7S fraction is also heterogeneous and contains β-conglycinin (βCG), α-amylase, lipoxygenase, and haemagglutinin. The 11S fraction contains only glycinin. Glycinin (11S-globulin) and β-conglycinin (7S-globulin) make up 70–80% of the total protein. The 15S fraction is a minor component accounting for 10% of the soy protein and is considered to be a dimer of glycinin (Sui, Zhang, and Jiang 2021). Depending on the proteins present, the digestibility may vary (Qin, Wang, and Luo 2022), and a lower ratio of glycinin: β-conglycinin favours better LDL homeostasis in vitro (Rebollo-Hernanz, Bringe, and de Mejia 2023). In addition, some peptides, ranging from 2 to 20 amino acids in length, become bioactive when released from their original proteins (Chatterjee, Gleddie, and Xiao 2018).

Other Compounds May Be Present in Soy Protein Fraction

There are several methods for extracting soy protein, such as alkaline, acid, enzyme-assisted, NaCl-assisted, and, more recently, basic or acid electroactivation (Ovando, Rodríguez-Sifuentes, Martínez, and Chuck-Hernández 2022). Little attention has been paid to the chemical composition of the bioactive compounds in soy protein extracts after different processing methods. This is particularly relevant for isoflavones, phytosterols (Nakai, Fujita, and Kamei 2020), or hydrolysed peptides and their chemical modifications (Chatterjee, Gleddie, and Xiao 2018).

TABLE 26.2
Major Groups of Soy Proteins by Ultracentrifugation Preparation

Fraction	Percentage	Main Protein Constituents
2S	20%	Albumin, 2S globulin, cytochrome C, and Kunitz and Bowman–Birk protease inhibitors
7S	40%	β-conglycinin (βCG), α-amylase, lipoxygenase, and haemagglutinin
11S	30%	Glycinin
15S	10%	Glycinin dimer

Source: Adapted from Sui, Zhang, and Jiang (2021).

DIETARY SOY PROTEIN AND ATHEROSCLEROSIS IN APOLIPOPROTEIN E-DEFICIENT MICE

Pioneering work by Ni et al. investigated the effects of protein source on the development of atherosclerotic lesions (Ni, Tsuda, Sakono, and Imaizumi 1998). The authors used male ApoE-deficient mice on the C57BL/6J genetic background, feeding them purified diets containing 1% cholesterol and 0.25% cholate and soy protein isolate or casein, depending on the experimental group, for 6 weeks. They observed no changes in serum total cholesterol concentration but found lower thoracic aortic lesions in the soy protein group compared to the casein group. When they repeated the experiments with cholesterol- and cholate-deficient diets for longer periods (9 and 24 weeks), they observed no changes in serum total cholesterol or homocysteine concentrations between the soy protein isolate and casein-fed groups and confirmed the previous finding regarding thoracic aortic lesions. Adding an ethanol extract of soy protein to the casein-containing diet abolished these differences when compared with the ethanol-extracted soy protein isolate diet. These results indicate that the antiatherogenic effect of soy protein isolate was independent of plasma lipids or homocysteine, but they could not distinguish whether the effect was due to the protein component or to the ethanol-extracted soy protein isolate (Ni, Tsuda, Sakono, and Imaizumi 1998).

Researchers used ApoE-deficient mice or mice lacking LDL receptors and overproducing apolipoprotein B to compare the effects of dietary soy protein (total isoflavone content of 1.72 mg/g) and alcohol-washed soy protein isolate (total isoflavones equal to 0.04 mg/g) with casein/lactalbumin as a control diet. Both the alcohol-washed and the intact soy protein isolate diets showed reduced atherosclerosis in both groups of mice compared to the control group. The anti-atherosclerotic effect was more pronounced in LDL receptor-deficient, apoB-overproducing mice compared to ApoE-deficient mice and less pronounced in mice receiving alcohol-washed soy protein isolate. Atherosclerotic changes were not related to plasma LDL, VLDL, or HDL cholesterol concentrations. These results provide further evidence that dietary soy protein isolate inhibits atherosclerosis independently of plasma lipoproteins (Adams, Golden, Anthony et al. 2002) and highlight the additional effect of soy isoflavones.

The effect of certain soy fractions or peptides on the development of atherosclerosis was also studied in the same groups of mice fed with casein/lactalbumin, isoflavone-containing soy protein isolate, β-conglycinin, glycinin (11S-globulin), β-conglycinin-depleted soy protein, or a peptide fraction produced by hydrolysis and precipitation of soy protein isolate. All soy protein-containing diets reduced atherosclerosis compared to the group fed a casein/lactalbumin-based diet. Only the β-conglycinin-containing diet reduced atherosclerosis compared to the isoflavone-containing soy protein isolate diet. These changes were not associated with variation in isoflavone content and only minimally related to plasma lipoproteins. These results suggest that β-conglycinin is responsible for the atheroprotective effects, which are not ascribable to plasma lipoproteins (Adams et al. 2004) (Figure 26.2). When Ishihara et al. used an amino acid mixture simulating dietary soy protein in KK-Ay mice, they observed an increased postprandial energy metabolism compared to those receiving a mixture simulating casein (Ishihara et al. 2003). Studies on the effects of soy β-conglycinin (7S-globulin) and glycinin (11S-globulin) on serum lipid levels and liver metabolism in normal (ICR) and genetically obese (KK-Ay) mice showed lower serum triglyceride, glucose, and insulin levels were lower in beta-conglycinin-fed mice than in casein- and glycinin-fed mice of both strains. The soy beta-conglycinin diet reduced serum TAG levels by accelerating beta-oxidation, suppressing fatty acid synthase and/or increasing faecal TAG excretion, and also reduced serum glucose and insulin levels. Thus, soy beta-conglycinin may offer a potentially useful dietary protein source for preventing hypertriglyceridaemia, hyperinsulinaemia, and hyperglycaemia (Moriyama et al. 2004). These findings suggest that amino acids or specific soy protein fractions alone may be responsible for the observed atherosclerotic findings, independently of plasma cholesterol or its transport in lipoproteins.

To investigate the atheroprotective effect of soy phyto-oestrogenic isoflavones through oestrogen receptor-dependent processes and determine which oestrogen receptor subtype (α or β) might be involved, researchers crossed ApoE-deficient mice with oestrogen receptor α- or β-deficient mice, comparing these double mutants to apolipoprotein E-deficient mice. They fed these groups of mice two different diets for 16 weeks: one enriched in soy protein with a low isoflavone content and one with a high isoflavone content. The high isoflavone diet reduced atherosclerosis in double mutant mice lacking ApoE and oestrogen receptor β and in ApoE-deficient mice, but not in double ApoE and oestrogen receptor α-deficient mice (Figure 26.2).

These results suggest that oestrogen receptor α mediates the effect of soy isoflavones on the development of atherosclerosis, independent of plasma total, VLDL, LDL, and HDL cholesterol concentrations (Adams, Golden, Register et al. 2002). When this experiment was carried out in other experimental backgrounds, such as ovariectomised mice heterozygous for the human CETP transgene and deficient for the LDL receptor, soy protein-containing isoflavones did not modify aortic atherosclerotic lesions (Asakura et al. 2006). Therefore, the genetic background represents an important aspect of these actions. A role for sex in the susceptibility to the development of atherosclerosis was also found when comparing ApoE-deficient mice receiving Western diets with different protein sources (Martínez-Beamonte et al. 2021). In summary, genetic background and sex are important modulators of responses.

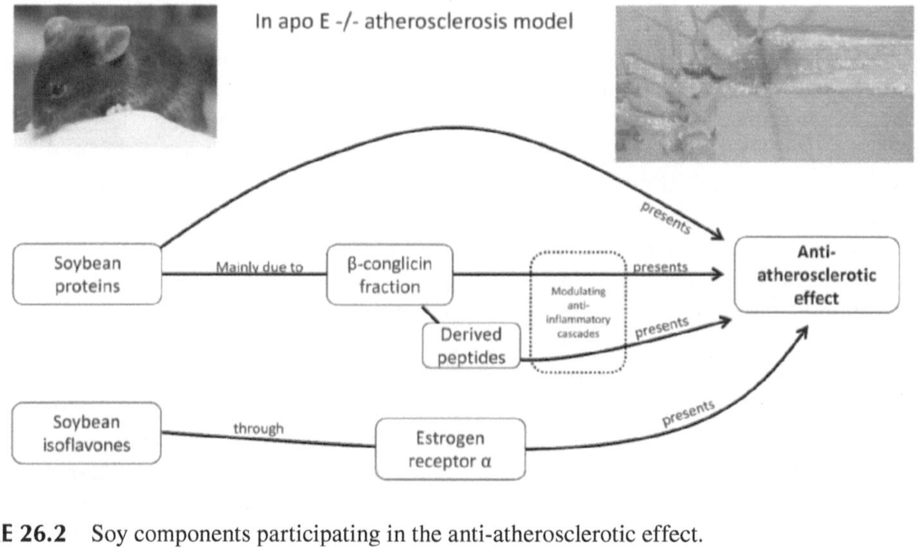

FIGURE 26.2 Soy components participating in the anti-atherosclerotic effect.

Although unrelated to soy protein, it is worth mentioning the influence of branched-chain amino acids (BCAA) on the development of atherosclerosis since soy protein is relatively poor in these amino acids (Martínez-Beamonte et al. 2021). Their influence was tested using a high-fat diet supplemented with BCAA. ApoE-deficient mice fed this diet showed reduced atherosclerotic lesion areas and significantly decreased total serum and LDL cholesterol levels compared to mice fed the high-fat diet. The supplemented diet also reduced macrophage infiltration and serum levels of inflammatory factors such as monocyte chemoattractant protein-1 (MCP-1), tumour necrosis factor-α (TNF-α), interleukin-1β (IL-1β), and interleukin-6 (IL-6). In addition, the BCAA supplementation influenced the gut microbiota by reducing harmful bacteria, promoting bile acid excretion, and increasing cecal and colonic levels of primary 12α- and non-12α-hydroxylated bile acids (Li et al. 2022).

L-arginine, well represented in soy protein (Martínez-Beamonte et al. 2021), serves as a substrate for the formation of nitric oxide (NO) by the NO synthase (NOS) enzymes. Dietary supplementation with L-arginine has been shown to reduce atherosclerosis by restoring NO release (Böger et al. 1997). Other authors have shown that L-arginine supplementation at 25 g/L had no effect on lesion formation in Western chow-fed ApoE-deficient mice but abolished the protective effect of inducible NOS gene deficiency. This was associated with an increase in thiobarbituric acid-reactive malondialdehyde adducts, nitrotyrosine staining within lesions, and a decrease in the ratio of reduced tetrahydrobiopterin to total biopterins (Chen et al. 2003). This suggests a proatherogenic effect of L-arginine supplementation via mechanisms involving lipid oxidation, peroxynitrite formation, and NOS uncoupling. It is clear that certain isolated amino acids may not reflect the complexity of soybean proteins.

As shown in Table 26.3, despite all the different experimental approaches, soy protein consistently demonstrates an anti-atherosclerotic effect of soy protein compared with casein or casein/lactalbumin. The absence of changes in plasma lipids was also a consistent finding.

DIETARY SOY PROTEIN AND INFLAMMATION

As mentioned above, an isoflavone-free soy protein diet has been shown to reduce atherosclerotic lesions in a hyperlipidaemic mouse model compared to casein-fed mice despite unchanged serum lipid levels. As inflammation is a component of atherosclerosis, its contribution to the athero-protective effect of isoflavone-free soy protein was explored in ApoE-deficient mice fed this diet or a casein-containing diet and then challenged with LPS. The isoflavone-free soy protein-containing diet significantly reduced aortic VCAM-1 mRNA and protein expression compared to casein-fed mice (Figure 26.3).

This effect was also observed in LPS-treated mice, accompanied by reduced monocyte adhesion to the vascular endothelium. The isoflavone-free soy protein diet also inhibited LPS-induced NF-κB activation and upregulation of its pro-inflammatory cytokines (TNF-α, IL-6, IL-1β, and MCP-1) (Figure 26.3). NF-κB activation was blocked by phosphorylation of I-κB and activation of protein kinase B, without involvement of mitogen-activated protein kinase. Researchers also investigated in vitro incubation of human vascular endothelial cells with soy peptides, two of which (KNPQLR and EITPEKNPQLR, both from the α- and β-subunits of β-conglycinin) strikingly reproduced the anti-inflammatory effect (Burris, Ng, and Nagarajan 2014). These results demonstrate that soy protein and certain peptides may modulate anti-inflammatory cascades, thus explaining the observed reduction in atherosclerosis.

The effects of isoflavones on atherosclerosis were studied in ApoE-deficient mice subjected to ovarian resection. Feeding ovariectomised mice an isoflavone-containing diet reduced the size of atherosclerotic lesions, aortic MCP-I expression, and NO secretion by in vitro macrophages compared to an isoflavone-free diet. No effect on plasma cholesterol was observed (Sato et al. 2007). Dietary isoflavones show an antiatherogenic effect by preventing macrophage activation following ovariectomy.

TABLE 26.3
Effects of Soy-Containing Diets on Atherosclerosis In ApoE-Deficient Mice

Study Characteristics	Experimental Details	Atherosclerotic Outcomes	Plasma Lipids	Analysis of Plaque Composition	Other Atherosclerotic Components	Reference
Model: ApoE-deficient **Sex:** Both **Diet:** Basal* or 1% cholesterol + 0.25% cholate **Protein:** 20%	Cross-sectional and *en face* analyses	Decreased in soy group vs. casein	No change	Yes	No	Ni et al. (1998)
Model: ApoE-deficient **Sex:** Males, ovariectomised females **Diet:** Basal + 0.15% cholesterol **Protein:** 20% + methionine	Aortic cholesterol content	Decreased with soy protein vs. casein/lactoalbumin	No change	No	No	Adams, Golden, Anthony, et al. (2002)
Model: ApoE-deficient **Sex:** Males, ovariectomised females **Diet:** Basal + 0.15% cholesterol **Protein:** 20% + methionine	Aortic cholesterol content	Decreased with soy protein and β-conglycinin vs. casein/lactoalbumin	No change	No	No	Adams et al. (2004)
Model: ApoE-deficient × ERα- or ERβ-deficient **Sex:** Males, ovariectomised females **Diet:** Basal **Protein:** 20% + methionine + isoflavones	Aortic cholesterol content	ERα mediates soy isoflavone effect	No change	No	No	Adams, Golden, Register, et al. (2002)

(*Continued*)

TABLE 26.3 (CONTINUED)
Effects of Soy-Containing Diets on Atherosclerosis In ApoE-Deficient Mice

Study Characteristics	Experimental Details	Atherosclerotic Outcomes	Plasma Lipids	Analysis of Plaque Composition	Other Atherosclerotic Components	Reference
Model: ApoE-deficient **Sex:** Males **Diet:** Basal + 0.05% cholesterol + 20% lard/butter **Protein:** 23%	*En face* analysis	Decreased in soy group vs. casein	Not analysed	No	Yes	Sawashita et al. (2006)
Model: ApoE-deficient **Sex:** Ovariectomised females **Diet:** Basal* **Protein:** 20%	Cross-sectional analysis	Decreased in isoflavone group vs. casein	No change	No	Yes	Sato et al. (2007)
Model: ApoE-deficient **Sex:** Females **Diet:** Basal* **Protein:** 20%	Cross-sectional and *en face* analyses	Decreased in soy group vs. casein; isoflavones enhance effect	No change	Yes	Yes	Nagarajan et al. (2008)
Model: ApoE-deficient **Sex:** Females **Diet:** Basal* **Protein:** 20%	Cross-sectional analysis	Smallest lesion area with soy + exercise	No change	No	Uraemia-associated CVD	Tomayko et al. (2011)
Model: ApoE-deficient **Sex:** Females **Diet:** Basal* **Protein:** 20%	Monocyte adhesion, VCAM-1, mRNA	Soy protein/peptides may prevent chronic inflammation in atherosclerosis	No change	Yes	Inflammatory cytokines	Burris et al. (2014)
Model: ApoE-deficient **Sex:** Males, females **Diet:** Basal + 0.15% cholesterol + 20% palm fat **Protein:** 11%	Cross-sectional and *en face* analyses	Soy comparable to avian proteins; sex modifies response	No change	Yes	Paraoxonase activity	Martínez-Beamonte et al. (2021)

*Basal diet composition was based on the AIN-93G formulation (Reeves, Rossow, and Lindlauf 1993), except that the source of 10% fat was olive oil.

ER, oestrogen receptor; VCAM-1, vascular cell adhesion molecule 1.

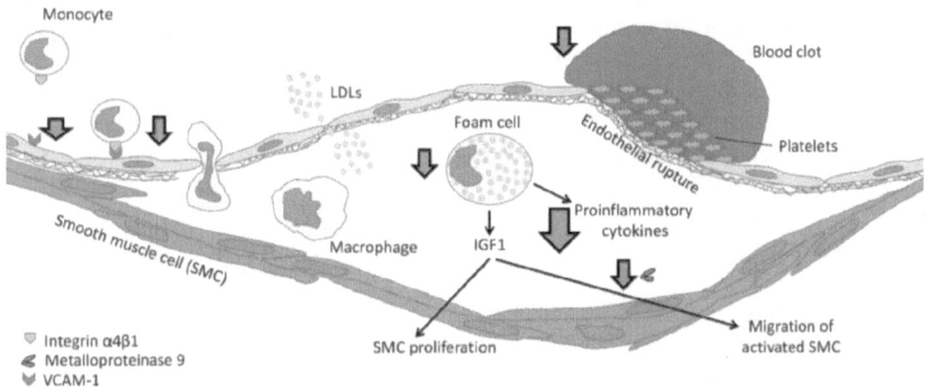

FIGURE 26.3 Atherosclerosis setting and action of soy proteins.

Comparing soy protein isolates with or without phytochemicals to casein-containing diets in ApoE-deficient mice revealed reduced atherosclerotic lesions in the aortic sinus and *en face* analyses of the descending aorta. The inclusion of phytochemicals further reduced the observed lesions. The atheroprotective effect of the soy-based diet was independent of plasma lipid profiles, suggesting alternative mechanisms. To investigate the inflammatory component of atherosclerosis, the authors examined the expression of monocyte chemoattractant protein-1 and the number of macrophages in the proximal aorta, finding that both parameters were reduced in mice fed both soy-based diets compared to casein-fed mice (Figure 26.3). When they incubated macrophages in vitro with soy isoflavones (genistein, daidzein, and equol alone or in combination) at different doses, lipopolysaccharide-induced MCP-1 secretion was inhibited in a dose-dependent manner. In light of these results, the reduction in atherosclerotic lesions observed in mice fed the soy-based diet may be due to inhibition of MCP-1, which could result in reduced monocyte migration, an early event in atherogenesis (Nagarajan et al. 2008).

The effects of isolated genistein were also investigated in ApoE-deficient mice fed an atherogenic diet containing this isoflavone at doses of 15 and 45 mg/kg/day. In a dose-dependent manner, genistein significantly reduced atherosclerotic plaque formation and serum levels of pro-inflammatory cytokines (IL-1β, IL-6, IL-17A, IFN-γ, and TNF-α). It also promoted plaque stability by reducing necrotic core areas in atherosclerotic lesions and metalloproteinase-9 protein expression in primary smooth muscle cells. In addition, genistein reduced the increased expression of tumour necrosis factor receptor superfamily member 4 (OX40) in blood and spleen mononuclear cells induced by the atherogenic diet (Wei et al. 2019). Thus, genistein itself has an important anti-atherosclerotic effect by modulating inflammatory cells through the OX40 pathway. In conclusion, isoflavone-free soy protein reduced the inflammatory response, enhanced by the inclusion of isoflavones, which also showed this effect *per se*.

SOY PROTEIN CONSUMPTION AND THROMBOSIS

The intertwined links between atherosclerosis and thrombosis have led authors to speak of a single entity called atherothrombosis (Libby 2021; Bonacina et al. 2023).

With this in mind, the effect of long-term consumption of purified vegetable and animal proteins (casein, pork, egg white, chicken, white and red fish, soybean, and potato) and powders of whole vegetable and animal meats (soybean, pork, chicken, and horse mackerel) on thrombotic tendency was studied in ApoE and low-density lipoprotein receptor-deficient mice. Both mice types were fed a Western-style high-fat diet with different protein sources for more than 8 months, and their thrombotic tendency was monitored via an *in vivo* assay. There was no difference in thrombotic tendency between the vegetable and animal protein diets, except for pork protein, which had a prothrombotic effect. This effect was not observed in animals fed a high-protein diet. The thrombotic tendency was not affected by the preparation of dietary powders from whole pork, chicken, or horse mackerel meat and casein as a control, all containing the same percentages of protein and lipid. In contrast, soy powder showed an antithrombotic effect (Figure 26.3), mainly attributed to inhibition of atherogenesis rather than platelet inhibition (Sawashita et al. 2006). Further studies are needed to clarify this aspect.

SOY PROTEIN CONSUMPTION AND EXERCISE IN CHRONIC KIDNEY DISEASE

Chronic kidney disease is a risk factor for cardiovascular disease (Moe and Chen 2004) and fractures (Moe et al. 2006). Researchers simulated the benefits of soy protein consumption and exercise training on these risk factors in chronic kidney disease patients using ApoE-deficient mice that underwent a surgical procedure to induce uraemia.

These mice were randomly assigned to one of four experimental groups that received a control diet or a diet containing soy protein and exercised or did not exercise. The intervention did not alter atherosclerotic lesion areas or calcium deposits in the aorta. However, both diet and exercise significantly increased relative bone volume, trabecular number, and trabecular density, decreased trabecular separation, and did not change trabecular thickness in the proximal femur. The soy diet alone decreased plasma urea levels (Tomayko, Chung, and Wilund 2011). Thus, soy protein intake and exercise training have a synergistic effect on bone properties in mice with renal failure.

EFFECT OF SOYBEAN PROTEIN-DERIVED PEPTIDES

New findings in cell culture deserve a few comments. First, the soybean protein tripeptide Leu-Ser-Trp (LSW), originally identified as a potent inhibitor of angiotensin-converting enzyme, has been reported to exert a protective effect against angiotensin II-induced endothelial dysfunction (Song et al. 2021). Recently, incubation with extracellular vesicles released from LSW-treated vascular smooth muscle cells attenuated oxidised low-density lipoprotein-induced endothelial dysfunction in vascular endothelial cells. These extracellular vesicles were particularly enriched for miRNA-145 (Song et al. 2022). It is therefore tempting to suggest that this miRNA may modulate the effect of the LSW tripeptide on endothelial dysfunction. As mentioned above, a direct effect of soy peptides (KNPQLR and EITPEKNPQLR, both from the α- and β-subunits of β-conglycinin) was found to reduce the inflammatory effect in human vascular endothelial cells (Burris, Ng, and Nagarajan 2014).

The second line of research involves the effect of soy protein-derived peptides on the inhibition of lipopolysaccharide (LPS)-induced changes in inflammatory cells. Indeed, soy protein-derived peptides inhibited the release of pro-inflammatory cytokines (TNF-α, IL-6, and IL-1β) induced by LPS incubation of the murine macrophage cell line RAW264.7. The proposed mechanisms for this finding include an increase in toll-like receptor 4 activity by limiting lymphocyte antigen 96 (LY96), inhibition of the mitogen-activated protein kinase c-Jun N-terminal kinase pathway in cells, degradation of nuclear factor of kappa light polypeptide gene enhancer in B cells inhibitor, alpha (IκBβ), and blockade of NF-κB activation (Yi et al. 2020).

As both endothelial dysfunction and inflammation are involved in atherosclerosis, further research into these peptides' potential application is warranted. Compared to soy protein, the derived peptides are more soluble and absorbable, making their use as dietary supplements for the treatment of chronic diseases more feasible.

SOYBEAN PREPARATIONS

The field is not limited to current soybeans but is also open to the discovery of new varieties and their potential, along with innovative processing. Yak-Kong is a small black Korean soybean that has been shown to contain higher concentrations of antioxidants than green or yellow soybeans (Lee et al. 2017). Fermented derived Yak-Kong showed increased antioxidant capacity due to increased p-coumaric acid. Furthermore, this fermented Yak-Kong extract significantly inhibited lipopolysaccharide-induced THP-1 monocyte–endothelial cell adhesion and suppressed vascular cell adhesion molecule (VCAM-1) expression in human umbilical vein endothelial cells (Kim et al. 2019). These new cultivars and technological formulations may provide improved ways to enhance the anti-atherosclerotic potential of soybeans and merit new studies.

THE EFFECTS OF OTHER PROTEINS

The effect of whey protein on atherosclerosis has also been studied in ApoE-deficient mice. Zhang et al. analysed the effect of this protein source at two levels (10 or 20%, w/w of the diet) in males of this genetic background fed a high-fat/cholesterol diet for 18 weeks. Despite no changes in body weight or food consumption among the groups studied, the whey protein-supplemented groups showed reduced hepatic steatosis. Similarly, whey protein supplementation was associated with a dose-dependent reduction in aortic atherosclerotic lesions both en face and cross-sectionally. At the same time, serum high-density lipoprotein cholesterol levels increased. The highest concentration of whey protein decreased serum levels of pro-inflammatory cytokine (interleukin-6) and increased levels of anti-inflammatory cytokine (interleukin-10). Decreased levels of NF-κB in the liver and aorta were also observed (Zhang et al. 2018).

Recently, Wang et al. tested the effect of whey protein hydrolysate (WPH) on atherosclerosis and fatty liver in these mice fed a Western diet for 15 weeks. They also found it inhibited the development of aortic atherosclerosis and reduced fatty liver severity. The WPH-fed group showed reduced plasma lipids and inflammatory markers. These authors also found that this group of mice had reduced expression of genes involved in cholesterol biosynthesis and increased expression of those involved in hepatic secretion and uptake. They also observed an increased ratio of n-3/n-6 polyunsaturated fatty acids in both serum and liver (Wang et al. 2022). Both studies suggest that whey protein supplementation improves atherosclerosis independent of diet.

Martínez-Beamonte et al. studied the effect of avian (chicken and turkey) proteins on atherosclerosis and fatty liver disease in this experimental model fed purified Western diets with different protein sources for 12 weeks. They observed sex differences in the response. Specifically, females consuming the turkey protein diet showed reduced *en face* atherosclerosis. The anti-atherosclerotic activity of paraoxonase increased in the latter group (Martínez-Beamonte et al. 2021). These results indicate that the influence of protein source on atherosclerosis is a fertile area of research and that researchers should include sex as a factor in studies.

MINI DICTIONARY OF TERMS

- **C57BL/6J:** Strain of mice employed in metabolic studies.
- **Cross-sectional:** Lipid staining of transverse sections of the aorta and quantification of areas.
- ***En face*:** Lipid staining of whole dissected aorta and quantification of areas.
- **Intercellular adhesion molecule-1 (ICAM-1):** Endothelial molecule involved in recruitment of monocytes.
- **Institute of Cancer Research (ICR):** Strain of albino mice.
- **KK-Ay:** Mouse strain with metabolic abnormalities useful for diabetes and obesity research.
- **Nuclear factor-kappa B (NF-κB):** A transcription factor involved in the activation of the inflammatory response.

- **Restricting lymphocyte antigen 96 (LY96):** Protein associated with toll-like receptor 4 on the cell membrane involved in responsiveness to lipopolysaccharide.
- **THP-1:** An immortalised monocyte cell line.
- **Vascular cell adhesion molecule-1 (VCAM-1):** An endothelial molecule involved in the recruitment of monocytes.

SUMMARY POINTS

- In ApoE-deficient mice, soybean proteins display anti-atherosclerotic effects, which are mainly due to β-conglycinin and some specific peptides.
- This effect is reinforced by the presence of isoflavones.
- The anti-atherosclerotic properties were independent of plasma lipoproteins.
- Soybean protein and its derived peptides have shown anti-inflammatory and immunoregulatory properties.
- The existence of natural or engineered soybean varieties with enhanced anti-atherosclerotic potential may be a fertile aspect of research. Likewise, the development of technological formulations to reinforce these properties.

ACKNOWLEDGEMENTS

The research of this group was funded by grants from *Ministerio de Ciencia e Innovación* (MCIN/AEI/10.13039/501100011033, PID2019-104915RB-I00 and PID2022-104915RB-I00), "ERDF A way of making Europe," the European Union, and the *Fondo Social Europeo-Gobierno de Aragón* (B16_23R). CIBER *de Fisiopatología de la Obesidad y Nutrición* (CIBEROBN, CB06/03/1012) is an initiative of FEDER-ISCIII.

REFERENCES

Adams, M. R., D. L. Golden, M. S. Anthony, T. C. Register, and J. K. Williams. 2002. "The inhibitory effect of soy protein isolate on atherosclerosis in mice does not require the presence of LDL receptors or alteration of plasma lipoproteins." *J Nutr* 132 (1):43–9. doi: 10.1093/jn/132.1.43.

Adams, M. R., D. L. Golden, A. A. Franke, S. M. Potter, H. S. Smith, and M. S. Anthony. 2004. "Dietary soy beta-conglycinin (7S Globulin) inhibits atherosclerosis in mice." *J Nutr* 34 (3):511–6. doi: 10.1093/jn/134.3.511.

Adams, M. R., D. L. Golden, T. C. Register, M. S. Anthony, J. B. Hodgin, N. Maeda, and J. K. Williams. 2002. "The atheroprotective effect of dietary soy isoflavones in apolipoprotein E-/- mice requires the presence of estrogen receptor-alpha." *Arterioscler Thromb Vasc Biol* 22 (11):1859–64. doi: 10.1161/01.atv.0000042202.42136.d0.

Asakura, L., P. M. Cazita, L. M. Harada, V. S. Nunes, J. A. Berti, A. G. Salerno, D. F. Ketelhuth, M. Gidlund, H. C. Oliveira, and E. C. Quintao. 2006. "Soy protein containing isoflavones favorably influences macrophage lipoprotein metabolism but not the development of atherosclerosis in CETP transgenic mice." *Lipids* 41 (7):655–62. doi: 10.1007/s11745-006-5016-7.

Böger, R. H., S. M. Bode-Böger, R. P. Brandes, L. Phivthong-ngam, M. Böhme, R. Nafe, A. Mügge, and J. C. Frölich. 1997. "Dietary L-arginine reduces the progression of atherosclerosis in cholesterol-fed rabbits: comparison with lovastatin." *Circulation* 96 (4):1282–90. doi: 10.1161/01.cir.96.4.1282.

Bonacina, F., A. Di Costanzo, V. Genkel, X. Y. Kong, J. Kroon, E. Stimjanin, D. Tsiantoulas, and M. O. Grootaert. 2023. "The heterogeneous cellular landscape of atherosclerosis: Implications for future research and therapies. A collaborative review from the EAS young fellows." *Atherosclerosis* 372:48–56. doi: 10.1016/j.atherosclerosis.2023.03.021.

Burris, R. L., H. P. Ng, and S. Nagarajan. 2014. "Soy protein inhibits inflammation-induced VCAM-1 and inflammatory cytokine induction by inhibiting the NF-kappaB and AKT signaling pathway in apolipoprotein E-deficient mice." *Eur J Nutr* 53 (1):135–48. doi: 10.1007/s00394-013-0509-7.

Chatterjee, Cynthia, Stephen Gleddie, and Chao-Wu Xiao. 2018. "Soybean bioactive peptides and their functional properties." *Nutrients* 10 (9):1211. doi: 10.3390/nu10091211.

Chen, J., P. Kuhlencordt, F. Urano, H. Ichinose, J. Astern, and P. L. Huang. 2003. "Effects of chronic treatment with L-arginine on atherosclerosis in apoE knockout and apoE/inducible NO synthase double-knockout mice." *Arterioscler Thromb Vasc Biol* 23 (1):97–103. doi: 10.1161/01.atv.0000040223.74255.5a.

Hofker, M. H., B. J. van Vlijmen, and L. M. Havekes. 1998. "Transgenic mouse models to study the role of APOE in hyperlipidemia and atherosclerosis." *Atherosclerosis* 137 (1):1–11. doi: 10.1016/s0021-9150(97)00266-9.

Imaizumi, K. 2011. "Diet and atherosclerosis in apolipoprotein E-deficient mice." *Biosci Biotechnol Biochem* 75 (6):1023–35. doi: 10.1271/bbb.110059.

Ishihara, K., Y. Fukuchi, W. Mizunoya, Y. Mita, Y. Fukuya, T. Fushiki, and K. Yasumoto. 2003. "Amino acid composition of soybean protein increased postprandial carbohydrate oxidation in diabetic mice." *Biosci Biotechnol Biochem* 67 (12):2505–11. doi: 10.1271/bbb.67.2505.

Kim, J. S., J. H. Kim, S. A. Palaniyandi, C. C. Lee, J. W. You, H. Yang, J. H. Yoon Park, S. H. Yang, and K. W. Lee. 2019. "Yak-Kong soybean (Glycine max) fermented by a novel pediococcus pentosaceus inhibits the oxidative stress-induced monocyte-endothelial cell adhesion." *Nutrients* 11 (6). doi: 10.3390/nu11061380.

Lee, Charles C., Stéphanie Dudonné, Pascal Dubé, Yves Desjardins, Jong Hun Kim, Ji Seung Kim, Jong-Eun Kim, Jung Han Yoon Park, Ki Won Lee, and Chang Yong Lee. 2017. "Comprehensive phenolic composition analysis and evaluation of Yak-Kong soybean (Glycine max) for the prevention of atherosclerosis." *Food Chemistry* 234:486–93. doi: 10.1016/j.foodchem.2017.05.012.

Li, Z., R. Zhang, H. Mu, W. Zhang, J. Zeng, H. Li, S. Wang, X. Zhao, W. Chen, J. Dong, and R. Yang. 2022. "Oral administration of branched-chain amino acids attenuates atherosclerosis by inhibiting the inflammatory response and regulating the gut microbiota in ApoE-deficient mice." *Nutrients* 14 (23):5065. doi: 10.3390/nu14235065.

Libby, P. 2021. "The changing landscape of atherosclerosis." *Nature* 592 (7855):524–533. doi: 10.1038/s41586-021-03392-8.

Martínez-Beamonte, R., J. Sanchez-Marco, G. Lazaro, M. Barco, T. Herrero-Continente, M. Serrano-Megias, D. Botaya, C. Arnal, C. Barranquero, J. C. Surra, J. Osada, and M. A. Navarro. 2021. "Dietary avian proteins are comparable to soybean proteins on the atherosclerosis development and fatty liver disease in apoe-deficient mice." *Nutrients* 13 (6):1838. doi: 10.3390/nu13061838.

Moe, S., T. Drüeke, J. Cunningham, W. Goodman, K. Martin, K. Olgaard, S. Ott, S. Sprague, N. Lameire, and G. Eknoyan. 2006. "Definition, evaluation, and classification of renal osteodystrophy: a position statement from Kidney Disease: Improving Global Outcomes (KDIGO)." *Kidney Int* 69 (11):1945–53. doi: 10.1038/sj.ki.5000414.

Moe, S. M., and N. X. Chen. 2004. "Pathophysiology of vascular calcification in chronic kidney disease." *Circ Res* 95 (6):560–7. doi: 10.1161/01.Res.0000141775.67189.98.

Moriyama, T., K. Kishimoto, K. Nagai, R. Urade, T. Ogawa, S. Utsumi, N. Maruyama, and M. Maebuchi. 2004. "Soybean beta-conglycinin diet suppresses serum triglyceride levels in normal and genetically obese mice by induction of beta-oxidation, downregulation of fatty acid synthase, and inhibition of triglyceride absorption." *Biosci Biotechnol Biochem* 68 (2):352–9. doi: 10.1271/bbb.68.352.

Mukherjee, P., S. Roy, D. Ghosh, and S. K. Nandi. 2022. "Role of animal models in biomedical research: a review." *Lab Anim Res* 38 (1):18. doi: 10.1186/s42826-022-00128-1.

Nagarajan, S., R. L. Burris, B. W. Stewart, J. E. Wilkerson, and T. M. Badger. 2008. "Dietary soy protein isolate ameliorates atherosclerotic lesions in apolipoprotein E-deficient mice potentially by inhibiting monocyte chemoattractant protein-1 expression." *J Nutr* 138 (2):332–7. doi: 10.1093/jn/138.2.332.

Nakai, S., M. Fujita, and Y. Kamei. 2020. "Health promotion effects of soy isoflavones." *J Nutr Sci Vitaminol (Tokyo)* 66 (6):502–7. doi: 10.3177/jnsv.66.502.

Nakashima, Y., A. S. Plump, E. W. Raines, J. L. Breslow, and R. Ross. 1994. "ApoE-deficient mice develop lesions of all phases of atherosclerosis throughout the arterial tree." *Arterioscler Thromb* 14 (1):133–140. doi: 10.1161/01.atv.14.1.133.

Ni, W., Y. Tsuda, M. Sakono, and K. Imaizumi. 1998. "Dietary soy protein isolate, compared with casein, reduces atherosclerotic lesion area in apolipoprotein E-deficient mice." *J Nutr* 128 (11):1884–9. doi: 10.1093/jn/128.11.1884.

Osada, J., J. Joven, and N. Maeda. 2000. "The value of apolipoprotein E knockout mice for studying the effects of dietary fat and cholesterol on atherogenesis." *Curr Opin Lipidol* 11 (1):25–29. doi: 10.1097/00041433-200002000-00004.

Ovando, Emilio, Lucio Rodríguez-Sifuentes, Luz María Martínez, and Cristina Chuck-Hernández. 2022. "Optimization of soybean protein extraction using by-products from NaCl electrolysis as an application of the industrial symbiosis concept." *Applied Sciences* 12 (6):3113. doi: 10.3390/app12063113.

Plump, A. S., J. D. Smith, T. Hayek, K. Aalto-Setala, A. Walsh, J. G. Verstuyft, E. M. Rubin, and J. L. Breslow. 1992. "Severe hypercholesterolemia and atherosclerosis in apolipoprotein E- deficient mice created by homologous recombination in ES cells." *Cell* 71 (2):343–53. doi: 10.1016/0092-8674(92)90362-g.

Preece, K. E., N. Hooshyar, and N. J. Zuidam. 2017. "Whole soybean protein extraction processes: A review." *Inn Food Sci Emer Tech* 43:163–172. doi: 10.1016/j.ifset.2017.07.024.

Qin, Pingxu, Taoran Wang, and Yangchao Luo. 2022. "A review on plant-based proteins from soybean: Health benefits and soy product development." *J Agric Food Res* 7:100265. doi: 10.1016/j.jafr.2021.100265.

Rebollo-Hernanz, M., N. A. Bringe, and E. G. de Mejia. 2023. "Selected soybean varieties regulate Hepatic LDL-Cholesterol homeostasis depending on their Glycinin:beta-Conglycinin ratio." *Antioxidants* 12 (1):20. doi: 10.3390/antiox12010020.

Reddick, R. L., S. H. Zhang, and N. Maeda. 1994. "Atherosclerosis in mice lacking apo E. Evaluation of lesional development and progression [published erratum appears in Arterioscler Thromb 1994 May;14(5):839]." *Arterioscler Thromb* 14 (1):141–7. doi: 10.1161/01.atv.14.1.141.

Reeves, P. G., K. L. Rossow, and J. Lindlauf. 1993. "Development and testing of the AIN-93 purified diets for rodents: results on growth, kidney calcification and bone mineralization in rats and mice." *J Nutr* 123 (11):1923–31. doi: 10.1093/jn/123.11.1923.

Sato, M., H. Sato, A. Ogawa, R. Nomura, S. Takashima, H. J. Bang, H. Matsuoka, and K. Imaizumi. 2007. "Antiatherogenic effect of isoflavones in ovariectomized apolipoprotein e-deficient mice." *J Agric Food Chem* 55 (22):8967–71. doi: 10.1021/jf071771q.

Sawashita, N., A. Naemura, M. Shimizu, F. Morimatsu, Y. Ijiri, and J. Yamamoto. 2006. "Effect of dietary vegetable and animal proteins on atherothrombosis in mice." *Nutrition* 22 (6):661–667. doi: 10.1016/j.nut.2006.02.002.

Song, T., M. Lv, M. Zhou, M. Huang, L. Zheng, and M. Zhao. 2021. "Soybean-derived antihypertensive peptide LSW (Leu-Ser-Trp) antagonizes the damage of Angiotensin II to vascular endothelial cells through the trans-vesicular pathway." *J Agric Food Chem* 69 (36):10536–10549. doi: 10.1021/acs.jafc.1c02733.

Song, T., M. Zhou, W. Li, L. Zheng, J. Wu, and M. Zhao. 2022. "Tripeptide Leu-Ser-Trp regulates the vascular endothelial cells phenotype switching by mediating the vascular smooth muscle cells-derived small extracellular vesicles packaging of miR-145." *Molecules* 27 (20):7025. doi: 10.3390/molecules27207025.

Sui, X., T. Zhang, and L. Jiang. 2021. "Soy protein: Molecular structure revisited and recent advances in processing technologies." *Annu Rev Food Sci Tech* 12 (1):119–47. doi: 10.1146/annurev-food-062220-104405.

Tamminen, M., G. Mottino, J. H. Qiao, J. L. Breslow, and J. S. Frank. 1999. "Ultrastructure of early lipid accumulation in ApoE-deficient mice." *Arterioscler Thromb Vasc Biol* 19 (4):847–53. doi: 10.1161/01.atv.19.4.847.

Tomayko, E. J., H. R. Chung, and K. R. Wilund. 2011. "Soy protein diet and exercise training increase relative bone volume and enhance bone microarchitecture in a mouse model of uremia." *J Bone Miner Metab* 29 (6):682–90. doi: 10.1007/s00774-011-0278-4.

van Ree, J. H., W. J. van den Broek, V. E. Dahlmans, P. H. Groot, M. Vidgeon-Hart, R. R. Frants, B. Wieringa, L. M. Havekes, and M. H. Hofker. 1994. "Diet-induced hypercholesterolemia and atherosclerosis in heterozygous apolipoprotein E-deficient mice." *Atherosclerosis* 111 (1):25–37. doi: 10.1016/0021-9150(94)90188-0.

Wang, K., Z. Fu, X. Li, H. Hong, X. Zhan, X. Guo, Y. Luo, and Y. Tan. 2022. "Whey protein hydrolysate alleviated atherosclerosis and hepatic steatosis by regulating lipid metabolism in apoE(-/-) mice fed a Western diet." *Food Res Int* 157:111419. doi: 10.1016/j.foodres.2022.111419.

Wei, J., Z. Yao, H. Li, J. Lin, Z. Cui, and L. Zhang. 2019. "Genistein alleviates atherosclerosis in apolipoprotein E-deficient mice by interrupting the OX40/OX40L pathway." *Int J Clin Exp Pathol* 12 (5):1658–65.

Yi, G., H. Li, M. Liu, Z. Ying, J. Zhang, and X. Liu. 2020. "Soybean protein-derived peptides inhibit inflammation in LPS-induced RAW264.7 macrophages via the suppression of TLR4-mediated MAPK-JNK and NF-kappa B activation." *J Food Biochem* 44 (8):e13289. doi: 10.1111/jfbc.13289.

Zhang, S. H., R. L. Reddick, J. A. Piedrahita, and N. Maeda. 1992. "Spontaneous hypercholesterolemia and arterial lesions in mice lacking apolipoprotein E." *Science* 258 (5081):468–71. doi: 10.1126/science.1411543.

Zhang, Z., R. Zhang, Z. Z. Qin, J. P. Chen, J. Y. Xu, and L. Q. Qin. 2018. "Effects of Chronic Whey Protein Supplementation on Atherosclerosis in ApoE(-/-) Mice." *J Nutr Sci Vitaminol (Tokyo)* 64 (2):143–50. doi: 10.3177/jnsv.64.143.

27 Soy Protein Ingestion and Its Effect on Organelles Involved in Skeletal Muscle Contraction after Exercise

Keita Kanzaki, Daiki Watanabe, and Masanobu Wada

ABBREVIATIONS

ATP	Adenosine triphosphate
[Ca^{2+}]	Ca^{2+} concentration
DHRP	Dihydropyridine receptor
EC	Excitation-contraction
ECC	Eccentric contraction
G-actin	Globular actin
HMB	Beta-hydroxy beta-methylbutyrate
JP	Junctophilin
mTORC1	Mechanistic/mammalian target of rapamycin complex 1
NO	Nitric oxide
PLAS	Plasmalemma
RNS	Reactive nitrogen species
ROS	Reactive oxygen species
RyR	Ryanodine receptor
SR	Sarcoplasmic reticulum
T-tubule	Transverse tubule

INTRODUCTION

"Living systems are worn by inactivity and developed by use." This quote, attributed to Professor Szent-Györgyi, one of the greatest biochemists of the 20th century, succinctly captures the essence of physiology. Skeletal muscle, which accounts for ~40% of human body weight, exemplifies this concept. Extensive research has been dedicated to enhancing muscle function and mitigating muscle deterioration. These investigations have led to various forms of physical exercise tailored to individual needs (Kenney et al. 2015).

Skeletal muscle contractions can be categorized into three types based on changes in muscle length during contraction: concentric, isometric, and eccentric. Following intense physical activity, such as lifting heavy weights repeatedly, individuals often experience muscle soreness and weakness. This phenomenon is primarily caused by eccentric contraction (ECC), in which muscles generate force while lengthening (Kanzaki et al. 2022). ECC can produce greater force than concentric or isometric contractions (Allen 2001), making it a crucial component of training regimens for competitive athletes. Additionally, the high force and low energy cost associated with ECC makes

DOI: 10.1201/9781003597926-27

it suitable for various applications, including injury rehabilitation for athletes and health maintenance for older individuals. However, ECC typically induces more substantial and prolonged force depression than concentric and isometric contractions, resulting in extended recovery periods. This may hinder training progress for athletes and reduce motivation for individuals engaged in exercise.

Strategies aimed at expediting the recovery of post-exercise force production have garnered significant interest and investigation. These strategies include electrostimulation (Lambert et al. 2002; Hiroshige et al. 2018), nutritional supplementation (Kanzaki et al. 2018; Markus et al. 2021), drug administration (Kanzaki et al. 2017), and cryotherapy (Machado et al. 2017). Research findings in these areas have yielded conflicting results. For instance, although some studies suggest that muscle electrostimulation positively impacts force recovery (Lambert et al. 2002; Hiroshige et al. 2018), others have shown no such effect (Weber et al. 1994). Additionally, even if stimulation is effective, its accessibility remains limited due to the requirement for specialized equipment.

Soybeans are legumes native to East Asia that are widely cultivated as edible beans. Soy foods are inexpensive sources of protein consumed worldwide. Recently, soy protein ingestion was shown to benefit ECC-induced muscle damage by protecting intracellular organelles involved in excitation-contraction (EC) coupling, an essential process in muscle physiology (Kanzaki et al. 2019). Without a doubt, this nutritional supplementation is practical for many people. The first part of this chapter provides an overview of the roles of various organelles in skeletal muscle contraction. The following part discusses the mechanisms underlying ECC-induced muscle damage. Finally, the effects of soy protein ingestion on ECC-induced muscle damage are discussed.

EXCITATION-CONTRACTION COUPLING IN SKELETAL MUSCLE: UNDERSTANDING THE BASIS

Opening of Ryanodine Receptor

EC coupling is an essential process in muscle contraction. The term EC coupling was used as early as the 1950s (Sandow 1952). This process was named because it begins with the excitation of the plasmalemma (action potential generation) and results in muscle fiber contraction (Sandow 1952). Acetylcholine, released from the axon terminal of the α-motoneuron, binds to receptors on the plasmalemma of the muscle cells, triggering an action potential. The action potential propagates along the plasmalemma and into specialized invaginations called transverse tubules (T-tubules) (Westerblad et al. 2000). The sarcoplasmic reticulum (SR) is a membranous structure surrounding each myofibril with two distinct compartments: the longitudinal tubule and the terminal cisternae. The longitudinal tubule is located in the middle of each SR segment and connects the terminal cisternae (Figure 27.1). The T-tubules are flanked on either side by terminal cisternae, forming a triad structure. The membranes of the T-tubules and terminal cisternae are separated by only about 12 nm; this space is termed the triad junction. The action potential is detected by the dihydropyridine receptor (DHPR), a T-tubule voltage sensor (Westerblad et al. 2000). This detection leads to a structural change, which, in turn, causes the opening of the ryanodine receptor (RyR), an SR calcium ion (Ca^{2+}) release channel. Although the signaling mechanism from DHPR to RyR was unknown until a few years ago, recent studies have shown that the opening is triggered by the mechanical interaction between these two organelles through STAC3 (Figure 27.1) (Shishmarev 2020). When the RyR opens, the Ca^{2+} stored in the lumen of the SR is released into the triad junction and diffuses into the myoplasm, increasing the myoplasmic Ca^{2+} concentration ($[Ca^{2+}]$) from approximately 50 nM to ~4–5 μM.

Myofibril Shortening and Relaxing

In the mid-19th century, excellent studies of muscle structure were conducted using light microscopy (Brucke 1858). However, these remarkable results were largely forgotten in the first half of

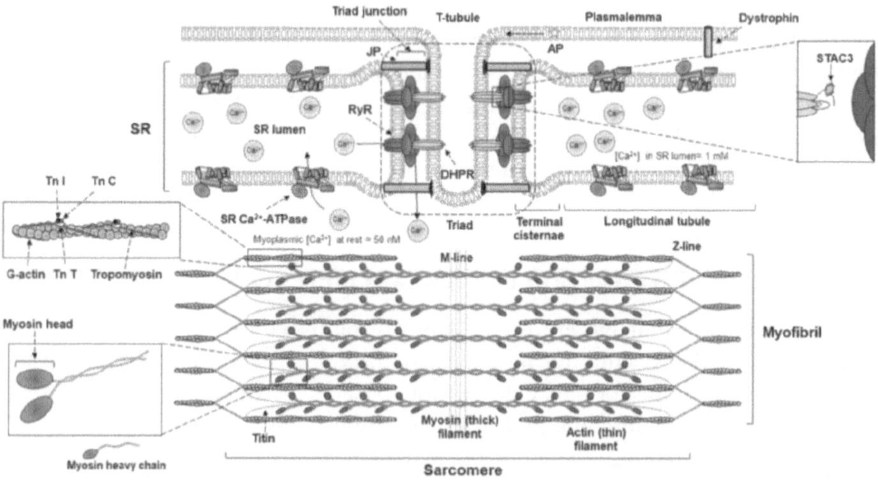

FIGURE 27.1 A diagram of the structures involved in skeletal muscle contraction. The action potential (AP) propagates along the plasmalemma and into the T-tubules. Detection of the AP by the DHPR triggers the opening of the RyR. Calcium ions stored in the SR lumen are then released from the RyR, increasing myoplasmic [Ca^{2+}]. As [Ca^{2+}] increases, the myosin head binds to the G-actin and pulls the actin filament toward the center of the sarcomere. The SR Ca^{2+}-ATPase translocates Ca^{2+} from the myoplasm into the SR lumen. AP, action potential; ATP, adenosine triphosphate; [Ca^{2+}], Ca^{2+} concentration; DHPR, dihydropyridine receptor; G-actin, globular actin; JP, junctophilin; RyR, ryanodine receptor; SR, sarcoplasmic reticulum; Tn, troponin; T-tubule, transverse tubule (adapted from Kanzaki et al. 2022).

the 20th century. One of the reasons for this loss of knowledge was the prevailing belief among scientists at the beginning of the 20th century that life functions were governed by molecules that could not be observed under a light microscope, leading to the neglect of earlier microscopic studies (Galler 2015). The study of muscles saw a resurgence in the mid-20th century with the advent of electron microscopes, which were invented in the 1930s. Most of the findings presented below are based on research using electron microscopy.

The muscle fiber contains several thousand myofibrils with a diameter of 1–2 μm (Figure 27.1). Two types (myofilaments) of small filaments exist within the myofibril. The thicker ones (~14 nm in diameter) are called myosin filaments, whereas the thinner (~7 nm in diameter) ones are called actin filaments (Figure 27.1). The primary component of myosin filaments is a strand-shaped protein called the myosin heavy chain, which has one end connected to a globular head, referred to as the myosin head. In contrast, the actin filament consists of three major protein molecules: globular actin (G-actin), tropomyosin, and the troponin complex (comprising troponin I, T, and C). The segment between one Z-line and the next, known as a sarcomere, serves as the fundamental contractile unit of the muscle (McComas 1996).

Since the groundbreaking proposal by two different Huxleys, A. F. Huxley and H. E. Huxley, in 1954, it has been widely accepted that the shortening of a muscle fiber involves the sliding of myosin and actin filaments past each other (Galler 2015). At rest, tropomyosin covers the myosin-binding site on G-actin, thus preventing the binding of the myosin head. When the myoplasmic [Ca^{2+}] increases, stemming from the Ca^{2+} release from the SR, Ca^{2+} binds to troponin C. This causes tropomyosin to move away from the myosin-binding site, allowing the myosin heads to attach to the binding site, forming a cross-bridge. Subsequently, the myosin heads tilt and pull the actin filament toward the center of the sarcomere, resulting in sarcomere shortening. When adenosine triphosphate (ATP) is hydrolyzed by ATPase to adenosine diphosphate and inorganic phosphate, a significant amount of free energy is released. In the late 1930s and early 1940s, it was discovered that myofibrils enzymatically cleave ATP, which serves as the energy source for muscle contraction (Kenny et al. 2015). The myosin head, in addition to its structural role, acts as an ATPase (referred to as myosin ATPase), and the energy required for the tilting motion is released from ATP hydrolysis (Saltin and Gollnick 1983). Ca^{2+} uptake from the myoplasm is regulated by SR Ca^{2+}-ATPase, located in the longitudinal tubules of the SR (Figure 27.1). SR Ca^{2+}-ATPase transports 2 mol of Ca^{2+} into the SR lumen with the hydrolysis of 1 mol of ATP. The reduction in the myoplasmic [Ca^{2+}] by SR Ca^{2+}-ATPase allows the myosin head to detach from G-actin, resulting in muscle fiber relaxation (Tupling 2004).

SKELETAL MUSCLE SUBJECTED TO ECC IS EXPOSED TO SEVERAL STRESSES

Muscle fatigue and muscle damage are commonly distinguished. Muscle fatigue is a reversible performance depression that occurs during contraction, typically recovering within a few hours. Muscle damage also leads to performance depression, but this recovery process spans several days (Allen et al. 2008). Muscles undergoing ECC (hereafter referred to as "ECC muscles") are particularly susceptible to muscle damage, which explains the substantial and enduring force depression resulting from ECC. Extensive research has indicated that ECC muscles are exposed to multiple stresses contributing to muscle damage (Allen 2001; Peake et al. 2017; Hody et al. 2019; Kanzaki et al. 2022).

Mechanical Stress

The fact that ECC results in structural indications of muscle damage, such as Z-line broadening and streaming, overstretched half-sarcomeres, myofibril disorganization, and triad disruption (Figure 27.1 and Table 27.1), is no longer a subject of debate (Allen 2001; Proske and Morgan 2001). These changes are likely attributed to the mechanical stress caused by the stretching and contraction of myofibrils during ECC. According to a proposal by Morgan (1990), weaker half-sarcomeres absorb myofibrillar stretching during ECC, leading to overstretching beyond the myofilament overlap. As the muscle relaxes, the myofilaments in some overstretched sarcomeres fail to reinterdigitate, resulting in disrupted sarcomeres. If the region of disruption is large enough, it leads to membrane damage of the T-tubule, contributing to reduced SR Ca^{2+}-release (Proske and Morgan 2001; Hody et al. 2019). The magnitude of mechanical stress primarily depends on sarcomere length and the extent of myofilament activation during ECC. Mechanical stress-induced muscle damage progresses during ECC, making it challenging to mitigate unless ECC is performed with shorter muscle length and/or less myofilament activation.

TABLE 27.1
Various Stress-Induced Changes in Skeletal Muscles Subjected to Eccentric Contraction

Mechanical Stress	Oxidative Stress	Ca^{2+} Stress
Ca^{2+} entry	Increased permeability of plasmalemma	Proteolysis of titin, desmin, dystrophin, RyR,
Disruption of triad structure	Decreased SR Ca^{2+}-ATPase activity	DHPR JP, and myosin heavy chain
Broadening and streaming of Z-line		
Overstretch of sarcomere		

Muscles undergoing eccentric contraction are subjected to mechanical, oxidative, and Ca^{2+} stress. These stresses lead to muscle damage. RyR, ryanodine receptor; DHPR, dihydropyridine receptor; JP, junctophilin.

Oxidative Stress

Inflammation is defined as the biological response of the body to harmful stimuli, followed by repair and regeneration. One of its functions is the removal of damaged proteins. Leukocytes include neutrophils, eosinophils, basophils, lymphocytes, and monocytes, with macrophages differentiating from monocytes. In ECC muscles, inflammation often occurs as neutrophils and macrophages invade muscle cells to remove tissue debris generated by mechanical stress (Neubauer et al. 2014; Peake et al. 2017). Macrophages and neutrophils release reactive nitrogen species (RNS) and reactive oxygen species (ROS), respectively. ROS are highly reactive oxygen compounds, whereas RNS are highly reactive nitrogen compounds. In skeletal muscle, the primary compounds produced are superoxide, hydrogen peroxide, hydroxyl radicals for ROS, and nitric oxide (NO) for RNS. Both ROS and RNS can modify the proteins and lipids composing muscle cell organelles, impairing the function of some organelles (Table 27.1) (Peake et al. 2017; Kanzaki et al. 2022).

Calcium Stress

Although Ca^{2+} is essential for muscle contraction, it can also lead to muscle damage. Stretch-activated channels are present in the plasmalemma (Guharay and Sachs 1984; Zhang et al. 2012). When these channels open during ECC, Ca^{2+} enters the muscle cell from the outside, elevating resting myoplasmic $[Ca^{2+}]$ from ~50 nM to ~250 nM, and this elevation can last for days (Lynch et al. 1997).

Calpains are non-lysosomal, Ca^{2+}-regulated cysteine proteases. Skeletal muscle expresses calpain-1, 2, and 3 (Murphy 2010). Increases in resting myoplasmic $[Ca^{2+}]$ trigger calpain activation. Calpain targets in ECC muscles include titin, dystrophin, desmin, RyR, DHPR, and junctophilin (Figure 27.1 and Table 27.1) (Zhang et al. 2008; Kanzaki et al. 2010, 2017). Similar to calpains, caspases are also myoplasmic proteases. To date, 14 caspase isoforms have been identified in mammalian cells (Primeau et al. 2002). Of these, caspase-3 is indirectly activated by Ca^{2+}. One of the targets of caspase-3 is the myofibril (Peake et al. 2017). Calpain-1, calpain-3, and caspase-3 are likely involved in degrading target proteins in ECC muscle. The *de novo* synthesis of degraded proteins and their incorporation into the original organelle is necessary to restore normal function, which explains the long-lasting force deficit in the ECC muscle.

EFFECTS OF SOY PROTEIN INGESTION IN EXERCISED MUSCLE

As mentioned above (in the mechanical stress section), mitigating ECC-induced mechanical stress is challenging. Therefore, the primary approach to inhibit ECC-induced muscle damage is to alleviate oxidative and/or Ca^{2+} stress, and nutritional supplementation plays a vital role in achieving this goal. Antioxidants commonly ingested by humans include vitamins C and E, *N*-acetylcysteine, and taurine. Despite extensive research, there is no consensus regarding the efficacy of these antioxidants (Childs et al. 2001; Kerksick et al. 2010; Silva et al. 2011; He et al. 2015). For example, He et al. (2015) demonstrated that the ingestion of vitamins C and E before downhill running in humans inhibited the delayed onset of muscle soreness and increased serum creatine kinase (an indicator of membrane damage; see effects on humans). In contrast, Childs et al. (2001) showed that ingestion of vitamin C and *N*-acetylcysteine transiently increased serum creatine kinase and lipid hydroperoxide levels after downhill running. There is limited information regarding whether dietary supplementation can inhibit ECC-induced proteolysis. Kanzaki et al. (2018, 2019) demonstrated in rodent skeletal muscle that the ingestion of soy protein or arginine mitigates the ECC-related degradation of organelles involved in EC coupling. This section will delve into this topic further.

TABLE 27.2
Macronutrient Profile of Proteins

Nutrient	Soy Protein	Whey Protein	Casein
Carbohydrate (g/100 g)	4.0	6.6	0.1
Protein (g/100 g)	85.8	79.3	91.4
Fat (g/100 g)	0.2	5.9	0.7
Energy (kcal/100 g)	361.0	396.7	372.3

Soy protein contains less energy and fat than whey protein and casein. Adapted from Kanda et al. (2016).

Amino Acid Composition of Soy Protein

Proteins are the major structural components of cells and are composed of amino acids linked by peptide bonds (Kenney et al. 2015). A total of 20 amino acids exist. Of these, eight are classified as essential amino acids because they cannot be synthesized within the human body. Generally, the daily protein requirement (0.8 g/kg per day) for normal activities can be obtained from a regular diet. However, for certain individuals, such as athletes training for muscle hypertrophy or aerobic endurance, this amount may be insufficient, necessitating protein supplementation. Common supplements include whey protein, casein, and soy protein.

Soy protein has been suggested to offer a variety of health benefits, particularly in preventing chronic diseases (Messina 2016), primarily because it contains less energy and fat than whey protein and casein (Table 27.2) (Kanda et al. 2016). The ingestion of protein shortly after exercise is well known to stimulate protein synthesis in skeletal muscles. Leucine plays a central role in muscle protein synthesis by activating the mechanistic/mammalian target of rapamycin complex 1 (mTORC1), a key anabolic signaling molecule. Glutathione, an antioxidant found at high levels in mammalian cells, contributes to muscle resistance against atrophy by protecting organelles from oxidative damage caused by ROS (Powers et al. 2007). Cysteine supplementation provides the thiols necessary for glutathione synthesis. Whey protein contains more leucine and cysteine than soy protein (Table 27.3). In contrast, soy protein has the highest arginine content, which is crucial for inhibiting ECC-induced proteolysis.

SOY PROTEIN INGESTION AND ECC-INDUCED PROTEOLYSIS

Effects on Ca^{2+} Release-Regulating Proteins

As mentioned earlier (see Ca^{2+} stress), resting [Ca^{2+}] in ECC muscles is elevated to ≥200 nM. Prolonged high resting [Ca^{2+}] causes autolysis of calpains from a full-length form to a smaller form (Murphy and Lamb 2009). Autolysis can be used as an indicator of calpain activation, as it reduces the [Ca^{2+}] required for calpain activation (to 0.5–20 μM, 20–150 μM, and < 1 μM for calpain 1, 2, and 3, respectively). It has been shown that *(1)* calpain-1 autolysis and the degradation of Ca^{2+}-regulating organelles occur nearly simultaneously in ECC muscle (a few days after ECC) (Kanzaki et al. 2014); *(2)* the extent of Ca^{2+}-induced impairment of EC coupling is similar in muscles from wild-type and calpain-3-deficient mice (Verburg et al. 2009); and *(3)* extremely high [Ca^{2+}], a rare occurrence in normal muscle cells, is required for calpain-3 activation even after autolysis, suggesting that calpain-1 plays a central role in ECC-related proteolysis.

Kanzaki et al. (2018, 2019) investigated the efficacy of soy protein or arginine ingestion in rat ECC muscle and found that ingestion prior to ECC facilitated force recovery and partially or completely inhibited the degradation of RyR, DHPR, and JP (Figure 27.2A shows the results 3 days after ECC. Only the RyR results are shown in Figure 27.2B and 27.2C). They also observed that soy

TABLE 27.3
Amino Acid Composition of Proteins (g/100 g)

Amino Acid	Soy Protein	Whey Protein	Casein
Essential Amino Acids			
Isoleucine	4.55	5.31	4.86
Leucine	7.84	11.89	8.81
Lysine	6.20	9.39	7.57
Methionine	1.27	2.15	2.72
Phenylalanine	5.23	3.61	4.82
Threonine	3.81	5.19	4.09
Tryptophan	1.36	2.27	1.14
Valine	4.72	5.27	6.19
Nonessential Amino Acids			
Alanine	4.15	4.69	2.81
Arginine	7.58	2.73	3.50
Aspartic acid + Asparagine	11.66	11.22	6.73
Cysteine	1.25	2.99	0.32
Glutamic acid + Glutamine	19.50	16.27	21.25
Glycine	4.12	1.97	1.71
Histidine	2.63	2.31	2.89
Proline	5.27	4.60	10.31
Serine	5.09	4.52	5.26
Tyrosine	3.74	3.61	5.22

Soy protein has the most arginine, whereas whey protein has the most leucine and cysteine. Adapted from Kanda et al. (2016).

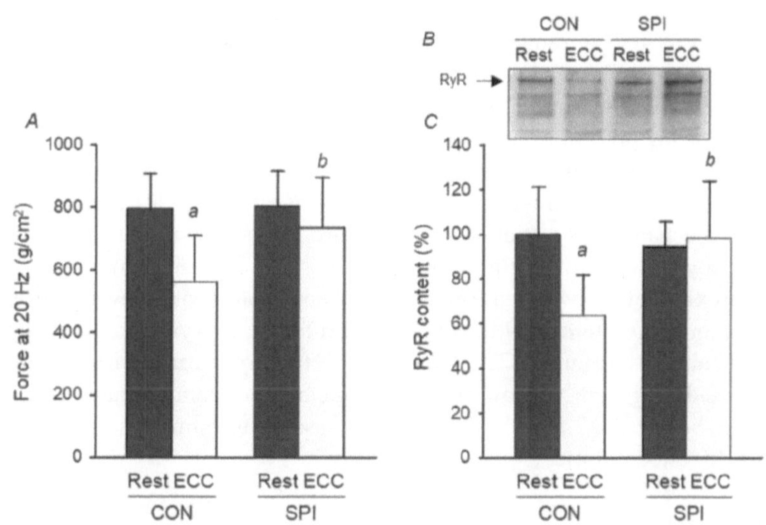

FIGURE 27.2 Effect of SPI ingestion and ECC on force production and RyR content. Rats were fed a diet containing 20% soy protein isolate (SPI) for 4 weeks before ECC. A) Isometric force at 20 Hz in extensor digitorum longus. B) Immunoblot analysis of RyR. C) RyR content. Values are means ± SD. [a]$P < 0.05$, vs. resting muscles within rats. [b]$P < 0.05$, vs. ECC muscles from CON. CON, control rat; ECC, muscle subjected to eccentric contraction; RyR, ryanodine receptor; Rest, resting muscle; SPI, soy protein isolate-fed rat (adapted from Kanzaki et al. 2019).

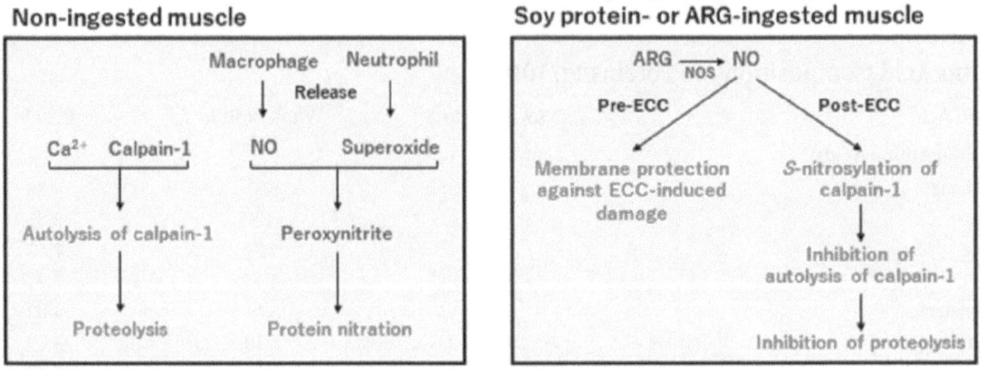

FIGURE 27.3 Reaction of nitric oxide (NO) in soy protein or arginine-ingested muscle and non-ingested muscle subjected to eccentric contraction (ECC). In non-ingested muscle, where macrophages and neutrophils infiltrate the muscle cells, more NO interacts with superoxide to form peroxynitrite. In contrast, in soy protein- or ARG-ingested muscle, elevated NO levels are responsible for S-nitrosylation of calpain-1. ARG, arginine; NOS, NO synthase (adapted from Kanzaki et al. 2022).

protein or arginine ingestion increased muscle NOx (nitric oxide and nitrate) concentrations and *S*-nitrosylation (*S*-nitrosylation is a covalent attachment of NO to a thiol: $SH + NO \rightarrow SNO + H^+$) of calpain-1 and inhibited ECC-induced calpain-1 autolysis. The application of L-NAME, an inhibitor of NO synthase, negated the effects of soy protein or arginine ingestion (Kanzaki et al. 2018, 2019). Based on these results, the following mechanism was proposed for the efficacy of soy protein and arginine ingestion (Figure 27.3) (Kanzaki et al. 2022):

(1) Soy protein or arginine ingestion leads to an increase in intracellular arginine concentration.
(2) Arginine is a precursor of NO, and NO synthase synthesizes NO from it. Therefore, the pre-ECC NO levels are elevated.
(3) Increased NO levels lead to *S*-nitrosylated calpain-1, which, in turn, inhibits Ca^{2+}-induced calpain-1 autolysis and subsequent proteolysis in ECC muscles.

As mentioned above (oxidative stress), NO levels are also elevated in ECC muscles from individuals who do not ingest soy protein or arginine (muscle from non-ingested individuals is referred to as non-ingested muscle), as macrophages that have invaded the cell release NO (oxidative stress). Why does *S*-nitrosylation of calpain-1 not occur in non-ingested muscles despite elevated NO levels? Although the mechanism is a matter of conjecture, the reaction of NO may differ between non-ingested and soy protein- or arginine-ingested muscles. In non-ingested muscles, not only NO but also superoxide levels, which are released by neutrophils, are elevated after ECC. Under these conditions, more NO interacts with superoxide to form peroxynitrite, resulting in decreased *S*-nitrosylation of calpain-1 (Figure 27.3). Conversely, NO levels are elevated in ingested muscle prior to ECC. Considering that NO can protect the membrane from damage (Szelid et al. 2010), elevated NO levels before ECC may inhibit the ECC-associated infiltration of macrophages and neutrophils in the ingested muscle.

Effects on Other Organelles

Does the ingestion of soy protein or arginine impact other organelles involved in EC coupling in the ECC muscles? Apart from RyR, DHPR, and JP, ECC also leads to the proteolysis of titin, desmin, dystrophin, STAC3, SR Ca^{2+}-ATPase, and myosin heavy chain. Notably, it has been shown that proteolysis of titin, desmin, dystrophin, and myosin heavy chain does not involve calpain-1 activation (Zhang et al. 2008; Kanzaki et al. 2010). Moreover, the administration of a calpain-1 inhibitor does not seem to suppress ECC-related proteolysis of SR Ca^{2+}-ATPase, suggesting that soy protein or arginine ingestion may not inhibit the proteolysis of these organelles (Kanzaki et al. 2017). Considering that titin, desmin, and dystrophin degradation occurs concurrently with calpain-3 activation, it is likely that calpain-3 plays a role in the breakdown of these organelles (Kanzaki et al. 2014; Zhang et al. 2008, 2012). The degradation of SR Ca^{2+}-ATPase and myosin heavy chain may result from oxidative modification and caspase-3 activity, respectively, as suggested by previous findings (Matsunaga et al. 2001; Peake et al. 2017). Further studies are required to investigate the mechanism behind the degradation of STAC3 in ECC muscles.

Effects on Humans

Human studies on the effects of soy protein or arginine at the molecular level remain limited. One challenge is the need for biopsy samples for biochemical analyses of ECC muscle. Some studies examining serum enzyme activity have demonstrated that soy protein ingestion before eccentric exercise can inhibit the increase in serum creatine kinase activity (Shenoy et al. 2016). Creatine kinase is an enzyme present only in muscle cells, suggesting that ingestion may mitigate ECC-induced membrane damage.

In a study by Kanzaki et al. (2018), rats consumed 611 mg/kg body weight^{-1} day^{-1} of arginine. This supplemental dose is equivalent to 98 mg/kg body weight/day in humans, assuming a conversion of 1:0.16 (rat vs. human), and it has been demonstrated to be safe (Cynober et al. 2016).

THE EFFECT OF OTHER PROTEINS

Are proteins other than soy protein effective in relieving ECC-induced muscle damage? Whey protein and casein contain lower levels of arginine than soy protein (Table 27.3). Therefore, these proteins may offer some protection against muscle damage, albeit to a lesser degree than soy protein. Additionally, it is plausible that whey protein and casein have no effect, given the possibility of an arginine threshold required to ameliorate muscle damage. However, these ideas remain speculative. To date, no animal or human studies have been conducted to compare the effects of soy protein, whey protein, and casein in this context. Addressing this issue is likely to be an important area of focus for future investigation.

As previously discussed, leucine promotes muscle protein synthesis by activating mTORC1. Leucine is metabolized to alpha-ketoisocaproate, which possesses anti-catabolic properties (Wilson et al. 2008). Alpha-ketoisocaproate is further converted to beta-hydroxy-beta-methylbutyrate (HMB), which also activates mTORC1. Similar to calpain, the ATP-dependent proteasome serves as a cytosolic protease. Increased activity of the proteasome pathway occurs not only during various exercise conditions but also in circumstances such as cancer, antigravity environments, and periods of reduced physical activity (i.e., disuse). An *in vitro* study conducted on mouse myotubes revealed that applying HMB can inhibit proteasome activation (Smith et al. 2004). Considering these findings in conjunction with the fact that the branched-chain amino acids (i.e., leucine, isoleucine, and valine) constitute approximately 35% of muscle protein, it becomes plausible that protein sources rich in branched-chain amino acids, such as whey protein, may be more suitable for promoting muscle hypertrophy and maintaining muscle mass compared to soy protein.

CONCLUDING REMARKS

The significance of ECC in muscle adaptation is widely recognized. For instance, regular ECC exercises have been shown to facilitate muscle hypertrophy, increase force production, and induce neural adaptations (Reeves et al. 2009; Hody et al. 2019), surpassing other contraction modes. The adaptability of ECC, coupled with its low energy costs, holds great promise for various individuals, including competitive athletes. In older individuals, eccentric exercise improves mobility and independence, reduces the risk of falls, and helps prevent sarcopenia (Hody et al. 2019). However, the muscle pain and weakness that accompany such benefits may deter the adoption of eccentric exercises and diminish training efficiency. Widespread adoption could increase if physiological methods to alleviate muscle damage were available. In this regard, the ingestion of soy protein appears to be an effective strategy. Nonetheless, it is important to recognize that treatments that significantly inhibit muscle damage might also suppress the desirable effects of ECC, as muscle damage serves as a necessary stimulus for specific muscle adaptations.

MINI DICTIONARY OF TERMS

- **Autolysis:** Digestion of an enzyme by the action of its own enzyme.
- **Calpain:** Non-lysosomal proteases in the cell.
- **Dihydropyridine receptor:** T-tubule voltage sensor that detects the action potential.
- **Eccentric contraction:** A contraction during which skeletal muscles are stretched.
- **Excitation-contraction coupling:** Processes that begin with the excitation of the plasmalemma and result in the contraction of the muscle fiber.
- **Muscle damage:** Force depression that takes several days to recover from.
- **Muscle fatigue:** Force depression that takes a few hours to recover from.
- **Nitric oxide:** Highly reactive nitrogen compound synthesized from arginine by nitric oxide synthase in living organisms.
- **Ryanodine receptor:** A Ca^{2+} release channel of the sarcoplasmic reticulum.
- **Sarcoplasmic reticulum:** An organelle that stores large amounts of Ca^{2+} in its lumen.
- **S-nitrosylation:** A covalent attachment (SNO) of nitric oxide (NO) to a thiol (SH).

SUMMARY POINTS

- Soy foods are inexpensive sources of protein that are consumed worldwide.
- Soy protein contains more arginine than other proteins, such as whey protein and casein.
- Eccentric contraction (ECC) is a muscle contraction during which the skeletal muscle is stretched during daily activities.
- ECC often leads to large and prolonged force depression caused by muscle damage, characterized by delayed-onset muscle soreness, triad deformation, increased membrane permeability, overstretched sarcomeres, and organelle degradation.
- ECC-induced proteolysis is primarily mediated by calpains, which are non-lysosomal, Ca^{2+}-regulated cysteine proteases.
- Nitric oxide (NO) is synthesized from arginine by the enzyme NO synthase.
- Ingestion of arginine-rich soy protein increases NO levels in muscle cells.
- Increased NO levels lead to *S*-nitrosylation of calpain-1, which, in turn, attenuates Ca^{2+}-induced calpain-1 activation and subsequent ECC-induced muscle damage.
- Soy protein ingestion is likely an effective strategy for inhibiting muscle damage and promoting the recovery of force production after exercise, especially exercises involving a substantial eccentric phase.

REFERENCES

Allen, D. G. 2001. Eccentric muscle damage: mechanisms of early reduction of force. *Acta Physiologica Scandinavica* 171: 311–9.

Allen, D. G., G. D. Lamb, and H. Westerblad. 2008. Skeletal muscle fatigue: cellular mechanisms. *Physiological Review* 88: 287–332.

Brucke, E. 1858. Untersuchungen über den Bau der Muskelfasern mit Hilfe des polarisierten Lichtes. *Math Naturwiss Cl* 15: 69–84.

Childs, A., C. Jacobs, T. Kaminski, B. Halliwell, and C. Leeuwenburgh. 2001. Supplementation with vitamin C and *N*-acetyl-cysteine increases oxidative stress in humans after an acute muscle injury induced by eccentric exercise. *Free Radical Biology and Medicine* 31: 745–53.

Cynober, L., D. M. Bier, M. Kadowaki, S. M. Morris, Jr., R. Elango, and M. Smriga. 2016. Proposals for upper limits of safe intake for arginine and tryptophan in young adults and an upper limit of safe intake for leucine in the elderly. *The Journal of Nutrition* 146: 2652S–4S.

Galler, S. 2015. Forgotten research from 19th century: science should not follow fashion. *Journal of Muscle Research and Cell Motility* 36: 5–9.

Guharay, F. and F. Sachs. 1984. Stretch-activated single ion channel currents in tissue-cultured embryonic chick skeletal muscle. *The Journal of Physiology* 352: 685–701.

He, F., J. A. Hockemeyer, and D. Sedlock. 2015. Does combined antioxidant vitamin supplementation blunt repeated bout effect? *International Journal of Sports and Medicine* 36: 407–13.

Hiroshige, Y., D. Watanabe, C. Aibara, K. Kanzaki, S. Matsunaga, and M. Wada. 2018. The efficacy of microcurrent therapy on eccentric contraction-induced muscle damage in rat fast-twitch skeletal muscle. *Open Journal of Applied Science* 8: 89–102.

Hody, S., J. L. Croisier, T. Bury, B. Rogister, and P. Leprince. 2019. Eccentric muscle contractions: risks and benefits. *Frontiers in Physiology* 10: 536.

Kanda, A., K. Nakayama, C. Sanbongi, M. Nagata, S. Ikegami, and H. Itoh. 2016. Effects of whey, caseinate, or milk protein ingestion on muscle protein synthesis after exercise. *Nutrients* 8: http://www.ncbi.nlm.nih.gov/pubmed/27271661.

Kanzaki, K., M. Kuratani, S. Matsunaga, N. Yanaka, and M. Wada. 2014. Three calpain isoforms are autolyzed in rat fast-twitch muscle after eccentric contractions. *Journal of Muscle Research and Cell Motility* 35: 179–89.

Kanzaki, K., M. Kuratani, T. Mishima, S. Matsunaga, N. Yanaka, S. Usui, and M. Wada. 2010. The effects of eccentric contraction on myofibrillar proteins in rat skeletal muscle. *European Journal of Applied Physiology* 110: 943–52.

Kanzaki, K., D. Watanabe, C. Aibara, Y. Kawakami, T. Yamada, Y. Takahashi, and M. Wada. 2018. L-arginine ingestion inhibits eccentric contraction-induced proteolysis and force deficit via *S*-nitrosylation of calpain. *Physiological Reports* 6: e13582. http://www.ncbi.nlm.nih.gov/pubmed/29368397.

Kanzaki, K., D. Watanabe, C. Aibara, Y. Kawakami, T. Yamada, Y. Takahashi, and M. Wada. 2019. Ingestion of soy protein isolate attenuates eccentric contraction-induced force depression and muscle proteolysis via inhibition of calpain-1 activation in rat fast-twitch skeletal muscle. *Nutrition* 58: 23–9.

Kanzaki, K., D. Watanabe, M. Kuratani, T. Yamada, S. Matsunaga, and M. Wada. 2017. Role of calpain in eccentric contraction-induced proteolysis of Ca^{2+}-regulatory proteins and force depression in rat fast-twitch skeletal muscle. *Journal of Applied Physiology (1985)* 122: 396–405.

Kanzaki, K., D. Watanabe, J. Shi, and M. Wada. 2022. Mechanisms of eccentric contraction-induced muscle damage and nutritional supplementations for mitigating it. *Journal of Muscle Research and Cell Motility* 43: 147–56.

Kenney, W. L., J. H. Wilmore, and D. L. Costill. 2015. *Physiology of sport and exercise* (6th ed). Champaign: Human Kinetics.

Kerksick, C. M., R. B. Kreider, and D. S. Willoughby. 2010. Intramuscular adaptations to eccentric exercise and antioxidant supplementation. *Amino Acids* 39: 219–32.

Lambert, M. I., P. Marcus, T. Burgess, and T. D. Noakes. 2002. Electro-membrane microcurrent therapy reduces signs and symptoms of muscle damage. *Medicine and Science in Sports and Exercise* 34: 602–7.

Lynch, G. S., C. J. Fary, and D. A. Williams. 1997. Quantitative measurement of resting skeletal muscle $[Ca^{2+}]_i$ following acute and long-term downhill running exercise in mice. *Cell Calcium* 22: 373–83.

Machado, A. F., A. C. Almeida, J. K. Micheletti, F. M. Vanderlei, M. F. Tribst, J. Netto Junior, and C. M. Pastre. 2017. Dosages of cold-water immersion post exercise on functional and clinical responses: a randomized controlled trial. *Scandinavian Journal of Medicine and Science in Sports* 27: 1356–63.

Markus, I., K. Constantini, J. R. Hoffman, S. Bartolomei, and Y. Gepner. 2021. Exercise-induced muscle damage: mechanism, assessment and nutritional factors to accelerate recovery. *European Journal of Applied Physiology* 121: 969–92.

Matsunaga, S. S. Harmon, B. Gohlsch, K. Ohlendieck, and D. Pette. 2001. Inactivation of sarcoplasmic reticulum Ca^{2+}-ATPase in low-frequency stimulated rat muscle. *Journal of Muscle Research and Cell Motility* 22: 685–91.

McComas, J. A. 1996. *Skeletal muscle: form and function*. Champaign: Human Kinetics.

Messina, M. 2016. Soy and health update: evaluation of the clinical and epidemiologic literature. *Nutrients* 8: https://www.ncbi.nlm.nih.gov/pubmed/27886135.

Morgan, D. L. 1990. New insights into the behavior of muscle during active lengthening. *Biophysical Journal* 57: 209–21.

Murphy, R. M. 2010. Calpains, skeletal muscle function and exercise. *Clinical and Experimental Pharmacology and Physiology* 37: 385–91.

Murphy, R. M. and G. D. Lamb. 2009. Endogenous calpain-3 activation is primarily governed by small increases in resting cytoplasmic [Ca^{2+}] and is not dependent on stretch. *Journal of Biological Chemistry* 284: 7811–9.

Neubauer, O., S. Sabapathy, K. J. Ashton, B. Desbrow, J. M. Peake, R. Lazarus, B. Wessner, D. Cameron-Smith, K. H. Wagner, L. J. Haseler, and A. C. Bulmer. 2014. Time course-dependent changes in the transcriptome of human skeletal muscle during recovery from endurance exercise: from inflammation to adaptive remodeling. *Journal of Applied Physiology (1985)* 116: 274–87.

Peake, J. M., O. Neubauer, P. A. Della Gatta, and K. Nosaka. 2017. Muscle damage and inflammation during recovery from exercise. *Journal of Applied Physiology (1985)* 122: 559–70.

Powers, S. K., A. N. Kavazis, and J. M. McClung. 2007. Oxidative stress and disuse muscle atrophy. *Journal of Applied Physiology* 102: 2389–97.

Primeau, A. J., P. J. Adhihetty, and D. A. Hood. 2002. Apoptosis in heart and skeletal muscle. *Canadian Journal of Applied Physiology* 27: 349–95.

Proske, U. and D. L. Morgan. 2001. Muscle damage from eccentric exercise: mechanism, mechanical signs, adaptation and clinical applications. *The Journal of Physiology* 537: 333–45.

Reeves, N. D., C. N. Maganaris, S. Longo, and M. V. Narici. 2009. Differential adaptations to eccentric versus conventional resistance training in older humans. *Experimental Physiology* 94: 825–33.

Saltin, B. and P. D. Gollnick. 1983. Skeletal muscle adaptability: significance for metabolism and performance. In *Handbook of physiology: skeletal muscle*, ed. L. D. Peachey, R. H. Adrian, and S. R. Geiger, 555–631. Baltimore: Waverly Press Inc.

Sandow, A. 1952. Excitation-contraction coupling in muscular response. *Yale Journal of Biology and Medicine* 25: 176–201.

Shenoy, S., M. Dhawan, and J. S. Sandhu. 2016. Four weeks of supplementation with isolated soy protein attenuates exercise-induced muscle damage and enhances muscle recovery in well trained athletes: a randomized trial. *Asian Journal of Sports and Medicine* 7: e33528.

Shishmarev, D. 2020. Excitation-contraction coupling in skeletal muscle: recent progress and unanswered questions. *Biophysical Review* 12: 143–53.

Silva, L. A., P. C. Silveira, M. M. Ronsani, P. S. Souza, D. Scheffer, L. C. Vieira, M. Benetti, C. T. De Souza, and R. A. Pinho. 2011. Taurine supplementation decreases oxidative stress in skeletal muscle after eccentric exercise. *Cell Biochemistry and Function* 29: 43–9.

Smith, H. J., S. M. Wyke, and M. J. Tisdale. 2004. Mechanism of the attenuation of proteolysis-inducing factor stimulated protein degradation in muscle by beta-hydroxy-beta-methylbutyrate. *Cancer Research* 64: 8731–5.

Szelid, Z., P. Pokreisz, X. Liu, P. Vermeersch, G. Marsboom, H. Gillijns, M. Pellens, E. Verbeken, F. Van de Werf, D. Collen, and S. P. Janssens. 2010. Cardioselective nitric oxide synthase 3 gene transfer protects against myocardial reperfusion injury. *Basic Research in Cardiology* 105: 169–79.

Tupling, A. R. 2004. The sarcoplasmic reticulum in muscle fatigue and disease: role of the sarco(endo)plasmic reticulum Ca^{2+}-ATPase. *Canadian Journal of Applied Physiology* 29: 308–29.

Verburg, E., R. M. Murphy, I. Richard, and G. D. Lamb. 2009. Involvement of calpains in Ca^{2+}-induced disruption of excitation-contraction coupling in mammalian skeletal muscle fibers. *American Journal of Physiology* 296: C1115–22.

Weber, M. D., F. J. Servedio, and W. R. Woodall. 1994. The effects of three modalities on delayed onset muscle soreness. *Journal of Orthopaedic and Sports Physical Therapy* 20: 236–42.

Westerblad, H., J. D. Bruton, D. G. Allen, and J. Lännergren. 2000. Functional significance of Ca^{2+} in long-lasting fatigue of skeletal muscle. *European Journal of Applied Physiology* 83: 166–74.

Wilson, G. J., J. M. Wilson, A. H. Manninen. 2008. Effects of beta-hydroxy-beta-methylbutyrate (HMB) on exercise performance and body composition across varying levels of age, sex, and training experience: a review. *Nutrition and Metabolism* 5. https://doi.org/10.1186/1743-7075-5-1.

Zhang, B. T., N. P. Whitehead, O. L. Gervasio, T. F. Reardon, M. Vale, D. Fatkin, A. Dietrich, E. W. Yeung, and D. G. Allen. 2012. Pathways of Ca^{2+} entry and cytoskeletal damage following eccentric contractions in mouse skeletal muscle. *Journal of Applied Physiology* 112: 2077–86.

Zhang, B. T., S. S. Yeung, D. G. Allen, L. Qin, and E. W. Yeung. 2008. Role of the calcium-calpain pathway in cytoskeletal damage after eccentric contractions. *Journal of Applied Physiology* 105: 352–7.

28 Pea (*Pisum sativum* L.) Protein and Its Effects on Human Health

Aubree L. Hawley, Jamie I. Baum, and Chetanjot Kaur Romana

ABBREVIATIONS

4e-BP1	Eukaryotic initiation factor 4E binding protein 1
AA	Amino acid
BCAA	Branched-chain amino acids
BMR	Basal metabolic rate
CCK	Cholecystokinin
DIAAS	Digestible indispensable amino acid score
EAA	Essential amino acids
FAO	Food and Agriculture Organization
GIP	Glucose-dependent insulinotropic polypeptide
GLP-1	Glucagon-like peptide 1
HDL	High-density lipoprotein
IAA	Indispensable amino acids
LBM	Lean body mass
LDL	Low-density lipoprotein
MPS	Muscle protein synthesis
mTORC1	Mechanistic target of rapamycin complex 1
p70S6K	Ribosomal protein S6 kinase beta-1
PPC	Pea protein concentrate
PPH	Pea protein hydrolysate
PPI	Pea protein isolate
PYY	Peptide YY
TEE	Total energy expenditure
TEF	Thermic effect of food
WPI	Whey protein isolate

INTRODUCTION

Chronic conditions, including obesity, cardiovascular disease, type 2 diabetes, and cancer, cause over 41 million deaths annually, accounting for 74% of all deaths globally (World Health Organization 2023). Nutrition, specifically dietary protein intake, serves as an important modifiable factor to support skeletal muscle mass and improve metabolic health throughout an individual's lifespan (Hawley and Baum 2023). Plant-based protein has risen in popularity in recent years, driven largely by concerns over the environmental impact of animal agriculture and the health benefits of plant foods (Singh, Jain, Ujinwal, and Langyan 2022).

DOI: 10.1201/9781003597926-28

The environmental impact of animal agriculture has become a major concern, with livestock estimated to account for 14.5% of global greenhouse gas emissions (Gerber 2013). Shifting toward plant-based diets is increasingly seen as a sustainable strategy to mitigate climate change and other environmental issues like water scarcity, pollution, and biodiversity loss (Saget et al. 2021). Replacing animal proteins with plant proteins like pea offers sustainability advantages, given the substantially lower land, water, and energy requirements of legume crops compared to meat production (de Boer and Aiking 2011; Singh, Jain, Ujinwal, and Langyan 2022). Furthermore, legumes such as peas can enrich soil through nitrogen fixation, reducing the need for synthetic fertilizers (Saget et al. 2021). This shift toward more ecologically friendly plant-based eating patterns has accelerated the demand for high-quality plant-based protein sources. While animal proteins like meat, eggs, and dairy contain highly bioavailable complete amino acid profiles, the protein in many plants has limited bioavailability and is low in one or more essential amino acids (EAAs). Consuming a variety of plant proteins can compensate for their individual deficiencies. Still, interest has grown in identifying single plant protein sources with more complete, digestible EAA profiles that can support metabolic health.

Cultivated peas (*Pisum sativum* L.) are a class of legumes that include two classification types: (1) common/garden peas (*Pisum sativum* ssp. *hortense*), identified by the wrinkled nature of their seed and cotyledon and higher starch accumulation, and (2) field peas (*Pisum sativum* ssp. *arvense*), identified by their smooth seed surface and characterized by a lower sugar content (Grdeń and Jakubczyk 2023). Peas are one of the oldest domesticated crops cultivated for human food or livestock feed. As a major legume crop, global pea production has steadily increased over the past 30 years (Lu et al. 2020). Driven by high demand and relatively low production costs, the global pea protein market was valued at $1.7 billion in 2022 and is expected to reach $2.9 billion by 2027 (MarketsandMarkets Research Pvt. Ltd 2023). Pea protein has emerged as one of the most promising plant-based proteins due to its high protein content (20–25%), essential amino acid profile, high digestive and metabolic amino acid bioavailability, sustainability, and hypoallergenic properties (Gorissen and Witard 2018; Lu et al. 2020). Furthermore, several studies identify pea protein as a protein source that may improve human health through improvements in body composition, physical performance, and cardiometabolic markers (Figure 28.1)

The purpose of this chapter is to comprehensively review the nutritional aspects and metabolic effects of pea protein on human health.

Pea Nutritional Composition

The common pea, specifically the yellow field pea, is commonly fractionated into protein, fiber, and starch and incorporated into various food ingredients and products. In general, pea seeds contain 20–30% protein, 10–20% fiber, and 40–50% starch (Shanthakumar et al. 2022). Pea protein is characterized by its high digestibility, hypoallergenic properties, and complete amino acid (AA) profile. It contains all nine EAAs and high levels of lysine, which may help compensate for lysine shortages in cereal-based diets (Singh et al. 2022). Pea protein contains high and balanced amounts of leucine, isoleucine, and valine, the three essential branched-chain amino acids (BCAAs) that promote muscle growth (Lu et al. 2020). Peas also have good arginine content but limited amounts of the sulfur-containing AAs (methionine and cysteine) (see Table 28.1) compared to other plant proteins (Singh et al. 2022). Furthermore, the approximately 30% EAA content of pea protein meets the WHO/FAO/UNO-recommended EAA requirements based on a dietary protein intake of 0.8 g/kg body weight/day (Gorissen and Witard 2018; WHO/FAO/UNO 2007).

Pea protein is primarily consumed in four forms: whole pea, pea protein isolate (PPI), pea protein concentrate (PPC), and pea protein hydrolysate (PPH), sourced from either yellow pea (lathryus aphaca L.), chickpea (Cicer arietinum L.), or lentils (Lens culinaris). The form of pea protein significantly affects its amino acid composition and digestibility (Table 28.1).

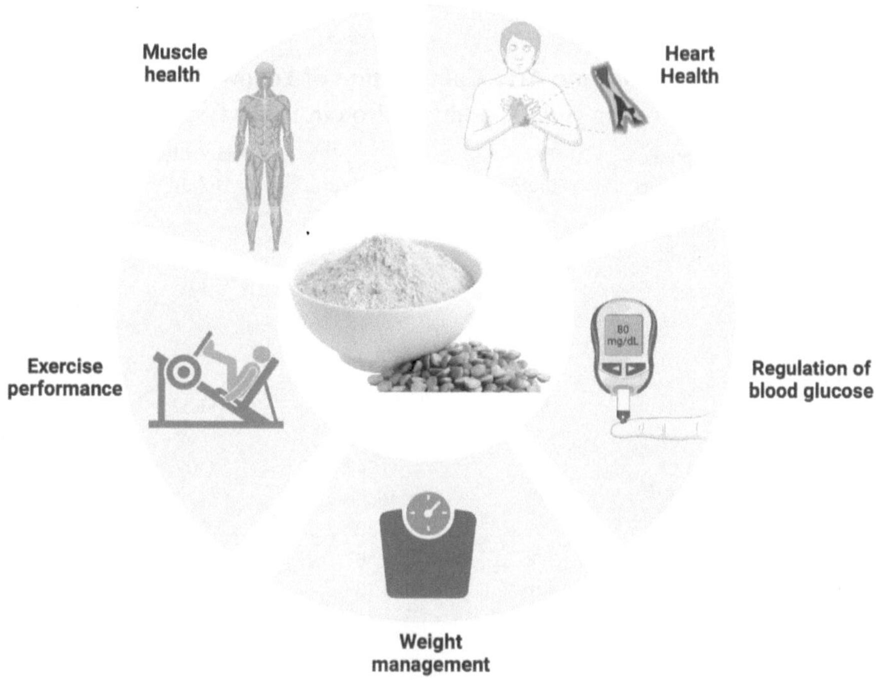

FIGURE 28.1 A schematic representation of pea protein's effect on metabolic health. This figure shows the potential health benefits of pea proteins in sustaining muscular health, improving exercise performance, managing weight, regulating blood glucose levels, and improve cardiovascular health.

Table 28.1 summarizes the nutritional components and amino acid composition of yellow pea, pea flour, pea protein concentrate, pea protein isolate, and pea protein hydrolysate. Moreover, the dietary nitrogen kinetics and 12% nitrogen content of PPI are comparable to those of milk protein (Guillin et al. 2022). In addition to protein content, peas contain vitamins and minerals like zinc, copper, manganese, iron, nickel, vitamin C, and vitamin E (Singh et al. 2022). However, the mineral content varies significantly with genotype and processing (Harmankaya et al. 2010; Shanthakumar et al. 2022).

Pea protein can further be classified into four groups based on chemical structure: albumin, globulin, glutelin, and prolamin. Of these, 65–80% are globulins, and 10–20% are albumins. Globulins are the main storage proteins, soluble in salt solutions, whereas albumin is water-soluble. As a metabolic and enzymatic protein, albumin shows cytosolic function and contains molecules that play roles in seedling growth. Albumin also contains anti-nutrients such as enzymes, protease inhibitors, amylase inhibitors, and lectins. While these anti-nutrients bind micronutrients and reduce macronutrient digestibility, the correct ratio of anti-nutrients to nutrients can reduce the negative impact on digestibility and enhance cellular processes via antioxidant and anti-inflammatory mechanisms (Millar et al. 2019). The ratio of globulin to albumin in pea protein products, specifically PPI, varies due to differences in genotypes and processing methods, which can influence the physicochemical properties of PPI (Shanthakumar et al. 2022; Lu et al. 2020). Of the different forms of pea protein, PPI sourced from yellow peas is the most widely studied and preferred for supporting metabolic health through modifications in body composition (Guillin et al. 2022).

Pea Protein Quality

Protein quality is determined by the digestibility, amount, and diversity of EAAs according to physiological needs. To evaluate protein quality, the Food and Agriculture Organization of the United

TABLE 28.1
Nutritional Components and Amino Acid Composition of Yellow Pea, Pea Flour, Pea Protein Concentrate, Pea Protein Isolate, and Pea Protein Hydrolysate

Component	Yellow Pea (Lathyrus aphaca)[1]	Pea Flour[2]	Pea Protein Concentrate[3]	Pea Protein Isolate[3]	Pea Protein Hydrolysate[5]
Protein (g/100 g)	21.85	24.20	48.5	89.6	83.4
Lipid (g/100 g)	1.87	1.03	0.9	1.6	**
Fiber (g/100 g)	9.11	26.7	**	0	**
Amino Acids (g/100 g protein)					
Aspartine Acid	**	**	11.58	11.52	0.03
Threonine	0.81	3.82	3.12	3.69	0.06
Serine	1.05	4.41	4.96	6.09	0.03
Glutamic acid	**	**	16.39	17.03	0.21
Proline	0.70	**	4.30	5.01	0.007
Glycine	0.84	3.96	4.50	4.68	0.01
Alanine	0.92	4.05	4.13	4.41	0.09
Valine	0.77	4.10	5.13	4.81	0.04
Methionine	0.18	1.01	0.85	0.78	0.10
Isoleucine	0.67	3.56	3.48	3.68	0.11
Leucine	1.34	6.53	6.94	8.16	0.45
Tyrosine	0.39	3.10	3.35	3.79	0.16
Phenylalanine	0.88	4.44	4.67	5.18	0.14
Lysine	1.28	8.88	8.12	8.96	0.09
Histidine	0.50	2.96	3.39	3.81	0.007
Tryptophan	**	1.21	0.51	0.51	0.03
Arginine	1.45	7.20	14.22	7.15	0.06
Cysteine	0.29	1.56	**	**	0.14

[1] Ma, Boye, and Hu (2017); Xu et al. (2019). [2] Martineau-Côté et al. (2023). [3] Tömösközi et al. (2001). [4] Xia et al. (2022); García Arteaga et al. (2022). ** Not detected. All values are expressed in g/100 g of protein.

Nations (FAO) recommends using the digestible indispensable amino acid score (DIAAS) (Food and Agriculture Organization 2013) based on the indispensable amino acid (IAA) composition of the proteins and their individual ileal digestibility. Measuring IAA digestibility in humans is challenging, and studies on pea protein are limited. In a seminal 1996 study, Gausserès et al. (1996) determined the gastro-ileal behavior of pea protein in twenty healthy volunteers. The study found pea protein had an 89.4% true gastro-ileal absorption. More recently, Guillin et al. (2022), used naso-ileal intubation and 15N-labeled proteins to determine the IAA real ileal digestibility of casein and pea protein. They found a DIAAS of 1.00 for pea protein compared to 1.45 for casein. They also found high digestibility (94.6%) and a DIAAS of 0.88 for PPI in rats. When supplemented with methionine, pea protein quality equaled that of casein. These studies confirm the high digestibility of pea protein. However, other pea protein forms like extruded chickpea, yellow pea, pea flour, and pea protein concentrate had lower DIAAS scores of 89.0%, 88.0% (Devi et al. 2020), 71.6% (Kashyap et al. 2019), and 62.0% (Mathai, Liu, and Stein 2017), respectively, indicating the robust effect of processing on digestibility.

Muscle Health and Physical Performance

Muscle health refers to the overall condition and performance of skeletal muscle tissue, which influences cardiometabolic health, physical function, exercise performance, recovery, and well-being (Hawley and Baum 2023). Dietary protein supports muscle health partly via increases in skeletal muscle protein synthesis (MPS) (Baum and Wolfe 2015). The anabolic action of the BCAA leucine activates independent intracellular signaling pathways, which converge at mechanistic target of rapamycin complex 1 (mTORC1), promoting translation initiation and elongation (Gordon, Kelleher, and Kimball 2013). Downstream targets of mTORC1, eukaryotic initiation factor 4E binding protein 1 (4E-BP1) and ribosomal protein S6 kinase beta-1 (p70S6K), play key roles in initiating mRNA translation. The muscle's anabolic response depends on protein digestion and absorption kinetics, AA profile, and postprandial EAA availability, particularly leucine (Baum and Wolfe 2015).

Plant proteins like soy, wheat, and rice elicit weaker anabolic responses compared to dairy proteins (Wolfe et al. 2018). However, PPI may elicit a similar anabolic response to animal proteins, although increasing plasma EAA concentration to a lesser extent (Table 28.2) (Pinckaers et al. 2023; Lanng et al. 2023; Salles et al. 2021; West et al. 2023)

In a seminal study conducted by Lanng et al. (2023), 0.25 g/kg (approximately 14 g) of whey protein concentrate and PPI activated mTORC1 signaling equivalently via mTORC1, p70s6k, p-S6, and peIF4e phosphorylation at rest and post-exercise, although plasma EAAs were lower following PPI intake.

In some instances, lower EAA bioavailability from pea protein may be relevant if protein quantity is insufficient or in older adults and individuals where maintenance of muscle mass and function is difficult due to anabolic resistance or increased need (e.g., illness). For example, studies show older adults digest and absorb protein more slowly in mixed meals containing plant-based foods such as rolled oats and peanut butter than younger adults (Milan et al. 2015). Although the absorption kinetics of PPI within a mixed meal are unknown, delayed absorption of EAAs following a mixed meal may suppress or delay protein synthesis in older muscle. Research shows maximal MPS stimulation with 15 g EAA in older adults (reviewed in Wolfe (2002)). Plant protein blends can increase pea protein's EAA content to meet the 15 g requirement without needing a higher dose. For example, Pinckaers et al. (2023) showed a pea/corn/wheat blend elicited similar MPS to milk protein in young, healthy males. Therefore, blended isolates may compensate for PPI's compositional limitations when required in young, healthy adults. However, for many healthy people, PPI alone may achieve maximum MPS and not pose a health risk.

Few studies have evaluated the effect of pea protein ingestion on strength, physical function, and muscle damage (Table 28.3).

Overall, when coupled with exercise, pea protein and whey protein elicit similar effects on muscle thickness and mass (Babault et al. 2015; Banaszek et al. 2019; Spoelder et al. 2023), muscle strength (Babault et al. 2015; Banaszek et al. 2019; Spoelder et al. 2023), muscle soreness (Nieman et al. 2020; Spoelder et al. 2023), physical performance (Nieman et al. 2020), and muscle damage (Nieman et al. 2020; Loureiro et al. 2023; Spoelder et al. 2023). This may be attributed to sufficient EAAs/leucine in PPI eliciting comparable MPS, degradation rates, mitochondrial activity, and inflammation (Salles et al. 2021).

Weight Management

Appetite, Satiety, and Energy Expenditure

Obesity, defined as an excessive accumulation of fat that may result in adverse metabolic health outcomes (WHO 2021), is a leading cause of chronic disease and all-cause mortality (Global et al. 2016). Dietary protein has been identified as a tool to help individuals lose weight or maintain weight loss, partly through improvements in appetite control and satiety, while protecting skeletal muscle mass (Drummen et al. 2018). However, research on the effect of protein quality on appetite

TABLE 28.2
The Effect of Pea Protein Supplementation on Muscle Protein Synthesis in Clinical Trials

Reference	Study Design	Duration	Population	Exposure/ Intervention	Dose	Outcome Measure	Results and Percent Change
Lanng et al. (2023)	Randomized parallel controlled trial	Acute	Males; mean age: 22.1 years; $n = 50$	One-legged resistance exercise followed by ingestion of pea protein isolate (LinusPro Aps, Aarhus, Denmark) vs cricket vs whey protein concentrate mixed with water	0.25 g/kg fat-free mass (approximately 14.1 g protein)	Plasma EAA concentrations; mTORC1 activation	Plasma EAA concentrations increased more following whey consumption compared to pea and cricket . No differences in activation of mTORC1 signaling pathway (p-Akt, p-mTOR, p-p70s6k, p-S6, p-eIF4E, atrogin) at rest or post-exercise.
Pinckaers et al. (2023)	Randomized, double-blind, parallel-group design	Acute	Males; mean age: 24 years; $n = 24$	Milk protein vs plant protein blend (15 g wheat, 7.5 g corn, and 7.5 g pea protein concentrate) with measurements taken 5 hours postprandial	30 g protein	Plasma EAA concentrations; myofibrillar protein synthesis rates (FSRs)	Plasma EAA concentrations increased more following milk protein consumption. Milk and plant proteins elicit similar MPS responses. Plant blend: 0.064 ± 0.016%/h; milk blend: 0.053 ± 0.013%/h

(Continued)

TABLE 28.2 (CONTINUED)
The Effect of Pea Protein Supplementation on Muscle Protein Synthesis in Clinical Trials

Reference	Study Design	Duration	Population	Exposure/ Intervention	Dose	Outcome Measure	Results and Percent Change
West et al. (2023)	Randomized, double-blind, parallel-group design	Acute	Resistance-trained males and females; mean age: 21 years; *n* = 33	Pea protein vs mycoprotein vs blend post-exercise	25 g protein	Myofibrillar protein fractional synthetic rates (FSRs)	Plasma EAA and leucine concentrations increased more following pea and blend composition compared to mycoprotein. No differences in FSR were observed.

EAA: essential amino acid; mTORC1: mammalian target of rapamycin complex 1; p-Akt: phosphorylated Akt; p-mTOR: phosphorylated mammalian target of rapamycin; p-p70s6k: phosphorylated p70 ribosomal S6 kinase; p-S6: phosphorylated S6; p-eIF4E: phosphorylated eukaryotic initiation factor 4E; MPS: muscle protein synthesis.

TABLE 28.3
The Effect of Pea Protein Supplementation on Performance Outcomes in Clinical Trials

Reference	Study Design	Duration	Population	Exposure/ Intervention	Dose	Outcome Measure	Results and Percent Change
Babault et al. (2015)	Randomized double-blind placebo-controlled clinical trial	12 weeks	Resistance-trained men; mean age: 22 years; $n = 161$	Carbohydrate vs pea protein (Nutralys) vs whey protein concentrate	25 g protein	Muscle thickness, strength	Pea protein and whey protein have similar effects on muscle thickness and strength.
Banaszek et al. (2019)	Parallel design pilot study	8 weeks	High-intensity functional trained men; mean age: 38 years; $n = 15$	Whey vs pea protein (True Nutrition, Vista, CA, USA) with ~350 mL water	25 g protein`	Muscle thickness, strength, force production, workout of the day performance	Pea protein and whey protein result in similar body composition and strength.
Loureiro et al. (2023)	Randomized double-blind crossover study	10 days	Professional soccer players; Male; mean age: 18 years	0.5 g/kg protein from either pea protein (Cosucra, Peqc, Belgium) or whey protein (Nutrata, SC, Brazil) mixed with 350 mL of water	18.68 g protein	Muscle damage	Pea protein lowered creatine kinase levels 24 and 48h post-game compared to whey protein. Conversely, whey protein increased levels of glutamate and sarcosine (indicating oxidative stress) and decreased levels of taurine, serine, betaine, ketoisoisoleucine, and proline.

(Continued)

TABLE 28.3 (CONTINUED)
The Effect of Pea Protein Supplementation on Performance Outcomes in Clinical Trials

Reference	Study Design	Duration	Population	Exposure/ Intervention	Dose	Outcome Measure	Results and Percent Change
Nieman et al. (2020)	Randomized double-blind parallel design study	5 days	Non-athletic, non-obese males	PPI (NUTRALYS S85 Plus, Roquette, Lestrem, France) vs WPI (biPro, Eden, Prairie, MN, USA) vs water	0.9 g protein/kg divided into three doses/ day	Physical performance; delayed-onset muscle soreness; muscle damage	No differences were observed between WPI and PPI.
Spoelder et al. (2023)	Randomized double-blind placebo-controlled trial	13 days	Physically active older adults; mean age: 70 years	Pea protein vs whey protein vs iso-caloric placebo dissolved in water or juice; variables measured 1, 2, and 3 days following a 20–30 km walking bout	12.5 g AM, 12.5 g PM protein	Skeletal muscle mass, muscle strength, muscle soreness, muscle damage	Whey protein decreased creatine kinase compared to pea and placebo groups. No differences in muscle strength, skeletal muscle mass, or muscle soreness.

WPI: whey protein isolate; PPI: pea protein isolate.

and satiety has yielded mixed results. The effects of pea protein on weight management indices via appetite, satiety, and food intake have only been investigated in an acute manner (Table 28.4).

Appetite and satiety are quantified via perceived sensations of hunger and satiety, along with key peripheral hormonal signals that initiate hunger (i.e., ghrelin) or satiety, such as cholecystokinin (CCK), peptide YY (PYY), and glucagon-like peptide 1 (GLP-1) (Leidy 2014). Appetite and satiety have been widely investigated, and PPI elicits similar effects in young and older healthy men (Hawley et al. 2020) and superior effects to WPI in overweight females and males aged 18–60 years (Diepvens, Häberer, and Westerterp-Plantenga 2008) and young, healthy males (Abou-Samra et al. 2011). This may be attributed to the anorexigenic response via hormones CCK, GLP-1, and PYY due to the adequate BCAA content of PPI (Braden, Gwin, and Leidy 2023). Pea protein has further been identified as an intermediate fast protein that moderately and transiently aggregates in the stomach and becomes intestinally available for satiety signaling slightly later than WPI, improving its satiety effect (Overduin et al. 2015). Lastly, pea protein reportedly has lower palatability and higher viscosity compared to whey, casein, and soy (Braden, Gwin, and Leidy 2023; Hawley et al. 2020), further enhancing its appetite and satiety effects.

Furthermore, energy expenditure is a critical component of weight management. High protein diets increase total energy expenditure (TEE) by increasing the thermic effect of food (TEF) or basal metabolic rate (BMR). TEF refers to the energy required for intestinal absorption of nutrients, early stages of nutrient metabolism, and nutrient storage (Hawley and Baum 2023). TEF also increases with higher calorie and protein content. Typically, TEF accounts for 0–3% of total energy intake for fat, 5–10% for carbohydrates, and 20–30% for proteins. Although the effects of PPI on TEF have yet to be widely investigated, PPI exerts similar effects as WPI (15 young men: 25.2 ± 2.8 years; 15 older men: 67.7 ± 4.5 years) (Hawley et al. 2020) and soy protein isolate (8 young men: 28.5 ± 3.6 years) (Claessens et al. 2007) in healthy subjects. Beyond TEF, dietary protein preserves BMR by preventing LBM loss during weight loss interventions. Although the long-term effects of pea protein on weight loss have yet to be elucidated, it is likely PPI elicits similar benefits as WPI due to the comparable effects on the mTORC1, MPS, and physical function reviewed above.

Acute, whole, or partial supplement replacement of animal protein by pea protein does not weaken gastrointestinal satiety signaling, appetite response, or energy expenditure despite pea protein's different amino acid composition and altered gastrointestinal processing. Pea protein can be used as a tool to support weight management interventions. However, as only acute data are available, long-term intervention studies are needed to make conclusions regarding long-term efficacy.

Pea Protein and Cardiometabolic Health

Glycemic Response and Insulin Resistance

Diets higher in protein improve glycemic control by modulating insulin signaling, stimulating the glucose-alanine cycle, and aiding glycemic control indirectly by improving body composition, satiety, and TEF (Layman and Baum 2004). In acute studies, pea protein shows insulinotropic properties in healthy subjects (Lang et al. 1998; Abou-Samra et al. 2011; Diepvens, Häberer, and Westerterp-Plantenga 2008; Re et al. 2016; Claessens et al. 2009). PPI doses of ≥15 g enhance carbohydrate-induced insulin and glucose responses compared to carbohydrate controls similarly to whey protein in healthy male subjects ($n = 8$, 32 ± 13 years) (Claessens et al. 2009) and in animal models *in vivo* (Re et al. 2016). In addition, pea protein-derived bioactive peptides reportedly suppress hepatic glucose production by regulating glucagon and/or insulin signaling pathways (Liu et al. 2021). This may occur through the suppression of glucose production via inhibition of the cAMP response element-binding protein (CREB)-mediated signaling in the gluconeogenic pathway (Liao et al. 2022). The incretin hormones glucose-dependent insulinotropic polypeptide (GIP) and GLP-1 appear to play a minor role in the insulinotropic effect of pea protein (Markova et al. 2018). PPI stimulates the release of GIP similar to WPI (Re et al. 2016) and more substantially than intact pea.

TABLE 28.4
The Effect of Pea Protein Supplementation on Appetite, Satiety, and Energy Intake Outcomes in Clinical Trials

Reference	Study Design	Duration	Population	Intervention	Protein Dose	Outcome Measures	Results
Hawley et al. (2020)	Randomized, single-blind crossover design	Acute	Healthy young males (mean age: 25.2 years; $n = 15$) and older males (mean age: 67.7 years; $n = 15$)	Isocaloric volume-matched WPI vs PPI. Meal response study 4 hours postprandial	40 g	• Appetite • Food intake • Postprandial biomarkers of appetite • Energy expenditure	WPI and PPI exert similar effects on appetite, energy expenditure, and 24-hour energy intake
Mollard et al. (2014)	Crossover design	Acute	Males (mean age: 21.5 years; $n = 16$)	Pea hull fiber (7 g), pea protein (10 g), pea hull fiber + pea protein (7 g + 10g), yellow peas (406 g) provided by Nutri-Pea Limited (Portage la Prairie, Man., Canada) in a pizza meal	10 g	• Appetite • Food intake	No differences in appetite or food intake
Lang et al. (1998)	Randomized single-blind crossover design	Acute	Males (mean age: 22.6 years; $n = 12$)	Protein-manipulated lunches with pea protein, wheat protein (gluten), soy protein, egg white protein (albumin), casein, or pig gelatin	40.1–57.5 g	• Appetite • Food intake (24 hours) • Glucose response (7.5 hours)	No effect of protein source observed

(*Continued*)

TABLE 28.4 (CONTINUED)
The Effect of Pea Protein Supplementation on Appetite, Satiety, and Energy Intake Outcomes in Clinical Trials

Reference	Study Design	Duration	Population	Intervention	Protein Dose	Outcome Measures	Results
Abou-Samra et al. (2011)	Randomized single-blind crossover design	Acute	Males (mean age: 25 years; $n = 32$)	Casein, whey, pea protein, egg albumin, or maltodextrin dissolved in water with additives vs water 30 min before the meal	20 g	Study 1: • Subjective appetite • Food intake Study 2: • Ad libitum meal and food intake	Study 1: Pea protein and casein increased satiety, decreased energy intake Study 2: No differences between protein sources
Smith et al. (2012)	Randomized single-blind crossover design	Acute	Males (mean age: 23 years; $n = 19$)	Tomato soup with or without yellow PPI or fiber followed by an albidum pizza meal	10 g or 20 g	• Appetite • Food intake • Blood glucose	10 g and 20 g yellow PPI suppressed food intake and reduced glycemic response at 30 minutes vs fiber and control
Diepvens, Häberer, and Westerterp-Plantenga (2008)	Randomized single-blind crossover design	Acute	Males and females (20/19; mean age: 42.3 years; $n = 39$)	WPI, PPH, WP + PPH, or milk protein control (80% casein and 20% WP)	15 g	• Subjective appetite • Appetite biomarkers • Food intake	PPH: modest satiety enhancement, longer inter-meal interval, trend for a higher satiety index
Braden, Gwin, and Leidy (2023)	Randomized crossover design	3-day acclimation to beverage and acute testing on day 4	Males and females (mean age: 25 years; $n = 32$)	PPI, WPI, SPI, or micellar casein (250 kcal)	24 g	• Subjective appetite • Appetite biomarkers • Food intake	PPI and micellar casein (not whey): greater acute changes in appetite and satiety vs SPI; no effect on energy intake; PPI increased PYY vs SPI

(Continued)

TABLE 28.4 (CONTINUED)
The Effect of Pea Protein Supplementation on Appetite, Satiety, and Energy Intake Outcomes in Clinical Trials

Reference	Study Design	Duration	Population	Intervention	Protein Dose	Outcome Measures	Results
Re et al. (2016)	Four-arm double-blind, randomized, crossover, pilot study	Acute	Males and females (mean age: 36–44; $n = 33$ for satiety, $n = 9$ for blood collection)	Preload powdered vegetable soup (~200 kcal): Control (no protein) vs 15 g PPI vs 30 g PPI vs 30 g WPC. Not matched for carbohydrates. Yellow pea protein powder (NUTRALYS S85 Plus pea protein)	15 g or 30 g	• Appetite and satiety (VAS) • Objective appetite via biomarkers • Energy intake • Glucose regulation	PPI reduced food intake, glycemic and insulinemic responses vs control; 30 g of PPI and WPC reduced glycemia and insulinemia; no effect on CCK, GLP-1, PYY

WPI: whey protein isolate; PPI: pea protein isolate; SPI: soy protein isolate; PPH: pea protein hydrolysate; PYY: peptide YY; WPC: whey protein concentrate; CCK: cholecystokinin; GLP-1: glucagon-like peptide 1; VAS: visual analog scale.

As GIP is associated with inflammation and insulin resistance (Gögebakan et al. 2015), pea protein in conjunction with pea fiber or whole yellow peas may be an appropriate option to improve insulin resistance and glycemic response in healthy and diabetic populations (Marinangeli and Jones 2011; Yoshimoto et al. 2020).

Blood Lipids

The effect of pea protein on lipid metabolism has not been well-studied. However, consuming pulses (i.e., beans, peas, chickpeas, and lentils) (Abeysekara et al. 2012) or combining pea protein with soluble fiber decreases total cholesterol concentration compared to protein supplementation alone (Sirtori et al. 2012). Sirtori et al. (2012) found pea protein coupled with oat fiber or apple pectin reduced total cholesterol levels in male and female adults ($n = 25$, 52.3 ± 12.4 years) by 4.7% and 6.4% and low-density lipoprotein (LDL) cholesterol by 5.8% and 6.4%, respectively. Furthermore, when nutritionally balanced, caloric-restricted, fiber-fortified diets were supplemented with partial meal replacements rich in soy, pea, and wheat protein in obese subjects (BMI >27; $n = 50$, male 23, female 27) for 8 weeks, pea improved total serum cholesterol, LDL, high-density lipoprotein (HDL), and insulin resistance (Lu et al. 2019). As the data on pea protein is scarce, the mechanism of pea protein's hypocholesterolemic activity may be deduced from animal studies. Rodent and *in vitro* studies have established a link between gene regulation of hepatic metabolism and activation and depression of liver LDL (Rigamonti et al. 2010), stimulation of bile acid excretion, and modulation of the gut microbiota and metabolites (Tong et al. 2021).

Blood Pressure

Partially replacing dietary carbohydrates with protein benefits blood pressure management. A meta-analysis of forty randomized controlled trials (including 3,277 participants) found that plant and animal proteins similarly reduce systolic and diastolic blood pressure in adults with and without chronic disease (Rebholz et al. 2012), although little data on the effects of pea protein exist. In acute studies, when test meals consisted of 0.6 g protein/kg body mass, pea protein reduced blood pressure comparably to a milk-protein meal and more than an egg white protein meal. The acute antihypertensive effects of pea protein may result from increased nitric oxide levels, a potent vasodilator, due to glycine and arginine availability and induction of the hormones insulin, glucagon, and GLP-1 (Teunissen-Beekman et al. 2014).

Thermoase-digested yellow field pea PPH consists of low molecular weight bioactive peptides (2 to 6 amino acid residues) saturated with hydrophilic amino acids (Girgih et al. 2016). Human, *in vivo*, and *in vitro* research suggests the low molecular weight peptides found in yellow peas effectively reduce systolic blood pressure via the renin-angiotensin system, which helps regulate the key enzymes renin and angiotensin I-converting enzyme, which are responsible for increases in blood pressure (Li et al. 2011; Girgih et al. 2016). In humans (Li et al. 2011), the overall maximum systolic blood pressure reduction of 10 mmHg was observed following 3 g/day of PPH, comparable to a single dose of an antihypertensive drug. However, more clinical trials are needed to confirm the safety and efficacy of PPH as an antihypertensive agent.

THE EFFECTS OF OTHER PROTEINS

In addition to pea protein, it is important to consider other protein sources in the diet, such as WPI, casein, soy protein isolate, and insect protein.

Studies have shown that whey and casein have a higher proportion of EAAs and BCAAs compared to pea protein (Gorissen et al. 2018). Although PPI has a relatively high DIAAS of 1, WPI has a higher DIAAS of 1.09 (Rutherfurd and Moughan 2012). With a DIAAS of 1, WPI can complement lower-quality proteins if nitrogen intake is adequate, thereby improving diet quality (Food and Agriculture Organization 2013). Unlike pea protein, long-term studies (>12 weeks) have evaluated the effects of WPI on metabolic health outcomes. These show beneficial or neutral effects of WPI on body composition, satiety, physical function, inflammation, energy expenditure, lipid profiles, and glycemic control (Griffen, Duncan, et al. 2022; Pal, Ellis, and Dhaliwal 2010; Griffen, Renshaw, et al. 2022).

Soy protein, a widely studied plant protein, has a lower EAA content compared to pea protein (Gorissen et al. 2018) and is allergenic, although research indicates that long-term soy consumption provides metabolic health benefits in both young and older adults, with and without chronic disease (Messina et al. 2022).

Moreover, insect protein has emerged as a novel, sustainable, and high-quality protein source. Like plant proteins, insect protein provides an alternative, nutritious protein with anti-inflammatory properties due to its high phenolic content (Quinteros et al. 2022). Research suggests beneficial effects on muscle health due to its comparable anabolic potential to PPI and WPI (Lanng et al. 2023).

Therefore, while pea protein appears to offer comparable benefits to other high-quality protein sources, incorporating a variety of protein sources within a healthy eating pattern may promote metabolic health.

CONCLUSION

In summary, pea protein is a promising plant-based, sustainable protein source that appears comparable to animal proteins for supporting muscle health and exercise recovery when consumed in adequate amounts. Early research also indicates beneficial effects on appetite regulation and cardiometabolic parameters. However, more studies are needed to determine long-term health impacts. Pea protein is a quality, sustainable protein option that may provide health benefits and contribute to environmental sustainability through its incorporation into dietary recommendations and food products.

MINI DICTIONARY OF TERMS

- **Energy expenditure:** The sum of calories utilized by the body's metabolic processes.
- **Muscle health:** The overall condition and performance of skeletal muscle tissue.
- **Muscle protein synthesis:** The metabolic process by which amino acids are synthesized into skeletal muscle proteins.
- **Pea protein:** A plant-based food product and protein supplement typically derived from the yellow field pea that contains all nine essential amino acids.
- **Protein quality:** An index of the digestibility, amount, and diversity of EAAs according to physiological needs.

SUMMARY POINTS

- This chapter focuses on pea protein as a dietary source.
- Pea protein is primarily consumed in four forms, including whole pea, pea protein isolate, concentrate, and hydrolysate.
- Pea protein's anabolic effects are comparable to those of whey protein.
- Pea protein supports weight management in the short term.
- Long-term data evaluating the efficacy of pea protein are limited.
- Including pea protein in the diet acutely supports metabolic health in humans.

REFERENCES

Consultation, J.F. 2007. "Protein and amino acid requirements in human nutrition." *World Health Organization Technical Report Series* (935):1–265, back cover.

Abeysekara, S., P. D. Chilibeck, H. Vatanparast, and G. A. Zello. 2012. "A pulse-based diet is effective for reducing total and LDL-cholesterol in older adults." *Br J Nutr* 108 (Suppl 1):S103–10. doi: 10.1017/s0007114512000748.

Abou-Samra, R., L. Keersmaekers, D. Brienza, R. Mukherjee, and K. Macé. 2011. "Effect of different protein sources on satiation and short-term satiety when consumed as a starter." *Nutr J* 10:139. doi: 10.1186/1475-2891-10-139.

Babault, N., C. Païzis, G. Deley, L. Guérin-Deremaux, M. H. Saniez, C. Lefranc-Millot, and F. A. Allaert. 2015. "Pea proteins oral supplementation promotes muscle thickness gains during resistance training: a double-blind, randomized, Placebo-controlled clinical trial vs. Whey protein." *J Int Soc Sports Nutr* 12 (1):3. doi: 10.1186/s12970-014-0064-5.

Banaszek, A., J. R. Townsend, D. Bender, W. C. Vantrease, A. C. Marshall, and K. D. Johnson. 2019. "The effects of whey vs. Pea protein on physical adaptations following 8-weeks of high-intensity functional training (HIFT): a pilot study." *Sports (Basel)* 7 (1). doi: 10.3390/sports7010012.

Baum, J. I., and R. R. Wolfe. 2015. "The link between dietary protein intake, skeletal muscle function and health in older adults." *Healthcare (Basel)* 3 (3):529–43. doi: 10.3390/healthcare3030529.

Braden, M. L., J. A. Gwin, and H. J. Leidy. 2023. "Protein source influences acute appetite and satiety but not subsequent food intake in healthy adults." *J Nutr* 153 (6):1825–33. doi: 10.1016/j.tjnut.2023.04.001.

Claessens, M., W. Calame, A. D. Siemensma, W. H. Saris, and M. A. van Baak. 2007. "The thermogenic and metabolic effects of protein hydrolysate with or without a carbohydrate load in healthy male subjects." *Metabolism* 56 (8):1051–9. doi: 10.1016/j.metabol.2007.04.001.

Claessens, M., W. Calame, A. D. Siemensma, M. A. van Baak, and W. H. Saris. 2009. "The effect of different protein hydrolysate/carbohydrate mixtures on postprandial glucagon and insulin responses in healthy subjects." *Eur J Clin Nutr* 63 (1):48–56. doi: 10.1038/sj.ejcn.1602896.

de Boer, Joop, and Harry Aiking. 2011. "On the merits of plant-based proteins for global food security: marrying macro and micro perspectives." *Ecological Economics* 70 (7):1259–65. doi: 10.1016/j.ecolecon.2011.03.001.

Devi, S., A. Varkey, M. Dharmar, R. R. Holt, L. H. Allen, M. S. Sheshshayee, T. Preston, C. L. Keen, and A. V. Kurpad. 2020. "Amino acid digestibility of extruded chickpea and yellow pea protein is high and comparable in moderately stunted south indian children with use of a dual stable isotope tracer method." *J Nutr* 150 (5):1178–85. doi: 10.1093/jn/nxaa004.

Diepvens, K., D. Häberer, and M. Westerterp-Plantenga. 2008. "Different proteins and biopeptides differently affect satiety and anorexigenic/orexigenic hormones in healthy humans." *Int J Obes (Lond)* 32 (3):510–8. doi: 10.1038/sj.ijo.0803758.

Drummen, M., L. Tischmann, B. Gatta-Cherifi, T. Adam, and M. Westerterp-Plantenga. 2018. "Dietary protein and energy balance in relation to obesity and co-morbidities." *Front Endocrinol (Lausanne)* 9:443. doi: 10.3389/fendo.2018.00443.

Food and Agriculture Organization. 2013. Dietary protein quality evaluation in human nutrition. In *Report of an FAO Expert Consultation*. Food and Nutrition Paper n92: FAO.

García Arteaga, V., V. Demand, K. Kern, A. Strube, M. Szardenings, I. Muranyi, P. Eisner, and U. Schweiggert-Weisz. 2022. "Enzymatic hydrolysis and fermentation of pea protein isolate and its effects on antigenic proteins, functional properties, and sensory profile." *Foods* 11 (1):118. doi: 10.3390/foods11010118.

Gausserès, N., S. Mahè, R. Benamouzig, C. Luengo, H. Drouet, J. Rautureau, and D. Tomè. 1996. "The gastro-ileal digestion of 15N-labelled pea nitrogen in adult humans." *Br J Nutr* 76 (1):75–85. doi: 10.1079/bjn19960010.

Gerber, P. J., H. Steinfeld, B. Henderson, A. Mottet, C. Opio, J. Dijkman, A. Falcucci, and G. Tempio. 2013. "Tackling climate change through livestock – A global assessment of emissions and mitigation opportunities." Food and Agriculture Organization of the United Nations (FAO), Rome.

Girgih, A. T., I. D. Nwachukwu, J. O. Onuh, S. A. Malomo, and R. E. Aluko. 2016. "Antihypertensive properties of a pea protein hydrolysate during short- and long-term oral administration to spontaneously hypertensive rats." *J Food Sci* 81 (5):H1281–7. doi: 10.1111/1750-3841.13272.

Global, B. M. I. Mortality Collaboration, E. Di Angelantonio, N. Bhupathiraju Sh, D. Wormser, P. Gao, S. Kaptoge, A. Berrington de Gonzalez, B. J. Cairns, R. Huxley, L. Jackson Ch, G. Joshy, S. Lewington, J. E. Manson, N. Murphy, A. V. Patel, J. M. Samet, M. Woodward, W. Zheng, M. Zhou, N. Bansal,

A. Barricarte, B. Carter, J. R. Cerhan, G. D. Smith, X. Fang, O. H. Franco, J. Green, J. Halsey, J. S. Hildebrand, K. J. Jung, R. J. Korda, D. F. McLerran, S. C. Moore, L. M. O'Keeffe, E. Paige, A. Ramond, G. K. Reeves, B. Rolland, C. Sacerdote, N. Sattar, E. Sofianopoulou, J. Stevens, M. Thun, H. Ueshima, L. Yang, Y. D. Yun, P. Willeit, E. Banks, V. Beral, Zh Chen, S. M. Gapstur, M. J. Gunter, P. Hartge, S. H. Jee, T. H. Lam, R. Peto, J. D. Potter, W. C. Willett, S. G. Thompson, J. Danesh, and F. B. Hu. 2016. "Body-mass index and all-cause mortality: individual-participant-data meta-analysis of 239 prospective studies in four continents." *Lancet* 388 (10046):776–86. doi: 10.1016/s0140-6736(16)30175-1.

Gögebakan, Ö., M. A. Osterhoff, R. Schüler, O. Pivovarova, M. Kruse, A. C. Seltmann, A. S. Mosig, N. Rudovich, M. Nauck, and A. F. Pfeiffer. 2015. "GIP increases adipose tissue expression and blood levels of MCP-1 in humans and links high energy diets to inflammation: a randomised trial." *Diabetologia* 58 (8):1759–68. doi: 10.1007/s00125-015-3618-4.

Gordon, B. S., A. R. Kelleher, and S. R. Kimball. 2013. "Regulation of muscle protein synthesis and the effects of catabolic states." *Int J Biochem Cell Biol* 45 (10):2147–57. doi: 10.1016/j.biocel.2013.05.039.

Gorissen, S. H. M., J. J. R. Crombag, J. M. G. Senden, W. A. H. Waterval, J. Bierau, L. B. Verdijk, and L. J. C. van Loon. 2018. "Protein content and amino acid composition of commercially available plant-based protein isolates." *Amino Acids* 50 (12):1685–95. doi: 10.1007/s00726-018-2640-5.

Gorissen, S. H. M., and O. C. Witard. 2018. "Characterising the muscle anabolic potential of dairy, meat and plant-based protein sources in older adults." *Proceedings of the Nutrition Society* 77 (1):20–31. doi: 10.1017/S002966511700194X.

Grdeń, P., and A. Jakubczyk. 2023. "Health benefits of legume seeds." *J Sci Food Agric* 103 (11):5213–20. doi: 10.1002/jsfa.12585.

Griffen, C., M. Duncan, J. Hattersley, M. O. Weickert, A. Dallaway, and D. Renshaw. 2022. "Effects of resistance exercise and whey protein supplementation on skeletal muscle strength, mass, physical function, and hormonal and inflammatory biomarkers in healthy active older men: a randomised, double-blind, placebo-controlled trial." *Exp Gerontol* 158:111651. doi: 10.1016/j.exger.2021.111651.

Griffen, C., D. Renshaw, M. Duncan, M. O. Weickert, and J. Hattersley. 2022. "Changes in 24-h energy expenditure, substrate oxidation, and body composition following resistance exercise and a high protein diet via whey protein supplementation in healthy older men." *Physiol Rep* 10 (11):e15268. doi: 10.14814/phy2.15268.

Guillin, F. M., C. Gaudichon, L. Guérin-Deremaux, C. Lefranc-Millot, G. Airinei, N. Khodorova, R. Benamouzig, P. H. Pomport, J. Martin, and J. Calvez. 2022. "Real ileal amino acid digestibility of pea protein compared to casein in healthy humans: a randomized trial." *Am J Clin Nutr* 115 (2):353–63. doi: 10.1093/ajcn/nqab354.

Guillin, F. M., C. Gaudichon, L. Guérin-Deremaux, C. Lefranc-Millot, D. Azzout-Marniche, N. Khodorova, and J. Calvez. 2021. "Multi-criteria assessment of pea protein quality in rats: a comparison between casein, gluten and pea protein alone or supplemented with methionine." *Br J Nutr* 125 (4):389–97. doi: 10.1017/s0007114520002883.

Harmankaya, Mustafa, Mehmet Özcan, Serdar Karadaş, and Ercan Ceyhan. 2010. "Protein and mineral contents of pea (Pisum sativum L.) genotypes grown in central anatolian region of turkey." *South Western Journal of Horticulture, Biology and Environment* 1:159–65.

Hawley, A. L., and J. I. Baum. 2023. "Nutrition as the foundation for successful aging: a focus on dietary protein and omega-3 polyunsaturated fatty acids." *Nutr Rev.* doi: 10.1093/nutrit/nuad061.

Hawley, A. L., E. Gbur, A. M. Tacinelli, S. Walker, A. Murphy, R. Burgess, and J. I. Baum. 2020. "The short-term effect of whey compared with pea protein on appetite, food intake, and energy expenditure in young and older men." *Curr Dev Nutr* 4 (2):nzaa009. doi: 10.1093/cdn/nzaa009.

Kashyap, S., A. Varkey, N. Shivakumar, S. Devi, B. H. R. Reddy, T. Thomas, T. Preston, S. Sreeman, and A. V. Kurpad. 2019. "True ileal digestibility of legumes determined by dual-isotope tracer method in Indian adults." *Am J Clin Nutr* 110 (4):873–82. doi: 10.1093/ajcn/nqz159.

Lang, V., F. Bellisle, J. M. Oppert, C. Craplet, F. R. Bornet, G. Slama, and B. Guy-Grand. 1998. "Satiating effect of proteins in healthy subjects: a comparison of egg albumin, casein, gelatin, soy protein, pea protein, and wheat gluten." *Am J Clin Nutr* 67 (6):1197–204. doi: 10.1093/ajcn/67.6.1197.

Lanng, S. K., M. Oxfeldt, S. S. Pedersen, F. T. Johansen, J. Risikesan, T. Lejel, H. C. Bertram, and M. Hansen. 2023. "Influence of protein source (cricket, pea, whey) on amino acid bioavailability and activation of the mTORC1 signaling pathway after resistance exercise in healthy young males." *Eur J Nutr* 62 (3):1295–308. doi: 10.1007/s00394-022-03071-y.

Layman, Donald K., and Jamie I. Baum. 2004. "Dietary protein impact on glycemic control during weight loss." *The Journal of Nutrition* 134 (4):968S–73S. doi: https://doi.org/10.1093/jn/134.4.968S.

Leidy, H. J. 2014. "Increased dietary protein as a dietary strategy to prevent and/or treat obesity." *Mo Med* 111 (1):54–8.

Li, H., N. Prairie, C. C. Udenigwe, A. P. Adebiyi, P. S. Tappia, H. M. Aukema, P. J. Jones, and R. E. Aluko. 2011. "Blood pressure lowering effect of a pea protein hydrolysate in hypertensive rats and humans." *J Agric Food Chem* 59 (18):9854–60. doi: 10.1021/jf201911p.

Liao, W., X. Cao, H. Xia, S. Wang, and G. Sun. 2022. "Pea protein-derived peptides inhibit hepatic glucose production via the gluconeogenic signaling in the AML-12 cells." *Int J Environ Res Public Health* 19 (16). doi: 10.3390/ijerph191610254.

Liu, J. P., Y. F. Qian, G. Y. Qin, L. Y. Zhao, and G. T. Chen. 2021. "Antidiabetic activities of glycoprotein from pea (Pisum sativum L.) in STZ-induced diabetic mice." *Food Funct* 12 (11):5087–95. doi: 10.1039/d1fo00535a.

Loureiro, L. L., T. J. Ferreira, F. L. C. Cahuê, V. Z. Bittencourt, A. P. Valente, and Aptr Pierucci. 2023. "Comparison of the effects of pea protein and whey protein on the metabolic profile of soccer athletes: a randomized, double-blind, crossover trial." *Front Nutr* 10:1210215. doi: 10.3389/fnut.2023.1210215.

Lu, T. M., H. F. Chiu, Y. M. Chen, Y. C. Shen, Y. C. Han, K. Venkatakrishnan, and C. K. Wang. 2019. "Effect of a balanced nutrition meal replacement diet with altered macromolecular composition along with caloric restriction on body weight control." *Food Funct* 10 (6):3581–8. doi: 10.1039/c9fo00192a.

Lu, Z. X., J. F. He, Y. C. Zhang, and D. J. Bing. 2020. "Composition, physicochemical properties of pea protein and its application in functional foods." *Crit Rev Food Sci Nutr* 60 (15):2593–605. doi: 10.1080/10408398.2019.1651248.

Ma, Zhen, Joyce I. Boye, and Xinzhong Hu. 2017. "In vitro digestibility, protein composition and techno-functional properties of Saskatchewan grown yellow field peas (Pisum sativum L.) as affected by processing." *Food Res Int* 92:64–78. doi: 10.1016/j.foodres.2016.12.012.

Marinangeli, C. P., and P. J. Jones. 2011. "Whole and fractionated yellow pea flours reduce fasting insulin and insulin resistance in hypercholesterolaemic and overweight human subjects." *Br J Nutr* 105 (1):110–7. doi: 10.1017/s0007114510003156.

MarketsandMarkets Research Pvt. Ltd. 2023. "Global pea protein market size, value & industry growth analysis report." https://www.globenewswire.com/news-release/2023/08/31/2735252/0/en/Global-Pea-Protein-Market-Size-Value-Industry-Growth-Analysis-Report.html.

Markova, M., S. Hornemann, S. Sucher, K. Wegner, O. Pivovarova, N. Rudovich, R. Thomann, R. Schneeweiss, S. Rohn, and A. F. H. Pfeiffer. 2018. "Rate of appearance of amino acids after a meal regulates insulin and glucagon secretion in patients with type 2 diabetes: a randomized clinical trial." *Am J Clin Nutr* 108 (2):279–91. doi: 10.1093/ajcn/nqy100.

Martineau-Côté, D., A. Achouri, M. Pitre, J. Wanasundara, S. Karboune, and L. L'Hocine. 2023. "Investigation of the nutritional quality of raw and processed Canadian faba bean (Vicia faba L.) flours in comparison to pea and soy using a human in vitro gastrointestinal digestion model." *Food research international* 173:113264. doi: 10.1016/j.foodres.2023.113264.

Mathai, J. K., Y. Liu, and H. H. Stein. 2017. "Values for digestible indispensable amino acid scores (DIAAS) for some dairy and plant proteins may better describe protein quality than values calculated using the concept for protein digestibility-corrected amino acid scores (PDCAAS)." *Br J Nutr* 117 (4):490–99. doi: 10.1017/S0007114517000125.

Messina, M., A. Duncan, V. Messina, H. Lynch, J. Kiel, and J. W. Erdman, Jr. 2022. "The health effects of soy: A reference guide for health professionals." *Front Nutr* 9:970364. doi: 10.3389/fnut.2022.970364.

Milan, A. M., R. F. D'Souza, S. Pundir, C. A. Pileggi, E. B. Thorstensen, M. P. Barnett, J. F. Markworth, D. Cameron-Smith, and C. J. Mitchell. 2015. "Older adults have delayed amino acid absorption after a high protein mixed breakfast meal." *J Nutr Health Aging* 19 (8):839–45. doi: 10.1007/s12603-015-0500-5.

Millar, K. A., E. Gallagher, R. Burke, S. McCarthy, and C. Barry-Ryan. 2019. "Proximate composition and anti-nutritional factors of fava-bean (Vicia faba), green-pea and yellow-pea (Pisum sativum) flour." *J Food Compos Anal* 82:103233. doi: 10.1016/j.jfca.2019.103233.

Mollard, R. C., B. L. Luhovyy, C. Smith, and G. H. Anderson. 2014. "Acute effects of pea protein and hull fibre alone and combined on blood glucose, appetite, and food intake in healthy young men – a randomized crossover trial." *Appl Physiol Nutr Metab* 39 (12):1360–5. doi: 10.1139/apnm-2014-0170.

Nieman, D. C., K. A. Zwetsloot, A. J. Simonson, A. T. Hoyle, X. Wang, H. K. Nelson, C. Lefranc-Millot, and L. Guérin-Deremaux. 2020. "Effects of whey and pea protein supplementation on post-eccentric exercise muscle damage: a randomized trial." *Nutrients* 12 (8). doi: 10.3390/nu12082382.

Overduin, J., L. Guérin-Deremaux, D. Wils, and T. T. Lambers. 2015. "NUTRALYS(®) pea protein: characterization of in vitro gastric digestion and in vivo gastrointestinal peptide responses relevant to satiety." *Food Nutr Res* 59:25622. doi: 10.3402/fnr.v59.25622.

Pal, S., V. Ellis, and S. Dhaliwal. 2010. "Effects of whey protein isolate on body composition, lipids, insulin and glucose in overweight and obese individuals." *Br J Nutr* 104 (5):716–23. doi: 10.1017/s0007114510000991.

Pinckaers, P. J. M., I. W. K. Kouw, S. H. M. Gorissen, L. H. P. Houben, J. M. Senden, Wkhw Wodzig, Lcpgm de Groot, L. B. Verdijk, T. Snijders, and L. J. C. van Loon. 2023. "The muscle protein synthetic response to the ingestion of a plant-derived protein blend does not differ from an equivalent amount of milk protein in healthy young males." *J Nutr* 152 (12):2734–43. doi: 10.1093/jn/nxac222.

Quinteros, M. F., J. Martínez, A. Barrionuevo, M. Rojas, and W. Carrillo. 2022. "Functional, antioxidant, and anti-inflammatory properties of cricket protein concentrate (Gryllus assimilis)." *Biology (Basel)* 11 (5). doi: 10.3390/biology11050776.

Re, R., S. Pombo, W. Calame, C. Lefranc-Millot, and L. Guérin-Deremaux. 2016. "The satiating effect of NUTRALYS® Pea protein leads to reduced energy intake in healthy humans." *Journal of Nutritional Health & Food Science* 4 (3):1–10. doi: http://dx.doi.org/10.15226/jnhfs.2016.00165.

Rebholz, C. M., E. E. Friedman, L. J. Powers, W. D. Arroyave, J. He, and T. N. Kelly. 2012. "Dietary protein intake and blood pressure: a meta-analysis of randomized controlled trials." *Am J Epidemiol* 176 Suppl 7:S27–43. doi: 10.1093/aje/kws245.

Rigamonti, E., C. Parolini, M. Marchesi, E. Diani, S. Brambilla, C. R. Sirtori, and G. Chiesa. 2010. "Hypolipidemic effect of dietary pea proteins: Impact on genes regulating hepatic lipid metabolism." *Mol Nutr Food Res* 54 Suppl 1:S24–30. doi: 10.1002/mnfr.200900251.

Rutherfurd, S. M., and P. J. Moughan. 2012. "Available versus digestible dietary amino acids." *Br J Nutr* 108 Suppl 2:S298–305. doi: 10.1017/s0007114512002528.

Saget, S., M. Costa, C. Sancho Santos, M. Wilton Vasconcelos, J. Gibbons, D. Styles, and M. Williams. 2021. "Substitution of beef with pea protein reduces the environmental footprint of meat balls whilst supporting health and climate stabilisation goals." *J Clean Prod* 297:126447. doi: https://doi.org/10.1016/j.jclepro.2021.126447.

Salles, J., C. Guillet, O. Le Bacquer, C. Malnero-Fernandez, C. Giraudet, V. Patrac, A. Berry, P. Denis, C. Pouyet, M. Gueugneau, Y. Boirie, H. Jacobs, and S. Walrand. 2021. "Pea proteins have anabolic effects comparable to milk proteins on whole body protein retention and muscle protein metabolism in old rats." *Nutrients* 13 (12). doi: 10.3390/nu13124234.

Shanthakumar, P., J. Klepacka, A. Bains, P. Chawla, S. B. Dhull, and A. Najda. 2022. "The current situation of pea protein and its application in the food industry." *Molecules* 27 (16). doi: 10.3390/molecules27165354.

Singh, N., P. Jain, M. Ujinwal, and S. Langyan. 2022. "Escalate protein plates from legumes for sustainable human nutrition." *Front Nutr* 9:977986. doi: 10.3389/fnut.2022.977986.

Sirtori, C. R., M. Triolo, R. Bosisio, A. Bondioli, L. Calabresi, V. De Vergori, M. Gomaraschi, G. Mombelli, F. Pazzucconi, C. Zacherl, and A. Arnoldi. 2012. "Hypocholesterolaemic effects of lupin protein and pea protein/fibre combinations in moderately hypercholesterolaemic individuals." *Br J Nutr* 107 (8):1176–83. doi: 10.1017/s0007114511004120.

Smith, C. E., R. C. Mollard, B. L. Luhovyy, and G. H. Anderson. 2012. "The effect of yellow pea protein and fibre on short-term food intake, subjective appetite and glycaemic response in healthy young men." *Br J Nutr* 108 Suppl 1:S74–80. doi: 10.1017/s0007114512000700.

Spoelder, M., L. Koopmans, Y. A. W. Hartman, Ccwg Bongers, M. C. A. Schoofs, T. M. H. Eijsvogels, and M. T. E. Hopman. 2023. "Supplementation with whey protein, but not pea protein, reduces muscle damage following long-distance walking in older adults." *Nutrients* 15 (2). doi: 10.3390/nu15020342.

Teunissen-Beekman, K. F., J. Dopheide, J. M. Geleijnse, S. J. Bakker, E. J. Brink, P. W. de Leeuw, J. Serroyen, and M. A. van Baak. 2014. "Differential effects of proteins and carbohydrates on postprandial blood pressure-related responses." *Br J Nutr* 112 (4):600–8. doi: 10.1017/s0007114514001251.

Tömösközi, S, R Lásztity, Reka Haraszi, and O Baticz. 2001. "Isolation and study of the functional properties of pea proteins." *Food/Nahrung* 45 (6):399–401.

Tong, L. T., T. Xiao, L. Wang, C. Lu, L. Liu, X. Zhou, A. Wang, W. Qin, and F. Wang. 2021. "Plant protein reduces serum cholesterol levels in hypercholesterolemia hamsters by modulating the compositions of gut microbiota and metabolites." *iScience* 24 (12):103435. doi: 10.1016/j.isci.2021.103435.

West, S., A. J. Monteyne, G. Whelehan, I. van der Heijden, D. R. Abdelrahman, A. J. Murton, T. J. A. Finnigan, F. B. Stephens, and B. T. Wall. 2023. "Ingestion of mycoprotein, pea protein, and their blend support comparable postexercise myofibrillar protein synthesis rates in resistance-trained individuals." *Am J Physiol Endocrinol Metab* 325 (3):E267–79. doi: 10.1152/ajpendo.00166.2023.

WHO. 2021. "Obesity and overweight." https://www.who.int/news-room/fact-sheets/detail/obesity-and-overweight. Accessed 09/16/22.

Wolfe, R. R. 2002. "Regulation of muscle protein by amino acids." *J Nutr* 132 (10):3219S–24S.

Wolfe, R. R., J. I. Baum, C. Starck, and P. J. Moughan. 2018. "Factors contributing to the selection of dietary protein food sources." *Clin Nutr* 37 (1):130–138. doi: 10.1016/j.clnu.2017.11.017.

World Health Organization. 2023. "Noncommunicable diseases." https://www.who.int/news-room/fact-sheets/detail/noncommunicable-diseases.

Xia, Yixuan, Ling Zhu, Gangcheng Wu, Tongtong Liu, Xiaojing Li, Xingguo Wang, and Hui Zhang. 2022. "Comparative study of various methods used for bitterness reduction from pea (Pisum sativum L.) protein hydrolysates." *Food Sci Tech*159:113228. doi: 10.1016/j.lwt.2022.113228.

Xu, Minwei, Zhao Jin, Senay Simsek, Clifford Hall, Jiajia Rao, and Bingcan Chen. 2019. "Effect of germination on the chemical composition, thermal, pasting, and moisture sorption properties of flours from chickpea, lentil, and yellow pea." *Food Chem* 295:579–87. doi: 10.1016/j.foodchem.2019.05.167.

Yoshimoto, J., Y. Kato, M. Ban, M. Kishi, H. Horie, C. Yamada, and Y. Nishizaki. 2020. "Palatable noodles as a functional staple food made exclusively from yellow peas suppressed rapid postprandial glucose increase." *Nutrients* 12 (6). doi: 10.3390/nu12061839.

29 Pigeon Pea (*Cajanus cajan*) Protein and Potential in the Human Diet

Rabia Syed and Ying Wu

ABBREVIATIONS

ACE	Angiotensin-I converting enzyme
DIAAS	Digestible indispensable amino acid score
IL-1β	Interleukin-1β
IL-6	Interleukin-6
IP6	Inositol hexaphosphate
NSP	Non-starch polysaccharide
OAC	Oil absorption capacity
PDCAAS	Protein digestibility-corrected amino acid score
TNFα	Tumor necrosis factor α
WAC	Water absorption capacity

INTRODUCTION

Growing population, water shortage, and climate change are driving global food production challenges. With the rise of suburbanization, healthy diets are being replaced with refined sugars, high fats, and meats, leading to an increase in global agricultural greenhouse gas emissions, land clearing, and chronic non-communicable diseases (Tilman and Clark 2014). Global greenhouse gas emissions from animal-based foods are estimated to be twice those of plant-based foods (Xu et al. 2021). One possible way to simultaneously increase and conserve food availability while reducing the environmental footprint and biodiversity loss is through dietary shifts away from animal-based foods (de Boer and Aiking 2021, Scarborough et al. 2023). By 2050, swapping half of the meat and milk products with plant-sourced substitutes is projected to reduce agriculture and land greenhouse gas emissions by 31% and preserve forest and land area (Kozicka et al. 2023). A mounting body of evidence has drawn attention to consuming plant-based proteins while avoiding simple carbohydrates to reduce the risk of heart disease, diabetes, and cancer (Dinu et al. 2017). Using crops with multiple bioactive components is a viable and sustainable way to meet nutritional needs, promote health, and avoid disease. Diets comprising whole grains, vegetables, fruits, nuts, and legumes help maintain a healthy lifestyle (Hu 2003; Orlich and Fraser 2014). Bioactive components in pulse seeds have been getting increased attention in recent years, including proteins (Boye et al. 2010), dietary fiber (Tosh and Yada, 2010), and minor components (Campos-Vega et al. 2013). Pulses are edible dry seeds of legumes belonging to the Leguminosae or Fabaceae family, and they are packed with the indispensable amino acid lysine, accompanied by vital micronutrients, including potassium, magnesium, folate, iron, and zinc (Duranti 2006; Messina 2014). Pulse proteins are also gaining popularity as commercial proteins in alternative meat and food industries due to higher yield, accessibility, and cost-effectiveness (Ge et al. 2020). Functional foods not only provide basic dietary

DOI: 10.1201/9781003597926-29

needs, but they also offer health benefits for overall well-being. There is an upward trend to prefer snacks that deliver health benefits beyond nutrition, with an estimated USD 90.62 billion market in 2022 and anticipated growth of 6.7% from 2023 to 2030 (Grand View Research 2019). Legumes are affordable and significant protein sources, making them nutritious and valuable candidates in different food systems. Pulse flour can be added to baked food, pasta, and extruded snacks as an affordable, natural, and attractive source for the gluten-free market (Sozer et al. 2017).

Pigeon pea (*Cajanus cajan* (L.) Millsp.) is an essential perennial legume crop of sub-tropical and tropical regions that originated from the northern part of the Indian sub-continent at least 3,500 years ago (Fuller and Harvey 2006; Van der Maeson 1995). As a member of the Leguminosae family, it is commonly named red gram, congo pea, gungo pea, and no-eye pea. This distinct crop is tolerant to low and high temperatures and ranks sixth in the world in dryland annual legume production (Nene et al. 1990; Wu et al. 2009). Pigeon pea is an adaptable crop cultivated mainly as a vegetable in the Caribbean and South America and as a multi-use grain crop in India and some parts of Africa. Vegetable products include immature pods, fresh leaves, and pea-like seeds, while mature, dry seeds are cooked whole or split and eaten commonly as a pulse, just like any other edible dried beans.

Nutritionally, this pulse is a good source of protein, fiber, and minerals. Conventional seed consumption includes green vegetables and dry pulses, but different parts of the pigeon pea plant were part of folk and traditional medicine in India, China, and South America (Morton, 1976). The successful use of plant-based proteins depends on utilizing their beneficial properties in the food system. Functional and physicochemical properties of proteins, such as water absorption, viscosity, and hydration, are vital in determining their potential in product development (Kaushal et al. 2012).

PIGEON PEA SEED

Pigeon pea seed, as shown in Figure 29.1, is 85% cotyledon, 14% seed coat, and about 1% embryo. More than half of the protein is in the embryo, while cotyledon is high in carbohydrates, calcium, and iron (Saxena et al. 2010). This pulse is a wholesome source of protein, fiber, and vitamins like B-complex, making it a good contender for fortifying staple foods. Its protein content ranges between 18 and 25%, carbohydrates between 51.4 and 58.8%, crude fiber between 1.2 and 8.1%, and lipids between 0.6 and 3.8% (Table 29.1). Starch in pigeon pea seed is resistant to digestion due to the high molecular weight of amylopectin and amylose, making it suitable for diabetic patients (Sandhu and Lim 2008). Water-insoluble, water-soluble non-starch polysaccharides (NSPs) and cellulosic fractions of whole seed are composed of uronic acid, hexoses, and pentoses. Total NSPs range between 18.72 and 19.84% and cellulosic content from 8.37 to 9.56%. Seed husk is rich in arabinose, xylose, galacturonic acid, and glucuronic acid (Swamy et al. 1991). Hemicelluloses constitute a substantial part of non-cellulosic polysaccharides. Arabinose is the main constituent (48.5%) of water-soluble NSP fraction, followed by galacturonic acid (32.3%) (Syed et al. 2022).

PIGEON PEA PROTEIN

Fundamental proteins within pulse seeds are storage proteins classified as globulins, albumins, and glutelins (Boye et al. 2010). Globulins comprise about 60% of the total protein in pigeon peas and are soluble in dilute saline solution (Shewry et al. 1995). Vicilin constitutes approximately 30% of the proteins, along with cajanin subfractions (Bravo et al. 2022). The total protein content of pigeon peas is around 22–28% on a dry weight basis (Adenekan et al. 2017; Oshodi and Ekperigin 1989). Pigeon pea protein isolate is composed of essential amino acids, including histidine (3.5%), isoleucine (4.6%), leucine (8.5%), lysine (6.2%), methionine (1.2%), phenylalanine (8.7%), threonine (3.9%), and valine (4.3%) (Syed et al. 2022) (Table 29.2).

Close homology is reported between soy and pigeon pea amino acid profiles, with a balance of hydrophobic, hydrophilic, and charged amino acids. Pulse protein isolates in their purest form are

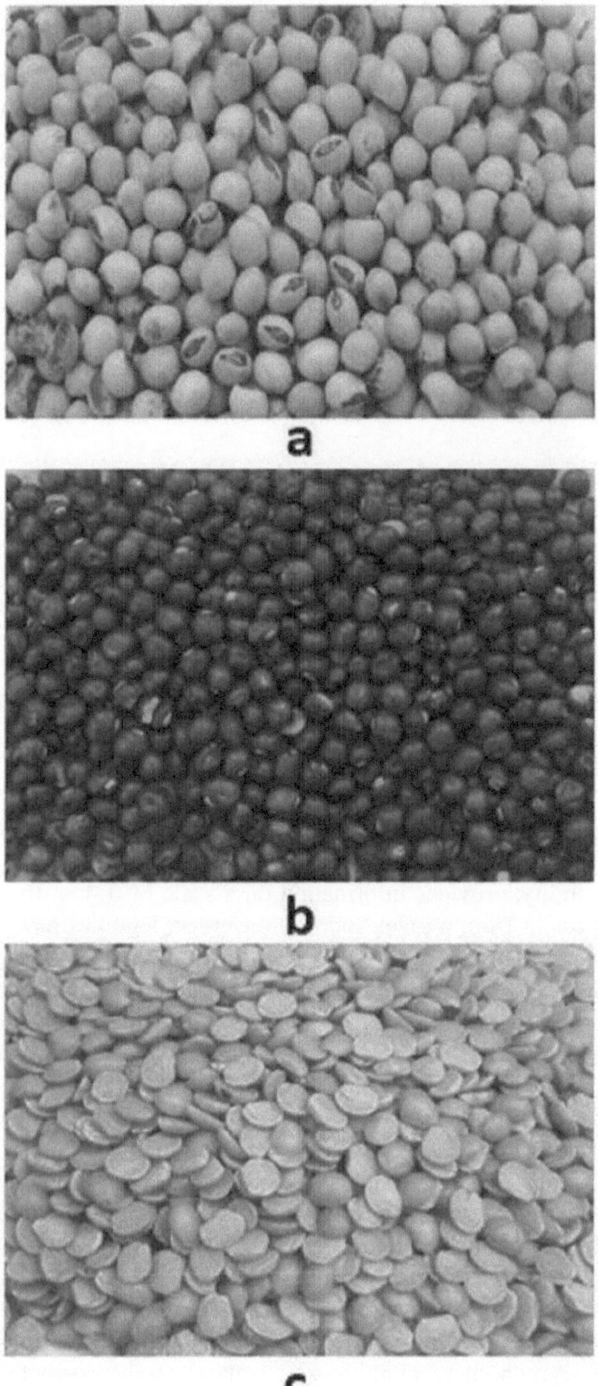

FIGURE 29.1 Pigeon pea seeds. a) whole white seeds; b) whole red seeds; c) split legume.

commonly produced by the wet alkaline extraction method, while dry fractionation is an alternative technique. Protein isolates are gaining popularity as a cost-effective dietary supplement with good digestibility and enormous potential in the food industry for nutritive and physicochemical properties (Adenekan et al. 2017). The protein digestibility-corrected amino acid score (PDCAAS),

TABLE 29.1
Distribution of Nutrients in Mature Pigeon Pea Seeds

Nutrients	Amount
Macronutrients	**(g/100 g)**
Protein	21.7
Carbohydrate	62.8
Total dietary fiber	15
Total lipid (fat)	1.49
Micronutrients	**(mg/100 g)**
Calcium (Ca)	130
Iron (Fe)	5.23
Magnesium (Mg)	183
Phosphorus (P)	367
Potassium (K)	1390
Sodium (Na)	17
Zinc (Zn)	2.76
Niacin	2.96
Thiamin	0.643
Riboflavin	0.187
Vitamin B5	1.27
Vitamin B6	0.283

US Department of Agriculture, Agricultural Research Service, 2016. USDA National Nutrient Database for Standard Reference, release 28. https://fdc.nal.usda.gov/fdc-app.html.

a measurement scale that evaluates dietary protein's ability to meet the body's amino acid needs and actual fecal digestibility, provides information on a scale of 0–1 of the human body's ability to absorb and digest protein from a given food. On average, legumes have a PDCAAS rating of 0.5–0.7, while soy protein scores are high with 0.91. A revised method, the digestible indispensable amino acid score (DIAAS), replaces the PDCAAS and calculates individual amino acid digestibility or bioavailability. A DIAAS score of 100 ranks the protein's quality as equivalent to that of reference animal protein (FAO 2011). Pigeon pea protein's true digestibility, or the proportion of a given food absorbed from the digestive tract into the bloodstream, is reported as 0.788 (Schaafsma 2000; Semba et al. 2021). Antinutritional factors, such as polyphenols, phytic acid, saponins, protease inhibitors, oligosaccharides, and non-physiological proteins like lectins, can limit the utilization of nutrients and protein digestibility in human nutrition. Employing different processing techniques, including germination, fermentation, soaking, thermal processing, and microwave radiation, enhances the bioavailability and functionality of legume proteins (Singh 1988; Torres et al. 2007). Microwave treatment is a promising approach for increasing flour protein quality and utilization; in one study, it significantly increased *in vitro* protein digestibility from $54.4 \pm 2.5\%$ to $71.6 \pm 4.2\%$, possibly due to changes in protein secondary structures and particle size (Sun et al. 2020). Enzyme hydrolysis is another technique used to alter legume protein properties. Alcalase and bromelain hydrolysis improved the functional and biological properties of pigeon pea, lentil, and chickpea protein isolates (Xu et al. 2021).

MINOR BIOACTIVE COMPONENTS IN PIGEON PEA

Bioactive components are not just limited to drugs but are also vital to food components with health benefits. Besides macronutrients such as protein and carbohydrates, pigeon pea's minor components

TABLE 29.2
Amino Acid Composition of Pigeon Pea and Soy Protein Isolates

Amino acid	Pigeon Pea Isolate*a*	Soy Protein Isolate*b*
Alanine	4.5	4.2
Argininc	6.7	8.0
Aspartic acid	11.6	12.0
Glutamic acid	18.7	20.0
Glycine	3.6	4.2
Histidine*	3.5	2.7
Isoleucine*	4.6	4.3
Leucine*	8.5	7.8
Lysine*	6.2	6.5
Methionine*	1.2	1.4
Phenylalanine*	8.7	5.4
Proline	5.1	5.3
Serine	5.9	5.7
Threonine*	3.9	3.6
Tyrosine	3.0	4.1
Valine*	4.3	4.5

Note: Values represent percentage composition by weight. Duplicate analysis (n = 2, standard deviation <5%).
a Data from Syed et al. 2022.
b Data from Mohsen et al. (2009); Tang et al. (2006).
* Essential amino acids.

exhibit bioactive effects. These molecules are reported to have antioxidant, anti-inflammatory, and bioactive properties against diseases like cancer, hypertension, and diabetes (Wu et al. 2009). Campos-Vega et al. (2010) summarized pulses' minor components, including phenolic compounds, enzyme inhibitors, lectins, fatty acids, phytosterols, phytic acid, and saponins, which are major contributors to antioxidant activity. In recent studies, most of the so-called antinutrients have health-promoting properties if used appropriately. Different processing methods might have various effects on phytochemical profiles and bioactivities. The most extensively investigated ones include phenolic compounds, phytic acid, and saponins. Among the 30 varieties of commonly consumed legumes in India, pigeon peas showed moderate antioxidant activity evaluated using DPPH, ABTS, and FRAP assays. The antioxidant activity correlated with total phenolic and phytochemical content (Xu and Chang, 2011; Marathe et al. 2011; Campos-Vega et al. 2010). So far in the literature, seven flavonoids in pigeon peas have been identified, with 27 different types recorded (Nix et al. 2015). Pigeon pea seed extract is reported to have advantageous effects on sickle cell disease, with active molecules contributing to this property, including cajaminose, phenylalanine, and hydroxybenzoic acid (Mathew et al. 2017). Soaked and sliced pigeon pea seeds tested positive for the phytoalexins cajanol, cajanin, and two unidentified isoprenylated flavones after incubation (Dahiya et al. 1984). Saponins are low-molecular-weight plant glycosides found in many edible legumes. After working on four genotypes of pigeon peas, Vasishtha and Srivastava (2011) concluded that pigeon peas have saponin glycosides and sapogenol A and B of the triterpene type. Phytic acid, or myo-inositol hexaphosphate (IP6), occurs in many seed plants, usually soluble as sodium or potassium salts, contributing 66–75% of phosphorus in pigeon peas (Ene-Obong, 1995). Hassan et al. 2015 observed that hexane extract (predominantly high in diterpene alcohol, phenolic compounds, and steroidal compounds) from pigeon pea seeds inhibited carrageenan-induced inflammation in rats by lowering the serum tumor necrosis factor-α (TNF-α) and interleukin-6 (IL-6) levels. Phytic acid and saponins have long been termed antinutrients due to their ability to block the absorption of nutrients, but emerging scientific findings indicate that these unfavorable factors do not outweigh their medicinal and therapeutic properties. The protective and therapeutic effect of phytic acid against colon cancer is attributed to its capacity to control the immune function of colon epithelium through the regulation of cytokines such as IL-1β and IL-6 (Kapral et al. 2012; Shamsuddin, 2002). Saponins display diverse anticancer properties by targeting several cancer-related proteins and pathways, including cell cycle arrest, apoptosis induction, and invasion inhibition (Xu et al. 2016).

BIOACTIVE PROPERTIES OF PIGEON PEA PROTEIN

The bioactive properties of proteins and peptides sourced from pulse seeds have gained increased interest in food science and nutrition for their potential to treat and prevent diseases (Campos-Vega et al. 2010). Pigeon pea protein has been found to possess bioactive properties such as antioxidant, antihypertensive, hypolipidemic, and antidiabetic effects as shown in Table 29.3.

The presence of bioactive peptides, essential amino acids, and increased antioxidant capacity in the *ex vivo* digest of pepsin-treated pigeon pea protein isolates makes it a potential nutraceutical protein (Tapal et al. 2019). Pigeon pea protein hydrolysates obtained from pepsin and pancreatin hydrolysis were high in hydrophobic amino acids, including isoleucine, phenylalanine, and leucine. They exhibited potent antioxidant and angiotensin-I converting enzyme (ACE) inhibition (61.82%) activity by reducing systolic blood pressure (–26.12 mmHg) within two hours of administration in rats (Olagunju et al. 2018). Alpha-amylase and alpha-glucosidase are key carbohydrate digestion enzymes facilitating intestinal glucose absorption. Alpha-amylase breaks down long-chain carbohydrates, while alpha-glucosidase hydrolyzes starch and disaccharides to glucose. Legumes possess a low glycemic index (<50), and alpha-amylase inhibitors are found specifically in legumes. One of the isoforms (alpha-amylase inhibitor 1) is unique to the germ and seeds (Gętek et al. 2014). Either the globulin protein fraction or an indirect consequence of antioxidant activity in pigeon peas is responsible for α-amylase inhibition activity (Uchegbu and Ishiwu 2016; Amalraj and Ignacimuthu 1998; Prema and Kurup 1973). A functional drink prepared with boiled, dried, and powdered pigeon pea seeds was administered to diabetic-hypercholesterolemic rats at doses equivalent to human consumption of 30 g/day. The drink proved effective in reducing plasma glucose and total cholesterol levels and elevating antioxidant status by 33.86% (Ariviani et al. 2018). The enhanced α-glucosidase inhibition observed in germinated pigeon pea seeds may be attributed to the release of small bioactive peptides (Uchegbu and Ishiwu 2016; Ohanenye et al. 2021). An interaction between bioactive peptides and minor constituents in pigeon pea seeds is likely responsible for the nutraceutical and therapeutic activity.

APPLICATION OF PIGEON PEA IN FOODS

Product development using pulse flour generally involves mixing it with other grains. Typically, pulse flour is incorporated into wheat flour to increase the nutritional value of cereal-based foods. While plant-derived protein isolates have been successfully incorporated into finished products, the addition of whole-pulse flour also increases the fiber, mineral, and phenolic content (Table 29.4). Successfully incorporating legume flour as a food ingredient depends on its functional and sensory characteristics responsible for an acceptable product.

TABLE 29.3
Key Bioactivities of Pigeon Pea Seeds

Therapeutic Activity	Experimental Findings	Reference
Hypoglycemic effect	Germinated pigeon pea meal inhibited carbohydrate-digesting enzymes, reducing hyperglycemia and associated hyperlipidemia in a rat model.	Uchegbu and Ishiwu (2016)
	Germinated seeds enhanced the *in vitro* inhibitory activity of the seed digest against α-glucosidase.	Ohanenye et al. (2021)
	A single dose of unroasted seeds (60% and 80%) significantly reduced the serum glucose level after 1–2 hours, followed by a rise after 3 hours in mice.	Amalraj and Ignacimuthu (1998)[a]
	The blood glucose response of healthy human volunteers to cooked pigeon peas (30.99 ± 4.1 glycemic index) was significantly lower than that of bread.	Panlasigui, Panlilio, and Madrid (1995)[b]
Hypolipidemic effect	Total and free cholesterol in serum, aorta, and liver of rats fed a high-fat diet supplemented with globulin fraction from *Cajanus cajan* were much lower than in the control.	Prema and Kurup (1973)[c]
	Pigeon pea administration promoted cholesterol conversion to bile acid in a high fat-induced hamster model, accompanied by elevated antioxidant enzymes in the liver. The dyslipidemia effect was more significant than β-sitosterol administration.	Dai et al. (2013)
Antioxidant, anti-hypertensive, and antisickling effect	Protein hydrolysate demonstrated antioxidant properties and a robust antihypertensive effect by lowering systolic blood pressure within 2 hours of administration *in vitro* and in a rat model.	Olagunju et al. (2018)
	The protein from *C. cajan* exhibited hepatoprotective antioxidant properties by downregulating free radicals, improving hepatorenal marker enzymes and liver/kidney functions, reducing signs of acetaminophen-induced hepatic (APAP) damage, and normalizing hepatic cell architecture in rats.	Aly et al. (2013)
	Water extracts of *B. subtilis*-fermented pigeon pea significantly improved systolic and diastolic blood pressure, elevated antioxidant levels, nattokinase activity, and angiotensin-converting enzyme inhibitory activity in spontaneously hypertensive rats. An in-silico analysis of purified and proteolyzed main globulin fraction, cajanin, showed 41 antihypertensive and nine antioxidant peptides.	Lee, Lai, and Wu (2015)*d*; Bravo et al. (2022)
	Seed extract exhibited 70% of the *in vitro* antisickling potency due to a high phenylalanine amino acid concentration (26.3%).	Ekeke and Shode (1990)
Anti-inflammatory effect	Pigeon pea extracts and cyanidin-3-monoglucoside exhibited anti-inflammatory activity by suppressing the production of inflammatory (TNF-α, IL-1β, and IL-6) cytokines in lipopolysaccharide-treated macrophages.	Lai et al. (2012)[e]

[a] Amalraj, T., and S. Ignacimuthu. 1998. Hypoglycemic Activity of Cajanus Cajan (Seeds) in Mice. *Indian Journal of Experimental Biology* 36 (10): 1032–33.

[b] Panlasigui, Leonora N., Lourdes M. Panlilio, and June C. Madrid. 1995. Glycemic Response in Normal Subjects to Five Different Legumes Commonly Used in the Philippines. *International Journal of Food Sciences and Nutrition* 46 (2): 155–60.

[c] Prema, L., and P. A. Kurup. 1973. Effect of Protein Fractions from Cajanus Cajan (Redgram) and Dolichos Biflorus (Horsegram) on the Serum, Liver and Aortic Lipid Levels in Rats Fed a High-Fat-High-Cholesterol Diet. *Atherosclerosis* 18 (3): 369–77.

[d] Lee, Bao-Hong, Yi-Syuan Lai, and She-Ching Wu. 2015. Antioxidation, Angiotensin Converting Enzyme Inhibition Activity, Nattokinase, and Antihypertension of Bacillus Subtilis (Natto)-Fermented Pigeon Pea. *Journal of Food and Drug Analysis* 23 (4): 750–57.

[e] Lai, Yi-Syuan, Wei-Hsuan Hsu, Jan-Jeng Huang, and She-Ching Wu. 2012. Antioxidant and Anti-Inflammatory Effects of Pigeon Pea (Cajanus Cajan L.) Extracts on Hydrogen Peroxide- and Lipopolysaccharide-Treated RAW264.7 Macrophages. *Food & Function* 3 (12): 1294–1301.

TABLE 29.4
Application of Pigeon Pea in Foods

Food Category	Application	Results	Reference
Functional Properties of Flour	Unripe cooking banana, pigeon pea, and sweet potato flours were mixed in 17 combinations. These blends and individual pigeon pea/rice/taro flours were tested for physicochemical and functional properties.	Protein, carotenoid content, fiber, ash, foaming, emulsion, least gelation capacity, pasting temperature, and time of the blends increased with the pigeon pea flour level. Pigeon pea flour exhibited excellent foam stability (>80 ml/100 ml) after 2 hours of storage.	Ohizua et al. (2017);[a] Kaushal et al. (2012)
	The functional properties of raw and processed pigeon pea flour were compared with soy flour.	The fat absorption capacity of pigeon pea flour improved compared to raw soy flour with processing (soaking/blanching in water).	Mamah (2001)[b]
Pasta/Noodles	Pigeon pea flour from germinated seeds was used to make pasta products in the proportions of 5%, 10%, and 12%.	Pasta with a 10% substitution of pigeon pea flour had improved protein, fat, fiber, and mineral content compared to the control (100% semolina) with similar sensory acceptability.	Torres et al. (2007)
	Semolina flour was supplemented with fermented and germinated pigeon pea flour in pasta.	Incorporation of the processed flour into semolina improved the protein quality of pasta.	Martínez-Villaluenga et al. (2010)
	Noodles were prepared with pigeon pea and rice starches.	A 70% pigeon pea and 30% rice starch blend produced good quality noodles with a higher overall acceptability score and increased cooked noodles' weight.	Yadav, Yadav, and Kumar 2011)[c]
Biscuits/Cookies	14 flour blends of cooking banana, pigeon pea, and sweet potato flour were tested. The various ratios (100:0, 75:25, 65:35, and 50:50) of millet and pigeon pea flour were used to bake biscuits.	Biscuits prepared from a flour blend of 21.67% unripe cooking banana, 21.67% pigeon pea, and 56.67% sweet potato were high in protein, fiber, and Mg and favored for mouthfeel. 65:35 blend resulted in the maximum scores for flavor, texture, and general acceptability with up to 15.2% protein content.	Adeola and Ohizua (2018); Eneche (1999)

(*Continued*)

TABLE 29.4 (CONTINUED)
Application of Pigeon Pea in Foods

Food Category	Application	Results	Reference
	Ten formulations of germinated pigeon pea, fermented sorghum, and cocoyam flour blends were used to prepare cookies. Baked snacks were formulated with integrated pigeon pea and cassava flour.	Cookies prepared with a higher proportion of germinated pigeon pea flour were favorable in taste, highest in protein content (19.89%), energy (376.56 kcal/100g), and least in fragility. Adding pigeon pea flour resulted in a deep yellow color, higher protein content, water absorption index, bulk density, and moderate taste acceptability.	Okpala, Okoli, and Udensi (2013); Rampersad, Badrie, and Comissiong (2003)[d]

[a] Ohizua, Ehimen R., Abiodun A. Adeola, Micheal A. Idowu, Olajide P. Sobukola, T. Adeniyi Afolabi, Raphael O. Ishola, Simeon O. Ayansina, Tolulope O. Oyekale, and Ayorinde Falomo. 2017. Nutrient Composition, Functional, and Pasting Properties of Unripe Cooking Banana, Pigeon Pea, and Sweetpotato Flour Blends. *Food Science & Nutrition* 5 (3): 750–62.

b Mamah, L. C. and E. N. Okpala. 2001. Functional Properties of Raw and Processed Pigeonpea (Cajanus Cajan) Flour. *International Journal of Food Sciences and Nutrition* 52 (4): 343–46. *c* Yadav, Baljeet S., Ritika B. Yadav, and Mahesh Kumar. 2011. Suitability of Pigeon Pea and Rice Starches and Their Blends for Noodle Making. *LWT – Food Science and Technology* 44 (6): 1415–21. *d* Rampersad, R., N. Badrie, and E. Comissiong. 2003. Physico-Chemical and Sensory Characteristics of Flavored Snacks from Extruded Cassava/Pigeonpea Flour. *Journal of Food Science* 68 (1): 363–67.

Incorporating pulse flour in bread making is challenging since gluten plays an essential role in structural development. Recent studies indicate that factors critical to the integration and percentage of pulse flour depend on the seed type and pre-treatments (Boukid et al. 2019). Pigeon pea flour can be incorporated into food formulations to increase protein and fiber content due to its favorable functional properties. Key functional characteristics include emulsification, foaming, gelation, texture, viscosity, and water and oil absorption capacities (Adebowale and Lawal 2004).

Water absorption capacity (WAC) and oil absorption capacity (OAC) measure a food material's ability to absorb water and oil, respectively. These properties in food proteins depend on factors like amino acid composition, hydrophobicity, and protein conformation. Flour samples with high WAC are prone to amylose leaching and loss of crystalline structure but are preferred for use in bakery products requiring hydration, such as dough and sausages. The high protein content in legumes and beans may cause starch granules to become embedded within a rigid protein matrix, limiting water access to starch and curbing swelling. While proteins have hydrophilic and hydrophobic groups, in some cases, hydrophilic polysaccharides can increase WAC. OAC refers to the capacity of flour protein to physically bind fat by capillary action, and it is vital since fats act as flavor retainers and improve the mouthfeel of foods.

Pigeon pea flour outperforms soy flour in WAC (138% vs. 130%), OAC (89.7% vs. 84.4%), foaming capacity (68% vs. 66%), and foam stability (20% vs. 14.6%) (Oshodi and Ekperigin 1989; Kaushal et al. 2012). Its high OAC makes pigeon pea suitable for food systems requiring oil absorption, especially bread and other baked foods (Kinsella and Melachouris 1976). High protein flours can physically entrap oil and favor non-covalent attractions such as hydrophobic, electrostatic, and hydrogen bonding (Adebowale and Lawal 2004).

Processing techniques also influence the physical and nutritional properties of the flour. Using germinated and fermented pigeon pea seeds to formulate pasta increased its nutritional value while reducing cooking time and antinutritional factors (Torres et al. 2007; Martínez-Villaluenga et al. 2010). Formulating cookies/biscuits with pigeon pea flour is advantageous in increasing their nutritional profile and achieving gluten-free products without significantly impacting texture (Eneche 1999; Okpala et al. 2013). Studies have shown that the viscosity and emulsion stability of pigeon pea protein solutions were significantly higher than those of soy protein solutions (Syed et al. 2022), making pigeon pea a good contender for application in commercial food products. Pigeon pea protein exhibited desirable and better functional properties, particularly gelation capacity, compared to soy and yellow pea proteins (Tang et al. 2021).

THE EFFECTS OF OTHER PROTEINS

Nutritionally, plant and animal-sourced proteins differ in amino acid profile, structure, and digestibility. Dietary proteins are critical for the synthesis of body tissues (muscle protein synthesis), nitrogenous compounds like hormones, and energy production. The optimal quantity and bioavailability of the essential amino acids are important in regulating skeletal muscle mass. Proteins from animal sources have all nine essential amino acids in the appropriate quantities that the human body requires. Lysine and leucine play important roles in muscle growth and collagen production, while most cereal proteins are typically low in these two amino acids. These differences are important factors when picking protein sources to fulfill the needs of infants and growing children (Day et al. 2022).

Studies suggest that soy and wheat-sourced proteins have a less profound effect on muscle synthesis than casein, whey, beef, and egg proteins and are more likely to be used for oxidation rather than protein synthesis of muscles (Vliet et al. 2015; Berrazaga et al. 2019). In a study by Phillips (2012), beef was a superior source of muscle protein synthesis compared to soy protein meat. Conversely, a meta-analysis by Messina et al. (2018) found no difference in the effects of supplementing with soy protein vs. whey protein on gains in muscle mass and strength in response to resistance exercise.

The sulfur-containing amino acid methionine is a primary methyl donor in the body and is involved in the synthesis of creatinine and phosphatidylcholine during vigorous growth periods. Cereals like rice (4.4%), wheat (4.1%), and corn (4.4%) are good sources of methionine and cysteine (Day et al. 2022). The amino acid profile of pigeon pea protein is in close homology to soy protein (Table 29.2), with a moderate proportion of lysine (6.2%) and leucine (8.5%) and a low quantity of methionine (1.3%) (Syed et al. 2022). Pigeon pea, especially when combined with cereals like wheat and rice, is a promising alternative for fulfilling nutritional requirements (Boye et al. 2010).

Factors responsible for plant-based proteins' lower digestibility include the presence of polyphenols, protease inhibitors, antinutrients, and a high proportion of β-sheet conformations, which may reduce the accessibility of digestive enzymes (Sun et al. 2020). As consumers increasingly seek sustainable and healthy protein alternatives, ongoing research and technological advancements may enable plant-based proteins to become an integral part of diets.

MINI DICTIONARY OF TERMS

- **Bioactive:** Any compound/molecule that has beneficial effects on living cells.
- **Globulins:** Primary storage and high-molecular-weight proteins in pulse seeds.
- **Phytochemicals:** Chemicals produced by plants through primary or secondary metabolism as a defense mechanism and possessing beneficial properties.
- **Protein isolates:** Pure and processed protein powder free from fats, carbohydrates, and other impurities.
- **Pulses:** Dried seeds of legume plants like beans, peas, and lentils.

SUMMARY POINTS

- Pigeon peas in whole food systems can satisfy human food and protein needs.
- This pulse is a good source of protein, fiber, and minerals, with bioactive phytochemicals and peptides, possessing antioxidant, antihypertensive, hypolipidemic, antidiabetic, and anti-inflammatory properties.
- Pigeon pea protein isolates contain essential amino acids and can be utilized in food industries due to their unique functional properties.
- Different processing techniques, including germination, fermentation, soaking, thermal processing, and microwave radiation, can enhance the bioavailability and functionality of pigeon pea protein.
- Whole pigeon pea flour can be used to develop functional foods that provide benefits beyond essential nutrition.

REFERENCES

Adebowale, K. O., and Lawal, O. S. 2004. Comparative Study of the Functional Properties of Bambarra Groundnut (Voandzeia Subterranean), Jack Bean (Canavalia Ensiformis) and Mucuna Bean (Mucuna Pruriens) Flours. *Food Research International* 37 (4): 355–65.

Adenekan, M. K., Fadimu, G. J., Odunmbaku, L. A., and Oke, E. K. 2017. Effect of Isolation Techniques on the Characteristics of Pigeon Pea (Cajanus Cajan) Protein Isolates. *Food Science & Nutrition* 6 (1): 146–52.

Adeola, A. A., and Ohizua, E. R. 2018. Physical, Chemical, and Sensory Properties of Biscuits Prepared from Flour Blends of Unripe Cooking Banana, Pigeon Pea, and Sweet Potato. *Food Science & Nutrition* 6 (3): 532–40.

Aly, H. F., Rizk, M. Z., Abo-Elmatty, D. M., Desoky, M., Ibrahim, N., and Younis, E. A. 2013. Therapeutic and Protective Effects of Caesalpinia gilliesii and Cajanus cajan Proteins against Acetaminophen Overdose-Induced Renal Damage. *Toxicology and Industrial Health* 32 (4): 753–68.

Amalraj, T., and Ignacimuthu, S. 1998. Hypoglycemic Activity of Cajanus Cajan (seeds) in Mice. *Indian Journal of Experimental Biology*, 36 (10): 1032–3.

Ariviani, S. Affandi, D., Listyaningsih, E., and Handajani, S. 2018. The Potential of Pigeon Pea (Cajanus Cajan) Beverage as an Anti-Diabetic Functional Drink. *IOP Conference Series: Earth and Environmental Science* 102 (January): 012054.

Berrazaga, I., Micard, V., Gueugneau, M., and Walrand, S. 2019. The Role of the Anabolic Properties of Plant-versus Animal-Based Protein Sources in Supporting Muscle Mass Maintenance: A Critical Review. *Nutrients* 11 (8): 1825.

Boukid, F., Zannini, E., Carini, E., and Vittadini, E. 2019. Pulses for Bread Fortification: A Necessity or a Choice? *Trends in Food Science & Technology* 88 (June): 416–28.

Boye, J., Zare, F., and Alison Pletch, A. 2010. Pulse Proteins: Processing, Characterization, Functional Properties and Applications in Food and Feed. *Food Research International* 43 (2): 414–31.

Bravo, R. K. D., Angelia, M. R. N., Uy, L. Y. C., Garcia, R. N., and Torio, M. A. O. 2022. Isolation, Purification and Characterization of the Antibacterial, Antihypertensive and Antioxidative Properties of the Bioactive Peptides in the Purified and Proteolyzed Major Storage Protein of Pigeon Pea (Cajanus Cajan) Seeds. *Food Chemistry: Molecular Sciences* 4 (July): 100062.

Campos-Vega, R., Loarca-Piña, G., and Oomah, B. D. 2010. Minor Components of Pulses and Their Potential Impact on Human Health. *Food Research International* 43 (2): 461–82.

Campos-Vega, R., Oomah, B. D., Loarca-Piña, G., and Vergara-Castañeda, H. A. 2013 Common Beans and Their Non-Digestible Fraction: Cancer Inhibitory Activity – An Overview. *Foods* 2 (3): 74–392.

Dahiya, J. S., Strange, R. N., Bilyard, K. G., Cooksey, C. J., and Garratt, P. J. 1984. Two Isoprenylated Isoflavone Phytoalexins from *Cajanus Cajan*. *Phytochemistry* 23 (4): 871–73.

Day, Li., Cakebread, J. A., and Loveday, S. M. 2022. Food Proteins from Animals and Plants: Differences in the Nutritional and Functional Properties. *Trends in Food Science & Technology* 119: 428–42.

de Boer, J., and Aiking, H. 2021. Exploring Food Consumers Motivations to Fight Both Climate Change and Biodiversity Loss: Combining Insights from Behavior Theory and Eurobarometer Data. *Food Quality and Preference* 94: 1–10.

Dietary Protein Quality Evaluation in Human Nutrition Report of an FAO Expert Consultation. n.d. https://www.fao.org/ag/humannutrition/35978-02317b979a686a57aa4593304ffc17f06.pdf.

Dinu, M., Abbate, R., Gensini, G. F., Casini, A., and Sofi, F. 2017. Vegetarian, Vegan Diets and Multiple Health Outcomes: A Systematic Review with Meta-Analysis of Observational Studies. *Critical Reviews in Food Science and Nutrition* 57 (17): 3640–49.

Duranti, M. 2006. Grain Legume Proteins and Nutraceutical Properties. *Fitoterapia* 77 (2): 67–82.

Eneche, E. H. 1999. Biscuit-making Potential of Millet/pigeonpea Flour Blends. *Plant Foods for Human Nutrition* 54 (1): 21–27.

Ene-Obong, H. N. 1995. Content of Antinutrients and in Vitro Protein Digestibility of the African Yambean, Pigeon and Cowpea. *Plant Foods for Human Nutrition* 48 (3): 225–33.

FAO. 2011. https://www.fao.org/news/archive/news-by-date/2011/en/

Fuller, D. Q., and Harvey, E. L. 2006. The Archaeobotany of Indian Pulses: Identification, Processing and Evidence for Cultivation. *Environmental Archaeology* 11 (2): 219–46.

Ge, J., Sun, C. X., Corke, H.,Gul, K., Gan, R. Y., and Fang. Y. 2020. The Health Benefits, Functional Properties, Modifications, and Applications of Pea (Pisum *Sativum* L.) Protein: Current Status, Challenges, and Perspectives. *Comprehensive Reviews in Food Science and Food Safety* 19 (4): 1835–76.

Gętek, M., Czech, N., Muc-Wierzgoń, M., Grochowska-Niedworok, E., Kokot, T., and Nowakowska-Zajdel, E. 2014. The Active Role of Leguminous Plant Components in Type 2 Diabetes. *Evidence-Based Complementary and Alternative Medicine* 2014: 1–12.

Grand View Research. 2019. Healthy Snacks Market Size & Trends Report, 2030. https://www.grandviewresearch.com/industry-analysis/healthy-snack-market

Hassan, E. M., Matloub, A., Aboutabl, M. E., Ibrahim, N. A., and Mohamed, S. 2015. Assessment of Anti-Inflammatory, Antinociceptive, Immunomodulatory, and Antioxidant Activities of *Cajanus Cajan* L. Seeds Cultivated in Egypt and Its Phytochemical Composition. *Pharmaceutical Biology* 54 (8): 1380–9.

Hu, F. B. 2003. Plant-Based Foods and Prevention of Cardiovascular Disease: An Overview. *The American Journal of Clinical Nutrition* 78 (3): 544S551S.

Kapral, M., Wawszczyk, J., Jurzak, M., Hollek, A., and Węglarz, L. 2012. The Effect of Inositol Hexaphosphate on the Expression of Selected Metalloproteinases and Their Tissue Inhibitors in IL-1β-stimulated Colon Cancer Cells. *International Journal of Colorectal Disease* 27 (11): 1419–28.

Kaushal, P., Kumar, V., and Sharma, H. K. 2012. Comparative Study of Physicochemical, Functional, Antinutritional and Pasting Properties of Taro (Colocasia Esculenta), Rice (Oryza Sativa) Flour, Pigeonpea (Cajanus Cajan) Flour and Their Blends. *LWT – Food Science and Technology* 48 (1): 59–68

Kinsella, J. E., and Melachouris, N. 1976. Functional Properties of Proteins in Foods: A Survey. *C R C Critical Reviews in Food Science and Nutrition* 7 (3): 219–80.

Kozicka, M., Havlík, P., Valin, H., Wollenberg, E., Andre Deppermann, A., Leclère, D., Lauri, P., et al. 2023. Feeding Climate and Biodiversity Goals with Novel Plant-Based Meat and Milk Alternatives. *Nature Communications* 14 (1): 5316.

Marathe, S. A., Rajalakshmi, V., Jamdar, S. N., and Sharma, A. 2011. Comparative Study on Antioxidant Activity of Different Varieties of Commonly Consumed Legumes in India. *Food and Chemical Toxicology* 49 (9): 2005–12.

Martínez-Villaluengaa, C., Torres, A., Friasa, J., and Vidal-Valverde, C. 2010. Semolina Supplementation with Processed Lupin and Pigeon Pea Flours Improve Protein Quality of Pasta. *LWT – Food Science and Technology* 43 (4): 617–22.

Mathew, D., Lidiya John, P., Manila, T.M. Divyasree, P., and Sandhya Rajan, V. T. K. 2017. Therapeutic Molecules for Multiple Human Diseases Identified from Pigeon Pea (Cajanus cajan L. Millsp.) through GC–MS and Molecular Docking. *Food Science and Human Wellness* 6 (4): 202–16.

Messina, M., Lynch, H., Dickinson, J. M., and Reed, K. E. 2018. No Difference Between the Effects of Supplementing With Soy Protein Versus Animal Protein on Gains in Muscle Mass and Strength in Response to Resistance Exercise. *International Journal of Sport Nutrition and Exercise Metabolism* 28 (6): 674–85.

Messina, V. 2014. Nutritional and Health Benefits of Dried Beans. *The American Journal of Clinical Nutrition* 100 (Suppl_1): 437S442S.

Mohsen, S. M., Fadel, H. H., Bekhit, M. A., Edris, A. E., and Ahmed, M. Y. 2009. Effect of Substitution of Soy Protein Isolate on Aroma Volatiles, Chemical Composition and Sensory Quality of Wheat Cookies. *International Journal of Food Science & Technology* 44 (9): 1705–12.

Morton, J. F. 1976. The Pigeonpea (*Cajanus cajan* (L) Millspaugh), a High Protein Tropical Bush Legume. *Horticulture Science* 11: 11–19.

Nene, Y. L., Hall, S. D., and Sheila, V. K. 1990. *The Pigeonpea: Google Books*. CAB International, University Club, Cambridge, 1–14.

Nix, A., Paull, C. A., and Colgrave, M. 2015. The Flavonoid Profile of Pigeonpea, Cajanus Cajan: A Review. *SpringerPlus* 4 (1): 1–6.

Ohanenye, I. C., Sun, X., Sarteshnizi, R. A., and Udenigwe, C. C. 2021. Germination Alters the Microstructure, in Vitro Protein Digestibility, α -Glucosidase and Dipeptidyl Peptidase-IV Inhibitory Activities of Bioaccessible Fraction of Pigeon Pea (Cajanus Cajan) Seeds. *Legume Science* 3 (1): e79.

Okpala, L., Okoli, E., and Udensi, E. 2013. Physico-Chemical and Sensory Properties of Cookies Made from Blends of Germinated Pigeon Pea, Fermented Sorghum, and Cocoyam Flours. *Food Science & Nutrition* 1 (1): 8–14.

Olagunju, A. I., Omoba, O. S., Enujiugha, V. N., Alashi, A. M., and Aluko, R. E. 2018. Antioxidant Properties, ACE/Renin Inhibitory Activities of Pigeon Pea Hydrolysates and Effects on Systolic Blood Pressure of Spontaneously Hypertensive Rats. *Food Science & Nutrition* 6 (7): 1879–89.

Orlich, M. J., and Fraser, G. E. 2014. Vegetarian Diets in the Adventist Health Study 2: A Review of Initial Published Findings. *The American Journal of Clinical Nutrition* 100 (suppl_1): 353S–358S.

Oshodi, A. A., and Ekperigin, M. M. 1989. Functional Properties of Pigeon Bean Pea (*Cajanus cajan*) Flour. *Food Chemistry* 34: 187–99.

Phillips, S. M. 2012. Nutrient-Rich Meat Proteins in Offsetting Age-Related Muscle Loss. *Meat Science* 92 (3): 174–78.

Prema, L., and Kurup, P. A. 1973. Effect of Protein Fractions from Cajanus Cajan (redgram) and Dolichos biflorus (Horsegram) on the Serum, Liver and Aortic Lipid Levels in Rats Fed a High-fat-cholesterol Diet. *Atherosclerosis* 18 (3): 369–77.

Sandhu, K. S., and Lim, S.T. 2008. Digestibility of Legume Starches as Influenced by Their Physical and Structural Properties. *Carbohydrate Polymers* 71 (2): 245–52.

Saxena, K., Kumar, R. V., and Sultana, R. 2010. Quality Nutrition through Pigeonpea – a Review. *Health* 2 (11): 1335–44.

Scarborough, P., Clark, M., Cobiac, L., Papier, K., Knuppel, A., Lynch, J., Harrington, R., Key, T., and Springmann, M. 2023. Vegans, Vegetarians, Fish-Eaters and Meat-Eaters in the UK Show Discrepant Environmental Impacts. *Nature Food* 4 (7): 565–74.

Schaafsma, G. 2000. The Protein Digestibility–Corrected Amino Acid Score. *The Journal of Nutrition* 130 (7): 1865S1867S.

Semba, R. D., Ramsing, R., Rahman, N., Kraemer, K., and Bloem, M. W. 2021. Legumes as a Sustainable Source of Protein in Human Diets. *Global Food Security* 28: Article 100520.

Shamsuddin, A. M. 2002. Anti-cancer Function of Phytic Acid. *International Journal of Food Science and Technology* 37: 769–82.

Shewry, P. R., Napier, J. A., and Tatham, A. S. 1995. Seed Storage Proteins: Structures and Biosynthesis. *The Plant Cell* 7 (7): 945.

Singh, U. 1988. Antinutritional Factors of Chickpea and Pigeonpea and Their Removal by Processing. *Plant Foods for Human Nutrition* 38 (3): 251–6.

Sozer, N., Holopainen-Mantila, U., and Poutanen, K. 2017. Traditional and New Food Uses of Pulses. *Cereal Chemistry Journal* 94 (1): 66–73.

Sun, X., Ohanenye, I. C., Ahmed, T., and Udenigwe, C. C. 2020. Microwave Treatment Increased Protein Digestibility of Pigeon Pea (Cajanus Cajan) Flour: Elucidation of Underlying Mechanisms. *Food Chemistry* 329 (November): 127196.

Swamy, N. R., Ramakrishnaiah, N., Kurien, P. P., and Salimath, P. V. 1991. Studies on Carbohydrates of Red Gram (Cajanus Cajan) in Relation to Milling. *Journal of the Science of Food and Agriculture* 57 (3): 379–90.

Syed, R., Ding, H.H., Hui, D., and Wu, Y. 2022. Physicochemical and Functional Properties of Pigeon Pea (Cajanus Cajan) Protein and Non-Starch Polysaccharides. *Bioactive Carbohydrates and Dietary Fibre* 28 (November): 100317.

Tang, C. H., Ten, Z., Wang, X. S., and Yang, X. Q. 2006. Physicochemical and Functional Properties of Hemp (Cannabis sativa L) Protein. *Journal of Agricultural and Food Chemistry* 54: 8945–50.

Tang, X, Shen, Y., Zhang, Y. M., Schilling, W., and Li, Y. 2021. Parallel Comparison of Functional and Physicochemical Properties of Common Pulse Proteins. *LWT* 146: 111594.

Tapal, A., Vegarud, G. E., Sreedhara, A., and Kaul Tiku, P. 2019. Nutraceutical Protein Isolate from Pigeon Pea (*Cajanus Cajan*) Milling Waste By-Product: Functional Aspects and Digestibility. *Food & Function* 10 (5): 2710–19.

Tilman, D., and Clark, M. 2014. Global Diets Link Environmental. Global Diets Link Environmental Sustainability and Human Health. *Nature* 515 (7528): 518–22.

Torres, A., Frias, J., Granito, M., and Vidal-Valverde, C. 2007. Germinated Cajanus Cajan Seeds as Ingredients in Pasta Products: Chemical, Biological and Sensory Evaluation. *Food Chemistry* 101 (1): 202–11.

Tosh, S. M., and Yada, S. 2010. Dietary Fibers in Pulse Seeds and Fractions: Characterization, Functional Attributes and Applications. *Food Research International* 43: 617–26A.

Uchegbu, N. N., and Ishiwu, C. N. 2016. Germinated Pigeon Pea (Cajanus cajan): A Novel Diet for Lowering Oxidative Stress and Hyperglycemia. *Food Science & Nutrition* 4 (5): 772–7.

Van der Maeson, L. J. G. 1995. Pigeonpea Cajanus Cajan. In Smartt, J. and Simmonds, N. W. (eds.), *Evolution of Crop Plants*. Essex: Longman, pp. 251–5.

Van Vliet, S., Burd, N. A., and van Loon, L. J. 2015. The Skeletal Muscle Anabolic Response to Plant- versus Animal-Based Protein Consumption. *The Journal of Nutrition* 145 (9): 1981–91.

Vasishtha, H. and Srivastava, R. P. 2011. Effect of Dehusking and Cooking on Sapogenols of Pigeon Pea (Cajanus cajan) Genotypes. *Indian Journal of Agricultural Biochemistry* 24: 60–4.

Wu, N., Fu, K., Fu, Y-J., Zu, Y-G., Chang, F-R., Chen, Y-H., Liu, X-L., Kong, Y., Liu, W., and Gu, C-B. 2009. Antioxidant Activities of Extracts and Main Components of Pigeonpea [Cajanus Cajan (L.) Millsp.] Leaves. *Molecules* 14 (3): 1032–43.

Xu, B., and Chang, S. K. C. 2011. Reduction of Antiproliferative Capacities, Cell-Based Antioxidant Capacities and Phytochemical Contents of Common Beans and Soybeans upon Thermal Processing. *Food Chemistry* 129 (3): 974–81.

Xu, X., Sharma, P., Shu, S., Lin, T. S., Ciais, P., Tubiello, F. N., Smith, P., Campbell, N., and Jain, A. K. 2021. Global Greenhouse Gas Emissions from Animal-based Foods Are Twice Those of Plant-based Foods. *Nature Food* 2(9): 724–32.

Xu, X. H., Li, T., Fong, C. M. V., Chen, X., Chen, X., Wang, Y. T., Huang, M. Q., and Lu, J. J. 2016. Saponins from Chinese Medicines as Anticancer Agents. *Molecules* 21: 1326.

30 Chickpea (*Cicer arietinum*) Protein Hydrolysates as Functional Components

Potential Use in Type 2 Diabetes

Subhiksha Chandrasekaran and Elvira Gonzalez de Mejia

ABBREVIATIONS

CCK	Cholecystokinin
DPP-IV	Dipeptidyl peptidase-IV
GI	Gastrointestinal
GLP-1	Glucagon-like peptide-1
GPCR	G-protein coupled receptor
T2D	Type 2 diabetes
T2R	Bitter taste receptor
TRPM5	Transient receptor potential cation channel subfamily M member 5

INTRODUCTION

Chickpea is the world's second most widely produced legume (Food and Agriculture Organization of the United Nations 2020). The protein content in chickpeas ranges from 15 to 20%, which makes them an excellent source of plant-based proteins (Aisa et al. 2019). Chickpea protein has also been shown to have high bioavailability compared to other pulses and contains essential fatty acids (Wang et al. 2021; Madurapperumage et al. 2021).

Chickpea protein hydrolysis through the action of enzymatic systems has also been studied for its antidiabetic properties over the last ten years. The release of peptides by proteases contributes to their increased bioactive properties since peptides can be easily absorbed in the small intestine, thereby increasing their efficacy in managing different chronic diseases (Cruz-Casas et al. 2021).

The processing methods for legumes play a vital role in determining their bioactive potential (Acquah et al. 2021). Processing techniques, such as boiling, high-pressure systems, fermentation, and germination, have been studied for chickpeas. Germination is particularly interesting because it is cost-effective and requires no energy sources such as heat or pressure. Germination also improves protein digestibility through the action of endoproteases, which can remove the beany taste often associated with legumes, as well as enhance its bioactive properties (Sofi et al. 2020; Newton and Majumder 2023; Pérez-Ramirez et al. 2023).

However, despite well-established evidence supporting the bioactive properties of chickpea, chickpea protein hydrolysates have limited commercialization because of their bitter taste (Li-Chan 2015).

Bitterness is one of the five taste types that humans can recognize. Bitter taste receptors are believed to have evolved in humans to detect and prevent ingesting harmful and potentially

DOI: 10.1201/9781003597926-30

poisonous substances. Extraoral bitter taste receptors have been identified in the brain, intestines, lungs, heart, and respiratory tract (Bloxham et al. 2020). Antidiabetic effects through the activation of bitter receptor cascades have been observed in multiple studies (Chou 2021). Although there is evidence that protein hydrolysates may taste bitter, few studies have explored this characteristic concerning extraoral bitter receptors.

Thus, this chapter aims to summarize the latest information on the effect of germinating chickpeas and the hydrolysis of chickpea protein, their antidiabetic properties, and their relationship with bitterness.

ANTIDIABETIC PROPERTIES OF CHICKPEA PROTEIN HYDROLYSATES, GERMINATED CHICKPEA, GERMINATED CHICKPEA PROTEINS, AND GERMINATED CHICKPEA PROTEIN HYDROLYSATES

Type 2 Diabetes (T2D) is characterized by the body's decreased response to insulin, which in turn results in hyperglycemia. The antidiabetic potential of food-derived peptides is well established (Jahandideh et al. 2022). Dipeptidyl peptidase (DPP-IV) cleaves glucagon-like peptide-1 (GLP-1), which is responsible for approximately 50% of insulin secretion. This, in turn, affects glucose homeostasis and results in increased blood glucose levels. Both α-amylase and α-glucosidase cleave starch into glucose, thus allowing for easier absorption by enterocytes. Inhibition of DPP-IV, α-amylase, and α-glucosidase by chickpea protein hydrolysate as a functional ingredient can therefore ensure sustained levels of blood glucose and regular insulin production in humans (Jahandideh et al. 2022).

Chickpea Protein Hydrolysates

In Silico Studies

A recent study of *in silico* hydrolysis of chickpea proteins legumin and provicilin found 191 legumin and 190 provicilin sequences with potential DPP-IV inhibitory properties (Mora-Melgem et al. 2023). Of these, only 92 unique peptides were identified. Legumin contained more peptides than provicilin with potential DPP-IV inhibitory activity. *In silico* hydrolysis with alcalase and pepsin released more peptides with DPP-IV inhibitory activity compared to in silico digestion with papain, ficin and bromelain. Of the peptides identified, 46 had tridimensional structures available in PubChem and were therefore used for further analysis. Absorption, distribution, metabolism, excretion, and toxicity (ADMET) were used to predict the toxicity and bioavailability of peptides (Mora-Melgem et al. 2023). Of 46 peptides, 45 were found to be non-toxic and could reach systemic circulation. In molecular docking, 30 peptides formed hydrophobic interactions with the active site (S1) of DPP-IV. S1 includes hydrophobic residues such as Tyr547, Tyr631, Val656, Trp659, Tyr662, and Val711. Thirty-two peptides were found to interact with the catalytic site containing hydrophilic residues, including Ser630, Asp708, Asn710, and His740.

Biochemical Studies

Different varieties of chickpeas were compared for their dipeptidyl peptidase (DPP)-IV inhibition. An IC_{50} of 0.2 mg/mL was found with raw chickpea protein hydrolysate of the Billy bean variety, using a 1:30 E/S ratio and a 60-minute hydrolysis time. The authors found that only one variety of the five inhibited α-amylase by greater than 50% (Billy bean, 0.1 mg/mL). Maximum inhibition of α-glucosidase (66%) was achieved in precooked chickpea hydrolysates in Billy bean (10 mg/mL) (Acevedo Martínez and Gonzalez de Mejia 2021).

Raw chickpea protein hydrolysate produced with gastrointestinal (GI) enzymes had an IC_{50} of 0.3 mg/mL for DPP-IV inhibition (Chandrasekaran et al. 2020). In comparison, bromelain hydrolysate had an IC_{50} of 0.8 mg/mL. The simulated GI system also produced a more potent hydrolysate inhibitor of α-amylase, with 38% inhibition at 10 mg/mL. The bromelain hydrolysate at the same concentration inhibited α-amylase by 11%. Molecular docking of DPP-IV with peptides identified in the simulated GI hydrolysate showed binding with S1 residues of DPP-IV (the active site), including Tyr547 and Tyr662, and with the catalytic site (S2) of DPP-IV, including Ser209 and His740. In comparison, bromelain hydrolysates did not bind to these sites, resulting in reduced inhibitory potency of DPP-IV.

Chickpea protein hydrolysates produced with alcalase using albumin and globulin fractions of raw chickpea protein have also been evaluated for their antidiabetic potential (Quintero-Soto et al. 2021). A mixture of three peptides (FEI, FEL, FIE) from the best hydrolysate showed an IC_{50} of 4.2 μg/mL for DPP-IV inhibition. Three other peptides, FGKG, MEE, and FKN, were also evaluated, resulting in IC_{50} values of 7.3 μg/mL, 7.7 μg/mL, and 12.1 μg/mL, respectively.

Another peptide, FGKG, showed the highest inhibition values for both α-amylase (37%) and α-glucosidase (17%) when evaluated at 0.1 mg/mL (Quintero-Soto et al. 2021).

Chickpea protein hydrolysate produced with subtilisin and subsequent hydrolysis with trypsin, obtaining a degree of hydrolysis (DH) of 20%, showed inhibition of α-glucosidase (IC_{50} 1.4 mg/mL); the fraction with molecular weight of 0.5–1.1 kDa was the most potent (IC_{50} 0.5 mg/mL) inhibiting α-glucosidase (Rivero-Pino et al. 2021). Hydrolysates prepared with either subtilisin or trypsin showed IC_{50} values ranging from 10–14 mg/mL.

A peptide identified in chickpea alcalase hydrolysate, namely Leu-Gly-Glu-Phe-Val-Leu-Thr-Arg, showed an IC_{50} of 123.0 μg/mL for α-amylase and an IC_{50} of 101.3 μg/mL for α-glucosidase (Gupta et al. 2022).

In Vitro Studies

Chickpea protein hydrolysis was performed using Protamex®, Neutrase, Alcalase, and Papain. It was then evaluated for its antidiabetic properties *in vitro* in Caco-2 cells, using DPP-IV as a marker. Protamex® is a proprietary blend of microbial endo-proteases. Neutrase is a broad-spectrum endoprotease isolated from bacteria. The authors found that biochemical inhibition of DPP-IV with the Neutrase hydrolysate was significantly higher (48%) at 1 mg/mL in comparison to other enzymes at the same concentration, specifically 30% (Protamex®), 31% (Alcalase), and 32% (papain). Hydrolysis time was further optimized for Neutrase, and it was found that 60 min of hydrolysis had the highest DPP-IV inhibition (51% at 1 mg/mL). Four peptides were identified in the Neutrase hydrolysate, which had IC_{50} values of 25.8 μM (PPGIPYW), 58.0 μM (AAWPGHPEF), 110.5 μM (LAFP), and 12.4 μM (IAIPPGIPYW). Pure peptides IAIPPGIPYW and PPGIPYW were tested *in vitro* in Caco-2 cells for their DPP-IV inhibition and found to have IC_{50} values of 138.6 μM (IAIPPGIPYW) and 270.6 μM (PPGIPYW). Peptide IAIPPGIPYW formed hydrogen bonds with Tyr547 and Lys554 in molecular docking, which are involved in the active site of DPP-IV. Similarly, peptide PPGIPYW formed hydrogen bonds with Lys554, Tyr547, and Ser209, which are involved in the active site of DPP-IV. However, IAIPPGIPYW formed more hydrogen bonds overall, resulting in a more potent peptide, as seen in Figure 30.1 (Zan et al. 2023).

Chickpea protein hydrolysates have been primarily investigated using biochemical and *in silico* models, particularly DPP-IV, α-glucosidase, and α-amylase as T2D markers of interest. Future studies may focus on *in vitro* and *in vivo* studies to better understand the mechanism of action of different chickpea protein hydrolysates and their constituents.

Germinated Chickpea

Whole chickpeas were germinated for 3–5 days, hydrolyzed, and evaluated with a simulated GI system for their antidiabetic potential (Di Stefano et al. 2019). DPP-IV inhibition values were 57–60% with 100 mg/mL of germinated chickpea. No significant difference was observed between non-germinated and germinated chickpeas. For α-glucosidase inhibition, 3-day and 5-day germination displayed 75% and 70% inhibition of α-glucosidase at 25 mg/mL. Based on current evidence, as

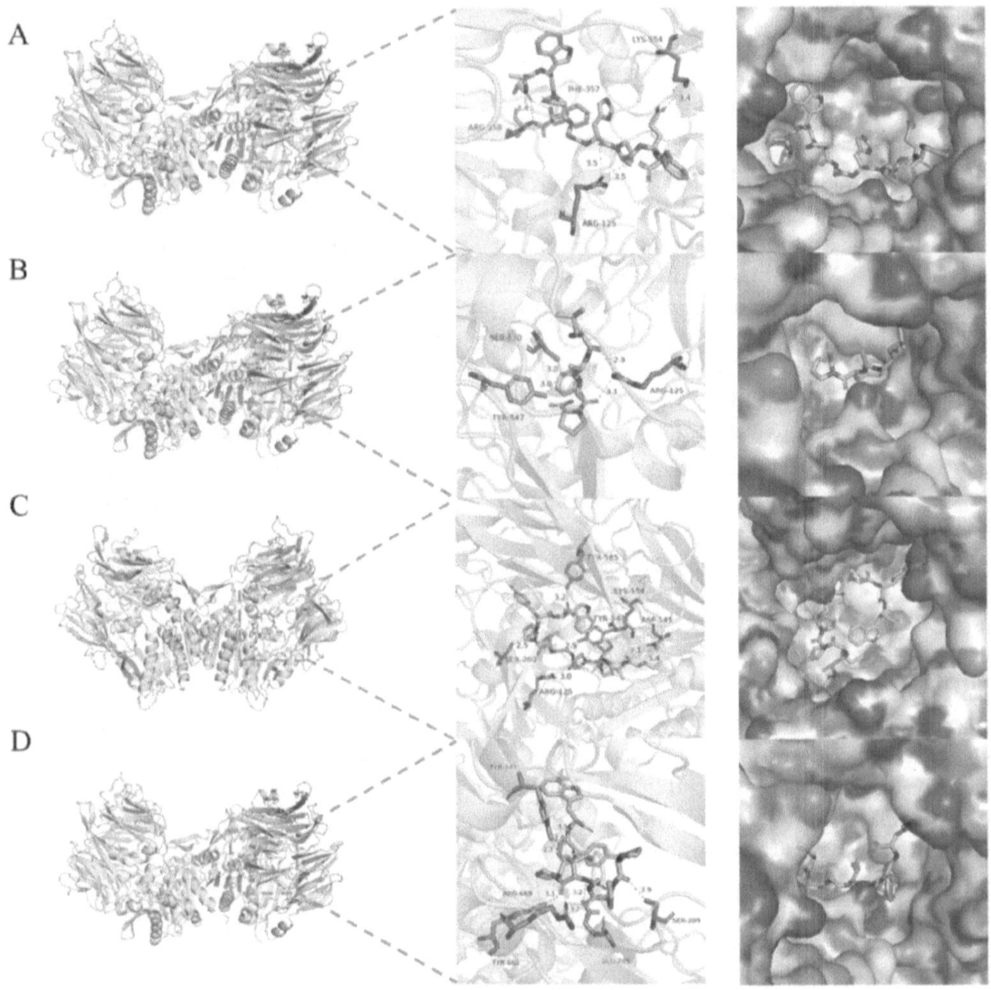

FIGURE 30.1 Molecular docking of peptides (A) AAWPGHPEF, (B) LAFP, (C) IAIPPGIPYW, and (D) PPGIPYW to DPP-IV. This figure shows the 3D pink (peptides) stick models and the purple (DPP-IV residues) stick models. Hydrogen bonds are shown with yellow dotted lines. Reprinted with permission from Zan, R., Wu, Q., Chen, Y., Wu, G., Zhang, H., and Zhu, L. 2023. Identification of Novel Dipeptidyl Peptidase-IV Inhibitory Peptides in Chickpea Protein Hydrolysates. *Journal of Agricultural and Food Chemistry* 71 (21): 8211–8219. Copyright (2023) American Chemical Society.

seen in the studies mentioned earlier, chickpea protein hydrolysate is a more potent inhibitor of both DPP-IV and α-glucosidase compared to germinated chickpeas.

However, studies on the antidiabetic potential of germinated chickpeas are limited. Future studies may explore other germination times, using *in vitro* and *in vivo* models, as well as "enriched" germination by adding selenium or hydrogen peroxide during germination.

Germinated Chickpea Protein Hydrolysate

Biochemical Studies

Germinated chickpea proteins were hydrolyzed with either papain or ficin and optimized for DPP-IV inhibition. The optimum conditions (6-day germination, 1:10 E/S ratio, and 30 min hydrolysis time with ficin) had an IC_{50} value of 49 μg/mL (Chandrasekaran and Gonzalez de Mejia 2022).

Additionally, α-glucosidase inhibition of 47% was seen at 1 mg/mL in a hydrolysate produced after four days of germination, 1:30 E/S ratio, and 30 min hydrolysis time with ficin. Two pure peptides (SPGAGKG and GLAR) were evaluated for their DPP-IV inhibition and potential α-glucosidase inhibition. SPGAGKG and GLAR had an IC_{50} of 0.3 mg/mL and 12.7 mg/mL for DPP-IV inhibition, respectively. For α-glucosidase inhibition, pure peptides SPGAGKG and GLAR had an IC_{50} of 1.8 mg/mL and 8.7 mg/mL, respectively. Peptides with molecular masses of 362.4–572.3 g/mol were found in the optimum hydrolysate.

In Vitro Studies

Germinated chickpea proteins were hydrolyzed with ficin, which reduced glucose absorption in Caco-2 cells through the reduced expression of GLUT2 (Chandrasekaran and Gonzalez de Mejia 2023). Compared to the non-treated sample, germinated chickpea protein hydrolysate presented significant GLUT2 inhibition, with a maximum of 32% inhibition at 2.5 mM. Pure peptides FDLPAL, GEAGR, and VVFW, identified in the hydrolysate, showed 25%, 22%, and 39% GLUT2 inhibition at 50 μM. Sucrase-isomaltase, which converts sucrose, maltose, and isomaltose into glucose for absorption, was also inhibited by both the hydrolysate and peptides identified in the hydrolysate. Maximum inhibition of sucrase and isomaltase was achieved at 500 μM, with 59% inhibition and 65% inhibition, respectively. Germinated chickpea protein hydrolysate showed the maximum maltase inhibition at 46% (1 mM). Compared to the pure peptides tested, pure peptide FDLPAL showed maximum inhibition of sucrase (44%) and maltase (64%) at 100 μM. Peptide FDLPAL at 50 μM showed the maximum inhibition of isomaltase (52%). Pure peptides did not show high DPP-IV inhibitory activity *in vitro,* but the germinated chickpea protein hydrolysate inhibited DPP-IV by 52% at 2.5 mM (Chandrasekaran and Gonzalez de Mejia 2023). The authors concluded that synergistic interactions between multiple peptides in germinated chickpea protein hydrolysate contributed to higher DPP-IV inhibition.

Inhibition of sucrase-isomaltase and glucose absorption helps manage T2D by reducing overall glucose absorption. This, in turn, reduces blood glucose levels, which are often elevated in T2D patients (Ninomiya et al. 2022).

COMPARISON OF THE EFFECTS OF GERMINATION AND ENZYMATIC HYDROLYSIS ON CHICKPEAS' ANTIDIABETIC PROPERTIES

The highest inhibition of DPP-IV (IC_{50} 4.2 μg/mL) in biochemical assays has been found with peptides FEI, FIE, FEL (Quintero-Soto et al. 2021). However, the concentration of DPP-IV used in different studies has not been specified, and it would be helpful to compare different peptides in future studies.

With DPP-IV inhibition, the composition of the hydrolysate played a more vital role than the length of the peptide, as observed with peptides GLAR (IC_{50} 12.7 mg/mL) and FGKG (7.3 μg/mL). Previously, it was shown through molecular docking that longer peptides have different types of bonding associated with DPP-IV than smaller peptides (Power et al. 2014). This bonding ultimately determines the DPP-IV inhibitory potential and is heavily influenced by the peptide composition. Hydrophobic amino acids in peptide sequences have also previously contributed to DPP-IV inhibitory potential (Nongonierma and FitzGerald 2017). This was likely a result of their ability to bind to the S1 subsite of DPP-IV.

The highest inhibition of α-glucosidase in studies presented thus far was one peptide (FGKG) found in chickpea albumin hydrolysate produced with alcalase. The α-glucosidase inhibition of hydrolysate prepared using subtilisin was comparable to the germinated chickpea protein hydrolysate (Rivero-Pino et al. 2021). In whole germinated chickpeas that were hydrolyzed with a simulated GI system, the resulting product had lower inhibitory potency of α-glucosidase compared to chickpea protein hydrolysates. Hydrolysates produced using bromelain and precooked chickpea proteins were, in comparison to germinated chickpea protein hydrolysates, relatively less effective inhibitors of α-glucosidase. As with DPP-IV, the composition of the protein hydrolysates is a critical factor in determining the α-glucosidase inhibitory properties of protein hydrolysates. This has also been concluded previously in a review focusing on α-glucosidase inhibitory peptides from different sources (Carroll et al. 2018).

Chickpea protein hydrolysates have been studied to a minimal extent in *in vitro* studies. To our knowledge, only a few studies have evaluated antidiabetic markers in Caco-2 cells. In these investigations, the germinated chickpea protein hydrolysate was less potent in inhibiting DPP-IV, with 52% inhibition at 1.3 mg/mL (2.5 mM), compared to an IC_{50} of 0.2 mg/mL (138.6 μM) with peptide IAIPPGIPYW. However, this was the only measured marker *in vitro* that allowed for comparison. Future studies may focus on exploring alternative markers of T2D, such as sucrase-isomaltase, GLP-1, and glucose absorption. Different cell models are also available to explore multiple mechanisms of action involved in T2D (Rozengurt and Sternini 2007).

In silico evaluation methods such as molecular docking in future studies may help understand the role of different amino acids and their position on the peptide sequence regarding inhibiting α-glucosidase. The antidiabetic properties of chickpea protein hydrolysates and germinated chickpea protein hydrolysates are summarized in Table 30.1.

Both germination and protein hydrolysis are effective processing methods for enhancing the bioactive properties of chickpeas. However, there is a gap in knowledge regarding the combination of the two processes and their collective effect on different biomarkers. Future studies should focus on filling this gap while understanding the role of the composition of hydrolysates, the role of the enzyme used, and the degree of hydrolysis.

EXTRAORAL BITTER TASTE RECEPTORS AND T2D

Bitter-tasting compounds activate bitter taste receptors (T2Rs), which are G-protein-coupled receptors (GPCRs) (Lu et al. 2017). When a bitter compound binds to a bitter taste receptor, the subunits of the associated G-protein, gustducin, dissociate. The subunits activate a cascade of reactions, leading to calcium influx through the inositol triphosphate-sensitive calcium stores (Lu et al. 2017). This effect results in sodium influx through the transient receptor potential cation channel subfamily M member 5 (TRPM5), releasing ATP through calcium homeostasis modulator one and activating the sensory nerve associated with bitterness. This mechanism is illustrated in Figure 30.2 (Lu et al. 2017).

On the other hand, extraoral bitter taste receptors have been identified in the human brain, intestines, lungs, heart, and respiratory tract (Yang et al. 2021). Consequently, various functions of these receptors have been evaluated. Multiple detailed reviews have highlighted the potential role of extraoral bitter taste receptors in various physiological processes (Wang, Liszt, and Depoortere 2020; Bloxham, Foster, and Thomas 2020).

Extraoral bitter receptors have primarily been explored for their relationship with the hormones ghrelin, cholecystokinin (CCK), and GLP-1, which play vital roles in managing hunger and satiety. As mentioned previously, GLP-1 is responsible for approximately 50% of insulin secretion, which is impaired in T2D patients (Jahandideh et al. 2022). Additionally, the role of α-gustducin and TRPM5, which are involved in the GPCR mechanism of bitter taste transduction, has also been explored in pancreatic β-cells, which secrete insulin and are often impaired in T2D.

GHRELIN, CHOLECYSTOKININ (CCK), AND T2D

Ghrelin is a hormone that regulates appetite (Prior et al. 2017). It stimulates appetite and has a strong inverse correlation with insulin resistance (Churm et al. 2017). Epicatechin gallate, a monomeric flavanol, has been shown to stimulate ghrelin secretion, and the corresponding mechanism involves bitter taste receptors hTAS2R14 and hTAS2R39 (Serrano et al. 2016).

TABLE 30.1
Antidiabetic Properties of Chickpea Protein Hydrolysates and Germinated Chickpea Protein Hydrolysates

	Model	Results	Inhibition	Reference
		Chickpea Protein Hydrolysate		
Chickpea proteins legumin and provicilin hydrolyzed	In silico	↑ DPP-IV inhibition	Peptides produced with alcalase or pepsin, and identified in legumin showed more DPP-IV inhibitory potential	Mora-Melgen et al 2023
Raw, pre-cooked and cooked chickpea proteins from five varieties hydrolyzed with bromelain	Biochemical	↑ DPP-IV inhibition	0.2 mg/mL (raw chickpea protein hydrolyzed with bromelain)	Acevedo Martínez and Gonzalez de Mejia 2021
		↑ α-amylase inhibition	50% at 0.1 mg/mL (Billy bean variety)	
		↑ α -glucosidase inhibition	66% at 10 mg/mL (pre-cooked Billy bean hydrolysate)	
Chickpea protein hydrolysate produced with bromelain or by a simulated GI system		↑ DPP-IV inhibition	Simulated GI system - IC_{50} 0.3 mg/mL	Chandrasekaran et al 2020
			Bromelain - IC_{50} 0.8 mg/mL	
		↑ α-amylase inhibition	Simulated GI system -38% inhibition at 10 mg/mL	
			Bromelain - 11% inhibition at 10 mg/mL	
Peptide LGEVLTR from chickpea alcalase hydrolysate		↑ α-amylase inhibition	IC_{50} 123.0 µg/mL	Gupta et al 2022
		↑ α -glucosidase inhibition	IC_{50} 101.3 µg/mL	
Chickpea protein hydrolysates produced with alcalase, using albumin and globulin fractions of raw chickpea protein from 8 varieties		↑ DPP-IV inhibition	IC_{50} 4.2 µg/mL (peptides FEI, FEL, FIE mixed)	Quintero-Soto et al 2021
		↑ α -amylase inhibition	37% at 0.1 mg/mL (peptide FGKG)	
		↑ α -glucosidase inhibition	17% at 0.1 mg/mL (peptide FGKG)	

(Continued)

TABLE 30.1 (CONTINUED)
Antidiabetic Properties of Chickpea Protein Hydrolysates and Germinated Chickpea Protein Hydrolysates

	Model	Results	Inhibition	Reference
Chickpea protein hydrolysates produced with subtilisin and/or trypsin		↑ α -glucosidase inhibition	IC_{50} 1.4 mg/mL with hydrolysis using subtilisin followed by trypsin	Rivero-Pino et al 2021
Pure peptides from chickpea protein hydrolysates produced with Neutrase	In vitro (Caco-2 cells)	↑f DPP-IV inhibition	IC_{50} values of 138.6 μM (IAIPPGIPYW) and 270.6 μM (PPGIPYW).	Zan et al 2023
	Germinated Chickpea Protein Hydrolysate			
Chickpeas germinated for 3-5 days and hydrolyzed with a simulated GI system	Biochemical	↑ DPP-IV inhibition	60% inhibition with 100 mg/mL	Di Stefano et al 2019
		↑ α -glucosidase inhibition	75% inhibition with 25 mg/mL	
Germinated chickpea protein hydrolysate				
Chickpeas germinated for 2-6 days and hydrolyzed with ficin or papain	Biochemical	↑ DPP-IV inhibition	IC_{50} 49 μg/mL	Chandrasekaran and Gonzalez de Mejia 2022
		↑ α -glucosidase inhibition	47% inhibition at 1 mg/mL	
Chickpeas germinated for 6 days and hydrolyzed with ficin, and pure peptides identified in the hydrolysate	In vitro (Caco-2 cells)	↑ DPP-IV inhibition	Germinated chickpea protein hydrolysate inhibited DPP-IV by 87% at 2.5 mM	Chandrasekaran and de Mejia 2023
		↓ glucose absorption	Germinated chickpea protein hydrolysate presented 31.6% inhibition at 2.5 mM. Pure peptides FDLPAL, GEAGR showed 25%, 22% and 39% inhibition respectively at 50 μM.	

This table presents the results of germinated and non-germinated chickpea hydrolyzed protein on antidiabetic properties. DPP-IV: Dipeptidyl-peptidase-IV; IC50: inhibitory concentration for 50% target inhibition.

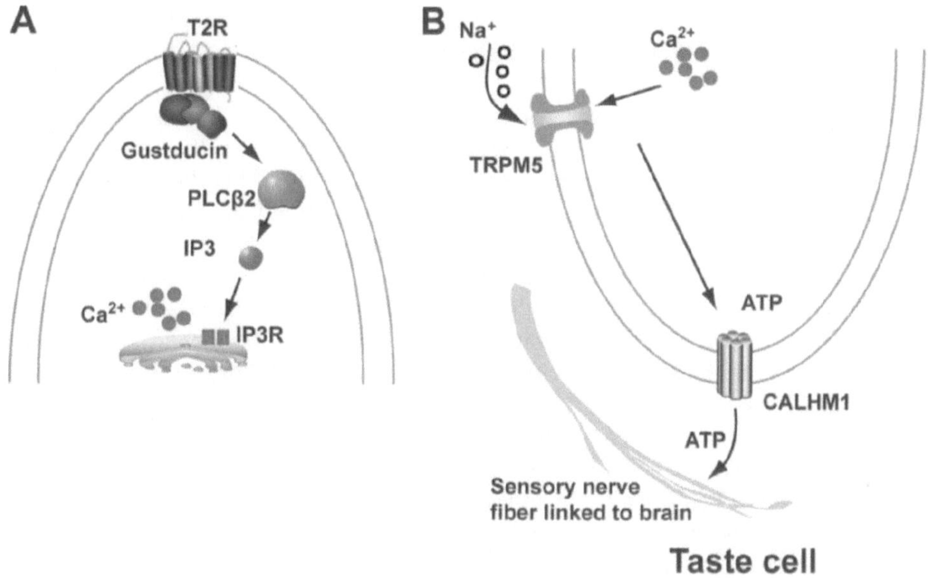

FIGURE 30.2 Canonical T2R signaling pathway. This figure presents (A) The invariant portion of T2R-mediated signaling in the tongue and extraoral cells/tissues, involving the binding of bitter compounds (outside the cell; not depicted) with the receptors to increase the intracellular calcium levels. (B) The remaining components of the T2R pathway in the taste buds. TRPM5, transient receptor potential cation channel subfamily M member 5; PLCβ2, phospholipase Cβ2; IP3, inositol triphosphate; CALHM1, calcium homeostasis modulator 1; ATP, adenosine triphosphate. From Lu et al. (2017). "Extraoral bitter taste receptors in health and disease." *Journal of General Physiology*, 149 (2): 181–197. https://doi.org/10.1085/jgp.201611637. Reprinted with permission under Creative Commons License (Attribution-Noncommercial-Share Alike 4.0 International License).

An extract from the plant *Hoodia gordonii* was evaluated for its effects on CCK secretion (Le Nevé et al. 2010). CCK is a hormone that is a key regulator of appetite by suppressing the desire to eat. Diet plays a vital role in the management of T2D, and through suppressing appetite, CCK can help with portion control. In HuTu-80 cells, a steroid glycoside from *Hoodia gordonii* increased CCK secretion by 1.4x compared to the control while simultaneously activating TAS2R14. In the same study, a bitter receptor antagonist reduced CCK secretion, indicating that CCK secretion may be induced by the activation of bitter receptors (Jeruzal-Świątecka, Fendler, and Pietruszewska 2020).

GLP-1 AND T2D

An analog of an extract of the hop plant (*Humulus lupulus*), KDT501, stimulated increased secretion of GLP-1 by activating mTAS2R108 when tested at 20 μM (1.4 times higher than the control cells) in STC-1 cells (Kok et al. 2018). Using functional gene expression analysis, KDT501 was profiled against 34 mice and 25 human bitter receptors. The signaling pathway involving mTAS2R108 and TAS2R1 was the only pathway activated. In response to mTAS2R108 knockdown in STC-1 cells, GLP-1 secretion was significantly reduced (3 times lower). In the same study, GLP-1 plasma levels increased (490 pg/mL) compared to the control (20 pg/mL) (Kok et al. 2018).

Cucurbitacin B, a compound found in bitter melon (*Momordica charantia*), stimulates GLP-1 release *in vitro* and *in vivo* (Kim et al. 2018). The knockdown of hTAS2R10 in NCI-H716 cells significantly reduced GLP-1 secretion (2 times reduction). In comparison, treatment of cells with 100 μM cucurbitacin B resulted in increased GLP-1 levels (6500 pg/mL, 3.25x higher than the control), indicating that bitter receptor activation may be helpful in the management of T2D through GLP-1 secretion. In a mouse model, cucurbitacin B significantly stimulated GLP-1 release (80 pg/mL) compared to the control (30 pg/mL).

A similar mechanism leading to the release of GLP-1 through TAS2R38 was observed with berberine treatment *in vitro* (Yu et al. 2015). Specifically, in NCI-H716 cells, a significant increase in GLP-1 secretion was observed when cells were treated with 100 μM berberine (1.5 times higher than that in non-treated cells). The expression of TAS2R38 was significantly higher when cells were treated with at least 100 μM berberine (2 times higher than that in non-treated cells). Cells with siRNA-mediated knockdown of TAS2R38 and treated with 100 μM berberine exhibited 0.6 times lower GLP-1 secretion compared to cells with basal expression of TAS2R38. When NCI-H716 cells were simultaneously treated with an antagonist of TAS2R38 and berberine, GLP-1 levels were 0.8 times lower compared to those in cells with basal expression of TAS2R38. Therefore, ample evidence exists that GLP-1 secretion can be increased by activating extraoral bitter receptors.

Isosinensetin, a compound present in *Bupleurum falcatum* L., was found to stimulate the secretion of GLP-1 in NCI-H716 cells by activating TAS2R50 (Lee et al. 2023). *Bupleurum falcatum* L. is a herbal plant described in ancient Chinese medicinal texts (Li et al. 2022). The secretion of GLP-1 increased 2-fold when cells were treated with 40 μM isosinensetin. Simultaneously, siRNA of hTAS2R50 decreased by 0.4-fold, indicating the involvement of hTAS2R50 activation in the increased secretion of GLP-1 (Lee et al. 2023). Increased GLP-1 secretion may be achieved through activating hTAS2R50, leading to greater insulin production and better management of T2D.

In NCI-H716 cells, cucurbitacin B appeared to be a more potent compound in producing GLP-1 through bitter receptor activation compared to berberine and isosinensetin. However, NCI-H716 cells were transfected with TAS2R10 siRNA, whereas the cell line expressed TAS2R38. Future studies may focus on profiling cell lines used in T2D and obesity research to understand which bitter receptors are expressed. Evaluations of T2D and obesity multiple markers and their association with bitter taste receptor activation are needed.

α-Gustducin and T2D

Apart from bitter taste receptors, other markers involved in bitter taste receptor activation have been assessed for their role in T2D. *α*-Gustducin, a G-protein involved in bitter taste receptor induction, was characterized in pancreatic β-cells (Udagawa et al. 2020). Secreted insulin levels significantly increased upon *α*-gustducin knockdown (0.4–2% of total insulin content). The cAMP levels also increased with *α*-gustducin knockdown, from 550 pmol/μg to 900 pmol/μg of protein. Intracellular calcium levels also increased by 20 units of fluorescence intensity.

TRPM5 and T2D

The expression of TRPM5 increases in pancreatic β-cells subjected to glucose-stimulated insulin secretion, and an increase in ATP levels increases the Ca^{2+} influx within cells, thereby promoting insulin secretion (Vennekens et al. 2018). During glucose-stimulated insulin secretion, an increase in ATP levels increases Ca^{2+} influx within cells. As mentioned, both bitter taste receptors and GLP-1 operate via a GPCR mechanism, which is activated in response to a Ca^{2+} influx. Thus, increased glucose uptake has been associated with increased TRPM5 activation, which, in turn, increases the Ca^{2+} influx and GLP-1 production.

Overall, the activation of bitter receptors and their effect on GLP-1 production have predominantly been explored, resulting in increased intracellular calcium. Limited studies have explored the complete bitter receptor mechanism and its relationship with T2D. Most studies have focused only on one taste receptor or one downstream product of bitter receptor activation.

BITTER PEPTIDES

The bitterness of some peptides has limited the acceptability and commercialization of protein hydrolysates (Aluko 2017). Several bitter peptides have been identified in plant-based protein sources (Ying et al. 2021). The determinants of bitterness include hydrophobicity, amino acid position, isomeric configuration, peptide length, and amino acid type. Extensive enzymatic hydrolysis has been highlighted as an effective method to reduce bitterness.

Studies have shown that peptides can also block bitter taste receptors in humans (Zhang et al. 2019). Notably, beef protein hydrolysates were found to be bitter taste modifiers, with the ability to reduce the bitter taste of quinine by up to 38% (Zhang et al. 2019). Specifically, the release of calcium by the bitter taste receptor T2R4 was reduced by hydrolysates of HEK293 cells. Hen protein-derived peptides such as AGFAGDDAPR, AGGATAAQLE, ALGQNPTNAEINK, ASNPYSTVT, FTQQIE, GDDAPR, ILGNPSKEE, ITTNPY, ITTNPYD, KALQEAHQQTLDD, KNLQEE, LEGSLE, LELNQ, PIGNIN, SMQSTLD, and TDISQIQS have also been identified as inhibitors of T2R4, as well as those of the receptors T2R7 and T2R14 (Xu et al. 2019). Like beef protein hydrolysates, these peptides significantly inhibited quinine bitterness.

Bitter Peptides Identified in Chickpea Proteins

Chickpea albumin hydrolyzed with Alcalase and Flavourzyme® was evaluated for bitterness using a sensory panel (Kou et al. 2013). The bitterness of the hydrolysate was higher when it was prepared with Alcalase (4.5/5). With the addition of Flavourzyme®, the score decreased to a value close to 0.5. The bitter peptide RQSHFANAQP was identified in this hydrolysate.

In raw chickpea protein hydrolysates produced using either GI enzymes or bromelain, bitter fragments were found in all peptide sequences and were potential activators of multiple bitter receptors (Chandrasekaran et al. 2020). In germinated chickpea protein hydrolysates, two out of three peptides identified in the protein hydrolysate were found to contain bitter fragments, and all three peptides had the potential to activate bitter receptors (Chandrasekaran and Gonzalez de Mejia 2022).

Theoretical hydrolysis of chickpea legumin was performed using ficin and bromelain (Real Hernandez and Gonzalez de Mejia 2019). A total of 17 bitter fragments were detected during the theoretical hydrolysis with bromelain, and these fragments were also associated with bioactive properties. In comparison, only three of these fragments were detected in the presence of ficin.

Bitter peptides have been predicted to activate hTAS2R38 and hTAS2R10 in the studies mentioned above, thereby showing potential to be explored in NCI-H716 cells regarding GLP-1 production, like berberine and cucurbitacin.

The structures of known bitter compounds with antidiabetic effects were compared with that of a known bitter peptide described by Kou et al. (2013), shown in Figure 30.3. The primary similarity between the different bitter compounds, such as isosinensetin and epicatechin gallate, and the peptide is the presence of a benzene ring in the structure. Carbonyl groups were common between known bitter antidiabetic compounds and the bitter peptide identified in chickpea protein hydrolysates. One of the many factors affecting a peptide's bitterness is its net hydrophobicity (Aluko 2017). The presence of a benzene ring contributes to its net hydrophobicity and may be a key determinant of bitter taste. Additionally, proline at the C-terminus correlates with bitterness (Aluko 2017).

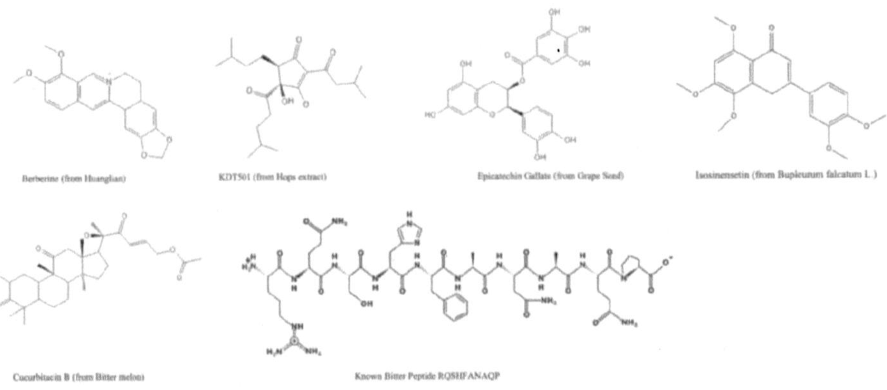

FIGURE 30.3 Chemical structure comparison of known bitter compounds with antidiabetic effects. This figure presents structural differences among bitter compounds present in bitter melon, hops extracts, grape seeds, huanglian, *Bupleurum falcatum L.*, and chickpeas. Structures were obtained from ChemSpider.

Correlation between Antidiabetic Properties and Bitterness of Chickpea Peptides *In Silico*

Chickpea peptides from other studies that have not been evaluated for bitterness were analyzed in this review using the BioPep database (Table 30.2).

The bioactive properties of the peptides were also determined using the same database to compare these properties and associated bitterness. Multiple bitter fragments are associated with their bioactive properties. A correlation plot was constructed between the different bioactive properties analyzed and the bioactive bitter fragments found in previously identified peptides from chickpea protein hydrolysates using the R program (Table 30.3). A moderate positive relationship was observed between DPP-IV inhibition and bioactive bitter fragments (0.59) and α-glucosidase inhibition (0.40) ($p < 0.05$). Given that there is evidence that bitter receptor activation plays a role in increasing GLP-1, it is vital to understand if this mechanism also involves inhibition of DPP-IV.

The other bioactive properties, such as α-amylase inhibition and glucose uptake, did not appear to be affected by bitterness. Further investigation into the role of bitterness in inhibiting α-glucosidase and DPP-IV in *in vitro* and *in vivo* models is required to understand the mechanism of action. Specifically, pure peptides and the role of the associated bitter fragments in the exertion of bioactive properties need to be further investigated to better understand the role of bitterness in chickpea protein hydrolysates when used to manage metabolic disorders.

In summary, the bioactive properties of chickpea protein germination and subsequent hydrolysis have yet to be largely explored. Limited but promising information is available regarding the bioactive properties of germinated chickpea protein hydrolysates, which incentivizes future studies to investigate whether germination may increase the efficacy of chickpea protein hydrolysates. *In vitro* models investigating the effects of chickpea protein hydrolysates on extraoral bitter taste receptor activation have been minimally studied despite *in silico* evidence that these hydrolysates may have bitter fragments and might activate bitter receptors. A mechanistic view of the bioactive properties of germinated chickpea protein hydrolysates, the role of hydrolysate compositions in determining the bioactive properties, and their association with bitterness is needed.

TABLE 30.2
Bioactive and Bitter Peptides Fragments Identified in Chickpea Protein Hydrolysates

Peptide	Bioactive Properties	Bioactive Fragments	Bitter Fragments	Reference
SPKAGGF	DPP-IV inhibitor	KA, SP, AG, GF, GG, PK	P, F, PK, GF, GGF, K	Acevedo Martínez and Gonzalez de Mejia 2021
HAAGGKG	DPP-IV inhibitor	HA, AA, AG, GG, KG	K, KG	
GKGSAT	DPP-IV inhibitor	AT, KG	K, KG	
LALPV	DPP-IV inhibitor	LA, LP, AL, PV	P, V, L, LA	
NGGPPA	DPP-IV inhibitor	GP, PA, GG, NG, PP	P, PP, GP, GGP, PA	
VLDGPA	DPP-IV inhibitor	GP, PA, GPA, VL	P, GP, V, VL, LD, L, DG, PA	
	Glucose uptake stimulating	VL		
LVVPQ	Glucose uptake stimulating	LV	P, V, L, LV, VV	
	DPP-IV inhibitor	VP, VV, LV, PQ		
SVKSPPGGSK	DPP-IV inhibitor	PP, SP, PPG, GG, KS, PG, SK, SV, VK	P, PP, PPG, PGG, V, K, PG	
	α-glucosidase inhibitor	PP		
SPKGAGF	DPP-IV inhibitor	SP, GA, AG, GF, KG, PK	P, F, PK, GF, K, KG	
SPKGGAF	DPP-IV inhibitor	SP, GA, AF, GG, KG, PK	P, F, PK, AF, K, KG	
KGGSAT	DPP-IV inhibitor	AT, GG, KG	K, KG	
NPGGPA	DPP-IV inhibitor	GP, PA, GPA, NP, GG, PG	P, GP, PGG, GGP, PA, PG	
KSPPGAGSSR	α-glucosidase inhibitor	PP	R, P, PP, PPG, K, PG	
	DPP-IV inhibitor	PP, SP, GA, PPG, AG, KS, PG		
NKGPG	DPP-IV inhibitor	GP, KG, PG	P, GP, GPG, K, KG, PG	
TKGAAGP	DPP-IV inhibitor	GP, GA, AA, AG, KG, TK	P, GP, K, KG	
VPGGGKG	DPP-IV inhibitor	VP, GG, KG, PG	P, PGG, V, K, KG, PG	
NGPGPA	DPP-IV inhibitor	GP, PA, GPA, NG, PG	P, GP, PGP, GPG, PA, PG	
TTKPPGAGSK	DPP-IV inhibitor	PP, KP, GA, PPG, AG, PG, SK, TK, TT	P, PP, KP, PPG, K, PG	
	α-glucosidase inhibitor	PP		

(*Continued*)

TABLE 30.2 (CONTINUED)
Bioactive and Bitter Peptides Fragments Identified in Chickpea Protein Hydrolysates

Peptide	Bioactive Properties	Bioactive Fragments	Bitter Fragments	Reference
LLASPAGCNLVPPRS	DPP-IV inhibitor	PP, LA, PA, VP, LL, SP, AG, AS, LV, NL	R, P, PP, PR, V, LL, L, LV, LA, PA	
	Glucose uptake stimulating	LV, LL		
	α-glucosidase inhibitor	PP		
VTGPNPVATLA	DPP-IV inhibitor	GP, VA, LA, NP, AT, PN, PV, TG, TL, VT	P, GP, V, L, VA, LA	
EVLSEVSF	DPP-IV inhibitor	EV, SF, VL, VS	F, V, VL, L, EV	
	Glucose uptake stimulating	VL		
FDLPALR	DPP-IV inhibitor	PA, LP, AL	R, P, F, L, DL, PA	
FDLPAL	DPP-IV inhibitor	PA, LP, AL	P, F, L, DL, PA	
VVFW	DPP-IV inhibitor	VV, VF	F, VV, VF, FW, W, V	
SFDLPAL	DPP-IV inhibitor	PA, LP, AL, SF	P, F, L, DL, PA	
HPPVGGVS	α-glucosidase inhibitor	PP	P, PP, V, GV, GGV, VG	
	DPP-IV inhibitor	PP, HP, GG, GV, PV, VG, VS		
LR	DPP-IV inhibitor	LR	L, R	Chandrasekaran et al. 2020
PLLVE	α-glucosidase inhibitor	VE	P, V, L, VE, LL, LV, PL	
	Glucose uptake stimulating	LV, LL		
	DPP-IV inhibitor	LL, PL, LV, VE		
SPKAGAGK	DPP-IV inhibitor	KA, SP, GA, AG, PK	P, K, PK	
HATGGGSGR	DPP-IV inhibitor	HA, AT, GG, TG	R, GR	
PHPATSGGGL	DPP-IV inhibitor	PA, HP, GL, AT, GG, PH, TS	P, L, GL, PA, GGL, GGGL	
TPKASATAAL	DPP-IV inhibitor	KA, TP, TA, AL, AA, AS, AT, PK	P, K, L, PK	
TLTTGTGGLL	DPP-IV inhibitor	LL, GL, GG, LT, TG, TL, TT	L, LL, GL, GLL, GGL	
	Glucose uptake stimulating	LL		
YVDGSGTPLT	DPP-IV inhibitor	TP, PL, LT, VD, PV	P, V, L, VD, PL, DG	
TKTPGAGTSAGL	DPP-IV inhibitor	TP, GA, GL, AG, KT, PG, TK, TS	P, K, L, GL, PG	
KEGGGTGTGAAR	DPP-IV inhibitor	GA, AA, EG, GG, KE, TG	R, K, EG, EGG	

(Continued)

TABLE 30.2 (CONTINUED)
Bioactive and Bitter Peptides Fragments Identified in Chickpea Protein Hydrolysates

Peptide	Bioactive Properties	Bioactive Fragments	Bitter Fragments	Reference
STGPNAGGGAGGY	DPP-IV inhibitor	GP, GA, AG, GG, GY, NA, PN, TG	P, GP, GY, GGY	
TLLFTELLF	DPP-IV inhibitor	LL, TE, TL	F, L, LF, LL, EL, ELL	
	Glucose uptake stimulating	LL		
KNGAAGPSTVAR	DPP-IV inhibitor	GP, VA, GA, AA, AG, NG, PS, TV	R, P, K, V, GP, VA	
LASEGASAATGAF	DPP-IV inhibitor	LA, GA, AA, AF, AS, AT, EG, TG, LA	F, L, LA, EG, AF	
VLTSGAGSGAAALT	Glucose uptake stimulating	VL	V, L, VL	
	DPP-IV inhibitor	GA, AL, AA, AG, LT, TS, VL		
KNGLGAGAGAGSAR	DPP-IV inhibitor	GA, GL, AG, NG, AGA	R, K, L, LG, GL, GLG	
LSAHAGGTGATLW	DPP-IV inhibitor	HA, GA, LW, AG, AH, AT, GG, TG, TL	L, W, LW	
LDLARAGGCPTKN	DPP-IV inhibitor	LA, RA, AG, GG, PT, TK	R, P, L, L, LD, DL, LA	
SPQSPPFATPLW	DPP-IV inhibitor	PP, FA, TP, SP, PL, LW, AT, PF, PQ, QS	P, F, L, W, PP, PF, LW, PL, PPF	
	α-glucosidase inhibitor	PP		
LLSASMGSQLLSF	Glucose uptake stimulating	LL	F, L, LL	
	DPP-IV inhibitor	LL, AS, MG, QL, SF		
GKGSGAF	DPP-IV inhibitor	GA, AF, KG	F, K, AF, KG	
TRGTGGR	DPP-IV inhibitor	GG, RG, TG, TR	R, RG, GR	
KMTAGSGVT	DPP-IV inhibitor	TA, AG, GV, VT	V, K, GV	
KSGGGGGGTAVT	DPP-IV inhibitor	TA, AV, GG, KS, VT	V, K	
GKAAPGSGGGTKA	DPP-IV inhibitor	KA, AP, APG, AA, GG, PG, TK	P, K, PG	
RASAAGGGGGGVSSR	DPP-IV inhibitor	RA, AA, AG, AS, GG, GV, VS	R, V, GV, GGV	
GKGSSGTGAGGASVSGVT	DPP-IV inhibitor	GA, AG, AS, GG, GV, KG, SV, TG, VS, VT	V, K, GV, KG	
NKKSGAGGGSGAGKGGVA	DPP-IV inhibitor	VA, GA, AG, GG, GV, KG, KK, KS	V, K, GV, KG, VA, GGV	
LLGELCGSGNTVVEL	Glucose uptake stimulating	LL	V, L, VE, GE, LL, LG, EL, VV, LLG	
	DPP-IV inhibitor	LL, VV, GE, NT, TV, VE		
	α-glucosidase inhibitor	VE		

(Continued)

TABLE 30.2 (CONTINUED)
Bioactive and Bitter Peptides Fragments Identified in Chickpea Protein Hydrolysates

Peptide	Bioactive Properties	Bioactive Fragments	Bitter Fragments	Reference
QNPLSSAAPTGAGKPY	DPP-IV inhibitor	AP, KP, GA, NP, AA, PL, AG, PT, PY, QN, TG	P, L, K, KP, PL	
GLTQGASLAGSGAPSPLF	DPP-IV inhibitor	LA, AP, SP, GA, SL, PL, AG, AS, LT, PS, QG, TQ	P, F, L, LF, GL, PL, LA, SLA	
AMMELGWSTSGEFLL	DPP-IV inhibitor	LL, FL, WS, GE, GW, ME, MM, TS	F, L, W, FL, GE, LL, LG, EL, EF, FLL	
	Glucose uptake stimulating	LL		
SPGAGKG	DPP-IV inhibitor	SP, GA, AG, KG, PG	P, K, KG, PG	Chandrasekaran and Gonzalez de Mejia 2022
GLAR	DPP-IV inhibitor	LA, GL	R, GL, L, LA	
STSA	DPP-IV inhibitor	TS	N/A	
FGKG	DPP-IV inhibitor	KG	F, FG, K, KG	Quintero-Soto et al. 2021
FEI	DPP-IV inhibitor	EI	F, EI	
FEL	N/A	N/A	F, L, EL	
FIE	N/A	N/A	F, FI	
MEE	DPP-IV inhibitor	ME	EE	
TNDR	DPP-IV inhibitor	DR, ND, TN	R	Rivero-Pino et al. 2021
EGDIIA	Glucose uptake stimulating	II	II, EG, IA	
	DPP-IV inhibitor	IA, EG, II		
QNQL	DPP-IV inhibitor	NQ, QL, QN	L	
QPHR	N/A	N/A	N/A	
NPQAGR	DPP-IV inhibitor	NP, AG, PQ, QA	R, P, GR	
NDQDTP	DPP-IV inhibitor	TP, DQ, ND, QD	P	
QQEGS	DPP-IV inhibitor	EG, QE, QQ	EG	
QGR	N/A	N/A	R, GR	
NAMF	DPP-IV inhibitor	MF, NA	F	
TAPF	DPP-IV inhibitor	AP, TA, PF	P, F, PF	
NHPQF	DPP-IV inhibitor	HP, NH, PQ, QF	P, F	
NPL	DPP-IV inhibitor	NP, PL	P, L, PL	
QHNIGF	DPP-IV inhibitor	GF, QH	F, GF, IG	
TNTDDS	DPP-IV inhibitor	NT, TD, TN	N/A	
TAAK	DPP-IV inhibitor	TA, AA	K	
QQEER	DPP-IV inhibitor	QE, QQ	R, EE	
TIDQL	DPP-IV inhibitor	DQ, QL, TI	L, ID	
HAAM	DPP-IV inhibitor	HA, AA	N/A	
ATEIA	DPP-IV inhibitor	IA, AT, EI, TE	EI, IA	
NAL	DPP-IV inhibitor	AL, NA	L	
TMES	DPP-IV inhibitor	ES, ME, TM	N/A	
TTNQY	DPP-IV inhibitor	NQ, QY, TN, TT	N/A	
TNGF	DPP-IV inhibitor	GF, NG, TN	F, GF	
NPTQN	DPP-IV inhibitor	NP, PT, QN, TQ	P	

(*Continued*)

TABLE 30.2 (CONTINUED)
Bioactive and Bitter Peptides Fragments Identified in Chickpea Protein Hydrolysates

Peptide	Bioactive Properties	Bioactive Fragments	Bitter Fragments	Reference
QTDCF	DPP-IV inhibitor	QT, TD	F	
TQGEPS	DPP-IV inhibitor	EP, GE, PS, QG, TQ	P, GE	
TINS	DPP-IV inhibitor	IN, TI	IN	
GAA	DPP-IV inhibitor	GA, AA	N/A	
NTS	DPP-IV inhibitor	NT, TS	N/A	
NITR	DPP-IV inhibitor	TR	R	
QGL	DPP-IV inhibitor	GL, QG	GL, L	
NGF	DPP-IV inhibitor	GF, NG	F, GF	
TAS	DPP-IV inhibitor	TA, AS	N/A	
TPL	DPP-IV inhibitor	PL, TP	P, L, PL	
TADAIF	DPP-IV inhibitor	TA, AD	F, IF, AD, DA	
	α-glucosidase inhibitor	AD		
THMAGS	DPP-IV inhibitor	MA, AG, TH	N/A	
QAAF	DPP-IV inhibitor	AA, AF, QA	F, AF	
NGIF	DPP-IV inhibitor	GI, NG	F, IF, GI	
TGEF	DPP-IV inhibitor	GE, NG	F, GE, EF	
TEF	DPP-IV inhibitor	TE	F, EF	
NGGR	DPP-IV inhibitor	GG, NG	R, GR	
QGS	DPP-IV inhibitor	QG	N/A	
TGS	DPP-IV inhibitor	TG	N/A	
NTK	DPP-IV inhibitor	NT, TK	K	
TGF	DPP-IV inhibitor	GF, TG	F, GF	
TDF	DPP-IV inhibitor	TD	F	
GEY	DPP-IV inhibitor	GE, EY	GE, EY	
TNEAY	DPP-IV inhibitor	AY, NE, TN	EA	
	α-glucosidase inhibitor	EA		
TPGS	DPP-IV inhibitor	TP, PG	P, PG	
NTL	DPP-IV inhibitor	NT, TL	L	
AAWPGHPEF	DPP-IV inhibitor	WP, HP, AA, AW, GH, PG	P, F, EF, WP, W, PG	Zan et al. 2023
	α-glucosidase inhibitor	PE	P, F, FP, AF	
LAFP	DPP-IV inhibitor	LA, FP, AF		
IAIPPGIPYW	α-amylase inhibitor	IPP	P, PP, PPG, PGI, GI, W, PG, IA, IP, PY	
	α-glucosidase inhibitor	IPP		
	DPP-IV inhibitor	PP, IP, IA, PPG, GI, PG, PY, YW		
PPGIPYW	α-glucosidase inhibitor	PP	P, PP, PPG, PGI, GI, W, PG, IA, IP, PY	
	DPP-IV inhibitor	IP, PPG, GI, PG, PY, YW		

This table shows the specific amino acid sequences of peptides with bioactive and bitter properties suggested and identified in chickpea protein hydrolysates from antidiabetic studies. N/A indicates that no data is available regarding the property of the given peptide in the specific column. DPP-IV: dipeptidyl-peptidase-IV.

TABLE 30.3
R Values among Peptide Fragments with Antidiabetic and Bitter Properties

	DPP-IV Inhibition	α-Glucosidase Inhibition	Glucose Uptake Stimulating	α-Amylase Inhibition	Bioactive Bitter Properties
DPP-IV inhibition	1				
α-Glucosidase inhibition	0.3	1			
Glucose uptake stimulating	0.18	0.14	1		
α-Amylase inhibition	0.11	0.26*	–0.02	1	
Bioactive bitter properties	0.59*	0.40*	0.29*	0.14	1

This table presents the correlations among peptide fragments with antidiabetic properties such as DPP-IV inhibition, glucose uptake stimulation, α-amylase inhibition, and α-glucosidase inhibition, and the presence of bioactive bitter properties. Asterisks (*) indicate significance at $p < 0.05$; DPP-IV: Dipeptidyl-peptidase-IV.

MINI DICTIONARY OF TERMS

- **Bitterness:** One of five tastes humans can sense.
- **Chickpea:** Round, white seeds that are rich in protein but are an incomplete protein source due to reduced methionine content.
- **Germination:** Hydrated seeds form "sprouts" similar to those growing in soil.
- **Peptides:** Peptides typically refer to the primary structure of a short amino acid sequence.
- **Type 2 diabetes (T2D):** A disease characterized by a reduced response of the body to insulin, resulting in dysregulated glucose metabolism.

SUMMARY POINTS

- The highest inhibition of DPP-IV in biochemical assays thus far has been found in peptides FEI, FIE, and FEL (IC_{50} 4.2 μg/mL).
- Increased bitterness contributed to increased GLP-1 release through the activation of bitter receptors hTAS2R38, hTAS2R10, and hTAS2R1.
- The composition of protein hydrolysates generated during germination and enzymatic hydrolysis played a vital role in determining the hydrolysate's ability to inhibit the activity of T2D markers such as dipeptidyl peptidase-IV and α-glucosidase.
- In *in vitro* models, the only marker measured with both chickpea protein hydrolysate and germinated chickpea protein hydrolysate was DPP-IV. Germinated chickpea protein hydrolysate was less potent in inhibiting DPP-IV, with 52% inhibition at 1.3 mg/mL (2.5 mM), compared to an IC_{50} of 0.2 mg/mL (138.6 μM) with peptide IAIPPGIPYW from chickpea protein hydrolysate.
- Germinated chickpea protein hydrolysate and pure peptides identified in germinated chickpea protein hydrolysate significantly inhibited glucose absorption and sucrase-isomaltase activity.
- A moderate positive correlation was found between DPP-IV inhibition and bioactive bitter fragments, indicating that future research should focus on understanding the mechanism of action involving both markers.

REFERENCES

Acquah, Caleb, Godfred Ohemeng-Boahen, Krista A. Power, and Susan M. Tosh. "The effect of processing on bioactive compounds and nutritional qualities of pulses in meeting the sustainable development goal 2." *Frontiers in Sustainable Food Systems* 5 (2021): 681662

Aisa, Haji Akber, Yanhua Gao, Abulimiti Yili, Qingling Ma, and Zhen Cheng. "Beneficial role of chickpea (*Cicer arietinum* L.) functional factors in the intervention of metabolic syndrome and diabetes mellitus." In *Bioactive food as dietary interventions for diabetes*, editors: Ronald Ross Watson, Victor R Preedy, pp. 615–627. Academic Press, 2019.

Aluko, R. E. Structural characteristics of food protein-derived bitter peptides. In *Bitterness: Perception, chemistry and food processing*, editors: M. Aliani, M. N. A. Eskin, pp. 105–129. Wiley, 2017.

Berberine. 2023. CSID:2263. http://www.chemspider.com/Chemical-Structure.2263.html

Bloxham, Conor J., Simon R. Foster, and Walter G. Thomas. "A bitter taste in your heart." *Frontiers in Physiology* 11 (2020): 431.

Carroll, Richard G., Zbigniew Zasłona, Silvia Galván-Peña, Emma L. Koppe, Daniel C. Sévin, Stefano Angiari, Martha Triantafilou, Kathy Triantafilou, Louise K. Modis, and Luke A. O'Neill. "An unexpected link between fatty acid synthase and cholesterol synthesis in proinflammatory macrophage activation." *Journal of Biological Chemistry* 293, no. 15 (2018): 5509–5521.

Chandrasekaran, Subhiksha, and Elvira Gonzalez de Mejia. "Optimization, identification, and comparison of peptides from germinated chickpea (*Cicer arietinum*) protein hydrolysates using either papain or ficin and their relationship with markers of type 2 diabetes." *Food Chemistry* 374 (2022): 131717.

Chandrasekaran, Subhiksha, and Elvira Gonzalez de Mejia. "Germinated chickpea protein ficin hydrolysate and its peptides inhibited glucose uptake and affected the bitter receptor signaling pathway *in vitro*." *Food & Function* 14 (2023): 8467.

Chandrasekaran, Subhiksha, Diego Luna-Vital, and Elvira Gonzalez de Mejia. "Identification and comparison of peptides from chickpea protein hydrolysates using either bromelain or gastrointestinal enzymes and their relationship with markers of type 2 diabetes and bitterness." *Nutrients* 12, no. 12 (2020): 3843.

Chou, Wen-Ling. "Therapeutic potential of targeting intestinal bitter taste receptors in diabetes associated with dyslipidemia." *Pharmacological Research* 170 (2021): 105693.

Churm, Rachel, Jaimes S. Davies, Jeffrey W. Stephens, Sarah L. Prior. "Ghrelin function in human obesity and type 2 diabetes: A concise review." *Obesity Reviews* 18, no. 2 (2017): 140–148.

Cruz-Casas, Dora Elisa, Cristóbal N. Aguilar, Juan A. Ascacio-Valdés, Raúl Rodríguez-Herrera, Mónica L. Chávez-González, and Adriana C. Flores-Gallegos. "Enzymatic hydrolysis and microbial fermentation: The most favorable biotechnological methods for the release of bioactive peptides." *Food Chemistry: Molecular Sciences* 3 (2021): 100047.

Cucurbitacin, B. 2023. CSID:4444693. http://www.chemspider.com/Chemical-Structure.4444693.html

Di Stefano, Elisa, Apollinaire Tsopmo, Teresa Oliviero, Vincenzo Fogliano, and Chibuike C. Udenigwe. "Bioprocessing of common pulses changed seed microstructures, and improved dipeptidyl peptidase-IV and α-glucosidase inhibitory activities." *Scientific Reports* 9, no. 1 (2019): 15308.

Epicatechin Gallate. 2023. CSID:97034. http://www.chemspider.com/Chemical-Structure.97034.html

"Food and Agriculture Organization of the United Nations." 2020. *International organization*. https://www.fao.org/home/en

Gupta, Neha, Sameer Quazi,Saurabh Kumar Jha, Mohammad Khursheed Siddiqi, Kanika Verma, Swapnil Sharma, Rizwan Hassan Khan, Sameer Suresh Bhagyawant. "Chickpea peptide: A nutraceutical molecule corroborating neurodegenerative and ACE-I inhibition." *Nutrients* 14 (2022): 4824.

Isosinensetin. 2023. CSID:548876. http://www.chemspider.com/Chemical-Structure.548876.html

Jahandideh, Forough, Stephane L. Bourque, and Jianping Wu. "A comprehensive review on the glucoregulatory properties of food-derived bioactive peptides." *Food Chemistry: X* 13 (2022): 100222.

Jeruzal-Świątecka, Joanna, Wojciech Fendler, and Wioletta Pietruszewska. "Clinical role of extraoral bitter taste receptors." *International Journal of Molecular Sciences* 21, no. 14 (2020): 5156.

KDT501. 2023. CSID:32701818. http://www.chemspider.com/Chemical-Structure.32701818.html

Kim, Kang-Hoon, In-Seung Lee, Ji Young Park, Yumi Kim, Eun-Jin An, and Hyeung-Jin Jang. "Cucurbitacin B induces hypoglycemic effect in diabetic mice by regulation of AMP-activated protein kinase alpha and glucagon-like peptide-1 via bitter taste receptor signaling." *Frontiers in Pharmacology* 9 (2018): 1071.

Kok, Bernard P., Andrea Galmozzi, Nicole K. Littlejohn, Verena Albert, Cristina Godio, Woojoo Kim, Sean M. Kim et al. "Intestinal bitter taste receptor activation alters hormone secretion and imparts metabolic benefits." *Molecular Metabolism* 16 (2018): 76–87.

Kou, Xiaohong, Jie Gao, Zhaohui Xue, Zhijun Zhang, Hua Wang, and Xu Wang. "Purification and identification of antioxidant peptides from chickpea (*Cicer arietinum* L.) albumin hydrolysates." *LWT-Food Science and Technology* 50, no. 2 (2013): 591–598.

Le Nevé, Boris, Martin Foltz, Hannelore Daniel, and Robin Gouka. "The steroid glycoside Hg-12 from Hoodia gordonii activates the human bitter receptor TAS2R14 and induces CCK release from HuTu-80 cells." *American Journal of Physiology – Gastrointestinal and Liver Physiology* 299, no. 6 (2010): G1368–G1375.

Lee, Seung-Hyeon, Hyun Min Ko, Wona Jee, Hyungsuk Kim, Won-Seok Chung, and Hyeung-Jin Jang. "Isosinensetin stimulates glucagon-like peptide-1 secretion via activation of hTAS2R50 and the Gβ γ-mediated signaling pathway." *International Journal of Molecular Sciences* 24, no. 4 (2023): 3682.

Li-Chan, Eunice CY. "Bioactive peptides and protein hydrolysates: research trends and challenges for application as nutraceuticals and functional food ingredients." *Current Opinion in Food Science* 1 (2015): 28–37.

Li, Yuchan, Jun Zhao, Hua Chen, Yanping Mao, Yuping Yang, Liang Feng, Chuanxin Mo, Lin Huang, Dabin Hou, and Ma Yu. "Transcriptome level reveals the triterpenoid saponin biosynthesis pathway of bupleurum falcatum L." *Genes* 13, no. 12 (2022): 2237.

Lu, Ping, Cheng-Hai Zhang, Lawrence M. Lifshitz, and Ronghua ZhuGe. "Extraoral bitter taste receptors in health and disease." *Journal of General Physiology* 149, no. 2 (2017): 181–197.

Madurapperumage, Amod, Leung Tang, Pushparajah Thavarajah, William Bridges, Emerson Shipe, George Vandemark, and Dil Thavarajah. "Chickpea (*Cicer arietinum* L.) as a source of essential fatty acids – a biofortification approach." *Frontiers in Plant Science* 12 (2021): 734980.

Martínez, Karla A. Acevedo, and Elvira Gonzalez de Mejia. "Comparison of five chickpea varieties, optimization of hydrolysates production and evaluation of biomarkers for type 2 diabetes." *Food Research International* 147 (2021): 110572.

Mora-Melgem, José Antonio, Jesús Gilberto Arámburo-Gálvez, Feliznando Isidro Cárdenas-Torres, Jhonatan Gonzalez-Santamaria, Giovanni Isaí Ramírez-Torres, Aldo Alejandro Arvizu-Flores, Oscar Gerardo Figueroa-Salcido, and Noé Ontiveros. "Dipeptidyl peptidase IV inhibitory peptides from chickpea proteins (*Cicer arietinum* L.): pharmacokinetics, molecular interactions, and multi-bioactivities." *Pharmaceuticals* 16, no. 8 (2023): 1109.

Newton, Ashley, and Kaustav Majumder. "Germination and simulated gastrointestinal digestion of chickpea (*Cicer arietinum* L.) in exhibiting in vitro antioxidant activity in gastrointestinal epithelial cells." *Antioxidants* 12, no. 5 (2023): 1114.

Ninomiya, Kazumi, Yusuke Yamaguchi, Fumie Shinmachi, Hitoshi Kumagai, and Hitomi Kumagai. "Suppression of postprandial blood glucose elevation by buckwheat (*Fagpopyrum esculentum*) albumin hydrolysate and identification of the peptide responsible to the function." *Food Science and Human Wellness* 11, no. 4 (2022): 992–998.

Nongonierma, Alice B., and Richard J. FitzGerald. "Strategies for the discovery and identification of food protein-derived biologically active peptides." *Trends in Food Science & Technology* 69 (2017): 289–305.

Pérez-Ramírez, Iza Fernanda, Diana E. Escobedo-Alvarez, Magdalena Mendoza-Sánchez, Nuria E. Rocha-Guzmán, Rosalía Reynoso-Camacho, Jorge A. Acosta-Gallegos, and Minerva Ramos-Gómez. "Phytochemical profile and composition of chickpea (*Cicer arietinum* L.): Varietal differences and effect of germination under elicited conditions." *Plants* 12, no. 17 (2023): 3093.

Power, Orla, A. B. Nongonierma, P. Jakeman, and R. J. FitzGerald. "Food protein hydrolysates as a source of dipeptidyl peptidase IV inhibitory peptides for the management of type 2 diabetes." *Proceedings of the Nutrition Society* 73, no. 1 (2014): 34–46.

Prior, Sarah, Stephens, Jeffrey, Davis, Jeffrey and Churm, Rachel. "Ghrelin function in human obesity and type 2 diabetes: a concise review." *Obesity Reviews* 18, no. 2 (2017): 140–148.

Quintero-Soto, María F., Jeanett Chávez-Ontiveros, José A. Garzón-Tiznado, Nancy Y. Salazar-Salas, Karen V. Pineda-Hidalgo, Francisco Delgado-Vargas, and José A. López-Valenzuela. "Characterization of peptides with antioxidant activity and antidiabetic potential obtained from chickpea (*Cicer arietinum* L.) protein hydrolyzates." *Journal of Food Science* 86, no. 7 (2021): 2962–2977.

Real Hernandez, Luis M., and Elvira Gonzalez de Mejia. "Enzymatic production, bioactivity, and bitterness of chickpea (Cicer arietinum) peptides." *Comprehensive Reviews in Food Science and Food Safety* 18, no. 6 (2019): 1913–1946.

Rivero-Pino, Fernando, F. Javier Espejo-Carpio, and Emilia M. Guadix. "Unravelling the α-glucosidase inhibitory properties of chickpea protein by enzymatic hydrolysis and in silico analysis." *Food Bioscience* 44 (2021): 101328.

Rozengurt, Enrique, and Catia Sternini. "Taste receptor signaling in the mammalian gut." *Current Opinion in Pharmacology* 7, no. 6 (2007): 557–562.

Serrano, Joan, Àngela Casanova-Martí, Inge Depoortere, Maria Teresa Blay, Ximena Terra, Montserrat Pinent, and Anna Ardévol. "Subchronic treatment with grape-seed phenolics inhibits ghrelin production despite a short-term stimulation of ghrelin secretion produced by bitter-sensing flavanols." *Molecular Nutrition & Food Research* 60, no. 12 (2016): 2554–2564.

Sofi, Sajad Ahmad, Jagmohan Singh, Shabir Ahmad Mir, and B. N. Dar. "In vitro starch digestibility, cooking quality, rheology and sensory properties of gluten-free pregelatinized rice noodle enriched with germinated chickpea flour." *LWT* 133 (2020): 110090.

Udagawa, Haruhide, Masaki Hiramoto, Miho Kawaguchi, Takashi Uebanso, Mica Ohara-Imaizumi, Takao Nammo, Wataru Nishimura, and Kazuki Yasuda. "Characterization of the taste receptor-related G-protein, α -gustducin, in pancreatic β -cells." *Journal of Diabetes Investigation* 11, no. 4 (2020): 814–822.

Vennekens, Rudi, Margot Mesuere, and Koenraad Philippaert. "TRPM5 in the battle against diabetes and obesity." *Acta Physiologica* 222, no. 2 (2018): e12949.

Wang, Junyu, Yonghui Li, Ang Li, Rui Hai Liu, Xin Gao, Dan Li, Xiaohong Kou, and Zhaohui Xue. "Nutritional constituent and health benefits of chickpea (*Cicer arietinum* L.): a review." *Food Research International* 150 (2021): 110790.

Wang, Qiaoling, Kathrin I. Liszt, and Inge Depoortere. "Extra-oral bitter taste receptors: new targets against obesity?" *Peptides* 127 (2020): 170284.

Xu, Qingbiao, Nisha Singh, Hui Hong, Xianghua Yan, Wenlin Yu, Xu Jiang, Prashen Chelikani, and Jianping Wu. "Hen protein-derived peptides as the blockers of human bitter taste receptors T2R4, T2R7 and T2R14." *Food Chemistry* 283 (2019): 621–627.

Yang, Moon Young, Amirhossein Mafi, Soo-Kyung Kim, William A. Goddard, and Brian Guthrie. "Predicted structure of fully activated human bitter taste receptor TAS2R4 complexed with G protein and agonists." *QRB Discovery* 2 (2021): e3.

Ying, Xin, Dominic Agyei, Chibuike Udenigwe, Benu Adhikari, and Bo Wang. "Manufacturing of plant-based bioactive peptides using enzymatic methods to meet health and sustainability targets of the sustainable development goals." *Frontiers in Sustainable Food Systems* 5 (2021): 769028.

Yu, Yunli, Gang Hao, Quanying Zhang, Wenyan Hua, Meng Wang, Wenjia Zhou, Shunlin Zong, Ming Huang, and Xiaozhou Wen. "Berberine induces GLP-1 secretion through activation of bitter taste receptor pathways." *Biochemical Pharmacology* 97, no. 2 (2015): 173–177.

Zan, Rong, Qiming Wu, Yiling Chen, Gangcheng Wu, Hui Zhang, and Ling Zhu. "Identification of novel dipeptidyl peptidase-IV inhibitory peptides in chickpea protein hydrolysates." *Journal of Agricultural and Food Chemistry* 71, no. 21 (2023): 8211–8219.

Zhang, Chunlei, Adeola M. Alashi, Nisha Singh, Prashen Chelikani, and Rotimi E. Aluko. "Glycated beef protein hydrolysates as sources of bitter taste modifiers." *Nutrients* 11, no. 9 (2019): 2166.

31 Gluten and Gluten-Free Diets

Hayrullah Yazar and Yıldırım Kayacan

ABBREVIATIONS

AB	Abdominal bloating
ABH	Alternating bowel habits
AP	Abdominal pain
CD	Celiac disease
CMA	Cow's milk allergy
CU	Contact urticaria
DH	Dermatitis herpetiformis
DM	Diabetes mellitus
EU	European Union
FA	Food allergy
FAO	Food and Agriculture Organization
GA	Gluten ataxia
GD	Gastrointestinal discomfort
GF	Gluten-free
GFD	Gluten-free diet
GIS	Gastrointestinal system
GRD	Gluten-related disorders
GMO	Genetically modified organisms
HDL	High-density lipoproteins
HLA	Human leukocyte antigens
HPLC	High-performance liquid chromatography
IBS	Irritable bowel syndrome
IL-17	Interleukin-17
MetS	Metabolic syndrome
mRNA	Messenger ribonucleic acid
NCGS	Non-celiac gluten sensitivity
NCWS	Non-celiac wheat sensitivity
NGMO	Non-genetically modified organisms
RA	Respiratory allergy
WD	Western diet
WDEIA	Wheat-dependent induced anaphylaxis
WHO	World Health Organization

INTRODUCTION

Throughout history, gluten-containing products have been a primary source of human nutrition and are still widely consumed today. Wheat and its products are particularly popular worldwide, leading to extensive research on gluten. However, studies have shown that gluten is associated with gastro-intestinal (GI)-based diseases and many other diseases (Vaquero et al. 2015). The first things that

DOI: 10.1201/9781003597926-31

come to mind are celiac disease, non-celiac gluten sensitivity (NCGS) and wheat allergy (Aljada et al. 2021).

Gastrointestinal system symptoms caused by gluten are non-specific (bloating, abdominal discomfort, diarrhoea). As can be seen, the symptoms of NCGS are similar to other gluten-related diseases, irritable bowel syndrome and Crohn's disease. Of course, this similarity, as expected, has made it very difficult for physicians to make a correct diagnosis. As a matter of fact, in a review, a total of 67 clinical studies published between 1989 and 2019 were scanned and data that could help physicians were summarised in this respect (Roszkowska et al. 2019). However, all these data aside, the dough quality of wheat flour, which has a high gluten content, continued to be preferred, especially by those who make commercial pastries (Li et al. 2023). Additionally, Gong et al. (2023) revealed that the amount of gluten in wheat flour is essential factor improving water retention capacity and dough quality. On the other hand, gluten, which commercial wheat flour dough manufacturers cannot abandon, poses a severe risk with its adverse effects on the GIS (Croall et al. 2021; Wu et al. 2021).

The most effective treatment for gluten-related health problems is undoubtedly a gluten-free or low-gluten diet. In this context, traditional non-genetically modified organisms (NGMO) wheat flours introduced to the market have become popular recently, especially since they contain less Gluten (Nye-Wood et al. 2021). However, the fact that gluten-free or low-gluten products have lower nutritional quality and are more expensive also reveals that these foods need to be developed.

Another issue that should be emphasised is the relationship between gluten and obesity. As it is known, obesity is considered a significant health problem all over the world (Caballero 2019). Consuming gluten-rich foods leads to obesity, severe systemic diseases and various risk factors. These include metabolic syndrome (MetS), diabetes mellitus (DM), asthma, unhealthy pregnancy, etc. Additionally, obesity is a risk factor for increased mortality from COVID-19 (Catalano and Shankar 2017; Piché et al. 2020; Peters et al. 2018; Soeroto et al. 2020). As can be seen, although foods containing gluten are of higher quality (protein), they threaten a healthy life in terms of the problems they cause.

SOME BASIC FACTS ABOUT GLUTEN

Main Source of Gluten: Wheat

Along with corn and rice, wheat is one of the world's three strategically valuable products. Wheat grows at every geographical altitude, albeit with different productivity, which is one factor that makes it widespread (Shewry 2002). As a result of its high consumption and general use, the need for wheat increased and ultimately paved the way for the emergence of commercial varieties. Of course, the structure and function of gluten in wheat, which continues to be a strategic global food source, is also worth examining. In a study, intact functional gluten polymers were biochemically examined down to their monomeric subunits (Bacala et al. 2022). According to them, the number of gluten polymers and the ratios between gluten proteins are essential because the timing of events occurring within the cell will determine the strength and effectiveness of gluten. As a result of the research, it was stated that gluten protein structures can be examined as a whole with proteomic technologies.

On the other hand, traditional wheat varieties' natural and organic properties and gluten content raised the question of whether they could be an alternative to commercial wheat. Based on this, many new researchers have become interested in the subject. In a study, "High-Performance Liquid Chromatography" (HPLC) analyses of five different wheat varieties, which are the raw materials of bread wheat dough, were performed (Takač et al. 2021). An examination of wheat grown with organic and traditional methods in Hungary and Serbia showed exceptionally high molecular weight glutenin subunits in spelt wheat bread (Takač et al. 2021). Concerns about a severe increase in gluten-related health problems have recently reduced wheat consumption. In a study investigating the predisposing effect of genetic manipulation of wheat on intestinal inflammation, the impact of the modern Gallagher variety and two heirloom varieties (Turkey and Kharkof) on intestinal inflammation was compared. The study was performed in C57BL/6 mice under Western diet (WD) conditions. The study found that heirloom wheat moderately reduced interleukin-17 (IL-17) in the context of WD, while the modern variety improved the villus structure. In addition, mRNA and tight junction proteins and serum lipopolysaccharide-binding proteins were observed to be unchanged. As a result, the study concluded that the modern wheat variety did not contribute to intestinal inflammation compared to heirloom wheat (Keirns et al. 2019).

Gluten

Gluten is an essential component that gives dough its structure and strength. Commercially, dough with high gluten content is preferred because it is more durable and flexible. Gluten makes the dough strong, flexible and durable (Shewry et al. 2002). Due to this feature, flour and bakery products with high gluten content are becoming increasingly important in restaurants and other food service establishments.

Gluten has a structure in which all protein molecules consist of large amounts of small molecules and are connected by S-S (disulfide) bonds. This structure makes gluten the most essential main component of flour. While gluten is effective in solubility in slightly aqueous conditions, it is effective in bread making with dried fractions. (Schofield 1986). It has also been determined that the gluten structure has more than one DQ2 haplotype. The HLA-DQ2 haplotype, which has two genes, called DQ2.5, was selected in studies associated with celiac patients (up to 95%) (Balakireva and Zamyatnin 2016).

As shown in Figure 31.1, gluten has a very complex structure. Gluten contains mainly glutenin and gliadin and consists of starch, other proteins, lipids and sugars (Lockhart et al. 1993). Gliadin, one of the main components of this complex, is found only in grain seeds and has a heterogeneous structure containing peptide chains that resemble each other and have the chemical characteristics of simple proteins (Pyler 1988). The main protein that affects the viscosity and elasticity increase that the gluten structure adds to bread dough is gliadin, which has a lower molecular weight than gluten (Tapucu 1996).

Gluten is a mixture of many proteins, including gliadin and glutenin (Biesiekierski 2017; Lavoignat et al. 2022). Gluten, the viscoelasticity (elasticity and extensibility) of wheat dough, is primarily used in bread making, pasta, cakes, biscuits, etc. Gluten serves as the primary raw material in many bakery products. Many food producers choose elastic and firm dough flour with a high gluten content because it stretches more. The most important structural protein complex that gives dough this feature is gluten, and research has been carried out on it for hundreds of years (Schofield

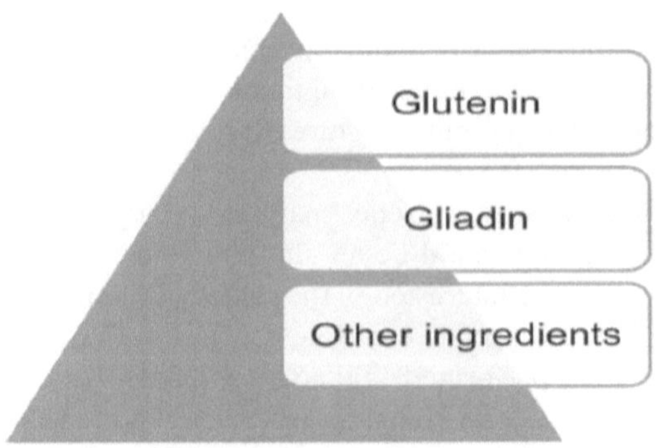

FIGURE 31.1 Structure of gluten (Adapted from Mosleth and Uhlen 1991; Lookhart et al. 1993).

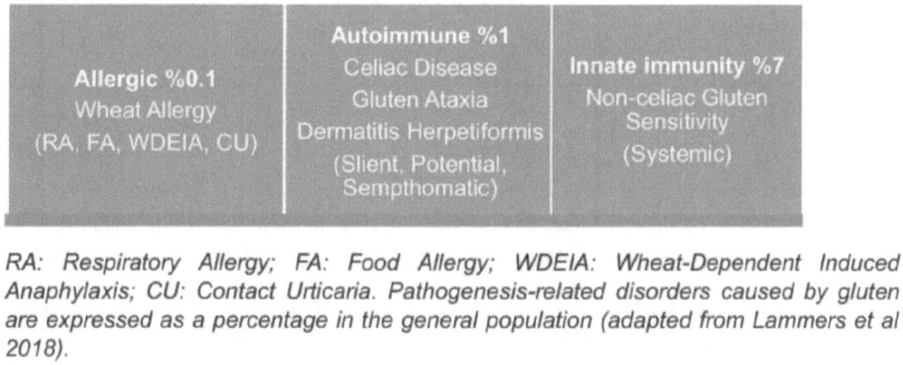

FIGURE 31.2 Pathogenetic disorders affected by gluten. Pathogenesis-related disorders caused by gluten are expressed as a percentage in the general population (Adapted from Lammers et al. 2018).

1994; Shewry et al. 1995). On the other hand, studies on producing quality gluten-free bread are ongoing (Vacca 2023).

Pathogenetic Disorders Affected by Gluten

When humans consume foods (wheat, barley, oats) and products (flour and bakery products) containing gluten, complete breakdown does not occur. Subsequently, many diseases that arise due to gluten intake reveal a complex situation that is triggered by the immune system and includes an immune response. The most researched of these is celiac disease, with a prevalence of 1%. However, non-celiac gluten sensitivity, which has recently accounted for 7%, also stands out (Lammers et al. 2018). Moreover, pathological conditions less associated with gluten, such as wheat allergy, gluten ataxia (GA) and dermatitis herpetiformis (DH), are also significant, as shown in Figure 31.2.

Gluten and Celiac Disease

The pathological condition that occurs with the deterioration of the immune response in the GI mucosa in individuals with a genetic predisposition as a result of oral ingestion of gliadin, one of the essential parts of gluten, is called celiac disease (CD) (Sánchez et al. 2021). Table 31.1 presented in Balakireva and Zamyatnin's 2016 study compares the baseline characteristics of CD, allergy, and non-celiac gluten sensitivity (NCGS).

Furthermore, CD is well-understood in terms of immunopathogenesis, and its association with human leukocyte antigens (HLA) is depicted in Figure 31.3. The resulting pathological condition is associated with hypersensitivity to the gluten protein contained in grains and subsequent localised intestinal lesion formation. However, the definitive diagnosis is made by detecting antibodies against transglutaminase 2 in the blood (Rosinach et al. 2016). At this point, information has been obtained on how HLA-DQ molecules, which create the appropriate environment for celiac disease, are linked to the formation of post-translationally modified gluten peptides and autoantibodies (Iversen and Sollid 2023). Additionally, the pathogenetic mechanisms of CD and its effects on the microbiota have recently been examined. Studies have focused on the impact of antigens formed against consumed foods by microbes and their components.

Some Symptoms: Gluten-Related Diseases, Crohn's Disease, and IBS

Gluten-related diseases may be similar to IBS and NCGS in their symptoms. Undoubtedly, these similarities make the job of clinicians complex in terms of differential diagnosis. This is why some cases have not received the correct treatment for years (Roszkowska et al. 2019). Gluten-related

TABLE 31.1
The Main Characteristics of Gluten Intolerance

Characteristic	Celiac Disease	Allergy	Non-Celiac Gluten Sensitivity
Laboratory Biomarkers	[1]Genetic	Atopy (100%)	[2]Probably, genetic.
Underlying Causes	[3]Antibodies	[4]Specific IgE	[5]IgG antibodies
Histopathological Intestine Symptoms	[6]Atrophy of villi	[7]Mucosal damage	[8]Mucosal damage

[1]*Genetic:* HLA-DQ2 or/and–DQ8 haplotype. [2]Probably genetic: DQ2 and/or DQ8 (up to 50% of patients). [3]IgA (IgG) anti-tTG, IgA(IgG) anti-endomysium (anti-EMA), anti-deamidated gliadin peptides antibodies.[4]Specific IgE for wheat, specific IgE for ω-5 gliadin, specific IgE for non-specific lipid transfer proteins.[5]IgG antigliadin antibodies (only in some patients).Atrophy of villi, crypt hyperplasia, increased infiltration by intraepithelial lymphocytes.[7]Any mucosal damage or increased infiltration by intraepithelial lymphocytes or atrophy of villi and crypt hyperplasia. [8]Any mucosal damage or increased infiltration by intraepithelial lymphocytes.

Comparison of essential features for Celiac Disease (CD), Allergy and Non-Celiac Gluten Sensitivity (NCGS) (Balakireva and Zamyatnin 2016).

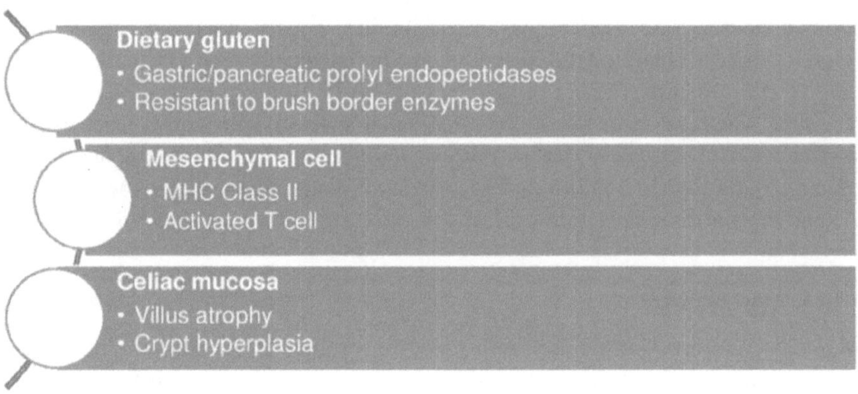

FIGURE 31.3 Diagram of celiac disease involving the possible interaction between intestinal protein processing and the specific immune system. When gluten is ingested in the diet, it is processed by intraluminal digestive enzymes, including prolyl endopeptidases (Adapted from Burtis et al. 2006, Chapter 48, Figure 48.6).

diseases may have common symptoms, as shown in Figure 31.4. Although celiac disease is a chronic disease with a genetic predisposition, patients may present to outpatient clinics with symptoms of diarrhoea and developmental delay, which are seen in many GI disorders (Posner and Haseeb 2024).

Gluten and Obesity

Is there a relationship between gluten and obesity? Before answering this question, let's briefly draw attention to the danger of obesity because obesity has become one of the alarming and rapidly growing epidemics in all age groups today (Bluher 2019; Doreswamy et al. 2020). Additionally, diet and nutrition play an essential role in everyone's life because proper nutrition helps build a healthy body and a strong mind. However, obesity leads to the opposite effects, that is, to an unhealthy life. At this point, we should point out that studies investigating the relationship between gluten, nutrition and obesity are remarkable. One was done by considering the body mass index of patients diagnosed

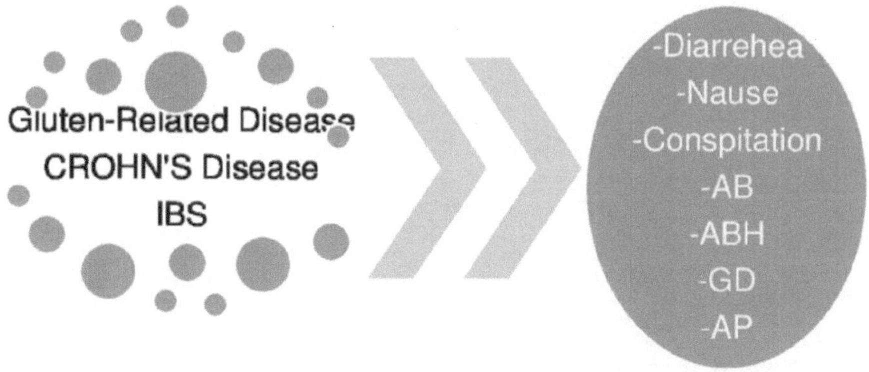

FIGURE 31.4 Overlapping symptoms in gluten-related diseases, Crohn's disease, and IBS.

with celiac disease. The diagnosis of 1,018 patients participating in the study was confirmed by biopsy, and a specialist dietitian prepared gluten-free diets. A gluten-free diet lasted an average of 39.5 months, and BMI values were measured. Additionally, the findings were compared with regional data. As a result, the probability of being obese was significantly lower in the celiac cohort in this study (Kabbani et al. 2012).

The relationship between gluten and obesity has attracted the attention of researchers, leading to numerous scientific studies being conducted on the topic. The EU-funded Stance4Health project has this feature. The study investigating the pathogenesis of metabolic diseases, gluten-related diseases and obesity was also evaluated (Dello Russo et al. 2022). In another study, the relationship between gluten and obesity was assessed through leptin-insulin resistance and beta cell volume (Haupt-Jorgensen et al. 2018). On the other hand, as stated in Figure 31.5, although non-GMO wheat products are considered a healthier diet, the low amount of gluten (67%) in their content produces a low amount of protein (Nye-Wood et al. 2021). The opposite situation exists in GMO products, especially regarding the increase in protein content. In other words, although commercial GMO wheat is a quality food, it is an important triggering factor for gastrointestinal diseases.

Gluten and Diabetes Mellitus

Glutenin peptides enter the pancreas and can trigger stress in beta cells and increase insulin secretion. As a result, gluten may be an essential determinant in type 1 and type 2 diabetes. The fact that components of grain products containing gluten affect the microbiota and increase intestinal permeability is one reason for this situation. Studies have shown that the GF diet during pregnancy reduces the risk of T1DM in humans and animals. Although current information indicates that gluten may be an etiopathogenic factor for developing T1D and T2D, confirmation of this information requires further human studies (Haupt-Jorgensen et al. 2018).

SOME BASIC FACTS ABOUT GLUTEN-FREE DIETS

Gluten-Free Diet

Complete removal of gluten from diets used for nutritional purposes is called a gluten-free diet (GFD). So, can consumers identify flour and products containing gluten? The answer to this question was the subject of a study. Volunteers with gastrointestinal symptoms without celiac disease used a GFD in a prospective, randomised, double-blind, placebo-controlled study. In the survey, the participants evaluated gluten-containing and gluten-free flour for 6 months, and their scores were determined. As a result, only 34% of individuals correctly identified flour containing gluten (Zanini

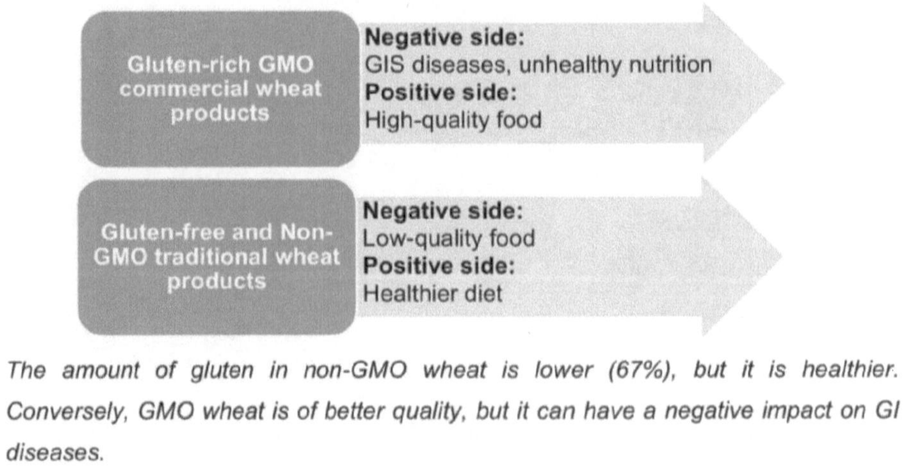

FIGURE 31.5 Nutrition with wheat products rich and poor in gluten: Evaluation of gluten amounts in GMO and non-GMO wheat products and their relation to gastrointestinal diseases (Nye-Wood et al. 2021).

et al. 2015). Although this rate shows a severe increase in awareness, it also reflects the need for consumers to be completely selective about gluten.

Although gluten proteins are one of the main determinants of wheat used in bread making, they are also associated with various digestive disorders. Based on this, studies on developing immunological gluten-free wheat lines using RNAi and genetic technologies continue rapidly. This issue was discussed in a review (García-Molina et al. 2019). Their results showed that wheat with shallow gluten content had a reduced capacity to stimulate T cells in celiac patients. Again, their study stated that consumption of bread made with wheat flour containing low gliadin caused positive changes in the intestinal microbiota in patients with non-celiac wheat sensitivity (NCWS) (García-Molina et al. 2019).

Gluten triggers immune reactions that cause GI malabsorption and enteropathic symptoms in CD; this is a known mechanism. However, the mechanisms leading to clinical manifestations in NCGWS are unknown. Therefore, for GRD applications, it is recommended to use it with caution in cases other than CD due to the risks of nutritional deficiencies. According to recommendations, long-term management of nutrition for those who qualify as GRD should involve a multidisciplinary team, including a doctor and dietitian for monitoring (Abdi et al. 2023). Additionally, the pathogenetic mechanisms of CD and increases in immunity to foods are also examined in terms of microbes and their components. The effectiveness of microbiota in CD and NCGS patients was determined, as indicated in Table 31.2.

Gluten-Free Diet and Celiac

When the GFD comes to the agenda, the first disease that comes to mind will undoubtedly be celiac. The GFD is still considered the most effective and safest treatment method for celiac patients (Bascuñán et al. 2017). A gluten-free oligoantigenic diet reduces proteinuria, especially in patients with conditions such as celiac disease and nephrotic syndrome (Uy et al. 2015). It is also stated that a GFD will balance the intestinal microbiota and even reduce IL-10 cytokine production caused by bacteria (Uy et al. 2015).

In a study, 80 children were examined in two groups between the ages of 7 and 18 in the gastroenterology, hepatology and child nutrition services. The celiac and control groups consisted of 40 children each. The celiac group was placed on a strict GFD for two years. According to their results, a GFD may be sufficient to reduce oxidative stress in celiac patients (Diaz-Castro et al. 2020). So, is

TABLE 31.2
Evaluation of Some Research on the Gluten-Free Diet

Study	Methods	Findings	Study Group
Defeudis et al. 2023	Examined GFD and glycometabolic parameters	Effects of GFD on MetS are unclear; only improvement in HDL observed.	Individuals with dysmetabolic disorders
García-Molina et al. 2019	Studied GFW type E82, conducted linical review	Positive changes in intestinal microbiota	Individuals with celiac disease and NCWS
Elli et al. 2016	Conducted a two-stage study lasting 21 days	50% of patients with NCGS responded to GFD	Individuals with gastroenterology symptoms
Rosinach et al. 2016	Examined transglutaminase	Clinical relapse on a gluten diet was 91%	Individuals in clinical remission after GFD
Zanini et al. 2015	Focused on identifying gluten-containing flour	Accuracy in identifying gluten content: 34%	Individuals on GFD by own initiative

GFD: gluten-free diet; GFW: gluten-free wheat; NCGS: non-celiac gluten sensitivity; MetS: metabolic syndrome; HDL: high-density lipoprotein.

healthy and proper nutrition important only for those with food sensitivities? Of course not, because unhealthy nutrition is a common problem. A detailed examination of the nutritional components of individuals with NCGS can be given as an example because research on this subject emphasises the need to analyse nutritional diets (Zingone et al. 2017). In another study that will contribute to the results obtained from this study, a relationship was found between GFD and anti-inflammatory activity at the cellular level. Namely, The immunological effect and safety of the gluten-free and dairy-free (GF/DF) diet were investigated prospectively in children diagnosed with steroid-resistant nephrotic syndrome (SRNS). The study applied a strict GF/DF diet, and blood, urine and stool samples were collected for four weeks. The results showed that the GF/DF diet had a significant anti-inflammatory effect at all participants' protein and cellular levels (Pérez-Sáez et al. 2021).

Gluten triggers immune reactions that cause GI malabsorption and enteropathic symptoms in CD; this is a known mechanism. The intestinal microbiota is positively affected by GFD. Maybe that's why healthy individuals have recently shown an increase in the preference for GFDs by healthy individuals recently. However, when making these choices, nutritional counselling control is recommended. As it is known, GFD is the primary option in the treatment of patients with celiac disease, wheat allergy and non-celiac gluten (Campaniello et al. 2022).

Gluten-Free Diet and Metabolic Syndrome

The effect of gluten on the inflammatory response to MetS components is also among the researched topics. Especially in recent years, the impact of a GFD on hypometabolic markers and its relationship with diabetes has been investigated. In addition, these studies have also shown that a GFD causes improvement in HDL levels that are impaired in MetS (Defeudis et al. 2023).

A gluten-free oligoantigenic diet reduces proteinuria, especially in patients with celiac disease and nephrotic syndrome (Uy et al. 2015). It is also stated that a GFD will balance the intestinal microbiota and even reduce IL-10 cytokine production caused by bacteria (Uy et al. 2015). In another study that will contribute to the results obtained from this study, a relationship was found between GFD and anti-inflammatory activity at the cellular level. Namely, The immunological effect and safety of the gluten-free and dairy-free (GF/DF) diet were investigated prospectively in children diagnosed with SRNS. The study applied a strict GF/DF diet, and blood, urine and stool samples were collected for four weeks. The results showed that the GF/DF diet had a significant anti-inflammatory effect at all participants' protein and cellular levels (Pérez-Sáez et al. 2021).

GIS disorders, especially in individuals with genetic gluten sensitivity, effectively reveal the symptoms of many systemic autoimmune disorders, particularly celiac disease. In such cases, nutritional diets need to be replaced with low- or gluten-free products to eliminate or alleviate symptoms. A gluten-free diet is the most effective treatment. On the other hand, the low-protein, low-salt and high-fat nature of GF processed foods is a matter of debate. In this respect, GFDs need further development and serious content regulation (Melini and Melini 2019). If additionally stated, When applying the GFD, attention should be paid to vitamin and mineral deficiencies because the primary purpose of the diet should be not only gluten-free but also healthy (Bascuñán et al. 2017). In this regard, it is essential to provide training on correct diet practices by trained nutritionists.

ALLERGENIC EFFECTS OF PROTEINS OTHER THAN GLUTEN

Proteins in the food you consume usually cause food allergies. However, this only applies to certain types of food. For an allergic reaction to occur, the body must produce IgE in response to the food, which can result in complex medical problems arising from the allergenic protein (Bannon 2004). The effects of proteins other than gluten, on human life can be examined under three headings. it is important to note that even though proteins of animal origin are not the main topic of this section, they should not be disregarded.

Vegetable-Derived Proteins

Legumes, such as peanuts and soy, contain allergenic structures and can cause allergic reactions. Peanut allergy, in particular, tends to increase in both adults and children worldwide and can result in life-threatening anaphylaxis reactions (Połomska et al. 2023). Nuts and seeds obtained from trees may also contain allergenic plant proteins. Grains like wheat and similar grains contain prolamin proteins that can cause clinical problems like anaphylaxis and atopic dermatitis (Mills and Breiteneder 2005). Fresh fruits and vegetables are another frequently consumed food group but can also cause allergies. Tree and grass pollens are associated with fruit allergy, while vegetables such as celery are also known to cause allergies. Allergic reactions to peach and kiwi fruit have also increased recently (Kallen et al. 2023; Bringheli et al. 2023).

Allergenic Effects of Industrial Proteins

Today, products are available for consumers to use for food or cosmetics. It's worth noting that contact dermatitis, which can occur due to contact with many industrial products, including cosmetics, has an allergic basis. Although contact dermatitis (CD) is often an occupational disease among healthcare workers, hairdressers and other workers, it's essential to be cautious about potential allergens (Karagounis and Cohen 2023). On the other hand, it's also evident that awareness is increasing among consumers in the European Union, the USA and other countries. As a result of this awareness, companies selling prepackaged industrial products and cosmetics containing allergenic foods have had to comply with regulations set forth by the FAO or WHO and indicate the allergenic product on their labels (Mills and Breiteneder 2005). This step was crucial for the consumers' self-control system.

Proteins of Animal Origin

Proteins from animal sources can be found in foods of animal origin; some may have allergenic properties. For example, cow's milk is a widely consumed food that can cause cow's milk allergy (CMA) (Vandenplas et al. 2023). It was demonstrated years ago that whey and casein are allergenic

(Mills and Breiteneder 2005). Another source of allergenic protein is fish (Añibarro et al. 2023). Eggs are another frequently consumed animal protein with allergenic effects, and egg allergy is the second most common food allergy in children (Leau et al. 2023). Finally, shellfish contains the heat-stable muscle protein tropomyosin, which can cause allergic reactions (Mills and Breiteneder 2005).

Mini Dictionary of Terms

- **Celiac disease:** An autoimmune, systemic, chronic disease that causes permanent intolerance in individuals with genetic sensitivity to gluten proteins.
- **Contact dermatitis:** A type of skin inflammation caused by direct or indirect contact with a substance, followed by itching, rashes and blisters.
- **Diabetes mellitus:** A metabolic and systemic disease whose incidence increases with unhealthy lifestyle and unhealthy nutrition, it affects all humanity and has reached epidemic levels. There is also a genetic predisposition, especially to Type 2 diabetes.
- **Food allergies:** A chain reaction where sensitive individuals produce IgE against certain foods, leading to clinical reactions.
- **Gluten:** Gluten, which has a very complex structure, mainly contains glutenin and gliadin and consists of starch, other proteins, lipids and sugars.
- **Gluten-free diet (GFD):** The complete removal of gluten from diets used for nutrition. GFD is generally accepted as the most effective treatment method for celiac patients and is also considered the safest diet.
- **HLA-DQ antibodies:** The most common antibodies associated with gluten enteropathies.
- **Metabolic syndrome (MetS):** A prevalent condition, the incidence of which has increased in recent years. MetS involves at least three of five risk factors. These include obesity (central), increased fasting glucose, high blood pressure and lipid profile disorder.
- **Non-celiac gluten sensitivity:** A condition in which various physiopathological conditions, especially GI disorders, are observed when foods containing gluten are consumed. Moreover, these people do not have celiac disease or wheat allergy.
- **Obesity:** Excessive fat accumulation in the body that impairs health.

SUMMARY POINTS

- This chapter explores gluten's source, structure, related diseases and connection to obesity and metabolic syndrome.
- The chapter also mentions other diseases indirectly linked to gastrointestinal symptoms, particularly celiac disease, which is directly related to gluten.
- The text provides information about the gluten-free diet, emphasising that, for now, it remains the only option for people with celiac disease. It also highlights the insufficient protein content of gluten-free diets and recommends multidisciplinary implementation under the supervision of a dietitian.
- This chapter also describes the allergenic properties of gluten-free foods. Although many allergenic yet gluten-free animal and plant foods are still consumed today, attention is drawn to them here.
- In addition, attention is drawn to food or cosmetic products that are industrially produced and offered to consumers.

REFERENCES

Abdi, F., Zuberi, S., Blom, J.J., Armstrong, D., Pinto-Sanchez M.I. 2023. Nutritional considerations in celiac disease and non-celiac gluten/wheat sensitivity. *Nutrients* 15(6):1475.

Aljada, B., Zohni, A., El-Matary, W. 2021. The gluten-free diet for celiac disease and beyond. *Nutrients* 13;11:3993:1–56.

Añibarro, B., Feijoo, L., de Las Cuevas, N., Seoane, F.J.2023. Occupational asthma induced by fish exposure. *Occup Med (Lond)* 30;73(9):581–3.

Bacala, R., Hatcher, D.W., Perreault, H., Fu, B.X. 2022. Challenges and opportunities for proteomics and the improvement of bread wheat quality. *J Plant Physiol* 275;153743:1–16.

Balakireva, A.V., Zamyatnin, A.A. 2016. Properties of gluten intolerance: gluten structure, evolution, pathogenicity and detoxification capabilities. *Nutrients* 18;8(10):644.

Bannon, G.A. 2004. What makes a food protein an allergen? *Curr Allergy Asthma Rep* 4(1):43–6.

Bascuñán, K.A., Vespa, M.C., Araya, M. 2017. Celiac disease: understanding the gluten-free diet. *Eur J Nutr* 56;2:449–59.

Biesiekierski, J.R. 2017. What is gluten? *J Gastroenterol Hepatol* 32;1:78–81.

Blüher, M. 2019. Obesity: global epidemiology and pathogenesis. *Nat Rev Endocrinol* 15;5:288–98.

Bringheli, I., Brindisi, G., Morelli, R., Marchetti, L., Cela, L., Gravina, A., Pastore, F., Semeraro, A., Cinicola, B., Capponi, M., Gori, A., Pignataro, E., Piccioni, M.G., Zicari, A.M, Anania, C. 2023. Kiwifruit's allergy in children: what do we know? *Nutrients* 15(13):3030.

Burtis, C.A., Ashwood, E.R., Bruns, D.E 2006. *Tietz Textbook of Clinical Chemistry and Molecular Diagnostics, Chapter 48*, 1860–1861. 4th edition, Section VI. Elsevier Saunders Press.

Caballero, B. 2019. Humans against obesity: who will win? *Adv Nutr* 1;10:54–9.

Campaniello, D., Corbo, M.R., Sinigaglia, M., Speranza, B., Racioppo, A., Altieri, C., Bevilacqua, A. 2022. How diet and physical activity modulate gut microbiota: evidence, and perspectives. *Nutrients* 14;14(12):2456.

Catalano, P.M., Shankar, K. 2017. Obesity and pregnancy: mechanisms of short term and long term adverse consequences for mother and child. *BMJ* 8;356:1:1–44.

Croall, I.D., Hoggard, N., Hadjivassiliou, M. 2021. Gluten and autism spectrum disorder. *Nutrients* 13;2:572:1–19.

Defeudis, G., Massari, M.C., Terrana, G., Coppola, L., Napoli, N., Migliaccio, S. 2023. Gluten-free diet and metabolic syndrome: could be a not benevolent encounter? *Nutrients* 15(3):627.

Dello Russo, M., Russo, P., Rufián-Henares, JÁ., Hinojosa-Nogueira, D., Pérez-Burillo, S., de la Cueva, S.P., Rohn, S., Fatouros, A., Douros, K., González-Vigil, V., Epstein, D., Francino, M.P., Siani, A., Lauria, F. 2022. The Stance4Health project: evaluating a smart personalised nutrition service for gut microbiota modulation in normal- and overweight adults and children with obesity, gluten-related disorders or allergy/intolerance to cow's milk. *Foods* 11(10):1480.

Diaz-Castro, J., Muriel-Neyra, C., Martin-Masot, R., Moreno-Fernandez, J., Maldonado, J., Nestares, T. 2020. Oxidative stress, DNA stability and evoked inflammatory signaling in young celiac patients consuming a gluten-free diet. *Eur J Nutr* 59;4:1577–84.

Doreswamy, S., Bashir, A., Guarecuco, J.E., Lahori, S., Baig A., Narra, LR., Patel, P., Heindl, S.E. 2020. Effects of diet, nutrition, and exercise in children with autism and autism spectrum disorder: a literature review. *Cureus* 22;12(12):e12222.

Elli, L., Branchi, F., Tomba, C., Villalta, D., Norsa, L., Ferretti, F., Roncoroni, L., Bardella, M.T. 2015. Diagnosis of gluten related disorders: celiac disease, wheat allergy and non-celiac gluten sensitivity. *World J Gastroenterol* 21;21(23):7110–9.

García-Molina, M.D., Giménez, M.J., Sánchez-León, S., Barro, F. 2019. Gluten free wheat: are we there? *Nutrients* 26;11:487:1–13.

Gong, W., Wang, X., Wang, F., Wang, J. 2023. Correlation analysis between wheat flour solvent retention capacity and gluten aggregation characteristics. *Foods* 12;9:1879:1–11.

Haupt-Jorgensen, M., Holm, L.J., Josefsen, K., Buschard, K. 2018. Possible prevention of diabetes with a gluten-free diet. *Nutrients* 10(11):1746.

Iversen, R., Sollid, LM. 2023. The immunobiology and pathogenesis of celiac disease. *Annu Rev Pathol* 18:47–70.

Kabbani TA., Goldberg, A., Kelly, C.P., Pallav, K., Tariq, S., Peer, A., Hansen, J., Dennis, M., Leffler, D.A. 2012. Body mass index and the risk of obesity in coeliac disease treated with the gluten-free diet. *Aliment Pharmacol Ther* 35(6):723–9.

Kallen, E.J.J., Revers, A., Fernández-Rivas, M., Asero, R., Ballmer-Weber, B., Barreales, L., Belohlavkova, S., de Blay, F., Clausen, M., Dubakiene, R., Ebisawa, M., Fernández-Perez, C., Fritsche, P., Fukutomi, Y., Gislason, D., Hoffmann-Sommergruber, K., Jedrzejczak-Czechowicz, M., Knulst, A.C., Kowalski, M.L., Kralimarkova, T., Lidholm, J., Metzler, C., Mills, E.N.C., Papadopoulos, N.G., Popov, T.A., Purohit, A., Reig, I., Seneviratne, S.L., Sinaniotis, A., Takei, M., Versteeg, S.A., Vassilopoulou, A.E., Vieths, S., Welsing, P.M.J., Zwinderman, A.H., Le, T.M., Van, Ree R. 2023. A European-Japanese study on peach allergy: IgE to Pru p 7 associates with severity. *Allergy* 78(9):2497–509.

Karagounis, T.K, Cohen, D.E. 2023. Occupational hand dermatitis. *Curr Allergy Asthma Rep* 23(4):201–12.

Keirns, B.H., Anderson, K.L., Ojo, B.A., Washburn, K.F., El-Rassi, G.D., Lightfoot, S.A., Carver, B.F., Lucas, E.A., Smith, B.J. 2019. A comparative study of modern and heirloom wheat on indicators of gastrointestinal health. *J Agric Food Chem* 26;67:14027–37.

Lavoignat, M., Bancel, E., Rimbert, H., Bagnon, S., Benigna, M., Chassin, A., Berges, S., Faye, A., Heumez, E., Perrochon, S., Rhazi, L., Valluis, B., Souply, F., Leroux, M.C., Giraudeau, P., Ravel, C. 2022. Bread wheat (T. aestivum) variability: Phenotypic and genotypic data from 75 varieties. *Data Brief* 46:108807:1–8.

Lammers KM, Herrera MG, Dodero VI. 2018. Translational chemistry meets gluten-related disorders. *ChemistryOpen* 27;7(3):217–32.

Leau, A., Denery-Papini, S., Bodinier, M., Dijk, W. 2023. Tolerance to heated egg in egg allergy: explanations and implications for prevention and treatment. *Clin Transl Allergy* 13(12):e12312.

Li, L., Liu, Z., Li, X., Chu, X., Yang, W., Wang, B., Xie, Y., Li, X. 2023. Superior gluten structure and more small starch granules synergistically confer dough quality for high amylose wheat varieties. *Front Nutr* 10:1195505:1–10.

Lookhart, G.L., Martin, M.L., Mosleth, E., Uhlen, A.K., Hoseney, R.C. 1993. Comparison of highmolecular-weight subunits of glutenin and baking performance of flours varying in bread-making quality. *Lebensm. Wiss Technology* 26;4:301–6.

Melini, V., Melini, F. 2019. Gluten-free diet: gaps and needs for a healthier diet. *Nutrients* 11;170:1–21.

Mills, E.N, Breiteneder, H. 2005. Food allergy and its relevance to industrial food proteins. *Biotechnol Adv* 23(6):409–14.

Mosleth, E., Uhlen, A.K. 1991. Associations between the Composition of Gliadins and HMW Glutenin Subunits and the Gluten Quality in Wheat (T. aestivum L.). In *Gluten Proteins 1990*, eds. W. Bushuk and R. Tkachuk, 112–28, American Association of Cereal Chemists Inc., St. Paul, Minnesota.

Nye-Wood, M.G., Juhász, A., Bose, U., Colgrave, M.L. 2021. Proteome analysis and epitope mapping in a commercial reduced-gluten wheat product. *Front Nutr* 8;705822:1–11.

Pérez-Sáez, M.J, Uffing, A., Leon, J., Murakami, N., Watanabe, A., Borges, T.J., Sabbisetti, V.S., Cureton, P., Kenyon, V., Keating, L., Yee, K., Fernandes Satiro, C.A., Serena, G., Hildebrandt, F., Riella, C.V., Libermann, T.A., Wang, M., Pascual, J., Bonventre, J.V, Cravedil, P., Fasano, A., Riella, L.V. 2021. Immunological impact of a gluten-free dairy-free diet in children with kidney disease: a feasibility study. *Front Immunol* 12:624821.

Peters, U., Dixon, A.E., Forno, E. 2018. Obesity and asthma. *J Allergy Clin Immunol* 141;4:1169–79.

Piché, M.E., Tchernof, A., Després, J.P. 2020. Obesity phenotypes, diabetes, and cardiovascular diseases. *Circ Res* 22;126:1477–500.

Połomska, J., Dydak, P., Sozańska, B., Sikorska-Szaflik, H. 2023. Peanut allergy and component-resolved diagnostics possibilities-what are the benefits? *Nutrients* 18;15(24):5132.

Posner, E.B., Haseeb, M. 2024. Celiac disease. 2023 Aug 8. In *StatPearls* [Internet]. StatPearls Publishing PMID: 28722929.

Pyler, E.J. 1988. *Baking Science and Technology*. U.S.A. Sosland Pub. Co., Kansas. Publishing Company Press. https://www.scirp.org/reference/referencespapers?referenceid=1680832

Roszkowska, A., Pawlicka, M., Mroczek, A., Bałabuszek, K., Nieradko-Iwanicka, B. 2019. Non-celiac gluten sensitivity: a review. *Medicina* (Kaunas) 28;55:1–19.

Rosinach, M., Fernández-Bañares, F., Carrasco, A., Ibarra, M., Temiño, R., Salas, A., Esteve, M. 2016. Double-blind randomized clinical trial: gluten versus placebo rechallenge in patients with lymphocytic enteritis and suspected celiac disease. *PLoS One* 11(7):e0157879.

Sánchez, D., Hoffmanová, I., Szczepanková, A., Hábová, V., Tlaskalová-Hogenová, H. 2021. Contribution of infectious agents to the development of celiac disease. *Microorganisms* 6;9(3):547.

Schofield, J.D. 1994. Wheat proteins: structure and functionality in milling and breadmaking. In *Wheat Production, Properties and Quality*, eds. W. Bushuk, V. F. Rasper, 72–106. https://link.springer.com/book/10.1007/978-1-4615-2672-8

Schofield, J.D. 1986. Flour proteins: Structure and functionality in baked products. In *Chemistry and Physics of Baking*, eds. J.M.V. Blanshard, P.J. Frazier, T. Galliard, 14–29. The Royal Society of Chemistry, England, Press.

Shewry, P.R., Halford, N.G., Belton, P.S., Tatham, A.S. 2002. The structure and properties of gluten: an elastic protein from wheat grain. *Philos Trans R Soc Lond B Biol Sci* 28;357(1418):133–42.

Shewry, P.R., Tatham, A.S., Barro, F., Barcelo, P., Lazzeri, P. 1995 Biotechnology of breadmaking: unravelling and manipulating the multi-protein gluten complex. *BioTechnology* 13:1185–90.

Soeroto, A.Y., Soetedjo, N.N., Purwiga, A., Santoso, P., Kulsum, I.D., Suryadinata, H., Ferdian, F. 2020. Effect of increased BMI and obesity on the outcome of COVID-19 adult patients: A systematic review and meta-analysis. *Diabetes Metab Syndr* 14:1897–904.

Takač, V., Tóth, V., Rakszegi, M., Mikić, S., Mirosavljević, M., Kondić-Špika, A. 2021. Differences in processing quality traits, protein content and composition between spelt and bread wheat genotypes grown under conventional and organic production. *Foods* 13;10:156:1–26.

Tapucu B.Ş.K.1996. Effects of vital wheat gluten, ascorbic acid and DATEM on bread quality by using response surface methodology. Middle East Technical University Institute of Science, Department of Food Engineering, Master's Thesis, Ankara, Thesis Number: 56786 https://tez.yok.gov.tr/UlusalTezMerkezi/tezSorguSonucYeni.jsp

Uy, N., Graf, L., Lemley, K.V, Kaskel, F. 2015. Effects of gluten-free, dairy-free diet on childhood nephrotic syndrome and gut microbiota. *Pediatr Res* 77(1–2):252–5.

Vacca, M., Pinto, D., Annunziato, A., Ressa, A., Calasso, M., Pontonio, E., Celano, G., De Angelis, M. 2023. Gluten-free bread enriched with artichoke leaf extract in vitro exerted antioxidant and anti-inflammatory properties. *Antioxidants* 12:845:1–18.

Vaquero, L., Alvarez-Cuenllas, B., Rodríguez-Martín, L., Aparicio, M., Jorquera, F., Olcoz, J.L, Vivas, S. 2015. Revısiön de las patologías relacionadas con la ıngesta de gluten [A review of diseases related to the intake of gluten]. *Nutr Hosp* 31:2359–71.

Vandenplas, Y., Meyer, R., Nowak-Wegrzyn, A., Salvatore, S., Venter, C., Vieira, M.C. 2023. The remaining challenge to diagnose and manage cow's milk allergy: an opinion paper to daily clinical practice. *Nutrients* 13;15(22):4762.

Wu, X., Qian, L., Liu, K., Wu, J., Shan Z. 2021. Gastrointestinal microbiome and gluten in celiac disease. *Ann Med* 53:1797–805.

Zanini, B., Baschè, R., Ferraresi, A., Ricci, C., Lanzarotto, F., Marullo, M., Villanacci, V., Hidalgo, A., Lanzini, A. 2015. Randomised clinical study: gluten challenge induces symptom recurrence in only a minority of patients who meet clinical criteria for non-coeliac gluten sensitivity. *Aliment Pharmacol Ther* 42(8):968–76.

Zingone, F., Bartalini, C., Siniscalchi, M., Ruotolo, M., Bucci, C., Morra, I., Iovino, P., Ciacci, C. 2017. Alterations in diets of patients with nonceliac gluten sensitivity compared with healthy individuals. *Clin Gastroenterol Hepatol* 15:63–8.

32 Nutritional Aspects of Dietary Protein

Gluten-Free Diets and Vitamin Status—Focus on Vitamins D and B12

Michele Di Stefano and Cristina Capittini

ABBREVIATIONS

CD	Coeliac disease
FAO	Food and Agriculture Organisation
GFD	Gluten-free diet
PTH	Parathyroid hormone
RDA	Recommended dietary allowance
SNP	Single nucleotide polymorphisms

INTRODUCTION

Coeliac disease (CD) is a chronic inflammatory disorder of the small bowel caused in genetically predisposed subjects by the ingestion of gluten, a protein complex contained in cereals such as wheat, rye and barley and rich in glutamine and proline moieties (Green and Cellier 2007; Di Sabatino et al. 2009). The term "gluten" pertains to the whole protein component; on the contrary, the term "gliadin" pertains to the alcohol-soluble gluten fraction, containing a large part of the toxic components. The most characterised toxic peptide is a fragment of 33 amino acids of α-gliadin, resistant to gastric, pancreatic and intestinal degradation, crossing the mucosal barrier during conditions that increase intestinal permeability and evoke an immunological response in the lamina propria.

Clinical Presentation of CD

CD is characterised by a broad clinical polymorphism, ranging from patients with asymptomatic/paucisymptomatic disease diagnosed because of the presence of minor, apparently unrelated symptoms or first-degree kinship with known patients, to subjects with severe disease, suffering from severe intestinal malabsorption and its clinical consequences and severe complications. On the contrary, intestinal lesions are always characterised by the presence of different degrees of villous atrophy, crypt hyperplasia, and an increase in intraepithelial lymphocyte count, which frequently configures the presence of flat mucosa (Green and Cellier 2007; Di Sabatino et al. 2009) (Figure 32.1).

CD is generally a benign condition: both histological alterations and clinical manifestations revert after the complete withdrawal of gluten from the diet. However, the frequent association with autoimmune disorders results in increased morbidity. Additionally, the higher risk of T-cell clonal

DOI: 10.1201/9781003597926-32

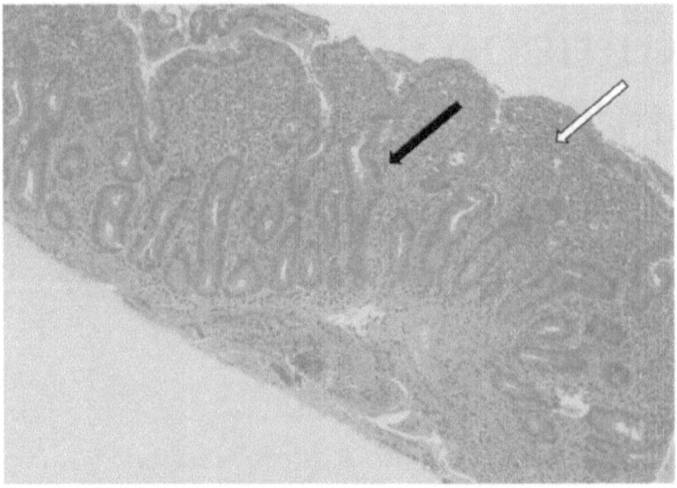

FIGURE 32.1 Histology of duodenal mucosa in untreated coeliac disease. There is a lack of villi, crypt hyperplasia (black arrow), and an increase of intraepithelial lymphocytes (white arrow).

proliferations, which predispose to enteropathy-type T-cell lymphoma, and the increased risk for neoplastic diseases raise the mortality (Di Sabatino et al. 2009).

CD and Gluten-Free Diet

Even if a large body of research has improved our understanding of the molecular basis of CD pathophysiology, enhancing the identification of new targets for future treatments, a rigorous gluten-free diet (GFD) remains the mainstay of the treatment. Gluten withdrawal from diet allows the progressive extinguishing of the immunological response against gluten epitopes and the progressive improvement of lesions. Accordingly, a normal absorptive mucosa is restored, and nutrient absorption is guaranteed (Green and Cellier 2007).

CD History

During evolution, the nomadic life of humans permitted the procurement of food by hunting or fishing and by fruit and vegetable collection. Humans were not yet involved in cultivation, and we can deduce that the Palaeolithic diet was gluten-free. In Southwestern Asia, in an area including Iraq, Palestine, Syria, Lebanon, and South of Turkey, called the "Fertile Crescent," the cultivation of some wild grains started, and humans began to adapt their lives to a non-migratory model, preferring a resident life in villages (Figure 32.2).

We can, therefore, deduce that CD appeared after such a lifestyle and dietary modification occurred. Even if the first description of CD appeared in the 1st and 2nd centuries (Losowsky 2008), the nosology of the disease dates back to the 19th century, with its description in England and the United States (Gee 1888; Davidson et al. 1950). The condition, initially named Gee-Herter syndrome, was described in children as a severe malabsorption syndrome, causing diarrhoea, steatorrhea and weight loss and symptom onset was correlated with a modification of dietary habits, including the intake of gluten. For many years, CD was considered a paediatric condition, severely symptomatic, causing an important impact on caloric intake and nutritional status, characterised by severe nutrient deficiencies.

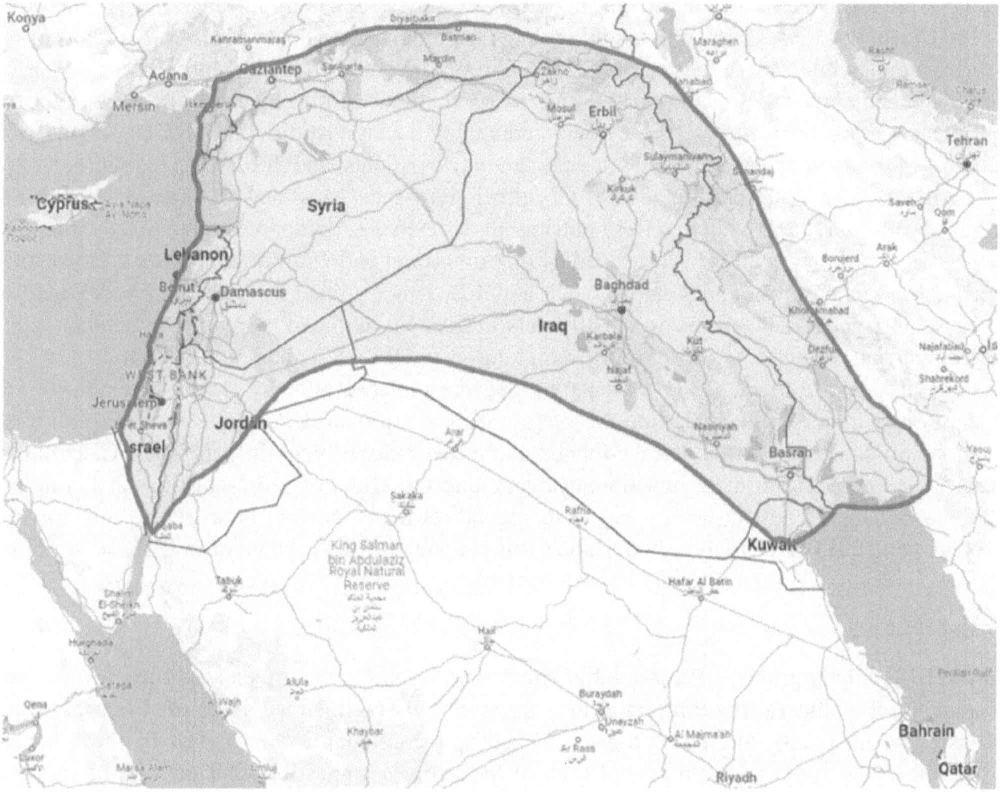

FIGURE 32.2 In the Fertile Crescent area (shaded area), the cultivation of wild grains started, and humans began to prefer non-migratory lifestyle.

Epidemiological Studies and the Prevalence of CD

The first epidemiological studies were conducted in 1950, when typical malabsorption symptoms guided CD diagnosis, and a prevalence of 1:8000 in England and 1:4000 in Scotland was reported (Davidson et al. 1950). The availability of a system for intestinal biopsy collection improved our knowledge of CD epidemiology, and the prevalence was set at 1:450 in Ireland, Scotland and Switzerland (Van Stirum et al. 1982; Mylotte et al. 1973). The availability of accurate serological tests revolutionised the history of CD epidemiology, and prevalences of 1:99 and 1:106 were detected in Finnish (Maki et al. 2003) and Italian (Tommasini et al. 2004) schoolchildren, respectively. Similar rates of CD-associated serum autoantibody positivity were detected also in adults in the UK and the US (West et al. 2003; Fasano et al. 2003), with prevalences of 1:87 and 1:105, respectively.

Epidemiological Studies and Clinical Issues of CD

Besides the discussion of epidemiological issues, these studies provided important clinical information as they showed that a large proportion of CD patients had not yet been diagnosed due to the presence of asymptomatic/paucisymptomatic disease. Terms like "subclinical," "minor" and "silent," in contrast to "classical," began circulating in the medical literature reporting clinical aspects of CD, and the symbolic representation of "the CD iceberg" was depicted, highlighting the large number of patients in the submerged portion while a smaller number in the emerged portion of an allegorical iceberg (Catassi et al. 1994; Corazza et al. 1997; Catassi et al. 1996). Accordingly, in the last decades, CD has been diagnosed more and more frequently, thanks to a radical change in the diagnostic paradigm: physicians have developed an increased awareness of the importance of the relationship between CD and associated conditions, rather than frank malabsorption symptoms (Rampertab et al. 2006). The most important of these conditions are iron-deficiency anaemia, autoimmune thyroiditis, type I diabetes, early-onset osteoporosis, and, in particular, familial history. The most important consequences have been, firstly, the evident reduction in diagnostic delay for CD; secondly, the awareness of the presence of adult and not only paediatric patients; and thirdly, the recognition of less severe patients. This latter point is pivotal for nutritional issues. Most newly diagnosed patients are generally well-nourished, without severe nutritional deficiencies, compared to previously diagnosed patients, who were frequently characterised by macronutrient and vitamin deficiencies. However, an extensive modification of dietary habits, such as GFD, if not guided by dedicated personnel, may also cause nutritional deficiencies and insufficient nutritional intake of many micronutrients in both newly diagnosed patients and those following a long-term GFD (Shepherd et al. 2013).

Although it is rare to encounter patients with severe malabsorption syndrome secondary to CD nowadays, it is important to underline the literature on nutritional deficiencies in this condition, to refresh the possibility of both a disease-related and a diet-induced vitamin deficiency. GFD must be tailored to each patient to meet nutritional targets, and the effect of a pre-existing or diet-induced intake inadequacy on patient health may help specialists in the general approach to this condition (Shepherd et al. 2013). Due to their importance, this chapter will focus on vitamin B12 and vitamin D.

Vitamin B12

Vitamin B12, cobalamin, is a water-soluble vitamin with a highly complex structure. Multicellular animals cannot synthesise this compound, as none have a gene coding for cobalamin. Microorganisms such as bacteria, yeasts, and some algae can synthesise cobalamin, and some of these bacteria are present in the upper gastrointestinal tract of herbivores, suggesting why these animals do not develop cobalamin insufficiency despite a negligible dietary intake. Besides some algae, Asiatic mushrooms, and some yeast products, cobalamin is contained in foods of animal origin, such as meat, liver, kidney, eggs, milk, fish, and shellfish.

Assimilation and Transport of Vitamin B12

Three proteins and their membrane receptors are involved in the complex mechanism of assimilation and transport of cobalamin: haptocorrin, intrinsic factor, and transcobalamin. Cobalamin is released from food proteins in the stomach and binds to endogenous carriers. Haptocorrin derives from saliva and binds 10–40% of cobalamin in the gastric juice. At a very low gastric pH, the affinity of haptocorrin for cobalamin is higher than that of the intrinsic factor. When pancreatic enzymes metabolise haptocorrin, cobalamin is transferred to the intrinsic factor in the duodenum. The complex cobalamin-intrinsic factor allows the assimilation of more than 98% of this vitamin in the ileum by receptor-mediated endocytosis. A small proportion is also absorbed passively along the entire small bowel (Kuzminski et al. 1998). Transcobalamin conveys cobalamin to the liver, where it is stored, but enterohepatic circulation is also evident (Figure 32.3).

Vitamin B12 in Untreated Adult CD Patients

It was previously shown that serum levels of cobalamin are inadequate in up to 41% of CD patients at diagnosis (Bode and Gudmand-Hoyer 1996; Harper et al. 2007; Dahele and Ghosh 2001; Dickey 2002; Bledsoe et al. 2019). However, the reported prevalence of cobalamin deficiency in these studies ranges from 5 to 12% in the majority of them (Bode and Gudmand-Hoyer 1996; Harper et al. 2007; Dickey 2002; Bledsoe et al. 2019) and proved to be very high only in the Scottish paper (Dahele and Ghosh 2001), reporting 41% of cases with cobalamin deficiency. A severe clinical presentation, without autoimmune gastritis, was considered the main reason for this discrepancy.

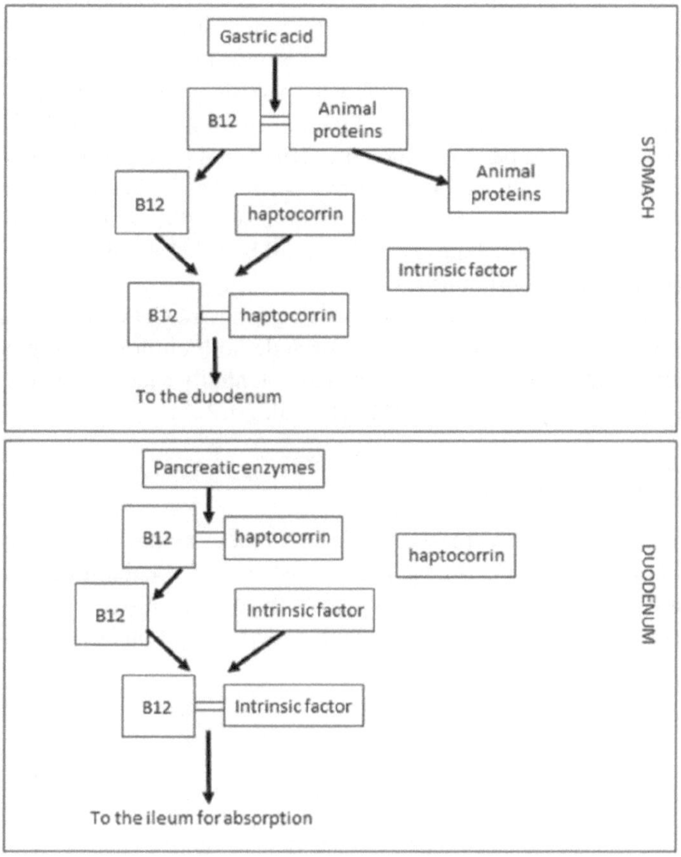

FIGURE 32.3 Haptocorrin is the vitamin B12 carrier in the stomach, and the intrinsic factor is the carrier from the duodenum to the ileum.

However, stool characteristics, abdominal symptoms, and weight loss did not predict cobalamin deficiency (Bledsoe et al. 2019). Clinical guidelines underline the high frequency of micronutrient deficiencies in CD at diagnosis (Rubio-Tapia et al. 2013) and the need for additional nutritional supplements, mainly in the early stages after diagnosis.

Vitamin B12 in Treated Adult CD Patients

In CD, micronutrient deficiencies may persist in subjects following a strict, long-term GFD. In a group of patients diagnosed in adult age, despite a strict GFD for a median period of 16 months, the complete reversal of mucosal lesions occurred in only 8% of cases. Moreover, in 65% of patients, remission was associated with intraepithelial lymphocytosis, and in 27% of cases, a lack of histological response was evident (Lanzini et al. 2009). Even if this slow response seems frequent in adult patients over 50 years (Lebwohl et al. 2014), it may occur in one child out of five after 1 year of GFD (Leonard et al. 2017).

However, persistent alterations of serum levels of cobalamin are infrequent in patients with CD on a strict GFD. In a group of 30 adults on long-term GFD, ranging from 8 to 12 years, no one showed cobalamin deficiency, and all of them had cobalamin intake higher than the recommended (Hallert et al. 2002). The supplementation of cobalamin, as expected, increased serum levels of this vitamin, but an improvement in clinical conditions was also evident, suggesting that the lower limit of normality was rather ambiguous. (Hallert et al. 2009). An adequate intake of cobalamin was detected in all enrolled patients on GFD in three Spanish studies (Churruca et al. 2015; Gonzalez et al. 2018; Ballestero-Fernández et al. 2021) and one Canadian study (Jivraj et al. 2022). In this latter study, only one patient on GFD for less than 2 years showed reduced serum levels of cobalamin. Similarly, a study from Norway on CD patients with persistent gastrointestinal symptoms showed an insufficient intake of cobalamin in only one patient (van Megen et al. 2023). The very low prevalence of cobalamin deficiency in patients following GFD could be explained, at least in part, by the significantly higher cobalamin content of gluten-free corn flakes, bread, and pasta in comparison to the corresponding gluten-containing products (Larretxi et al. 2019). Moreover, cobalamin intestinal absorption through a passive route along the entire small bowel (Kuzminski et al. 1998) may facilitate the maintenance of normal serum levels.

Accordingly, when the persistence of cobalamin deficiency in CD patients on a rigorous GFD is detected, further investigations are mandatory to exclude both unintentional gluten intake and the coexistence of other conditions not yet diagnosed and potentially causing impaired vitamin absorption, such as autoimmune atrophic gastritis (Miceli et al. 2012).

Homocysteinaemia in CD Patients

In untreated adult CD patients, increased levels of homocysteinaemia rapidly improve after a few months of GFD (Saibeni et al. 2005). The coexistence of cobalamin and folate deficiencies, both implicated in hyperhomocysteinaemia, suggests the causative role of these alterations in the pathogenesis of vascular complications, typical of disorders of the homocysteine metabolic pathway (Figure 32.4).

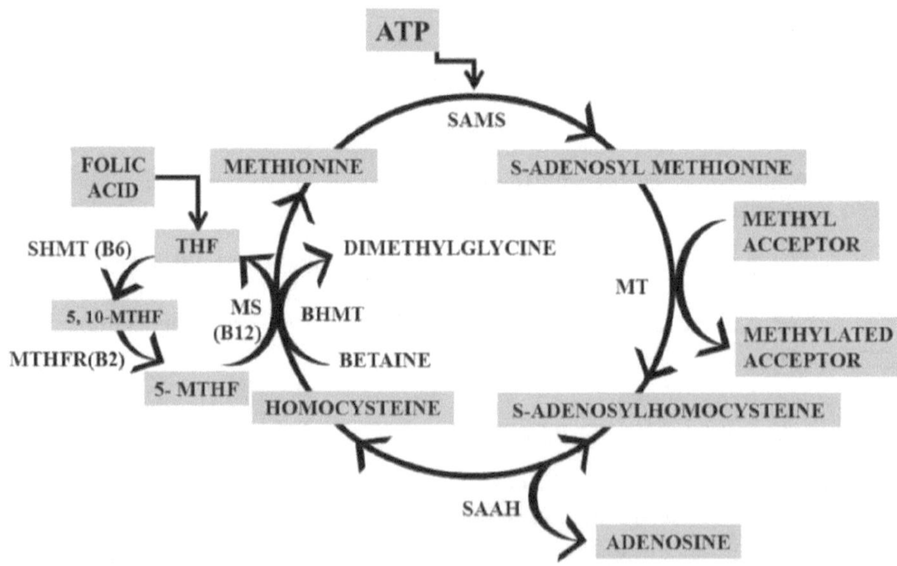

FIGURE 32.4 Homocysteine (HCy) is synthesised from methionine by S-adenosylmethionine synthetase (SAMS), methyltransferase (MT), and S-adenosylhomocysteine hydrolase (SAHH) in sequence. Homocysteine is remethylated to methionine by methionine synthase (MS), which needs folate and vitamin B12, and betaine homocysteine S-methyltransferase (BHMT), which needs betaine, a metabolite of choline. Remethylation of homocysteine via MS needs 5-methyltetrahydrofolate (5-MTHF), which is derived from 5,10-methylenetetrahydrofolate (5,10-MTHF) in a reaction catalysed by MTHFR with vitamin B2 as a cofactor. 5-MTHF is transformed into tetrahydrofolate (THF), which in turn is transformed into 5,10-MTHF by serine hydroxymethyltransferase (SHMT) with vitamin B6 as a cofactor to complete the folate cycle.

The catabolism of homocysteine requires both cobalamin and folate; consequently, hyperhomocysteinaemia may reflect a deficit of both nutrients. In adult CD, a reduced folate intake should be considered the main responsible for persistent hyperhomocysteine, as suggested by several papers on treated patients, even in long-term GFD (Unalp-Aride et al. 2022; Ballestero-Fernández et al. 2021; Churruca et al. 2015; Gonzalez et al. 2018; Bascunan et al. 2019; Jivraj et al. 2022; van Megen et al. 2023; Shepherd et al. 2013; Bledsoe et al. 2019). It should be emphasised that gluten-free cereal products contain lower amounts of folate compared to their gluten-containing counterparts (Thompson 2000).

Vitamin D

Bone Loss, GFD, and CD

Alterations of bone mass and mineral metabolism are very frequent in adult CD. At diagnosis, calcium metabolism is impaired in all the patients, and bone loss is present in three-quarters of patients with overt malabsorption and half of patients with minor CD (Di Stefano et al. 2013). A strict GFD in childhood normalises both BMD and anthropometric parameters, with a significant bone mass improvement after the first six months of treatment (Gerenli et al. 2021). Unfortunately, this is not the case for patients diagnosed in adulthood: GFD improves bone and mineral metabolism (Di Stefano et al. 2013), confirming its therapeutic role, but does not normalise bone mass. Very limited data are available on the effect of drug treatment in patients with CD (Meyer et al. 2001; Mulder et al. 2011; Kumar et al. 2013) making it hard to revert the increased fracture risk characterising postmenopausal status. Hence, preventing bone loss through early diagnosis and an active search for this clinical consequence is mandatory (Figure 32.5).

Despite severe malabsorption syndrome, hypocalcaemia is very rare in untreated CD (Corazza et al. 1995), as serum calcium is finely regulated, being a key actor in muscular and cardiac contraction. Moreover, adopting serological screening for conditions conferring an elevated risk for CD diagnosis elicited the recognition of patients in an early phase of the disease. Together with serum calcium levels, parathyroid hormone (PTH) and vitamin D take part in both the regulation of bone and mineral metabolism and the pathophysiology of bone loss. Vitamin D is a secosteroid circulating in blood in two main forms: 25-hydroxyvitamin D, reflecting the entity of vitamin D storage,

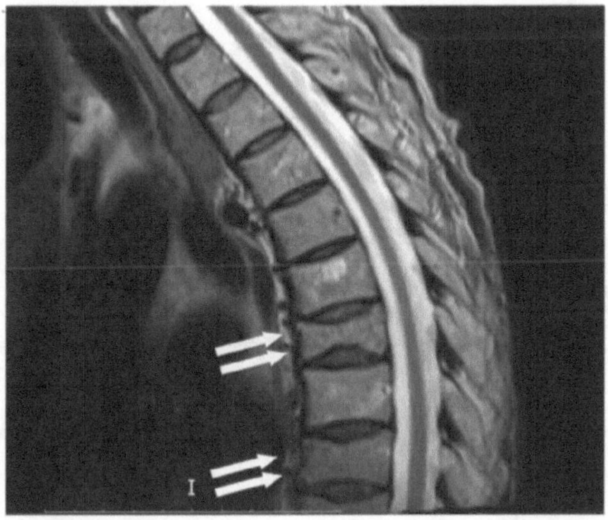

FIGURE 32.5 Lateral magnetic resonance (MR) scan in a 45-year-old untreated female patient with CD showing two vertebral fractures of the dorsal spine.

and 1,25-dihydroxyvitamin D, the active metabolite, regulating calcium balance and also modulating the immune system.

Alterations of Bone Metabolism and Vitamin D

In untreated CD patients, reduced serum calcium, mainly due to faecal losses, is promptly rebalanced by activating a complex reactive network (Di Stefano et al. 2013), as shown in Figure 32.2. The stimulation of renal 1-α-hydroxylase by the release of PTH enhances the conversion of 25-vitamin D into 1,25-vitamin D, improving intestinal calcium absorption through increased vitamin D-dependent active transport. However, the intestinal compensation for calcium faecal losses is frustrated by the enterocyte, which expresses a normal number of vitamin D receptors (Di Stefano et al. 2013), but contains negligible levels of vitamin D-dependent calcium-binding protein (Di Stefano et al. 2013). The activation of this complex network causes only negative consequences on bone mineralisation due to the direct pro-resorptive effect of increased levels of both PTH and excessive levels of 1,25-vitamin D (Maierhofer et al. 1983) (Figure 32.6).

Therefore, untreated CD patients show low serum levels of 25-vitamin D but high serum levels of 1,25-vitamin D as a consequence of hyperparathyroidism-induced hyperconversion. Increased levels of 1,25-vitamin D at diagnosis are associated with increased levels of PTH (Taranta et al. 2004; Molteni et al. 1995), and a strict GFD normalises these alterations (Keaveny et al. 1996; Corazza et al. 1996; Valdimarsson et al. 2000) when mucosal lesions are reverted. In patients with refractory CD or those with low compliance to a GFD (Mautalen et al. 1997), hyperparathyroidism may persist and alteratins in vitamin D metabolism can still be detected (Corazza et al. 1996). Undiagnosed patients on calcium and vitamin D supplementation may mask these pivotal alterations and present to physicians a misleading bone and mineral metabolism condition (Selby et al. 1999).

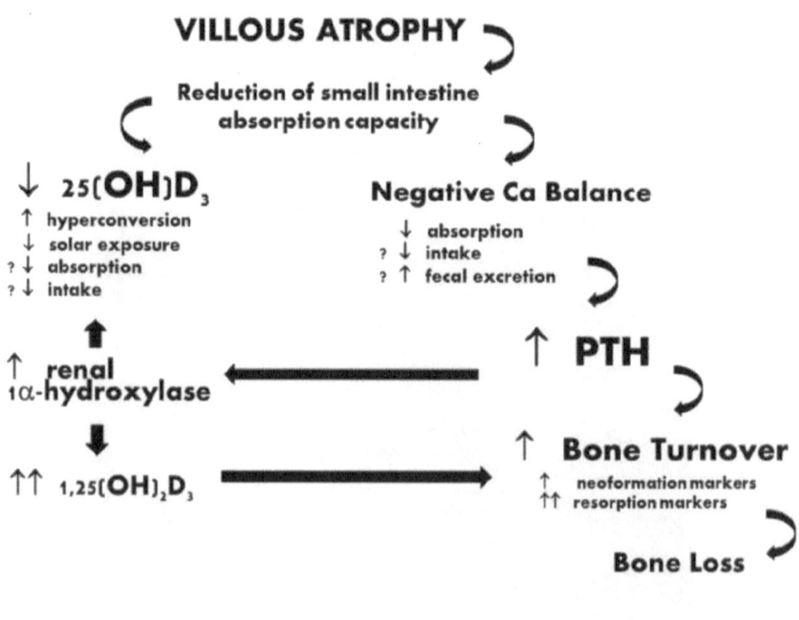

FIGURE 32.6 Endocrine reaction to hypocalcaemia in untreated CD. The release of PTH stimulates 1-α-hydroxylase activation, enhancing the conversion of 25 vitamin D into 1,25 vitamin D. Consequently, activated vitamin D increases intestinal calcium absorption through vitamin D-dependent active transport.

Duration of GFD and Bone Metabolism Improvement

The normalisation of mineral metabolism generally requires a GFD period longer than one year (Taranta et al. 2004; Molteni et al. 1995; Keaveny et al. 1996; Corazza et al. 1996; Mautalen et al. 1997; Stein et al. 2015). Serum 1,25-vitamin D levels directly correlate to PTH levels due to renal 1-α-hydroxylase activity. This correlation is evident in untreated patients, in patients on GFD for a median 2-year period (Molteni et al. 1995; Di Stefano et al. 2019), in patients on GFD for longer periods (Taranta et al. 2004; Corazza et al. 1996; Stein et al. 2015) and in patients on long-term GFD (Corazza et al. 1997). Interestingly, the reduction of serum levels of 1,25-vitamin D is very rapid, beginning after just three months of GFD (Lemieux et al. 2001). Moreover, the progressive normalisation of calcium balance improves 25-vitamin D levels, which increase after the introduction of GFD, as shown in a group of CD patients on long-term GFD independently of the presence of bone loss (Davies et al. 1980).

Prevalence of Vitamin D Deficiency in CD Patients

Based on previous pathophysiological issues, in untreated CD, vitamin D deficiency should be considered very rare, as the PTH-related reduction of 25-vitamin D levels is always accompanied by increased levels of 1,25-vitamin D. On the contrary, the prevalence of vitamin D deficiency in patients following GFD represents a more important clinical issue, deserving specific diagnostic and therapeutic approaches. However, very few papers report on this information. It is expected that a strict GFD reduces the prevalence of low 25-vitamin D. In a longitudinal study of untreated patients followed for 5 years after beginning a GFD, the prevalence was 68% at baseline and 54% after one year of GFD, falling to 8% after 5 years of diet (Kempainnen et al. 1999). Moreover, two recent papers described a low prevalence of 25-vitamin D in treated patients, at 25% (Tavakkoli et al. 2013) and 28% (Ciacci et al. 2020), but information on both age and duration of GFD at the measurement, two important parameters for a correct interpretation of the results, is lacking.

Vitamin D Receptor Genotypes

The role of vitamin D receptor genotypes was suggested in the pathophysiology of bone loss and vitamin D serum alterations in patients with CD. Among the numerous single nucleotide polymorphisms (SNPs), Fok I (SNP rs2228570), Bsm I (SNP rs1544410), Apa I (SNP rs7975232), and Taq I (SNP rs731236) are the most studied. However, a recent meta-analysis disproved a causal relationship between VDR polymorphism and bone alterations (Lu et al. 2021).

Vitamin D Supplementation

There is much interest regarding nutritional supplementation in CD patients, and differences often characterise guidelines. An up-to-date Consensus Conference highlighted the necessity for additional studies designed to explain the role of vitamin D in the pathophysiology of CD and the necessity for nutritional supplementation (Giustina et al. 2020). Nevertheless, similar considerations could be given to calcium supplementation. The age of the subjects is the key factor in defining the correct calcium intake to maintain mineral metabolism balance and bone health. Older people need a high amount of calcium due to reduced intestinal calcium absorption, while adolescents need a high amount of calcium due to rapid growth. Nonetheless, in women and men over 50, FAO recommends a calcium intake of 800–1,000 mg per day (Dai et al. 2021). The Institute of Medicine of the United States National Academy of Sciences recommends a calcium intake of 1,200 mg/day for men over 70 and post-menopausal women and an intake of 1,000 mg for 19–70-year-old men and 19–50-year-old women. Increasing pharmacological calcium supplementation beyond 1,200 mg/day may induce an increased risk of urinary stones; however, the risk of this problem must be checked in all subjects following calcium supplementation.

Serum 25-vitamin D levels below 30 nmol/L are related to an increased risk of bone disorders, and values above 50 nmol/L, or 20 ng/mL, are considered proper for bone health (Sempos et al.

2018; Bouillon et al. 2019; Amrein et al. 2020). There is, however, a lack of standardisation for vitamin D measurement (Elsenberg et al. 2017) hindering clinical research; all attempts to overcome this serious shortcoming are welcome.

Age, gender, skin type, geographical area, and season should be considered for adequate vitamin D supplementation. The US Institute of Medicine and the European Food Safety Authority agreed to settle on 15 µg of vitamin D as the optimal recommended dietary allowance (RDA) (Thomas et al. 2008; EFSA Panel, 2016; Dai et al. 2021). An RDA of 600 IU/day is recommended for 50–70-year-old subjects, and 800 IU/day is recommended for subjects over 70 years. The aim of pharmacological vitamin D supplementation should be to attain serum 25-vitamin D levels equal to 50 nmol/L; this value was shown to be effective in maintaining bone health in over 97% of North Americans (Holick et al. 2011; Ross et al. 2011).

Vitamin D Supplementation in Untreated CD

In CD patients, the increased conversion of 25-vitamin D to 1.25-vitamin D is a crucial topic that should be emphasised. In untreated CD, low levels of 25-vitamin D should not be considered a manifestation of vitamin deficiency; hyperconversion to 1.25-vitamin D, due to hyperparathyroidism, causes low levels of 25-vitamin D. Thus, in CD patients, 25-vitamin D pharmacological supplementation at diagnosis may be not only needless but also a detrimental therapy, since severely increased serum levels of 1.25-vitamin D have a pro-resorptive effect, worsening bone loss (Bouillon et al. 1980).

Pharmacological vitamin D supplementation in untreated adult CD should be started based on the assessment of serum levels of the two vitamin D metabolites, together with PTH. In patients showing high levels of 1,25-vitamin D and PTH associated with low 25-vitamin D levels, the administration of pharmacological preparations to increase serum 25-vitamin D levels is nonsensical: the increased PTH levels will further increase the hyperconversion to 1,25-vitamin D and further increase the risk of 1,25-vitamin D-mediated bone resorption. Furthermore, it was clearly shown that pharmacological supplementation of 25-vitamin D as an additional treatment to GFD does not improve bone mass compared to GFD alone (Lemieux et al. 2001), making this therapy even more needless.

On the contrary, two different approaches could be recommended. Since a fast GFD-related modification of vitamin D metabolite levels was observed (Lemieux et al. 2001), to verify the effect of GFD, a reassessment of serum 25-vitamin D, 1,25-vitamin D, and PTH levels after 3 months of GFD (Di Stefano et al. 2019) is recommended. Otherwise, as the modifications of serum vitamin D and PTH levels in untreated CD express an altered calcium balance, oral calcium supplementation could be a suitable initial therapy. Villous atrophy may hinder the effectiveness of this therapy because untreated CD patients display lower calcium absorption that improves with GFD (Molteni et al. 1995). However, the fast increase in serum levels of both 25-vitamin D and 1,25-vitamin D after three months of GFD (Lemieux et al. 2001) suggests that the effect of calcium supplementation on improving secondary hyperparathyroidism may be low at the beginning of GFD, improving with the continuation of GFD. Furthermore, normal vitamin D and PTH levels during calcium and vitamin D pharmacological supplementation initiated before diagnosis in untreated CD patients suggest a helpful effect of this therapy beyond the presence of villous atrophy (Selby et al. 1999).

Vitamin D Supplementation in Treated CD

In treated CD patients showing a progressive improvement in calcium balance on GFD, the rationale for vitamin D supplementation has a different purpose. Recently, in a group of CD patients on GFD and a group of non-CD adult volunteers, vitamin D intake, as well as energy, calcium, folate, iodine, magnesium, and zinc intakes, did not reach the recommended levels, with no differences between females and males (Kim 2017). One out of three patients showed vitamin D levels between 10 and 30 ng/ml, which was not dissimilar in the group of non-CD volunteers. Accordingly, the need to assess serum vitamin D to select patients with vitamin D deficiency and refer them for a nutritional intake evaluation is evident.

The age of patients is a pivotal point. Before the age of 45 years, before the peri-menopausal age, the persistence of vitamin D deficiency will indicate low compliance to GFD and also the coexistence of disorders responsible for vitamin D deficiency. Among them, thyroid diseases (Sarela et al. 2016), which are very often associated with CD, are the main actors. Reduced vitamin D levels were described in patients with Graves' disease and Hashimoto's thyroiditis (Amrein et al. 2020; Kim 2017). Vitamin D deficiency is responsible for the reduced suppression of T cells, which causes the release of pro-inflammatory cytokines and the consequent inflammatory-related morphological and functional alterations of the thyroid (Moscogiuri et al. 2014). Lymphocytes, macrophages and dendritic cells express vitamin D receptors and transform 25-vitamin D into 1,25 vitamin D (Lucas et al. 2014), which prevent Th1 cell proliferation and Th1 cell cytokine production, reduces B cell apoptosis and HLA class II antigen surface expression (Moscogiuri et al. 2014; Guillot et al. 2010; Vanoirbeek et al. 2011). Pharmacological oral supplementation of 2000 IU/day of vitamin D, more than twice the RDA, decreases anti-thyroid autoantibodies, indicating a protective effect (Krysiak et al. 2017). Moreover, patients with CD and intestinal malabsorption often show iron deficiency, aggravating thyroid function and causing an impairment of heme-dependent TPO (O'Kane et al. 2018). If the alterations in calcium balance do not depend on gluten toxicity, another disease to be excluded is sarcoidosis (Bell et al. 1979). A recent systematic review with meta-analysis reported that the risk of sarcoidosis in CD patients is higher than in subjects without CD, with a pooled OR greater than 7 (Wijarnpreecha et al. 2019).

THE EFFECTS OF OTHER PROTEINS

Alternative alimentary sources of vitamin B12 are strongly needed due to the complex absorption pathway of this metabolite. Vitamin B12 deficiency represents a causative factor for the development of anaemia, a condition characterised by a very high frequency at diagnosis in patients with coeliac disease. Some evidence suggests that administering whey proteins improves serum vitamin B12 levels. A crossover study on healthy adults with vitamin B12 deficiency found that daily supplementation with 50 g of whey proteins (equivalent to 2.8 mg of cyanocobalamin) for 8 weeks improved vitamin B12 status, while soy protein supplementation did not show the same effect. Notably, administering whey proteins reduces hyperhomocysteinaemia levels in patients with vitamin B12 deficiency (Dhillon et al. 2017). On the contrary, a subsequent paper on the same cohort of subjects showed that whey proteins did not improve cognitive functions (Zajac et al. 2019).

Unfortunately, in patients with coeliac disease, evidence suggesting an improvement of vitamin B12 status after these types of protein supplementation is lacking. It could be argued that secondary lactose intolerance due to a reduced expression of lactase at the apex of intestinal villi is a frequent finding in patients with coeliac disease. However, a strict gluten-free diet can restore normal intestinal structure, which in turn normalises lactase expression in the intestines, thereby improving lactose digestion. Accordingly, the administration of whey protein isolates could also represent an effective supplementation in these patients.

Similarly, in patients with coeliac disease, evidence suggesting an improved vitamin D status after administering other proteins is not yet available.

GLUTEN-FREE DIET AND VITAMIN STATUS: FOCUS ON VITAMIN D AND VITAMIN B12

In this chapter, we reported on the prevalence of vitamin B12 and vitamin D deficiencies in adult CD and the effect of GFD. Vitamin deficiencies are a frequent complication of CD due to the associated malabsorption syndrome, but they typically improve once patients begin following a GFD, which is the primary treatment of CD. Vitamin B12 deficiency is significant as it worsens haemocoagulative balance and, therefore, predisposes patients to thromboembolic consequences. Vitamin D deficiency should be accurately investigated, and determining vitamin metabolites is mandatory in CD. Unfortunately, in clinical practice, it is a frequent habit to determine only 25-vitamin D, as commonly used in the follow-up of post-menopausal osteoporosis. However, in CD, this could induce clinical mistakes, particularly in untreated patients. An exogenous supplementation is mandatory in this condition only when a clear insufficiency is detected at diagnosis and persists after the introduction of GFD. The administration of cholecalciferol is frequently useless in untreated patients due to the hyperconversion of 25-vitamin D into 1,25-vitamin D, secondary to hyperparathyroidism.

MINI DICTIONARY OF TERMS

- **Gliadin:** The alcohol-soluble gluten fraction, containing a large part of the toxic component.
- **Gluten-free diet:** A dietary regimen excluding gluten-containing cereals.
- **Haptocorrin:** Saliva-derived protein binding vitamin B12.
- **Intrinsic factor:** Stomach-derived protein binding vitamin B12.

SUMMARY POINTS

- This chapter focuses on vitamin B12 and vitamin D deficiency in patients with untreated and treated adult CD.
- CD is characterised by broad clinical polymorphism, ranging from asymptomatic to severe disease.
- Malabsorption causes secondary vitamin deficiency.
- Vitamin B12 deficiency worsens haemocoagulative alterations in CD.
- Vitamin D deficiency should be diagnosed after determine 25-vitamin D, 1,25-vitamin D, and parathyroid hormone serum levels in CD.

REFERENCES

Amrein, K.; Scherkl, M.; Hoffmann, M.; Neuwersch-Sommeregger, S.; Kostenberger, M.; Berisha, A. T.; Martucci, G.; Pilz, S.; Malle, O. 2020. Vitamin D deficiency 2.0: an update on the current status worldwide. *Eur J Clin Nutr* 74:1498–1513.

Ballestero-Fernández, C.; Varela-Moreiras, G.; Úbeda, N.; Alonso-Aperte, E. 2021. Nutritional status in spanish adults with celiac disease following a long-term gluten-free diet is similar to non-celiac. *Nutrients* 13(5):1626.

Bascuñán, K. A.; Elli, L.; Pellegrini, N.; Scricciolo, A.; Lombardo, V.; Doneda, L.; Vecchi, M.; Scarpa, C.; Araya, M.; Roncoroni, L. 2019. Impact of FODMAP content restrictions on the quality of diet for patients with celiac disease on a gluten-free diet. *Nutrients* 11(9):2220.

Bell, N. H.; Stern, P. H.; Pantzer, E.; Sinha, T. K.; DeLuca, H. F. 1979. Evidence that increased circulating 1-alpha, 25-dihydroxyvitamin D is the probable cause for abnormal calcium metabolism in sarcoidosis. *J Clin Invest* 64:218–225.

Bledsoe, A. C.; King, K. S.; Larson, J. J.; Snyder, M.; Absah, I.; Choung, R. S.; Murray, J. A. 2019. Micronutrient deficiencies are common in contemporary celiac disease despite lack of overt malabsorption syndrome. *Mayo Clin Proc* 94:1253–1260.

Bode, S. and E. Gudmand-Hoyer. 1996. Symptoms and haematological features in consecutive adult coeliac patients. *Scand J Gastroenterol* 31:54–60.

Bouillon, R.; Marcocci, C.; Carmeliet, G.; Bikle, D.; White, J. H.; Dawson-Hughes, B.; Lips, P.; Munns, C. F.; Lazaretti-Castro, M.; Giustina, A.; Bilezikian, J. 2019. Skeletal and extraskeletal actions of vitamin D: current evidence and outstanding questions. *Endocr Rev* 40:1109–1151.

Bouillon, R.; Muls, E.; De Moor, P. 1980. Influence of thyroid function on the serum concentration of 1,25-dihydroxyvitamin D3. *J Clin Endocrinol Metab* 51:793–797.

Catassi, C.; Fabiani, E.; Rätsch, I. M.; Coppa, G. V.; Giorgi, P. L.; Pierdomenico, R.; Alessandrini, S.; Iwanejko, G.; Domenici, R.; Mei, E.; Miano, A.; Marani, M.; Bottaro, G.; Spina, M.; Dotti, M.; Montanelli, A.; Barbato, M.; Viola, F.; Lazzari, R.; Vallini, M.; Guariso, G.; Plebani, M.; Cataldo, F.; Traverso, G.; Ughi, C.; Chiaravallotti, G.; Baldassarre, M.; Scarcella, P.; Bascietto, F.; Ceglie, L.; Valenti, A.; Paolucci, P.; Caradonna, M.; Bravi, E.; Ventura, A. 1996. The coeliac iceberg in Italy. A multicentre antigliadin antibodies screening for coeliac disease in school-age subjects. *Acta Paediatr Suppl* 412:29–35.

Catassi, C.; Rätsch, I. M.; Fabiani, E.; Rossini, M.; Bordicchia, F.; Candela, F.; Coppa, G. V.; Giorgi, P. L. 1994. Coeliac disease in the year 2000: exploring the iceberg. *Lancet* 343(8891):200–203.

Churruca, I.; Miranda, J.; Lasa, A.; Bustamante, M. Á.; Larretxi, I.; Simon, E. 2015. Analysis of body composition and food habits of spanish celiac women. *Nutrients* 7(7):5515–5531.

Ciacci, C.; Bilancio, G.; Russo, I.; Iovino, P.; Cavallo, P.; Santonicola, A.; Bucci, C.; Cirillo, M.; Zingone, F. 2020. 25-hydroxyvitamin D, 1,25-dihydroxyvitamin D, and peripheral bone densitometry in adults with celiac disease. *Nutrients* 12:929.

Corazza, G. R.; Andreani, M. L.; Biagi, F.; Corrao, G.; Pretolani, S.; Giulianelli, G.; Ghironzi, G.; Gasbarrini, G. 1997. The smaller size of the coeliac iceberg in adults. *Scand J Gastroienterol* 32:917–919.

Corazza, G. R.; Di Sario, A.; Cecchetti, L.; Jorizzo, A.; Di Stefano, M.; Minguzzi, L.; Brusco, G.; Bernardi, M.; Gasbarrini, G. 1996. In-fluence of pattern of clinical presentation and of gluten-free diet on bone mass and metabolism in adult coeliac disease. *Bone* 18:525–530.

Corazza, G. R.; Di Sario, A.; Cecchetti, L.; Tarozzi, C.; Corrao, G.; Bernardi, M.; Gasbarrini, G. 1995. Bone mass and metabolism in patients with celiac disease. *Gastroenterology* 109(1):122–128.

Corazza, G. R.; Di Stefano, M.; Jorizzo, R. A.; Cecchetti, L.; Minguzzi, L.; Gasbarrini, G. 1997. Propeptide of type I procollagen is predictive of post-treatment bone mass gain in adult celiac disease. *Gastroenterology* 113:67–71.

Dahele, A. and S. Ghosh. 2001. Vitamin B12 deficiency in untreated celiac disease. *Am J Gastroenterol* 96:745–750.

Dai, Z.; McKenzie, J. E.; McDonald, S.; Baram, L.; Page, M. J.; Allman-Farinelli, M.; Raubenheimer, D.; Bero, L. A. 2021. Assessment of the methods used to develop vitamin D and calcium recommendations. A systematic review of bone health guidelines. *Nutrients* 13:2423.

Davidson, L.S.P. and J.R. Fountain. 1950. Incidence of the sprue syndrome: with some observations on the natural history. *BMJ* 1:1157–1161.

Davies, M.; Mawer, E. B.; Krawitt, E. L. 1980. Comparative absorption of vitamin D3 and 25-hydroxyvitamin D3 in intestinal disease. *Gut* 21:287–292.

Dhillon, V. S.; Zabaraz, D.; Almond, T.; Cavuoto, P.; James-Martin, G.; Fenech, M. 2017. Whey protein isolatesì improves vitamin B12 and folate status in elderly Australians with subclinical deficiency of vitamin B12. *Mol Nutr Food Res* 61:1600915.

Di Sabatino, A. and G. R. Corazza. 2009. Coeliac disease. *Lancet* 373:1480–1493

Di Stefano, M.; Bergonzi, M.; Benedetti, I.; De Amici, M.; Torre, C.; Brondino, N.; Miceli, E.; Pagani, E.; Marseglia, G.L.; Corazza, G. R.; Di Sabatino, A. 2019. Alterations of inflammatory and matrix production indices in celiac disease with low bone mass on long-term gluten-free diet. *J Clin Gastroenterol* 53(6):e221–e226.

Di Stefano, M.; Mengoli, C.; Bergonzi, M.; Corazza, G. R. 2013. Bone mass and mineral metabolism alterations in adult celiac disease: pathophysiology and clinical approach. Nutrients 5:4786–4799

Dickey, W. 2002. Low serum vitamin B12 is common in coeliac disease and is not due to autoimmune gastritis. *Eur J Gastroenterol Hepatol* 14:425–427.

EFSA Panel on Dietetic Products, Nutrition and Allergies (NDA). Dietary reference values for vitamin D. *EFSA J* doi: 10.2903/j.efsa.2016.4547.

Elsenberg, E. H. A. M.; Ten Bockel, E.; Huijgen, H.; Heijboer, A. C. 2017. Standardization of automated 25-hydroxyvitamin D assays: how successful is it? *Clin Biochem* 50:1126–1130.

Fasano, A.; Berti, I.; Gerarduzzi, T.; Not, T.; Colletti, R. B.; Drago, S.; Elitsur, Y.; Green, P. H.; Guandalini, S.; Hill, I. D.; Pietzak, M.; Ventura, A.; Thorpe, M.; Kryszak, D.; Fornaroli, F.; Wasserman, S. S.; Murray, J. A.; Horvath K. 2003. Prevalence of celiac disease in at-risk and not-at-risk groups in the United States: a large multicenter study. *Arch Intern Med* 163(3):286–292.

Gee, S. J. 1888. On the celiac affection. *St Bartholomew's Hosp Rep* 24:17–20.

Gerenli, N.; Dursun, F.; Celtik, C.; Kirmizibekmez, H. 2021. Significant improvement in bone mineral density in pediatric celiac disease: even at six months with gluten-free diet. *J Ped Endocrinol Metab* 34:341–348.

Giustina, A.; Adler, R. A.; Binkley, N.; Bollerslev, J.; Bouillon, R.; Dawson-Hughes, B.; Ebeling, P. R.; Feldman, D.; Formenti, A. M.; Lazzaretti-Castro, M.; Marcocci, C.; Rizzoli, R.; Sempos, C. T.; Bilezikian, J. P. 2020. Consensus statements from 2nd International Conference on controversies in Vitamin D. *Rev Endocr Metab Dis* 21:89–116.

González, T.; Larretxi, I.; Vitoria, JC.; Castaño, L.; Simón, E.; Churruca, I.; Navarro, V.; Lasa, A. 2018. Celiac male's gluten-free diet profile: comparison to that of the control population and celiac women. *Nutrients* 10:1713.

Green, P. H. R. and C. Cellier. 2007. Celiac disease. *NEJM* 357:1731–1743.

Guillot, X.; Semerano, L.; Saidenberg-Kermanach, N.; Falgarone, G.; Boissier M.C. 2010. Vitamin D and inflammation. *Joint Bone Spine* 77:552–557

Hallert C.; Grant C.; Grehn S.; Grännö C.; Hultén S.; Midhagen G.; Ström M.; Svensson H.; Valdimarsson T. 2002. Evidence of poor vitamin status in coeliac patients on a gluten-free diet for 10 years. *Aliment Pharmacol Ther* 16(7):1333–1339.

Hallert, C.; Svensson, M.; Tholstrup, J.; Hultberg, B. 2009. Clinical trial: B vitamins improve health in patients with coeliac disease living on a gluten-free diet. *Aliment Pharmacol Ther* 29:811–816.

Harper, J. W.; Holleran, S. F.; Ramakrishnan, R.; Bhagat, G.; Green, P. H. R. 2007. Anemia in celiac disease is multifactorial in etiology. *Am J Hematol* 82:996–1000

Holick, M. F.; Binkley, N. C.; Bischoff-Ferrari, H. A.; Gordon, C. M.; Hanley, D. A.; Heaney, R. P.; Murad, M. H.; Weaver, C. M.; Endocrine Society. 2011. Evaluation, treatment, and prevention of vitamin D deficiency: an Endocrine Society clinical practice guidelines. *J Clin Endocrinol Metab* 96:1911–1930.

Human Vitamin and Mineral Requirements. Report of a joint FAO/WHO expert consultation. Bangkok, Thailand. https://www.fao.org/3/y2809e/y2809e.pdf

Jivraj, A.; Hutchinson, J. M.; Ching, E.; Marwaha, A.; Verdu, E. F.; Armstrong, D.; Pinto-Sanchez, M. I. 2022. Micronutrient deficiencies are frequent in adult patients with and without celiac disease on a gluten-free diet, regardless of duration and adherence to the diet. *Nutrition* 103–104:111809.

Keaveny, A. P.; Freaney, R.; McKenna, M. J.; Masterson, J.; O'Donoghue, D. P. 1996. Bone remodeling indices and secondary hyperparathyroidism in celiac disease. *Am J Gastroenterol* 91:1226–1231.

Kempainnen, T.; Kroger, H.; Janatuinen, E.; Arnala, I.; Lamberg-Allardt, C.; Karkkainen, M.; 1999. Bone recovery after a gluten-free diet: a 5-year follow-up study. *Bone* 25:355–360.

Kim, D. 2017. The role of vitamin D in thyroid disease. *Int J Mol Sci* 18:1949.

Krysiak, R.; Szkróbka, W.; Okopień, B. 2017. The effect of vitamin d on thyroid autoimmunity in levothyroxine-treated women with hashimoto's thyroiditis and normal vitamin D status. *Exp Clin Endocrinol Diabetes* 125:229–233.

Kumar, M.; Rastogi, A.; Bhadada, SK.; Bhansali, A.; Vaiphei, K.; Kochhar, R. 2013. Effect of zoledronic acid on bone mineral density in patients of celiac disease: a prospective, randomized, pilot study. *Indian J Med Res* 138:882–887.

Kuzminski, A. M.; Del Giacco, E. J.; Alle, R. H.; Stabler, S. P.; Lindenbaum, J. 1998. Effective treatment of cobalamin deficiency with oral cobalamin. *Blood* 92:1191–1198.

Lanzini, A.; Lanzarotto, F.; Villanacci, V.; Mora, A.; Bertolazzi, S.; Turini, D.; Carella, G.; Malkagoli, A.; Ferrante, G.; Cesana, B. M.; Ricci, C. 2009. Complete recovery of intestinal mucosa occurs very rarely in adult coeliac patients despite adherence to gluten-free diet. *Aliment Pharmacol Ther* 29:1299–1308.

Larretxi, I.; Txurruka, I.; Navarro, V.; Lasa, A.; Bustamante, M. Á.; Fernández-Gil, M. D. P.; Simón, E.; Miranda, J. 2019. Micronutrient analysis of gluten-free products: their low content is not involved in gluten-free diet imbalance in a cohort of celiac children and adolescent. *Foods* 8:321.

Lebwhol, B.; Murray, J. A.; Rubio-Tapia, A.; Green, P. H. R.; Ludvigsson, J. F. 2014. Predictors of persistent villous atrophy in coeliac disease: a population-based study. *Aliment Pharmacol Ther* 39:488–495.

Lemieux, B.; Boivin, M.; Brossard, J. H.; Lepage, R.; Picard, D.; Rousseau, L.; D'Amour, P. 2001. Normal parathyroid function with decreased bone mineral density in treated celiac disease. *Can J Gastroenterol* 15:302–307.

Leonard, M. M.; Weir, D. C.; DeGroote, M. Mitchell, P. D.; Singh, P.; Silvester, J. A.; Leichtner, A. M.; Fasano, A. 2017, Value of IgA tTG in predicting mucosal recovery in children with celiac disease on a gluten-free diet. *J Pediatr Gastroenterol Nutr* 64:286–291.

Losowsky, M. S. 2008. A history of coeliac disease. *Dig Dis* 26:112–120

Lu, C.; Zhou, W.; He, X.; Zhou, X.; Yu, C. 2021. Vitamin D status and vitamin D receptor genotypes in celiac disease: a meta-analysis. *Crit Rev Food Sci Nutr* 61:2098–2106.

Lucas, R. M.; Gorman, S.; Gedenhuys, S.; Hart, P. H. 2014. Vitamin D and immunity. *F1000 Prime Rep* 6:118

Maierhofer, W. J.; Gray, R. W.; Cheung, H. S.; Lemann, J. Jr. 1983. Bone resorption stimulated by elevated serum levels of 1,25-(OH)2-vitamin D concentrations in healthy men. *Kidney Int* 24:555–560.

Mäki, M.; Mustalahti, K.; Kokkonen, J.; Kulmala, P.; Haapalahti, M.; Karttunen, T.; Ilonen, J.; Laurila, K.; Dahlbom, I.; Hansson, T.; Höpfl, P.; Knip, M. 2003. Prevalence of Celiac disease among children in Finland. *N Engl J Med* 348(25):2517–2524.

Mautalen, C.; Gonzalez, D.; Mazure, R.; Vazquez, H.; Lorenzetti, M. P.; Maurino, E.; Niveloni, S.; Pedreira, S.; Smecuol, E.; Boerr, L. A.; Bai, J. C. 1997. Effect of treatment on bone mass, mineral metabolism, and body composition in untreated celiac disease patients. *Am J Gastroenterol* 92:313–318.

Meyer, D.; Stavropolous, S.; Diamond, B.; Shane, E.; Green, P. H. 2001. Osteoporosis in a north american adult population with celiac disease. *Am J Gastroenterol* 96:112–119.

Miceli, E.; Lenti, M.V.; Padula, D.; Luinetti, O.; Vattiato, C.; Monti, C. M.; Di Stefano, M.; Corazza, G. R. 2012. Common features of patients with autoimmune atrophic gastritis. *Clin Gastroenterol Hepatol* 10:812–814.

Molteni, N.; Bardella, M. T.; Vezzoli, G.; Pozzoli, E.; Bianchi, P. 1995. Intestinal calcium absorption as shown by stable strontium test in celiac disease before and after gluten-free diet. *Am J Gastroenterol* 90:2025–2028.

Molteni, N.; Caraceni, M.P.; Bardella, M.T.; Ortolani, S.; Gandolini, G. G.; Bianchi, P. A. 1990. Bone mineral density in adult celiac patients and the effect of gluten-free diet from childhood. *Am. J. Gastroenterol* 85:51–53.

Moscogiuri, G.; Tirabassi, G.; Bizzarro, G.; Orio, F.; Paschou, S.; Vryonidou, A.; Balercia, G.; Shoenfeld, Y.; Colao, A. 2014. Vitamin D and thyroid disease: to D or not to D? *Eur J Clin Nutr* 69:291–296.

Mulder, CJ.; Cardile, AP.; Dickert, J. 2011. Celiac disease presenting as severe osteopenia. *Hawaii Med J* 70:242–244.

Mylotte, M.; Egan-Mitchell, B.; McCarthy, CF.; McNicholl, B. 1973. Incidence of coeliac disease in the West of Ireland. *BMJ* 1:703–705.

O'Kane, M.; Mulhern, M. S.; Pourshahidi, L. K.; Strain, J. J.; Yeates, A. J. 2018. Micronutrients, iodine status and concentrations of thy-roid hormones: a systematic review. *Nutr Rev* 76:418–431.

Rampertab, S. D.; Pooran, N.; Brar, P.; Singh, P.; Green, P. H. 2006. Trends in the presentation of celiac disease. *Am J Med* 11:355.e9–14.

Ross, A. C.; Manson, J. E.; Abrams, S. A.; Aloia, J. F.; Brannon, P. M.; Clinton, S. K.; Durazo-Arvizu, R. A.; Gallagher, J. C.; Gallo, R. L.; Jones, G.; Kovacs, C. S.; Mayne, S. T.; Rosen, C. J.; Shapses, S. A. 2011. The 2011 report on dietary reference intakes for calcium and vitamin D from the Institute of Medicine: what clinicians need to know. *J Clin Endocrino Metab* 96:53–58.

Rubio-Tapia, A.; Hill, I. D.; Kelly, C. P.; Calderwood, A. H.; Murray, J. A. 2013. ACG clinical guidelines: diagnosis and management of celiac disease. *Am J Gastroenterol* 108:656–676.

Saibeni, S.; Lecchi, A.; Meucci, G.; Cattaneo, M.; Tagliabue, L.; Rondonotti, E.; Formenti, S.; De Franchis, R.; Vecchi, M. 2005. Prevalence of hyperhomocysteinemia in adult gluten-sensitive enteropathy at diagnosis: role of B12, folate, and genetics. *Clin Gastroenterol Hepatol* 3:574–580.

Sarela, S.; Thompson, D. V.; Nagrant, B.; Thakkar, P.; Clarke, K. 2016. A retrospective chart review evaluating the association of psychological disorders and vitamin D deficiency with celiac disease. *Minerva Gastroenterol Dietol* 62:240–244.

Selby, P. L.; Davies, M.; Adams, J. E.; Mawer, E. B. 1999. Bone loss in celiac disease is related to secondary hyperparathyroidism. *J Bone Miner Res* 14:652–657.

Sempos, C. T.; Heijboer, A. C.; Bikle, D. D.; Bollerslev, J.; Bouillon, R.; Brannon, P. M.; DeLuca, H. F.; Jones, G.; Munns, C. F.; Bilezikian, J. P.; Giustina, A.; Binkley, N. 2018. Vitamin D assays and the definition of hypovitaminosis D: results from the First International Conference on Controversies in Vitamin D. *Br J Clin Pharmacol* 84:2194–2207.

Shepherd, SJ. and P.R. Gibson. 2013. Nutritional inadequacies of the gluten-free diet in both recently-diagnosed and long-term patients with coeliac disease. *J Hum Nutr Diet* 26(4):349–358.

Stein, E. M.; Rogers, H.; Leib, A.; McMahon, D. J.; Young, P.; Nishijama, K.; Guo, X. E.; Lewis, S.; Green, P.; Shane, E. 2015. Abnormal skeletal strength and microarchitecture in women with celiac disease. *J Clin Endocrinol Metab* 100(6):2347–2353.

Taranta, A.; Fortunati, D.; Longo, M.; Rucci, N.; Iacomino, E.; Aliberti, F.; Facciuto, E.; Migliaccio, S.; Bardella, M. T.; Dubini, A.; Borghi, M. O.; Saraifoger, S.; Teti, A.; Bianchi, M. L. 2004. Imbalance of osteoclastogenesis-regulating factors in patients with celiac disease. *J Bone Miner Res* 19:1112–1121.

Tavakkoli, A.; DiGiacomo, D.; Green, P. H.; Lebwohl, B. 2013. Vitamin D status and concomitant autoimmunity in celiac disease. *J Clin Gastroenterol* 47:515–519.

Thomas, S. D. C; Need, A. G.; Tucker, G.; Slobodian, P. O.; O'Loughlin, P. D.; Nordin, B. E. C. 2008. Suppression of parathyroid hormine and bone resorption by calcium carbonate and calcium citrate in postmenopausal women. *Calcif Tissue Int* 83:81–84.

Thompson, T. 2000. Folate, iron, and dietary fiber contents of the gluten-free diet. *J Am Diet Ass* 100:1389–1396.

Tommasini, A.; Not, T.; Kiren, V.; Baldas, V.; Santon, D.; Trevisiol, C.; Berti, I.; Neri, E.; Gerarduzzi, T.; Bruno, I.; Lenhardt, A.; Zamuner, E.; Spanò, A.; Crovella, S.; Martellossi, S.; Torre, G.; Sblattero, D.; Marzari, R.; Bradbury, A.; Tamburlini, G.; Ventura, A. 2004. Mass screening for coeliac disease using antihuman transglutaminase antibody assay. *Arch Dis Child* 89(6):512–515.

Unalp-Arida, A.; Liu, R.; Ruhl, CE. 2022. Nutrient intake differs among persons with celiac disease and gluten-related disorders in the United States. *Sci Rep* 12(1):5566.

Valdimarsson, T.; Toss, G.; Lofman, O.; Strom, M. 2000. Three years' follow up of bone density in adult coeliac disease: significance of secondary hyperparathyroidism. *Scand J Gastroenterol* 35:274–280.

van Megen, F.; Fossli, M.; Skodje, G. I.; Carlsen, M. H.; Andersen, L. F.; Veierød, M. B.; Lundin, K. E. A.; Henriksen, C. 2023. Nutritional assessment of women with celiac disease compared to the general population. *Clin Nutr ESPEN* 54:251–257.

Van Stirum, J.; Baerlocher, K.; Fanconi, A.; Gugler, E.; Tonz, O.; Shmerling, DH. 1982. The incidence of coeliac disease in children in Switzerland. *Helv Pediatr Acta* 37:421–430.

Vanoirbeek, E.; Krishnan, A.; Eelen, G.; Verlinden, L.; Bouillon, R.; Feldman, A.; Verstuyf, A. 2011. The anti-cancer and an-ti-inflammatory actions of 1,25(OH)2D3. *Best Pract Res Clin Endocrinol Metab* 25:593–604

West, J.; Logan, RF.; Hill, PG.; Lloyd, A.; Lewis, S.; Hubbard, R.; Reader, R.; Holmes, GK.; Khaw, KT. 2003. Seroprevalence, correlates, and characteristics of undetected coeliac disease in England. *Gut* 52(7):960–965.

Wijarnpreecha, K.; Panjawatanan, P.; Corral, J. E.; Lukens, F. J.; Ungprasert, P. 2019. Celiac disease and risk of sarcoidosis: A systematic review and meta-analysis. *J Evid Based Med* 12:194–199.

Zajac, I. T.; Herrenn, D.; Bastiaans, K.; Dhillon, V. S.; Fenech, M. 2019. The effect of whey and soy protein isolates on cognitive function in older Australians with low vitamin B12: a randomized controlled cross-over trial. *Nutrients* 11:19.

33 Dipeptidyl Peptidase IV (DPP-IV) Inhibitory Peptides in Vegetable Protein and Potential for Functional Foods

Fernando Rivero-Pino

ABBREVIATIONS

DPP-IV	Dipeptidyl peptidase IV
GIP	Gastric inhibitory polypeptide
GLP-1	Glucagon-like peptide-1
HDL-C	High-density lipoprotein-cholesterol
LDL-C	Low-density lipoprotein-cholesterol
SGID	Simulated gastrointestinal digestion

INTRODUCTION

Globalisation, along with novel consumer patterns and the increased availability and revalorisation of natural resources, has sparked a never-before-seen revolution in food science and technology. In recent years, traditional proteins (i.e., milk, fish or beef) have been extensively investigated and consumed. However, Western eating patterns are gradually shifting, emphasising plant-based sources over meat (Alfieri et al. 2023).

Compared to animal protein, vegetable-derived protein offers numerous health benefits for consumers and the environment, which are among the main priorities in current society. Western diets heavy in meat, processed sugar and fat have been linked to an increased risk of certain diseases and are considered less health-promoting than plant-based diets. Consequently, authorities are promoting the consumption of foods such as legumes (EFSA NDA Panel 2022). On top of that, the amino acid composition and absorption rate are the two main limitations for plant proteins (e.g., pea protein lacking methionine), but consuming varied plant sources could overcome these issues (Nadathur, Wanasundara, and Scanlin 2017). Additionally, compared to animal-based diets, vegetable cultivation helps to minimise agricultural greenhouse gas emissions, land destruction, and subsequent species extinctions. For instance, plant protein production uses fewer resources, such as water, compared to the production of an equivalent amount of animal protein (Tilman and Clark 2014).

Among the most consumed and investigated vegetable proteins currently, soy, wheat or oat are noteworthy, as well as lupin, whose benefits beyond its high quantity and quality protein include dietary fibre or polyunsaturated fatty acids. Protein sources can be employed to manufacture concentrates or isolates, to which treatment to release peptides can be applied. The most employed techniques are enzymatic hydrolysis (using food-grade proteases such as alcalase, trypsin, or Flavourzyme) and fermentation (by specific microorganisms). The cleavage of proteins into peptides

DOI: 10.1201/9781003597926-33

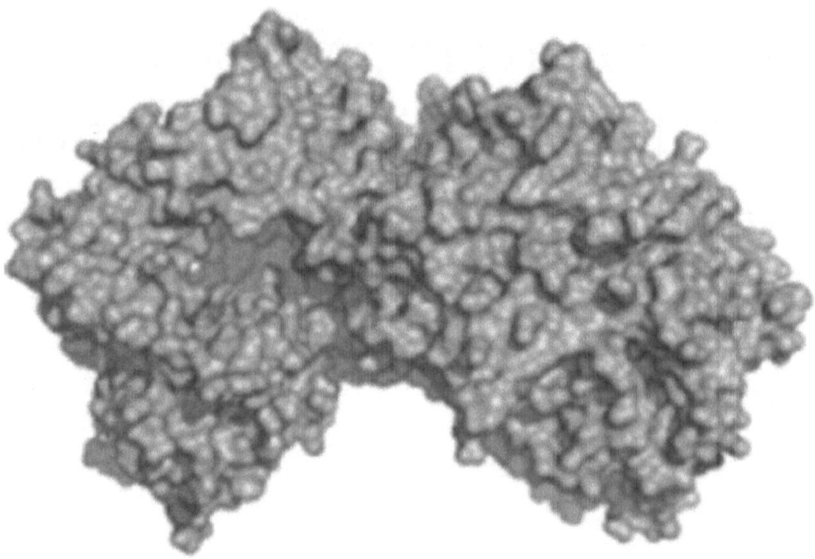

FIGURE 33.1 Dimeric representation of DPP-IV: the structure of the enzyme DPP-IV (PDB code: 4A5S).

liberates sequences, which, based on their molecular characteristics, might exert bioactivity by targeting and inhibiting enzymes (Cruz-Casas et al. 2021). One of the most studied bioactivities is the inhibition of dipeptidyl peptidase IV (DPP-IV) (Figure 33.1), a key enzyme involved in the regulation of blood glucose levels in the postprandial period, as it negatively modulates incretin levels (Mills et al. 2022).

The inhibition of DPP-IV is directly correlated with an increased half-life of these incretins (GLP-1 and GIP), restoring the insulinotropic effects and regulating blood glucose levels (Figure 33.2). Nutritional interventions using proteins and their derivatives as strategies to manage the development of these diseases, potentially preventing diabetes, show promising results. Research on DPP-IV inhibitory peptides derived from vegetable sources is still scarce at present, and considering the wide variety of substrates and processing conditions that might be applied, this field opens new lines of research (Chan-Zapata, Sandoval-Castro, and Segura-Campos 2022).

These vegetable-derived peptides could be used as food supplements (directly as produced, as powder or encapsulated), or they could be incorporated into a food matrix to produce a so-called functional food. The inclusion of peptides into food matrices has been described for several types of peptides, although research on DPP-IV vegetable peptides is limited. No human studies have been reported on the inhibition of DPP-IV by vegetable peptides (as protein hydrolysate), while the consumption of vegetable proteins, either native or as hydrolysates, and their impact on other closely related parameters (e.g., metabolic syndrome or inflammation) has been described in some reports.

DPP-IV INHIBITORY PROTEIN HYDROLYSATES

Vegetable sources encompass a wide variety of substrates, including legumes (e.g., chickpea, lupin, lentil), cereals (e.g., barley, oat, wheat), nuts (e.g., almond, peanut, pistachio), seeds (from sunflower, hemp or flax), pseudo cereals (e.g., amaranth, quinoa) and others (Alfieri et al. 2023). The protein content in different vegetable sources is highly variable, but through different processing methods, concentrates and isolates can be obtained to produce high-protein products that can be used to create protein hydrolysates (Jia et al. 2021). For obtaining peptides, the most common aids, according to the technique, are: i) alcalase, trypsin, Flavourzyme and/or pepsin (sequentially or simultaneously)

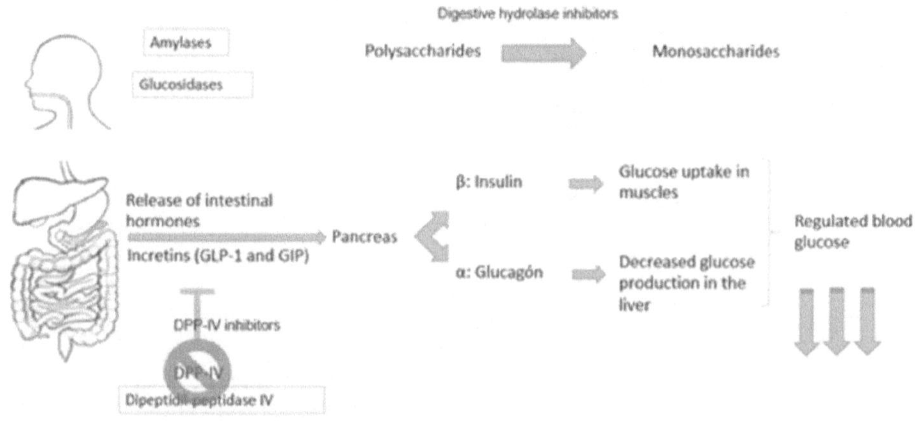

FIGURE 33.2 Schematic explanation of how the inhibition of DPP-IV promotes the regulation of the glycaemic index. The incretin hormones glucose-dependent insulinotropic polypeptide (GIP) and glucagon-like peptide-1 (GLP-1) are quickly inactivated by DPP-IV. DPP-IV inhibition prolongs and enhances the effects of endogenous GLP-1 and GIP, which are crucial postprandial stimulators of insulin production and regulators of blood glucose homeostasis.

in enzymatic hydrolysis; and ii) lactic acid bacteria (*Lactobacillus* species) in the fermentation process (Rivero-Pino 2023).

FERMENTATION

Few studies have reported on peptides' ability to inhibit the enzyme DPP-IV obtained by fermentation. Sharma et al. (2021) employed *Lactobacillus plantarum* strain NCDC 374 for the fermentation of flaxseed and released bioactive peptides. The authors reported half-maximal inhibitory concentration (IC_{50}) values of 0.58, 0.64 and 0.42 mg/mL for 5 kDa, 10 kDa and non-filtrated protein hydrolysate, respectively. In addition, Sato et al. (2018) fermented soybean previously fermented with *B. subtilis* (i.e., natto) with *Aspergillus oryzae* to release bioactive peptides. The hydrolysate had an IC_{50} value of 5.35 mg/mL and two highly bioactive sequences were characterised (Table 33.1). Ramírez et al. (2021) reported that fermentation of spent coffee grounds by *Bacillus clausii* induced the release of bioactive peptides, and among the sequences identified, based on prediction analyses, the sequence YGF was proposed as highly capable of inhibiting DPP-IV. A recent review has explored the relevance of bioactive peptides in fermented foods and their application (Chourasia et al. 2023).

On the other hand, the use of food-grade proteases has been more extensively studied in the release of DPP-IV inhibitory peptides, including plant sources. As previously indicated and shown in Figure 33.3, quinoa and soy are among the most evaluated sources (Farias et al. 2022).

ENZYMATIC HYDROLYSIS OF SOY PROTEIN

Soybean (*Glycine max*) is one of the most consumed proteins worldwide, with an appropriate quantity and quality, making it suitable for human consumption.

A sequential hydrolysis with alcalase-trypsin and Flavourzyme over a total reaction time of seven hours released a soy hydrolysate with an IC_{50} value of 2.39 mg/mL, from which peptides <3 kDa, after purification, had a reduced IC_{50} of 1.16 mg/mL (Rivero-Pino, Espejo-Carpio, and Guadix 2021). Similarly, hydrolysis using the digestive proteases pepsin and pancreatin released a bioactive pool of peptides with an IC_{50} value of 1.49 mg/mL (Gonzalez-Montoya et al. 2018). Nongonierma

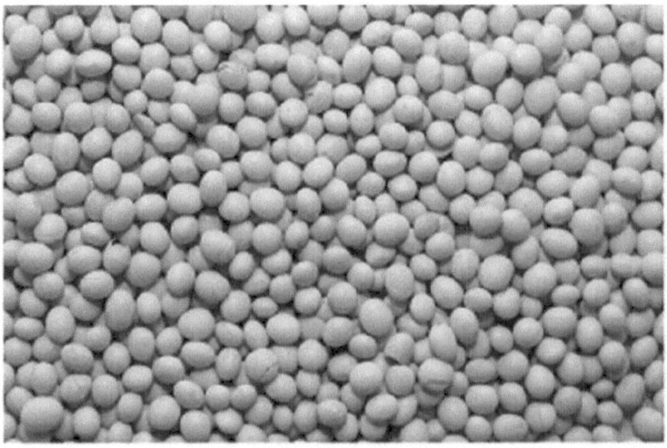

A)

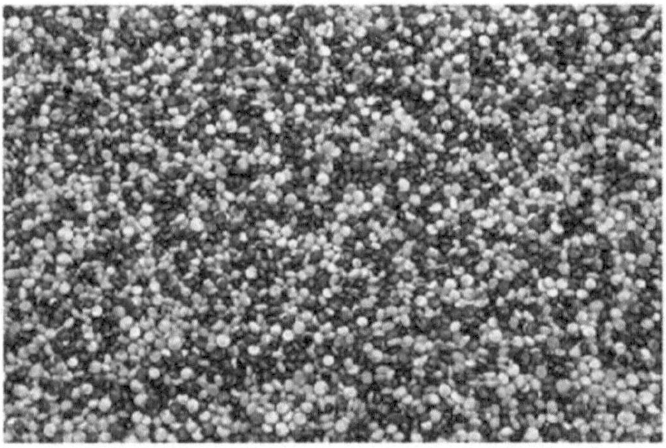

B)

FIGURE 33.3 Vegetable sources of DPP-IV inhibitory peptides. A) Soybean, B) Quinoa.

and Fitzgerald (2015) evaluated the enzymatic hydrolysis of soy with Protamex, Promod 144MG, and Corolase L10 hydrolysates and found that the samples obtained with Protamex and Promod 144MG had IC_{50} values ranging from 0.85 to 2.21 mg/mL, depending on the time, while the hydrolysates obtained with Corolase showed no activity. Bollati et al. (2022) reported an IC_{50} value of 1.15 mg/mL for a soybean protein hydrolysate, which also reduced the activity of DPP-IV expressed on the surface of human intestinal Caco-2 cells.

Soybean protein appears to be an adequate source of peptides due to its content of alanine and proline (Samaranayaka 2017), widely reported as relevant in sequences able to inhibit the target enzyme (Berraquero-García et al. 2023).

ENZYMATIC HYDROLYSIS OF QUINOA PROTEIN

Quinoa (*Chenopodium quinoa*) as a source of DPP-IV inhibitory peptides has been investigated using proteases such as bromelain, chymotrypsin, and Pronase E, which resulted in highly bioactive hydrolysates, with IC_{50} values ranging from 0.72 to 1.12 mg/mL (Mudgil et al. 2020). Additionally, peptides obtained by in vitro simulated gastrointestinal digestion (SGID) and fractionated by ultrafiltration reported high bioactivity (Vilcacundo, Martínez-Villaluenga, and Hernández-Ledesma 2017), especially in the <5 kDa fraction compared to the >5 kDa fraction. These results were also supported by the inhibitory values exerted by the fractions obtained by Rivero-Pino, Espejo-Carpio, and Guadix (2021), emphasising the relevance of medium molecular weight peptides as DPP-IV inhibitors. Recently, the use of papain, alcalase, Neutrase, Flavourzyme and pepsin-trypsin digestion on quinoa hydrolysis has been reported, highlighting the effect of the last treatment. From this sample, the fraction with a molecular weight of less than 1 kDa exhibited DPP-IV inhibitory activity with an IC_{50} of 3.40 mg/mL (You, Wu, et al. 2022). Overall, the potential of quinoa as a source of bioactive peptides inhibiting DPP-IV is promising, but in vivo studies are required.

ENZYMATIC HYDROLYSIS OF OAT PROTEIN

Oat (*Avena sativa* L.), as well as buckwheat (*Fagopyrum esculentum*) and highland barley (*Hordeum vulgare trifurcatum* L. Trofim), peptides have been released by the action of alcalase, trypsin and SGID, showing IC_{50} values ranging from 0.13 mg/mL to 8.15 mg/mL. From these samples, peptides were identified and tested to validate the activity (Table 33.1) (F. Wang et al. 2015).

Oat hydrolysate obtained with alcalase was also recently reported to be highly bioactive (Ramírez Fuentes, Richard, and Chen 2021), as well as hydrolysates obtained with Flavourzyme, papain, Neutrase, SGID and alcalase. The sample obtained with Neutrase, as occurred in other substrates, was the most active, with an IC_{50} value of 2.55 mg/mL (W. Wang et al. 2022).

ENZYMATIC HYDROLYSIS OF CHICKPEA AND PEA PROTEIN

Peptides from chickpea (*Cicer arietinum* L.) have been obtained by different enzymatic treatments, such as the sequential hydrolysis with alcalase-trypsin-Flavourzyme previously indicated, leading to an IC_{50} value of 2.68 mg/mL (Rivero-Pino, Espejo-Carpio, and Guadix 2021) or through Neutrase, Protamex, alcalase, and papain, of which the most active was the sample obtained with Neutrase (IC_{50} value of 0.86 mg/mL), although the activity decreased after SGID. The activity of identified peptides was also verified (Table 33.1).

Similarly, DPP-IV inhibitory hydrolysates were obtained from pea (*Pisum sativum* L.) using alcalase 2.4 L, trypsin, papain, bromelain, and Protamex. Although no IC50 values were calculated for these samples, values were calculated for the fractions obtained after purifying the Protamex-derived sample, showing values of around 0.75–1 mg/mL. (M. Zhang et al. 2022).

ENZYMATIC HYDROLYSIS OF NOVEL SOURCES

Researchers are exploring novel plant-based protein sources to produce protein hydrolysates. For example, *Phoenix dactylifera* L. seed hydrolysates were obtained using different proteases (e.g., alcalase, bromelain, papain and protease) over hydrolysis times of up to six hours. Mostafa et al. (2022) reported that enzymatic hydrolysis with bromelain produced the most bioactive hydrolysate for inhibiting DPP-IV, with an IC_{50} value of 48.56 µg/mL. They described these results as some of the most active compared to similar products. This finding highlights the need for further research into new protein sources that could yield novel ingredients with enhanced techno-functional and bioactive properties.

In another study, hydrolysates derived from dehulled hard-to-cook beans, obtained with alcalase and bromelain, presented adequate DPP-IV inhibition, though IC_{50} values could not be quantified for the original samples. However, these values could be quantified for the low molecular weight peptides, which were obtained using an ultrafiltration membrane system (values around 100 µg/mL, depending on the treatment applied and the bean variety) (Oseguera-Toledo, Gonzalez de Mejia, and Amaya-Llano 2015).

Agustia et al. (2023) evaluated the release of peptides from jack bean sprouts (*Canavalia ensiformis* L. DC.) during simulated digestion and absorption using the everted gut sac method. They reported high levels of inhibition after 2.5 hours of digestion, attributed to the increase of low

TABLE 33.1
Peptides Identified as DPP-IV Inhibitory Agents and Their IC_{50} Values

Source	Sequence	Treatment	IC_{50} Value (μM)	Reference
Brewers' spent grain	VPIP	Alcalase and Flavourzyme	54.69	Cermeño et al. (2019)
	IPVP		38.67	
	IPLQP		105.45	
	LPY		87.15	
	IPIPQ		75.7	
	PAIP		111.18	
	IPY		52.15	
	LPVP		105.25	
	APLP		122.45	
	LPIA		45.07	
	LAVP		98.76	
Broccoli	VPLVM	Trypsin	99.7	Zhou et al. (2021)
	LPGVLPVA)		392	
	YLYSPAY		181	
Carioca bean	KTYGL	Pepsin/pancreatin digestion	1084.3	Mojica, Chen, and de Mejía (2015)
	CPGNK		1679.5	
	GGGLHK		1073.9	
	KKSSG		1264.8	
Dark tea protein	QGQELLPSDFK	Trypsin	3084.8	Zhao et al. (2020)
	MSLYPR		1762.4	
Lupin	LTFPGSAED	Pepsin	228	Lammi et al. (2016)
Oat	LQAFEPLR	Trypsin	103.5	F. Wang et al. (2015)
Picrorhiza kurroa	ASGLCPEEAVPRR	Trypsin	2.2	Thakur et al. (2021)
Rapeseed napin	IPQVS	Alcalase and trypsin	52.16	Xu et al. (2019)
	KTMPGP		162.73	
	ELHQEEPL		78.46	
	PAGPF		135.7	
	IPK	Simulated gastrointestinal digestion	44.4	You, Zhang, et al. (2022)
Soybean protein	IAVPTGVA	Pepsin	106	Lammi et al. (2016)
	KL	Fermentation with *A. oryzae*	0.16	Sato et al. (2018)
	LR		2	
Wheat gluten	LPQ	Ginger protease	56.7	Taga et al. (2017)
	QPG		70.9	
	SPQ		78.9	
	QPF		71.7	
	QPQ		79.8	

(*Continued*)

TABLE 33.1 (CONTINUED)
Peptides Identified as DPP-IV Inhibitory Agents and Their IC_{50} Values

Source	Sequence	Treatment	IC_{50} Value (μM)	Reference
Hemp	LPQNIPP	Trypsin/chymotrypsin, pepsin, proteinase K, and thermolysin	80	Chen et al. (2023)
	YPYY		18.	
	YPW		180	
	LPYPY		200	
	WWW		220	
	YPY		290	
	YPF		420	
	WS		440	
African yam	AVIAIMF	Simulated gastrointestinal digestion	139	Ibrahim et al. (2023)
	GPADPF		246.4	
Taro	NGDF		96.5	
	NGNW		178.2	
Sorghum	LSICGEESFGTGSDHIR	Simulated gastrointestinal digestion	73.5	Majid et al. (2022)
	SLGESLLQEDVEAHK		82.5	
	QLRDIVDK		8.55	
Sacha inchi	GPSRGF	Protamex and alkaline proteases	75.75	A. Zhang et al. (2023)
	WPYH		128.40	
	APVYWVQ		23.43	
	APESKPVGV		53.11	
	LLMWPY		79.92	
Pea	IPYWTY	Protamex	11.04	M. Zhang et al. (2022)
Chickpea	IAIPPGIPYW	Neutrase	12.43	Zan et al. (2023)
Quinoa	IPI	Pepsin-trypsin	5.25	You, Wu, et al. (2022)
	IPV		26.15	
	VAYPL		42.93	
	IPIN		56.58	

The table shows the DPP-IV inhibitory activity of vegetable-derived peptides, indicating the source, the treatment applied to the native protein and the quantitative value of the bioactivity. Treatments, unless specified, refer to the name of the protease as indicated by the authors.

molecular weight peptides (<1 kDa). Their results showed that after 180 minutes of digestion simulation, the inhibitory activity persisted after absorption, highlighting the activity of the sequences KAVGDPI and QGVVLRP. Researchers observed similar results when subjecting *Sorghum bicolor* to SGID, which led to a highly bioactive protein hydrolysate (IC_{50} value of 27.3 μg/mL). From this hydrolysate, three sequences could be identified (Table 33.1) (Majid et al. 2022).

Studies have also demonstrated that dark tea (*Camellia sinensis* L.) protein is an adequate source of DPP-IV peptides in vitro and in vivo in the spleen–brain axis of diabetic mice. Researchers identified sequences (Table 33.1) able to inhibit DPP-IV in vitro and reported that the extract could exert glucose-lowering effects by modulating the spleen–brain axis (Zhao et al. 2020; Su, Mao, and Zhang 2021).

ENZYMATIC HYDROLYSIS OF BYPRODUCTS AND COMMODITIES

As a byproduct of the brewing process, brewer's spent grain shows potential as a valuable source of bioactive peptides. Treatment with alcalase and Flavourzyme produced to highly DPP-IV inhibitory pool of peptides, although SGID reduced the bioactivity (Cermeño et al. 2019). In spite of that, researchers identified and characterised highly bioactive peptides (Table 33.1).

Recent studies have examined other commodity-derived proteins, such as lentil and potato (Rivero-Pino, Espejo-Carpio, and Guadix 2021; Ibrahim et al. 2019). Researchers have investigated potato peptides through in silico analyses (Ibrahim et al. 2019) and in vitro assays (Rivero-Pino et al. 2021). Treatment with alcalase, trypsin and Flavourzyme yielded less bioactive results compared to hydrolysates derived from other sources subjected to the same enzymatic treatment. However, when applied to lentil protein, this treatment led to a highly bioactive sample, with a reported IC_{50} value of 2.92 mg/mL.

DPP-IV lupin-derived peptides produced by hydrolysis with alcalase-trypsin-Flavourzyme showed an IC_{50} value of 3.42 mg/mL (Rivero-Pino, Espejo-Carpio, and Guadix 2021), though other reports have yielded different results (Lammi et al. 2016). Researchers have also evaluated the efficacy of lupin peptides in humans, although without reporting on the inhibition of DPP-IV, as will be described later.

Generally, the IC_{50} values of protein hydrolysates derived from plant sources are comparable to those obtained in animal-derived protein hydrolysates, typically ranging from 0.5 to 10 mg/mL. These findings imply that, along with serving as healthier and more environmentally friendly protein sources than those derived from animals, plant-based proteins' hydrolysis into bioactive peptides exhibits appropriate and equivalent outcomes to these conventional sources. The specificity of the proteases employed, as well as the state of the native protein, are the main parameters affecting the release of peptides during the reaction.

IDENTIFICATION OF PEPTIDES

Identifying the bioactive sequences enables the characterisation of obtained peptides to ensure their functionality for nutrition. The typical workflow involves enzymatic hydrolysis of the protein, concentration of low molecular weight peptides (by membranes having a cut-off <1 or 3 kDa, or via size exclusion chromatography) and purification by reverse-phase chromatography. Researchers then analyse the resulting sample using mass spectrometry, enabling the identification of specific sequences de novo. In addition, they can directly identify peptides in a hydrolysate by comparing it with the source's proteome.

Table 33.1 presents recent examples of active peptides identified as DPP-IV inhibitors with IC_{50} values determined in vitro. Validating the bioactivity with the pure peptide is crucial for understanding each peptide's contribution to the hydrolysate's bioactivity. Consequently, the relative abundance of the sequences is also relevant for understanding these mechanisms.

USE AS INGREDIENTS IN FOOD MATRICES

Using vegetable-derived peptides as functional ingredients is a recent priority, in line with societal concerns and food business operators' desire to manufacture appealing, nutritious and sustainable products. However, few studies examined the fortification of food matrices with vegetable peptides demonstrating DPP-IV inhibitory activity (Fan et al. 2022). This topic is important for understanding how amino acids interact with other components based on processing conditions (temperature, humidity, etc.), potentially producing new compounds which may be safe or concerning (Rivero-Pino 2023).

Acevedo-Martinez and de Mejia (2021) fortified a maize tortilla with DPP-IV inhibitory peptides from chickpea at levels ranging from 5 to 15%. They applied a heat treatment of 232°C for 2 minutes, which led to changes only in colour and texture and increased bioactivity from 11 to 26% (controls) to 91–95% in the 15% fortified sample. After SGID, they found no significant differences, indicating that the matrix helps maintain the structure of the bioactive peptides. Similarly, Felix et al. (2019) used a chickpea protein isolate to generate sunflower oil-in-water emulsions, which had DPP-IV inhibitory activity in vitro. This activity decreased during storage but increased when subjected to SGID, likely due to the release of smaller peptides from the isolate. Samaei et al. (2021) fortified an apple juice with a faba bean protein hydrolysate, demonstrating DPP-IV inhibitory peptides, though they did not report an experimental assay on the functional food's efficacy.

On top of that, researchers should assess the effect of heat treatments on these bioactive peptides' efficacy, as such temperature applications are common processes for ensuring microbiological safety in products. For example, the DPP-IV inhibitory effect of *Amaranthus hypochondriacus* L. peptides may be conserved or improved, depending on their processing conditions (López-Sánchez et al. 2016).

CHALLENGES AND PERSPECTIVES

PRODUCTION

Current literature suggests that using vegetable protein as a source of bioactive peptides is a promising research field with potential socioeconomic and environmental impact. Despite these advantages and the apparent health-promoting properties of these peptides, based on the assays reported here, many gaps and challenges remain.

Producing vegetable protein hydrolysates can be challenging, considering the protein's behaviour in production facilities, as solubility and/or viscosity can cause problems in some sources (Rivero-Pino, Espejo-Carpio, and Guadix 2021). In addition, researchers must evaluate the efficacy of the enzymatic hydrolysis and fermentation, and ensure consistency among batches at pilot plant and industrial levels, as most current studies are conducted at the laboratory level. In line with this, coupling these processes with pre-treatments such as non-thermal technologies (i.e., ultrasound or high-pressure processing) could be a key factor in improving current techno-functional challenges, while also promoting the release of bioactive peptides. Once researchers identify the protein containing the DPP-IV inhibitory peptides, they may optimise the generation of bioactive peptides by, for instance, removing other proteins prior to enzymatic hydrolysis based on their isoelectric point. This would prevent the production of non-bioactive peptides. Additionally, considering the molecular weight of the peptides after hydrolysis, separation via membranes could concentrate the bioactive peptides, which are usually smaller than 3 kDa.

SAFETY AND FEASIBILITY

It must be emphasised that new foods must undergo a safety evaluation before being put on the market, depending on regional regulations. This process may include microbiological examination or testing for toxins, aspects that have received limited attention in studies thus far. For protein hydrolysates intended as food ingredients, it is necessary to consider how bioactive peptides may alter a food's texture, colour, solubility, or viscosity. Therefore, assessing their impact on technological properties is crucial when creating the food (Rivero-Pino 2023).

EFFICACY IN ANIMAL STUDIES

While food-derived peptides appear promising, well-designed in vivo studies are necessary, as in vitro studies have limited relevance, not accounting for bioavailability, plasma stability, and the actual ability to inhibit the enzyme under physiological conditions (Table 33.2). Well-designed animal model studies (e.g., with rats) could be useful in understanding the in vivo fate of peptides

TABLE 33.2
Levels of Evidence Supporting the DPP-IV Inhibitory Activity of Peptides

Type of Study	Purpose	Limitations
In vitro	Screening of different compounds	No biological relevance
Animal	Mechanisms of action	Ethics and costs Not extrapolable to humans
Clinical trials	Causality	Ethics and costs Interindividual variability
Nutritional epidemiology	Statistical associations	Not easy to compare the results

Different types of studies that which can be used to demonstrate the DPP-IV inhibitory activity of peptides, highlighting the usefulness and limitations.

and whether they have an impact on the glucose homeostasis of the subjects. Some reports have shown benefits, but with specific peptides, such as the efficacy of the sequence GFAGDDAPR from black tea (*Camellia sinensis*). Its administration (400 mg/day) for 57 days to streptozotocin-induced hyperglycaemic mice resulted in increased GLP-1 and insulin blood levels, improved pancreatic β-cell function and suppressed proliferation of pancreatic α-cells (Lu et al. 2019). Similarly, Pei et al. (2022) showed that the broccoli-derived peptide VPLVM exerted an excellent hypoglycaemic effect 30 minutes after administration in the oral glucose tolerance test. The peptide also showed gastrointestinal enzyme resistance, could be transported through the Caco-2 cell monolayer via paracellular diffusion and demonstrated adequate in vitro plasma stability. Furthermore, it has been reported that the peptidic fraction from *Aloe vera* had beneficial effects in the alleviation of diabetes by maintaining intestinal permeability through regulating zonulin and GLP-1 levels, which was related to its inhibitory activity towards DPP-IV in diabetic rats, with a reported increase in GLP-1, among other changes (Babu et al. 2021).

Plant-derived peptides improving lipid and glucose metabolism through in vivo studies have been reported, but these are related to other activities, such as cholesterol lowering, triglyceride lowering, anti-obesity or inhibition of fatty acid synthase (Nagaoka, Takeuchi, and Banno 2021).

Human Studies

As indicated previously, most of the studies employing peptides/protein hydrolysates are in vitro studies or animal assays. The evidence in human studies remains scarce. A search of clinicaltrials.gov revealed no clinical trials related to interventions using vegetable-derived peptides to manage diabetes development by targeting DPP-IV. Thus, human studies assessing the safety and efficacy of DPP-IV inhibitory peptides are still a pending issue in evaluating the effectiveness of these protein hydrolysates. Some studies have aimed to demonstrate the benefits of plant peptides related to metabolic syndrome, but without measuring DPP-IV levels. For instance, it has been reported that a plant-based meal could increase gastrointestinal hormones (i.e., GLP-1, amylin, and peptide YY) and satiety more efficiently than a processed-meat meal in T2DM, obese, and healthy men in the postprandial period (up to 180 minutes). While DPP-IV levels were not measured, the changes in other hormones suggest possible effects due to the plant-derived components (Klementova et al. 2019).

Similarly, acute ingestion of different vegetable proteins (buckwheat, fava bean, pea, hemp, and lupin) showed a significant increase in GLP-1 plasma, especially with hemp consumption, compared to other plant-based meals, along with a decrease in plasma ghrelin concentrations. The peptides released after the ingestion of the protein might be responsible for this behaviour (Neacsu et al. 2022). Recently, a study reported on the efficacy of a drink fortified with lupine peptides on the immune, oxidative and lipid status in healthy subjects. A dose of 1 g for 1 month led to variations in many biochemical parameters in fasting peripheral blood and urine samples. The authors reported a decrease in the LDL-C/HDL-C atherogenic index and total cholesterol levels in the male cohort (Cruz-Chamorro et al. 2021).

Research

Evaluating protein hydrolysates presents challenges in drawing conclusions, as tracking the fate of each specific peptide is difficult, considering peptide degradation, absorption and distribution. Improving methodologies to assess the toxicokinetics of compounds is also crucial in the field of precision nutrition. While several products on the market assert health benefits because they include peptides, these benefits are often associated with improved digestibility or sensory factors.

A promising and increasingly popular methodological approach is the use of in silico tools, which enable simulation of enzymatic hydrolysis and identification and characterisation of peptides.

Functional foods can prevent or treat diseases at a lower cost than medical care, demonstrating a favourable effect on society's socioeconomic conditions. For this reason, investments in research and development in this field are necessary, and further investigations in the near future are needed to fully exploit vegetable protein-derived peptides for manufacturing antidiabetic ingredients capable of inhibiting DPP-IV in humans.

CONCLUSIONS

In recent times, various concerns (such as health risks, environmental issues, manufacturing costs, etc.) have led the food industry to prioritise plant-based components over animal sources. The enhancement of these sustainable proteins' bioactivity is being assessed to improve their potential health-promoting properties, which could benefit human physiology. Diabetes, one of the most prevalent diseases in society, is characterised by high blood glucose levels. Glucose homeostasis can potentially be regulated by inhibiting DPP-IV, an enzyme that affects the half-life of hormones related to insulin secretion. Studies have reported vegetable-derived peptides released by enzymatic hydrolysis or fermentation as efficient DPP-IV inhibitory peptides, mainly through in vitro assays and some animal studies.

MINI DICTIONARY OF TERMS

- **Dipeptidyl peptidase IV:** A protein exerting enzymatic activity, which degrades the incretin hormones GLP-1 and GIP.
- **Enzymatic hydrolysis:** The process of cleaving peptidic bonds, which allows the release of peptides from proteins with the aid of proteases.
- **Gastric inhibitory polypeptide:** A hormone that stimulates insulin secretion, exerts anti-apoptotic effects and induces beta cell growth in the pancreas.
- **Glucagon-like peptide-1:** An endogenous hormone produced in response to glucose. When released, it increases insulin secretion and reduces glucagon production.

SUMMARY POINTS

- This chapter focuses on dipeptidyl peptidase IV inhibitory peptides from vegetables.
- The bioactivity values of the hydrolysates range from 0.5 to 10 mg/mL.
- Low-molecular-weight peptides are more likely to be bioactive.
- Several peptides have been identified in vegetable sources.
- Soy and quinoa are among the most studied sources.

- The inhibitory activity of numerous peptides has been validated using synthetic peptides.
- Animal studies have shown the potential of peptides in vivo.
- Human studies demonstrating this bioactivity with vegetable peptides are lacking.
- Research on the functionality of peptides within food matrices is limited.
- Several industrial challenges need to be addressed to market vegetable-derived peptides.

REFERENCES

Acevedo-Martinez, Karla A., and Elvira Gonzalez de Mejia. 2021. "Fortification of Maize Tortilla with an Optimized Chickpea Hydrolysate and Its Effect on Dppiv Inhibition Capacity and Physicochemical Characteristics." *Foods* 10 (8). doi:10.3390/foods10081835.

Agustia, Friska Citra, Supriyadi, Agnes Murdiati, and Retno Indrati. 2023. "Formation of Dipeptidyl Peptidase-IV (DPP-IV) Inhibitory Peptides from Jack Bean (Canavalia Ensiformis (L.) DC.) Sprout in Simulated Digestion." *Food Science and Biotechnology* 0123456789. Springer Nature Singapore. doi:10.1007/s10068-023-01343-9.

Alfieri, Fabio, Fernando Rivero-Pino, Panagiota Zakidou, Antonio Fernandez-Dumont, and Ruth Roldán-Torres. 2023. "Processes for Obtaining Plant-Based Dairy and Meat Substitutes." In *Sustainable Food Science – A Comprehensive Approach*, 75–99. Elsevier. doi:10.1016/b978-0-12-823960-5.00051-2.

Babu, Spoorthy N., S. Govindarajan, M. A. Vijayalakshmi, and Ayesha Noor. 2021. "Role of Zonulin and GLP-1/DPP-IV in Alleviation of Diabetes Mellitus by Peptide/Polypeptide Fraction of Aloe Vera in Streptozotocin- Induced Diabetic Wistar Rats." *Journal of Ethnopharmacology* 272. Elsevier B.V.: 113949. doi:10.1016/j.jep.2021.113949.

Berraquero-García, Carmen, Fernando Rivero-Pino, Lizeth Ospina, Raul Perez-Galvez, F. Javier Espejo-Carpio, Antonio Guadix, Pedro J. García-Moreno, and Emilia M. Guadix. 2023. "Activity, Structural Features and in Silico Digestion of Antidiabetic Peptides." *Food Bioscience* 102954. doi:10.1016/j.fbio.2023.102954.

Bollati, Carlotta, Ruoxian Xu, Giovanna Boschin, Martina Bartolomei, Fabrizio Rivardo, Jianqiang Li, Anna Arnoldi, and Carmen Lammi. 2022. "Integrated Evaluation of the Multifunctional DPP-IV and ACE Inhibitory Effect of Soybean and Pea Protein Hydrolysates." *Nutrients* 14 (12): 1–14. doi:10.3390/nu14122379.

Cermeño, Maria, Alan Connolly, Martina B. O'Keeffe, Cal Flynn, Adeola M. Alashi, Rotimi E. Aluko, and Richard J. FitzGerald. 2019. "Identification of Bioactive Peptides from Brewers' Spent Grain and Contribution of Leu/Ile to Bioactive Potency." *Journal of Functional Foods* 60. Elsevier Ltd: 103455. doi:10.1016/j.jff.2019.103455.

Chan-Zapata, Ivan, Carlos Sandoval-Castro, and Maira Rubí Segura-Campos. 2022. "Proteins and Peptides from Vegetable Food Sources as Therapeutic Adjuvants for the Type 2 Diabetes Mellitus." *Critical Reviews in Food Science and Nutrition* 62 (10). Taylor & Francis: 2673–82. doi:10.1080/10408398.2020.1857331.

Chen, Hai-Hong Hong, Wei Li, Yi Wang, Bing Xu, Xi Hu, Xiao-Bing Bing Li, Jun-Yu Yu Liu, Chong Can-Yang Yang Zhang, Chong Can-Yang Yang Zhang, and Xin-Hui Hui Xing. 2023. "Mining and Validation of Novel Hemp Seed-Derived DPP-IV-Inhibiting Peptides Using a Combination of Multi-Omics and Molecular Docking." *Journal of Agricultural and Food Chemistry*, April. American Chemical Society. doi:10.1021/acs.jafc.3c00535.

Chourasia, Rounak, Loreni Chiring Phukon, Md Minhajul Abedin, Srichandan Padhi, Sudhir P. Singh, and Amit Kumar Rai. 2023. "Bioactive Peptides in Fermented Foods and Their Application: A Critical Review." *Systems Microbiology and Biomanufacturing* 3 (1). Springer Nature Singapore: 88–109. doi:10.1007/s43393-022-00125-4.

Cruz-Casas, Dora Elisa, Cristóbal N. Aguilar, Juan A. Ascacio-Valdés, Raúl Rodríguez-Herrera, Mónica L. Chávez-González, and Adriana C. Flores-Gallegos. 2021. "Enzymatic Hydrolysis and Microbial Fermentation: The Most Favorable Biotechnological Methods for the Release of Bioactive Peptides." *Food Chemistry: Molecular Sciences* 3: 100047. doi:10.1016/j.fochms.2021.100047.

Cruz-Chamorro, Ivan, Nuria Álvarez-Sánchez, Ana Isabel Álvarez-Ríos, Guillermo Santos-Sánchez, Justo Pedroche, Francisco Millán, Cecilio Carrera Sánchez, et al. 2021. "Safety and Efficacy of a Beverage Containing Lupine Protein Hydrolysates on the Immune, Oxidative and Lipid Status in Healthy Subjects: An Intervention Study (the Lupine-1 Trial)." *Molecular Nutrition and Food Research* 65 (14): 1–10. doi:10.1002/mnfr.202100139.

EFSA NDA Panel. 2022. "Scientific Advice Related to Nutrient Profiling for the Development of Harmonised Mandatory Front-of-pack Nutrition Labelling and the Setting of Nutrient Profiles for Restricting Nutrition and Health Claims on Foods." *EFSA Journal* 20 (4). doi:10.2903/j.efsa.2022.7259.

Fan, Hongxiu, Hongcheng Liu, Yanrong Zhang, Shanshan Zhang, Tingting Liu, and Dawei Wang. 2022. "Review on Plant-Derived Bioactive Peptides: Biological Activities, Mechanism of Action and Utilizations in Food Development." *Journal of Future Foods* 2 (2). Elsevier B.V.: 143–59. doi:10.1016/j.jfutfo.2022.03.003.

Farias, Ticiane Carvalho, Thaiza Serrano Pinheiro de Souza, Ana Elizabeth Cavalcante Fai, and Maria Gabriela Bello Koblitz. 2022. "Critical Review for the Production of Antidiabetic Peptides by a Bibliometric Approach." *Nutrients* 14 (20): 1–19. doi:10.3390/nu14204275.

Felix, Manuel, Maria Cermeño, Alberto Romero, and Richard J. FitzGerald. 2019. "Characterisation of the Bioactive Properties and Microstructure of Chickpea Protein-Based Oil in Water Emulsions." *Food Research International* 121. Elsevier: 577–85. doi:10.1016/j.foodres.2018.12.022.

Gonzalez-Montoya, Marcela, Blanca Hernández-Ledesma, Rosalva Mora-Escobedo, and Cristina Martinez-Villaluenga. 2018. "Bioactive Peptides from Germinated Soybean with Anti-Diabetic Potential by Inhibition of Dipeptidyl Peptidase-IV, a-Amylase, and a-Glucosidase Enzymes." *International Journal of Molecular Sciences* 19: 2883. doi:10.3390/ijms19102883.

Ibrahim, Mohammed Auwal, Megan J. Bester, Albert W. Neitz, and Anabella R. M. Gaspar. 2019. "Tuber Storage Proteins as Potential Precursors of Bioactive Peptides: An In Silico Analysis." *International Journal of Peptide Research and Therapeutics* 25. Springer Netherlands: 437–46. doi:10.1007/s10989-018-9688-7.

Ibrahim, Mohammed Auwal, June Cheptoo Serem, Aliyu Dantani Abdullahi, Suleiman Aminu, Abubakar Babando Aliyu, Aliyu Muhammad Musa, Bashir Musa, Megan J. Bester, and Anabella R. M. Gaspar. 2023. "Bioactive Peptides from African Yam (AVIAIMF and GPADPF) and Taro (NGDF and NGNW) Reveal Multifunctional Antidiabetic Effects Using Biochemical and Cellular Models." *International Journal of Peptide Research and Therapeutics* 29 (3). Springer Netherlands. doi:10.1007/s10989-023-10518-1.

Jia, Wanqing, Elvira Rodriguez-Alonso, Marine Bianeis, Julia K. Keppler, and Atze Jan van der Goot. 2021. "Assessing Functional Properties of Rapeseed Protein Concentrate versus Isolate for Food Applications." *Innovative Food Science and Emerging Technologies* 68. Elsevier Ltd: 102636. doi:10.1016/j.ifset.2021.102636.

Klementova, Marta, Lenka Thieme, Martin Haluzik, Renata Pavlovicova, Martin Hill, Terezie Pelikanova, and Hana Kahleova. 2019. "A Plant-Based Meal Increases Gastrointestinal Hormones and Satiety More than an Energy-and-Macronutrient-Matched Processed-Meat Meal in T2d, Obese, and Healthy Men: A Three-Group Randomized Crossover Study." *Nutrients* 11 (1): 1–10. doi:10.3390/nu11010157.

Lammi, Carmen, Chiara Zanoni, Anna Arnoldi, and Giulio Vistoli. 2016. "Peptides Derived from Soy and Lupin Protein as Dipeptidyl-Peptidase IV Inhibitors: In Vitro Biochemical Screening and in Silico Molecular Modeling Study." *Journal of Agricultural and Food Chemistry* 64: 9601–6. doi:10.1021/acs.jafc.6b04041.

López-Sánchez, J., E. Ponce-Alquicira, R. Pedroza-Islas, A. de la Peña-Díaz, and J. Soriano-Santos. 2016. "Effects of Heat and PH Treatments and in Vitro Digestion on the Biological Activity of Protein Hydrolysates of Amaranthus Hypochondriacus L. Grain." *Journal of Food Science and Technology* 53 (12): 4298–307. doi:10.1007/s13197-016-2428-0.

Lu, Y., P. Lu, Y. Wang, X. Fang, J. Wu, and X. Wang. 2019. "A Novel Dipeptidyl Peptidase IV Inhibitory Tea Peptide Improves Pancreatic β-Cell Function and Reduces α-Cell Proliferation in Streptozotocin-Induced Diabetic Mice." *International Journal of Molecular Sciences* 20 (2): 322.

Majid, Abdul, M. Lakshmikanth, N. K. Lokanath, and C. G. Poornima Priyadarshini. 2022. "Generation, Characterization and Molecular Binding Mechanism of Novel Dipeptidyl Peptidase-4 Inhibitory Peptides from Sorghum Bicolor Seed Protein." *Food Chemistry* 369. Elsevier Ltd: 130888. doi:10.1016/j.foodchem.2021.130888.

Mills, Hilla, Ronald Acquah, Nova Tang, Luke Cheung, Susanne Klenk, Ronald Glassen, Magali Pirson, Alain Albert, Duong Trinh Hoang, and Thang Nguyen Van. 2022. "Type 2 Diabetes Mellitus (T2DM) and Carbohydrate Metabolism in Relation to T2DM from Endocrinology, Neurophysiology, Molecular Biology, and Biochemistry Perspectives." *Evidence-Based Complementary and Alternative Medicine* 2022. doi:10.1155/2022/1708769.

Mojica, Luis, Karen Chen, and Elvira González de Mejía. 2015. "Impact of Commercial Precooking of Common Bean (Phaseolus Vulgaris) on the Generation of Peptides, After Pepsin-Pancreatin Hydrolysis, Capable to Inhibit Dipeptidyl Peptidase-IV." *Journal of Food Science* 80 (1): H188–98. doi:10.1111/1750-3841.12726.

Mostafa, Hussein, Noura Al-Ahbabi, Oladipupo Qudus Adiamo, Priti Mudgil, and Sajid Maqsood. 2022. "Phoenix Dactylifera L. Seed Protein Hydrolysates as a Potential Source of Peptides with Antidiabetic and Anti-Hypercholesterolemic Properties: An in Vitro Study." *Food Bioscience* 49. Elsevier Ltd: 101916. doi:10.1016/j.fbio.2022.101916.

Mudgil, Priti, Bhanu Priya, Hina Kamal, Olusegun Abayomi, Richard J Fitzgerald, Chee-yuen Gan, and Sajid Maqsood. 2020. "Multifunctional Bioactive Peptides Derived from Quinoa Protein Hydrolysates : Inhibition of α-Glucosidase, Dipeptidyl Peptidase-IV and Angiotensin I Converting Enzymes." *Journal of Cereal Science* 96. Elsevier Ltd: 103130. doi:10.1016/j.jcs.2020.103130.

Nadathur, S. R., J. P.D. Wanasundara, and L. Scanlin. 2017. "Proteins in the Diet: Challenges in Feeding the Global Population." In *Sustainable Protein Sources*, 1–19. Elsevier Inc. doi:10.1016/B978-0-12-802778-3.00001-9.

Nagaoka, Satoshi, Asahi Takeuchi, and Arata Banno. 2021. "Plant-Derived Peptides Improving Lipid and Glucose Metabolism." *Peptides* 142. Elsevier Inc.: 170577. doi:10.1016/j.peptides.2021.170577.

Neacsu, Madalina, Nicholas J. Vaughan, Salvatore Multari, Elisabeth Haljas, Lorraine Scobbie, Gary J. Duncan, Louise Cantlay, et al. 2022. "Hemp and Buckwheat Are Valuable Sources of Dietary Amino Acids, Beneficially Modulating Gastrointestinal Hormones and Promoting Satiety in Healthy Volunteers." *European Journal of Nutrition* 61 (2). Springer Berlin Heidelberg: 1057–72. doi:10.1007/s00394-021-02711-z.

Nongonierma, Alice B., and Richard J. FitzGerald. 2015. "Investigation of the Potential of Hemp, Pea, Rice and Soy Protein Hydrolysates as a Source of Dipeptidyl Peptidase IV (DPP-IV) Inhibitory Peptides." *Food Digestion* 6: 19–29. doi:10.1007/s13228-015-0039-2.

Oseguera-Toledo, Miguel Eduardo, Elvira Gonzalez de Mejia, and Silvia L. Amaya-Llano. 2015. "Hard-to-Cook Bean (Phaseolus Vulgaris L.) Proteins Hydrolyzed by Alcalase and Bromelain Produced Bioactive Peptide Fractions That Inhibit Targets of Type-2 Diabetes and Oxidative Stress." *Food Research International* 76: 839–51. doi:10.1016/j.foodres.2015.07.046.

Pei, Jingyan, Zhu Liu, Daodong Pan, Yufen Zhao, Yali Dang, and Xinchang Gao. 2022. "Transport, Stability, and in Vivo Hypoglycemic Effect of a Broccoli-Derived DPP-IV Inhibitory Peptide VPLVM." *Journal of Agricultural and Food Chemistry* 70 (16): 4934–41. doi:10.1021/acs.jafc.1c08191.

Ramírez Fuentes, Lourdes, Caroline Richard, and Lingyun Chen. 2021. "Sequential Alcalase and Flavourzyme Treatment for Preparation of α-Amylase, α-Glucosidase, and Dipeptidyl Peptidase (DPP)-IV Inhibitory Peptides from Oat Protein." *Journal of Functional Foods* 87. Elsevier Ltd: 104829. doi:10.1016/j.jff.2021.104829.

Ramírez, Karina, Karen V. Pineda-Hidalgo, and Jesús J. Rochín-Medina. 2021. "Fermentation of Spent Coffee Grounds by Bacillus Clausii Induces Release of Potentially Bioactive Peptides." *Lwt* 138. Elsevier Ltd: 110685. doi:10.1016/j.lwt.2020.110685.

Rivero-Pino, Fernando. 2023. "Bioactive Food-Derived Peptides for Functional Nutrition: Effect of Fortification, Processing and Storage on Peptide Stability and Bioactivity within Food Matrices." *Food Chemistry* 406. Elsevier Ltd: 135046. doi:10.1016/j.foodchem.2022.135046.

Rivero-Pino, Fernando, F. Javier Espejo-Carpio, and Emilia M. Guadix. 2021. "Identification of Dipeptidyl Peptidase IV (DPP-IV) Inhibitory Peptides from Vegetable Protein Sources." *Food Chemistry* 354. Elsevier Ltd: 129473. doi:10.1016/j.foodchem.2021.129473.

Samaei, Seyedeh P, Serena Martini, Davide Tagliazucchi, Andrea Gianotti, and Elena Babini. 2021. "Antioxidant and Angiotensin I – Converting Enzyme (ACE) Inhibitory Peptides Obtained from Alcalase Protein Hydrolysate Fractions of Hemp (Cannabis Sativa L.) Bran." *Journal of Agricultural and Food Chemistry*. doi:10.1021/acs.jafc.1c01487.

Samaranayaka, A. 2017. "Lentil: Revival of Poor Man's Meat." In *Sustainable Protein Sources*, 185–96. Elsevier Inc. doi:10.1016/B978-0-12-802778-3.00011-1.

Sato, Kousuke, Syogo Miyasaka, Akira Tsuji, and Hiroshi Tachi. 2018. "Isolation and Characterization of Peptides with Dipeptidyl Peptidase IV (DPPIV) Inhibitory Activity from Natto Using DPPIV from Aspergillus Oryzae." *Food Chemistry* 261. Elsevier: 51–56. doi:10.1016/j.foodchem.2018.04.029.

Sharma, Poorva, Deepansh Sharma, Sawinder Kaur, and Anjan Borah. 2021. "Optimization of Flaxseed Milk Fermentation for the Production of Functional Peptides and Estimation of Their Bioactivities." *Food Science and Technology International* 27 (7): 585–97. doi:10.1177/1082013220973815.

Su, Keying, Xinliang Mao, and Xuewu Zhang. 2021. "Glucose-Lowering Activity of Dark Tea Protein Extract by Modulating Spleen–Brain Axis of Diabetic Mice." *British Journal of Nutrition* 126: 961–69. doi:10.1017/S0007114520005012.

Taga, Yuki, Osamu Hayashida, Masashi Kusubata, Kiyoko Ogawa-Goto, and Shunji Hattori. 2017. "Production of a Novel Wheat Gluten Hydrolysate Containing Dipeptidyl Peptidase-IV Inhibitory Tripeptides Using Ginger Protease." *Bioscience, Biotechnology, and Biochemistry* 81 (9). Oxford Academic: 1823–28. doi :10.1080/09168451.2017.1345615.

Thakur, Shweta, Jyoti Chhimwal, Robin Joshi, Manglesh Kumari, Yogendra Padwad, and Rajiv Kumar. 2021. "Evaluating Peptides of Picrorhiza Kurroa and Their Inhibitory Potential against ACE, DPP-IV, and Oxidative Stress." *Journal of Proteome Research* 20 (8): 3798–813. doi:10.1021/acs.jproteome.1c00081.

Tilman, David, and Michael Clark. 2014. "Global Diets Link Environmental Sustainability and Human Health." *Nature* 515. Nature Publishing Group: 518–22. doi:10.1038/nature13959.

Vilcacundo, Rubén, Cristina Martínez-Villaluenga, and Blanca Hernández-Ledesma. 2017. "Release of Dipeptidyl Peptidase IV, α-Amylase and α-Glucosidase Inhibitory Peptides from Quinoa (Chenopodium Quinoa Willd.) during in Vitro Simulated Gastrointestinal Digestion." *Journal of Functional Foods* 35. Elsevier: 531–39. doi:10.1016/J.JFF.2017.06.024.

Wang, Feng, Guoyong Yu, Yanyan Zhang, Bolin Zhang, Junfeng Fan, Wang F, Yu G, Zhang Y, Zhang B, and Fan J. 2015. "Dipeptidyl Peptidase IV Inhibitory Peptides Derived from Oat (Avena Sativa L.), Buckwheat (Fagopyrum Esculentum), and Highland Barley (Hordeum Vulgare Trifurcatum (L.) Trofim) Proteins." *Journal of Agricultural and Food Chemistry* 63 (43): 9543–49. doi:10.1021/acs.jafc.5b04016.

Wang, Wei, Xiaoqing Liu, Yiju Li, Haixi You, Zhipeng Yu, Liying Wang, Xuebo Liu, and Long Ding. 2022. "Identification and Characterization of Dipeptidyl Peptidase-IV Inhibitory Peptides from Oat Proteins." *Foods* 11 (10): 1–11. doi:10.3390/foods11101406.

Xu, Feiran, Yijun Yao, Xiaoying Xu, Mei Wang, Mengmeng Pan, Shengyang Ji, Jin Wu, Donglei Jiang, Xingrong Ju, and Lifeng Wang. 2019. "Identification and Quantification of DPP-IV-Inhibitory Peptides from Hydrolyzed-Rapeseed-Protein-Derived Napin with Analysis of the Interactions between Key Residues and Protein Domains." *Journal of Agricultural and Food Chemistry* 67 (13). American Chemical Society: 3679–90. doi:10.1021/acs.jafc.9b01069.

You, Haixi, Tianliang Wu, Wei Wang, Yiju Li, Xuebo Liu, and Long Ding. 2022. "Preparation and Identification of Dipeptidyl Peptidase IV Inhibitory Peptides from Quinoa Protein." *Food Research International* 156. Elsevier Ltd: 111176. doi:10.1016/j.foodres.2022.111176.

You, Haixi, Yu Zhang, Tianliang Wu, Juanrui Li, Liying Wang, Zhipeng Yu, Jingbo Liu, Xuebo Liu, and Long Ding. 2022. "Identification of Dipeptidyl Peptidase IV Inhibitory Peptides from Rapeseed Proteins." *Lwt* 160. Elsevier Ltd: 113255. doi:10.1016/j.lwt.2022.113255.

Zan, Rong, Qiming Wu, Yiling Chen, Gangcheng Wu, Hui Zhang, and Ling Zhu. 2023. "Identification of Novel Dipeptidyl Peptidase-IV Inhibitory Peptides in Chickpea Protein Hydrolysates." *Journal of Agricultural and Food Chemistry* 12 (8). doi:10.1021/acs.jafc.3c00603.

Zhang, Aiyuan, Kai Wang, Xiaofei Liu, and Xuewu Zhang. 2023. "Isolation and Identification of Dipeptidyl Peptidase-IV Inhibitory Peptides from Sacha Inchi Meal." *Journal of the Science of Food and Agriculture* 103: 2926–38. doi:10.1002/jsfa.12464.

Zhang, Mingkai, Ling Zhu, Gangcheng Wu, Tongtong Liu, Xiguang Qi, and Hui Zhang. 2022. "Rapid Screening of Novel Dipeptidyl Peptidase-4 Inhibitory Peptides from Pea (Pisum Sativum L.) Protein Using Peptidomics and Molecular Docking." *Journal of Agricultural and Food Chemistry* 70 (33): 10221–28. doi:10.1021/acs.jafc.2c03949.

Zhao, Bingli, Keying Su, Xinliang Mao, and Xuewu Zhang. 2020. "Separation and Identification of Enzyme Inhibition Peptides from Dark Tea Protein." *Bioorganic Chemistry* 99 (June). Elsevier: 103772. doi:10.1016/j.bioorg.2020.103772.

Zhou, Tingyi, Zhu Liu, Jingyan Pei, Daodong Pan, Xinchang Gao, Yali Dang, and Yufen Zhao. 2021. "Novel Broccoli-Derived Peptides Hydrolyzed by Trypsin with Dual-Angiotensin I-Converting Enzymes and Dipeptidyl Peptidase-IV-Inhibitory Activities." *Journal of Agricultural and Food Chemistry* 69 (37): 10885–92. doi:10.1021/acs.jafc.1c02985.

34 Lupin as a Source of Dietary Protein in the Human Diet

Maria E. Martin Rubio, Ana Lemus Conejo, Fernando Rivero-Pino, and Maria C. Millan Linares

LUPIN AS AN ALTERNATIVE SOURCE OF DIETARY PROTEIN

In the new global economy, novel protein sources for the human diet have been attracting considerable interest due to the production costs and the environmental impact caused by animal protein manufacture. Plant proteins have emerged as major contributors in the effort to face the urgent need for healthy and sustainable food products for human consumption, where underutilized legumes of high protein content represent a potential source of low-cost and healthy protein alternatives (Colgrave et al. 2021).

The term legumes or pulses refers to the harvested crop of dried legume seeds, excluding legumes used to obtain oil, such as soybeans and peanuts, and green leafy plants, such as mung beans, peas and sprouts, which are considered vegetables (Kouris-Blazos and Belski 2016). These crops offer several advantages in terms of nutrition, health and sustainability, requiring less land, water or resources and becoming a cheaper and harmless alternative to meat (Hughes et al. 2022). Furthermore, legumes offer diverse culinary possibilities, and combining and fortifying them with grains, roots and tubers could be a way to alleviate poverty and malnutrition in developing countries (Herforth et al. 2019).

The genus *Lupinus* L. belongs to the *Fabaceae* or *Leguminosae* family and, within this, to the *Faboideae* subfamily (Ishaq et al. 2022) (Figure 34.1). There are about 200 varieties of *Lupinus* classified as "Old World" species, spread between the Mediterranean and North and East Africa, and "New World" species located in South and North America (Abreu et al. 2023). This cultivar presents high adaptability to different soil or climate conditions, low phosphorous requirements and an important nitrogen fixation ability, which avoids using nitrogen fertilizers and thus improves the quality of the crops. However, not all *Lupinus* species are suitable for human consumption due to the level of toxic alkaloids that the seeds can contain the seed. Lupines with a low content of alkaloids are called sweet lupine (Figure 34.2) (Osorio and Till 2022). Nowadays, only four of these species are cultivated for consumption: *Lupinus angustifolius* L. (Figure 34.2A), known as blue lupine or narrow-leaved lupin; *Lupinus luteus* L., known as yellow lupine (Figure 34.2B); *Lupinus albus* L. (Figure 34.2C), called white lupine; and *Lupinus mutabilis* L. (Figure 34.2D), known as Andean lupine (*USDA Plants Database* n.d.). *L. albus* is mainly produced in Europe, *L. angustifolius* is produced only in Australia, *L. luteus* is widely distributed in the Mediterranean region, and *L. mutabilis* is cultivated in South America (Lemus-Conejo et al. 2023; Magalhães et al. 2017; Mane et al. 2018).

LUPIN'S NUTRITIONAL POTENTIAL AND PROTEIN QUALITY

The Food and Agriculture Organization of the United Nations (FAO) classifies the genus *Lupinus* as part of the pulses group, which consists of protein-rich crops (FAO n.d.). Traditionally, lupins have been used as inexpensive legumes for soil improvement, animal feeding and human nutrition in

DOI: 10.1201/9781003597926-34

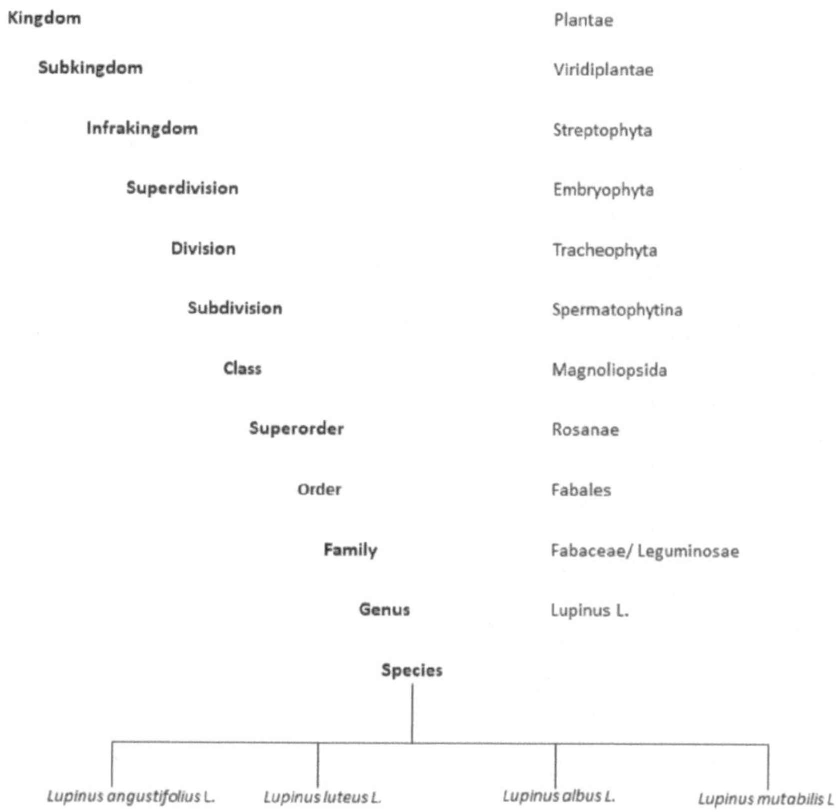

FIGURE 34.1 Taxonomy of the sweet *Lupinus* species. This figure shows the taxonomic levels from the Plantae kingdom to the edible *Lupinus* species. Figure compiled by the authors, based on information from the USDA-ARS Germplasm Resources Information Network (GRIN), accessed September 20, 2023.

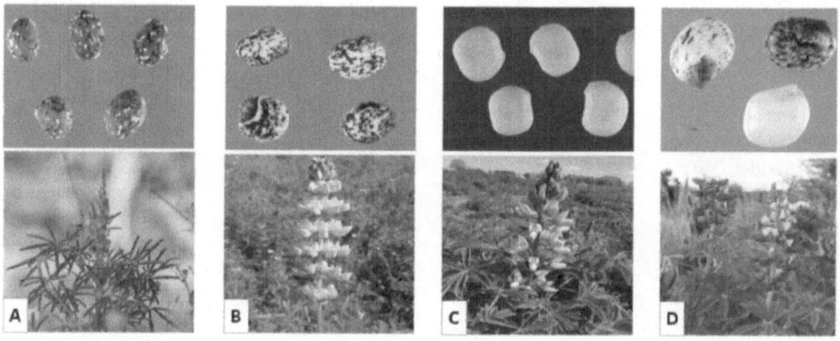

FIGURE 34.2 Pictures of sweet *Lupinus* species. This figure shows the plants and seeds of the four edible Lupinus. (A) *Lupinus angustifolius* L.; (B) *Lupinus luteus* L.; (C) *Lupinus albus* L.; (D) *Lupinus mutabilis* L. Figure compiled by the authors, based on information from Lemus-Conejo et al. (2023).

low-income countries, mainly in South America and the Mediterranean region. However, evidence suggests that lupin species may become a remarkable environmentally friendly protein source for underdeveloped and developed countries, replacing soybean as the main source of protein foods so far (Abraham et al. 2019).

On top of that, not only proteins but also other lupin components have been demonstrated to exert biological activities preventing current chronic diseases such as obesity, hypertension, hypercholesterolemia, diabetes, cancer or cardiovascular disease (Ferchichi et al. 2021; Lemus-Conejo et al. 2023).

Lupins have remarkable nutritional properties compared to other legumes due to their high protein content and dietary fibre, which are of high quality but have a low percentage of fat and scarce starch levels (Table 34.1). Lupin seeds' protein content ranges from 31% to 52% of their dry weight, depending on the cultivar conditions, in the four edible species. Moreover, the *in vivo* digestibility values are between 89% and 91%, largely due to their low content of lectins, saponins and protease inhibitors compared to beans and soybeans, among others (Monteiro et al. 2014).

Globulins are the most abundant proteins in lupin seeds, comprising nearly 90% of total content, followed by albumin, while gluten is absent in lupin plants. According to the sedimentation coefficient, lupin seed storage proteins are classified into 2S (generally termed albumin), 7S and 11S classes (sub-classes of the globulins). Nevertheless, there is evidence of the allergenic potential of some lupin proteins, such as conglutins, which is an important issue for many consumers (Shrestha et al. 2021).

The amino acid profile of these pulses is also important due to the presence of those essentials exceeding the standard requirements, although with low levels of sulphur amino acids, such as methionine (Table 34.2) (Carvajal-Larenas et al. 2016; Lemus-Conejo et al. 2023).

On the other hand, lupin proteins include short peptides of 2–20 amino acids in their structure, which may exert biological activities once released, depending on the amino acid sequence. Over the past decades, this has led to the optimization of protocols aimed at obtaining isolates and hydrolysates as protein-derived products of interest for the human diet. More recently, bioinformatic approaches (*in silico*) have helped search for the most suitable sequences of amino acids in available databases (Garmidolova et al. 2022). Biopeptides are inactive in the native protein but, after enzymatic cleavage in our digestive system, may reach systemic circulation and act as bioactive molecules (Millan-Linares et al. 2015), opening new perspectives in the search for new natural food

TABLE 34.1
Comparative Analysis of the Chemical Compositions of Edible *Lupinus* Species

Component	*L. albus*	*L. angustifolius*	*L. luteus*	*L. mutabilis*
Crude protein (% of DM*)	33–47	31–37	37–38	32–52
Crude ash (g)	3.4	3	3.8	3.9
Crude fibre (% of DM)	13–16	15–17	12–15	10
Oil (%)	6–13	6–7	5–9	13–24
Total oligosaccharides (% of DM)	7–8	8–9	NA	NA
Non-starch polysaccharides (%)	18	47–51	NA	NA
Metabolized energy (MJ/kg DM)	13–16	12–13	10	NA
Minerals (mg/100g DW)**				
Ca	200	232	210	147
Cu	0.5	0.5	0.9	1.0
Fe	2.6	6.1	9.3	5.9
K	NA	NA	NA	1265
Mg	NA	NA	NA	285
Mn	83.5	2.1	8.6	3.2
P	360	321	610	753

This table compares the general composition of sweet *Lupinus* species (Ishaq et al. 2022; Lemus-Conejo et al. 2023). *DM = dry matter; **DW = dry weight; NA = not available.

TABLE 34.2
Comparative Amino Acid Profile of Seeds, Flours, and Isolates from the Edible *Lupine* Genus (g/100 g protein)

Amino Acid	*L. albus*			*L. angustifolius*[a]			*L. luteus*			*L. mutabilis*			FAO Reference Values
	Seed[b,c]	Flour[d]	Protein Isolate[e]	Seed	Flour	Protein Isolate	Seed[b,f]	Flour[d,g]	Protein Isolate[g]	Seed[f]	Flour[d]	Protein Isolate[d]	
Essential													
Isoleucine	4.1	4.71	4.49	3.54	5.50	5.90	3.6	3.48	3.96	4.2	4.82	5.25	3.30
Histidine	2.0	2.38	2.09	3.75	2.70	2.70	3.1	2.56	2.54	3.5	2.95	2.72	1.50
Leucine	6.8	7.74	7.62	5.90	8.70	9.40	7.8	7.16	8.17	7	6.87	7.38	5.90
Lysine	4.5	5.02	4.25	5.26	5.40	4.30	4.5	4.51	4.60	5.8	5.93	5.59	4.50
Methionine	0.7	0.76	0.26	0.53	1.30	0.70	0.6	0.47	0.41	0.8	0.73	0.68	1.60
Phenylalanine	3.4	4.07	4.60	3.48	5.20	6.10	3.7	3.52	3.97	3.5	3.97	4.31	
Threonine	3.4	3.65	3.30	3.27	4.90	6.40	3.0	2.94	2.72	3.5	3.61	3.43	2.30
Valine	3.8	4.35	3.65	3.57	3.90	4.80	3.4	3.28	3.28	3.8	4.32	4.59	3.90
Cysteine	1.5	1.74	1.10	1.38	3.50	2.90	2.4	1.95	2.08	1.6	1.46	1.14	0.60
Tryptophan	0.9	0.76	0.57	0.60	0.60	0.60	0.9	0.72	0.66	0.8	0.97	1.00	0.60
Non-essential													
Alanine	2.69	3.45	2.94	3.03	3.80	3.00	3.6	2.95	2.70	3.3	3.73	3.53	
Arginine	12.4	10.86	11.60	12.17	11.50	13.50	9.1	11.1	11.4	10.2	10.67	11.19	
Aspartic acid	10.55	10.52	10.81	8.95	11.60	6.90	11.6	9.64	10.5	9.6	10.36	10.39	
Glutamic acid	27.40	21.66	23.13	22.74	25.60	19.90	23.7	21.6	26.1	24.3	22.45	22.03	
Glycine	3.68	4.07	3.79	3.98	4.60	5.30	4.5	3.56	3.53	3.8	4.25	4.04	
Proline	4.38	4.38	3.97	5.58	4.60	8.80	2.3	3.67	3.82	3.8	4.23	4.37	
Serine	5.35	4.63	5.57	4.39	7.10	7.70	6.5	4.64	5.11	4.9	4.04	4.22	
Tyrosine	4.8	4.32	5.23	3.47	5.9	7.5	2.9	2.65	2.80	4.0	4.20	4.26	

Data expressed as g/100 g protein. FAO: Reference amino acid values recommended by the Food and Agriculture Organization of the United Nations for evaluating protein quality in human nutrition (FAO, 2013). Sources: [a] Lemus-Conejo et al. (2023); [b] Carvajal-Larenas et al. (2016); [c] Duranti and Cerletti (1979); [d] Aguilar-Acosta et al. (2020); [e] Vogelsang-O'Dwyer et al. (2020); [f] Pastor-Cavada et al. (2009); [g] Burgos-Díaz et al. (2019).

byproducts for humans. So far, data from several studies show anti-inflammatory, antihypertensive, hypocholesterolemic, antidiabetic, antioxidant and antibacterial effects of peptides from lupin seeds (Garmidolova et al. 2022; Guo et al. 2018; Mathew et al. 2018).

RESEARCH REGARDING *LUPINUS* PROTEIN BYPRODUCTS IN HUMAN NUTRITION

The global population is expected to rise to 9.7 billion by 2050, necessitating over 70% more food than is currently being produced (Colgrave et al. 2021). Consequently, promoting a sustainable food system is a major issue for a future circular green economy approach, in line with objectives such as Zero Hunger (goal 2), Good Health and Well-Being (goal 3) and Responsible Consumption and Production (goal 12) included in the 2030 United Nations Agenda.

Lupin crops meet the needs of environmentally friendly, inexpensive cultivars, resulting in nutritional products and post-harvest biomass residues or byproducts with remarkable health-promoting potential due to their protein and bioactive peptide content. Thus, *Lupinus* species become a promising novel source of protein-enriched food products with healthy properties suitable for human consumption (Shrestha et al. 2021).

In line with this, previous research points to γ-conglutin, included in lupin globulins, as a glycaemia control agent both *in vitro* conditions and in rat models. There are many studies relating the ingestion of lupin protein with improvements in lipid metabolism, but these studies were mainly carried out in animals rather than in humans (Bryant et al. 2022; Rosa Lovati et al. 2012; Santos-Sánchez et al. 2022). In any case, several questions remain regarding the bioavailability and bioactivity of peptides from lupins. Thus, more *in vitro* and *in vivo* studies are needed to establish the potential of lupin byproducts rich in proteins and peptides in new nutritional strategies (Lemus-Conejo et al. 2023; Santos-Sánchez et al. 2022).

In addition, should lupin-based foods demonstrate a preventive role in chronic diseases, it would confer an advantage over other traditional protein crops such as soya cultivars.

Given all that has been mentioned so far, the genus *Lupinus* appears to be an inexpensive source of healthy protein for human consumption. The food industry has already leveraged lupin proteins due to their good solubility and techno-functional properties, such as emulsion, gelling and foaming abilities, as well as their water and fat absorption degree (Garmidolova et al. 2022; Khan et al. 2015; Mota et al. 2020; Shevkani et al. 2019; Villarino et al. 2015). So far, these products have shown wide consumer acceptance, including gluten-free food consumers. From now on, a greater focus on clinical trials and peptidome studies using proteases may help the agri-food industry design the most desirable proteins using profitable processes for human diets as functional foods, low-allergenic products or added ingredients (Abraham et al. 2019; Tahmasian et al. 2023).

In summary, during the following decades, lupins may play an outstanding role as a green crop, providing a more sustainable diet as an alternative to animal proteins with novel byproducts aimed at improving the nutrition of the global population using affordable food sources.

ISOLATES, PROTEIN HYDROLYSATES, AND BIOACTIVE PEPTIDES

Protein concentrates and isolates are considered high-value-added products due to their high protein content (over 80–90%) (Figure 34.3). Numerous studies have focused on obtaining these products, including some of the main lupin varieties (i.e., *Lupinus albus* and *Lupinus angustifolius*). Data from several sources have reported high protein extraction yield and solubility by different isolation techniques, with the most widespread method being extraction at alkaline pH (10–12) and subsequent precipitation to the isoelectric point or ultrafiltration, followed by micellization or acid extraction method (Boukid and Pasqualone 2022). The commercial application of these protein products is dependent on their functional properties. Lupine protein isolates and concentrates

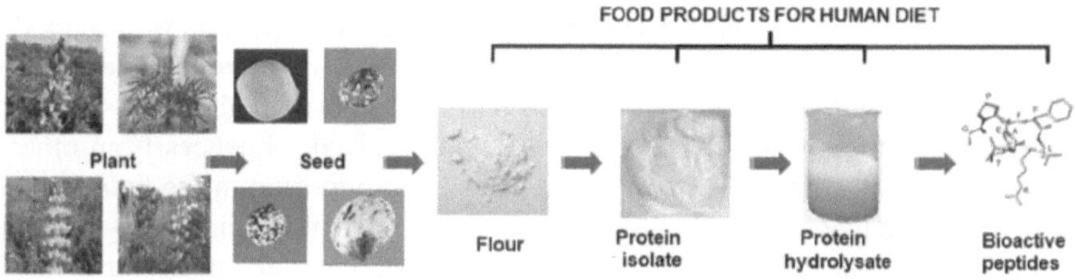

FIGURE 34.3 Obtention of products for human diet from *Lupin* species. This graphical abstract is a workflow of the processes to obtain enriched-protein products from the genus *Lupinus*. Figure compiled by the authors.

present interesting physical and functional properties (e.g., solubility, water and oil absorption, emulsifying capacity, foaming capacity and gelation capacity), making them valuable ingredients for the food and beverage industry. However, they are limited as manufactured foods, with a pH set at around 3–5. On the one hand, they have a low solubility; on the other hand, the intact proteins have regions known as antigenic epitopes responsible for food allergies. Protein hydrolysis alleviates these disadvantages.

Protein hydrolysates comprise the pool of peptides released after cleaving the native protein. This reaction can occur due to the action of enzymes (i.e., proteases) or microorganisms, among other techniques, releasing a pool of peptides with specific sequences and sizes depending on several parameters (i.e., catalyst, reaction time conditions, enzyme-to-substrate ratio, etc.). In this regard, peptides released upon the action of proteases have been investigated more than those released by fermentation, but both techniques have been shown to release low-molecular-weight peptides with enhanced techno-functional and biological properties (Schlegel et al. 2021). Among the peptides in a hydrolysate, some may exert biological activities, such as antioxidant, antidiabetic, antihypertensive, etc.

The active site of the enzyme or the properties of the microorganism employed would determine the peptidome obtained (Cruz-Casas et al. 2021). Consequently, the potential bioactivity of the hydrolysate can be exerted. These hydrolysates usually contain peptides ranging from 2 to 20 amino acids in length and can be identified using techniques such as liquid chromatography followed by mass spectrometry. In some cases, authors carry out a purification step consisting of size exclusion or reverse-phase chromatography to select sequences with specific features (i.e., size or hydrophobicity), as it has been demonstrated that peptides are usually small and hydrophobic (Acquah et al. 2018). The workflow usually includes, after identification, the chemical synthesis of the peptides to validate the activity of each single sequence.

Several studies have reported the efficacy of peptides from *Lupinus* spp. as bioactive agents. There is little evidence that *Lupinus* peptides positively impact human health (Garmidolova et al. 2022). It is impossible to generalize directly from research based on *in vitro* and/or cell-based tests to human response. Animal studies help examine probable chemical action mechanisms and modes of action (Lemus-Conejo et al. 2023).

In Vitro and *In Vivo* Studies

Animal studies have demonstrated that peptides from *Lupinus angustifolius* protein hydrolysate obtained using Alcalase (peptidome also reported) can modulate anxiety and spatial memory in ApoE−/− Western diet model mice, when administered intragastrically at a dose of 0.1 g/kg for 14 weeks (Santos-Sánchez et al. 2022). In the same vein, a human study running for four weeks reported the immune, oxidative and metabolic status of healthy subjects (n=33) after ingestion of 1 g per day in an open-label intervention. In addition to the demonstrated safety under the conditions used, modulation of the anti-/pro-inflammatory response of human peripheral blood mononuclear cells and improvement of the cellular antioxidant capacity were reported, as well as modifications in the low-density lipoprotein-cholesterol (LDL-C)/high-density lipoprotein-cholesterol (HDL-C) atherogenic index and serum total cholesterol levels (Cruz-Chamorro et al. 2021).

In addition to that, other authors have reported Lupine-derived sequences from other sources, as indicated in Table 34.3. One of the most studied sequences reported in the literature is derived from *L. angustifolius* octapeptide GPETAFLR, which has demonstrated bioactivity towards several targets (Millan-Linares et al. 2015). It is important to note that, the proteome of *L. mutabilis* has not been fully sequenced; consequently, some authors use BLAST to compare their findings with the *Lupinus* spp. proteome for more accurate protein identification (Muñoz et al. 2018).

In terms of the production process, different enzymes have been used to produce bioactive peptides from lupin, and overall, the diverse proteases employed have effectively released peptides that proved to exert bioactivity through *in vitro* assays (Millan-Linares et al. 2015).

In some cases, the bioactivity claimed for the peptides has been assessed using *in silico* techniques such as molecular docking or prediction tools, which might not be accurate and should not be used as evidence to state that a peptide is bioactive.

Moreover, it has been indicated that the previous step to the release of peptides, the extraction and isolation step with solvents, can have an impact on the lupin seed proteome coverage (Tahmasian et al. 2022); thus, the identification of peptides afterwards might be hindered by this limitation, highlighting the need for standardization of methods and improved analytical techniques.

IDENTIFICATION OF BIOACTIVE PEPTIDES

Table 34.3 summarizes the sequences identified from the four *Lupinus* species, indicating the substrate and protease employed and the bioactivity demonstrated by the authors. To the authors' knowledge, no specific sequences have been identified from yellow lupin (*Lupinus luteus*), although the bioactivity of hydrolysates derived from this species has been investigated (Garmidolova et al. 2022). The transepithelial transport, biostability, bioavailability and safety concerns of lupin-derived peptides were recently reviewed (Okagu et al. 2021). As can be seen in the table, peptides shorter than 20 amino acids, derived from different species of *Lupinus*, exhibit a range of biological activities, including antidiabetic, antihypertensive, and anti-inflammatory affects, among others. However, *in vivo* studies should be conducted to explore and validate these results.

Among the species hereby reported, *Lupinus albus* appears to be the most studied, as more sequences have been identified and assessed with different types of assays. Regarding the attribution of bioactivity to specific peptides, there are gaps, for instance, in evaluating other properties, such as antimicrobial activity. A *Lupinus angustifolius* hydrolysate obtained with Alcalase has demonstrated antibacterial activity towards *Staphylococcus aureus*, *Bacillus subtilis*, *Pseudomonas aeruginosa* and *Escherichia coli* bacteria, as well as proved to exert antibacterial activity in minced beef during storage at 4°C, but no identification was carried out (Osman et al. 2016).

On top of that, most of the studies suggest or assert that these peptides might be employed to produce supplements or fortify meals to prevent or treat illness. However, for this reason, the interaction of these peptides with the various food matrix constituents will affect their stability and, consequently, bioactivity, as well as whether or not this is maintained when the product is processed and stored. This is significant given the possibility of sequence degradation when employing bioactive peptides as nutraceuticals (Rivero-Pino 2023).

LUPIN PROTEIN IN THE FOOD MARKET

According to Future Market Insights, the global lupin protein industry is estimated to be worth USD 103.3 Million in 2024. Additionally, the market is expected to increase with a compound annual growth rate of 4.9% over the following ten years. The main use of lupin protein currently is flour,

TABLE 34.3
Identified Bioactive Peptides from *Lupinus* spp.: White Lupin (*L. albus*), Blue Lupin (*L. angustifolius*), and Pearl Lupin (*L. mutabilis*)

Source	Enzyme and Conditions	Sequence	Bioactivity (One or More Activities per Peptide)	Reference
L. angustifolius	Alcalase	GPETAFLR	Anti-inflammatory Antiosteoclastogenic Neuroprotective	Lemus-Conejoetal.(2022);Millan-Linares et al. (2015); Montserrat-de la Paz et al. (2019)
L. angustifolius	Alcalase	VPL, PGP, YL, GQ*	Anxiolytic/analgesic	Santos-Sanchez et al. (2022)
*L. mutabilis***	Pancreatin and pepsin	RLGN VNEGA, SEIGGA, NPDDC, SAPRST, GALGLGH, VVVVDE, PQNLDL, AGGPQQR, NVLSQL, PSELSGAAH, LPKHSDAD, LTFPGSAD, PQNLDL, PSELSGAAH,	ACE inhibitor, DPP-IV inhibitor, antioxidant, antiamnesic, anticancer	Muñoz et al. (2018)
L. albus	Alcalase, trypsin and Flavourzyme	RDDVPT, RNTSPQ, HDLPG, NPLL, APVPEM, APLAVR, APENPV	DPP-IV inhibitors	Rivero-Pino et al. (2021)
L. albus	*In vitro* gastrointestinal digestion	AKIQDKEGIPPDQQR, LIFAGKQLEDGR, LDDALRAEK, IQDKEGIPPDQQR, RRAIGK, RDDAASCLVR	Anti-inflammatory	Gao et al. (2020)
L. albus	Pepsin or trypsin	LTFPGSAED, LILPKHSDAD, GQEQSHQDEGVIVR, IPPGIPYWT, AVNELTFPGSAEDIER, ELTFPGSAEDIER	DPP-IV inhibitor, HMGCoAR inhibition, cholesterol-lowering activity, antiamnesic	Lammi et al. (2019); Lammi et al. (2016); Lammi, Zanoni et al. (2016)
L. albus	Alcalase, chymotrypsin, pancreatin, pepsin, neutrase, thermolysin/*Lactobacillus* spp. enzymes	GPSSSPDIYNPEAGRIK, LLHP, LLPHYN, GGLLLPH, FVPY, VKLPTL, MLLPK	Antioxidant	Babini et al. (2017)

This table shows the bioactive peptides from white lupin (*L. albus*), blue lupin (*L. angustifolius*) and pearl lupin (*L. mutabilis*) identified so far. *Principal motifs found from 58 identified peptides. **Homology found in *L. albus* and *L. angustifolius* for some sequences. ACE: Angiotensin-converting enzyme; DPP-IV: dipeptidyl peptidase IV; HMGCoAR: 3-hydroxy-3-methylglutaryl CoA reductase.

which has been considered a substitute for other flours due to its fibre content. Despite this, the industry is still investigating novel clean and economical protein separation procedures for producing high-protein isolates.

In general, the creation of novel plant-based foods is also being held back by a lack of large-scale manufacturing processes to convert plant-based ingredients into desirable end products to assess commercial viability. In this sense, technologies to enhance the efficiency of conversion of these byproduct streams into functional and nutritional food ingredients are needed.

Sweet lupines have been mainly used as food for humans and animals. However, they have recently been found to be an excellent candidate for the development of novel foods as a techno-functional ingredient in bakery products such as bread, biscuits, pasta and meat analogues (Chilón-Llico et al. 2022; Karoui et al. 2023) or as a nutraceutical in the health industry (Lima-Cabello et al. 2023). According to the authors, few companies produce lupin protein hydrolysates. While hydrolysis offers potential benefits such as reduced allergenicity, increased solubility, and bioactive peptides with health properties, industrial-scale production of isolated lupin-derived peptides from hydrolysates is currently not feasible.

In summary, *Lupinus* is valued for its edible seeds, which are an inexpensive and sustainable source of protein and other compounds that could be used to fortify products such as bread, breakfast cereals and snacks, or as foods such as meat or dairy alternatives like cheese or yoghurt. They also have potential applications in baby food formulation, improving the nutritional value and quality of manufactured foods as an effective alternative to ingredients of animal origin. However, the low-sulphur amino acid content in lupin protein needs to be addressed using, for example, methionine enrichment in the formulation (Shresta et al. 2021).

While the evidence for lupin protein products' health benefits is promising, more substantial research is required to include them in the functional food market.

THE EFFECTS OF OTHER PROTEINS

This chapter reviews the nutritional potential of edible *Lupinus* species, based on their protein content and quality.

Lupins are legume cultivars, which generally show high levels of protein (~40%) compared to other grains, such as wheat (12%) and soy (35%). However, a limiting factor for using lupins in human diets so far is the presence of quinolizidine alkaloids, especially in bitter species, and the content of other antinutrients (e.g., phytic acid, lectins and saponins). It has been shown that these compounds can affect the digestibility of proteins, the bioavailability of amino acids and the protein quality of foods.

Nevertheless, studies concerning consumable *Lupinus*, so-called "sweet lupins", with scarce alkaloid and high protein content, have highlighted their *in vivo* digestibility due to their low levels of undesirable or antinutritional components compared to other popular cultivars such as soy or beans (Monteiro et al. 2014).

Furthermore, regarding the amino acid content, sweet lupins show a balanced profile according to FAO (Food and Agriculture Organization of the United Nations) and FINUT (Ibero-American Foundation for Nutrition) recommendations, with higher levels of arginine than soy and lower values of sulphur-containing essential amino acids, in contrast to walnuts, rice or grapes. This limitation can be overcome with specific enrichments in food formulations (Lemus-Conejo et al. 2023).

Soybean is the most widely cultivated legume for protein production, and extensive research has shown its suitability for human consumption. However, novel plant protein sources must be considered to diminish our dependence on soy products, and the food industry may consider the improvement of extraction protocols that modulate the techno-functional properties of protein-rich products.

Thus, *Lupinus* appears to be a realistic alternative for human food enrichment and is still under-exploited in most countries. On the one hand, digestibility values support using lupin proteins in the food industry for humans. On the other hand, edible *Lupinus* crops exhibit more environmental benefits than soybean cultivation and lower production costs, providing agricultural opportunities for countries that may not produce soybeans because of unfavourable climate conditions or for deprived populations (Shrestha et al. 2021).

MINI DICTIONARY OF TERMS

- **Bioactive peptides:** Fragments of a specific protein composed of 2–20 amino acid residues that can exert biological activities, such as antioxidant, anti-inflammatory, antihypertensive or antimicrobial, influenced by the composition and the sequence of their amino acids. These activities occur when the peptides are released from the original protein, where they are encrypted and inactive.
- **Enzymatic hydrolysis:** The process of cleaving peptidic bonds, allowing the release of peptides from proteins, assisted by proteases.
- **Protein hydrolysates:** The pool of protein-derived products (free amino acids, small and medium peptides, polypeptides and even undigested protein) released after the action of proteases or by fermentation, breaking peptide bonds from an isolate/concentrate.
- **Protein isolate:** A protein matrix isolated from a natural source, such as food or other biological materials. The isolation process involves separating the target protein from other components in the source material, such as fats, carbohydrates and other proteins. This results in a product predominantly composed of the specific protein of interest with a concentration around 90% of the total product.

SUMMARY POINTS

- This chapter focuses on proteins obtained from *Lupinus* species as a novel source for a healthy human diet.
- The chemical composition of edible *Lupinus* is compared, with data from protein, carbohydrates, oil or fibre demonstrating their suitability for human consumption.
- The protein and amino acid content of *Lupinus* has shown healthy bioactivity.
- Several peptides have been identified in lupin species, with some data suggesting their potential bioactivity.
- The inhibitory activity of numerous peptides from *Lupinus* has been validated using synthetic peptides.
- Animal and human studies have shown the potential effectiveness of lupin peptides *in vivo*.
- Lupin protein products are promising ingredients for functional foods.

REFERENCES

Abraham, E. M., Ganopoulos, I., Madesis, P., Mavromatis, A., Mylona, P., Nianiou-Obeidat, I., Parissi, Z., Polidoros, A., Tani, E., Vlachostergios, D. 2019. The use of lupin as a source of protein in animal feeding: Genomic tools and breeding approaches. *International Journal of Molecular Sciences* 20: 851. https://doi.org/10.3390/IJMS20040851.

Abreu, B., Lima, J., Rocha, A. 2023. Consumer perception and acceptability of lupin-derived products: A systematic review. *Foods* 12: 1241.

Acquah, C., Di Stefano, E., Udenigwe, C. C. 2018. Role of hydrophobicity in food peptide functionality and bioactivity. *Journal of Food Bioactives* 4: 88–98. https://doi.org/10.31665/jfb.2018.4164.

Aguilar-Acosta, L. A., Serna-Saldivar, S. O., Rodríguez-Rodríguez, J., Escalante-Aburto, A., Chuck-Hernández, C. 2020. Effect of ultrasound application on protein yield and fate of alkaloids during lupin alkaline extraction process. *Biomolecules* 10: 292. https://doi.org/10.3390/BIOM10020292.

Babini, E., Tagliazucchi, D., Martini, S., Dei Più, L., Gianotti, A. 2017. LC-ESI-QTOF-MS identification of novel antioxidant peptides obtained by enzymatic and microbial hydrolysis of vegetable proteins. *Food Chemistry* 228: 186–196. https://doi.org/10.1016/j.foodchem.2017.01.143.

Boukid, F., Pasqualone, A. 2022. Lupine (*Lupinus* spp.) proteins: Characteristics, safety and food applications. *European Food Research and Technology* 248: 345–356. https://doi.org/10.1007/s00217-021-03909-5.

Bryant, L.; Rangan, A.; Grafenauer, S. 2022. Lupins and health outcomes: A systematic literature review. *Nutrients* 14: 327. https://doi.org/10.3390/nu1402032.

Burgos-Díaz, C., Opazo-Navarrete, M., Wandersleben, T., Soto-Añual, M., Barahona, T., Bustamante, M. 2019. Chemical and nutritional evaluation of protein-rich ingredients obtained through a technological process from yellow lupin seeds (Lupinus luteus). *Plant Foods for Human Nutrition* 74: 508–517. https://doi.org/10.1007/S11130-019-00768-0.

Carbonaro, M., Nucara, A. 2022. Legume proteins and peptides as compounds in nutraceuticals: A structural basis for dietary health effects. *Nutrients* 14. https://doi.org/10.3390/nu14061188.

Carvajal-Larenas, F. E., Linnemann, A. R., Nout, M. J. R., Koziol, M., van Boekel, M. A. J. S. 2016. *Lupinus mutabilis*: Composition, uses, toxicology, and debittering. *Critical Reviews in Food Science and Nutrition* 56: 1454–1487. https://doi.org/10.1080/10408398.2013.772089.

Chilón-Llico, R., Siguas-Cruzado, L., Apaza-Humerez, C. R., Morales-García, W. C., Silva-Paz, R. J. 2022. Protein quality and sensory perception of hamburgers based on quinoa, lupin and corn. *Foods* 11: 1–15. https://doi.org/10.3390/foods11213405.

Colgrave, M. L., Dominik, S., Tobin, A. B., Stockmann, R., Simon, C., Howitt, C. A., Vanhercke, T. 2021. Perspectives on future protein production. *Journal of Agricultural and Food Chemistry* 69: 15076–15083.

Cruz-Casas, D. E., Aguilar, C. N., Ascacio-Valdés, J. A., Rodríguez-Herrera, R., Chávez-González, M. L., Flores-Gallegos, A. C. 2021. Enzymatic hydrolysis and microbial fermentation: The most favorable biotechnological methods for the release of bioactive peptides. *Food Chemistry: Molecular Sciences* 3: 100047. https://doi.org/10.1016/j.fochms.2021.100047.

Cruz-Chamorro, I., Álvarez-Sánchez, N., Álvarez-Ríos, A. I., Santos-Sánchez, G., Pedroche, J., Millán, F., Carrera Sánchez, C., Fernández-Pachón, M. S., Millán-Linares, M. C., Martínez-López, A., Lardone, P. J., Bejarano, I., Guerrero, J. M., Carrillo-Vico, A. 2021. Safety and efficacy of a beverage containing lupine protein hydrolysates on the immune, oxidative and lipid status in healthy subjects: An intervention study (the Lupine-1 Trial). *Molecular Nutrition & Food Research* 65: 14. https://doi.org/10.1002/MNFR.202100139.

Duranti, M., Cerletti, P. 1979. Amino acid composition of seed proteins of *Lupinus Albus*. *Journal of Agricultural and Food Chemistry* 27: 977–978. https://doi.org/10.1021/JF60225A038/ASSET/JF60225A038.FP.PNG_V03.

FAO (Food and Agriculture Organization of the United Nations). n.d. ESS: Crops Statistics—Concepts, Definitions and Classifications. Retrieved August 8, 2023, from https://www.fao.org/economic/the-statistics-division-ess/methodology/methodology-systems/crops-statistics-concepts-definitions-and-classifications/en/.

FAO. 2013. Dietary protein quality evaluation in human nutrition: Report of an FAO expert consultation. FAO Food and Nutrition Paper 92. Rome.

Ferchichi, N., Toukabri, W., Vrhovsek, U., Nouairi, I., Angeli, A., Masuero, D., Mhamdi, R., Trabelsi, D. 2021. Proximate composition, lipid and phenolic profiles, and antioxidant activity of different ecotypes of *Lupinus albus, Lupinus luteus* and *Lupinus angustifolius*. *Journal of Food Measurement and Characterization* 15: 1241–1257. https://doi.org/10.1007/s11694-020-00722-8.

Gao, Y., Zhang, X., Ren, G., Wu, C., Qin, P., Yao, Y. 2020. Peptides from extruded lupin (*Lupinus albus* L.) regulate inflammatory activity via the p38 MAPK signal transduction pathway in RAW 264.7 cells. *Journal of Agricultural and Food Chemistry* 68: 11702–11709. https://doi.org/10.1021/acs.jafc.0c02476.

Garmidolova, A., Desseva, I., Mihaylova, D., Lante, A. 2022. Bioactive peptides from lupinus spp: Seed proteins-state-of-the-art and perspective. *Applied Sciences* 12: 3766. https://doi.org/10.3390/app12083766.

Guo, X., Shang, W., Strappe, P., Zhou, Z., Blanchard, C. 2018. Peptides derived from lupin proteins confer potent protection against oxidative stress. *Journal of the Science of Food and Agriculture* 98: 5225–5234. https://doi.org/10.1002/JSFA.9059.

Herforth, A., Arimond, M., Álvarez-Sánchez, C., Coates, J., Christianson, K., Muehlhoff, E. 2019. A global review of food-based dietary guidelines. *Advances in Nutrition* 10: 590–605. https://doi.org/10.1093/advances/nmy130.

Hodgson, J. M., Lee, Y. P., Puddey, I. B., Sipsas, S., Ackland, T. R., Beilin, L. J., Belski, R., Mori, T. A. 2010. Effects of increasing dietary protein and fibre intake with lupin on body weight and composition and blood lipids in overweight men and women. *International Journal of Obesity* 34: 1086–1094. https://doi.org/10.1038/ijo.2010.26.

Hughes, J., Pearson, E., Grafenauer, S. 2022. Legumes—A comprehensive exploration of global food-based dietary guidelines and consumption. *Nutrients* 14. https://doi.org/10.3390/nu14153080.

Ishaq, A. R., El-Nashar, H. A. S., Younis, T., Mangat, M. A., Shahzadi, M., Ul Haq, A. S., El-Shazly, M. 2022. Genus *Lupinus (Fabaceae)*: a review of ethnobotanical, phytochemical and biological studies. *Journal of Pharmacy and Pharmacology* 74: 1700–1717. https://doi.org/10.1093/jpp/rgac058.

Karoui, I. J., Terras, D. S., Yeddes, W., Hammami, M., Abderrabba, M. 2023. Formulation of pasta enriched with protein-rich lupine (*Lupinus mutabilis* Sweet) and wheat bran using mixture design approach. *Journal of Food Science* 1–14. https://doi.org/10.1111/1750-3841.16736.

Khan, M. K., Karnpanit, W., Nasar-Abbas, S. M., Huma, Z. e., Jayasena, V. 2015. Phytochemical composition and bioactivities of lupin: A review. *International Journal of Food Science and Technology* 50: 2004–2012. John Wiley & Sons, Ltd. https://doi.org/10.1111/ijfs.12796.

Kouris-Blazos, A., Belski, R. 2016. Health benefits of legumes and pulses with a focus on Australian sweet lupins. *Asia Pacific Journal of Clinical Nutrition* 25: 1–17. https://doi.org/10.6133/apjcn.2016.25.1.23.

Lammi, C., Aiello, G., Vistoli, G., Zanoni, C., Arnoldi, A., Sambuy, Y., Ferruzza, S., Ranaldi, G. 2016. A multidisciplinary investigation on the bioavailability and activity of peptides from lupin protein. *Journal of Functional Foods* 24: 297–306. https://doi.org/10.1016/j.jff.2016.04.017.

Lammi, C., Bollati, C., Lecca, D., Abbracchio, M. P., Arnoldi, A. 2019. Lupin peptide T9 (GQEQSHQDEGVIVR) modulates the mutant PCSK9D374Y pathway: *in vitro* Characterization of its dual hypocholesterolemic behavior. *Nutrients* 11: 1665. https://doi.org/10.3390/nu11071665.

Lammi, C., Zanoni, C., Arnoldi, A., Vistoli, G. 2016. Peptides derived from soy and lupin protein as dipeptidyl-peptidase IV Inhibitors: *In Vitro* biochemical screening and *in Silico* molecular modeling study. *Journal of Agricultural and Food Chemistry* 64: 9601–9606. https://doi.org/10.1021/acs.jafc.6b04041.

Lemus-Conejo, A., Millan-Linares M. del C., Toscano, R., Millan, F., Pedroche, J., Muriana, F. J. G., Montserrat-de-la-Paz, S. 2022. GPETAFLR, a peptide from *Lupinus angustifolius* L. prevents inflammation in microglial cells and confers neuroprotection in brain. *Nutritional Neuroscience* 25: 472–484. https://doi.org/10.1080/1028415X.2020.1763058.

Lemus-Conejo, A., Rivero-Pino, F., Montserrat-de la Paz, S., Millan-Linares, M. C. 2023. Nutritional composition and biological activity of narrow-leafed lupins (*Lupinus angustifolius* L.) hydrolysates and seeds. *Food Chemistry* 420: 136104. https://doi.org/10.1016/J.FOODCHEM.2023.136104.

Lima-Cabello, E., Escudero-Feliu, J., Peralta-Leal, A., Garcia-Fernandez, P., Siddique, K. H. M., Singh, K. B., Núñez, M. I., León, J., Jimenez-Lopez, J. C. 2023. β-Conglutins' unique mobile arm is a key structural domain involved in molecular nutraceutical properties of narrow-leafed lupin (*Lupinus angustifolius* L.). *International Journal of Molecular Sciences* 24: 7676. https://doi.org/10.3390/IJMS24087676/S1.

Magalhães, S. C. Q., Taveira, M., Cabrita, A. R. J., Fonseca, A. J. M., Valentão, P., Andrade, P. B. 2017. European marketable grain legume seeds: Further insight into phenolic compounds profiles. *Food Chemistry* 215: 177–184. https://doi.org/10.1016/J.FOODCHEM.2016.07.152.

Mane, S. P., Johnson, S. K., Duranti, M., Pareek, V. K., Utikar, R. P. 2018. Lupin seed γ-conglutin: Extraction and purification methods – A review. *Trends in Food Science & Technology* 73: 1–11. https://doi.org/10.1016/J.TIFS.2017.12.008.

Mathew, A. V., Li, L., Byun, J., Guo, Y., Michailidis, G., Jaiswal, M., Chen, Y. E., Pop-Busui, R., Pennathur, S. 2018. Therapeutic lifestyle changes improve HDL function by inhibiting myeloperoxidase-mediated oxidation in patients with metabolic syndrome. *Diabetes Care* 41: 2431–2437. https://doi.org/10.2337/DC18-0049.

Millán-Linares, M. del C., Millán, F., Pedroche, J., Yust, M. del M. 2015. GPETAFLR: A new anti-inflammatory peptide from *Lupinus angustifolius* L. protein hydrolysate. *Journal of Functional Foods* 18: 358–367. https://doi.org/10.1016/J.JFF.2015.07.016.

Monteiro, M. R. P., Costa, A. B. P., Campos, S. F., Silva, M. R., da Silva, C. O., Martino, H. S. D., Silvestre, M. P. C. 2014. Evaluation of the chemical composition, protein quality and digestibility of lupin (*Lupinus albus Lupinus angustifolius*). *O Mundo da Saúde, São Paulo* 38: 251–259.

Montserrat-De La Paz, S., Lemus-Conejo, A., Toscano, R., Pedroche, J., Millan, F., Millan-Linares, M. C. 2019. GPETAFLR, an octapeptide isolated from: *Lupinus angustifolius* L. Protein hydrolysate, promotes the skewing to the M2 phenotype in human primary monocytes. *Food and Function* 10: 3303–3311. https://doi.org/10.1039/c9fo00115h.

Mota, J., Lima, A., Ferreira, R. B., Raymundo, A. 2020. Lupin seed protein extract can efficiently enrich the physical properties of cookies prepared with alternative flours. *Foods* 9: 1064. https://doi.org/10.3390/FOODS9081064.

Muñoz, E. B., Luna-Vital, D. A., Fornasini, M., Baldeón, M. E., Gonzalez de Mejia, E. 2018. Gamma-conglutin peptides from Andean lupin legume (*Lupinus mutabilis* Sweet) enhanced glucose uptake and reduced gluconeogenesis *in vitro*. *Journal of Functional Foods* 45: 339–347. https://doi.org/10.1016/j.jff.2018.04.021.

Okagu, I. U., Ndefo, J. C., Aham, E. C., Obeme-Nmom, J. I., Agboinghale, P. E., Aguchem, R. N., Nechi, R. N., Lammi, C. 2021. Lupin-derived bioactive peptides: Intestinal transport, bioavailability and health benefits. *Nutrients* 13: 9. https://doi.org/10.3390/nu13093266.

Osman, A., El-araby, G. M., Taha, H. 2016. Potential use as a bio-preservative from lupin protein hydrolysate generated by alcalase in food system. *Journal of Applied Biology & Biotechnology* 4: 76–81. https://doi.org/10.7324/jabb.2016.40212.

Osorio, C. E., Till, B. J. 2022. A Bitter-Sweet Story: Unraveling the Genes Involved in Quinolizidine Alkaloid Synthesis in *Lupinus albus*. *Frontiers in Plant Science* 12: 1–8. https://doi.org/10.3389/fpls.2021.795091.

Pastor-Cavada, E., Juan, R., Pastor, J. E., Alaiz, M., Vioque, J. 2009. Analytical nutritional characteristics of seed proteins in six wild Lupinus species from Southern Spain. *Food Chemistry* 117: 466–469. https://doi.org/10.1016/J.FOODCHEM.2009.04.039.

Rivero-Pino, F. 2023. Bioactive food-derived peptides for functional nutrition: Effect of fortification, processing and storage on peptide stability and bioactivity within food matrices. *Food Chemistry* 406: 135046. https://doi.org/10.1016/J.FOODCHEM.2022.135046.

Rivero-Pino, F., Espejo-Carpio, F. J., Guadix, E. M. 2021. Identification of dipeptidyl peptidase IV (DPP-IV) inhibitory peptides from vegetable protein sources. *Food Chemistry* 354: 129473. https://doi.org/10.1016/j.foodchem.2021.129473.

Rosa Lovati, M., Manzoni, C., Castiglioni, S., Parolari, A., Magni, C., Duranti, M. 2012. Lupin seed γ-conglutin lowers blood glucose in hyperglycaemic rats and increases glucose consumption of HepG2 cells. *British Journal of Nutrition* 107: 67–73. https://doi.org/10.1017/S0007114511002601.

Santos-Sánchez, G., Cruz-Chamorro, I., Álvarez-Ríos, A. I., Álvarez-Sánchez, N., Rodríguez-Ortiz, B., Álvarez-López, A. I., Fernández-Pachón, M. S., Pedroche, J., Millán, F., Millán-Linares, M. D. C., Lardone, P. J., Bejarano, I., Carrillo-Vico, A. 2022. Bioactive Peptides from Lupin (*Lupinus angustifolius*) Prevent the Early Stages of Atherosclerosis in Western Diet-Fed ApoE-/-Mice. *Journal of Agricultural and Food Chemistry* 70: 8243–8253. https://doi.org/10.1021/ACS.JAFC.2C00809/ASSET/IMAGES/LARGE/JF2C00809_0006.JPEG.

Santos-Sánchez, G., Cruz-Chamorro, I., Bollati, C., Bartolomei, M., Pedroche, J., Millán, F., Millán-Linares, M. del C., Capriotti, A. L., Cerrato, A., Laganà, A., Arnoldi, A., Carrillo-Vico, A., Lammi, C. 2022. A *Lupinus angustifolius* protein hydrolysate exerts hypocholesterolemic effects in Western diet-fed ApoE-/- mice through the modulation of LDLR and PCSK9 pathways. *Food & Function* 13: 4158–4170. https://doi.org/10.1039/D1FO03847H.

Santos-Sánchez, G., Ponce-España, E., López, J. C., Álvarez-Sánchez, N., Álvarez-López, A. I., Pedroche, J., Millán, F., Millán-Linares, M. C., Lardone, P. J., Bejarano, I., Cruz-Chamorro, I., Carrillo-Vico, A. 2022. A Lupin (*Lupinus angustifolius*) protein hydrolysate exerts anxiolytic-like effects in Western diet-fed ApoE−/− Mice. *International Journal of Molecular Sciences* 23: 9828. https://doi.org/10.3390/IJMS23179828/S1.

Schlegel, K., Lidzba, N., Ueberham, E., Eisner, P., Schweiggert-Weisz, U. 2021. Fermentation of lupin protein hydrolysates—effects on their functional properties, sensory profile and the allergenic potential of the major lupin allergen lup an 1. *Foods* 10: 1–15. https://doi.org/10.3390/foods10020281.

Shevkani, K., Singh, N., Chen, Y., Kaur, A., Yu, L. 2019. Pulse proteins: secondary structure, functionality and applications. *Journal of Food Science and Technology* 56: 2787–2798. https://doi.org/10.1007/S13197-019-03723-8/FIGURES/4.

Shrestha, S., van't Hag, L., Haritos, V. S., Dhital, S. 2021. Lupin proteins: Structure, isolation and application. *Trends in Food Science & Technology* 116: 928–939.

Tahmasian, A., Broadbent, J. A., Juhász, A., Nye-Wood, M., Le, T. T., Bose, U., Colgrave, M. L. 2022. Evaluation of protein extraction methods for in-depth proteome analysis of narrow-leafed lupin (*Lupinus angustifolius*) seeds. *Food Chemistry* 367. https://doi.org/10.1016/j.foodchem.2021.130722.

Tahmasian, A., Drew, R., Broadbent, J. A., Juhász, A., Nye-Wood, M., Colgrave, M. L. 2023. Conventional solid-state fermentation impacts the white lupin proteome reducing the abundance of allergenic peptides. *Food Chemistry* 426: 136622. https://doi.org/10.1016/J.FOODCHEM.2023.136622.

USDA-ARS Germplasm Resources Information Network (GRIN). (n.d.). Retrieved October 12, 2023, from https://www.ars-grin.gov/.

USDA Plants Database. (n.d.). Retrieved October 12, 2023, from https://plants.usda.gov/home.

Villarino, C. B. J., Jayasena, V., Coorey, R., Chakrabarti-Bell, S., Johnson, S. K. 2015. Nutritional, health, and technological functionality of lupin flour addition to bread and other baked products: Benefits and challenges. *Critical Reviews in Food Science and Nutrition* 56: 835–857. https://doi.org/10.1080/10408398.2013.814044.

Vogelsang-O'Dwyer, M., Bez, J., Petersen, I. L., Joehnke, M. S., Detzel, A., Busch, M., Krueger, M., Ispiryan, L., O'Mahony, J. A., Arendt, E. K., Zannini, E. 2020. Techno-functional, nutritional and environmental performance of protein isolates from blue lupin and white lupin. *Foods* 9: 230. https://doi.org/10.3390/FOODS9020230.

35 Protein Quality of Maize (*Zea mays*) Crop and Leaves

Moattar Latif and Peter Uchenna Amadi

ABBREVIATIONS

BV	Biological value
DW	Dry weight
EAAI	Essential amino acid index
EAR	Estimated average requirement
GNA	*Galanthus nivalis* agglutinin
HIV	Human immunodeficiency virus
LDLc	Low-density lipoprotein cholesterol
PDCAAS	Protein digestibility-corrected amino acid score
PER	Protein efficiency ratio
RS2	Type 2-resistant starch

INTRODUCTION

Zea mays L., also known as corn or maize, is a vital annual grain crop member of the Poaceae family. The term "zea" traces its roots to ancient Greek, meaning "sustaining life," while "mays" is derived from the Taino language, meaning "life giver." The term maize itself originates in the Spanish word "maiz," providing a fitting description for the plant. Various alternative terms, like zea, silk maize, makka, barajovar, and more, are employed to denote this plant. Maize is acknowledged as a fundamental food source in various parts of the world, securing its position as the third most significant crop globally, trailing only behind rice and wheat. In American culture, maize is revered as the mother grain, playing a substantial role in propelling the US economy (Milind and Isha 2013). Despite being primarily used as animal feed, maize is extensively processed to produce a range of goods, including tortillas, snacks, starch, flour, and morning cereals.

Maize is abundant in carbohydrates and sugars, providing a substantial source of calories and energy. Moreover, it serves as an excellent reservoir of essential minerals and vitamins. Within the endosperm, the protein ranks as the second most abundant component, constituting 8–10% of the total weight of maize kernels, following starch. Saturated fatty acids, such as palmitic acid and stearic acid, are present in low concentrations. In contrast, corn showcases an abundance of unsaturated fatty acids, such as elevated linoleic acid, linolenic acid, and arachidonic acids. The specific types and quantities of these fatty acids vary with changing seasons. Additionally, maize boasts a significant presence of natural antioxidants, particularly in maize germ. Its oil, extracted by wet milling, is popularly used in salad dressings and cooking (Orthoefer et al. 2003).

A reasonable proportion of the plant, especially the leaf, is made up of polyunsaturated, monounsaturated, and saturated fatty acids. From our previous study, linoleic acid (15%), oleic acid (11%), palmitic acid (9%), stearic acid (1%), and linolenic acid (36%), in particular, are present in refined maize oil (Bob Chile-Agada and Amadi 2020). Within the human diet, they provide the primary forms of vitamin E: alpha and gamma tocopherols. Maize oil is notably abundant in tocopherols,

DOI: 10.1201/9781003597926-35

especially γ-tocopherol, with reported concentrations of 21.3 and 94.1 mg/100g (Kumar and Jhariya 2013).

The edible and nutritious components of maize include pollen and seeds. Seeds are a great source of carbohydrates and can be eaten raw or cooked. Corn is rich in niacin, thiamin, riboflavin, vitamin B-complex, pantothenic acid, and B6, making it good for heart and brain health, skin, hair, and digestion. Additionally, it contains significant amounts of vitamins C, A, and K, along with ample beta-carotene and a fair dose of selenium, which are beneficial for thyroid health and crucial for the proper functioning of the immune system. Maize exhibits a higher protein and fat content compared to other cereals. Both pollen and seeds stand out as nutritious and edible components of maize. Seeds, whether consumed in their raw or cooked form, serve as an excellent source of carbohydrates. Maizeric acid, fixed oils, resin, sugar, mucilage, salt, and fibres vital to our nutrition are all present in corn silk. Corn syrup is used as an alternative to cane sugar and maple syrup in making jams, jellies, and other sweets (Kopsell et al. 2009).

Phytochemicals are naturally occurring bioactive compounds found in plants, offering human health benefits and the capacity to lower the risk of significant chronic disorders. Maize is a crucial source of key phytochemicals, including phytosterols, phenolic compounds, and carotenoids (Lopez-Martinez et al. 2009). The concentrations of carotenoids, phenolic compounds, and phytosterols differ within maize. Yellow corn, especially in the floury and horny endosperm, exhibits a notable abundance of carotenoids. Carotenoids, belonging to a pigment family that includes yellow, orange, and red hues, are particularly prevalent in this variant of maize. These pigments fall into two classes: carotenes, which are purely hydrocarbons devoid of oxygen, and xanthophylls, which are hydrocarbons containing oxygen (Fieldor and Burda 2014).

In the kingdom of plants, phenolic compounds, which include stilbenes, coumarins, flavonoids, tannins, and phenolic acids, represent the most broadly disseminated class of phytochemicals. These chemicals are abundant in maize, especially in the husk. The primary phenolic compounds identified in maize are ferulic acid and anthocyanins. Among various sources, processed corn bran demonstrates the highest amount of FA, with wheat and barley following closely. The two main phenolic chemicals found in maize are anthocyanins and ferulic acid. Per 100 g of the edible component, refined corn bran contains: 71.88 g of carbohydrates, 8.82 g of protein, 4.57 g of fat, 2.12 g of fiber, 2.41 g of ash, 10.21 g of moisture, 343 mg of phosphorus, 15.5 mg of sodium, 116 mg of sulfur, 0.1 mg of riboflavin, 1.78 mg of amino acids, 1.5 g of minerals, 284 mg of potassium, 0.43 mg of thiamin, 0.15 mg of vitamin C, 9 mg of calcium, 136.5 mg of magnesium, and 0.13 of copper. According to Zhao and Moghadasian (2008), maize has the highest ferulic acid content among cereal grains, followed by wheat and barley.

Anthocyanins are members of the flavonoid class of phenolic compounds, constituting the most extensive category of water-soluble plant pigments with colors ranging from reddish to purple. Maize possesses the second-highest concentration of anthocyanins, making it the second-ranking crop in terms of anthocyanin content. Maize oil is particularly high in phytosterols, with sitosterol, stigmasterol, and campesterol being the most frequently encountered phytosterols in maize oil. The distribution of these phytosterols varies across different materials of the maize kernel, encompassing the pericarp, germ, and endosperm (Harrabi et al. 2008).

HUMAN HEALTH BENEFITS AND CONSTITUENT PHYTOCHEMICALS

Maize, also known as corn, offers numerous health benefits, particularly through its rich content of B-complex vitamins, which are highly advantageous for human health. These vitamins play a crucial role in maintaining the health of hair, skin, and heart, and facilitating proper digestion. Moreover, they are beneficial for individuals dealing with rheumatism, aiding in the mobility of limbs and joints. Additionally, maize plays a role in regulating blood pressure and promoting overall well-being. The fatty acids in maize contribute significantly to maintaining healthy blood pressure levels, managing cholesterol, and preventing obesity. Maize oil contains a substantial amount of vitamin E, known for its antioxidant activity. This property enhances the immune system, making it robust and responsive in the body.

Galanthus nivalis Agglutinin

Maize possesses an anti-HIV activity compound known as *Galanthus nivalis* agglutinin (GNA), proving to be beneficial in the treatment of HIV. Maize is considered a promising therapeutic option for HIV (Fouquaert et al. 2009). Additionally, the resistant starch in maize is a highly nutritious compound that, when consumed, helps prevent obesity and regulates cholesterol levels. Moreover, maize is used to address skin problems and combat certain types of cancers (Saeed and Saeed 2020). It functions effectively as a soothing agent for ulcers, swelling, and wounds. A decoction made from maize silk, roots, and leaves is employed to address issues related to the bladder, vomiting, and nausea. Similarly, a decoction of maize cob is used to alleviate stomach disorders.

Carotene

Carotene carries numerous health benefits. Different parts of maize contain varying concentrations of carotene: maize silage (21.58 mg/kg), stalklage (17.5 mg/kg), and yellow maize (6.57 mg/kg) (Shah et al. 2016). Both alpha (α) and beta (β) carotene exhibit pro-vitamin A activity. Elevated levels of β-carotene have been shown to function as a pro-antioxidant, inducing apoptosis in various cancer cells, including gastric cells, melanoma cancer cells, leukemia cells, and colon cancer cells, thereby imparting a powerful chemopreventive effect (Jang 2009).

Xanthophylls

Xanthophylls, specifically zeaxanthin and lutein in maize, play crucial and distinct adaptive roles. When supplemented in food in a dose-dependent manner, lutein exhibits various positive effects, including increasing tumor suppression, inhibiting mammary tumor growth, enhancing lymphocyte proliferation, and importantly protecting cells against damage induced by oxidants. Notably, lutein and zeaxanthin are the sole carotenoids in the macula of the retina accountable for acute and outgrowth vision. Additionally, they show a protective effect against phototoxic damage in humans and help prevent the development of age-related cataracts and macular degeneration. Subjects' macular pigment optical density significantly improved after adding lutein supplements to their diets over time, notably shielding the macula from damage caused by light. Additionally, lutein acts as a cancer chemopreventive agent, exerting repressive activity during the contingency of disease (Moreno et al. 2007).

Anthocyanins

Anthocyanins are widely recognized for their health-promoting advantages, including anticarcinogenic, antidiabetic, lipid-lowering, antimicrobial, antiatherogenic, and anti-inflammatory properties. Their powerful antioxidant characteristics reduce capillary permeability and fragility, stimulate the immune system, and inhibit platelet aggregation (Ghosh and Konishi 2007). The ingestion of anthocyanins from purple maize at a 5% dietary level over a 36-week administration period notably inhibited colorectal carcinogenesis in male rats, demonstrating a significant suppression of lesion development in the colon. Phytosterols offer various health advantages. The dietary intake of phytosterols is inversely related to cholesterol absorption, LDL cholesterol, and serum levels, attained by suppressing cholesterol absorption, promoting cholesterol synthesis, and impacting the intestine, ultimately leading to increased cholesterol excretion in stools.

Corn has various bioactive compounds in addition to the main ones mentioned above. The structures, natures, and sources of four types of resistant starches have been determined. The primary resistant starch in maize is type 2 resistant starch (RS2), which is more prevalent in high amylose corn and difficult for human digestion due to its natural granule shape. Of all the whole grains, high-amylose maize (70%) has the highest amylose content. According to the structure of starch granules, RS2 is resistant to intestinal digestion and positively colon health and blood sugar levels. All whole grains include lignins, common bioactive chemicals with anticancer and antioxidant properties. They go by different names: lariciresinol, matairesinol, pinoresinol, and secoisolariciresinol. In corn, there is 12 g/100 g dry weight (DW) of secoisolariciresinol and 11 g/100 g DW of lariciresinol; matairesinol and pinoresinol are absent (Siyuan et al. 2018). A research study assessed the influence of phytosterols in maize oil on cholesterol reduction, by analyzing the absorption of cholesterol between individuals who consumed regular maize oil and those who consumed commercialized maize oil with phytosterols removed. Prolonged consumption of corn oil has the potential to bring down cholesterol concentration and preclude atherosclerosis (Ostlund et al. 2002).

PROTEIN QUALITIES OF DIFFERENT MAIZE VARIETIES

To elaborate on the dietary protein obtainable from maize meals, this book chapterconsidered the protein qualities of different maize varieties. Yellow maize showed higher amino acid content than the white and black varieties, as presented in Table 35.1.

Furthermore, the protein quality of yellow maize was much higher than the other varieties. However, despite yellow maize being the most enriched in amino acids, still falls short of popular plant proteins like nuts or animal sources like eggs (Puglisi and Fernandez 2022). In Table 35.2, the leaves of *Zea mays* have been shown to contain appreciable amounts of leucine, valine, arginine, and lysine but lack adequate levels of tryptophan and methionine. However, the stalk and stem are very poor sources of amino acids.

From the results of Table 35.2, the protein qualities of *Zea mays* could match those of some vegetables like *S. macrocarpum* and *V. amygdalina* (Omoyeni et al. 2015). This implies that supplementing their tryptophan contents can sufficiently provide for the amino acid dietary requirements as much as the popularly consumed vegetables. Further, from the reports of Omoyeni et al. (2015), bitter leaf and scent leaf proteins contained lower amounts of non-essential amino acids when compared to those for *Zea mays*.

TABLE 35.1
Protein Qualities of Different Maize Varieties

Quality	White Maize	Yellow Maize	Black Maize
Total Amino Acid (g/100g)	89	94	82
Protein Quality Index			
P-PER I	3.6	4.2	3.0
P-PER II	3.8	4.1	2.7
P-PER IIII	3.3	3.8	2.6
EAAI	1.5	1.8	1.4
PDCAAS	0.47	0.59	0.40
Biological Value (%)	29	42	25

Values represent means of triplicate determinations. EAAI = essential amino acid index; P-PER = predicted protein efficiency ratio; PDCAAS = protein digestibility-corrected amino acid score.

TABLE 35.2
Protein Qualities of Maize Leaf, Stalk, and Stem

Quality	Leaf	Stalk	Stem
Total Amino Acid (g/100g)	85	69	58
Protein Quality Index			
P-PER I	2.1	1.9	1.8
P-PER II	2.5	2.3	2.0
P-PER IIII	1.7	1.7	1.2
EAAI	0.9	0.6	0.5
PDCAAS	0.2	0.2	0.1
Biological Value (%)	11	10	7

Values represent means of triplicate determinations. EAAI = essential amino acid index; P-PER = predicted protein efficiency ratio; PDCAAS = protein digestibility-corrected amino acid score.

IMPROVING PROTEIN QUALITY BY FERMENTATION

Some reports have shown the possibility of synthesizing nutraceuticals from the fermentation of fibrous wastes (Amadi et al. 2019; Carsanba et al. 2021). The leaf, stem, and stalk of *Zea mays* are major environmental wastes that could benefit from nutritional enrichment through simultaneous saccharification and fermentation. For instance, fermentation during cheese production prevents complications arising from lactose intolerance. Additionally, lactose maldigestion is avoided during yogurt production due to beta-glucosidase production from yogurt cultures (Savaiano 2014). According to Pessione and Cirrincinone (2016) and EFSA (2006), most dairy processes involving fermentation by lactic acid bacteria induce milk proteolysis, thereby enhancing the synthesis of polyamines and therapeutic peptides (Facioni et al. 2020). However, in some cases, toxic products such as biogenic amines are produced during these processes (Linares et al. 2016). Many bioactive peptides have been isolated from fermented foods like kefir and yogurt and have been applied for medicinal uses such as antidiabetic, antioxidant, and immunomodulatory (Pihlanto and Korhone 2015; Fekete et al. 2015). Filannino et al. (2015) observed that lactic acid bacteria-induced fermentation metabolizes phenolic compounds into therapeutically potent substances through phenolic acid esterase, reductase, and decarboxylases. The resultant intermediates are usually pyroanthocyanidins (Bai et al. 2014). In addition, the application of fermentation in food processing enhances the removal of antinutrients such as phytates and oxalates (Senger et al. 2016) and lowers food pH. This suggests that fermenting maize's leaf, stalk, and stem of maize could improve its nutritional value, especially its protein quality. Desirable changes in the food matrix, synthesis of therapeutic intermediates, or derivable nutrients from the fermenting organisms enhance the nutrient density of foods subjected to fermentation. The fermenting microbes extracellularly carry out enzyme-aided modification of food matrices that lead to total or partial degradation of macromolecules, thereby enhancing the nutritional value and digestibility. Fermentation is useful in poultry feeding as it promotes the digestion of complex polysaccharides into nutrient-dense products. The micronutrient enrichment obtained after fermentation and phytase activities also releases divalent minerals from complexes (Joudaki et al. 2023). Also, Hermans et al. (2010) showed that additional amino acids were synthesized from food products after fermentation. This implies that microbial fermentation improves the protein qualities of food materials.

PROTEIN QUALITY MEASUREMENTS OF THE LEAF, STALK, AND STEM OF THE *ZEA MAYS* PLANT

Table 35.3 shows the protein quality measurements of the leaf, stalk, and stem of the *Zea mays* plant. To bioprocess these materials, they must be ground, saccharified, and fermented for 72 hours using *Saccharomyces cerevisiae* in a submerged culture. The total amino acid levels increased after bioprocessing. The predicted protein efficiency ratios (P-PERs) almost doubled after the simultaneous saccharification and fermentation.

As evident in Table 35.3, the significantly low levels of the essential amino acid index (EAAI), PDCAAS, and biological value of the leaf, stalk, and stem were extensively improved by bioprocessing. Bob Chile-Agada and Amadi (2020) elucidated the essential oil composition of *Zea mays* leaf extract. They isolated 12 bioactive components in their study, and the sample showed an abundance of farnesene, hexadecanoic acid, caryophyllene, nonadecanoic acid, and phytol. Farnesene is a popular sesquiterpene with several therapeutic benefits (Celik et al. 2014), especially its potential to ameliorate various cancers and oxidative stress-induced ailments, thus it could become relevant in the orthodox management of such diseases (Sarikurkcu et al. 2013; Afoulous et al. 2013). Phytol and caryophyllene are both well documented for their strong antinociceptive, anti-inflammatory, and antioxidant properties (Guimarães-Santos et al. 2012; Katsuyama et al. 2013; Camila et al. 2013; Dahham et al. 2015), which expands the ethnomedicinal application of *Zea mays* leaves. To buttress other beneficial effects of the nutrients contained in *Zea mays* leaves, their fatty acid compositions were summarized in our earlier report (Bob Chile-Agada and Amadi 2020). A total of 19 fatty acids were quantified with eicosadienoic, dihomo-gamma-linolenic, and erucic acid undetected in *Zea mays* leaves. A total of 27.63% saturated fatty acids with a predominance of palmitic, arachidic, and myristic acids found in the leaves. In contrast, the most abundant unsaturated fatty acids were linolenic, linoleic, and oleic acids. With higher proportions of polyunsaturated fatty acids in the leaves, this unlikely source of fatty acids produces more than those reported for pumpkin, sesame, rapeseed (Orsavova et al. 2015), and sunflower and almond leaf oil (Sabudak 2007), which are popularly consumed for dietary needs. Hence, *Zea mays* leaves could be exploited for dietary and therapeutic purposes, especially for their heart health benefits.

TABLE 35.3
Protein Qualities of Different Maize Parts after Valorization by Simultaneous Saccharification and Fermentation

Quality	Leaf	Stalk	Stem
Total Amino Acid (g/100g)	87	92	80
Protein Quality Index			
P-PER I	4.6	4.9	4.4
P-PER II	4.1	4.6	4.1
P-PER IIII	4.2	4.5	4.3
EAAI	2.6	2.6	2.4
PDCAAS	1.3	1.2	1.3
Biological Value (5)	62	73	69

Values represent means of triplicate determinations. EAAI = essential amino acid index; P-PER = predicted protein efficiency ratio; PDCAAS = protein digestibility-corrected amino acid score.

EFFECT OF MAIZE ON THE LIVER

Furthermore, we have shown in a recent (unpublished) project that maize seed improves the total protein content of the liver using suitable experimental animal models. In the study, seven mice received either the maize seed, leaf, or stalk and were compared to a control group of similar sample size that only received normal chow. The experimental diets were provided as premixes with chow in a ratio of 80% diet and 20% commercial rat chow. As shown in Figures 35.1 and 35.2, the rats that

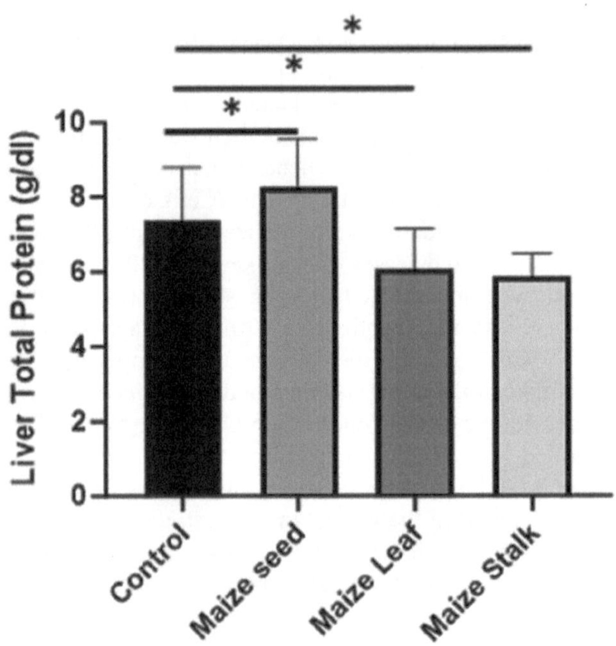

FIGURE 35.1 Total liver protein content of animals administered different parts of the maize plant. Values represent means of triplicate determinations. * Significant difference ($p < 0.05$) between two groups.

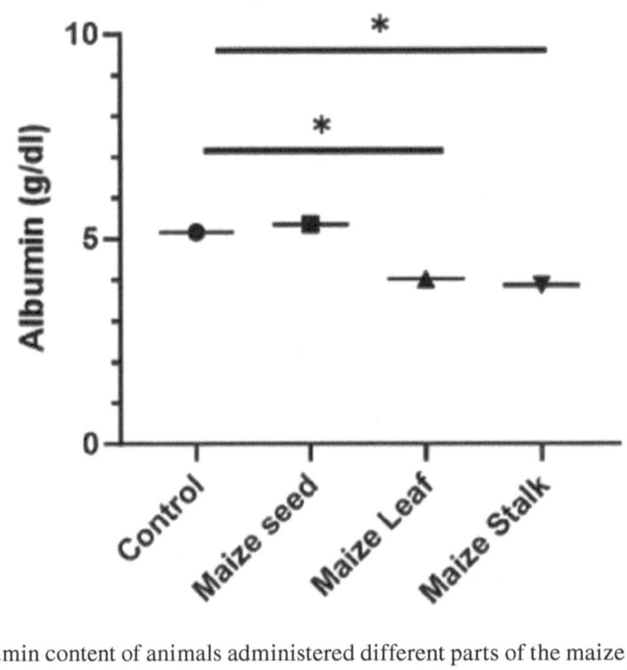

FIGURE 35.2 Albumin content of animals administered different parts of the maize plant. Values represent means of triplicate determinations. * Significant difference ($p < 0.05$) between two groups.

received the maize seeds produced significantly ($p < 0.05$) higher total protein content compared to the control. In contrast, whereas the rats that received other parts of the maize plant, such as the leaf and stem, showed significantly lower total protein and albumin.

The liver's total protein and albumin content is a direct measurement of the liver's functional status. Hepatocytes that populate the liver secrete albumin, which implies that increased albumin production directly mirrors the increase in these cells' populations and indirectly indicates an excellent functional condition of the liver. Taking this into account, Figure 35.3 and 35.4 compared the potentials of fermenting the leaves and stalks of *Zea mays*, to improve the functional status of the liver. Indeed, fermented leaves and stalk of *Zea mays* increased the rats' total protein and albumin levels compared to the control.

In addition, these other parts of *Zea mays* produced as much total protein and albumin as the seeds. This implies that the fermentation of these other parts of *Zea mays* may have detoxified them and improved their nutritional content compared the edible seeds of *Zea mays*. Thus, in summary, despite the popularity of the edible part of *Zea mays* being the seeds, other parts of *Zea mays* could be valorized for use in human and animal nutrition.

MINI DICTIONARY OF TERMS

- **Cereals:** Grass grown for use as food and contains an endosperm, a germ, and a bran.
- **Fermentation:** Anerobic transformation of glucose-rich substances into new products.
- **Phytochemicals:** Chemicals produced by plants that elicit biological effects.
- **Protein digestibility:** Potentials of a protein to hydrolyze to amino acids.
- **Protein efficiency ratio:** Measures how well a protein is utilized for growth.
- **Protein quality:** Amount and bioavailability of amino acids in a protein source.
- **Valorize:** To improve the quality of an underutilized product.

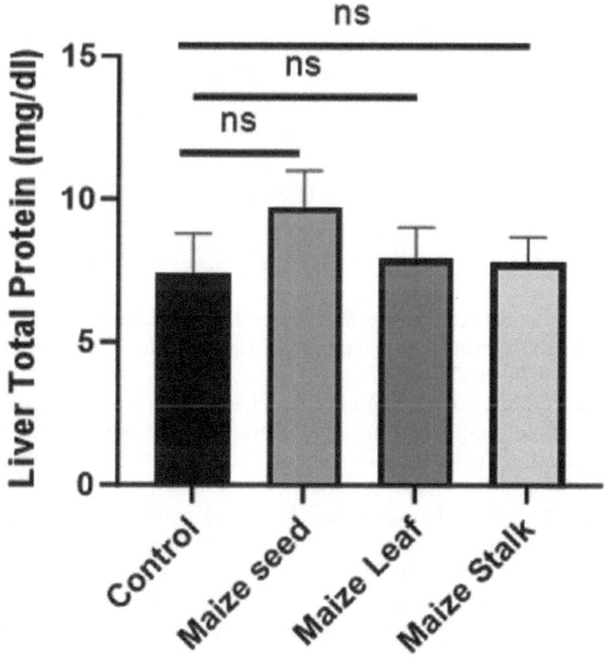

FIGURE 35.3 Total liver protein content of animals administered fermented parts of the maize plant. Values represent means of triplicate determinations. ns = no significant difference ($p > 0.05$) between the two groups.

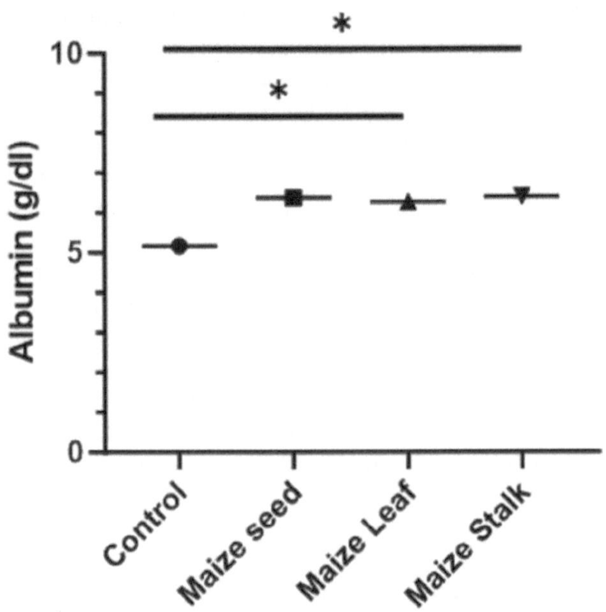

FIGURE 35.4 Albumin content of animals administered fermented parts of the maize plant. Values represent means of triplicate determinations. * Significant difference ($p < 0.05$) between two groups.

SUMMARY POINTS

- This review provides an overview of the nutritional properties of *Zea mays* with a special focus on its protein qualities.
- Despite the popularity of the edible seeds, other parts of the maize plant, such as the leaf and stalk, possess macro- and micronutrients that benefit human nutrition.
- *Zea mays* provides excellent protein content and fatty acids compared to other cereals.
- The other non-edible parts of the *Zea mays* contain proteins and fatty acids comparable to popular vegetables.
- The *Zea mays* leaves and stalk can be valorized by fermentation to improve their protein quality.
- Valorized maize stalk and leaves improve liver albumin content.

REFERENCES

Amadi, Peter Uchenna, Ogunka-Nnoka Charity, and Abbey Bene Willy. Effect of simultaneous snail slime-aided degradation and yeast fermentation on terpenoid composition of plantain pseudostem waste. *Curr Pharm Biotechnol.* 2019;20(6):459–464.

Afoulous, Samia, Hicham Ferhout, Emmanuel Guy Raoelison, Alexis Valentin, Béatrice Moukarzel, and François Couderc. Jalloul BouajilaChemical composition and anti-cancer, antiinflammatory, anti-oxidant and antimalarial activities of leaves essential oil of Cedrelopsis grevei. *Food Chem Toxicol.* 2013;56:352–362.

Bai, Yunpeng, Brandon Findlay, Alma Fernanda Sanchez Maldonado, Andreas Schieber, John C. Vederas, Michael G. Gänzle. Novel pyrano and vinylphenol adducts of deoxyanthocyanidins in sorghum sourdough. *J Agric Food Chem.* 2014;62:11536–11546.

Bob Chile-Agada, Adaeze, and Peter Amadi. Evaluation of bioactive component, free radical scavenging potentials and protein qualities of gomphrena celosoides and zea mays leaves. *Curr Bioact Compd.* 2020;16(7):1–7.

Camila, Carolina de Menezes Patrício Santos, Mirian Stiebbe Salvadori, Vanine Gomes Mota, Luciana Muratori Costa, Antonia Amanda Cardoso de Almeida, Guilherme Antônio Lopes de Oliveira, Jéssica Pereira Costa, Damião Pergentino de Sousa, Rivelilson Mendes de Freitas, and Reinaldo Nóbrega de Almeida. Antinociceptive and Antioxidant Activities of Phytol In vivo and In vitro Models. *Neuroscience J.* 2013;9:1–9.

Carsanba, Erdem, Pintado Manuela, and Oliveira Carla. Fermentation strategies for production of pharmaceutical terpenoids in engineered yeast. *Pharmaceuticals (Basel).* 2021;14(4):295.

Çelik, Kubra, Toğar Basak, Türkez Hasan, and Taşpinar Numan. In vitro cytotoxic, genotoxic, and oxidative effects of acyclic sesquiterpene farnesene. *Turk J Biol.* 2014;38:253–259.

Dahham Saad, Yasser Tabana, Muhammad Iqbal, Mohamed Ahamed, Mohammed Ezzat, Aman Majid, and Amin Majid. The anticancer, antioxidant and antimicrobial properties of the sesquiterpene β-caryophyllene from the essential oil of aquilaria crassna. *Molecules.* 2015;20(7):11808–11829.

Fouquaert, Elke, David Smith, Willy Peumans, Paul Proost, Jan Balzarini, Savvas Savvides, and Els Van Damme. "Lectins from snowdrop and maize differ in their carbohydrate-binding specificity. *Biochem Biophys Res Commun.* 2009;380(2):260–265.

Facioni, Sole Maria, Raspini Benedetta, Pivari Francesca, Dogliotti Elena, and Cena Hellas. Nutritional management of lactose intolerance: the importance of diet and food labelling. *J Transl Med.* 2020;18(1):260.

Fekete, Ágnes, Ian Givens, and Julie A Lovegrove. Casein-derived lactotripeptides reduce systolic and diastolic blood pressure in a meta-analysis of randomised clinical trials. *Nutrients.* 2015;7:659–681.

Fiedor, J. and K. Burda. Potential role of carotenoids as antioxidants in human health and disease. *Nutrients.* 2014;6(2):466–488.

Filannino Pasquale, Bai Yunpeng, Raffaela Di Cagno, Marco Gobbetti, and Michael G. Gänzle. Metabolism of phenolic compounds by Lactobacillus spp. during fermentation of cherry juice and broccoli puree. *Food Microbiol.* 2015;46:272–279.

Ghosh, Dilip, and Tetsuya Konishi. Anthocyanins and anthocyanin-rich extracts: role in diabetes and eye function. *Asia Pac J Clin Nutr.* 2007;16:200–208.

Guimarães-Santos, Adriano, Diego Siqueira Santos, Ijair Rogério Santos, Rafael Rodrigues Lima, Antonio Pereira, Lucinewton Silva de Moura, Raul Nunes Carvalho Jr, Osmar Lameira, and Walace Gomes-Leal. Copaiba oil-resin treatment is neuroprotective and reduces neutrophil recruitment and microglia activation after motor cortex excitotoxic injury. *Evid Based Complement Alternat Med.* 2012:2012918174.

Harrabi, Saoussem, Annik St-Amand, Faouzi Sakouhi, Khaled Sebei, Habib Kallel, Paul M. Mayer, and Sadok Boukhchina. Phytostanols and phytosterols distributions in corn kernel. *Food Chemistry.* 2008;111(1):115–120.

Hermans, N., P. Cos, L. Maes, T. De Bruyne, D. Vanden Berghe, A. Vlietinck, and L. Pieters. Challenges and pitfalls in antioxidant research. *Curr Med Chem.* 2010;14(4):417–430.

Jang, Sung Hee, Joo Weon Lim, and Hyeyoung Kim. Mechanism of β -carotene-induced apoptosis of gastric cancer cells: Involvement of ataxia-telangiectasia-mutated. *Ann NY Acad Sci.* 2009;1171:156–162.

Joudaki, Hanane, Negar Aria, Roya Moravej Mohamadreza Rezaei Yazdi, Zarrindokht Emami-Karvani, and Michael R. Hamblin. Microbial phytases: properties and applications in the food industry. *Curr Microbiol.* 2023;80(12):374.

Katsuyama, S., H. Mizoguchi, H. Kuwahata, T. Komatsu, K. Nagaoka, H. Nakamura, G. Bagetta, and T. S. Sakurada. SakuradaInvolvement of peripheral cannabinoid and opioid receptors in β-caryophyllene-induced antinociception. *Eur J Pain.* 2013;17(5):664–675.

Kopsell, Dean A., Gregory R. Armel, Thomas C. Mueller, Carl E. Sams, Dennis E. Deyton, J. Scott McElroy, and David E. Kopsell. Increase in nutritionally important sweet corn kernel carotenoids following mesotrione and atrazine applications. *J Agric Food Chem.* 2009;57(14):6362–6368.

Kumar, Dilip, and Aditya Narayan Jhariya. Nutritional, medicinal and economical importance of corn: a mini review. *Res J Pharm Sci.* 2013:555X.

Linares Daniel, Beatriz del Rio, Begoña Redruello, Victor Ladero, M. Cruz Martin, Maria Fernandez, Patricia Ruas-Madiedo, and Miguel A. Alvarez. Comparative analysis of the in vitro cytotoxicity of the dietary biogenic amines tyramine and histamine. *Food Chem.* 2016;197:658–663.

Lopez-Martinez, Leticia X., Rosa M. Oliart-Ros, Gerardo Valerio-Alfaro, Chen-Hsien Lee, Kirk L. Parkin, and Hugo S. Garcia. Antioxidant activity, phenolic compounds and anthocyanins content of eighteen strains of Mexican maize. *LWT-Food Sci Technol.* 2009;42(6):1187–1192.

Milind, P., and D. Isha. Zea maize: A modern craze. *Inter Res J Pharma.* 2013;4:39–43.

Moreno, Fernando Salvador, Luciana Passos Toledo, Aline de Conti, Renato Heidor, Alceu Jordão Jr, Helio Vannucchi, Monica Testoni Cardozo, and Thomas Prates Ong. Lutein presents suppressing but not blocking chemopreventive activity during diethylnitrosamine-induced hepatocarcinogenesis and this involves inhibition of DNA damage.*Chem Biol Interact.* 2007;168(3):221–228.

Omoyeni, Olubunmi, Olaofe Olorunfemi, and Akinyeye Odunayo. Amino acid composition of ten commonly eaten indigenous leafy vegetables of South-West Nigeria. *World J Nutr Health.* 2015;3(1):16–21.

Orsavova, Jana, Ladislava Misurcova, Jarmila Vavra Ambrozova, Robert Vicha, and Jiri Mlcek. Composition of vegetable oils and its contribution to dietary energy intake and dependence of cardiovascular mortality on dietary intake of fatty acids. *Int J Mol Sci.* 2015;16(6):12871–12890.

Orthoefer, F., Eastman, J., and List, G. Corn oil: composition, processing and utilization. In P. J. White and L. A. Johnson (eds.), *Corn: Chemistry and Technology* (2nd ed., pp. 671–693). St. Paul, MN: American Association of Cereal Chemists.

Ostlund Jr, Richard E., Susan B. Racette, Alfred Okeke, and William F. Stenson. Phytosterols that are naturally present in commercial corn oil significantly reduce cholesterol absorption in humans. *Am J Clin Nutr.* 2002;75(6):1000–1004.

Pessione, Enrica, and Simona Cirrincione. Bioactive molecules released in food by lactic acid bacteria: encrypted peptides and biogenic amines. Front Microbiol. 2016;87:6–21.

Pihlanto, Anne, and Hannu Korhonen. *Advances in Fermented Foods and Beverages.* Elsevier Ltd. 2015:23.

Puglisi, Michael, and Fernandez Maria. The health benefits of egg protein. *Nutrients.* 2022 15;14(14):2904.

Sabudak, Temine. Fatty acid composition of seed and leaf oils of pumpkin, walnut, almond, maize, sunflower and melon. *Chem Nat Compd.* 2007;43(4):465–467

Saeed, Muhammad Sulaman, and Ayesha Saeed. Health benefits of maize crop-an overview. *Curr Res Agric Farming.* 2020;1:5–8.

Sarikurkcu, Cengiz, Sabih Ozer, Ahmet Cakir, Mustafa Eskici, and Ebru Mete. GC/ MS evaluation and in vitro antioxidant activity of essential oil and solvent extracts of an endemic plant used as folk remedy in Turkey: Phlomis bourgaei Boiss. *Evid Based Complement Alternat Med.* 2013;1–9:2013293080.

Savaiano, D. A. Lactose digestion from yogurt: mechanism and relevance. *Am J Clin Nutr.* 2014;99(5 Suppl):1251S–5S.

Senger Donald, Dan Li, Shou-Ching Jaminet, and Shugeng Cao. Activation of the Nrf2 cell defense pathway by ancient foods: Disease prevention by important molecules and microbes lost from the modern western diet. *PLoS One* 2016;11(2):e0148042.

Shah, Tajamul Rouf, Kamlesh Prasad, and Pradyuman Kumar. Maize—A potential source of human nutrition and health: a review. *Cogent Food Agric.* 2016;2(1):1166995.

Siyuan, S., L. Tong, and R. H. Liu. Corn phytochemicals and their health benefits. *Food Sci Hum Well.* 2018;7:185–195.

Zhao, Zhaohui, and Mohammed H. Moghadasian. Chemistry, natural sources, dietary intake and pharmacokinetic properties of ferulic acid: A review. *Food Chemistry* 2008;109(4):691–702.

36 Peanut Flour as a Food Protein Source

Jianmei Yu

ABBREVIATIONS

ACE	Angiotensin-converting enzyme
CVD	Cardiovascular diseases
FDPF	Fully defatted peanut flour
HDL	High-density lipoprotein
LDL	Low-density lipoprotein
NTDs	Neglected tropical diseases
OTA	Ochratoxin A
PDPF	Partially defatted peanut flour
ROS	Reactive oxygen species
VLDL	Very-low-density lipoprotein

INTRODUCTION

In this chapter, the health benefits of peanut consumption, nutritional profiles, current and possible future applications of peanut flours of different fat contents, as well as challenges of using peanut flour as a protein source, were briefly reviewed. Peanut (*Arachis hypogaea, L.*), also called groundnut, is classified as a legume and an oil seed. As one of the most important oilseeds in the world, shelled raw peanut contains 42.64–57.47% of lipid, 3.8–7.99% moisture, 19.19–26.58% protein, 2–3% ash, and 11.54–19.65% carbohydrate, with high dietary fiber and low sugar content. The concentrations of these nutrients vary with the variety/cultivar and size of peanuts, as well as growing location and climate (Jonnala et al., 2005; Guy et al., 2013; Chowdhury et al., 2015; Muñoz-Arrieta et al., 2021). In addition, peanuts contain significant amounts of resveratrol and phytosterol (Sanders et al., 2000; Shin et al., 2010). Due to the high oil content, peanuts are widely used to produce cooking oil worldwide. Peanut oil extraction results in a large quantity of peanut cake, which is further processed into peanut flour or peanut meal depending on the oil extraction method used (Harris et al., 1972). In China alone, about 125,000 metric tons of peanut meal are produced each year (Liu et al., 2022). Such information in other countries was not found through internet searches. However, according to the peanut oil production data available, the top five peanut-flour producing countries are China, India, Nigeria, Myanmar, and Senegal. The United States ranked the seventh as of 2019 (NationMaster, 2020). Peanut flour and peanut meal are used interchangeably in most countries. However, they are different products in the United States, where the peanut flour is made for human consumption with high-quality roasted peanuts, using an all-natural oil-extracting process, such as extrusion followed by screw pressing. In contrast, peanut meal is produced for animal feed through a process consisting of screw press and solvent extraction with carefully controlled processing conditions (Harris et al., 1972). Figure 36.1 shows the process of peanut flour production. Based on the degree of defatting, peanut flour can be classified into fully defatted peanut flour (FDPF) and

DOI: 10.1201/9781003597926-36

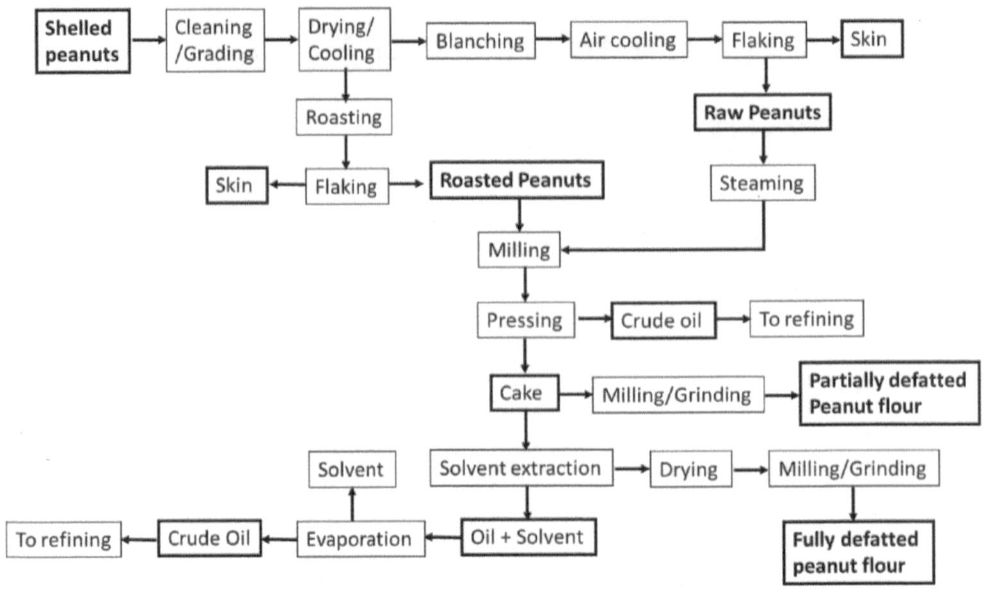

FIGURE 36.1 Flowchart of peanut flour production. This figure is self-constructed according to the description in the literature (Harris et al., 1975).

partially defatted peanut flour (PDPF), with PDPF containing 12% fat or higher. Based on the degree of roasting, peanut flour can be light roasted, medium roasted, and dark roasted. According to the Global Peanut Flour Market report, peanut flours with 28% and 12% fat, and organic peanut flour made from light, medium, or dark roasted peanuts, are avaialbe for international trade (Global Peanut Flour Market, 2023). The flavor, nutrient composition, and techno-functional properties of different types of peanut flour vary with peanut variety, degree of roasting, and degree of defatting.

HEALTH BENEFITS OF PEANUT CONSUMPTION

Both prospective and case-controlled studies have found that consuming peanuts (not peanut butter) and tree nuts is positively associated with reduced risks of different types of cancers (Yeh et al., 2006; van den Brandt and Nieuwenhuis, 2018; Zhao et al., 2018;), cardiovascular diseases (CVD) (Parilli-Moser et al., 2022), overweight and obesity (Moreno et al., 2013), type-2 diabetic (Jiang et al., 2002; Sapp et al., 2022), as well as mortalities caused by various diseases (Luu et al., 2015; van den Brandt and Schouten, 2015; Amba et al., 2019). Regularly consuming peanuts or peanut butter also contributes to improved cognitive health in elders and young adults (Li et al., 2019; Katzman et al., 2021; Parilli-Moser et al., 2021). These health benefits are because peanuts are packed with essential nutrients, including arginine-rich protein, heart-healthy monounsaturated fatty acids, dietary fiber-rich carbohydrates, important minerals, B vitamins, choline, and other health-promoting bioactive compounds such as phytosterols and resveratrol (Arya et al., 2016; Bonku and Yu, 2020). Full-fat peanut flour should retain all nutrients of peanuts, while the FDPF and PDPF have higher protein, dietary fiber, mineral, choline, and water-soluble vitamin contents but lower lipid and lipid-soluble components such as vitamin E than roasted peanuts. The nutrient compositions of peanut flours are shown in Tables 36.1–4. These tables were constructed obtained from data from the USDA's FoodData Central (USDA-NASS, 2019).

NUTRITIONAL COMPOSITION OF PEANUT FLOUR

Proximate Composition of Peanut Flour

Table 36.1 shows that peanut flour's calorie and fat contents decrease, while its protein content, ash, and carbohydrates, including dietary fiber, increase with degree of defatting (USDA-NASS, 2019). Peanut flour's protein and dietary fiber contents are 33.8–52.2% and 14.04–15.80%, respectively, significantly higher than the 24% protein and 8.4% dietary fiber in roasted peanuts. No information on the sugar content of PDPF is available from the database, but it is expected to be between 4.9% and 8.4% because it is not soluble in oil and cannot be removed through the oil-extraction process. Although the total carbohydrate content of peanut flour is higher than that of roasted peanuts, both peanut and peanut flour are classified as low glycemic index foods according to Glycemic Index Guide (https://glycemic-index.net/). The increased ash content implies a higher mineral concentration in peanut flour. Both saturated fatty acid and unsaturated fatty acid contents are lower in PDPF and FDPF. Consequently, the total calorie content of peanut flour is more than 100% lower than dry-roasted peanuts. The contribution of macronutrients to total calorie content in FDPF is in the order of protein > carbohydrate > fat, while in PDPF it isprotein > fat > carbohydrate. Therefore, peanut flour is a low-calorie protein source for vegans, vegetarians, and the regular population.

Amino Acid Composition of Peanut Flour Protein

As protein content increases, the contents of all amino acids in peanut flour increase with the increasing degree of defatting (Table 36.2). The richest amino acid in peanut flour is glutamic acid, followed by aspartic acid and arginine. Peanut protein has the highest arginine content among all food proteins, and defatting doubles the arginine content in peanut flour. "The arginine is an essential amino acid for birds, carnivores, and young mammals and a conditionally essential amino acid

TABLE 36.1
Proximate Composition of Roasted Peanuts and Partially Defatted and Fully Defatted Peanut Flour (Based on 100g of Peanut/Flour)

Nutrient	Unit	Dry-Roasted Peanuts	PDPF (21.9% fat)	PDPF (12% fat)*	FDPF
Water	g	1.81	7.80	2.50	7.80
Energy	kcal	857.00	428.00	364.44	327.00
Energy	kJ	3584.70	1790.00	1523.40	1370.00
Protein	g	24.35	33.80	46.30	52.20
Total lipid (fat)	g	49.66	21.90	13.00	0.55
Ash	g	2.92	5.23	6.10	4.75
Carbohydrate, by difference	g	21.26	31.30	32.1	34.70
Total dietary fiber	g	8.40	15.80	14.04	15.80
Sugars	g	4.90	N/A	N/A	8.22
Starch	g	4.39	N/A	N/A	N/A
Saturated Fatty Acids	g	7.72	3.04	2.16	0.06
Monounsaturated	g	26.20	10.9	6.18	0.23
Polyunsaturated	g	9.77	6.92	4.68	0.14

This table shows how the proximate composition of peanut flour changes based on the degree of defatting. The data are reconstructed from FoodData Central (USDA-NASS, 2019). No copyright permission is needed.

* Data for 12% fat PDPF are from the website of Protein Plus, LLC (https://proteinplusflour.com).

TABLE 36.2
Amino Acid Composition of Roasted Peanuts and Partially and Fully Defatted Peanut Flour (Based on 100g of Peanut/Flour)

Amino acids	Unit	Dry-Roasted Peanuts	PDPF (21.9% fat)	PDPF (12% fat)*	FDPF
Tryptophan	g	0.23	0.328	0.49	0.507
Threonine	g	0.811	1.158	1.75	1.788
Isoleucine	g	0.833	1.188	1.79	1.836
Leucine	g	1.535	2.191	3.3	3.384
Lysine	g	0.85	1.213	1.83	1.874
Methionine	g	0.291	0.415	0.63	0.641
Cystine	g	0.304	0.433	0.65	0.669
Phenylalanine	g	1.227	1.752	2.64	2.705
Tyrosine	g	0.963	1.374	2.07	2.122
Valine	g	0.993	1.418	2.14	2.189
Arginine	g	2.832	4.042	6.11	6.243
Histidine	g	0.599	0.854	1.29	1.319
Alanine	g	0.941	1.343	2.03	2.075
Aspartic acid	g	2.888	4.123	6.24	6.367
Glutamic acid	g	4.949	7.063	10.68	10.908
Glycine	g	1.427	2.037	3.08	3.145
Proline	g	1.045	1.492	2.25	2.304
Serine	g	1.167	1.665	2.52	2.572

This table shows the amino acid compositions of peanut flours with different fat contents. The data are reconstructed from FoodData Central (USDA-NASS, 2019). No permission is needed.

* Data for 12% fat PDPF are from the website of Protein Plus, LLC (https://proteinplusflour.com).

for adults" (Tapiero et al., 2002). Arginine supplementation has been found to lower blood pressure and keep arteries open and flexible even after a high-fat meal (Shiraseb et al., 2022). There is also growing evidence indicating that arginine is positively associated with improved immune function (Martí i Líndez and Reith, 2021). This may contribute to the lower incidence of hypertension among regular peanut consumers (Jones, 2014). Despite its high arginine content, peanut protein is more digestible than most plant proteins because of its low level of antinutritional factors (Arya et al., 2016). Although lysine, tryptophan, and methionine are considered the limiting essential amino acids of peanut protein, this issue can be easily resolved by incorporating peanut flour into rice and wheat-based products because wheat and rice are rich in these amino acids (Day et al., 2022).

Mineral Composition of Peanut Flours

Table 36.3 shows that peanut flour is a good source of iron (Fe), zinc (Zn), and potassium (K) and an excellent source of magnesium (Mg) and phosphorus (P). The defatting process enriches minerals in the peanut flour. Minerals are essential micronutrients for maintaining normal metabolism and tissue structure (Soetan et al., 2010). Potassium and magnesium are two nutrients that help maintain normal blood pressure (Houston and Harper, 2008). Deficiency of potassium in the diet has been reported to positively link to hypokalemia and kidney diseases, while a diet rich in potassium may help control chronic kidney diseases (Palmer et al., 2020). Cereal grains are the most important food staples worldwide, but they often have lower mineral content (Koehler and Wieser, 2012).

TABLE 36.3
Mineral Composition of Roasted Peanuts and Peanut Flours (Based on 100g of Peanut/Flour)

Minerals	Unit	Dry-Roasted Peanuts	PDPF (21.9% fat)	PDPF (12% fat)*	FDPF
Calcium, Ca	mg	58.00	130	69.60	140.00
Iron, Fe	mg	1.58	4.74	3.00	2.10
Magnesium, Mg	mg	178.00	48.00	309.00	370.00
Phosphorus, P	mg	363.00	508	628.07	760.00
Potassium, K	mg	634.00	1360	1154.40	1290.00
Sodium, Na	mg	6.00	1.00	10.53	180.00
Zinc, Zn	mg	2.77	5.99	5.81	5.10
Copper, Cu	mg	0.43	2.04	1.18	1.80
Manganese, Mn	mg	1.79	4.23	3.65	4.90
Selenium, Se	μg	9.30	7.10	13.16	7.10

This table shows the mineral compositions of peanut flours with different fat contents. The data are reconstructed from FoodData Central (USDA-NASS, 2019). No permission is needed.
* Data for 12% fat PDPF are from the website of Protein Plus, LLC (https://proteinplusflour.com/).

Thus, fortifying cereal-based food products with certain percentages of defatted or partially defatted peanut flour can significantly improve the mineral content of cereal products.

Vitamin Composition of Peanut Flours

According to the review of Bonku and Yu (2020), peanuts contain higher levels of tocopherols (vitamin E), B vitamins, and choline than most tree nuts and soybean. Table 36.4 shows that peanut flours have higher levels of thiamin, niacin (including nicotinic acid and nicotinamide), folate, and choline and lower levels of tocopherols levels (vitamin E) than roasted peanuts. Furthermore, the contents of these B vitamins and choline increased with the degree of defatting. The B vitamins are critical for energy metabolism, maintaining healthy nerve cells, and overall neurological functioning. They are cofactors for many essential enzymes involved in the energy metabolism and biosynthesis of RNA and DNA (Hanna et al., 2022). It is well known that niacin deficiency leads to pellagra, thiamin deficiency causes beriberi, while deficiency of folate in pregnant women increases the risk of giving birth to infants with various defects (Bonku and Yu, 2020). Although choline is not a vitamin, its biological importance led it being officially recognized as an essential nutrient in the United States in 1998. It is the precursor of two membrane lipids (phosphatidylcholine and sphingomyelin), two signaling lipids (platelet-activating factor and sphingosylphosphorylcholine), and one neurotransmitter (acetylcholine) (Blusztajn, 1998). Studies have continually unveiled that sufficient choline intake is needed to prevent liver disease, atherosclerosis, and possibly neurological disorders (Zeisel and da Costa, 2009). Thereby, regularly consuming peanut flour, which is rich in B vitamins and choline, may contribute to normal energy metabolism, healthy skin, improved cognitive function, healthy aging, and help fight diseases associated with vitamin B deficiency.

Phytochemical Composition of Peanut Flours

In addition to the macronutrients and micronutrients shown in the tables above, peanut flours contain significant amounts of phytochemicals such as phytosterols and resveratrol. Resveratrol has

TABLE 36.4
Vitamin Composition of Roasted Peanuts and Peanut Flours Containing Different Levels of Fat (Based on 100g of Peanut/Flour)

Vitamins	Unit	Dry-Roasted Peanuts	PDPF (21.9% fat)	PDPF (12% fat)*	FDPF
Vitamin C	mg	0.00	0.00	0.00	0.00
Thiamin	mg	0.15	0.457	0.77	0.70
Riboflavin	mg	0.20	0.172	0.17	0.48
Niacin	mg	14.36	11.5	23.73	27.00
Pantothenic acid	mg	1.01	1.54	2.45	2.74
Vitamin B6	mg	0.47	0.304	0.45	0.50
Folate, total	mg	97.00	133	254.91	248.00
Choline, total	μg	64.60	N/A	N/A	108.70
Vitamin E α-tocopherol	mg	4.93	N/A	2.03	0.05
β-Tocopherol	mg	0.36	3.04	N/A	0.00
γ-Tocopherol	mg	6.32	10.9	N/A	0.00
δ-Tocopherol	mg	0.61	6.92	N/A	0.00

This table shows the vitamin composition of peanut flours with different fat contents. The data are reconstructed from FoodData Central (USDA-NASS, 2019). No permission is needed.
*Data for 12% fat PDPF are from the website of Protein Plus, LLC (https://proteinplusflour.com).

been reported to reduce the risk and potentially improve the therapeutic outcome of cancer, multiple myeloma, metabolic syndrome, CVD, Alzheimer's disease, kidney diseases, and rhinopharyngitis (Singh et al., 2019). The resveratrol content of the edible part of major market types of peanuts ranges from 0.03 to 0.14μg/g (Sanders et al., 2000). The phytosterols are plant sterols, and they compete with cholesterol absorption in the digestive tract, thereby reducing the cholesterol absorption, improving serum lipid profiles, and reducing CVD risk (Arya et al., 2016). The major phytosterols in peanuts are campesterol, stigmasterol, β-sitosterol, and Δ5-avenasterol (Shin et al., 2010). Their chemical structures differ from animal cholesterol only on the side chain at position 17, as shown in Figure 36.2. Peanut flour contains 55–60mg/100g of phytosterols, with 78–83% being β-sitosterol (Awad et al., 2000; Zhou et al., 2018), which is higher than that in cereal grain and cereal-based food products (Normén et al., 2002). One study showed that feeding FDPF to hamsters on a high-cholesterol diet significantly lowered the plasma levels of total cholesterol, LDL, VLDL, and cholesteryl ester (CE), an indicator of the development of atherosclerosis, without significantly impacting HDL cholesterol (Stephens, 2010). β-sitosterol has also shown a preventive function against colorectal and breast cancer in both *in vitro* and *in vivo* studies (Baskar et al., 2010; Awad et al., 2008). A recent animal study (mouse model) discovered that a low dose of phytosterol improved the biomarkers of glucocorticoid-induced osteoporosis through the regulation of gut microbes (Xiao et al., 2023). Thus, consuming peanut flour and its products may reduce the risks of CVD, cancer, and osteoporosis mortality caused by these diseases.

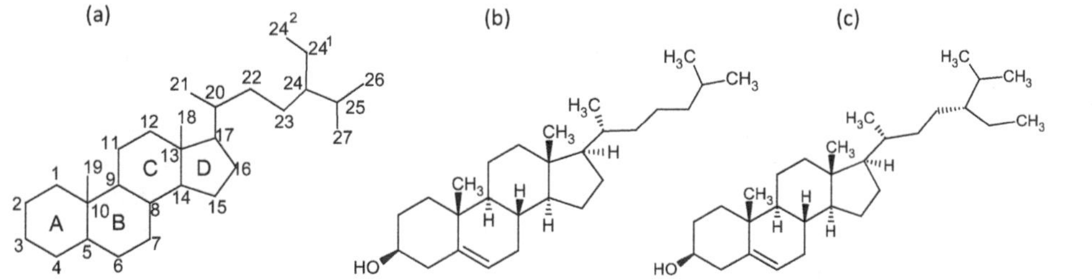

FIGURE 36.2 Chemical structure of (a) steroids, (b) cholesterol, and (c) β-sitosterol. This figure shows the structural similarity and difference between cholesterol and β-sitosterol. The chemical structures were made using ACD/ChemSketch Software. No copyright permission is needed

APPLICATIONS OF PEANUT FLOUR AS A PROTEIN SOURCE IN FOOD PRODUCT DEVELOPMENT

Traditional Application of Peanut Flour for Protein Improvement

Traditionally, peanut flour has been used as an ingredient in baked goods, crackers, protein-enhanced breakfast cereal, pasta, confection products, and nutrition bars for its high protein content and the unique flavor developed during roasting (Harris et al., 1972; Kulthe et al., 2014). In bread making, replacing 10% wheat flour with PDPF did not significantly affect the loaf volume and sensory quality. However, it significantly increased protein and lipid contents while reducing carbohydrate content. Consumers preferred the bread with 20% PDPF, although this substitution reduced microbial stability (Adeboye et al., 2018).

In the case of breakfast cereal, corn flakes produced by replacing 10–20% of corn cones with PDPF led to a product with reduced moisture content, lower bulk density, decreased hardness, shorter bowl life, and less water absorption. However, consumer acceptance remained similar to the control product (Cheewapramong et al., 2002). In pancake mix, replacing 30% of all-purpose white flour with PDPF (12% fat, light roasted) increased the crude fat, protein, and ash (mineral) contents of the resulting pancake from 5.77, 5.58, and 3.26% to 8.14, 9.87, and 4.34%, respectively, while the carbohydrate content decreased from 86.40% to 75.64%. The physicochemical properties of pancakes, including the reheating characteristics of frozen pancakes, remained acceptable (Yemmireddy et al., 2013). Similarly, supplementing PDPF at 10% in plain and egg cake, 15% in cupcakes, and 20% in multigrain cake did not significantly influence overall acceptability but noticeably increased protein, iron, and calcium contents of cakes (Seth and Kochhar, 2018). Pasta could be formulated by replacing up to 50% of durum wheat flour with light-roasted 12% fat peanut flour in the presence of 2.5–2.9% of λ-carrageenan, which served as an adhesive. Pasta containing 35–45% of PDPF showed the highest consumer preference, although it had a browner color (Howard et al., 2011). In addition to the higher protein, lipid, and mineral contents of peanut-flour-fortified baked and extruded food products, higher dietary fiber content was also evidenced in the crackers made with peanut flour (Howard et al., 2009). A study conducted in India demonstrated that nutritional bars developed with peanut flour had better nutrient composition, sensory quality, and higher consumer preference than commercially available products (Garg and Brar, 2017). In all products discussed above, the strong peanut flavor significantly contributed to good acceptability.

Innovative Application of Peanut Flour in Food Product Development

The health concern of consuming animal-based products (Abete et al., 2014; Neuenschwander et al., 2019) and the environmental impact of producing animal-based protein have driven the growth and demand for plant protein-based food products (Scanes, 2018). Cereals, legumes, and oil seeds have been the most used protein sources in the past two decades in plant-based product development. However, only a few studies have used peanut and peanut flour to develop plant-based meat analogs (Rehrah et al., 2009; Chen et al., 2023) and peanut-based dairy products, including milk, yogurt, and cheese (Zaaboul et al., 2019; Dai et al., 2022). Among 18 commercial brands of plant-based meat products, only two of them contain peanut protein (Shaghaghian et al., 2022). The peanut-based dairy products on the market are very limited, particularly in Western countries. Thus, peanut flour/protein is underutilized compared to other plant proteins, such as soy and pea proteins, in plant-based food product development.

Application of Peanut Flour as a Protein Source in Bioactive Peptide/Hydrolysate Production

In addition to being used as an ingredient in food product development, peanut flour also has great potential to be used to make protein isolate/concentrate, which can be further processed into multifunctional bioactive peptides/hydrolysates. Some studies have shown that protease hydrolysis of peanut protein isolate or peanut flour could produce hydrolysates with antioxidant activities through scavenging reactive oxygen species (ROS), reducing power, metal-chelating, and inhibiting lipid oxidation (Chen et al., 2007; Dong et al., 2019; Yu et al., 2020). Fermentation of peanut flour with non-pathogenic molds or bacteria such as *Bacillus subtilis* and *Lactobacillus* also resulted in products with increased *in vitro* antioxidant activity (Zhang et al., 2011; Wang et al., 2011). These hydrolysates also exhibited both *in vitro* and *in vivo* anti-hypertensive activity by inhibiting the activities of renin and angiotensin-converting enzyme (ACE), lowering blood cholesterols and increasing antioxidant activity (Quist et al. 2009; Yu et al., 2021; Zeng et al., 2013; Shi et al., 2014). The bioactivities of peanut flour/protein hydrolysates or fermented peanut flour are due to the formation of multifunctional bioactive peptides during protease hydrolysis or fermentation. Because of the high content of allergenic proteins, peanut flour has also been used as an effective antigen for oral immunotherapy to induce tolerance to peanuts in children who are allergic to peanuts (Berglund et al., 2017).

CHALLENGES OF PEANUT FLOUR APPLICATION IN FOOD

Peanut Allergy and Method of Mitigation

Despite the high protein content and well-accepted flavor, peanut flour/meal is mainly used as an animal feed ingredient, with limited application in foods and dietary supplements in Western countries due to peanut allergy, which is an IgE-mediated allergic reaction triggered by peanut protein. In the US, the rate of self-reported peanut allergy among adults is 2.9% (95% CI, 2.7%–3.1%), and more than 17% of them developed a peanut allergy in their adulthood (Warren et al., 2021). Overall, approximately 2% of the general population of Western nations is affected by peanut allergy, with 7%–14% of cases caused by accidental peanut exposure annually, and one-third to half may experience anaphylaxis (Lieberman et al., 2021). As a result, the portion of peanuts consumed as a food ingredient in 2023 was only 2% of total peanuts consumed in the United States, according to the American Peanut Council (2023). Many efforts have been made to reduce the allergenicity of peanuts and peanut flour and to desensitize peanut-allergic patients. Previous studies have repeatedly confirmed that extensive protease hydrolysis of peanuts/peanut flour tremendously reduced the allergenicity of peanut flour/kernels without significantly affecting the sensory quality and consumer acceptance of the product (Cabanillas et al., 2012; Yu et al., 2015; Yu et al., 2021). Other methods that may reduce the allergenicity of peanut protein, such as genetic modification and physical and chemical treatments, can be found in the review by Yu (2016). The use of oral immunotherapy to induce tolerance to peanut proteins has been evaluated in many clinical trials and the results have been promising (Berglund et al., 2017). Despite various desensitizing approaches, the eye-catching sign of peanut flour on the product label is extremely important to avoid accidental exposure for those with peanut anaphylaxis.

Mycotoxins in Peanuts and Peanut Flour

Mycotoxins are the secondary metabolites produced by pathogenic molds. Several mycotoxins, including aflatoxins, ochratoxin A, and cyclopiazonic acid, were detected in peanuts and peanut-derived products, with aflatoxins being the major health concern (Er Demirhan and Demirhan, 2022). In Western countries, mycotoxins were managed by Good Agricultural Practice, Good Manufacturing Practice, and the enforcement of strict mycotoxin regulations throughout peanut production, processing, and marketing. Further, peanut flour for human consumption is typically made from high-quality roasted peanuts. The roasting could destroy 60–90% of aflatoxin, depending on the initial load of aflatoxin and roasting condition (Lee et al., 1969; Dhanshetty et al., 2021), extrusion for peanut flour production can further destroy aflatoxin (Zheng et al., 2015); thus, mycotoxin is not a major concern. In developing countries, the incidence and level of aflatoxin contamination in peanuts are high, posing a significant food safety issue. In Africa, peanut flour is often used in baby formula and for nutrient enrichment to combat malnutrition. However, peanuts in African markets typically contain higher levels of aflatoxins compared to other regions of the world (Siwela et al., 2011; Ankwasa et al., 2021). Consequently, African consumers of peanuts and peanut-flour-fortified food products may face a higher risk of aflatoxicosis. Removing moldy peanut kernels and blanching to remove peanut skin before roasting and oil extraction will significantly reduce aflatoxin levels. In addition, quantification of aflatoxin content in the peanuts can help determine whether a lot of peanuts can be used to produce peanut flour for human consumption. If the total aflatoxin content is below the regulation limit (for example, 20 ug/kg), the peanuts can be directly used as a food ingredient in most countries.

MINI DICTIONARY OF TERMS

- **Aflatoxicosis:** Also called aflatoxin poisoning. Diseases caused by consuming food or feed contaminated by aflatoxins.
- **Anaphylaxis:** Severe allergic reaction to an allergen/antigen such as peanuts, with symptoms of impaired breathing, swelling in the throat, a sudden drop in blood pressure, pale skin or blue lips, fainting, and dizziness.

SUMMARY POINTS

- The nutritional composition of peanuts, partially defatted peanut flour, and fully defatted peanut flour are compared.
- The protein contents of peanut flour products range from 24–52%, depending on the degree of defatting.
- The contents of minerals, B vitamins, and choline in peanut flour increased with decreasing fat content.
- Including 10–20% defatted or partially defatted peanut flour in most traditional food products significantly increased the protein, dietary fiber, mineral, and B vitamin contents without affecting the consumer acceptability of those products.
- Peanut flour also has great potential to be used to make plant-based meat, dairy alternatives, and bioactive peptides.
- The major challenges of using peanut flour as a dietary protein source are peanut allergy in Western countries and mycotoxin contamination in developing countries.

- Due to heat instability and chemical and biochemical reactions among food components during food processing/cooking, the retention of B vitamins and phytosterols in different food products fortified with peanut flour needs to be investigated.

REFERENCES

Abete, I., Romaguera, D., Vieira, A. R., de Munain, A. L., and Norat, T. 2014. Association between total, processed, red and white meat consumption and all-cause, CVD and IHD mortality: a meta-analysis of cohort studies. *British Journal of Nutrition* 112(5):762–775.

Adeboye, A. S., Fayemi, O. E., Bamgbose, A., Adewunmi, A., and Sobowale, S. S. 2018. Towards the development of peanut–wheat flour composite dough: Influence of reduced-fat peanut flour on bread quality. *Journal of Food Processing and Preservation* 42(1):e13385.

Amba, V., Murphy, G., Etemadi, A., Wang, S., Abnet, C. C., and Hashemian, M. 2019. Nut and peanut butter consumption and mortality in the national institutes of health-AARP diet and health study. *Nutrients* 11(7):1508.

American Peanut Council. Peanut industry. https://peanutsusa.com/industry-info/the-peanut-industry.html. (Accessed on August 31, 2023).

Ankwasa, E. M., Francis, I., and Ahmad, T. 2021. Update on mycotoxin contamination of maize and peanuts in East African Community Countries. *Journal of Food Science and Nutrition Therapy* 7:1–10.

Arya, S. S., Salve, A. R., and Chauhan, S. 2016. Peanuts as functional food: a review. *Journal of Food Science and Technology* 53:31–41.

Awad, A. B., Barta, S. L., Fink, C. S., and Bradford, P. G. 2008. β -Sitosterol enhances tamoxifen effectiveness on breast cancer cells by affecting ceramide metabolism. *Molecular Nutrition and Food Research* 52(4):419–426.

Awad, A. B., Chan, K. C., Downie, A. C., and Fink, C. S. 2000. Peanuts as a source of β-sitosterol, a sterol with anticancer properties. *Nutrition and Cancer* 36(2):238–241.

Baskar, A. A., Ignacimuthu, S., Paulraj, G. M., and Al Numair, K. S. 2010. Chemopreventive potential of β-sitosterol in experimental colon cancer model-an in vitro and in vivo study. *BMC Complementary and Alternative Medicine*, 10:1–10.

Berglund, J. P., Szczepanski, N., Penumarti, A., Beavers, A., Kesselring, J., Orgel, K., ... and Kulis, M. 2017. Preparation and analysis of peanut flour used in oral immunotherapy clinical trials. *The Journal of Allergy and Clinical Immunology: In Practice* 5(4):1098–1104.

Blusztajn, J. K. 1998. Choline, a vital amine. *Science* 281(5378):794–795.

Bonku, R. and Yu, J. 2020. Health aspects of peanuts as an outcome of its chemical composition. *Food Science and Human Wellness* 9(1):21–30.

Cabanillas, B., Pedrosa, M. M., Rodríguez, J., Muzquiz, M., Maleki, S. J., Cuadrado, C., Burbano, C., and Crespo, J. F. 2012. Influence of enzymatic hydrolysis on the allergenicity of roasted peanut protein extract. *International Archives of Allergy and Immunology* 157(1):41–50.

Cheewapramong, P., Riaz, M. N., Rooney, L. W., and Lusas, E. W. 2002. Use of partially defatted peanut flour in breakfast cereal flakes. *Cereal Chemistry 79*(4):586–592.

Chen, G. T., Zhao, L., Zhao, L. Y., Cong, T., and Bao, S. F. 2007. In vitro study on antioxidant activities of peanut protein hydrolysate. *Journal of the Science of Food and Agriculture* 87(2):357–362.

Chen, Y., Lan, D., Wang, W., Zhang, W., and Wang, Y. 2023. Quality characteristics of peanut protein-based patties produced with pre-emulsified olive oil as a fat replacer: Influence of acylglycerol type. *International Journal of Biological Macromolecules* 252:126262.

Chowdhury, F. N., Hossain, D., Hosen, M., and Rahman, S. (2015). Comparative study on chemical composition of five varieties of groundnut (Arachis hypogaea). *World Journal of Agricultural Science* 11(5):247–254.

Dai, T., Shuai, X., Chen, J., Li, C., Wang, J., Liu, W., ... Wang, R. 2022. Whole peanut milk prepared by an industry-scale microfluidization system: Physical stability, microstructure, and flavor properties. *LWT* 171:114140.

Day, L., Cakebread, J. A., and Loveday, S. M. 2022. Food proteins from animals and plants: differences in the nutritional and functional properties. *Trends in Food Science and Technology* 119:428–442.

Dhanshetty, M., Elliott, C. T., and Banerjee, K. 2021. Decontamination of aflatoxin B1 in peanuts using various cooking methods. *Journal of Food Science and Technology* 58:2547–2554.

Er Demirhan, B., and Demirhan, B. 2022. Investigation of twelve significant mycotoxin contamination in nut-based products by the LC–MS/MS method. *Metabolites* 12(2):120.

Dong, X. H., Li, J., Jiang, G. X., Li, H. Y., Zhao, M. M., and Jiang, Y. M. 2019. Effects of combined high pressure and enzymatic treatments on physicochemical and antioxidant properties of peanut proteins. *Food Science and Nutrition* 7(4):1417–1425.

Garg, P., and Brar, J. K. 2017. Development and organoleptic evaluation of nutritious bars by using defatted peanut flour, roasted soybean seeds for gym trainees. *Chemical Science Review and Letters* 6(23):2051–2057.

Global Peanut Flour Market: Industry Analysis and Forecast (2019–2027). https://www.maximizemarketresearch.com/market-report/global-peanut-flour-market/72734/ (Accessed on August 20, 2023).

Guy, E., Emmanuel, A. A., and John, B. 2013. Nutrients content and lipid characterization of seed pastes of four selected peanut (*Arachis hypogaea*) varieties from Ghana. *African Journal of Food Science* 7(10):375–381.

Hanna, M., Jaqua, E., Nguyen, V., and Clay, J. B. 2022. Vitamins: Functions and Uses in Medicine. *Perm Journal*, 26:89–97.

Harris, H., Davis, E. Y., Van De Mark, M. S., Rymal, K. S., and Spadaro, J. J. 1972. Development and use of defatted peanut flours., meals, and grits. Bulletin 431, Alabama Agricultural Experiment Station. http://hdl.handle.net/11200/2367 (Accessed on August 21, 2023).

Houston, M.C. and Harper, K.J. 2008. Potassium, magnesium, and calcium: their role in both the cause and treatment of hypertension. *The Journal of Clinical Hypertension* 10(7):3–11.

Howard, B. M., McWatters, K. H., Saalia, F., and Hashim, I. 2009. Formulation and evaluation of snack crackers made with peanut flour. *Cereal Foods World (CFW)* 54(4):166.

Howard, B. M., Hung, Y. C., and McWatters, K. 2011. Analysis of ingredient functionality and formulation optimization of pasta supplemented with peanut flour. *Journal of Food Science* 76(1): E40–E47.

IUPAC. 1989. The nomenclature of steroids. https://iupac.qmul.ac.uk/steroid (Accessed on October 31, 2023).

Jiang, R., Manson, J. E., Stampfer, M. J., Liu, S., Willett, W. C., and Hu, F. B. 2002. Nut and peanut butter consumption and risk of type 2 diabetes in women. *JAMA* 288(20):2554–2560.

Jones, J. B., Provost, M., Keaver, L., Breen, C., Ludy, M. J., and Mattes, R. D. 2014. A randomized trial on the effects of flavorings on the health benefits of daily peanut consumption. *The American Journal of Clinical Nutrition* 99(3):490–496.

Jonnala, R. S., Dunford, N. T., and Chenault, K. 2005. Nutritional composition of genetically modified peanut varieties. *Journal of Food Science* 70(4):S254–S256.

Katzman, E. W., and Nielsen, S. J. 2021. The association between peanut and peanut butter consumption and cognitive function among community-dwelling older adults. *The Journal of Prevention of Alzheimer's Disease* 8(4):436–441.

Koehler, P., and Wieser, H. 2012. Chemistry of cereal grains. In *Handbook on sourdough biotechnology*, eds M. Gobbetti and M. Gänzle, 11–45. New York, NY: Springer.

Kulthe, A. A., Pawar, V. D., Kotecha, P. M., Chavan, U. D., and Bansode, V. V. 2014. Development of high protein and low-calorie cookies. *Journal of Food Science and Technology* 51:153–157.

Lee, L. S., Cucullu, A. F., Franz Jr, A. O., and Pons Jr, W. A. 1969. Destruction of aflatoxins in peanuts during dry and oil roasting. *Journal of Agricultural and Food Chemistry* 17(3):451–453.

Lieberman, J. A., Gupta, R. S., Knibb, R. C., Haselkorn, T., Tilles, S., Mack, D. P., and Pouessel, G. 2021. The global burden of illness of peanut allergy: a comprehensive literature review. *Allergy* 76(5):1367–1384.

Li, M., Shi, Z. A. 2019. Prospective association of nut consumption with cognitive function in chinese adults aged 55+ – China health and nutrition survey. *Journal of Nutrition, Health and Aging* 23:211–216.

Liu, Y., Hu, H., Liu, H., and Wang, Q. 2022. Recent advances for the developing of instant flavor peanut powder: generation and challenges. *Foods* 11(11):1544.

Luu, H. N., Blot, W. J., Xiang, Y. B., Cai, H., Hargreaves, M. K., Li, H., … Shu, X. O. 2015. Prospective evaluation of the association of nut/peanut consumption with total and cause-specific mortality. *JAMA Internal Medicine* 175(5):755–766.

Martí i Líndez, A. A., and Reith, W. 2021. Arginine-dependent immune responses. *Cellular and Molecular Life Sciences* 78(13):5303–5324.

Moreno, J. P., Johnston, C. A., El-Mubasher, A. A., Papaioannou, M. A., Tyler, C., Gee, M., and Foreyt, J. P. 2013. Peanut consumption in adolescents is associated with improved weight status. *Nutrition Research* 33(7):552–556.

Muñoz-Arrieta, R., Esquivel-Alvarado, D., Alfaro-Viquez, E., Alvarez-Valverde, V., Krueger, C. G., and Reed, J. D. 2021. Nutritional and bioactive composition of Spanish, Valencia, and Virginia type peanut skins. *Journal of Food Composition and Analysis* 98:103816.

NationMaster. 2020. Top countries in groundnut oil production. https://www.nationmaster.com/nmx/ranking/groundnut-oil-production (Accessed on September 2023).

Neuenschwander, M., Ballon, A., Weber, K. S., Norat, T., Aune, D., Schwingshackl, L., and Schlesinger, S. 2019. Role of diet in type 2 diabetes incidence: umbrella review of meta-analyses of prospective observational studies. *BMJ* 366:l2368.

Nieuwenhuis, L., and van den Brandt, P. A. 2018. Total nut, tree nut, peanut, and peanut butter consumption and the risk of pancreatic cancer in the Netherlands Cohort Study. *Cancer Epidemiology, Biomarkers and Prevention* 27(3):274–284.

Normen, L., Bryngelsson, S., Johnsson, M., Evheden, P., Ellegård, L., Brants, H., ... Dutta, P. 2002. The phytosterol content of some cereal foods commonly consumed in Sweden and in the Netherlands. *Journal of Food Composition and Analysis* 15(6):693–704.

Palmer, B. F., Colbert, G., and Clegg, D. J. 2020. Potassium homeostasis, chronic kidney disease, and the plant-enriched diets. *Kidney360* 1(1):65.

Parilli-Moser, I., Domínguez-López, I., Trius-Soler, M., Castellví, M., Bosch, B., Castro-Barquero, S., ... and Lamuela-Raventós, R. M. 2021. Consumption of peanut products improves memory and stress response in healthy adults from the ARISTOTLE study: A 6-month randomized controlled trial. *Clinical Nutrition* 40(11):5556–5567.

Parilli-Moser, I., Hurtado-Barroso, S., Guasch-Ferré, M., and Lamuela-Raventós, R. M. 2022. Effect of peanut consumption on cardiovascular risk factors: a randomized clinical trial and meta-analysis. *Frontiers in Nutrition* 9:853378.

Quist, E. E., Phillips, R. D., and Saalia, F. K. 2009. Angiotensin converting enzyme inhibitory activity of proteolytic digests of peanut (Arachis hypogaea L.) flour. *LWT-Food Science and Technology* 42(3):694–699.

Rehrah, D., Ahmedna, M., Goktepe, I., and Yu, J. 2009. Extrusion parameters and consumer acceptability of a peanut-based meat analogue. *International Journal of Food Science and Technology* 44(10):2075–2084.

Sanders, T. H., McMichael, R. W., and Hendrix, K. W. 2000. Occurrence of resveratrol in edible peanuts. *Journal of Agricultural and Food Chemistry* 48(4):1243–1246.

Sapp, P. A., Kris-Etherton, P. M., and Petersen, K. S. 2022. Peanuts or an isocaloric lower fat, higher carbohydrate nighttime snack have similar effects on fasting glucose in adults with elevated fasting glucose concentrations: a 6-week randomized crossover trial. *The Journal of Nutrition* 152(1):153–162.

Scanes, Colin G. 2018. Impact of agricultural animals on the environment. In *Animals and human society*, ed C.G. Scanes and S. Toukhsati, 427–449. Academic Press.

Seth, K., and Kochhar, A. 2018. Nutritional assessment of healthy cakes developed using partially defatted peanut flour. *Chemical Science Review and Letters* 7(25):244–249.

Shaghaghian, S., McClements, D. J., Khalesi, M., Garcia-Vaquero, M., and Mirzapour-Kouhdasht, A. (2022). Digestibility and bioavailability of plant-based proteins intended for use in meat analogues: A review. *Trends in Food Science and Technology* 129:646–656.

Shi, A., Liu, H., Liu, L., Hu, H., Wang, Q. et al. 2014. Isolation, purification and molecular mechanism of a peanut protein-derived ACE-inhibitory peptide. *PLoS One* 9(10):e111188.

Shin, E. C., Pegg, R. B., Phillips, R. D., and Eitenmiller, R. R. 2010. Commercial peanut (Arachis hypogaea L.) cultivars in the United States: phytosterol composition. *Journal of Agricultural and Food Chemistry* 58(16):9137–9146.

Shiraseb, F., Asbaghi, O., Bagheri, R., Wong, A., Figueroa, A., and Mirzaei, K. 2022. Effect of L-arginine supplementation on blood pressure in adults: A systematic review and dose–response meta-analysis of randomized clinical trials. *Advances in Nutrition* 13(4):1226–1242.

Singh, A. P., Singh, R., Verma, S. S., Rai, V., Kaschula, C. H., Maiti, P., and Gupta, S. C. 2019. Health benefits of resveratrol: Evidence from clinical studies. *Medicinal Research Reviews* 39(5):1851–1891.

Siwela, A. H., Mukaro, K. J., and Nziramasanga, N. 2011. Aflatoxin carryover during large scale peanut butter production. *Food and Nutrition Sciences* 2(2):4527.

Soetan, K. O., Olaiya, C. O., and Oyewole, O. E. 2010. The importance of mineral elements for humans, domestic animals and plants: A review. *African Journal of Food Science* 4(5):200–222.

Stephens, A. M., Dean, L. L., Davis, J. P., Osborne, J. A., and Sanders, T. H. 2010. Peanuts, peanut oil, and fat free peanut flour reduced cardiovascular disease risk factors and the development of atherosclerosis in Syrian golden hamsters. *Journal of Food Science* 75(4):H116–H122.

Tapiero, H., Mathé, G., Couvreur, P. and Tew, K. D. 2002. I. arginine. *Biomedicine & Pharmacotherapy* 56(9):439–445.

USDA-NASS. 2019. FoodData central. USDA-NASS (usda.gov) (Accessed on August 9, 2023).

van den Brandt, P. A., and Nieuwenhuis, L. 2018. Tree nut, peanut, and peanut butter intake and risk of postmenopausal breast cancer: the Netherlands Cohort Study. *Cancer Causes and Control* 29:63–75.

van den Brandt, P. A., and Schouten, L. J. 2015. Relationship of tree nut, peanut and peanut butter intake with total and cause-specific mortality: a cohort study and meta-analysis. *International Journal of Epidemiology* 44(3):1038–1049.

Wang, N. F., Yan, Z., Li, C. Y., Jiang, N., and Liu, H. J. 2011. Antioxidant activity of peanut flour fermented with lactic acid bacteria. *Journal of Food Biochemistry* 35(5):1514–1521.

Warren, C., Lei, D., Sicherer, S., Schleimer, R., and Gupta, R. 2021. Prevalence and characteristics of peanut allergy in US adults. *Journal of Allergy and Clinical Immunology* 147(6):2263–2270.

Xiao, X., Wang, J., Zhu, Y., Deng, B., Liu, Y., Wang, S., ... Song, T. 2023. Phytosterols Protect against Osteoporosis by Regulating Gut Microbiota. *Journal of Agricultural and Food Chemistry* 71(40):14539–14549.

Yeh, C. C., You, S. L., Chen, C. J., and Sung, F. C. 2006. Peanut consumption and reduced risk of colorectal cancer in women: a prospective study in Taiwan. *World Journal of Gastroenterology* 12(2):222.

Yemmireddy, V. K., Chintagari, S., and Hung, Y. C. 2013. Physico-chemical properties of pancakes made from an instant mix containing different levels of peanut (Arachis hypogaea) flour. *Peanut Science* 40(2):142–148.

Yu, J. 2016. Methods for reducing allergenicity of peanuts and peanut derived products – Their efficacy, feasibility and safety. *Austin Food Sciences* 1(3):1012.

Yu, J., Hernandez, M., Li, H., Goktepe, I., Robinette, C., Auerbach, A., ... and Ahmedna, M. 2015. Allergenicity of roasted peanuts treated with a non-human digestive protease. *Food Research International* 69:341–347.

Yu, J., Mikiashvili, N., Bonku, R., and Smith, I. N. 2021. Allergenicity, antioxidant activity and ACE-inhibitory activity of protease hydrolyzed peanut flour. *Food Chemistry* 360:129992.

Yu, J., Smith, I. N., Idris, N., Gregory, N., and Mikiashvili, N. 2020. Oxidative stability of protease treated peanut with reduced allergenicity. *Foods* 9(6):762.

Zaaboul, F., Raza, H., Cao, C., and Yuanfa, L. 2019. The impact of roasting, high pressure homogenization and sterilization on peanut milk and its oil bodies. *Food Chemistry* 280:270–277.

Zeisel, S. H., and Da Costa, K. A. 2009. Choline: an essential nutrient for public health. *Nutrition Reviews* 67(11):615–623.

Zeng, Y., Wang, N., and Qian, W. 2013. Production of Angiotensin I Converting Enzyme inhibitory peptides from peanut meal fermented with lactic acid bacteria and facilitated with protease. *Advance Journal of Food Science and Technology* 5(9):1198–1203.

Zhang, Y., Zhang, H., Wang, L., Guo, X., Qi, X., and Qian, H. 2011. Influence of the degree of hydrolysis (DH) on antioxidant properties and radical-scavenging activities of peanut peptides prepared from fermented peanut meal. *European Food Research and Technology* 232: 941–950.

Zhao, Y., Zhao, L., Hu, Z., Wu, J., Li, J., Qu, C. ... Song, Q. 2018. Peanut consumption associated with a reduced risk of esophageal squamous cell carcinoma: A case–control study in a high-risk area in China. *Thoracic Cancer* 9(1):30–36.

Zheng, H., Wei, S., Xu, Y., and Fan, M. 2015. Reduction of aflatoxin B1 in peanut meal by extrusion cooking. *LWT-food Science and Technology* 64(2): 515–519.

Zhou, W., Branch, W. D., Gilliam, L., and Marshall, J. A. 2018. Phytosterol composition of *Arachis hypogaea* seeds from different maturity classes. *Molecules* 24:106.

37 Hemp Seed as a Novel Protein Source

Vermont P. Dia

ABBREVIATIONS

ACE	Angiotensin I converting enzyme
BDNF	Brain-derived neurotrophic factor
DPPH	2,2-diphenyl-1-picrylhydrazyl
HPI	Hemp protein isolate
IVD	*In vitro* digestibility
LPS	Lipopolysaccharide
ORAC	Oxygen radical absorbance capacity
PDCAAS	Protein digestibility-corrected amino acid score
SHRs	Spontaneously hypertensive rats

INTRODUCTION

Proteins are nitrogenous-containing substances required for the maintenance of life. They are needed for all body processes and provide structural and functional support to sustain life (Institute of Medicine 2002). In nature, 21 distinct amino acids serve as substrates for protein synthesis, of which 9 are considered essential and must be provided by the diet. The current dietary reference intakes for adults aged $\geq$19 years are 0.66 g protein/kg body weight/day (estimated average intake) and 0.80 g protein/kg body weight/day (recommended dietary allowance) (Institute of Medicine 2002). Negative nitrogen balance and a loss of functional body proteins are detrimental effects that result from not meeting the dietary reference intake for any of the nine essential amino acids (Kurpad et al. 2002; Borgonha et al. 2002). Hence, protein quality is an important consideration when evaluating alternative sources of dietary proteins.

Hemp (*Cannabis sativa* L.) is a crop that is traditionally used for industrial purposes, including the production of fiber, seeds, oil, and meal (Vonapartis et al. 2015) (Figure 37.1). It has gained attention as a sustainable agricultural crop with potential food applications. The interest in hemp food applications can be attributed to the unique chemical and nutritional composition of the different parts of the hemp plant. For instance, hemp seeds are rich in phytosterols and health-promoting omega fatty acids (Frassinetti et al. 2018; Anwar et al. 2006). In addition, hemp seed proteins contain all essential amino acids with a protein digestibility-corrected amino acid score (PDCAAS) similar to or better than other grains, nuts, and pulses (House et al. 2010). A recent report showed that hemp seed protein allergens could be removed during hemp seed protein isolate (HPI) production and gastrointestinal digestion (Mamone et al. 2019), making it an attractive alternative for individuals suffering from gastrointestinal sensitivities such as gluten intolerance and celiac disease. On average, whole hemp seeds contain about 30% crude fat, 24% crude protein, 33% neutral detergent fiber, 7% nitrogen-free extract, and 6% moisture (House et al. 2010). This proximate component analysis, as well as analysis of individual fatty acids and amino acids, shows that hemp seed is a potential source of high-quality food ingredients. In addition to an attractive macronutrient composition,

DOI: 10.1201/9781003597926-37

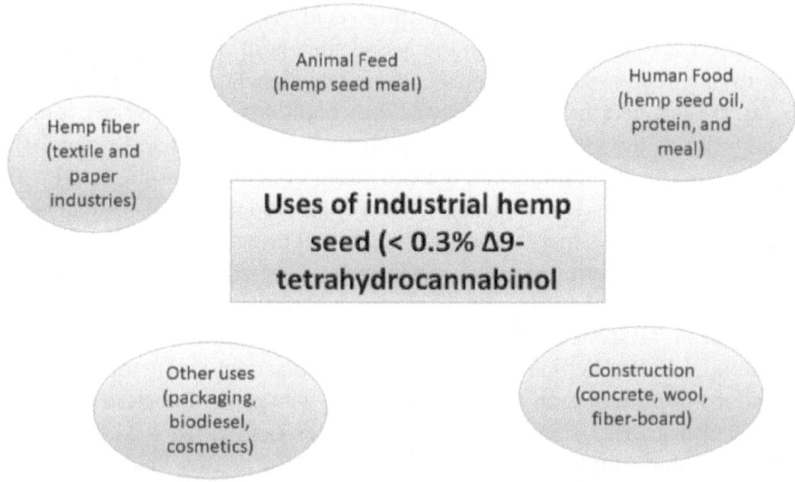

FIGURE 37.1 Different uses of industrial hemp seed: Hemp seed as a cultivated crop is used in different industries, including the textile and construction industries, animal feed, human food, and cosmetics, and is currently being studied for its other potential applications in biodiesel and pharmaceuticals.

hemp seed contains secondary metabolites with reported health properties (Yan et al. 2015; Wang et al. 2019; Pellati et al. 2018).

Due to its high-quality oils and proteins, hemp seed application in a variety of food preparations is currently being investigated. The residue after hemp seed oil extraction, known as hemp meal, can be made into hemp flour, which can be used in different food applications. The addition of hemp meal flour up to 50% in bread production led to increased protein content, increased total polyphenol concentration, and reduced staling, albeit with decreased overall acceptability, which may be associated with reduced volume and increased hardness and browning index (Kowalski et al. 2019). Moreover, hemp flour sourdough fermentation led to increased digestibility (Nionelli et al. 2018). Fortification of wheat bread with hemp sourdough increased the textural properties of wheat bread without adversely affecting the sensory characteristics of the final product (Nionelli et al. 2018). In starch-based gluten-free bread, hemp flour and hemp protein concentrate led to improved nutritional value by increasing levels of fibers as well as improved sensory acceptance associated with favorable crumb color, increased bread volume, and limited crumb hardening (Witczak et al. 2017). These studies clearly demonstrated the potential of hemp flour as a food ingredient with improved nutritional quality as well as acceptable sensory attributes. The purpose of this chapter is to discuss the role of hemp seed as a novel protein source with the potential to improve overall human health.

NUTRITIONAL QUALITY OF HEMP SEED PROTEIN

Proteins perform different functions in the body, ranging from building and maintaining body tissues to serving as enzymes and hormones to regulate body processes. As nutrients, the nutritional quality of proteins is measured by their digestibility and content of essential amino acids. Protein digestibility is affected by the structure of the proteins, the presence of antinutritional compounds, and processing (Sarwar 1997). House et al. (2010) evaluated the quality of protein from different hemp seed products using PDCAAS. In this study, 30 samples of hemp products, including whole hemp seed, hemp seed meals, and hemp seed hulls, were analyzed for their composition, amino acid concentration, and PDCAAS using a rat bioassay for protein digestibility. They reported that in comparison to casein with a PDCAAS of 100 and an amino acid score of 1.19, hemp seed, dehulled hemp seed, and hemp seed meal had lower PDCAAS and amino acid scores of 49–54% and 0.52–0.69, 53–66% and 0.54–0.69, and 46–51% and 0.50–0.64, respectively (House et al. 2010).

Further, lysine was reported as the first limiting amino acid, with leucine and tryptophan following, depending on the product. The limitation in the lysine content of the hemp seed products analyzed was comparable to other cereal grains such as corn and whole wheat (House et al. 2010).

Potin et al. (2019) evaluated the effect of extraction conditions (including pH, ionic strength, and press-cake/liquid ratio) on the yield and protein quality of hemp proteins. Among different factors, pH was reported to have the most impact on the extraction of hemp proteins, with an alkaline pH of 12 resulting in a significant 8-fold yield increase when compared to extraction at pH 8. Interestingly, the total nitrogen content in the supernatant, as a measure of protein solubilization (which can affect protein functionality and digestibility), was not improved by adding different concentrations of NaCl to proteins extracted at pH 10, 11, and 12 (Potin et al. 2019).

Alonso-Esteban et al. (2022) evaluated the chemical composition of eight hemp seed cultivars and eight commercial dehulled hemp seeds. They reported that dehulled hemp seed samples contain higher concentrations of protein than whole hemp seeds. The protein content of eight whole hemp seed cultivars ranged from 18.3–23.0%, while these values ranged from 24.6–28.4% for dehulled hemp seeds. Another study looking at the nutritional values of two Polish hemp seed cultivars reported that hemp seeds are rich in protein, fat, and dietary fiber (Teleszko et al. 2022). The authors concluded that the phenylalanine + tyrosine and histidine contents of the two hemp seed cultivars exhibited similarities to egg protein.

In vitro digestibility (IVD) studies are a common method to evaluate the potential nutritional quality of food ingredients. Reports on the IVD of hemp seed proteins as affected by cultivation, pre-processing, processing treatments, and sources have been reported. Khalesi et al. (2023) reported that organically cultivated hemp seed possessed higher total protein (with lower non-protein nitrogen content) than conventionally grown hemp seed. IVD of hemp seeds was evaluated by the degree of hydrolysis following simulated gastrointestinal digestion. The degree of hydrolysis among three hemp seed samples was not statistically different after gastric digestion, but organically cultivated hemp seed showed the lowest degree of hydrolysis after gastrointestinal digestion when compared to conventionally cultivated hemp seeds (Khalesi et al. 2023). The IVD of proteins isolated from hemp processing by-products (hemp seed cake and hemp seed hulls) was reported by Banskota et al. (2022). The *in vitro* protein digestibility values of protein isolates from hemp hearts, hemp whole seed, hemp cake, and hemp seed hulls were 98.5%, 94.6%, 91.1%, and 87.8%, respectively. Sharma et al. (2023) reported that dehulling yield was improved by 1.3–1.5-fold when hemp seeds were exposed to hydrothermal treatments. Further, they reported that steaming treatments at 14% moisture for 10 and 60 minutes resulted in improved *in vitro* protein digestibility of dehulled hemp seeds from 86.53% to 88.13–88.73% without impacting the protein nutritional composition of the dehulled hemp seeds (Sharma et al. 2023). Lin et al. (2020) reported that pre-heating of hemp protein isolates resulted in improved digestibility as measured by the degree of hydrolysis after pepsin-pancreatin digestion. The degree of hydrolysis increased from 1.66% for samples with no pre-heating to 10.56% for 10-minute pre-heating at 100°C and 15.76% for 30-minute pre-heating at 100°C after pepsin-pancreatin digestion. Another study reported the effect of drying methods on the *in vitro* protein digestibility of hemp seed meal, with protein content ranging from 76.42–79.72% (Lin et al. 2021). Among the three drying methods, freeze-drying resulted in the highest content of the limiting amino acid lysine, the highest total amino acid concentrations, and the highest *in vitro* protein digestibility of 88.22% (Lin et al. 2021). Another study on the effect of pre-processing on the nutritional properties of hemp seed investigated the impact of malting (Farinon et al. 2022). They reported that malting increased the protein content of the Futura 75 industrial hemp cultivar; germination for 2 days at 24°C in the dark with a relative humidity of 85%, followed by drying at 70°C for 6 hours, increased the protein content from 23.88% to 26.06% without affecting the fat content (Farinon et al. 2022).

BIOLOGICAL ACTIVITIES OF HEMP SEED PROTEIN HYDROLYSATES

Figure 37.2 presents the general steps involved in the production of hemp seed protein isolate and bioactive peptides from the isolate. Proteomics, the large-scale characterization of the entire protein components of cells, tissues, or organisms, has a wide range of applications in agriculture, including crop and animal health studies, resistance to stress, and improving yield and product quality. Two interesting studies have reported on the proteomic profiling and characterization of hemp seed proteins. Park et al. (2012) reported the proteome profile of hemp seed protein from the cultivar Cheungsam using two-dimensional gel electrophoresis and mass spectrometry. Of the 1102 protein spots resolved, 168 unique proteins were identified, belonging to proteins involved in energy regulation, metabolism, stress response, cytoskeleton, binding function, and protein synthesis, with 12% unclassified (Park et al. 2012). On the other hand, Aiello et al. (2016) identified a total of 181 expressed proteins utilizing combinatorial peptide ligand libraries, gel electrophoresis, mass spectrometry, and database search. Through the use of STRING software to perform protein-protein association network analysis, Aiello et al. (2016) were able to build the first interatomic map of hemp seed proteins. Further, they classified these proteins as belonging mostly to seed metabolic processes, response to stimulus, and biological processes. These proteomics studies can lay the groundwork for identifying proteins (and peptides) from hemp seed that can possess biological activities for the development of functional foods and beverages using hemp seed proteins as ingredients.

The concept of functional food started in Japan when epidemiological studies showed that certain populations consuming specific food groups and/or following particular types of diets had a lower risk of developing illnesses such as cancer and cardiovascular diseases. This concept has also been applied in the field of food protein ingredients, particularly the study of bioactive peptides. Bioactive peptides are short sequences of amino acids embedded in the protein's primary structure that can influence metabolic and regulatory processes in the body to promote overall health. They can be released during gastrointestinal digestion, food fermentation, and enzymatic hydrolysis of proteins during the preparation of food protein ingredients. In some cases, bioactive peptides may also be inherently present in the food. Prior to the determination of their biological activities, bioactive peptides are characterized to identify molecular features (as shown in Figure 37.3) that may contribute to their bioactive properties.

Antioxidant peptides have been produced and isolated from hemp seed proteins with varying mechanisms to explain their identified antioxidant properties. Girgih et al. (2013) performed gastrointestinal tract digestion followed by high-pressure liquid chromatographic fractionation to identify antioxidant peptides from HPI. They reported that some fractions had improved oxygen radical absorbance capacity (ORAC), while all fractions had increased their ability to scavenge the radical 2,2-diphenyl-1-picrylhydrazyl (DPPH). Girgih et al. (2013) attributed these improved antioxidant activities to increased concentrations of hydrophobic amino acids with concomitant reduction in the concentration of positively charged amino acids. Several studies have evaluated the effect of different enzymes on the generation of antioxidant peptides from hemp seed protein. Samaei et al. (2021) hydrolyzed protein from hemp bran with Alcalase and identified 12 antioxidant peptides that exhibited structural features related to their antioxidant properties. For instance, they reported that the presence of bulky tyrosine residue at the C-terminal of di- and tripeptides is important in determining their antioxidant properties. Teh et al. (2016) reported the effect of five enzymes on the generation of antioxidant peptides from hemp protein isolates. For instance, alkali-soluble hemp protein isolate hydrolyzed by HT proteolytic concentrate for 2 hours resulted in the highest ability to inhibit DPPH radical production at 73.33% (Teh et al. 2016). Saad and Dia (2023) reported that bromelain hydrolysis of hemp protein isolate improved DPPH scavenging and ORAC value.

Another common test for bioactive peptides is their ability to inhibit the enzyme angiotensin I converting enzyme (ACE). ACE accelerates the conversion of angiotensin I to the vasoconstrictor angiotensin II. Hence, peptides with the ability to inhibit ACE may be candidates for reducing high

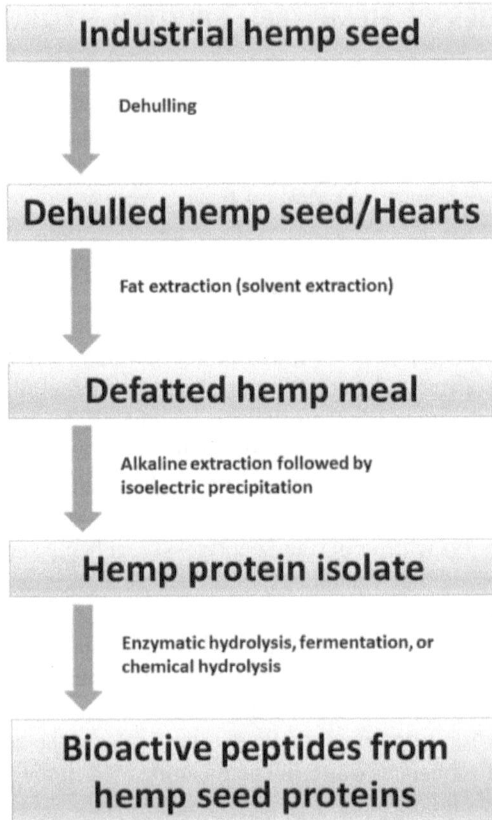

FIGURE 37.2 Generalized schematic steps in the production of hemp protein isolate and bioactive peptides from hemp seed proteins: Hemp seed undergoes a dehulling process followed by fat extraction. The defatted hemp seed, also known as meal, is a good source of proteins. Proteins are extracted from the meal by alkaline solubilization (pH ~10 or ~12), followed by isoelectric precipitation at pH ~5. The precipitate is dried and subjected to hydrolysis to generate bioactive peptides through enzymatic action, chemical action, fermentation, or their combination(s).

blood pressure. Orio et al. (2017) exposed HPI to extensive chemical hydrolysis and identified four bioactive peptides. Through solid-phase synthesis, they demonstrated that the tetrapeptide GVLY was the most potent, with an IC_{50} value of 16 μM (Orio et al. 2017). In spontaneously hypertensive rats (SHRs), Girgih et al. (2014) showed that hemp seed meal protein hydrolysate produced by simulated gastrointestinal digestion when fed to young growing SHRs attenuated normal increases in systolic blood pressure and also resulted in reduced systolic blood pressure in adult SHRs. These observations were accompanied by suppressed plasma ACE activity and reduced plasma renin levels (Girgih et al. 2014). The same group utilized an enzyme inhibition kinetics study combined with molecular docking to study the ACE-inhibitory activity of hemp seed purified peptides (Girgih et al. 2014). Their results showed that WVYY tetrapeptide inhibited ACE with an IC_{50} of 0.027 mM and inhibition constant of 0.06 mM, showing greater affinity to ACE active site residues through H-bonding (Girgih et al. 2014).

Other biological activities include the ability of peptic and tryptic hydrolysate of hemp seed protein concentrate to inhibit 3-hydroxy-methyl-coenzyme A reductase (Aiello et al. 2016; Zanoni et al. 2017; Li et al. 2022), modulation of low-density lipoprotein receptor (Cerrato et al. 2023), inhibition of acetylcholinesterase activity (Malomo and Aluko 2019), α-glucosidase inhibition activity (Cai et al. 2023), anti-inflammatory properties (Rodriguez-Martin et al. 2019; Rodriguez-Martin et al. 2020; Hong et al. 2022; Saad and Dia 2023), and inhibition of the enzyme dipeptidyl peptidase

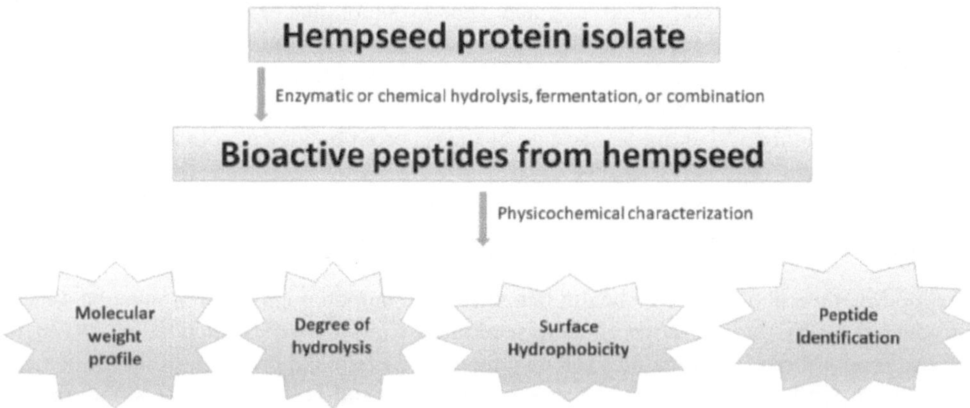

FIGURE 37.3 Typical physicochemical characterization of bioactive peptides from hemp seed protein is conducted prior to the evaluation of their biological activities. Before the bioactive properties of hemp seed-derived peptides are assessed, they undergo physicochemical characterization to potentially relate their physicochemical properties to their biological activities.

IV involved in diabetes (Chen et al. 2023; Aiello et al. 2016). Although the majority of these studies on the bioactivity of hemp protein hydrolysates utilized *in vitro* and *in vivo* designs, these pre-screening studies could serve as supporting information to validate the health-promoting effects of hemp seed proteins in human clinical settings.

HUMAN STUDIES LOOKING AT THE HEALTH BENEFITS OF HEMP SEED

Human studies on the health benefits of hemp seed protein consumption are limited. This is not surprising given industrial hemp seed's association with the psychoactive plant marijuana. For instance, cultivation of industrial hemp seed was only allowed in the United States through the Agricultural Improvement Act of 2018. Nevertheless, there are some studies looking at this, and it will be interesting to see how this area will proceed in the future.

Mollard et al. (2021) looked at the effects of hemp protein consumption on glycemic and satiety control. In this study, two acute randomized crossover experiments were conducted comparing hemp seed protein, soybean protein, and a carbohydrate control. Blood glucose, insulin, and satiety were measured as markers of glycemic response. In both experiments, protein consumption lowered overall mean blood glucose levels pre-pizza meal. In the experiment providing a fixed meal based on body weight consumption, both 40 g of hemp protein and 40 g of soy protein lowered overall mean insulin concentrations. Another study compared the effect of hemp seed alone and in combination with aerobic exercise on metabolic markers, oxidative stress, and neurotrophic factors in sedentary young men (Mohammadrezaei et al. 2022). Hemp seed supplements were given in two 1 g capsules and consumed daily. The results showed that hemp seed consumption alone resulted in a significant increase in high-density lipoproteins while combining hemp seed with aerobic exercise led to significant differences in body weight, body mass index, fat mass, high-density lipoprotein, catalase, and brain-derived neurotrophic factor (BDNF) (Mohammadrezaei et al. 2022). The authors concluded that aerobic physical activity combined with hemp seed consumption may improve anthropometric indices, lipid profile, and BDNF.

A study by Samsamikor et al. (2020) was designed as a double-blind, randomized crossover trial comparing the effect of consuming whole hemp seed protein to hemp seed protein hydrolysate, published as a study protocol in 2020. In this trial, the goal was to study the hypotensive effects of hemp seed protein in 35 hypertensive individuals, defined as having a systolic blood pressure between 130 and 160 mm Hg and a diastolic blood pressure of $\leq$110 mm Hg. The study compared the effect of casein, hemp seed protein, and hemp seed protein plus hemp hydrolysate on 24-hour systolic blood pressure as the primary outcome. In addition, body composition was assessed using dual X-ray absorptiometry. As of this writing, no publications of results have been reported (https://clinicaltrials.gov/study/NCT03508895).

Table 37.1 and Figure 37.4 summarize some of the reported biological activities of peptides isolated from hemp seed.

FUNCTIONAL PROPERTIES OF HEMP SEED PROTEIN

For any food ingredient to confer its health benefits to the human population, it must be added to a food product. As such, the utilization of hemp seed protein in food will be dictated by its functional properties. Food protein functionalities refer to the physicochemical properties that influence their performance in food products during processing, storage, and consumption (Damodaran 2017). These range from their ability to dissolve in water to their ability to stabilize interfacial tension, as shown in Figure 37.5.

Tang et al. (2006) were among the first to report on the functional properties of hemp protein isolate and compare it to soy protein isolate. They reported a lower protein solubility of hemp protein isolate than soy protein isolate when evaluated at a pH less than 8. Further, they reported that the emulsification and water-holding properties of hemp protein isolate were lower than those of soy protein isolate, with similar fat adsorption capacity. In the study by Malomo et al. (2014), the functional properties of HPI were compared to defatted hemp seed protein meal. They showed that hemp protein isolate has better foaming capacity at pH 3, while defatted hemp seed protein meal had higher quality emulsions at 10 and 25 mg/mL (Malomo et al. 2014). The differences in the functional properties were attributed to specific structural transformations of protein-based ingredients from hemp seed.

Wang et al. (2018) looked at the effect of heat and pH shifting on the structure, cross-linking, and emulsification of hemp seed protein. An alkaline pH of 12 and heating at 80°C for 60 min improved the solubility of hemp seed proteins, reaching 97.5% (Wang et al. 2018). A mild pH shift and heating combination conducted at pH 12 and 60°C for 5 min resulted in improved emulsifying properties associated with the dissociation of protein subunits and the exposure of hydrophobic groups due to the unraveling of hemp seed protein tertiary structure (Wang et al. 2018).

The effect of ultrasound treatment on the functional properties of HPI was reported by Karabulut and Yemis (2022). They reported that an acoustic intensity of 37 W/cm^2 for 7.8 min at a protein concentration of 6.9% was optimum in increasing hemp seed protein solubility, which resulted in enhanced functional properties, including emulsification, oil absorption, and foaming properties. A recent study compared the different fractions in HPI and concluded that the 2S hemp seed protein fraction has superior solubility, foaming capacity, and emulsifying activity compared to the 7S fraction, 11S fraction, and whole HPI (Ajibola and Aluko, 2022). Further, Li et al. (2022) reported that cultivars affected the functional properties of HPI. They reported that cultivars with more vicilin and albumin have higher protein solubility, impacting hemp seed protein functionality (Li et al. 2022). In addition, the protein isolation method affected the functionality of HPI. Fang et al. (2023) reported that salt-extracted HPI showed higher solubility, emulsion activity, and thermal stability than HPI prepared by the alkaline extraction–isoelectric precipitation method. These studies are highly important for understanding how hemp seed protein can be applied in food products to take advantage of its reported health benefits. For instance, pasta enriched with hemp flour has been studied, characterized by lower granularity and high nutritional value, which can be described as a high-protein and high-fiber product (Teterycz et al. 2021).

TABLE 37.1
Bioactive Properties of Hemp Seed Protein Hydrolysates and Peptides

Study Type	Bioactivity	Results	Reference
In vitro	Antioxidant	Gastrointestinal digestion of hemp seed proteins improved free radical scavenging activity	Khalesi et al. (2023)
		Fractionation of hemp seed hydrolysates enhanced antioxidant activity	Girgih et al. (2013)
		Alcalase hydrolysis improved the antioxidant activity of proteins from hemp seed bran	Samaei et al. (2021)
		Hydrolysis of hemp seed protein isolate by HT proteolytic concentrate improved antioxidation	Teh et al. (2016)
		Combined Alcalase and Flavourzyme hydrolysis improved antioxidant activity	Rodriguez-Martin et al. (2019)
	Inhibition of DPP-IV activity	16 peptides were identified with DPP-IV inhibitory activity with an IC_{50} of 0.08-246.47 mM	Chen et al. (2023)
		Short-chain peptides with MW 174.1-587.3 Da inhibited DPP-IV (IC_{50} = 0.82 mg/mL)	Cerrato et al. (2023)
	Inhibition of ACE activity	WVYY and WYT inhibited ACE activity with IC50 values of 0.027 mM and 0.574 mM, respectively	Girgih et al. (2014)
		Four peptides (GCLY, IEE, LGV, and RVR) were newly identified to inhibit ACE activity	Orio et al. (2017)
		Four enzymatic hydrolysates from two types of hemp protein isolate inhibited ACE activity from 45.48% to 70.61% after 4 h of incubation	Teh et al. (2016)
		35 peptides were identified to have ACE-inhibitory activity with IC_{50} of 0.5 to 2500 μM for peptides belonging to a fraction with MW of less than 1 kDa	Samaei et al. (2021)
	Modulation of cholesterol metabolism	Short-chain peptide mixtures modulated cholesterol metabolism by activating low-density lipoprotein receptor, increasing SREBP2 transcription factor, and decreasing PCSK9	Cerrato et al. (2023)
		Hemp seed peptide IGFLIIWV inhibited HMGCoA reductase activity, activated the AMPK pathway, reduced PCSK9 levels, and improved uptake of extracellular LDL	Li et al. (2022)
		Peptic hydrolysate of hemp seed proteins with 90 peptides identified inhibited HMGCoA reductase activity, activated AMPK pathway, and inactivated HMGCoA reductase phosphorylation	Zanoni et al. (2017)
	Antiproliferative	Pepsin-pancreatin digests of hemp protein isolate reduced the proliferation of colon cancer cells	Lin et al. (2020)
	Anti-inflammatory	Pepsin-pancreatin digests of hemp meal protein reduced the production of inflammatory molecules nitric oxide, TNF-α, and IL-6 in lipopolysaccharide (LPS)-induced RAW 264.7 macrophages	Lin et al. (2021)
		Hemp protein hydrolyzed by either Alcalase or bromelain reduced production of nitric oxide, TNF-α, and IL-6 in LPS-induced inflammation in RAW 264.7 macrophages	Hong et al. (2022)

(Continued)

TABLE 37.1 (CONTINUED)
Bioactive Properties of Hemp Seed Protein Hydrolysates and Peptides

Study Type	Bioactivity	Results	Reference
In vivo	Hypotensive	Hemp seed meal protein hydrolysate fed at 0.5 and 1.0% substitution for casein attenuated normal increases in systolic blood pressure (SBP) in young growing SHRs and significantly reduced SBP in adult SHRs	Girgih et al. (2014)
	Hypoglycemic	Peptides from non-dehulled hemp seed meal generated by alkaline protease 37,071 inhibited α-glucosidase activity *in* vitro and modulated blood glucose and blood lipids in hyperglycemic rats	Cai et al. (2023)
Human	Metabolic and oxidative stress	Hemp seed consumption in combination with physical activity caused significant differences in weight, body mass index, fat mass, high-density lipoprotein, catalase, and BDNF. Hemp seed consumption alone increased high-density lipoprotein levels	Mohammadrezaei et al. (2022)
	Glycemic and satiety control	Hemp seed protein concentrate treatment lowered 0–60-min blood glucose overall mean, lowered overall mean insulin concentration	Mollard et al. (2021)
	Study protocol for hypertension	Randomized, double-blind crossover clinical trial on 35 hypertensive participants with the primary outcome of 24-hour SBP and body composition	Samsamikor et al. (2020)

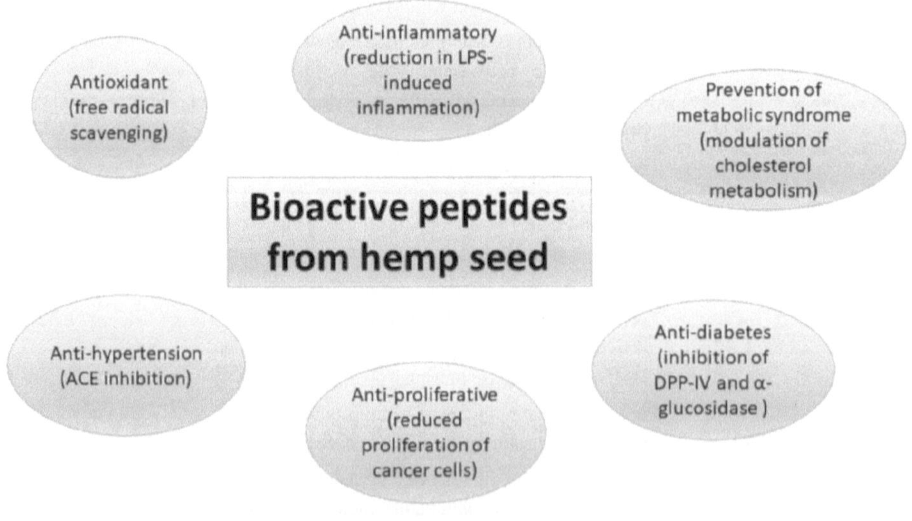

FIGURE 37.4 Reported *in vitro*, *in vivo*, and clinical-setting biological activities of hemp seed-derived bioactive peptides. Bioactive peptides derived from hemp seed proteins have shown a wide range of biological activities, including antioxidant, anti-inflammatory, antidiabetes, anticancer, and anticholesterol properties.

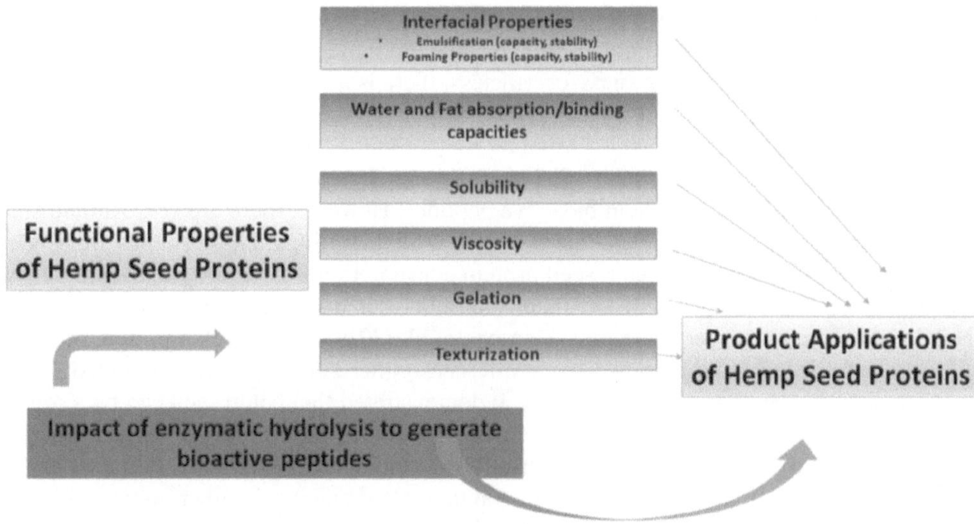

FIGURE 37.5 Functional properties of hemp seed proteins. These reported functional properties are significant for the potential applications of hemp seed proteins in different food products to take advantage of their reported health benefits.

THE EFFECT OF OTHER PROTEINS

Hemp seed protein is a relatively new food protein source that is currently being investigated as more countries allow cultivation and research of industrial hemp seed. Research on how hemp seed protein can be used in combination with other more commonly known food protein sources is ongoing. For instance, Zahari et al. (2020) studied the optimum ratio of hemp seed protein concentrate to soy protein isolate in the production of high-moisture meat analogue products. Their study showed that incorporating hemp protein at different levels (20, 40, and 60%) could be used in the production of texturized meat, but they noted that the nutritional composition and sensory acceptance of the resulting product need to be investigated. Further, they reported that a formulation with a higher concentration of soy protein isolate (up to 80%) resulted in a more compact meat analogue product. The same group studied the effect of adding wheat gluten and chickpea protein concentrate to high-moisture meat analogues from hemp seed protein concentrate (Zahari et al. 2023). The addition of wheat gluten to hemp seed protein concentrate resulted in meat analogue products that were less hard, less resilient, and less chewy. Further, incorporating 50% wheat gluten or 50% chickpea protein concentrate resulted in a meat analogue with promising physicochemical and sensory properties (Zahari et al. 2023). However, these studies did not look at how the combination of other proteins with hemp protein could impact the nutritional quality of the resulting product. In addition, the studies did not investigate the impact of other proteins on the gastrointestinal digestibility of the meat analogues. These are essential research questions that must be explored as they will likely impact the generation of bioactive peptides from these protein mixtures during digestion, thereby impacting the health benefits associated with industrial hemp seed protein.

SUMMARY AND FUTURE PERSPECTIVES

In this chapter, the nutritional quality, biological activities, and functional properties of hemp seed proteins were summarized. The nutritional quality of hemp seed proteins is dictated by their digestibility, which is similar to other cereal grain proteins. Furthermore, the essential amino acid content of hemp seed proteins is comparable to other plant proteins, with lysine as the first limiting amino acid. The biological activities of hemp seed proteins are mostly associated with bioactive peptides derived from hemp seed proteins that can be prepared through enzymatic digestion and, in some cases, by extensive chemical hydrolysis. Nevertheless, there is a scarcity of research on the role of fermentation in the generation of bioactive peptides from hemp seed proteins. This can be an avenue for future research.

Several *in vitro* and *in vivo* studies have shown the antioxidant, anti-inflammatory, and antihypertensive effects of hemp seed protein bioactive peptides. However, there are very limited studies on the health benefits of hemp seed proteins in human clinical settings. These studies are needed to substantiate the health benefits of hemp seed protein consumption. An important avenue for future research is the safety of hemp seed protein consumption. For instance, a few studies have shown that hemp seed proteins can be allergenic. Mamone et al. (2019) reported that proteomic analysis of HPI did not detect any of the known hemp allergens either before or after simulated gastrointestinal digestion. Recently, Beriziky et al. (2023) demonstrated that hemp seed can be a source of allergens with potential cross-reactivity to hazelnuts. It is therefore important to expand studies on the potential allergenicity of hemp seed proteins, their potential cross-reactivity with the "big nine" allergens, as well as the effect of food processing on their allergenicity. Another important aspect to consider when evaluating safety is the effect of prolonged ingestion of hemp seed proteins. Animal studies on hemp seed protein consumption mostly focused on its digestibility, and were conducted over a relatively short period of time. There is a need to investigate the effect of long-term hemp seed protein consumption on potential changes in the microbiota, metabolome, and proteome. In conclusion, hemp seed is a promising crop that can be a source of protein with the potential to feed the growing population and improve human health.

MINI DICTIONARY OF TERMS

- **Alkaline extraction–isoelectric precipitation:** A common method of isolating proteins from plant sources where ground plant materials are suspended at alkaline pH (8 to 12) and precipitated at their isoelectric points (pH 4 to 5).
- **Bioactive peptides:** Short sequences of amino acids embedded in the primary structure of the protein that can be released by enzymatic hydrolysis, fermentation, and/or chemical hydrolysis. These peptides demonstrate a wide range of biological activities when tested in vitro and in vivo, ranging from antioxidant to anticancer properties.
- **Functional properties of hemp seed proteins:** Characteristics that determine how hemp seed proteins would perform in a food product, indicating their potential application.
- **Hemp protein isolate:** A form of protein isolated from hemp seed with a protein content ranging from 85 to 95%.
- **Industrial hemp seed:** A form of cultivated hemp associated with low concentrations of Δ9-tetrahydrocannabinol, differentiating it from the psychoactive hemp.

SUMMARY POINTS

- This chapter focuses on hemp seed as a novel protein source.
- Hemp protein isolate can be derived from different hemp seed forms.
- Hemp protein isolate has a digestibility similar to cereal grain proteins.
- Hemp seed protein's first limiting amino acid is lysine.
- Hemp seed protein's health benefits are associated with bioactive peptides.
- Bioactive peptides from hemp seed proteins' biological activities include antioxidant, anti-inflammatory, antidiabetic, and antihypertensive activities.
- There are very few human studies on the health benefits of hemp seed proteins.
- Hemp seed proteins demonstrate important functional properties that can be taken advantage of for food product applications.

- Studies are needed to evaluate the safety of hemp seed proteins in terms of allergenicity and long-term consumption.

REFERENCES

Aiello G, Fasoli E, Boschin G, Lammi C, Zanoni C, Citterio A, Arnoldi A. 2016. Proteomic characterization of hempseed (*Cannabis sativa* L.). *Journal of Proteomics* 147: 187–196.

Aiello G, Lammi C, Boschin G, Zanoni C, Arnoldi A. Exploration of potentially bioactive peptides from the enzymatic hydrolysis of hempseed proteins. *Journal of Agricultural and Food Chemistry* 65: 10174–10184.

Ajibola CF, Aluko RE. 2022. Physocochemical and functional properties of 2S, 7S, and 11S enriched hemp seed protein fractions. *Molecules* 27: 1059.

Alonso-Esteban J, Pinela J, Ciric A, Clahelsa RC, Sokovic M, Ferreira IC, Barros L, Torija-Isasa E, Sanchez-Mata MC. 2022. Chemical composition and biological activities of whole and dehulled hemp (*Cannabis sativa* L.) seeds. *Food Chemistry* 374: 131754.

Anwar F, Latif S, Ashraf M. 2006. Analytical characterization of hemp (*Cannabis sativa*) seed oil from different agro-ecological zones of Pakistan. *Journal of the American Oil Chemists' Society* 4: 323–329.

Banskota AH, Tibbetts SM, Jones A, Stefanova R. Behnke J. 2022. Biochemical characterization and *in vitro* digestibility of protein isolates from hemp (*Cannabis sativa* L.) by-products for Salmonid feed applications. *Molecules* 97: 4794.

Beriziky P, Cherkaoui M, Linxe L, Perrin E, Rogniaux H, Denery-Papini S, Morisset M, Larre C, Dijk W. 2023. Hemp seed: An allergen source with potential cross-reactivity to hazelnut. *Food Research International* 169: 112932.

Borgonha S, Regan MM, Oh SH, Condon M, Young VR. 2002. Threonine requirement of healthy adults, derived with a 24-h indicator amino acid balance technique. *American Journal of Clinical Nutrition* 75(4): 698–704.

Cai L, Wu S, Jia C, Cui C, Sun-Waterhouse D. 2023. Active peptides with hypoglycemic effect obtained from hemp (*Cannabis sativa* L.) protein through identification, molecular docking, and virtual screening. *Food Chemistry* 429: 136912.

Cerrato A, Lammi C, Capriotti AL, Bollati C, Cavaliere C, Montone CM, Bartolomei M, Boschin G, Li J, Piovesana S, Arnoldi A, Lagana A. 2023. Isolation and functional characterization of hemp seed protein-derived short- and medium-chain peptide mixtures with multifunctional properties for metabolic syndrome prevention. *Food Research International* 163: 112219.

Chen H, Li W, Wang Y, Xu B, Hu X, Li X, Liu J, Zhang C, Zhang C, Xing X. 2023. Mining and validation of novel hemp seed-derived DPP-IV-inhibiting peptides using a combination of multi-omics and molecular docking. *Journal of Agricultural and Food Chemistry* 71: 9164–9174.

Damodaran S. 2017. Amino acids, peptides, and protein. In *Fennema's Food Chemistry*. 5th ed. CRC Press, Taylor & Francis Group, pp. 235–356.

Dia VP, Wang Z, Lin Y, Pangloli P. 2019. Comparative biological activities determination of aqueous extracts of hempseed oil and hempseed protein isolate production co-products. *Journal of American Oil Chemists' Society* 96(11): 1265–1274.

Fang B, Chang L, Ohm J, Chen B, Rao J. 2023. Structural, functional properties, and volatile profile of hemp protein isolate as affected by extraction method: Alkaline extraction–isoelectric precipitation vs salt extraction. *Food Chemistry* 405: 135001.

Farinon B, Costantini L, Molinari R, Di Matteo G, Garzoli S, Ferri S, Ceccantoni B, Mannina L, Merendino N. 2022. Effect of malting on nutritional and antioxidant properties of the seeds of two industrial hemp (*Cannabis sativa* L.) cultivars. *Food Chemistry* 370: 131348.

Frassinetti S, Moccia E, Caltavuturo L, Gabriele M, Longo V, Bellani L, Giorgetti L. 2018. Nutraceutical potential of hemp (Cannabis sativa L.) seeds and sprouts. *Food Chemistry* 262: 56–66.

Girgih AT, Alashi A, He R, Malomo S, Aluko RE. 2014. Preventive and treatment effects of a hemp seed (*Cannabis sativa* L.) meal protein hydrolysate against high blood pressure in spontaneously hypertensive rats. *European Journal of Nutrition* 53: 1237–1246.

Girgih AT, He R, Aluko RE. 2014. Kinetics and molecular docking studies of the inhibitions of angiotensin converting enzyme and renin activities by hemp seed (*Cannabis sativa* L.) peptides. *Journal of Agricultural and Food Chemistry* 62: 4135–4144.

Girgih AT, Udenigwe CC, Aluko RE. 2013. Reverse-phase HPLC separation of hemp seed (*Cannabis sativa* L.) protein hydrolysate produced peptide fractions with enhanced antioxidant capacity. *Plant Foods for Human Nutrition* 68: 39–46.

Hong S, Lin Y, Dia VP. 2022. Anti-inflammatory and antioxidant properties of hempseed protein enzymatic hydrolysates. *Food Hydrocolloids for Health* 2: 100082.

House JD, Neufeld J, Leson G. 2010. Evaluating the quality of protein from hemp seed (*Cannabis sativa* L.) products through the use of the protein digestibility-corrected amino acid score method. *Journal of Agricultural and Food Chemistry* 58: 11801–11807.

Institute of Medicine. 2002. *Dietary reference intakes for energy, carbohydrate, fiber, fat, fatty acids, cholesterol, protein, and amino acids.* Washington, DC: National Academies Press.

Karabulut G, Yemis O. 2022. Modification of hemp seed protein isolate (*Cannabis sativa* L.) by high-intensity ultrasound treatment. Part 1: Functional properties. *Food Chemistry* 375: 131843.

Khalesi M, Gcaza L, FitzGerald RJ. 2023. *In vitro* digestibility, biological activity, and physicochemical characterization of proteins extracted from conventionally and organically cultivated hempseed (*Cannabis sativa* L.). *Molecules* 28: 915.

Kowalski S, Sabat R, Skoczylas L, Tabaszewska M, Mikulec A. 2019. Hemp flour as a valuable component for enriching physicochemical and antioxidant properties of wheat bread. *LWT—Food Science and Technology* 102: 164–172.

Kurpad AV, Raj T, Regan MM, Vasudevan J, Caszo B, Nazareth D, Gnanou J, Young VR. 2002. Threonine requirements of healthy Indian men, measured by a 24-h indicator amino acid oxidation and balance technique. *American Journal of Clinical Nutrition* 76(4): 789–797.

Li J, Bollatti C, bartolomei M, Mazzolari A, Arnoldi A, Vistoli G, Lammi C. 2022. Hempseed (*Cannabis sativa*) peptide H3 (IGFLIIWV) exerts cholesterol-lowering effects in human hepatic cell line. *Nutrients* 14: 1804.

Lin Y, Pangloli P, Dia VP. 2021. Physicochemical, functional and bioactive properties of hempseed (Cannabis sativa L.) meal, a co-product of hempseed oil and protein production, as affected by drying process. *Food Chemistry* 350: 129188.

Lin Y, Pangloli P, Meng X, Dia VP. 2020. Effect of heating on the digestibility of isolated hempseed (*Cannabis sativa* L.) protein and bioactivity of its pepsin-pancreatin digests. *Food Chemistry* 314: 126198.

Liu M, Toth JA, Childs M, Smart LB, Abbaspourrad A. 2023. Composition and functional properties of hemp seed protein isolates from various hemp cultivars. *Journal of Food Science* 88: 942–951.

Malomo S, Aluko RE. 2019. Kinetics of acetylcholinesterase inhibition by hemp seed protein-derived peptides. *Journal of Food Biochemistry* 43: e12897.

Malomo SA, He R, Aluko RE. 2014. Structural and functional properties of hemp seed protein products. *Journal of Food Science* 79 (8): C1512–C1521.

Mamone G, Picariello G, Ramondo A, Nicolai MA, Ferranti P. 2019. Production, digestibility and allergenicity of hemp (Cannabis sativa L.) protein isolates. *Food Research International* 115: 562–571. doi: 10.1016/j.foodres.2018.09.017.

Mohammadrezaei A, Kavakeb A, Abbasalizad-Farhangi M, Mesgari-Abbsi M. 2022. Effects of hemp seed alone and combined with aerobic exercise on metabolic parameters, oxidative stress, and neurotrophic factors in young sedentary men. *Journal of Food Biochemistry* 46: e14417.

Mollard RC, Johnston A, Serrano Leon A, Wang H, Jones PJ, MacKay DS. 2021. Acute effects of hemp protein consumption on glycemic and satiety control: results of 2 randomized crossover trials. *Applied Physiology and Nutritional Metabolism* 46: 887–896.

Nionelli M, Pontonio V, Gobbetti R. 2018. Pro-technological and functional characterization of lactic acid bacteria to be used as starters for hemp (*Cannabis sativa* L.) sourdough fermentation and wheat bread fortification. *International Journal of Food Microbiology* 279: 14–25.

Orio LP, Boschin G, Recca T, Morelli CF, Ragona L, Francesco P, Arnoldi A, Speranza G. 2017. New ACE-inhibitory peptides from hemp seed (*Cannabis sativa* L.) proteins. *Journal of Agricultural and Food Chemistry* 65: 10482–10488.

Park S, Seo J, Lee M. 2012. Proteomic profiling of hempseed proteins Cheungsam. *Biochimica et Biophysica Acta* 2012: 374–382.

Pellati F, Borgonetti V, Brighenti V, Biagi M, Benvenuti S, Corsi L. 2018. *Cannabis sativa* L. and Nonpsychoactive Cannabinoids: Their Chemistry and Role against Oxidative Stress, Inflammation, and Cancer. *Biomed Research International* 2018: 1691428.

Potin F, Lubbers S, Husson F, Saurel R. 2019. Hemp (*Cannabis sativa* L.) protein extraction conditions affect extraction yield and protein quality. *Journal of Food Science* 84 (12): 3682–3690.

Rodriguez-Martin NM, Montserrat-de la Paz S, Toscano R, Grao-Cruces E, Villalueva A, Pedroche J, Millan F, Millan-Linares MC. 2020. Hemp (*Cannabis sativa* L.) protein hydrolysates promote anti-inflammatory response in primary human monocytes. *Biomolecules* 10: 803.

Rodriguez-Martin NM, Toscano R, Villalueva A, Pedroche J, Millan F, Montserrat-de la Paz S, Millan-Linares MC. 2019. Neuroprotective protein hydrolysates from hemp (*Cannabis sativa* L.) seeds. *Food & Function* 10: 6732–6739.

Saad JS, Dia VP. 2023. Bromelain hydrolysis modified the functionality, antioxidant, and anti-inflammatory properties of hempseed (*Candida sativa* L.) protein isolated at pH 12. *ACS Food Science and Technology*.

Samaei SP, Martini S, Tagliazucchi D, Gianotti A, Babini E. 2021. Antioxidant and angiotensin I-converting enzyme (ACE) inhibitory peptides obtained from Alcalase protein hydrolysate fractions of hemp (*Cannabis sativa* L.) bran. *Journal of Food and Agricultural Chemistry* 69: 9220–9228.

Samsamikor M, Mackay D, Mollard RC, Aluko RE. 2020. A double-blind, randomized, crossover trial protocol of whole hemp seed protein and hemp seed protein hydrolysate consumption for hypertension. *Trials* 21: 354.

Sarwar G. 1997. The protein digestibility-corrected amino acid score method overestimates quality of proteins containing antinutritional factors and of poorly digestible proteins supplemented with limiting amino acids in rats. *Journal of Nutrition* 127 (5): 758–764.

Sharma S, Tamilselvan T, Shakeb M, Prabhasankar P. 2023. Hydrothermal treatment of hemp seeds (*Cannabis sativa* L.): impact on its dehulling yield, fatty acid profile, and nutritional characteristics. *Journal of the Science of Food and Agriculture* 103: 2681–2689.

Tang C, Ten Z, Wang X, Yang X. 2006. Physicochemical and functional properties of hemp (*Cannabis sativa* L.) protein isolate. *Journal of Agricultural and Food Chemistry* 54: 8945–8950.

Teh SS, Bekhit AE, Carne A, Birch J. 2016. Antioxidant and ACE-inhibitory activities of hemp ((*Cannabis sativa* L.) protein hydrolysates produced by the proteases AFP, HT, Pro-G, actinidin and zingibain. *Food Chemistry* 203: 199–206.

Teleszko M, Zajac A, Rusak T. 2022. Hemp seeds of the Polish 'Biolobrzeskie' and 'Henola' varieties (*Cannabis sativa* L. var. *sativa*) as prospective plant sources for food production. *Molecules* 27: 1448.

Teterycz D, Sobota A, Prztgodzka D, Lysakowska P. 2021. Hemp seed (*Cannabis sativa* L.) enriched pasta: Physicochemical properties and quality evaluation. *PLOS One* 16(3): e0248790.

Vonapartis E, Aubin MP, Seguin P, Mustafa AF, Charron, JB. 2015. Seed composition often industrial hemp cultivars approved for production in Canada. *Journal of Food Composition and Analysis* 39: 8–12.

Wang Q, Jin Y, Xiong YL. 2018. Heating-aided pH shifting modified hemp seed protein structure, cross-linking, and emulsifying properties. *Journal of Agricultural and Food Chemistry* 66: 10827–10834.

Wang S, Luo Q, Fan P. 2019. Cannabis in F from Hemp (*Cannabis sativa*) Seed Suppresses Lipopolysaccharide-Induced Inflammatory Responses in BV2 Microglia as SIRT1 Modulator. *International Journal of Molecular Science* 20 (3). pii: E507.

Witczak M, Ziobro R, Juszczak L, Korus J. 2017. Hemp (*Cannabis sativa* subsp. *sativa*) flour and protein preparation as natural nutrients and structure forming agents in starch based gluten-free bread. *LWT—Food Science and Technology* 84: 143–150.

Yan X, Tang J, dos Santos Passos C, Nurisso A, Simões-Pires CA, Ji M, Lou H, Fan P. 2015. Characterization of Lignanamides from Hemp (Cannabis sativa L.) Seed and Their Antioxidant and Acetylcholinesterase Inhibitory Activities. *Journal of Agricultural and Food Chemistry* 63 (49): 10611–10619. doi: 10.1021/acs.jafc.5b05282.

Zahari I, Ferawati F, Helstad A, Ahsltrom C, Ostbring K, Rayner M, Puuhagen JK. 2020. Development of high-mositure meat analogues with hemp and soy protein using extrusion cooking. *Foods* 9 (6): 772.

Zahari I, Rinaldi S, Ahsltrom C, Ostbring K, Rayner M, Puuhagen J. 2023. High moisture meat analogues from hemp—the effect of co-extrusion with wheat gluten and chickpea proteins on the textural properties and sensorial attributes. *LWT—Food Science and Technology* 189: 115494.

Zanoni C, Aiello G, Arnoldi A, Lammi C. 2017. Hempseed peptides exert hypocholesterolemic effects with a statin-like mechanism. *Journal of Agricultural and Food Chemistry* 65 (40): 8829–8838.

38 Cereal By-Products, Proteins, and Amino Acids for Human Consumption: A New Narrative

Anca Corina Farcas, Oana Raluca Negrean, and Sonia Ancuta Socaci

ABBREVIATIONS

ABTS	2,2'-azino-bis (3-ethylbenzothiazoline-6-sulfonic acid)
ACE	Angiotensin-converting enzyme
AF	Alkaline protease + Flavourzyme
AFD	Gastrointestinal digested sample from AF-hydrolysate
ALK	Alkaline extraction
BSG	Brewer's spent grain
BSGP	Brewer's spent grain proteins
BSG-PI	Brewer's spent grain protein-enriched isolate
CDS	Condensed distiller's soluble components
CG	Corn germ
CSS	Coffee silver skin
DDGs	Corn distillers' dried grains
DFFF	Defatted durum wheat fine fraction
DH	Degrees of hydrolysis
DM	Dry matter
DPPH	2,2-diphenyl-1-picrylhydrazyl
EAI	Emulsifying activity index
FC	Foaming capacity
FRAP	Ferric reducing antioxidant power
HPLC	High-performance liquid chromatography
LC-MS/MS	Liquid chromatography-mass spectrometry
MAE	Microwave-assisted extraction
OH	Oat husk
ORAC	Oxygen radical absorbance capacity
PF	Neutral protease + Flavourzyme
PFD	Gastrointestinal digested sample from PF hydrolysate
PH	Protein hydrolysates
PP	Potato peel
RB	Rice bran
Sc-CO_2	Supercritical carbon dioxide extraction
SCP	Single-cell protein
WAC	Water absorption capacity

DOI: 10.1201/9781003597926-38

INTRODUCTION

The global market is currently experiencing an upward trend in consumer demand for enhanced dietary options, while the food industry is directing its efforts towards innovating novel functional components such as plant proteins. For decades, animal proteins have been the predominant dietary protein source. However, there has been a significant shift in recent years, with the general population moving towards plant-based food proteins (Qin et al., 2022). This trend has led to a considerable increase in plant protein production within the food industry. Proteins are indispensable for sustaining life, as they exist in all living organisms and perform vital functions within cells, tissues, organs, and systems. In addition to supplying essential amino acids, proteins offer numerous functional properties that are essential in making our food appealing and enjoyable to consume (Nadathur et al., 2016).

Cereal is the world's most significant food crop, and cereal products are of utmost importance as essential foods (Guerrieri and Cavaletto, 2018). Nine different kinds of cereal crops, including wheat (*Triticum*), rye (*Secale*), barley (*Hordeum*), oats (*Avena*), rice (*Oryza*), millet (*Pennisetum*), corn (*Zea*), sorghum (*Sorghum*), and triticale (a hybrid of wheat and rye), are known for supplying vital nutrients and energy for the average person's daily diet (Papageorgiou and Skendi, 2018). Cereals serve as both the main source of food for human consumption and feed for raising livestock. They are rich in carbohydrates, proteins, lipids, as well as vital phytochemicals, including ferulic acid, vitamins (particularly the B-complex and vitamin E), minerals, and other trace elements (Galanakis, 2020). The cereal food industry is increasingly focused on extracting valuable components from these grains, including proteins, lipids, dietary fiber, phenolic compounds, and other bioactive phytochemicals (Salazar-López et al., 2019). Depending on the species and variation, the protein content of cereal grains ranges from 7% to 18% of the dry mass (Poutanen et al., 2022).

Around the world, by-products are created during the harvesting and processing of various cereals, including wheat, rice, maize, barley, oats, millet, sorghum, and other cereal grains (Salazar-López et al., 2020). Different procedures are used to process cereals, including dry milling, pearling, wet milling, and malting (Galanakis, 2020). As the milling process takes place, the bran, germ, and the endospermic tissue's aleurone layer are separated from the cereal grain, forming the dry milling by-products. Also, during malting, enzymes break down the starches in the grain into simpler sugars, making them more accessible for fermentation. This process also involves the modification of proteins and other components, which contributes to the development of flavor and the nutritional profile of the final product (Papageorgiou and Skendi, 2018). In the alcoholic beverage production process, saccharification is essential for extracting sugars, leaving behind a spent grain by-product that is enriched in protein, with its amino acid content ranging from 30% to 85% of the total protein (Fărcaş et al., 2017).

PROTEINS AND AMINO ACIDS FROM CEREAL BY-PRODUCTS

Numerous plant-based protein sources have been widely consumed throughout the world for millennia. Protein sources that can be generated sustainably include grains (wheat, rice, millets, sorghum), seeds (chia, hemp), nuts (almond, walnut), pulses (beans, lentils, peas, lupins), and leaves (moringa, duckweed). In addition to nitrogen, plant-based diets offer the body's requirements for phytonutrients, vitamins, minerals, and fiber (Nadathur et al., 2016). The building blocks of human nutrition are proteins, which are also crucial for our bodies' natural cell growth and repair processes. The nutritional quality of a protein is determined not only by its total content but also by its digestibility, amino acid composition, and presence of antinutritive substances (Schweiggert-Weisz et al., 2020).

Cereal by-products offer substantial protein content, mainly sourced from outer grain layer components like the aleurone layer. Additionally, protein residues from the endosperm are also present in these by-products. It's noteworthy that protein compositions differ between the endosperm and outer grain layer: while glutenins and gliadins dominate as endosperm protein, albumins and globulins are prevalent in bran protein (Apprich et al., 2014). Moreover, cereal protein categorization hinges on distinct solubility profiles, resulting in four primary classes: albumins, soluble in water; globulins, soluble in saline solutions; prolamins, alcohol/water soluble; and glutelins, soluble in mild acidic or alkaline environments (Guerrieri and Cavaletto, 2018). Distinct nomenclatures have been assigned to the storage proteins of diverse cereals: gliadins for wheat prolamins, glutenins for wheat glutelins, zein for maize, secalins for rye, hordeins for barley, avenin for oats, oryzins for rice, and kafirin for millet and sorghum (Scherf et al., 2016). The main prolamins identified based on the type of cereal are exemplified in Figure 38.1, including glutenin and gliadin in wheat, zein in corn, kafirin in sorghum, hordein in barley, and secalin in rye.

The escalating global population heightens the need for cost-effective plant and microorganism-based dietary protein sources, which can potentially supplement or substitute the costly and finite reservoirs of animal protein. Wheat bran is obtained as a by-product of the milling process, which involves cleaning, conditioning, and sieving to produce white flour (Figure 38.2). Given its protein content ranging from 13% to 18%, wheat bran emerges as a promising candidate for protein extraction (Apprich et al., 2014). Laddmoda et al. (2015) also affirmed that the principal residue obtained during wheat milling contains more than 15% high-quality proteins and serves as a notable reservoir of minerals, B vitamins, and bioactive elements essential for human health (Laddomada, Caretto, et al., 2015). Moreover, the aleurone layer possesses proteins of superior biological and nutritional significance in comparison to the proteins found in the remaining parts of the wheat kernel (Prückler et al., 2014). In comparison to proteins found in the endosperm, those present in the bran showcase increased concentrations of lysine, arginine, alanine, asparagine, and glycine while exhibiting reduced levels of glutamine, proline, phenylalanine, and amino acids containing sulfur (Apprich et al., 2014). Moreover, wheat bran comprises a total of 18 amino acids, encompassing all the essential amino acids required by the human body (Cheng et al., 2022).

Another wheat by-product is represented by germs that have a high protein content between 26% and 35% (Brandolini et al., 2012). Defatted wheat germ has been proven to have a reasonably high protein content (more than 30%), making it an appealing source of vegetable protein. Albumin was the most abundant protein (32.02%), with globulin, glutenin, and prolamin accounting for 15.9%, 12.4%, and 4.3% of the total defatted wheat germ proteins (Wang et al., 2017).

In recent years, rye has received attention due to its nutritional properties (dietary fiber, high-quality proteins, source of minerals, vitamins, and other phytochemicals) as well as technological challenges in bran utilization (negative effects on dough rheology, texture, and sensory quality) (Kajala et al., 2016). Rye bran emerges as a by-product resulting from the refinement process of rye, with global production ranging between 17 and 36 million tons over the past ten years (Demirel et al., 2021). The predominant constituents of rye bran include dietary fiber (consisting of 33.4%

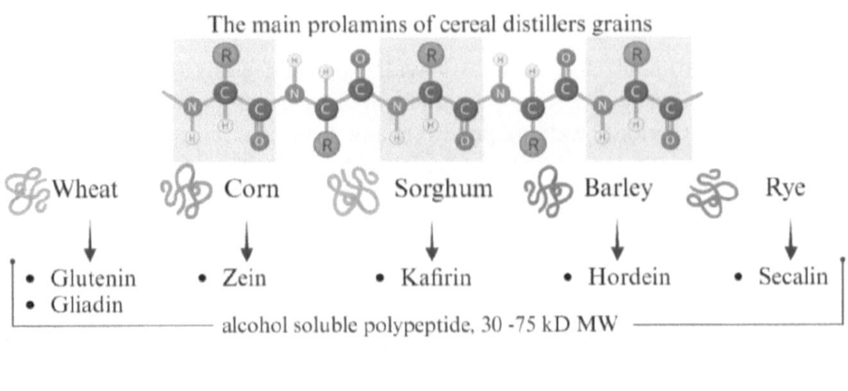

FIGURE 38.1 The main prolamins of cereal and by-products. Visual representation of the primary prolamin proteins found in various cereals and their by-products.

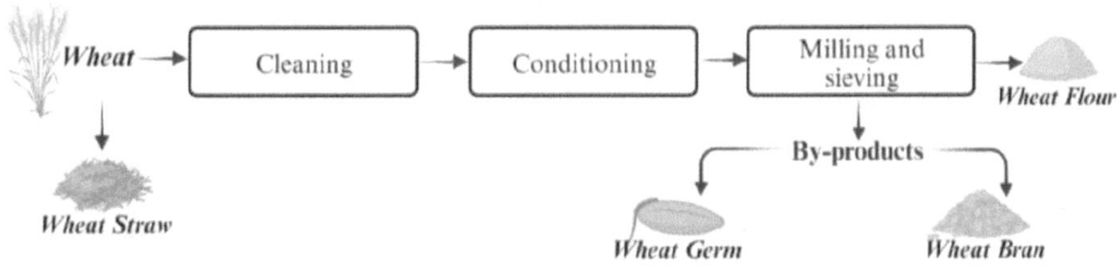

FIGURE 38.2 By-products of wheat processing: This figure succinctly illustrates the various by-products derived from the processing of wheat.

cellulose, 5.3% hemicellulose, and 3.3% lignin), starch (18.6%), protein (17.0%), and lipids (2.5%) (Juhnevica-Radenkova et al., 2021). Therefore, according to Kajala et al. (2016), the protein content in rye bran was 16.33±0.02 g/100 g bran, while in wheat bran it was 18.70±0.8 g/100 g bran.

Oats, a key component in human diets, contain essential nutrients and phytochemicals, many of which offer significant health benefits compared to other grain cereals. Their starch content varies from 27.3% to 50.0%, fibers from 13.6% to 30.2%, proteins from 9.7% to 17.3%, and unsaturated fatty acids from 5.2% to 12.4%. Among cereals, oats have the highest protein content, primarily composed of globulins (50–80%), with smaller amounts of albumins (1–12%), prolamins (4–15%), and glutenins (< 10%) (Sterna et al., 2016; Klose et al., 2012).

Recent reports have highlighted the presence of diverse valuable constituents within oat hulls, encompassing proteins (1–7% on a dry weight basis), cellulose (16–26%), hemicellulose (24–35%), and lignin (13–25%) (Schmitz et al., 2020). Research into alternative agro-industrial residues has shown that enzyme treatments can significantly increase protein extractability and enable the liberation of bioactive chemicals from residual matrices. In contrast to traditional methods employing strong alkalis or acids, the use of enzymes offers advantages by avoiding protein denaturation while also preventing decreased protein digestibility and critical amino acid levels (Schmitz et al., 2021; Tian et al., 2022).

Jing et al. (2016) characterized and analyzed the structure of proteins from oat bran. The findings indicated a relatively equilibrated distribution of amino acids across the four proteins (globulin, albumin, gluten, and gliadin), with notably elevated levels of essential amino acids in albumin (39.06%) and globulin (36.69%) (Jing et al., 2016).

Brewer's spent grain (BSG) is the primary by-product resulting from the beer-making process using cereal grains, with barley (*Hordeum vulgare L.*) being the most common raw material. BSG predominantly comprises various components, including protein, cell wall polysaccharides, lignin, lipids, and phenolic compounds (Yu et al., 2020). Because of their high proline and glutamine levels, the predominant proteins identified in BSG are known as hordeins. These account for 43% of the total protein composition and are conventionally separated using alcohols and a reducing agent (Ikram et al., 2017). Nonetheless, the insolubility of BSG proteins hinders their wider use in food. Protein hydrolysates offer bioactive benefits and potential as functional food ingredients, with key properties like emulsification, film formation, flavor binding, viscosity enhancement, and gelation for the food industry (Fărcaş et al., 2017).

BSG serves as a highly cost-effective alternative for acquiring protein intended for diverse industrial applications. However, it's essential to acknowledge that protein quantification relies on the total nitrogen content present in the sample, potentially incorporating non-protein nitrogen compounds like free amino acids resulting from protein degradation during the mashing process. Noteworthy is the substantial presence of essential amino acids – leucine, lysine, valine, phenylalanine, tyrosine, isoleucine, and threonine – in BSG, surpassing quantities found in foods such as beans, peas, wheat, maize, rice, potatoes, and cauliflower. These vital amino acids collectively contribute to about 30% of the total protein content, with particular attention drawn to lysine, which often assumes the role

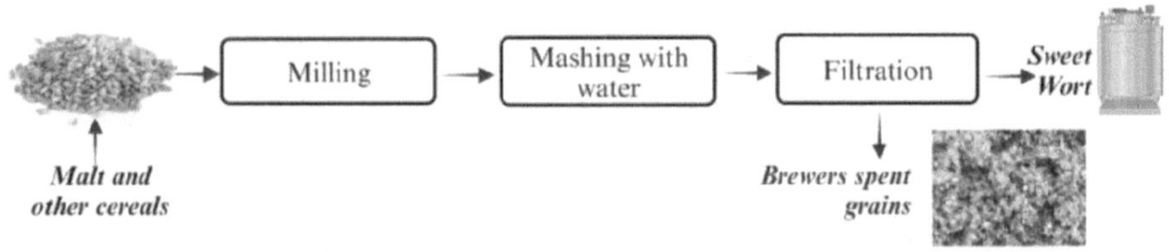

FIGURE 38.3 By-products generated during beer production include brewer's spent grain. The process of generating brewer's spent grain during the beer-brewing cycle involves the separation of the spent grain from the wort after the mashing process.

of the limiting amino acid in cereal-based foods designed for human consumption (Qin Fen et al., 2018; Jaeger et al., 2021) (Figure 38.3).

Zhang et al. (2021) conducted a comparative study involving the ultrasound treatment of coffee silver skin (CSS), BSG, and potato peel (PP) waste to extract phenolic compounds and amino acids. Regarding the amino acid content, concentrations were found to be 85, 42, and 247 mg/g in CSS, PP, and BSG, respectively. It's noteworthy that the highest concentration of essential amino acids, encompassing lysine, methionine, histidine, leucine, phenylalanine, threonine, valine, and isoleucine, was identified in BSG, reaching a total of 92 mg/g. Overall, BSG has been classified as a valuable source of essential amino acids (Zhang et al., 2021).

Corn, or maize (*Zea mays* L.), is a major crop used for food, animal feed, and industrial products such as cornstarch, cereals, adhesives, sweeteners, and alcohol (Ruan et al., 2019; Zhang et al., 2021). Corn harvesting and processing produce major by-products such as corn stover, corncob, corn germ, condensed distiller's soluble components (CDS), corn distiller's dried grains with solubles (DDGS), and processing effluent.

Zein, the main protein found in maize husk, is extracted using ethanol and then treated with an alkali acid solution. Due to its hydrophobic and hydrophilic components, it exhibits effective amphiphilicity. The zein protein aggregates quickly after the ethanol extraction, generating a fibrous structure that makes it easier to produce degradable zein film. Zein has a wide range of uses in the food sector, particularly in embedding agents, emulsifiers, gluten-free goods, and packaging materials, which contribute to its continuous and deliberate advancement (Jiao et al., 2022).

DDGS are widely marketed as livestock feed, valued for their 34% protein, 10% fat, and cost of 8–13 cents/kg. Recently, DDGS have served as a multifunctional filler in synthetic resin-bonded wood particle boards, enhancing their properties through hydrophobic zein proteins. Moreover, DDGS gains traction as a cost-effective alternative to pricier ingredients in animal feed, yet its amino acid content, affected by distinct heating conditions during production, can be variable despite its 30–32% crude protein content (Liaw et al., 2019; Sándor et al., 2021).

Kafirin, the prolamin found in sorghum, stands out as the most hydrophobic among prolamins, forming disulfide crosslinks due to its elevated cysteine levels. Its gradual digestibility is noteworthy, yet it remains non-reactive for individuals with celiac disease. These characteristics render kafirin potentially advantageous for a wide array of applications. Particularly, its potential as a bioplastic and encapsulating agent holds promise (Taylor and Taylor, 2018).

EFFECTS ON HUMAN HEALTH

Extraction and incorporation of proteins derived from cereal by-products into the human diet may confer a spectrum of health benefits attributable to the bioactive compounds intrinsic to these indispensable compounds that exert favorable physiological effects. The strategic integration of these protein-rich by-products into the human diet has the potential to significantly enhance overall

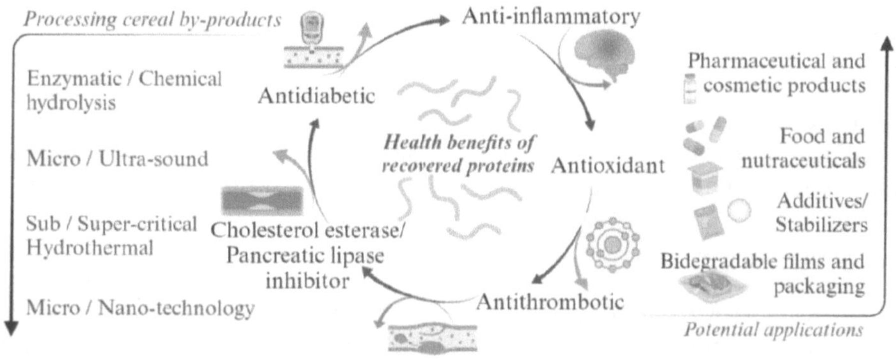

FIGURE 38.4 Health benefits of protein recovered from cereal by-products. Summarizes the main extraction techniques, health impacts, and applications of proteins from cereal by-products.

well-being, underpinned by the nutritional and functional properties of the bioactive compounds they contain (Figure 38.4).

ANTIOXIDANT AND ANTICANCER ACTIVITIES

Current scientific investigations are intensifying in the realm of cereal by-products, particularly focusing on their antioxidant activities. Researchers are developing advanced extraction techniques to isolate and utilize these bioactive compounds for their potential health benefits. Integrating these by-products into the human diet, either directly or as functional ingredients in various food formulations, presents a viable strategy to increase antioxidant sources, thereby potentially enriching overall dietary quality and healthfulness (Zhou et al., 2015).

Naibaho et al. (2022) investigated the protein properties and antioxidant activity of protease-treated BSG, along with its techno-functional characteristics. Protamex and a combination of protamex-flavourzyme were used for treatment, compared to a control. Enzymatic processing enhanced BSG proteins' (BSGPs') antioxidant activity, with a correlation between BSGP and ORAC/ABTS activities and FRAP with polyphenolic content. Treated BSGPs showed improved oil-holding and foaming capacities but lower emulsion properties. This suggests that enzyme treatment can enhance BSGPs' functionality, bioactivity, and potential for further applications (Naibaho et al., 2022). Exploring BSG for antioxidant peptides, researchers found protease hydrolysis improved protein solubility (94.4% at neutral pH) and enhanced DPPH scavenging activities (72.6% to 74.9%) with various enzyme combinations. Histidine played a key role in scavenging, with longer peptides effectively chelating ferrous ions. This positions BSG as a viable source of cost-effective natural antioxidants for food applications (Abeynayake et al., 2022).

Other researchers have directed their attention towards the antioxidant activity of oat by-product proteins. Vanvi et al. (2016) focused on optimizing pepsin hydrolysis of oat bran proteins to increase radical scavenging activity and identify active peptides. The best results were achieved with a 1:30 enzyme-substrate ratio over 2 hours, yielding hydrolysates with the highest activity (608 ± 17 μM TE/g). These were fractionated into eight HPLC fractions (F1–F8), with F3–F8 showing higher radical scavenging activities (447–874 μM TE/g). LC-MS/MS analysis identified fifty peptides in the most active F3 fraction (Vanvi et al., 2016).

Rodríguez-Restrepo et al. (2020) explored rice bran's (RB) valorization by extracting proteins and phenolics through enzymatic hydrolysis. They achieved efficient protein extraction with ethanol defatting, enhancing valorization without protein loss. The study found that phenolic compounds in protein fractions boosted extract activity, with protein hydrolysates showing increased antioxidant and ACE inhibitory activities post-trypsin digestion, thereby enhancing RB's industrial potential by improving protein digestibility and bioactivity (Rodríguez-Restrepo et al., 2020).

A study on papain-hydrolyzed sorghum kafirin revealed its antioxidant and anticancer capabilities. Optimal hydrolysis achieved with a 360 kU/g enzyme-to-substrate ratio for 4 hours yielded a 1–3 kDa fraction with significant antioxidative properties. In ground meat, 1.0 mg/g of this hydrolysate reduced lipid peroxidation by 32.1% and safely impeded HepG2 cancer cell growth, suggesting its potential as a food-based antioxidant with cancer-preventive benefits. (Xu et al., 2019).

ANTIDIABETIC ACTIVITY

Oxidative stress has been implicated in the development of prevalent human diseases such as diabetes. The potential of oat bran protein hydrolysates in the prevention and management of chronic conditions, notably diabetes, was investigated. Walters et al. (2020) conducted antidiabetic assessments, revealing a significant inhibition of α-amylase by 31.8%, along with a substantial 53.6% inhibition of dipeptidyl peptidase-4 (Walters et al., 2020).

Moreover, rice bran protein hydrolysates were another subject of study. Uraipong and Zhao (2016) studied the health effects of rice bran protein hydrolysates, focusing on their inhibitory activities against α-amylase, α-glucosidase, and ACE. Fractionated rice bran proteins underwent hydrolysis using Alcalase, Neutrase, Flavourzyme, and Protamax. Enhanced bioactivities were observed, particularly in albumin and glutelin hydrolysates, comparable to acarbose, a diabetic drug, indicating potential use in diabetic management (Uraipong and Zhao, 2016) (Figure 38.5).

BSG, another cereal by-product, has captured researchers' interest due to its potential role in diabetes prevention. The researchers investigated the potential of pale brewer's spent grain protein-enriched isolate (BSG-PI) hydrolysates to inhibit key enzymes involved in diabetes and hypertension management. Hydrolysates with degree-of-hydrolysis values from 1.15% to 14.67% were generated using various enzyme preparations. Notable variations in peptide composition were observed among BSG-PI and its hydrolysates, with tryptic digests showing the highest α-glucosidase inhibition. Corolase PP hydrolysates exhibited significant dipeptidyl peptidase IV inhibition (75% at 3.5 mg mL−1), while Prolyve 1000 hydrolysate demonstrated potent ACE inhibition (89.25% at 1 mg mL−1). These findings emphasize the potential role of BSG-PI hydrolysates as functional ingredients for managing type II diabetes and hypertension (Connolly et al., 2014).

ANTI-INFLAMMATORY ACTIVITY

Ferri et al. (2022) addressed modern challenges of a sustainable economy and agro-industrial by-product utilization in a study that showcased a biotechnological approach to extract bioactive peptides from rice starch production by-products. By employing enzymatic hydrolysis with Alcalase and Protamex, optimized in a 2 L bioreactor, promising digestates were identified based on peptide release and antioxidant capacity. Subsequent crossflow filtration generated fractions with varying molecular weights (10, 5, 1 kDa), revealing favorable nutritional traits alongside potential bitter

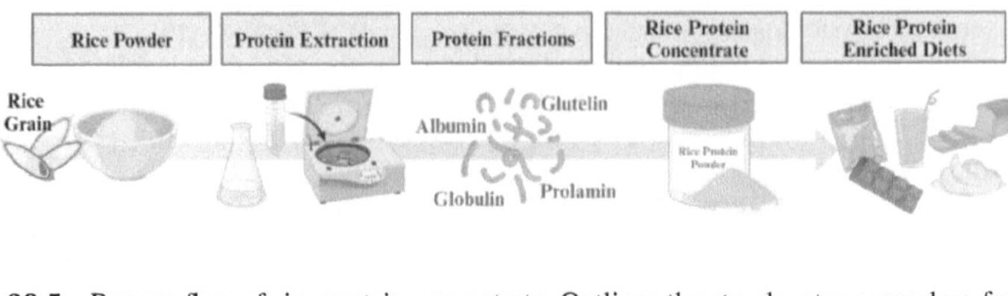

FIGURE 38.5 Process flow of rice protein concentrate. Outlines the step-by-step procedure for obtaining protein concentrate powder from rice.

taste. Notably, the Alcalase-derived 8 kDa retentate exhibited anti-inflammatory properties, while smaller fractions demonstrated potent tyrosinase inhibition.

McCarthy et al. (2013) also focused on the antioxidant and anti-inflammatory effects of brewer's spent grain protein-rich isolate and its associated hydrolysates. The findings of the conducted study indicated that protein preparations sourced from BSG did not exhibit antioxidant potential but demonstrated potential selective immunomodulatory effects. It was conceivable that the presence of phenolic compounds within these preparations played a role in the observed effects. Notably, the BSG protein isolate and its associated hydrolysates exhibited a significant capacity to decrease the production of the pro-inflammatory cytokine IFN-γ. This discovery holds promise for the potential use of these protein preparations in the treatment of inflammatory diseases.

ANTITHROMBOTIC ACTIVITY AND CHOLESTEROL ESTERASE INHIBITION

Cian et al. (2018) investigated the antithrombotic effects of brewer's spent grain peptides on blood coagulation pathways before and after simulated gastrointestinal digestion. They created two hydrolysates using different enzyme systems: alkaline protease + Flavourzyme (AF) and neutral protease + Flavourzyme (PF). These were then subjected to simulated digestion with porcine pepsin and pancreatin, resulting in digested forms AFD and PFD. Ultrafiltration of peptides showed a prevalence of medium and low molecular weight peptides, particularly after digestion, which also increased specific amino acids. These peptides, both in hydrolyzed and digested forms, demonstrated thrombin inhibitory activity, significantly delaying thrombin and thromboplastin times (by approximately 63%), indicating inhibition at the common pathway level (Cian et al., 2018).

Another study focused on the extraction and identification of cholesterol esterase (CE) and pancreatic lipase (PL) inhibitory peptides from BSG protein hydrolysate. Sequential fractionation steps, including anionic exchange, gel filtration, and reversed-phase HPLC, concentrated the inhibitory activities. The most potent fractions were analyzed via MALDI-TOF tandem mass spectrometry, revealing three peptides: one with high CE inhibition (WNIHMEHQDLTTME) and two with PL inhibition (DFGIASF and LAAVEALSTNG). These peptides shared hydrophobic and acidic residues (Asp, Glu) and amines (Asn, Gln), common among lipid-lowering peptides targeting CE and PL inhibition. The BSG by-product emerged as a valuable source of CE and PL inhibitory peptides, enhancing the utilization of this beer industry residue. This study confirmed the potential of BSG peptides to inhibit CE and PL enzymes (Garzón et al., 2020).

PROTEIN EXTRACTION TECHNIQUES

Research efforts are focused on improving protein extraction techniques, enhancing nutritional profiles, and ensuring cost-effectiveness and environmental sustainability. While advanced technologies promise better yield and functional outcomes, industrial adoption varies, and is influenced by the intended use, resources, and technical capacity. For example, enzyme-assisted extraction, though more environmentally friendly, requires more time and energy than alkaline extraction, which remains popular for its simplicity and cost-efficiency in deriving high-quality plant proteins (Pojić et al., 2018).

Microwave-assisted extraction (MAE) was used to optimize rice bran protein extraction, with ideal parameters being 1000 W microwave power, 90 s extraction duration, and a ratio of 0.89 g rice bran to 10 mL water. Compared to alkaline extraction (ALK), MAE yielded 1.54 times more protein with equivalent digestibility (Phongthai et al., 2016).

Yu et al. (2020) aimed to develop an eco-friendly, ultrasound-assisted enzymatic approach for extracting protein from BSG to create protein hydrolysates and analyze their properties. This emerging, non-thermal technology is notable for its energy efficiency and chemical-free nature. Moreover, elevating Alcalase enzyme loading from 1 to 20 μL per gram of BSG raised protein separation efficiency from 34.0% to 61.6%. Introducing ultrasound pretreatment further enhanced efficiency to 69.8%, reducing enzyme usage by 73% and incubation time by 56%.

Another team of researchers directed their attention towards utilizing ultrasound to process coffee silver skin, brewer's spent grain, and potato peel waste, targeting the extraction of phenolic compounds and amino acids. The findings unveiled that PP and CSS exhibited the most substantial content of umami free amino acids, both registering 0.13 mg/g. In contrast, BSG held the highest quantity of essential amino acids, reaching 92 mg/g (Zhang et al., 2021).

Qin et al. (2018) examined various methods for extracting protein from BSG, including alkaline, acid, enzymatic, and hydrothermal treatments. Key findings included a 90% protein extraction using a one-step dilute acid method and up to 95% extraction with combined alkaline-acid treatments. Hydrothermal pretreatment yielded 64–66% protein, demonstrating higher selectivity for protein recovery than chemical methods (Qin et al., 2018).

To extract compounds from oat husks (OH), Zhou et al. (2023) studied ultrasonication-assisted enzymatic bioprocessing. They used enzymes like Viscozyme®, Alcalase®, and feruloyl esterase, applying ultrasonication for efficient extraction. Enzyme type, ultrasonication frequency, and processing time influenced compound composition. Enzymatic treatments notably increased protein and phenolic acid content in the liquid fraction, while avenanthramides underwent degradation. The highest protein content (68.9 g/100 g DM) was achieved with feruloyl esterase treatment and 90 minutes of ultrasonication at 25 kHz (Zhou et al., 2023).

Espinosa-Pardo et al. (2020) conducted a study on protein recovery from corn germ, a by-product of flour processing. The research focused on extracting oil and protein, utilizing methods like ambient and 45°C hexane extraction, supercritical CO_2 extraction, and Soxhlet extraction with hexane and ethanol. Protein fractions analyzed showed content ranging from 19.9% to 48.5%, water absorption capacity from 1.34 to 2.79 g water/g, and varied solubility. Foaming capacity ranged from 25% to 84%, and emulsifying activity index from 84.8 to 246 m^2/g protein (Espinosa-Pardo et al., 2020).

Alzuwaid et al. (2020) developed a durum wheat bran protein concentrate using an alkaline-acid method and isoelectric precipitation, resulting in a product with approximately 61% protein, enriched in phytosterols, amino acids, and properties like solubility and absorption capacity (Alzuwaid et al., 2020).

APPLICATIONS OF CEREAL BY-PRODUCT PROTEINS

Upon successful identification and extraction, researchers have focused on incorporating proteins from cereal by-products into various food and supplement products, aiming to leverage their beneficial health effects for consumers. Regular consumption of dietary protein plays a crucial role in human nutrition, providing essential nutrients necessary for numerous physiological functions. Industries such as bakery, sports nutrition, infant formula, meat processing, and food additives have been primary areas of focus for improvement through the integration of these protein-rich by-products, reflecting a strategic approach to enhancing the nutritional quality and functional properties of food products.

Squeo et al. (2023) developed a protein and fiber-rich snack bar using dry-fractionated defatted Durum wheat cake (DFFF). The bar, containing 10% DFFF, 30% glucose syrup, and 60% puffed/rolled cereals, was notably firmer and had a more intense yellow color and caramel flavor compared to the DFFF-free control, attributed to DFFF's properties. This DFFF fortification resulted in a snack bar with enhanced nutritional quality, particularly in protein content (Squeo et al., 2023).

Zhou et al. (2013) studied rice protein hydrolysates as natural antioxidants to prolong meat product shelf-life. From enzymatic hydrolysis, two fractions, Val-F3 and AP-F3, showed potent antioxidant activity. Specifically, Val-F3 at 500 mg/g reduced lipid oxidation in meat by 19% and 15% after 8 and 15 days, respectively, indicating its potential to enhance meat preservation. (Zhou et al., 2013).

Muhiwa et al. (2017) conducted a study on the extraction of kafirin from coarse sorghum DDGS utilizing a percolation technique. Their findings indicated that this method effectively yields kafirin and zein, both exhibiting robust film-forming properties. The high protein concentration in DDGS contributes to substantial yields of high-purity kafirin. Notably, films derived from this kafirin demonstrate superior characteristics, such as reduced water absorption and lower digestibility, attributed to the heat-induced disulfide crosslinking inherent in the DDGS processing (Muhiwa et al., 2017).

THE EFFECTS OF OTHER PROTEINS

The production of single-cell proteins (SCP) represents an innovative approach to utilizing cereal by-products as substrates for the generation of high-value protein supplements. SCP, comprising dried cells of microorganisms like algae, fungi, yeast, and bacteria, serves as a protein supplement in human and animal diets. These microorganisms can be cultivated to produce biomass, protein concentrates, or amino acids, leveraging cost-effective feedstocks and waste products, including cereal by-products, as sources of carbon and energy. Cereal by-products, rich in carbohydrates and organic nitrogen, provide an ideal substrate for SCP production, especially for bacteria known for their rapid growth and cell mass doubling in short periods (Yunus et al., 2015; Singh et al., 2019).

Yunus et al. (2015) used wheat bran rich in carbohydrates for fermentation, producing microbial biomass. *Candida utilis* and *Rhizopus oligosporus* were tested for biomass production by optimizing various fermentation parameters (effect of inoculum size, age of inoculum, incubation period, moisture-to-substrate ratio, and incubation temperature). The best results were achieved with a 10% (v/w) inoculum size and a 48-hour-old culture, fermented for 48 hours at 30°C. This optimized process led to a remarkable increase in crude protein yield, reaching 41.02%, compared to the non-fermented wheat bran's 4.21% crude protein content (Yunus et al., 2015).

Thus, the integration of cereal by-products into SCP production presents a symbiotic solution, leveraging waste materials while producing valuable protein-rich supplements (Figure 38.6).

CONCLUSION

The incorporation of grain by-products into human diets is increasingly recognized as a viable strategy for enhancing well-being, owing to their high protein content and rich array of bioactive substances. These by-products, encompassing bran and husks remaining after grain processing, are abundant in beneficial bioactive chemicals. The acceptance and inclusion of proteins derived from these by-products in dietary practices offer promising avenues for improving overall health and wellness. This trend aligns with the shifting global market dynamics, where there is a growing demand for enhanced dietary options, particularly those that are more sustainable and health-conscious compared to traditional animal protein sources.

ACKNOWLEDGMENT

This work was supported by a grant from the Romanian Ministry of Education and Research, CCCDI-UEFISCDI, project number PN-III-P4-ID-PCE-2020-2306.

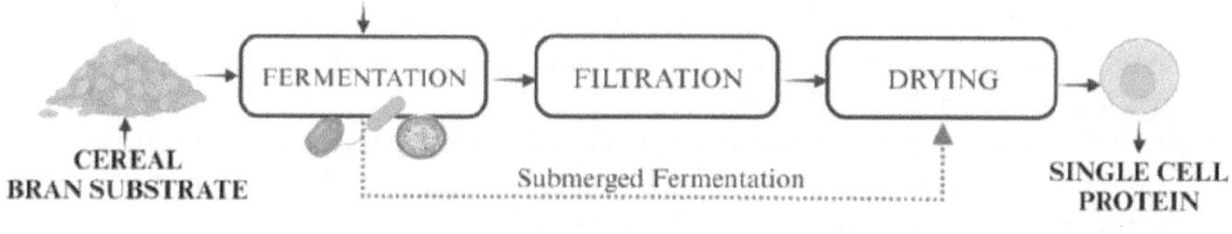

FIGURE 38.6 Processing steps for single-cell protein on cereal bran substrate: Displays the method for obtaining single-cell protein using cereal by-products as a substrate.

MINI DICTIONARY OF TERMS

- **Alcalase:** A commercial protease enzyme responsible for breaking proteins into smaller peptides and amino acids.
- **Brewer's spent grain:** The main by-product obtained from the mashing process of malted barley grains.
- **Distillers dried grains biomass:** A protein and fiber-rich by-product of ethanol production.
- **Hordeins:** Prolamin proteins from barley that can impact the brewing process.
- **Zein:** A prolamin protein found in corn kernels.

SUMMARY POINTS

- This chapter focuses on the effects of cereal by-product proteins and amino acids on human health.
- Due to its high protein content, incorporating cereal by-products into human diets is recommended.
- Rice and wheat bran are considered cost-effective cereal by-products due to their wide availability and versatile use in various applications, including animal feed and food products.
- Proteins derived from rice bran, brewer's spent grain, and oat bran offer health advantages, including antioxidant, antidiabetic, and anti-inflammatory effects.
- Recovered proteins can be integrated into various food sectors such as bakery, supplements, and functional products to meet essential dietary protein needs.
- Utilizing cereal by-products aligns with sustainable practices by providing an alternative protein source.

REFERENCES

Abeynayake, Ranithri, Sitian Zhang, Wenzhu Yang, and Lingyun Chen. "Development of antioxidant peptides from brewers' spent grain proteins." *LWT* 158 (2022): 113162.

Alzuwaid, Nabeel T., Mike Sissons, Barbara Laddomada, and Christopher M. Fellows. "Nutritional and functional properties of durum wheat bran protein concentrate." *Cereal Chemistry* 97, no. 2 (2020): 304–315.

Apprich, Silvia, Özge Tirpanalan, Johannes Hell, Michael Reisinger, Stefan Böhmdorfer, Susanne Siebenhandl-Ehn, Senad Novalin, and Wolfgang Kneifel. "Wheat bran-based biorefinery 2: Valorization of products." *LWT-Food Science and Technology* 56, no. 2 (2014): 222–231.

Brandolini, Andrea, and Alyssa Hidalgo. "Wheat germ: Not only a by-product." *International Journal of Food Sciences and Nutrition* 63, no. S1(2012): 71–74

Cheng, Wen, Yujie Sun, Mingcong Fan, Yan Li, Li Wang, and Haifeng Qian. "Wheat bran, as the resource of dietary fiber: A review." *Critical Reviews in Food Science and Nutrition* 62, no. 26 (2022): 1–28.

Cian, Raúl E., Antonela G. Garzón, Olga Martínez-Augustin, Cecilia C. Botto, and Silvina R. Drago. "Antithrombotic activity of brewers' spent grain peptides and their effects on blood coagulation pathways." *Plant Foods for Human Nutrition* 73 (2018): 241–246.

Connolly, Alan, Charles O. Piggott, and Richard J. FitzGerald. "In vitro α-glucosidase, angiotensin converting enzyme and dipeptidyl peptidase-IV inhibitory properties of brewers' spent grain protein hydrolysates." *Food Research International* 56 (2014): 100–107.

Demirel, Fadime, Mustafa Germec, and Irfan Turhan. "Fermentable sugars production from wheat bran and rye bran: response surface model optimization of dilute sulfuric acid hydrolysis." *Environmental Technology* 43, no. 24 (2022): 3779–3800.

Espinosa-Pardo, Faber Ariel, Raphaëlle Savoire, Pascale Subra-Paternault, and Christelle Harscoat-Schiavo. "Oil and protein recovery from corn germ: Extraction yield, composition and protein functionality." *Food and Bioproducts Processing* 120 (2020): 131–142.

Fărcaş, Anca Corina, Sonia Ancuţa Socaci, Elena Mudura, Francisc Vasile Dulf, Dan C. Vodnar, Maria Tofană, and Liana Claudia Salanţ ă. "Exploitation of brewing industry wastes to produce functional ingredients." In *Brewing Technology*, edited by Makoto Kanauchi, pp. 137–156. IntechOpen2017.

Ferri, Maura, Tullia Tedeschi, Barbara Prandi, Elisa Michelini, Maria Maddalena Calabretta, Elena Babini, Jürgen Graen-Heedfeld et al. "Looking for peptides from rice starch processing by-product: Bioreactor production, anti-tyrosinase and anti-inflammatory activity, and in silico putative taste assessment." *Frontiers in Plant Science* 13 (2022): 929918.

Galanakis, Charis. "Food waste valorization opportunities for different food industries." In *The interaction of food industry and environment*, edited by Charis Galanakis, pp. 341–422. Academic Press, 2020.

Garzón, Antonela Guadalupe, Raúl Esteban Cian, Marilin Estefanía Aquino, and Silvina Rosa Drago. "Isolation and identification of cholesterol esterase and pancreatic lipase inhibitory peptides from brewer's spent grain by consecutive chromatography and mass spectrometry." *Food & Function* 11, no. 6 (2020): 4994–5003.

Guerrieri, Nicoletta., and Maria Cavaletto. "Cereals proteins." In *Proteins in food processing*, edited by R. Y. Yada, pp. 223–244. Woodhead Publishing, 2018.

Ikram, Sana, LianYan Huang, Huijuan Zhang, Jing Wang, and Meng Yin. "Composition and nutrient value proposition of brewers spent grain." *Journal of Food Science* 82, no. 10 (2017): 2232–2242.

Jaeger, Alice, Emanuele Zannini, Aylin W. Sahin, and Elke K. Arendt. "Barley protein properties, extraction and applications, with a focus on brewers' spent grain protein." *Foods* 10, no. 6 (2021): 1389.

Jiao, Yan, Hao-Dong Chen, He Han, and Ying Chang. "Development and utilization of corn processing by-products: A review." *Foods* 11, no. 22 (2022): 3709.

Jing, Xuelian, Chen Yang, and Liping Zhang. "Characterization and analysis of protein structures in oat bran." *Journal of Food Science* 81, no. 10 (2016): C2337–C2343.

Juhnevica-Radenkova, Karina, Jorens Kviesis, Diego A. Moreno, Dalija Seglina, Fernando Vallejo, Anda Valdovska, and Vitalijs Radenkovs. "Highly-efficient release of ferulic acid from agro-industrial by-products via enzymatic hydrolysis with cellulose-degrading enzymes: Part i–the superiority of hydrolytic enzymes versus conventional hydrolysis." *Foods* 10, no. 4 (2021): 782.

Kajala, Ilkka, Jari Mäkelä, Rossana Coda, Shraddha Shukla, Qiao Shi, Ndegwa Henry Maina, Riikka Juvonen et al. "Rye bran as fermentation matrix boosts in situ dextran production by Weissella confusa compared to wheat bran." *Applied Microbiology and Biotechnology* 100 (2016): 3499–3510.

Klose, Christina, and Elke K. Arendt. "Proteins in oats; their synthesis and changes during germination: a review." *Critical Reviews in Food Science and Nutrition* 52, no. 7 (2012): 629–639.

Laddomada, Barbara, Sofia Caretto, and Giovanni Mita. "Wheat bran phenolic acids: Bioavailability and stability in whole wheat-based foods." *Molecules* 20, no. 9 (2015): 15666–15685.

Liaw, Joshua D., Dilpreet S. Bajwa, Jamileh Shojaeiarani, and Sreekala G. Bajwa. "Corn distiller's dried grains with solubles (DDGS) – A value added functional material for wood composites." *Industrial Crops and Products* 139 (2019): 111525.

McCarthy, Aoife L., Yvonne C. O'Callaghan, Alan Connolly, Charles O. Piggott, Richard J. FitzGerald, and Nora M. O'Brien. "In vitro antioxidant and anti-inflammatory effects of brewers' spent grain protein rich isolate and its associated hydrolysates." *Food Research International* 50, no. 1 (2013): 205–212.

Muhiwa, Peter J., Janet Taylor, and John RN Taylor. "Extraction and film properties of kafirin from coarse sorghum and sorghum DDGS by percolation." *Cereal Chemistry* 94, no. 4 (2017): 693–698.

Nadathur, Sudarshan, Janitha PD Wanasundara, and Laurie Scanlin, eds. *Sustainable protein sources.* Academic Press, 2016.

Naibaho, Joncer, Małgorzata Korzeniowska, Aneta Wojdyło, Hanif Muchdatul Ayunda, Maike Foste, and Baoru Yang. "Techno-functional properties of protein from protease-treated brewers' spent grain (BSG) and investigation of antioxidant activity of extracted proteins and BSG residues." *Journal of Cereal Science* 107 (2022): 103524.

Papageorgiou, Maria, and Adriana Skendi. "Introduction to cereal processing and by-products." In *Sustainable recovery and reutilization of cereal processing by-products*, edited by Charis M. Galanakis, pp. 1–25. Woodhead Publishing, 2018.

Phongthai, Suphat, Seung-Taik Lim, and Saroat Rawdkuen. "Optimization of microwave-assisted extraction of rice bran protein and its hydrolysates properties." *Journal of Cereal Science* 70 (2016): 146–154.

Pojić, Milica, Aleksandra Mišan, and Brijesh Tiwari. "Eco-innovative technologies for extraction of proteins for human consumption from renewable protein sources of plant origin." *Trends in Food Science & Technology* 75 (2018): 93–104.

Poutanen, Kaisa S., Anna O. Kårlund, Carlos Gómez-Gallego, Daniel P. Johansson, Nathalie M. Scheers, Ingela M. Marklinder, Anne K. Eriksen et al. "Grains – A major source of sustainable protein for health." *Nutrition Reviews* 80, no. 6 (2022): 1648–1663.

Prueckler, Michael, Susanne Siebenhandl-Ehn, Silvia Apprich, Stefan Hoeltinger, Cornelia Haas, Erwin Schmid, and Wolfgang Kneifel. "Wheat bran-based biorefinery 1: Composition of wheat bran and strategies of functionalization." *LWT-Food Science and Technology* 56, no. 2 (2014): 211–221.

Qin, Fen, Astrid Z. Johansen, and Solange I. Mussatto. "Evaluation of different pretreatment strategies for protein extraction from brewer's spent grains." *Industrial Crops and Products* 125 (2018): 443–453.

Qin, Pingxu, Taoran Wang, and Yangchao Luo. "A review on plant-based proteins from soybean: Health benefits and soy product development." *Journal of Agriculture and Food Research* 7 (2022): 100265.

Rodríguez-Restrepo, Yeimy A., P. Ferreira-Santos, C. E. Orrego, J. A. Teixeira, and Cristina MR Rocha. "Valorization of rice by-products: Protein-phenolic based fractions with bioactive potential." *Journal of Cereal Science* 95 (2020): 103039.

Ruan, Zhenhua, Xiaoqing Wang, Yan Liu, and Wei Liao. "Corn." In *Integrated processing technologies for food and agricultural by-products*, edited by Zhongli Pan, Ruihong Zhang, and Steven Zicari, pp. 59–72. Academic Press, 2019.

Salazar-López, Norma Julieta, Maribel Ovando-Martínez, and J. Abraham Domínguez-Avila. "Cereal/Grain By-products." In *Food Wastes and By-products: Nutraceutical and Health Potential*, edited by Rocio Campos-Vega, B. Dave Oomah, and Haydé Azeneth Vergara-Castañeda, pp. 1–34. John Wiley & Sons, 2019.

Sándor, Zsuzsanna J., Norbert Révész, Katalin Kinga Lefler, Radmilo Čolović, Vojislav Banjac, and Shivendra Kumar. "Potential of corn distiller's dried grains with solubles (DDGS) in the diet of European catfish (Silurus glanis)." *Aquaculture Reports* 20 (2021): 100653.

Scherf, Katharina Anne, Peter Koehler, and Herbert Wieser. "Gluten and wheat sensitivities – An overview." *Journal of Cereal Science* 67 (2016): 2–11.

Schmitz, Eva, Eva Nordberg Karlsson, and Patrick Adlercreutz. "Warming weather changes the chemical composition of oat hulls." *Plant biology* 22, no. 6 (2020): 1086–1091.

Schmitz, Eva, Eva Nordberg Karlsson, and Patrick Adlercreutz. "Ultrasound assisted alkaline pre-treatment efficiently solubilises hemicellulose from oat hulls." *Waste and Biomass Valorization* 12 (2021): 5371–5381.

Schweiggert-Weisz, Ute, Peter Eisner, Stephanie Bader-Mittermaier, and Raffael Osen. "Food proteins from plants and fungi." *Current Opinion in Food Science* 32 (2020): 156–162.

Singh, Rajni, Prerna Gautam, Mahek Fatima, Sonali Dua, and Jyoti Misri. "Microbes in foods and feed sector." *Microbial Interventions in Agriculture and Environment: Research Trends, Priorities and Prospects* 1 (2019): 329–352.

Squeo, Giacomo, Vittoria Latrofa, Francesca Vurro, Davide De Angelis, Francesco Caponio, Carmine Summo, and Antonella Pasqualone. "Developing a clean labelled snack bar rich in protein and fibre with Dry-Fractionated defatted durum wheat cake." *Foods* 12, no. 13 (2023): 2547.

Sterna, Vita, Sanita Zute, and Linda Brunava. "Oat grain composition and its nutrition benefice." *Agriculture and Agricultural Science Procedia* 8 (2016): 252–256.

Taylor, Janet, and John R. N. Taylor. "Making kafirin, the sorghum prolamin, into a viable alternative protein source." *Journal of the American Oil Chemists' Society* 95, no. 8 (2018): 969–990.

Tian, Ye, Marie Kriisa, Maike Föste, Mary-Liis Kütt, Ying Zhou, Oskar Laaksonen, and Baoru Yang. "Impact of enzymatic pre-treatment on composition of nutrients and phytochemicals of canola (Brassica napus) oil press residues." *Food Chemistry* 387 (2022): 132911.

Uraipong, Chatchaporn, and Jian Zhao. "Rice bran protein hydrolysates exhibit strong in vitro α -amylase, β -glucosidase and ACE-inhibition activities." *Journal of the Science of Food and Agriculture* 96, no. 4 (2016): 1101–1110.

Vanvi, Ariane, and Apollinaire Tsopmo. "Pepsin digested oat bran proteins: Separation, antioxidant activity, and identification of new peptides." *Journal of Chemistry* 4 (2016): ID 8216378.

Walters, Mallory E., William G. Willmore, and Apollinaire Tsopmo. "Antioxidant, physicochemical, and cellular secretion of glucagon-like peptide-1 properties of oat bran protein hydrolysates." *Antioxidants* 9, no. 6 (2020): 557.

Wang, Li, Yuanyuan Ding, Xinxia Zhang, Yongfu Li, Ren Wang, Xiaohu Luo, Yanan Li, Juan Li, and Zhengxing Chen. "Effect of electron beam on the functional properties and structure of defatted wheat germ proteins." *Journal of Food Engineering* 202 (2017): 9–17.

Xu, Shiwei, Yanting Shen, Jingwen Xu, Guangyan Qi, Gengjun Chen, Weiqun Wang, Xiuzhi Sun, and Yonghui Li. "Antioxidant and anticancer effects in human hepatocarcinoma (HepG2) cells of papain-hydrolyzed sorghum kafirin hydrolysates." *Journal of Functional Foods* 58 (2019): 374–382.

Yu, Dajun, Yewei Sun, Wenjun Wang, Sean F. O'Keefe, Andrew P. Neilson, Hao Feng, Zhiwu Wang, and Haibo Huang. "Recovery of protein hydrolysates from brewer's spent grain using enzyme and ultrasonication." *International Journal of Food Science & Technology* 55, no. 1 (2020): 357–368.

Zhang, Runyang, Sen Ma, Li Li, Minghui Zhang, Shuangqi Tian, Dongying Wang, Kunlun Liu, Huamin Liu, Wenxue Zhu, and Xuede Wang. "Comprehensive utilization of corn starch processing by-products: A review." *Grain & Oil Science and Technology* 4, no. 3 (2021): 89–107.

Zhang, Zhihang, Mahesha M. Poojary, Alka Choudhary, Dilip K. Rai, Marianne N. Lund, and Brijesh K. Tiwari. "Ultrasound processing of coffee silver skin, brewer's spent grain and potato peel wastes for phenolic compounds and amino acids: a comparative study." *Journal of Food Science and Technology* 58 (2021): 2273–2282.

Zhou, Cunshan, Jiali Hu, Haile Ma, Abu ElGasim A. Yagoub, Xiaojie Yu, John Owusu, Haiyan Ma, and Xiaopei Qin. "Antioxidant peptides from corn gluten meal: Orthogonal design evaluation." *Food Chemistry* 187 (2015): 270–278.

Zhou, Kequan, Corene Canning, and Shi Sun. "Effects of rice protein hydrolysates prepared by microbial proteases and ultrafiltration on free radicals and meat lipid oxidation." *LWT-Food Science and Technology* 50, no. 1 (2013): 331–335.

Zhou, Ying, Ye Tian, Gabriele Beltrame, Oskar Laaksonen, and Baoru Yang. "Ultrasonication-assisted enzymatic bioprocessing as a green method for valorizing oat hulls." *Food Chemistry* 426 (2023): 136658.

Yunus, Fakhar-un-Nisa, Muhammad Nadeem, and Farzana Rashid. "Single-cell protein production through microbial conversion of lignocellulosic residue (wheat bran) for animal feed." *Journal of the Institute of Brewing* 121, no. 4 (2015): 553–557.

39 Pulses as Sources of Protein
Considerations for Human Consumption

Cara L. Cargo-Froom, Christopher P.F. Marinangeli, Matthew G. Nosworthy, and Daniel A. Columbus

ABBREVIATIONS

AA	Amino acid
ANF	Anti-nutritional factors
DIAAS	Digestible indispensable amino acid score
IAA	Indispensable amino acid
IVPD	*In vitro* protein digestibility
PDCAAS	Protein digestibility-corrected amino acid score
PER	Protein efficiency ratio

INTRODUCTION

Pulses are a diverse group of leguminous crops integral to human diets and include, but are not limited to, common varieties such as chickpeas, kidney beans, lentils, and peas. They are high in protein, amino acids (AA), and other micronutrients and are a staple food source for millions worldwide. As societies increasingly embrace plant-based diets and sustainable food choices, pulses have garnered significant attention for their contributions to protein intake as the consumption of animal proteins decreases.

However, the true value of their protein content relies not only on quantity but also on nutritional quality, which is dependent on indispensable AA composition and digestibility. In addition to dietary fiber and the inherent food matrix, the latter can also be affected by the presence of antinutritional factors (ANF). Protein quality (PQ) can be measured by a variety of methods, which involve multiple steps, including evaluating the AA profile of the protein source and comparing it to human requirements, determining the overall protein digestibility, and identifying whether the protein source is capable of supporting growth. Multiple PQ indices, including the protein efficiency ratio (PER), protein digestibility-corrected amino acid score (PDCAAS), and the digestible indispensable amino acid score (DIAAS), have been developed to assess how effectively pulses can contribute to meeting the daily protein requirements of individuals (Nosworthy et al. 2023). While the specific calculations involved differ across methods, all PQ indicators attempt to characterize PQ based on the AA profile and bioavailability and how this relates to requirements for growth.

Overall, pulses are a valuable source of protein and AA in our diets; however, their utilization is influenced by the presence of ANF and the need for appropriate processing techniques to maximize nutritional value. Additionally, understanding PQ measurements is essential for evaluating the effectiveness of pulses in meeting our dietary protein needs, thereby contributing to a balanced diet. In the following sections, we will delve deeper into the ANFs associated with protein/AA, processing methods for pulses, and PQ of pulses.

DOI: 10.1201/9781003597926-39

PULSE PROTEIN-ASSOCIATED ANTI-NUTRITIONAL FACTORS

Anti-nutritional factors (ANFs) are compounds that reduce nutrient absorption, digestion, and/or utilization and can be naturally occurring or formed via chemical reactions during processing. For example, protease inhibitors are naturally occurring ANFs that result in impaired protein and amino acid digestion, whereas Maillard reactions, which occur during processing, reduce lysine bioavailability.

NATURALLY OCCURRING ANFS

Protease inhibitors function by inhibiting the action of enzymes utilized for protein digestion in the stomach and small intestine. Trypsin and chymotrypsin inhibitors have been measured in a variety of pulse crops, with their activity largely dependent on pulse species/cultivar (Guillamón et al. 2008; Roy et al. 2010). Tannins are water-soluble compounds that can bind and precipitate proteins (enzymes and dietary) in the gastrointestinal tract, forming insoluble resistant bonds (Reddy and Butler 1989; Jansman and Longstaff 1993). Phytic acid is reported to negatively influence the *in vitro* activity of digestive enzymes, including pepsin, trypsin, and chymotrypsin (Deshpande and Damodaran 1989). Phytic acid can either bind directly to proteins (enzymes and/or substrates) or indirectly bind to proteins through chelation with a mineral cofactor, impacting the function of digestive enzymes (O'Dell and De Boland 1976; Gilani et al. 2005). While naturally occurring ANF are a concern when pulses are consumed raw, humans do not consume raw pulses, and common processing methods are effective in inactivating and/or significantly reducing ANF content.

PROCESSING-INDUCED REDUCTIONS IN AA BIOAVAILABILITY

When pulses undergo heat or alkali treatment, amino acids (AA) can experience chemical changes, including Maillard reactions, oxidation of sulfur-containing AAs, racemization of AAs to D-enantiomers, and the formation of dehydroaminos and cross-linked AAs (Friedman 1999a, 1999b; Mauron 1981). The result of these chemical transformations renders AA unavailable for digestion and/or utilization. Although anti-nutritional factors limit the digestibility and availability of protein and AA, they are generally not of significant concern in human diets since pulses are not consumed raw. Formation of chemical compounds such as Maillard reaction products and cross-linked AAs should be considered during the processing of pulses; however, their generation is not a common concern with the majority of processed pulses currently consumed.

PULSE PROCESSING AND THE IMPACT ON PROTEIN AND AA CONTENT

Pulses must be processed prior to consumption in order to enhance palatability, digestibility, and nutrient availability, with the processing method used potentially affecting nutrient composition, digestibility, and availability, including both beneficial and adverse effects on protein and AA. Traditional methods of pulse processing include dehulling, grinding, soaking, and thermal cooking approaches such as boiling, pressure cooking/autoclaving, roasting, and extrusion. Additional processes, such as radiofrequency heating, microwave, and micronization (infrared heating), are being investigated as emerging processing technologies for pulses. The effects of various processes on protein and indispensable AA (IAA) content are summarized in Tables 39.1–39.7.

TRADITIONAL PROCESSING METHODS FOR PULSES AND EFFECTS ON NUTRIENT DENSITY

Soaking and Cooking (Boiling or Pressure Cooking)

Soaking is a common pre-treatment for pulses since the seeds are harvested dry and/or further dried prior to packaging. Generally, the most common approach to soaking pulses is in cold water for an extended period of time, ~8–12 hours, prior to additional processing (Table 39.1). Alternative soaking treatments, such as high-temperature soaking and soaking in salt or alkali solutions, can also be utilized (Khattab et al. 2009). Marginal increases in protein content have been reported for soaked black gram, peas, chickpeas, beans, and lentils (Candela et al. 1997; Rehman and Shah 2005; Wang et al. 2008, 2009, 2010). However, other studies have reported no changes or decrease in the protein content of black gram, chickpeas, peas, kidney beans, faba beans, and mung beans when soaked in cold water (El-Adawy 2002; Abd El-Hady and Habiba 2003; Mubarak 2005; Rehman and Shah 2005). When Canadian cowpeas, kidney beans, and peas were soaked for 18 h, increases and decreases in IAA content were observed, with changes in individual IAA differing between different pulse types (Geervani and Theophilus 1980).

In general, cooking in boiling water slightly decreases the protein content of pulses (0.3–1% unit change; Chitra et al. 1996; Clemente et al. 1998; Rehman and Shah 2005; Vadivel et al. 2010). Boiling and pressure cooking, including autoclaving, appear to impact individual IAA content differently across different pulses. For example, IAA increased in boiled cowpea but decreased lysine content in boiled chickpea (Candela et al. 1997; Khattab et al. 2009). Interestingly, across the majority of studies investigating changes in IAA content, methionine content consistently decreases when pulses are processed using boiling or pressure cooking (Table 39.2 and 39.3).

Dehulling

Pulses contain a seed coat, which can be consumed as part of the whole pulse or removed prior to consumption. Dehulling of pulses increases the protein content in a variety of pulses, including commonly consumed chickpeas, faba beans, kidney beans, and lentils (Table 39.4; Ghavidel and Prakash 2007; Alonso et al. 2000; Wang et al. 2008; Wang 2008). In mung beans, dehulling is reported to slightly increase IAA content (Mubarak 2005).

Roasting and Extrusion

Roasting or toasting (Table 39.5) of pulses involves cooking the seeds at a dry heat between 150 and 200°C (Malcolmson and Han 2019). Chitra et al. (1996), Vadivel et al. (2010), and Baik and Han (2012) reported no changes or decreases in the protein content of roasted chickpeas, mung beans, pigeon peas, sword beans, and urd beans, whereas Audu and Aremu (2011) and Baik and Han (2012) reported increases in the protein contents of pinto beans and chickpeas. Split pulses or dhal, which were roasted for 10 minutes at 160°C, consistently had slight decreases (0.06–0.7%) in cystine, methionine, lysine, threonine, and tryptophan content (Geervani and Theophilus 1980). Variable changes have been reported for IAA content in cowpeas, kidney beans, and peas that were roasted in a sand bath for 20 minutes at 180°C (e.g., a decrease of methionine in Egyptian kidney beans but an increase of methionine in Egyptian pea; Khattab et al. 2009).

Extrusion is another thermal treatment applied to pulses (Table 39.6), often when pulses are used as an ingredient in food products and/or to create single-ingredient snack foods. Extrusion is a high-temperature, high-pressure process that exposes the ingredient to a relatively short duration of heat. The effects of extrusion on protein and AA content vary. Although decreases and increases are reported in protein content in a variety of extruded pulses, these changes are small at 0.30–3% (Alonso et al. 2000; Abd El-Hady and Habiba 2003; Khattab et al. 2009; Nosworthy et al. 2017, 2018a, 2018b; Cargo-Froom et al. 2022). Changes in IAA content of extruded pulses

Emerging Processing Methods for Pulses

Micronization is a processing method that utilizes high-intensity infrared radiation to quickly heat and cook seeds (Malcolmson and Han 2019). Indispensable AA content increased in cowpea, kidney bean, and pea varieties, with the exception of a Canadian pea variety, when heated to 90°C (Khattab et al. 2009). In lentils tempered to 30% moisture and heated to 140°C, leucine content increased slightly (0.04%); however, this increase could be considered negligible (Laing et al. 2023). There were no reported changes in IAA content in heated chickpeas (Laing et al. 2023). Since changes in

TABLE 39.1
Effects of Soaking on Protein and Amino Acid Content, *In Vitro* Digestibility, and Protein Quality in a Variety of Pulses

	Effects of Processing				
Pulse	**Protein Content[1]**	**IAA Content[1,2]**	***In Vitro* Protein Digestibility[1]**	**PER[2]**	**Reference**
Chickpea	Decreased, 0.2	-	Increased, 1	-	Abd El-Hady and Habiba (2003)
Faba Bean	Decreased, 0.2	-	Increased, 1	-	
Kidney Bean	Decreased, 0.2	-	Increased, 1	-	
Pea	Decreased, 0.2	-	Increased, 1	-	
Faba Bean	No change	-	Increased, 0.5	-	Alonso et al. (2000)
Kidney Bean	No change	-	Increased, 3.3	-	
Canadian Cowpea	-	Decreased threonine, methionine, phenylalanine, and tryptophan. Increased valine, isoleucine, leucine, and lysine.	Increased 5	2.69	Geervani and Theophilus (1980)
Kidney Bean	-	Increased threonine, valine, isoleucine, and lysine. Decreased methionine, leucine, and tryptophan.	Increased 5.4	2.91	
Pea	-	Decreased threonine, methionine, leucine, and phenylalanine Increased valine, isoleucine, lysine and tryptophan.	Increased 5.3	2.22	
Cowpea	-	Increased total IAA.	Increased	-	Khattab et al. (2009)
Kidney Bean	-	Increased total IAA.	Increased	-	
Pea	-	Increased total IAA.	Increased	-	
Mung Bean	Decreased, 0.5	Decreased isoleucine, tryptophan, total sulfur AA, and lysine.	Increased, 7.2	-	Mubarak (2005)
Black Gram	No change	-	-	-	Rehman and Shah (2005)
Chickpea	No change	-	-	-	
Lentil	No change	-	-	-	
Red Kidney Bean	No change	-	-	-	
White Kidney Bean	No change	-	-	-	
Black Gram	Increased after most processing parameters	-	Increased	-	

(*Continued*)

TABLE 39.1 (CONTINUED)
Bioactive Properties of Hemp Seed Protein Hydrolysates and Peptides

	Effects of Processing				
Pulse	Protein Content[1]	IAA Content[1,2]	*In Vitro* Protein Digestibility[1]	PER[2]	Reference
Chickpea	Increased after most processing parameters	-	Increased	-	
Lentil	Increased after most processing parameters	-	Increased	-	
Red Kidney Bean	Increased after most processing parameters	-	Increased	-	
White Kidney Bean	Increased after most processing parameters	-	Increased	-	
Sword Bean	Increased after most processing parameters	-	-	-	Vadivel et al. 2010
Field Pea	Increased in 4/6 varieties, 0.5–1	-	-	-	Wang et al. 2008

This table was adapted and modified with permission from Cargo-Froom et al. (2020).

1 Numbers represent % value changed.

2 IAA = indispensable Amino Acid, PER = protein efficiency ratio, PDCAAS = protein digestibility-corrected amino acid score, DIAAS = digestible indispensable amino acid

the nutrient content of pulses are often variety-dependent, there is a need to generate datasets on the effects of micronization on protein and AA content in pulses (Table 39.7).

Microwave heating is a dielectric heating process that uses electromagnetic waves to heat and cook pulses (Ahmed 2020). Similar to other processes, changes in IAA content appear to be dependent on both processing parameters and pulse variety (Table 39.8). For example, threonine content decreased in microwaved peas but increased in cowpeas and kidney beans (Chung et al. 1981; Khattab et al. 2009).

EFFECTS OF PROCESSING ON PROTEIN DIGESTION

The overall goal of pulse processing is to improve nutrient bioavailability, including that of protein and AA. Protein and AA digestibility at the level of the terminal ileum is commonly used as a proxy for bioavailability. As *in vivo* determination of ileal digestibility in humans poses ethical issues, nutrient digestibility values determined in animal models are generally used as an estimate of nutrient bioavailability and PQ in humans. While the use of animal models is widespread, these studies are extremely complex and also pose ethical considerations. Therefore, many studies utilize *in vitro*

TABLE 39.2
Effects of Boiling on Protein and Amino Acid Content, *In Vitro* Digestibility, and Protein Quality in a Variety of Pulses

	Effects of Processing						
Pulse	**Protein Content[1]**	**IAA Content[1,2]**	***In Vitro* Protein Digestibility[1]**	**PER[2]**	**PDCAAS[2]**	**DIAAS[2]**	**Reference**
Chickpea	Increased, 1.0		Increased, 5.4	-	-	-	Baik and Han (2012)
Lentil	Increased, 0.8		Increased, 3	-	-	-	
Pea	No change		Increased, 3.8	-	-	-	
Chickpea	Increased, 4.51	Decreased lysine	-	-	-	-	Candela et al. (1997)
Kidney Bean	Increased, 4.83	Decreased all IAA, except histidine	-	-	-	-	
Lentil	No change	Decreased isoleucine, leucine, valine; Increased lysine, phenylalanine	-	-	-	-	
Colossus Pea	No change	Decreased histidine, isoleucine, leucine, lysine, methionine, phenylalanine, tyrosine, valine	-	-	-	-	Chung et al. (1981)
Chickpea	Decreased, 3.4	Decreased all IAA	Increased 11.7.	-	-	-	Clemente et al. (1998)
	No change	-	Increased, 4.91	-	-	-	El-Adawy (2002)
	No change	-	Increased, 5.79	-	-	-	
Bengal Gram Dhal	-	Decreased cystine, lysine, methionine, threonine, tryptophan	-	-	-	-	Geervani and Theophilus (1980)
Black Gram Dhal	-	Decreased cystine, lysine, methionine, threonine, tryptophan	-	-	-	-	
Green Gram Dhal	-	Decreased cystine, lysine, methionine, threonine, tryptophan	-	-	-	-	

(Continued)

TABLE 39.2 (CONTINUED)
Effects of Boiling on Protein and Amino Acid Content, *In Vitro* Digestibility, and Protein Quality in a Variety of Pulses

	Effects of Processing						
Pulse	Protein Content[1]	IAA Content[1,2]	*In Vitro* Protein Digestibility[1]	PER[2]	PDCAAS[2]	DIAAS[2]	Reference
Redgram Dhal	-	Decreased cystine, lysine, methionine, threonine, tryptophan	-	-	-	-	
Faba Bean	-	Increased leucine, tyrosine, threonine, and histidine. Decreased isoleucine, lysine, cystine, methionine, and valine.	Increased, 6	-	-	-	Khalil (1995)
Cowpea	-	Increased total IAA	Increased, 5	-	-	-	Khattab et al. 2009
Kidney Bean	-	Increased total IAA	Increased, 5	-	-	-	
Pea	-	Increased total IAA	Increased, 5	-	-	-	
Sword Bean	No change	-	-	-	-	-	Margier et al. (2018)
Mung Bean	Decreased, 0.7	Decreased isoleucine, tryptophan, total sulfur AA, and lysine; Increased leucine	Increased, 7.6	-	-	-	Mubarak (2005)
Mung Bean	Decreased, 0.8	Decreased isoleucine, tryptophan, total sulfur AA, and lysine; Increased leucine	Increased, 8.5	-	-	-	
Green Split Pea	-	-	-	1.4	72	0.67	Nosworthy et al. (2017)
Yellow Split Pea	-	-	-	1.7	69.19	0.66	
Black Bean	-	-	-	1.61	0.534	0.49	Nosworthy et al. (2017b)
Chickpea	-	-	-	2.32	0.519	0.67	
Kidney Bean	-	-	-	1.55	0.549	0.51	

(Continued)

TABLE 39.2 (CONTINUED)
Effects of Boiling on Protein and Amino Acid Content, *In Vitro* Digestibility, and Protein Quality in a Variety of Pulses

	Effects of Processing						
Pulse	Protein Content[1]	IAA Content[1,2]	*In Vitro* Protein Digestibility[1]	PER[2]	PDCAAS[2]	DIAAS[2]	Reference
Navy Bean	-	-	-	1.51	0.667	0.65	
Pinto Bean	-	-	-	1.64	0.59	0.6	
Green Lentil	-	-	-	1.3	0.628	0.58	
Red Split Lentil	-	-	-	0.98	0.538	0.5	
Green Split Pea	-	-	-	0.86	0.5	0.46	
Yellow Split Pea	-	-	-	1.42	0.643	0.73	
Green Lentil	-	-	Decreased	0.98	52.92	0.49	Nosworthy et al. (2018a)
Red Lentil	-	-	Decreased	1.14	57.4	0.53	
Black Bean	-	-	-	1.42	67.54	0.63	Nosworthy et al. (2018b)
Faba Bean	-	-	-	0.85	54.14	0.59	
Kidney Bean	-	-	-	1.47	62.4	0.58	
Navy Bean	-	-	-	1.52	61.23	0.57	
Pinto Bean	-	-	-	1.45	75.1	0.7	
Field Peas	Increased, 0.5–2	-	-	-	-	-	Wang et al. (2008)
Lentil	Increased all varieties, 0.5–1	-	-	-	-	-	Wang et al. (2009)
Chickpea	Increased, 0.5–1	-	-	-	-	-	Wang et al. (2010)
Great Northern Bean	Increased, 0.9	-	-	-	-	-	
Kidney Bean	Increased, 1	-	-	-	-	-	
Pinto Bean	Increased, 1.5	-	-	-	-	-	

This table was adapted and modified with permission from Cargo-Froom et al. (2020).
[1] Numbers represent % value changed.
[2] IAA = indispensable amino acid; PER = protein efficiency ratio; PDCAAS = protein digestibility-corrected amino acid score; DIAAS = digestible indispensable amino acid score.

TABLE 39.3
Effects of Pressure Cooking on Protein and Amino Acid Content, *In Vitro* Digestibility, and Protein Quality in a Variety of Pulses

	Effects of Processing				
Pulse	**Protein Content[1]**	**IAA Content[1,2]**	***In Vitro* Protein Digestibility[1]**	**PER[2]**	**Reference**
Chickpea	Decreased	-	Increased, 5.1	-	Chitra et al. (1996)
Pea	Decreased	-	Increased	-	
Sword Bean	Increased	-	Increased	-	
Lentil	-	Increased threonine, valine, isoleucine, leucine, phenylalanine, and lysine. Decreased methionine and tryptophan.	Increased, 8.42	3.02	Geervani and Theophilus (1980)
Faba Bean	-	Increased leucine, phenylalanine, threonine, and histidine. Decreased isoleucine, lysine, cystine, methionine, tyrosine, and valine.	Increased, 9	2.6	Khalil (1995)
Mung Bean	-	Decreased isoleucine and valine. Increased leucine and lysine.	Decreased	-	
Canadian Cowpea	-	Decreased threonine and tryptophan. Increased valine, isoleucine, leucine, phenylalanine, and lysine.	Increased, 7.9	2.99	Khattab et al. (2009)
Egyptian Cowpea	-	Increased threonine, valine, isoleucine, leucine, lysine, and tryptophan. Decreased methionine and phenylalanine.	Increased, 8.15	3.04	
Canadian Kidney Bean	-	Increased threonine, valine, isoleucine, leucine, lysine, and tryptophan. Decreased methionine and phenylalanine.	Increased, 8.15	3.04	

(*Continued*)

TABLE 39.3 (CONTINUED)
Effects of Pressure Cooking on Protein and Amino Acid Content, *In Vitro* Digestibility, and Protein Quality in a Variety of Pulses

	Effects of Processing				
Pulse	Protein Content[1]	IAA Content[1,2]	*In Vitro* Protein Digestibility[1]	PER[2]	Reference
Egyptian Kidney Bean	-	Decreased threonine, methionine, leucine, phenylalanine, and tryptophan. Increased isoleucine and lysine.	Increased, 8	2.72	
Canadian Pea	-	Decreased threonine, valine, methionine, leucine, and phenylalanine. Increased isoleucine, lysine, and tryptophan.	Increased, 8.15	2.8	
Egyptian Pea	-		Increased, 8.15	2.99	
Black Gram	Decreased at most temperatures/times.	-	Increased, 27–33	-	Rehman et al. (2005)
Chickpea	Decreased at most temperatures/times	-	Increased, 28–36	-	
Red Kidney Bean	Decreased at most temperatures/times	-	Increased, 28–34	-	
White Kidney Bean	Decreased at most temperatures/times	-	Increased, 27–36	-	
Lentil	Decreased at most temperatures/times	-	Increased, 30–38	-	
Chickpea	-	-	Increased, 5	-	Salazar-Villanea et al. (2016)
Faba Bean	-	-	Decreased, 4	-	
Kidney Bean	-	-	Increased, 7	-	
Lentil	-	-	Changed, 1–2	-	

This table was adapted and modified with permission from Cargo-Froom et al. (2020).

[1] Numbers represent % value changed.

[2] IAA = indispensable amino acid; PER = protein efficiency ratio; PDCAAS = protein digestibility-corrected amino acid score; DIAAS = digestible indispensable amino acid score.

TABLE 39.4
Effects of Dehulling on Protein and Amino Acid Content, *In Vitro* Digestibility, and Protein Quality in a Variety of Pulses

	Effects of Processing			
Pulse	**Protein Content[1]**	**IAA Content[1,2]**	***In Vitro* Protein Digestibility[1]**	**Reference**
Faba bean	Increased, 4	-	No change	Alonso et al. 2000
Kidney bean	Increased, 1.5	-	Increased, 3.5	
Chickpea	Increased, 5	-	Increased, 13.4	Ghavidel and Prakash 2007
Cowpea	Increased, 2.7	-	Increased, 13.4	
Green Gram	Increased, 2.2	-	Increased, 16.7	
Lentil	Increased, 3.1	-	Increased, 13.2	
Mung bean	No change	Slight increase all IAA	Increased, 4.1	Mubarak 2005
Horse gram	Increased 3/12 varieties			
	No change 9/12 varieties	-	-	Pal et al. 2016
Pea	Increased all varieties	-	-	Wang et al. 2008
Lentil	Increased all varieties	-	-	Wang et al. 2009
Lentil	Increased	-	-	Wang 2008

This table was adapted and modified with permission from Cargo-Froom et al. (2020).
[1] Numbers represent % value changed.
[2] IAA = Indispensable amino acid.

approaches to assess AA digestibility and PQ of pulses. The effects of various processes on *in vitro* protein digestibility (IVPD) content are summarized in Tables 39.1–39.7.

Thermal Processing on Protein Digestibility

Dehulling of chickpeas, cowpeas, green gram, kidney beans, lentils, and mung beans all resulted in an increase in IVPD (Alonso et al. 2000; Mubarak 2005; Ghavidel and Prakash 2007). Soaking of pulses for 18 hours resulted in an approximately 5% unit increase in IVPD in cowpeas, kidney beans, and peas (Geervani and Theophilus 1980). The majority of studies which cooked pulses using boiling or pressure cooking approaches reported increases in IVPD by up to 35% in a variety of pulses (Geervani and Theophilus 1980; Chitra et al. 1996; Clemente et al. 1998; Khattab et al. 2009; Rehman and Shah 2005; Vadivel et al. 2010; Salazar-Villanea et al. 2016); however, in faba beans and mung beans which were autoclaved, and lentils which were boiled, IVPD content was reported to decrease (Khalil and Mansour 1995; Salazar-Villanea et al. 2016; Nosworthy et al. 2018a).

Thermal methods, such as roasting and extrusion, have resulted in variable changes in IVPD and appear to be dependent on both processing parameters and pulse class. The IVPD of roasted chickpeas, mung beans, pigeon peas, and urd beans is reported to increase compared to unprocessed samples (Chitra et al. 1996; Vadivel et al. 2010), whereas the IVPD of roasted cowpeas, kidney beans, and peas is reported to decrease (~5%; Khattab et al. 2009). The effects of extrusion

TABLE 39.5
Effects of Roasting on Protein and Amino Acid Content, *In Vitro* Digestibility, and Protein Quality in a Variety of Pulses

	Effects of Processing				
Pulse	**Protein Content[1]**	**IAA Content[1,2]**	***In Vitro* Protein Digestibility[1]**	**PER[2]**	**Reference**
Chickpea	Slight increase	-	Increased 5.4	-	Baik and Han (2012)
Lentil	No change	-	No Change	-	
Pea	No change	-	No Change	-	
Chickpea	No change	-	Increased	-	Chitra et al. (1996)
Mung Bean	Decreased	-	Increased	-	
Pigeon Pea	Decreased	-	Increased	-	
Urd Bean	Decreased	-	Increased	-	
Bengal Gram Dhal	-	Decreased methionine 0.34, cystine 0.06, threonine 0.37, tryptophan 0.08, lysine 0.58.	-	1.91	Geervani and Theophilus (1980)
Black Gram Dhal	-	Decreased methionine 0.24, cystine 0.19, threonine 0.34, tryptophan 0.12, lysine 0.70.	-	1.48	
Green Gram Dhal	-	Decreased methionine 0.29, cystine 0.29, threonine 0.29, tryptophan 0.24, lysine 0.67.	-	0.95	
Red Gram Dhal	-	Decreased methionine 0.3, cystine 0.04, threonine 0.19, tryptophan 0.13, lysine 0.43.	-	1.77	
Canadian Cowpea	-	Decreased threonine, valine, phenylalanine, and tryptophan. Increased methionine, leucine, isoleucine, lysine,	Decreased 4.7	2.77	Khattab et al. (2009)
Egyptian Cowpea	-	Decreased threonine, Increased valine, methionine, and tryptophan. Increased isoleucine, leucine, phenylalanine, and lysine	Decreased 5	2.77	
Canadian Kidney Bean	-	Decreased leucine, phenylalanine, and tryptophan. Increased lysine.	Decreased 5.6	2.68	
Egyptian Kidney Bean		Decreased threonine and methionine. Increased valine, isoleucine, and lysine.	Decreased 5	2.78	

(*Continued*)

TABLE 39.5 (CONTINUED)
Effects of Roasting on Protein and Amino Acid Content, *In Vitro* Digestibility, and Protein Quality in a Variety of Pulses

	Effects of Processing				
Pulse	**Protein Content[1]**	**IAA Content[1,2]**	***In Vitro* Protein Digestibility[1]**	**PER[2]**	**Reference**
Canadian Pea	-	Decreased threonine, methionine, and phenylalanine. Increased isoleucine, lysine, and tryptophan.	Decreased 5.3	2.67	
Egyptian Pea	-	Decreased threonine. Increased valine, methionine, isoleucine, leucine, and lysine.	Decreased 5	2.34	
Sword Bean	No change	-	-	-	Vadivel et al. (2010)

This table was adapted and modified with permission from Cargo-Froom et al. (2020).
[1] Numbers represent % value changed.
[2] IAA = indispensable amino acid; PER = protein efficiency ratio; PDCAAS = protein digestibility-corrected amino acid score; DIAAS = Digestible indispensable amino acid score.

on IVPD vary depending on pulse and processing parameters. For example, kidney beans processed at 140°C/18% moisture or 140°C/22% moisture reported an increase and decrease in IVPD, respectively (Abd El-Hady and Habiba 2003). However, the degree to which IVPD is altered in extruded pulses when compared to other processes is generally smaller.

Emerging Processing Methods on Protein Digestibility

Micronization/infrared heating is reported to minimally affect (0.2–3%) IVPD of pulses, which increased in chickpeas, some lentil cultivars, and yellow peas and decreased in cowpea, kidney bean, and other pea cultivars (Khattab et al. 2009; Liu et al. 2022; Laing et al. 2023). Microwave cooking is reported to increase IVPD by up to 17% (Sun et al. 2020; Barpete et al. 2021). Similarly to many traditional methods, both micronization and microwave cooking can enhance the nutritive quality of pulses via increased protein digestion.

METHODS OF DETERMINING PQ

The methods required for quantifying the nutritional quality of a protein source, such as pulses, vary depending on the jurisdiction being considered. The most commonly used methods in North America, for example, are the PER and PDCAAS (Health Canada F0-1; FAO/WHO 1991), which are embedded in federal regulations to determine if foods can be identified as a source of protein in the marketplace. The most recent method for PQ assessment, the DIAAS, was developed by modifying PDCAAS but has yet to be incorporated into the regulatory assessment of proteins in any country (FAO/WHO 2013). Measurements of PQ for processed pulses are summarized in Tables 39.2–39.7.

TABLE 39.6
Effects of Extrusion on Protein and Amino Acid Content, *In Vitro* Digestibility, and Protein Quality in a Variety of Pulses

Pulse	Effects of Processing						Reference
	Protein Content[1]	IAA Content[1,2]	*In Vitro* Protein Digestibility[1]	PER[2]	PDCAAS[2]	DIAAS[2]	
Chickpea	Decreased, 0.35	-	Increased, 2.00	-	-	-	Abd El-Hady and Habiba (2003)
Faba Bean	Increased, 0.8	-	Increased, 2.00	-	-	-	
Kidney Bean	Decreased, 0.83	-	Increased, 2.49	-	-	-	
Pea	Decreased, 0.40	-	Increased, 0.22	-	-	-	
Chickpea	Increased, 0.88	-	Increased, 0.27	-	-	-	
Faba Bean	Increased, 0.94	-	Decreased, 0.34	-	-	-	
Kidney Bean	Increased, 0.69	-	Increased, 0.05	-	-	-	
Pea	Decreased, 1.23	-	Increased, 0.78	-	-	-	
Chickpea	Decreased, 0.81	-	Increased, 2.89	-	-	-	
Faba Bean	No change	-	Increased, 1.44	-	-	-	
Kidney Bean	Decreased, 2.15	-	Decreased, 0.07	-	-	-	
Pea	Decreased, 0.52	-	Increased, 1.83	-	-	-	
Chickpea	Decreased, 0.63	-	Increased, 0.95	-	-	-	
Faba Bean	Increased, 0.16	-	Increased, 0.32	-	-	-	
Kidney Bean	Increased, 0.17	-	Increased, 0.89	-	-	-	
Pea	Increased, 0.34	-	Increased, 1.17	-	-	-	
Pea	No change		Increased, 3.00	-	-	-	Alonso et al. (2000)
Chickpea	No change	Increased methionine 10	-	-	-	-	Cargo-Froom et al. (2022)
Faba Bean	No change	No change	-	-	-	-	
Lentil	Increased, ~3	Increased isoleucine, leucine, lysine, methionine, tryptophan, and valine	-	-	-	-	
Dun Pea	Increased, 1	No change	-	-	-	-	

(Continued)

TABLE 39.6 (CONTINUED)
Effects of Extrusion on Protein and Amino Acid Content, *In Vitro* Digestibility, and Protein Quality in a Variety of Pulses

	Effects of Processing						
Pulse	**Protein Content[1]**	**IAA Content[1,2]**	***In Vitro* Protein Digestibility[1]**	**PER[2]**	**PDCAAS[2]**	**DIAAS[2]**	**Reference**
Yellow Pea	Increased, 0.29	No change	No change	-	-	-	
Green Split Pea	-	-	Decreased	1.5	73.61	0.7	Nosworthy et al.
Yellow Split Pea	-	-	Decreased	1.5	65.44	0.67	(2017)
Green Lentil	-	-	Decreased	1.08	57.09	0.53	Nosworthy et al.
Red Lentil	-	-	Decreased	1.05	63.01	0.58	(2018a)
Black Bean	-	-	-	1.27	69.74	0.65	Nosworthy et al.
Faba Bean	-	-	-	0.45	58.01	0.54	(2018b)
Navy Bean	-	-	-	1.24	60.82	0.56	
Pinto	-	-	-	1.26	66.21	0.61	
Red Kidney Bean	-	-	-	1.23	64.98	0.60	

This table was adapted and modified with permission from Cargo-Froom et al. (2020).

[1] Numbers represent % value changed.

[2] IAA = indispensable amino acid; PER = protein efficiency ratio; PDCAAS = protein digestibility-corrected amino acid score; DIAAS = digestible indispensable amino acid score.

TABLE 39.7
Effects of Micronization on Protein and Amino Acid Content, *In Vitro* Digestibility, and Protein Quality in a Variety of Pulses

	Effects of Processing						
Pulse	**Protein Content**[1]	**IAA Content**[1,2]	***In Vitro* Protein Digestibility**[1]	**PER**[2]	**PDCAAS**[2]	**DIAAS**[2]	**Reference**
Grass Pea	-	-	Average increase of 2.49	-	-	-	Barpete et al. (2021)
Colossus Pea	No change	Decreased histidine 12.8, isoleucine 7.8, leucine 7.0, lysine 7.7, methionine 13, phenylalanine 8.5, threonine 9.6, valine 8.4	-	-	-	-	Chung et al. (1981)
Cowpea	-	Increased threonine, valine, isoleucine, and leucine. Decreased methionine, phenylalanine, lysine, and tryptophan	Increased, 10.51	-	-	2.76	Khattab et al. (2009)
Kidney Bean	-	Increased threonine, valine, isoleucine, phenylalanine, and lysine. Decreased methionine and tryptophan	Increased, 11	-	-	3.01	
Pea	-	Decreased threonine, methionine, leucine, and phenylalanine. Increased valine, isoleucine, lysine, and tryptophan	Increased, 10.68	-	-	2.48	
Pigeon Pea	-	-	Increased, 17	-	-	-	Sun et al. (2020)

This table was adapted and modified with permission from Cargo-Froom et al. (2020).

[1] Numbers represent % value changed.

[2] IAA = indispensable amino acid; PER = protein efficiency ratio; PDCAAS = protein digestibility-corrected amino acid score; DIAAS = digestible indispensable amino acid score.

TABLE 39.8
Effects of Microwave Cooking on Protein and Amino Acid Content, *In Vitro* Digestibility, and Protein Quality in a Variety of Pulses

	Effects of Processing				
Pulse	**Protein Content[1]**	**IAA Content[1,2]**	***In Vitro* Protein Digestibility[1]**	***In Vitro*-PDCAAS[2]**	**Reference**
Chickpea	No change		No change	Increased, 6 (tempered 20 moisture, 135°C)	Bai et al. (2018)
Cowpea	-	Increased total IAA	Decreased, 2	-	Khattab et al. (2009)
Kidney Bean	-	Increased total IAA	Decreased, 2–3	-	
Pea	-	Increased total IAA (except Canadian variety)	Decreased, 2–3	-	
Green Lentil	No change	Increased leucine 0.04	Increased, ~4–9	No change	Laing et al. (2023)
Yellow Pea	No change	No change	Increased, ~2–6	0.02 increase at 120°C/30 moisture	
Lentil	-	-	Increased, ~4–7	Increased ~1–5	Liu et al. (2022)
Mung Bean	No change	-	-	-	Padmashree et al. (2016)
Lentil	No change	-	-	-	Pathiratne et al. (2015)
Yellow Pea Flour	No change	-	-	-	Ribéreau et al. (2018)

[1] Numbers represent % value changed.
[2] IAA = indispensable amino acid; PER = protein efficiency ratio; PDCAAS = protein digestibility-corrected amino acid score; DIAAS = digestible indispensable amino acid score.

Different approaches are employed to determine PER and PDCAAS values (Figure 39.1 and Figure 39.2). It is notable that while PER is a measurement of growth, PDCAAS is a measurement of nutritional value and protein digestibility. Health Canada has recently adopted an equation to convert PDCAAS to PER values for content claims. For this conversion, the PDCAAS is multiplied by 2.5 to generate the estimated PER for the ingredient/food. The basis behind this calculation is that 100 is the highest value that PDCAAS can achieve, and a readily digestible protein source such as casein is set at a PER of 2.5. Therefore, $PER_{estimated} = PDCAAS \times 2.5$. As this is a relatively recent development, approved in December 2020, further investigation as to the validity of this conversion factor must be considered. As demonstrated in Figure 39.3 the relationship between PER and calculated PER is not linear when multiple different protein sources and processing methods are considered, presenting an $R^2 = 0.25$ (Nosworthy, unpublished). More appropriate regression equations should be considered based on the processing method and initial protein source, which would strengthen the relationship between PER and a calculated PER based on PDCAAS methodology.

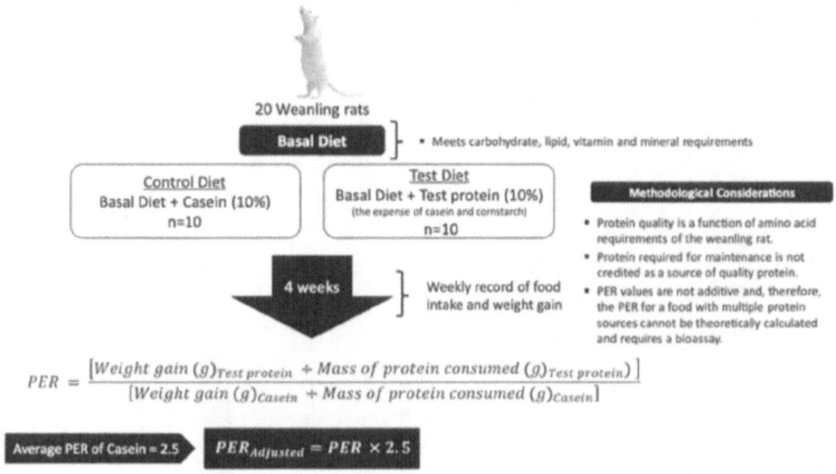

FIGURE 39.1 Summary of the determination of the protein efficiency ratio (PER) of a food. This figure is used with permission from Marinangeli and House (2017).

CONCLUSION

In conclusion, pulses play a role in our diets as a source of plant-based protein and amino acids (AA). Their nutritional value, however, is not solely determined by the quantity of protein but also by the quality of the protein, overall AA composition, and the presence of anti-nutritional factors. Appropriate processing techniques such as soaking, cooking, roasting, and extrusion can be employed to reduce these ANFs and unlock the full nutritional potential of pulses. Assessing the protein quality of pulses is another crucial aspect of understanding their nutritional value. Various PQ indices, including PER, PDCAAS, and DIAAS, have been developed to evaluate how effectively pulses can contribute to meeting daily protein requirements.

MINI DICTIONARY OF TERMS

- **Anti-nutritional factor:** Natural or processing-derived compounds that negatively affect digestion, absorption, and/or bioavailability of nutrients.
- **Digestible indispensable amino acid score:** A method of determining protein quality using true ileal amino acid digestibility.
- **Protein digestibility-corrected amino acid score:** A method of determining protein quality using true fecal nitrogen digestibility.
- **Protein efficiency ratio:** A method of determining protein quality using rat or chick growth assays.
- **Protein quality:** The ability of a protein source to meet the indispensable amino acid requirements of an individual and support physiological needs for metabolism, maintenance, and/or growth.

SUMMARY POINTS

- This chapter focuses on pulses and their ability to supply protein and AA as plant-based protein sources.

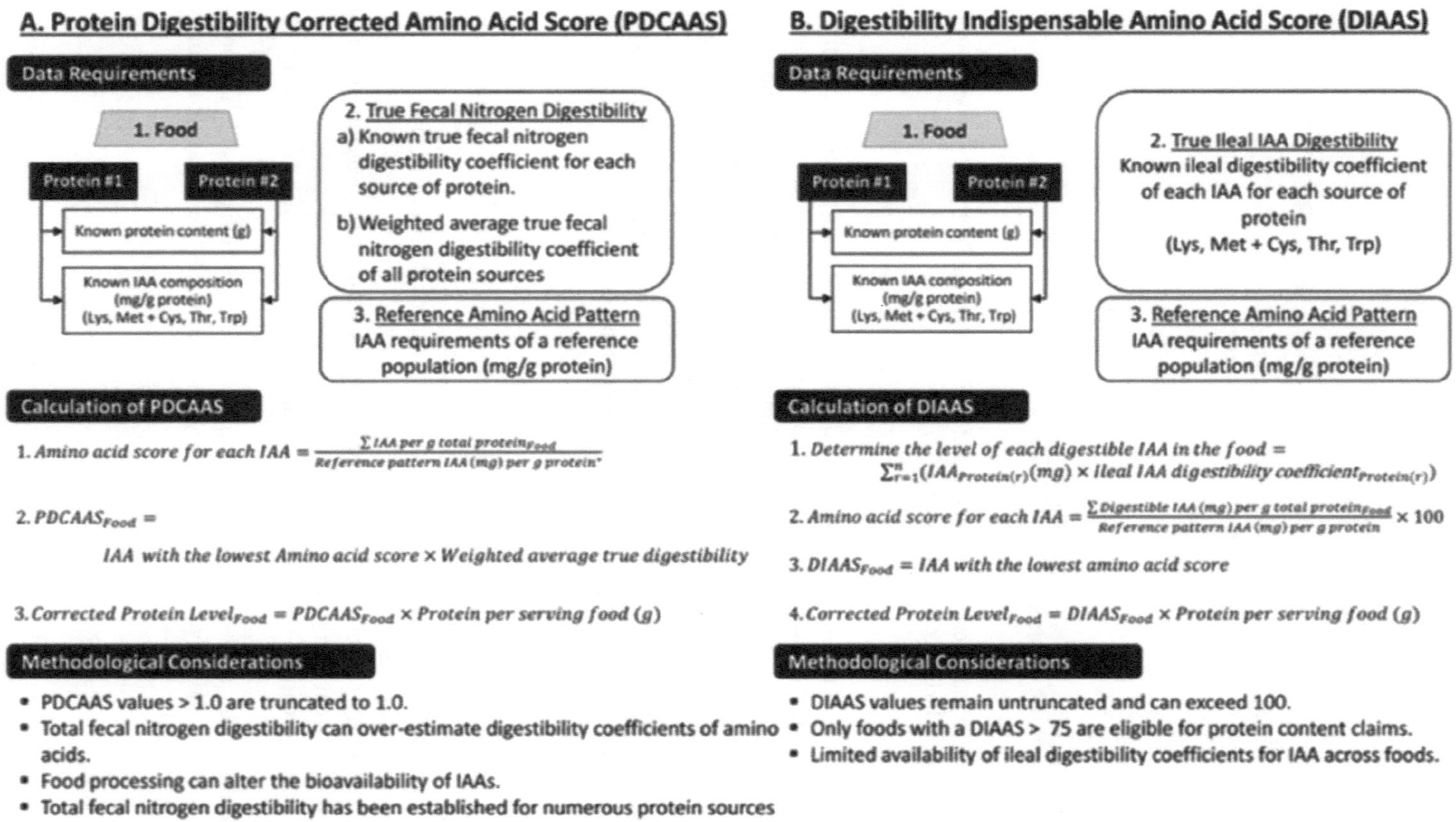

FIGURE 39.2 Summary and comparison of (A) the protein digestibility-corrected amino acid score (PDCAAS) and (B) the digestible indispensable amino acid score (DIAAS). This figure is adapted and used with permission from Marinangeli and House (2017). Abbreviations: Cys, cysteine; DIAAS, digestible indispensable amino acid score; IAA, indispensable amino acid; Lys, lysine; Met, methionine; PDCAAS, protein digestibility-corrected amino acid score; Thr, threonine; Trp, tryptophan.

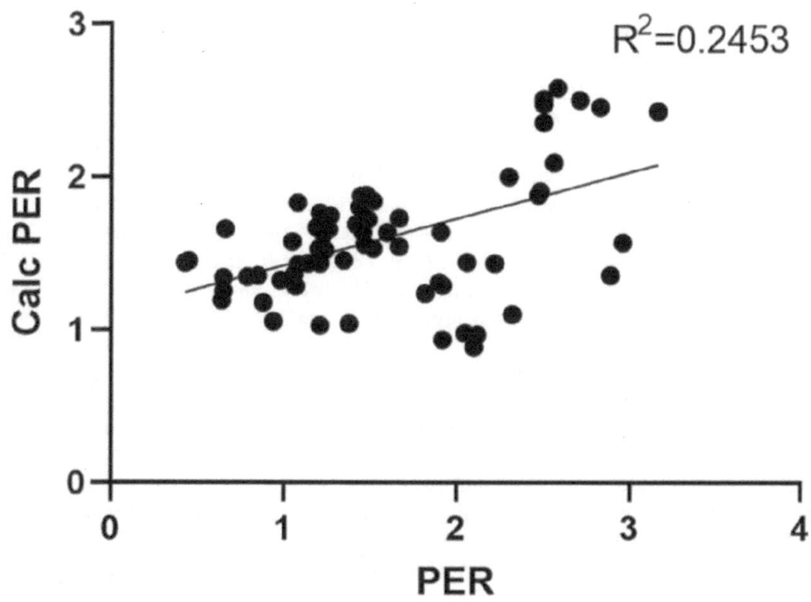

FIGURE 39.3 Relationship between protein efficiency ratio (PER) and calculated protein efficiency ratio.

- Due to the presence of ANFs, pulses must be cooked prior to consumption; however, this can cause changes in protein and AA content and/or protein and amino digestibility/availability.
- Dehulling increases the protein content of pulses consistently, while changes in protein and IAA content appear process- and pulse-dependent for various cooking methods.
- In general, IVPD increased significantly in processed pulses, with increases of 0.05–32% reported.
- Protein quality ratings of pulses can vary depending on the approach selected, i.e., PER/PDCAAS/DIAAS.

REFERENCES

Abd El-Hady, E.A., and R.A. Habiba. 2003. Effect of Soaking and Extrusion Conditions on Antinutrients and Protein Digestibility of Legume Seeds. *LWT—Food Science and Technology* 3 (36): 285–293. doi:10.1016/S0023-6438(02)00217-7.

Ahmed, J. 2020. Emerging Technologies for Pulse Processing. In *Pulse Foods: Processing, Quality and Nutraceutical Applications*, 2nd edition, ed. B.K Tiwari, A. Gowen, and B. McKenna, 265–293. Londog: Academic Press. doi:10.1016/B978-0-12-818184-3.00011-8.

Alonso, R., A. Aguirre, and F. Marzo. 2000. Effects of Extrusion and Traditional Processing Methods on Antinutrients and in Vitro Digestibility of Protein and Starch in Faba and Kidney Beans. *Food Chemistry* 68 (2): 159–165. doi:10.1016/S0308-8146(99)00169-7.

Audu, S.S. and M.O. Aremu. 2011. Nutritional Composition of Raw and Processed Pinto Bean (Phaseolus vulgaris L.) Grown in Nigeria. *Journal of Food, Agriculture, and Environment* 9 (3&4): 72–80.

Bai, T., A.K. Stone, and M.T. Nickerson. 2018. Effect of Tempering Moisture and Infrared Heating Temperature on the Functionality of Desi Chickpea and Hull-Less Barley Flours. *Cereal Chemistry* 95 (4): 508–517. doi:10.1002/cche.10054.

Baik, B.K., and I.H. Han. 2012. Cooking, Roasting, and Fermentation of Chickpeas, Lentils, Peas, and Soybeans for Fortification of Leavened Bread. *Cereal Chemistry* 89 (6): 269–275. doi:10.1094/CCHEM-04-12-0047-R.

Barpete, S., P. Gupta, K.M. Khawar, and S. Kumar. 2021. Effect of Cooking Methods on Protein Content and Neurotoxin (β-ODAP) Concentration in Grass Pea (Lathyrus Sativus L.) Grains. *CYTA—Journal of Food* 19 (1): 448–456. doi:10.1080/19476337.2021.1915879.

Candela, M., I. Astiasaran, and J. Bello. 1997. Cooking and Warm-Holding: Effect on General Composition and Amino Acids of Kidney Beans (Phaseolus Vulgaris), Chickpeas (Cicer Arietinum), and Lentils (Lens Culinaris). *Journal of Agricultural and Food Chemistry* 45 (12): 4763–4767. doi:10.1021/jf9702609.

Cargo-Froom, C.L., R.W. Newkirk, C.P.F. Marinangeli, A.K. Shoveller, Y. Ai, and D.A. Columbus. 2022. The Effects of Extrusion on Nutrient Content of Canadian Pulses with a Focus on Protein and Amino Acids. *Canadian Journal of Animal Science* 103 (1): 44–58. doi:10.1139/cjas-2022-0088.

Chitra, U., U. Singh, and V. Rao. 1996. Phytic Acid, in Vitro Protein Digestibility, Dietary Fiber, and Minerals of Pulses as Influenced by Processing Methods. *Plant Foods for Human Nutrition* 49: 307–316.

Chung, S.Y., C.V. Morr, and J.J. Jen. 1981. Effect of Microwave and Conventional Cooking on the Nutritive Value of Colossus Peas (Vigna Uniguiculata). *Journal of Food Science* 46 (1): 272–273. doi:10.1111/j.1365-2621.1981.tb14579.x.

Clemente, A.R. Sánchez-Vioque, J. Vioque, J. Bautista, and F. Millán. 1998. Effect of Cooking on Protein Quality of Chickpea (Cicer Arietinum) Seeds. *Food Chemistry* 62 (1): 1–6. doi:10.1016/S0308-8146(97)00180-5.

Deshpande, S.S., and S. Damodaran. 1989. Effect of Phytate on Solubility, Activity and Conformation of Trypsin and Chymotrypsin. *Journal of Food Science* 54 (3): 695–699.

El-Adawy, T.A. 2002. Nutritional Composition and Antinutritional Factors of Chickpeas (Cicer Arietinum L.) Undergoing Different Cooking Methods and Germination. *Plant Foods for Human Nutrition* 57 (1): 83–97. doi:10.1023/A:1013189620528.

FAO/WHO. 1991. *Protein Quality Evaluation*. Rome, Italy: Food and Agriculture Organization of the United Nations.

FAO/WHO. 2013. Dietary protein quality evaluation in human nutrition. *FAO Food Nutrition* 92: 1–66.

Friedman, M. 1999a. Chemistry, Biochemistry, Nutrition, and Microbiology of Lysinoalanine. *Lanthionine, and Histidinoalanine in Food and Other Proteins* 47 (4): 1295–1319. doi:10.1021/JF981000.

Friedman, M. 1999b. Chemistry, Nutrition, and Microbiology of D-Amino Acids. *Journal of Agricultural and Food Chemistry* 47 (9): 3457–3479. doi:10.1021/JF990080U/ASSET/IMAGES/LARGE/JF990080UF00009.JPEG.

Geervani, P., and F. Theophilus. 1980. Effect of Home Processing on the Protein Quality of Selected Legumes. *Journal of Food Science* 45 (3):707–710. doi:10.1111/j.1365-2621.1980.tb04138.x.

Ghavidel, R.A., and J. Prakash. 2007. The Impact of Germination and Dehulling on Nutrients, Antinutrients, in Vitro Iron and Calcium Bioavailability and in Vitro Starch and Protein Digestibility of Some Legume Seeds. *LWT* 40 (7):1292–1299. doi:10.1016/j.lwt.2006.08.002.

Gilani, G.S., K.A. Cockell, and E. Sepehr. 2005. Effects of Antinutritional Factors on Protein Digestibility and Amino Acid Availability in Foods. *Journal of AOAC International* 88 (3): 967–987. doi:10.1093/JAOAC/88.3.967.

Guillamón, E., M.M. Pedrosa, C. Burbano, C. Cuadrado, M. de Cortes Sánchez, and M. Muzquiz. 2008. The Trypsin Inhibitors Present in Seed of Different Grain Legume Species and Cultivar. *Food Chemistry* 107 (1): 68–74. doi:10.1016/j.foodchem.2007.07.029.

Health Canada. 1981. Determination of Protein Rating FO-1. http://www.hc-sc.gc.ca/fn-an/alt_formats/hpfb-dgpsa/pdf/res-rech/fo-1-eng.pdf

Jansman, A.J.M., and M. Longstaff. 1993. Nutritional Effects of Tannins and Vicine/Convicine in Legume Seeds. In *Recent Advances of Research in Antinutritional Factors in Legume Seeds*, ed. J. Huisman, A.F.B van Der Poel, and I.E. Liener, 301–316. Wageningen, EAAP, Wageningen Press.

Khalil, A.H., and E.H. Mansour. 1995. The Effect of Cooking, Autoclaving and Germination on the Nutritional Quality of Faba Beans. *Food Chemistry* 54 (2): 177–182. doi:10.1016/0308-8146(95)00024-D.

Khattab, R.Y., S.D. Arntfield, and C.M. Nyachoti. 2009. Nutritional Quality of Legume Seeds as Affected by Some Physical Treatments, Part 1: Protein Quality Evaluation. *LWT—Food Science and Technology* 42 (6): 1107–1112. Academic Press. doi:10.1016/J.LWT.2009.02.008.

Laing, E., A.K. Stone, D. Shi, M. Pickard, J.D. House, N. Wang, and M.T. Nickerson. 2023. Effect of Infrared Heating on the Nutritional Properties of Yellow Pea and Green Lentil Flours. *Cereal Chemistry* 100 (3): 601–613. doi:10.1002/cche.10653.

Liu, S., Y. Ren, H. Yin, M. Nickerson, M. Pickard, and Y. Ai. 2022. Improvement of the Nutritional Quality of Lentil Flours by Infrared Heating of Seeds Varying in Size. *Food Chemistry* 396: 133649. doi:10.1016/j.foodchem.2022.133649.

Malcolmson, L., and J. Han. 2019. *Pulse Processing and Utilization of Pulse Ingredients in Foods. Health Benefits of Pulses*, 129–149. Cham: Springer. doi:10.1007/978-3-030-12763-3_9.

Margier, M., S. George, N. Hafnaoui, D. Redmond, M. Nowicki, L. Du Chaffaut, M-J. Amiot, and E. Reboul. 2018. Nutritional Composition and Bioactive Content of Legumes: Characterization of Pulses Frequently Consumed in France and the Effect of the Cooking Method. *Nutrients* 10 (11): 1668. doi:10.3390/nu10111668.

Marinangeli, C.P. and J.D. House. 2017. Potential Impact of the Digestible Indispensable Amino Acid Score as a Measure of Protein Quality on Dietary Regulations and Health. *Nutrition Reviews* 75 (8): 658–667. doi:10.1093/nutrit/nux025.

Mauron, J. 1981. The Maillard Reaction in Food; a Critical Review from the Nutritional Standpoint. *Progress in Food and Nutrition Science* 5 (1–6): 5–35.

Mubarak, A.E. 2005. Nutritional Composition and Antinutritional Factors of Mung Bean Seeds (Phaseolus Aureus) as Affected by Some Home Traditional Processes. *Food Chemistry* 89 (4): 489–495. doi:10.1016/j.foodchem.2004.01.007.

Nosworthy, M.G., A.J. Franczyk, G. Medina, J. Neufeld, P. Appah, A. Utioh, P. Frohlich, and J.D. House. 2017. Effect of Processing on the in Vitro and in Vivo Protein Quality of Yellow and Green Split Peas (Pisum Sativum). *Journal of Agricultural and Food Chemistry* 65 (35): 7790–7796.

Nosworthy, M.G., G. Medina, A.J. Franczyk, J. Neufeld, P. Appah, A. Utioh, P. Frohlich, and J.D. House. 2018a. Effect of Processing on the in Vitro and in Vivo Protein Quality of Red and Green Lentils (Lens Culinaris). *Food Chemistry* 240: 588–593. doi:10.1016/J.FOODCHEM.2017.07.129.

Nosworthy, M.G., G. Medina, A.J. Franczyk, J. Neufeld, P. Appah, A. Utioh, P. Frohlich, and J.D. House. 2018b. Effect of Processing on the In Vitro and In Vivo Protein Quality of Beans (Phaseolus Vulgaris and Vicia Faba). *Nutrients* 10 (6): 671. doi:10.3390/NU10060671.

Nosworthy, M.G., G. Medina, Z.H. Lu, J.D. House. 2023. Plant Proteins: Methods of Quality Assessment and Human Health Benefits of Pulses. *Foods* 12 (15): 2816. doi:10.3390/foods12152816.

O'Dell, B.L., and A. De Boland. 1976. Complexation of Phytate with Proteins and Cations in Corn Germ and Oil Seed Meals. *Journal of Agricultural and Food Chemistry* 24 (4): 804–808.

Padmashree, A., A.D. Semwal, M.A. Khan, T. Govindaraj, and G.K. Sharma. 2016. Effect of Infrared Processing on Functional, Nutritional, Antinutritional and Rheological Properties of Mung Bean (Phaseolus Aereus) Seeds. *International Journal of Advanced Research* 4: 606–613.

Pal, R.S., A. Bhartiya, R. ArunKumar, L. Kant, J.P. Aditya, and J.K. Bisht. 2016. Impact of Dehulling and Germination on Nutrients, Antinutrients, and Antioxidant Properties in Horsegram. *Journal of Food Science and Technology* 53 (1): 337–347. doi:10.1007/s13197-015-2037-3.

Pathiratne, S.M., P.J. Shand, M. Pickard, and J.P.D. Wanasundara. 2015. Generating Functional Property Variation in Lentil (Lens Culinaris) Flour by Seed Micronization: Effects of Seed Moisture Level and Surface Temperature. *Food Research International* 76: 122–131. doi:10.1016/j.foodres.2015.03.026.

Reddy, V., and G. Butler. 1989. Incorporation of 14C from [14C]Phenylalanine into Condensed Tannin of Sorghum Grain. *Journal of Agricultural and Food Chemistry* 37 (2): 383–384. doi:10.1021/jf00086a024.

Rehman, Z.U., and W.H. Shah. 2005. Thermal Heat Processing Effects on Antinutrients, Protein and Starch Digestibility of Food Legumes. *Food Chemistry* 91 (2): 327–331. doi:10.1016/j.foodchem.2004.06.019.

Ribéreau, S., A.N.A. Aryee, S. Tanvier, J. Han, and J.I. Boye. 2018. Composition, Digestibility, and Functional Properties of Yellow Pea as Affected by Processing. *Journal of Food Processing and Preservation* 42 (1): e13375. doi:10.1111/JFPP.13375.

Roy, F., J.I. Boye, and B.K. Simpson. 2010. Bioactive Proteins and Peptides in Pulse Crops: Pea, Chickpea and Lentil. *Food Research International* 43 (2): 432–442. doi:10.1016/J.FOODRES.2009.09.002.

Salazar-Villanea, S., W.H. Hendriks, E.M.A.M. Bruininx, H. Gruppen, and A.F.B. Van Der Poel. 2016. Protein Structural Changes during Processing of Vegetable Feed Ingredients Used in Swine Diets: Implications for Nutritional Value. *Nutrition Research Reviews* 29 (1). doi:10.1017/S0954422416000056.

Sokhansanj, S.H., and R.T. Patil. 2003. Dehulling and Splitting Pulses. In *Handbook of Postharvest Technology: Cereals, Fruits, Vegetables, Tea, and Spices*, ed. A. Chakraverty, A.S. Mujumdar, G.S. Vijaya Raghavana, and H.S. Ramaswamy, 397. New York: Marcel Dekker Inc.

Sun, X., I.C. Ohanenye, T. Ahmed, and C.C. Udenigwe. 2020. Microwave Treatment Increased Protein Digestibility of Pigeon Pea (Cajanus Cajan) Flour: Elucidation of Underlying Mechanisms. *Food Chemistry* 329: 127196. doi:10.1016/j.foodchem.2020.127196.

Vadivel, V., A. Doss, and M. Pugalenthi. 2010. Evaluation of Nutritional Value and Protein Quality of Raw and Differentially Processed Sword Bean [Canavalia Gladiata] Seeds. *African Journal of Food, Agriculture, Nutrition and Development* 10 (7). doi:10.4314/ajfand.v10i7.59034.

Wang, N. 2008. Effect of Variety and Crude Protein Content on Dehulling Quality and on the Resulting Chemical Composition of Red Lentil (Lens Culinaris). *Journal of the Science of Food and Agriculture* 88 (5): 885–890. doi:10.1002/jsfa.3165.

Wang, N., D.W. Hatcher, and E.J. Gawalko. 2008. Effect of Variety and Processing on Nutrients and Certain Anti-Nutrients in Field Peas (Pisum Sativum). *Food Chemistry* 111 (1): 132–138. doi:10.1016/J.FOODCHEM.2008.03.047.

Wang, N., D.W. Hatcher, R. Toews, and E.J. Gawalko. 2009. Influence of Cooking and Dehulling on Nutritional Composition of Several Varieties of Lentils (Lens Culinaris). *LWT—Food Science and Technology* 42 (4): 842–848. doi:10.1016/j.lwt.2008.10.007.

Wang, N., D.W. Hatcher, R.T. Tyler, R. Toews, and E.J. Gawalko. 2010. Effect of Cooking on the Composition of Beans (Phaseolus Vulgaris L.) and Chickpeas (Cicer Arietinum L.). *Food Research International* 43 (2): 589–594. doi:10.1016/J.FOODRES.2009.07.012.

40 Recommended Resources for Plant and Animal Proteins in Health and Disease Prevention

Rajkumar Rajendram, Vinood B. Patel, and Victor R. Preedy

INTRODUCTION

Protein, an indispensable macronutrient, serves as a cornerstone of human health (Ardisson Korat et al., 2024). Thus, maintaining health and physical function requires adequate protein intake (Food and Agriculture Organization of the United Nations, 2017; Hruby et al., 2020; Phillips and Wolfe, 2009). Proteins derived from plant and animal sources are divergent in terms of compositional profiles, and substantial amounts of research have been conducted to determine the differences in outcomes of omnivorous or vegetarian individuals (Ferrari et al., 2022). The specific roles of plant and animal protein sources in health and disease prevention are, arguably, poorly defined.

A comprehensive comparison of plant and animal proteins reveals distinct nutritional profiles (Ferrari et al., 2022). Both sources offer essential amino acids. However, the specific amino acid composition varies (Ferrari et al., 2022). In simple terms, animal proteins generally provide a complete amino acid profile. Plant proteins may be deficient in one or more essential amino acids. However, combining different plant-based protein sources can compensate for this limitation. Additionally, food derived from plants is typically higher in fibre, while animal products tend to be higher in saturated fat and cholesterol.

Through a comprehensive understanding of plant and animal protein sources, healthcare professionals can guide patients towards an optimized dietary approach, fostering health and well-being across diverse populations. The type and quantity of protein we consume impact our health significantly across the lifespan. While the optimal protein intake varies based on age, activity level, and health status, a well-balanced approach incorporating both plant and animal sources offers distinct advantages (World Health Organization, 2007).

We have compiled a comprehensive directory to equip healthcare professionals and researchers with essential resources. This directory features over 100 organizations, scientific societies, regulatory bodies, and online platforms, drawing upon expert recommendations from the field. Additionally, a curated selection of books offers in-depth exploration of the subject matter.

It is crucial to note that this directory serves as a general informational resource. The inclusion of any organization, society, or resource does not constitute an endorsement or recommendation by the authors or editors.

This list of materials in these tables is included to provide general information only. It does not constitute any recommendation or endorsement of the activities of these sites, facilities, or other resources listed in this chapter by the authors or editors of this book.

Tables 40.1–40.5 list the most up-to-date information on the regulatory bodies (Table 40.1), professional societies (Table 40.2), books (Table 40.3), emerging technologies and platforms (Table 40.4), and other resources of interest (Table 40.5) that are relevant to an evidence-based approach to protein intake in health and disease. Some organizations are listed in more than one table as they occasionally fulfil multiple roles.

DOI: 10.1201/9781003597926-40

TABLE 40.1
Websites of Regulatory Bodies and Organizations Dealing with Plant and Animal Proteins in Health and Disease Prevention

Regulatory Body or Organization	Web Address
Agencia Española de Seguridad Alimentaria y Nutrición (AESAN; Spanish Agency for Food Safety and Nutrition)	www.aesan.gob.es/AECOSAN/web/home/aecosan_inicio.htm
Alternative Proteins Association	www.proteinreport.org/directory/alternative-proteins-association/
American Meat Science Association	https://meatscience.org/
Animal and Plant Health Agency	www.gov.uk/government/organisations/animal-and-plant-health-agency
Association for Nutrition	www.associationfornutrition.org/
Belgian Nutrition Society	www.belgiannutritionsociety.be/
BoMiProt	https://bomiprot.org/
Brazilian Society for Food and Nutrition	https://iuns.org/organisations/brazilian-society-for-food-and-nutrition/
Canadian Institute of Food Safety (CIFS)	www.foodsafety.ca/
Centers for Disease Control and Prevention (CDC)	www.cdc.gov/index.html
Cleveland Clinic	https://my.clevelandclinic.org/
Consiglio per la Ricerca in Agricoltura e l'Analisi dell'Economia Agraria (CREA; Council for Agricultural Research and Analysis of Agricultural Economics)	www.crea.gov.it/
CSIC – Instituto de Agroquímica y Tecnología de Alimentos (Institute of Agrochemistry and Food Technology)	www.iata.csic.es/es
CSIC – Instituto de la Grasa (Institute of Fats)	www.ig.csic.es/es/
Dietary Guidelines for Americans	www.dietaryguidelines.gov/
European Commission: Food, Farming, Fisheries	https://commission.europa.eu/food-farming-fisheries_en
European Food Safety Authority (EFSA)	www.efsa.europa.eu/en
European Medicines Agency (EMA)	www.ema.europa.eu/en/homepage
Faculty of Animal Productions Engineering and Management, University of Agronomic Sciences and Veterinary Medicine of Bucharest	www.usamv.ro/index.php/en/academics/faculties
Faculty of Food Science and Technology, University of Agronomic Sciences and Veterinary Medicine of Cluj-Napoca	https://inginerialimentara.usamvcluj.ro/
Federation of African Nutrition Societies	https://fanus.org/
Federation of Asian Nutrition Societies	https://fansnutrition.org/
Federation of European Nutrition Societies	https://fensnutrition.org/
Finnish Society for Nutrition Research	https://suomenravitsemustieteenyhdistys.fi/en/

(*Continued*)

TABLE 40.1 (CONTINUED)
Websites of Regulatory Bodies and Organizations Dealing with Plant and Animal Proteins in Health and Disease Prevention

Regulatory Body or Organization	Web Address
Food and Agriculture Organization	www.fao.org/home/en
Food Safety	www.foodsafety.gov/
Food Standards Agency United Kingdom	www.food.gov.uk/
Food Standards Scotland	www.foodstandards.gov.scot/
German Nutrition Society	www.dge.de/english/
Harvard T.H. Chan School of Public Health	www.hsph.harvard.edu/
International Livestock Research Institute (ILRI)	www.ilri.org/
Istituto Superiore di Sanità (ISS; Italian National Institute of Health)	www.iss.it/
Korean Society of Animal Science and Technology	www.e-ait.org/info/contact
Latin American Nutrition Society	www.slaninternacional.org/
Ministry of Agriculture, Food and Rural Affairs	www.mafra.go.kr/sites/home/index.do
National Institutes of Health (NIH) – National Institute of Diabetes and Digestive and Kidney Diseases (NIDDK)	www.niddk.nih.gov/
Nutrition Society	www.nutritionsociety.org/
Peanut Institute	https://peanut-institute.com/
PeptideAtlas	https://peptideatlas.org/#
Protein Society	www.proteinsociety.org/
Romanian Ministry of Education and Research, [CCCDI-UEFISCDI, project number PN-III-P4-ID-PCE-2020-2306]	https://uefiscdi.gov.ro/
Rural Development Administration	https://koreanfood.rda.go.kr
Spanish Nutrition Society	www.sennutricion.org/es/inicio
Swedish Association for Clinical Nutrition	www.sfkn.se/
The American College of Lifestyle Medicine (ACLM)	https://lifestylemedicine.org/
United Nations Environment Programme	www.unep.org/
United States Department of Agriculture (USDA)	www.usda.gov/

(Continued)

TABLE 40.1 (CONTINUED)
Websites of Regulatory Bodies and Organizations Dealing with Plant and Animal Proteins in Health and Disease Prevention

Regulatory Body or Organization	Web Address
University of Medicine and Pharmacy "Iuliu Hațieganu" Cluj-Napoca, Romania: Information on Nutrition and Dietetics	https://umfcluj.ro/farmacie/educatie/studii-de-licenta/nutritie-si-dietetica/
World Health Organization (WHO)	www.who.int/
World Organization for Animal Health (WOAH)	www.woah.org/en/home/

This table lists the regulatory bodies and organizations relevant to plant and animal proteins in health and disease prevention. The links were accurate when going to press but may move or change. In these cases, the "Search" tabs should be explored at the parent address or site. Dual-language sites often have pages for automatic translation into English. In some cases, links direct the reader to other pages (related to plant and animal proteins) within parent sites. Some societies and organizations prefer shortened terms, such as acronyms and abbreviations. Some organizations provide a dual role of imparting information on specific conditions (from diagnostics to epidemiology) and acting as professional or regulatory bodies. See also Table 40.2.

TABLE 40.2
Professional Societies Covering Plant and Animal Proteins in Health and Disease Prevention

Society Name	Web Address
Academic Society for Functional Foods and Bioactive Compounds (ASFFBC)	www.functionalfoodscenter.net/ASFFBC.html
Academy of Nutrition and Dietetics	www.eatright.org/
Agencia Española de Seguridad Alimentaria y Nutrición (AESAN)	www.aesan.gob.es/
Allergy UK	www.allergyuk.org/
American Heart Association (AHA)	www.heart.org/
American Society for Nutrition	https://nutrition.org/
American Society of Animal Science (ASAS)	www.asas.org/
American Veterinary Medical Association (AVMA)	www.avma.org/
Animal Health Australia	https://animalhealthaustralia.com.au/
Associazione Nazionale Specialisti in Scienza dell'Alimentazione (ANSISA)	www.ansisa.it/
British Dietetic Association	www.bda.uk.com/
British Heart Foundation	www.bhf.org.uk/
British Nutrition Foundation	www.nutrition.org.uk/
British Veterinary Association (BVA)	www.bva.co.uk/
Chinese Academy of Agricultural Sciences	www.caas.cn/en/
European Association for the Study of Diabetes (EASD)	www.easd.org
European Cooperation in Science and Technology (COST)	www.cost.eu/
European Food Information Council (EUFIC)	www.eufic.org/
European Food Safety Authority	www.efsa.europa.eu/en
European Plant Science Organisation (EPSO)	https://epsoweb.org/
European Vegetable Protein Association	https://euvepro.eu/
Food Allergy Research and Education	www.foodallergy.org/
Food and Agriculture Organisation of the United Nations (FAO)	www.fao.org/home/en
Food Foundation	https://foodfoundation.org.uk/
Food Frontier	www.foodfrontier.org/
Fundación Iberoamericana de Nutrición (FINUT)	www.finut.org/
Harvard Chan School of Public Health	www.hsph.harvard.edu/
Institute for the Advancement of Food and Nutrition Sciences	https://iafns.org/
Institute of Food Technologists (IFT)	www.ift.org/about-ift

(*Continued*)

TABLE 40.2 (CONTINUED)
Professional Societies Covering Plant and Animal Proteins in Health and Disease Prevention

Society Name	Web Address
International Society of Hypertension	https://ish-world.com/about-ish/
Korean Nutrition Society	www.kns.or.kr/english/
Korean Society of Community Nutrition	www.koscom.or.kr/
Korean Society of Dairy Science and Biotechnology	http://www.ksdst.org/
National Health and Medical Research Council Australia	www.nhmrc.gov.au/
National Institute of Animal Health (NIAH)	www.naro.go.jp/english/laboratory/niah/overview/index.html
Nutrition Australia	https://nutritionaustralia.org/
Nutrition Society	www.nutritionsociety.org/
Plant-Based Foods Association	www.plantbasedfoods.org/
Protein Society	www.proteinsociety.org/
Slow Food International	www.slowfood.com/
Sociedad Española de Cardiología (SEC)	https://secardiologia.es/
Società Italiana di Farmacologia	www.sifweb.org
Società Italiana di Nutraceutica (SINUT)	https://sinut.it/
Società Italiana di Nutrizione dello Sport e del Benessere (SINSeB)	www.sinseb.it/
Società Italiana di Nutrizione Umana (SINU)	https://sinu.it/
Società Italiana Nutrizione Artificiale e Metabolismo (SINPE)	www.sinpe.org/
Society of Nutrition and Food Science e.V.	www.snfs.org/
World Organisation for Animal Health	www.woah.org/en/home/

This table lists the professional societies and other organizations relevant to plant and animal proteins in health and disease prevention. See also Table 40.1.

TABLE 40.3
Books on Plant and Animal Proteins in Health and Disease Prevention

Book Title	Authors or Editors	Publisher	Year of Publication
Biochemistry, Essential Amino Acids	Lopez MJ	StatPearls Publishing	2023
Clinical Guide to Gluten-Related Disorders	Fasano A	Lippincott Williams and Wilkins	2013
Clinical Nutrition, 2nd Edition	Elia M, Ljungqvist O, Stratton RJ, Lanham-New SA	Wiley-Blackwell	2012
Current Advances for Development of Functional Foods Modulating Inflammation and Oxidative Stress	Hernández-Ledesma B, Martínez-Villaluenga C	AcademicPress, Elsevier	2022
Emerging Protein Sources for Food Production and Human Nutrition	Kitts D, Singh AP, Kowalczewski PL	MDPI Books	2023
Environmental, Health and Business Opportunities in the New Meat Alternatives Market	Bogueva D, Marinova D, Raphaely T, Schmidinger K	IGI Global	2019
Enzymes Beyond Traditional Applications in Dairy Science and Technology Foundations and Frontiers in Enzymology	Rajput YS, Sharma R	Academic Press	2023
Essentials of Medical Biochemistry: With Clinical Cases	Ha CE, Bhagavan NV	Elsevier	2022
Food in a Planetary Emergency	Marinova D, Bogueva D	Springer	2022
Food Preservation and Waste Exploitation	Sonia S, Anca F, Aussenac T, Laguerre J-C	IntechOpen	2021
Future Foods: How Modern Science Is Transforming the Way We Eat	McClements DJ	Springer	2019
Future Proteins	Tiwari BK, Healy LE	Elsevier	2023
Gluten-Free Food Science and Technology	Gallagher E	Eimear Gallagher	2009
Innovative Sources in Nutraceutical and Natural Products Pharmaceuticals	Galanakis C	AcademicPress, Elsevier	2019
Introduction to Human Nutrition, 3rd Edition	Lanham-New SA, Hill TR, Gallagher AM, Vorster HH	Wiley-Blackwell	2019
Introduction to Peptide Science	Hamley IW	Wiley	2020
Krause and Mahan's Food and the Nutrition Care Process	Raymond JL, Morrow K	Elsevier – Health Sciences Division	2022
Meat Less: The Next Food Revolution	McClements DJ	Springer	2023
Milk Proteins: From Expression to Food	Boland M, Singh H	Elsevier	2020
Novel Plant Protein Processing Developing the Foods of the Future	Khan ZS, Wani SA, Fayaz S	Routledge	2024
Nutrition, Food and Diet in Ageing and Longevity	Rattan SIS, Kaur G	Springer	2021

(*Continued*)

TABLE 40.3 (CONTINUED)
Professional Societies Covering Plant and Animal Proteins in Health and Disease Prevention

Book Title	Authors or Editors	Publisher	Year of Publication
Nutrition in the Prevention and Treatment of Disease	Coulston AM, Boushey CJ, Ferruzzi M, Delahanty D	Elsevier	2017
Olives and Olive Oil in Health and Disease Prevention	Preedy VR	Academic Press	2021
Plant Powered Protein: Nutrition Essentials and Dietary Guidelines for All Ages	Davis B, Melina V, Davis C	BPC	2023
Plant Protein Foods	Annamalai M	Springer Cham	2023
Probiotics: Advanced Food and Health Applications	Brandelli A	Academic Press	2022
Processing Technologies and Food Protein Digestion	Bhat ZF, Morton JD, Suleria HAR, Bekhit AE-DA	Elsevier	2023
Protein Interactions: The Molecular Basis of Interactomics	Helmes V, Kalinina OV	Wiley	2022
Protein Misfolding Diseases: Current and Emerging Principles and Therapies	Ramirez-Alvarado M, Kelly JW, Dobson CM	Wiley	2010
Proteins: Biochemistry and Biotechnology	Walsh G	John Wiley and Sons	2015
Proteins: Sustainable Source, Processing and Application	Galanakis CM	Academic Press	2019
Sourdough Innovations: Novel Uses of Metabolites, Enzymes, and Microbiota from Sourdough Processing	Garcia-Vaquero M, Rocha J	CRC Press	2023
Soybean Improvement: Physiological, Molecular and Genetic Perspectives	Wani SH, Sofi NuR, Bhat MA, Lin F	Springer	2022
Sustainable Food Science: A Comprehensive Approach	Ferranti P	Elsevier	2023
The China Study: The Most Comprehensive Study of Nutrition Ever Conducted and the Startling Implications for Diet, Weight Loss, and Long-Term Health	Campbell TC, Campbell II TM	Rodale Books	2005
Vegetarian and Plant-Based Diets in Health and Disease Prevention	François M	Elsevier	2017
Wheat Syndromes: How Wheat, Gluten and ATI Cause Inflammation, IBS and Autoimmune Diseases	Gisbert-Schuppan K, Schuppan D	Springer Nature	2019
Whey Protein Production, Chemistry, Functionality, and Applications	Guo M	Wiley	2019
Whey Proteins: From Milk to Medicine	Deeth HC, Bansal N	Academic Press	2019
Williams' Essentials of Nutrition and Diet Therapy, 13th Edition	Gilbert JA, Schlenker E	Elsevier	2022

TABLE 40.4
Emerging Techniques, Instruments, and Analytical Platforms or Devices for Investigating Plant and Animal Proteins in Health and Disease Prevention

Organization or Company Name	Web Address
American Society for Nutrition: Information on Nutritional Psychiatry	https://nutrition.org/food-and-mood-what-is-nutritional-psychiatry/
BIOPEP-UWM Database	https://biochemia.uwm.edu.pl/biopep/start_biopep.php
Bio-Rad	www.bio-rad.com/
British Heart Foundation: Information on Dietary Protein	www.bhf.org.uk/informationsupport/heart-matters-magazine/nutrition/protein
British Nutrition Foundation: Information on Protein	www.nutrition.org.uk/nutritional-information/protein/
Bruker: Information on ultrafleXtreme	www.bruker.com/en/products-and-solutions/mass-spectrometry/maldi-tof/ultraflextreme.html
Cleveland Clinic: Information on Integrative Medicine	https://my.clevelandclinic.org/health/treatments/21683-integrative-medicine
Deakin University: Information on Food and Mood Centre	https://foodandmoodcentre.com.au/team/felice-jacka/
EMBL's European Bioinformatics Institute: Various Online Resources and Tools	www.ebi.ac.uk/
Expasy Swiss Institute of Bioinformatics: Peptide Cutter	https://web.expasy.org/peptide_cutter/
Food Revolution	https://foodrevolution.org/
Foss: Kjeldahl Tecator Protein Microanalyser	www.fossanalytics.com/en/products/kjeltec-8400
Good Food Institute: The Science of Fermentation	https://gfi.org/science/the-science-of-fermentation/#:~:text=Precision%20fermentation%20targets%20specific%20molecules,already%20work%20in%20this%20space.
Institut Pasteur: Rapid Peptides Generator (RPG)	https://research.pasteur.fr/en/software/rapid-peptides-generator-rpg/
Institute de Cardiologie de Montréal: Information on Plant and Animal Proteins	https://observatoireprevention.org/en/2020/02/27/plant-or-animal-proteins-an-impact-on-health/#:~:text=Recent%20studies%20suggest%20an%20interesting,amount%20required%20to%20be%20healthy.
Labconco	www.labconco.com/

(*Continued*)

TABLE 40.4 (CONTINUED)
Emerging Techniques, Instruments, and Analytical Platforms or Devices for Investigating Plant and Animal Proteins in Health and Disease Prevention

Organization or Company Name	Web Address
Laboratory Equipment Company (LECO)	https://eu.leco.com/
Merckmillipore	www.merckmillipore.com/ES/es/20210416_153721
Milk Bioactive Peptide Database (MBPDB)	http://mbpdb.nws.oregonstate.edu/
Oregon State University	
Nanotempertech: Information on Prometheus	https://nanotempertech.com/prometheus/
National Center for Biotechnology Information (NCBI): Information on Protein	http://www.ncbi.nlm.nih.gov/protein
Nordic Co-operation: Information on Protein	https://pub.norden.org/nord2023-003/protein-.html
Nutrition Facts	https://nutritionfacts.org
PeptideAtlas	https://peptideatlas.org/#
PeptideRanker: PeptideLocator	http://bioware.ucd.ie/~compass/biowareweb/
Physicians Committee for Responsible Medicine: Information on Dietary Proteins	www.pcrm.org/good-nutrition/nutrition-information/protein
Promega	www.promega.co.uk/
Proteintech	www.ptglab.com/
PubChem	https://pubchem.ncbi.nlm.nih.gov/
Qiagen	www.qiagen.com/us
Rapidnovor	www.rapidnovor.com/
Thermofisher Ion Torrent	www.thermofisher.com/uk/en/home/life-science/sequencing/next-generation-sequencing/instruments/genexus-system.html
UniProt: Universal Protein Resource Knowledgebase (UniProtKB)	http://www.uniprot.org/
Waters: Amino Acid Determinations and Other Instruments	www.waters.com/
Waters: Xevo G2-XS QTof Quadrupole Time-of-Flight Mass Spectrometry	www.waters.com/waters/en_US/Xevo-G2-XS-QTof-Quadrupole-Time-of-Flight-Mass-Spectrometer/nav.htm

This table lists some emerging technologies, companies, and other sites relevant to investigating and studying plant and animal proteins. The links were accurate when going to press but may move or change. In these cases, the "Search" tabs should be explored at the parent address or site. In some cases, links direct the reader to pages related to plant and animal proteins within parent sites.

TABLE 40.5
Other Resources of Interest or Relevance for Healthcare Professionals or Patients Related to Plant and Animal Proteins in Health and Disease Prevention

Name of Resource or Organization	Web Address
American Heart Association (AHA): Information on Tofu	www.heart.org/en/news/2022/10/10/clearing-up-questions-on-whether-tofu-is-healthy
Associazione Colon Irritabile Nazionale Italiana (ACINI)	www.acini.info/
Associazione Italiana Celiachia (AIC)	www.celiachia.it/
Associazione Italiana Sindrome Fibromialgica (AISF)	https://sindromefibromialgica.it/
Australian Dietary Guidelines	www.eatforhealth.gov.au/guidelines/guidelines
British Heart Foundation: Information on Dietary Proteins	www.bhf.org.uk/informationsupport/heart-matters-magazine/nutrition/protein
Chinese Academy of Agricultural Sciences: Innovations in Agriculture	www.science.org/content/resource/agricultural-innovations-in-china-aid-countries-around-world
Cleveland Clinic: Information on Integrative Medicine	https://my.clevelandclinic.org/health/treatments/21683-integrative-medicine
Dietary Guidelines for Americans	www.dietaryguidelines.gov/
European Medicines Agency: Patients and Consumers Organisations	www.ema.europa.eu/en/partners-networks/patients-consumers/eligible-patients-consumers-organisations
Food and Agriculture Organization of the United Nations: One Health	www.fao.org/one-health/en
Food Science Society: Information for Students	https://engage.luu.org.uk/groups/34K/food-science-and-nutrition
Good Food Institute: Information on Cultivated Meat	https://gfi.org/science/the-science-of-cultivated-meat/
Harvard Chan School of Public Health: Information on Dietary Protein	www.hsph.harvard.edu/nutritionsource/what-should-you-eat/protein/#protein-research
Harvard T.H. Chan School of Public Health: The Nutrition Source	www.hsph.harvard.edu/nutritionsource/what-should-you-eat/protein/
Journal of Natural Life Medicine (JNLM)	https://dergipark.org.tr/en/pub/jnlm
Noakes Foundation	https://thenoakesfoundation.org/
Society of Nutrition and Food Science e.V.	www.snfs.org/
The Patients Association	www.patients-association.org.uk/
United States Department of Agriculture (USDA): Information of Biotechnology	www.usda.gov/topics/biotechnology/biotechnology-frequently-asked-questions-faqs
University of California, Los Angeles (UCLA) Health	www.uclahealth.org/news/is-plant-based-protein-for-you-heres-what-you-need-to-know
World Health Organization: Protein and Amino Acid Requirements for Human Nutrition	https://apps.who.int/iris/bitstream/handle/10665/43411/WHO_TRS_935_eng.pdf

(Continued)

TABLE 40.5 (CONTINUED)
Other Resources of Interest or Relevance for Healthcare Professionals or Patients Related to Plant and Animal Proteins in Health and Disease Prevention

Name of Resource or Organization	Web Address
World Organisation for Animal Health: Information on Swine Fever	www.woah.org/en/disease/african-swine-fever/

This table lists other resources and information relevant to plant and animal proteins in health and disease prevention. The links were accurate when going to press but may move or change. In these cases, the "Search" tabs should be explored at the parent address or site. In some cases, links direct the reader to pages related to plant and animal proteins in health and disease prevention within parent sites.

OTHER RESOURCES

Material on topics related to plant and animal proteins in health and disease prevention are held in The British Library (www.bl.uk/) and The Wellcome Collection (https://wellcomecollection.org/collections).

Other chapters on resources (recommended by eminent authors) may be relevant to plant and animal proteins in health and disease prevention (Alzaid et al., 2015; Rajendram et al., 2013a, 2013b, 2014, 2015, 2016, 2017, 2019a, 2019b, 2020, 2022a, 2022b, 2023).

The material contained in these tables is intended to provide general information only. The authors or editors of this book do not recommend or endorse the activities

ACKNOWLEDGEMENTS (IN ALPHABETICAL ORDER)

We thank the following authors for their contributions to developing this resource. We apologize if some of the suggested material was not included in this chapter or has been moved to different tables.

Ambatipudi, SK
Bogueva, D
Boşca, AB
Capanoglu, E
Di Stefano, M
Farcas, AC
Grammatikopoulou, M
Günal-Köröğlu, D
Kwon, Y-J
Lee, J-H
Lou-Bonafonte, J-M
Marinova, D
Martinez-Beamonte
Martin Rubio, ME
Matsunaga, M
Mattos Della Lucia, C
Montenegro, MA
Navarro, MA
Osada, J
Rivero-Pino, F
Siraj, N
Tulipano, G
Yazar, H
Yoon, J
Yu, J

REFERENCES

Alzaid, F., Rajendram, R., Patel, V.B., and Preedy, V.R. (2015). Expanding the knowledge base in diet, nutrition and critical care. Electronic and published resources. In Rajendram, R., Preedy, V.R., and Patel, V.B. (eds). *Diet and Nutrition in Critical Care*. Berlin, Germany: Springer.

Ardisson Korat, A.V., Shea, M.K., Jacques, P.F., Sebastiani, P., Wang, M., Eliassen, A.H., Willett, W.C., and Sun, Q. (2024). Dietary protein intake in midlife in relation to healthy aging – results from the prospective Nurses' Health Study cohort. *The American Journal of Clinical Nutrition*, 119(2), 271–282.

Ferrari, L., Panaite, S.A., Bertazzo, A., and Visioli, F. (2022). Animal- and plant-based protein sources: a scoping review of human health outcomes and environmental impact. *Nutrients*, 14(23), 5115. https://doi.org/10.3390/nu14235115

Food and Agriculture Organization of the United Nations. (2017). *Dietary Protein Quality for Human Life.* Food and Agriculture Organization of the United Nations. FAO Report, Rome, Italy.

Hruby, A., Sahni, S., Bolster, D., and Jacques, P.F. (2020). Protein intake and functional integrity in aging: the framingham heart study offspring. *The Journals of Gerontology. Series A, Biological Sciences and Medical Sciences*, 75(1), 123–130.

Phillips, S.M., and Wolfe, R.R. (2009). Dietary protein requirements and adaptations to dietary restriction. *Applied Physiology, Nutrition, and Metabolism*, 34(3), 899–909.

Rajendram, R., Gyamfi, D., Patel, V.B., and Preedy, V.R. (2022a). Recommended resources for biomarkers of nutrition. In Preedy, V.R., and Patel, V.B. (eds). *Biomarkers of Nutrition*. New York: Elsevier.

Rajendram, R., Gyamfi, D., Patel, V.B., and Preedy, V.R. (2022b). Recommended resources for biomarkers in diabetes: Methods, discoveries, and applications. In Patel, V.B., and Preedy, V.R. (eds). *Biomarkers in Diabetes: Biomarkers in Disease: Methods, Discoveries and Applications*. Berlin, Germany: Springer. https://doi.org/10.1007/978-3-030-81303-1_58-2

Rajendram, R., Gyamfi, D., Patel, V.B., and Preedy, V.R. (2023). Recommended resources on diabetes in relation to foods, plants, herbs and spices in human health. In Rajendram, R., Patel, V.B. and Preedy, V.R. (eds). *Ancient and Traditional Foods, Plants, Herbs and Spices Used in Diabetes*. Boca Raton: CRC Press.

Rajendram, R., Patel, V.B., and Preedy, V.R. (2014). Web based resources and suggested reading. In Rajendram, R., Patel, V.B., and Preedy, V.R. (eds). *Glutamine in Health and Disease* (pp. 527–532). New York: Springer.

Rajendram, R., Patel, V.B., and Preedy, V.R. (2015). Web based resources and suggested reading. In Rajendram, R., Patel, V.B., and Preedy, V.R. (eds). *Branched Chain Amino Acids in Health and Disease*. New York: Springer

Rajendram, R., Patel, V.B., and Preedy, V.R. (2016). Recommended resources on biomarkers in cardiovascular disease. In Patel, V. and Preedy, V. (eds). *Biomarkers in Cardiovascular Disease*. Dordrecht: Springer. https://doi.org/10.1007/978-94-007-7741-5_52-1

Rajendram, R., Patel, V.B., and Preedy, V.R. (2017). Recommended resources on maternal nutrition. In Rajendram, R., Patel, V.B., and Preedy, V.R. (eds). *Nutrition and Diet in Maternal Diabetes* (pp. 495–500). New York: Springer.

Rajendram, R., Patel, V.B., and Preedy, V.R. (2019a). Resources in famine, starvation, and nutrient deprivation. In Patel, V.B., and Preedy, V.R. (eds). *Famine, Starvation, and Nutrient Deprivation* (pp. 2399–2406). New York: Springer.

Rajendram, R., Patel, V.B., and Preedy, V.R. (2019b). Resources in diet, nutrition and epigenetics. In Patel, V.B., and Preedy, V.R. (eds). *Nutrition and Epigenetics* (pp. 2309–2314). New York: Springer.

Rajendram, R., Patel, V.B., and Preedy, V.R. (2020). Recommended resources for nutrition, oxidative stress, and dietary antioxidants. In Martin, C.R., and Preedy, V.R. (eds). *Nutrition, Oxidative Stress, and Dietary Antioxidants* (pp. 393–397). New York: Elsevier.

Rajendram, R., Rajendram, R., Patel, V.B., and Preedy, V.R. (2013a). Interlinking diet, nutrition, the menopause and recommended resources. In Hollins-Martin, C.J., Watson, R.R., and Preedy, V.R. (eds). *Nutrition and Diet in Menopause*. Berlin, Germany: Springer.

Rajendram, R., Rajendram, R., Patel, V.B., and Preedy, V.R. (2013b). Diet quality: What more is there to know? In Preedy, V.R., Hunter, L-A., and Patel, V.B. (eds). *Diet Quality: An Evidence-Based Approach* (pp. 397–401). Berlin, Germany: Springer.

World Health Organization. (2007). *Joint FAO/WHO/UNU Expert Consultation on Protein and Amino Acid Requirements in Human Nutrition ↑2002*. Geneva, Switzerland: Food and Agriculture Organization of the United Nations, World Health Organization and United Nations University. Protein and amino acid requirements in human nutrition: report of a joint FAO/WHO/UNU expert consultation. World Health Organization. Available at https://iris.who.int/handle/10665/43411 (Accessed 14/07/2024).

Index

D